Dermatology for Skin of Color

Dermatology for Skin of Color

A. PAUL KELLY
Professor of Medicine, Division of Dermatology
Charles Drew University of Medicine and Science
Chief Emeritus, Division of Dermatology
Former King/Drew Medical Center
Los Angeles, California
Clinical Professor of Medicine
Division of Dermatology
The David Geffen School of Medicine at UCLA
Los Angeles, California

SUSAN C. TAYLOR
Founding Director
Skin of Color Center
Division of Dermatology
St. Luke's-Roosevelt Hospital Center
New York, New York
Assistant Clinical Professor of Dermatology
College of Physicians and Surgeons
Columbia University Medical Center
New York, New York

McGraw Hill Medical

New York Chicago San Francisco Lisbon London Madrid Mexico City
Milan New Delhi San Juan Scoul Singapore Sydney Toronto

Dermatology for Skin of Color

1 2 3 4 5 6 7 8 9 0 CTP/CTP 0 12 11 10 9 8

ISBN 978-0-07-144671-6
MHID 0-07-144671-0

This book was set in StempelSchneidler by Aptara® Inc.
The editor was Anne M. Sydor.
The production supervisor was Sherri Souffrance.
Project management was provided by Sandhya Joshi, Aptara® Inc.
The interior designer was Alan Barnett.
The cover designer was Elizabeth Piscareta.
The index was prepared by Aptara® Inc.
China Translation & Printing, Ltd. was printer and binder.

This book is printed on acid-free paper.

Library of Congress Cataloging-in-Publication Data

Dermatology for skin of color / [edited by] A. Paul Kelly, Susan Taylor.
p. ; cm.
Includes bibliographical references and index.
ISBN-13: 978-0-07-144671-6 (hardcover : alk. paper)
ISBN-10: 0-07-144671-0 (hardcover : alk. paper)
1. Skin—Diseaeses—Treatment. 2. Black race. 3. Human skin color. I. Kelly, A. Paul. II. Taylor, Susan C.
[DNLM: 1. Skin Diseases. 2. Cosmetic Techniques. 3. Ethnic Groups—psychology. 4. Skin Diseases—ethnology. 5. Skin Pigmentation—physiology. WR 140 D435136 2008]
RL73.4.B63D47 2008
616.50089—dc22

2008052748

Dedication

A. Paul Kelly
To my wife, Beverly, my children, Traci and Kara, my parents Amanda and Paul and my granddaughters Keiley and Hayden, for their love, support, and wisdom.

Susan C. Taylor
To my wonderful family: my husband, Kemel Dawkins, my daughters, Morgan Elizabeth and Madison Lauren, my parents, Ethel and Charles and my sister, Flora.

CONTENTS

SECTION 4. Hair, Scalp, and Nail Disorders

SECTION 5. Sebaceous and Sweat Gland Disorders

SECTION 6. Skin Cancer

SECTION 7. Pigmentary Disorders

SECTION 8. Mucosal Disorders

SECTION 9. Dermatologic Infections

CONTRIBUTORS

A. Melvin Alexander, MD
Staff Dermatologist
Dermatology
Melbourne Internal Medicine Associates
Melbourne, Florida

Andrew F. Alexis, MD, MPH
Director
Skin of Color Center
St. Luke's Roosevelt Hospital
Assistant Clinical Professor of Dermatology
Columbia University College of Physicians & Surgeons
New York, New York

Marcy S. Alvarez DO
Private Practice
New York, New York

Ivonne Arellano-Mendoza, MD
Dermatology And Cutaneous Oncology Professor
Dermatology Department
Hospital General de Mexico, DO
Mexico City, Mexico

Saundrett G. Arrindell, MD
Assistant Professor, Division of Dermatology
Department of Medicine
Vanderbilt University School of Medicine
Nashville, Tennessee

Sonia Badreshia-Bansal MD, FAAD
Founder and Medical Director
Elite MD, Advanced Dermatology, Laser and Plastic Surgery Institute
Danville, California

Diane Baras
Typology Manager for Instrumental Make up Evaluation
L'Oréal Recherche
Chevilly-Larue, France

Elaine Bethell
Clinical Nurse Specialist
Smith & Nephew
Birmingham, United Kingdom

Michael Bigby, MD
Associate Professor
Dermatology
Harvard Medical School and Beth Israel Deaconess Medical Center
Boston, Massachusetts

Curley L. Bonds, MD
Adjunct Associate Professor & Chair
Psychiatry & Human Behavior
Charles R. Drew University of Medicine and Science
Associate Professor
Psychiatry & Biobehavioral Sciences
David Geffen School of Medicine at UCLA
Los Angeles, California

Khari H. Bridges, MD, MBA
Skin and Cancer Associates Center for Cosmetic Enhancement
Miami, Florida

Lorenzo Brown, MD
Assistant Professor
Otolaryngology/Head & Neck Surgery
Charles Drew School of Medicine and Science
Lost Angeles, California

Jimmy J. Brown, MD, DDS, FACS
Associate Professor
Department of Otolaryngology/Head & Neck Surgery
Stanford University
Palo Alto, California

Cheryl M. Burgess, MD, FAAD
Assistant Clinical Professor
Department of Dermatology
Georgetown University Hospital
Assistant Clinical Professor
Department of Dermatology
George Washington University Hospital
Washington, DC

Laurence Caisey
Worldwide Director for Make up Evaluation
L'Oréal Recherche
Chevilly-Larue, France

Valerie D. Callender, MD
Clinical Assistant Professor of Dermatology
Howard University College of Medicine
Washington, DC

Director
Callender Skin & Laser Center
Mitchellville, Maryland

Yuin-Chew Chan, MD
Consultant Dermatologist and Chief
Pediatric Dermatology Unit
National Skin Centre

Visiting Consultant Dermatologist
KK Women's and Children's Hospital
Singapore

Raechele Cochran Gathers, MD
Senior Physician
Henry Ford Health System
Department of Dermatology
Multicultural Dermatology Center
Detroit, Michigan

Fran E. Cook-Bolden, MD
Director and Founder
Skin Specialty Group and Ethnic Skin Specialty Group
Assistant Clinical Professor of Dermatology
Department of Dermatology
College of Physicians and Surgeons of Columbia University
New York, New York

C. Ralph Daniel III, MD
Clinical Professor
Medicine (Dermatolgy)
University of Mississipii—Jackson
Jackson, MS
Clinical Associate Professor
Dermatology
University of Alabama
Birmingham, Alabama

Vincent DeLeo, MD
Chairman
Dermatology
St. Luke's Roosevelt and Beth Israel Medical Centers
New York, New York

Kwame Denianke, MD
Department of Dermatopathology and Dermatology
Kaiser Permanente East Bay Medical Facility
Oakland, California

Nina Desai, MD
Dermatology Resident
Department of Dermatology
St. Luke's- Roosevelt Medical Center
New York, New York

Nicole DeYampert
Staff Dermatologist
DeWitt Army Community Hospital
Fort Belvoir, Virginia

Angela D. Dillard, PhD
Associate Professor
Center for Afroamerican & African Studies
University of Michigan
Ann Arbor, Michigan

Charles J. Dimitroff, MD
Assistant Professor of Dermatology
Department of Dermatology, Harvard Skin Disease Research Center
Brigham and Women's Hospital, Harvard Medical School
Boston, Massachusetts

Ncoza Dlova, MBChB, FCDerm S.A
Dermatology Department
Nelson R Mandela School of Medicine
University of Kwa-Zulu Natal
Durban, South Africa

Sean D. Doherty, MD
Resident
Department of Dermatology
Baylor College of Medicine
Houston, Texas

Christy B. Doherty, MD
Resident
Dermatology
Baylor College of Medicine
Houston, Texas

Jeanine B. Downie, MD
Assistant Attending
Dermatology
Overlook and Mountainside Hospitals

Director
Image Dermatology PC
Montclair, New Jersey

Osumane Faye, MD, MPH
Professor Assistant
Department of Dermatology
CNAM- EX Institut Marchoux
Faculty of Medecine, Bamako
Bamako.

Seth B. Forman, MD
Private Practice
Tampa, Florida
Chief Resident
Department of Dermatology
The Virginia Commonwealth University School of Medicine
Richmond, Virginia

Madeliene E. Gainers, MD
Washington University Dermatology Residency Program
St Louis, Missouri

Algin B. Garrett, MD
Chairman
Dermatology
Viriginia Commonwealth University Medical Center
Richmond, Virginia

Jorge I. Gaviria, MD
Medical Director
Hair Transplant Surgery and Research
Aderans/MHR
Boca Raton, FL
Scientifc & Medical Director
Hair Transplant Surgery and Research
Instituto Clinico Capilar
Barcelona, Spain

Amy Geng, MD
Dermatologist
Boston Dermatology and Laser Center
Boston, Massachusetts

Yvette Andree George, MD, FAAD
Hospital Staff
Internal Medicine
Northside Hospital
Atlanta, Georgia

Marcia J. Glenn, MD
Assistant Professor
Division of Dermatology
Internal Medicine
King-Drew Medical Center
Los Angeles, California
Private Practice
Odyssey MediSpa
Marina del Rey, California

Pearl E. Grimes, MD
Director
Vitiligo & Pigmentation Institute of Southern California
Clinical Professor
Division of Dermatology
David Geffen School of Medicine, UCLA
Los Angeles, California

Aditya K. Gupta, MD, PhD
Professor
Division of Dermatology
Department of Medicine
Sunnybrook and Women's College Health Sciences Center
University of Toronto
Toronto, Ontario
Mediprobe Research Inc.
London, Ontario

Jennifer C. Haley, MD
Associate Clinical Professor Dermatology
Co-Director Dermatopathology
David Geffen School of Medicine at UCLA
Los Angeles, California

Candrice R. Heath, MD
Clinical Research Fellow
Society Hill Dermatology
Philadelphia, Pennsylvania

Dóris Hexsel, MD
Former Professor of Dermatology
School of Medicine at the University of Passo Fundo, Brazil
Research Center
Brazilian Center for Studies in Dermatology
Porto Alegre, RS - Brazil

Shari Hicks-Graham, MD
Staff Physician
Internal Medicine, Dermatology
Grant Medical Center
Columbus, Ohio

Lori M. Hobbs, MD
Director of Dermatologic Lasers
Internal Medicine/Dermatology
King/MACC (Multi-Services Ambulatory Care Center)
Los Angeles, California

Marvi Iqbal, MD
Dermatology Resident
UCI Medical Center
Irvine, California

Gina D. Jefferson, MD
Resident Physician
Otolaryngology-Head & Neck Surgery
Charles R. Drew University
Los Angeles, California

Nathaniel J. Jellinek, MD
Assistant Professor
Department of Dermatology
Brown Medical School
Providence, Rhode Island

Elena Jones, MD
Associate Attending
Department of Dermatology
St. Luke's Roosevelt Hospital
New York, New York

Wilbert C. Jordan, MD, MPH
Director
OASIS Clinic
Los Angeles, California

Jacqueline M. Junkins-Hopkins, MD
Associate Professor
Dermatology
Univerity of Pennsylvania
Philadelphia, Pennsylvania
Associate Professor
Department of Dermatology
Johns Hopkins Univeristy
Baltimore, Maryland

Brittney Kaufman De Clerck, MD
Resident Physician
Dermatology
Los Angeles County & University of Southern California Medical Center
Los Angeles, California

A. PAUL KELLY, MD
Professor of Medicine, Division of Dermatology
Charles Drew University of Medicine and Science
Chief Emeritus, Division of Dermatology
Former King/Drew Medical Center
Los Angeles, California
Clinical Professor of Medicine
Division of Dermatology
The David Geffen School of Medicine at UCLA
Los Angeles, California

Lawrence S.W. Khoo, MD
Consultant Dermatologist
Dermatology Associates
Singapore

Tameka K. Lane, MD
Dermatology Service
William Jennings Bryan Dorn Veterans Affairs Medical Center
Department of Veterans Affairs, Columbia, South Carolina, USA

Anh Le, DDS, PhD
Associate Professor
Surgical, Therapeutic and Bioengineering Sciences
University of Southern California
Los Angeles, California

Barbara J. Leppard, DM, FRCP
Consultant Dermatologist (Retired)
Southampton University Hospitals NHS Trust
Southampton, United Kingdom
Associate Professor of Dermatology and Consultant Dermatologist
Regional Dermatology Training Centre, Kilimanjaro
Christian Medical Centre
Moshi, Tanzania

Joyce Teng Ee Lim, MD
Dermatologist
Joyce Lim Skin and Laser Clinic
Singapore
Visiting Consultant
National Skin Center
Singapore

Henry W. Lim, MD
Chariman and CS Livingood Chair of Dermatology
Henry Ford Hospital
Detroit, Michigan

Lindsay E. Lynch

Jason C. McBean, MD, FAAD
Fellow, Juva Skin and Laser Center
New York, New York

Halliday Craige McDonald, MD
Resident
Dermatology
University of Texas Southwestern
Dallas, Texas

Charles J. McDonald, MD
Professor of Medical Science and Chairman
Dermatology
The Warren Alpert Medical School of Brown University
Physician-in-Chief
Dermatology
Rhode Island Hospital
Providence, Rhode Island

Lynn McKinley-Grant, MD
Associate Clinical Professor
Dermatology
Washington Hospital Center
Washington, DC

Private Practice
Chevy Chase, Maryland

Amy J. McMichael, MD
Associate Professor of Dermatology
Department of Dermatology
Wake Forest University School of Medicine
Winston-Salem, North Carolina

Diana V. Messadi, DDS, MMSc, DMSc
Professor and Chair
Section of Oral Medicine and Orofacial Pain
UCLA School of Dentistry
Los Angeles, California

Ginat W. Mirowski, DMD, MD
Associate Professor
Department of Dermatology
Northwestern University
Chicago, Illinois
Adjunct Associate Professor
Oral Pathology, Medicine, Radiology
Indiana University
Indianapolis, Indiana

Richard S. Mizuguchi, MD
Director
Hair Restoration Surgery Center
Department of Dermatology
St. Luke's, Roosevelt and Beth Israel
New York, New York

Nilesh Morar, MBChB, MMedDerm, FCDerm
Consultant Dermatologist
Chelsea and Westminster Hospital
Honorary Senior Lecturer
Imperial College London
London, England

Gabriela Munhoz-da-Fontoura, MD
Resident of Dermatology
Sector of Dermatology and Post-Graduation Course in Dermatology
School of Medicine and HUCFF-UFRJ
Federal University of Rio de Janeiro
Rio de Janeiro, Brazil

Kim Nichols, MD
Private Practice
Skin Specialty Group
New York, New York

Edith Nkechi Nnoruka, MD
Senior Lecturer
Sub-Dept of Dermatology
College of Medicine
Consultant Physician/Dermato Venereologist
University of Nigeria Teaching Hospital
Enugu, Nigeria and
Parklane Specialist Hospital, Enugu, Nigeria

Anezi N. Okoro, MBChB, FRCP
Professor
Medicine
Ebonyi State University
Abakaliki, Ebonyi

Honorary Consultant
Medicine
Ebonyi State University Teaching Hospital
Abakaliki, Ebonyi

Mobolaji Opeola, MD
Center for Skin Cosmetic Dermatology
Fort Worth, Texas

Felix D. Oresanya, FMCP
Department of Medicine
General Hospital Lagos
Lagos, Nigeria

Amit G. Pandya, MD
Professor
Dermatology
University of Texas Southwestern Medical Center
Dallas, Texas

Jocelyne Papacharalambous, MD
Pfizer Pharmaceuticals Group
New York, New York

Justine H. Park, MD
Assistant Professor of Dermatology
University of Southern California
Director of Pediatric Dermatology, CHLA
Los Angeles, California

Frederick N. Quarles, MD, FAAD
Dermatologist
Private Practice
Virginia Beach, Virginia

Chemene R. Quinn, MD
Private Practice
Quinn Healthcare, PLLC
Ridgeland, Mississippi
Clinical Assistant Professor
Internal Medicine (Dermatology)
University of Mississippi Medical Center
Jackson, Mississippi

Shobita Rajagopalan, MD, FACP
Professor of Medicine
Internal Medicine/Infectious Disease
Charles R. Drew University of Medicine and Science
Los Angeles, California
Associate Medical Director
Office of the Medical Director
Los Angeles County Department of Public Health Office of AIDS Programs and Policy
Los Angeles, California

Marcia Ramos-e-Silva, MD, PhD
Associate Professor and Chair
Sector of Dermatology
School of Medicine and University Hospital
Federal University of Rio de Janeiro
Rio de Janeiro, Brazil

Marta I. Rendon, MD, FAAD, FACP
Clinical Associate Professor
Department of Dermatology
University of Miami
Miami, Florida
Medical Director
The Dermatology and Aesthetic Center
Boca Raton, Florida

Wendy E. Roberts, MD, FAAD
Medical Director
Desert Dermatology Skin Institute
Rancho Mirage, California

Assistant Clinical Professor of Medicine
Loma Linda University Medical Center
Loma Linda, California

Theodore Rosen, MD
Professor
Department of Dermatology
Baylor College of Medicine
Chief
Dermatology Services
Michael E. DeBakey VA Medical Center
Houston, Texas

Shirley B. Russell, PhD
Division of Dermatology and Center for Human Genetics Research
Department of Medicine
Vanderbilt University Medical Center
Research Service
VA Tennessee Valley Healthcare System
Nashville, Tennessee

Miguel R. Sanchez, MD
Associate Professor
New York University Department of Dermatology
New York University School of Medicine
Director of Dermatology
Department of Dermatology
Bellevue Hospital Center
New York, New York

Rashmi Sarkar, MD
Assistant Professor
Dermatology and Venereology
Maulana Medical College and LOK Nayar Hospital
New Delhi, India

Amado Saúl, MD
Dermatology Professor
Hospital General de Mexico, OD
Mexico City, Mexico

Richard K. Scher, MD, FACP
Professor of Dermatology
University of North Carolina
Chapel Hill, North Carolina
Professor Emeritus
Department of Dermatology
College of Physicians and Surgeons
Columbia University
New York, New York

Heddie O. Sedano, DDS, Dr. Odont
Lecturer
Oral Medicine and Orofacial Pain and also Clinical Especialties (Pediatric Dentistry and Craniofacial Clinic)
School of Dentistry UCLA
Los Angeles, California

Emeritus Professor
Oral Pathology and Genetics
School of Dentistry University of Minnesota
Minneapolis, Minnesota

Dwana R. Shabazz, MD
Dermatology Associates of Northern Virginia
Sterling, Virginia

Nanette B. Silverberg
Clinical Assistant Professor of Dermatology
Columbia University College of Physicians and Surgeons
Director, Pediatric Dermatology
Department of Dermatology
St. Luke's Roosevelt Hospital Center
New York, New York

Saurabh Singh, MD
Resident
Dermatology
Georgetown University/Washington Hospital Center
Washington, DC

Chandra Smart, MD
Department of Pathology and Laboratory Medicine
University of California, Los Angeles
Los Angeles, California

Seaver L. Soon, MD
Staff Physician
Division of Dermatology & Dermatologic Surgery
Scripps Clinic & The Scripps Research Institute
La Jolla, California

Pamela Summers, MD, MBA
Department of Dermatology
Case Western Reserve University, University Hospitals Case Medical Center
Cleveland, Ohio

Priya Swamy Zeikus, MD
Assistant Professor
University of Texas Southwestern Medical School
Dallas Texas

Flora N. Taylor, MD
Instructor of Group Processes
Wharton School of Business
University of Pennsylvania
Philadelphia, Pennsylvania

SUSAN C. TAYLOR, MD
Founding Director
Skin of Color Center
Division of Dermatology
St. Luke's-Roosevelt Hospital Center
New York, New York
Assistant Clinical Professor of Dermatology
College of Physicians and Surgeons
Columbia University Medical Center
New York, New York

Yemane-Berhan Tebebe, MD, PhD
Medicine
All Africa Leprosy Rehabilitation Training Center
Addis Ababa, Ethiopa

Ella L. Toombs
Assistant Professor of Dermatology Department of Dermatology
Rush University Medical Center Chicago Ill Aesthetic Dermatology Washington, DC

Gisela Torres-Bonilla, MD
Senior Instructor
Dermatology
Case Western Reserve University
Staff Dermatologist
Dermatology
MetroHealth Medical Center
Cleveland, Ohio

Andrea Trowers, MD
Voluntary Faculty
Department of Dermatology
University of Miami
Miami, Florida

Micole Tuchman, MD
Resident
Department of Dermatology
New York Medical College
New York, New York

Meredith Warnick, MD
Melanoma Fellow
Melanoma Center
Washington Cancer Institute, Washington Hospital Center
Washington, DC

Carl V. Washington, MD
Associate Professor of Dermatology
Emory University School of Medicine
Atlanta, Georgia

Jeffrey M. Weinberg, MD
Director, Clinical Research Center
Department of Dermatology
St. Luke's-Roosevelt Hospital Center
Assistant Clinical Professor of Dermatology
Department of Dermatology
Columbia University College of Physicians and Surgeons
New York, New York

Dakara Rucker Wright, MD
Henry Ford Medical Center
Dermatology Resident
Detroit, Michigan

Sharona Yashar, MD
Dermatologist,
Division of Dermatology, Department of Medicine
Ucla (David Geffen School of Medicine At UCLA)
Los Angeles, California

Cherie M. Young, MD
Director of Research
Callender Skin and Laser Center
Mitchellville, Maryland

Jasmine H. Yun, MD, PhD
Clinical Assistant Professor
Department of Dermatology
University of Southern California
Keck School of Medicine
Los Angeles, California

FOREWORD

The specialty and field of skin of color in dermatology has expanded greatly in recent years. In the United States, the proportion of the population with skin of color, including those of African descent as well as Latinos and Asians, is increasing. This trend will eventually lead to half of the U.S. population being composed of these groups by the middle of this century. The majority of the worldwide population is already composed of groups with skin of color.

Dermatological management and care can be vastly different in patients with skin of color. This is due to a number of differences in pathophysiology of skin disease, presentation of skin disease, and the presence of unique skin diseases in these patients. *Dermatology for Skin of Color* is inclusive of these differences. The textbook is important to the contemporary practice of dermatology, regardless of geographic locations, because patients with skin of color are encountered throughout the United States, as well as worldwide.

Rebat M. Halder, MD
Professor and Chairman
Department of Dermatology
Howard University
Washington, DC

INTRODUCTION

In the United States, as we begin the twenty-first century, great hope and promise fills the specialty of dermatology. New understandings of the genetic basis of illnesses, biological treatments for psoriasis, new devises for use in anti-aging, as well as other topical treatment for skin diseases have improved the lives of our patients.

The U.S. population is in the midst of a dramatic demographic shift. This population shift primarily involves increases in the number of people of color. Currently, the U.S. population is 12.7% black, 13% Hispanic, 4.6% Asian, and 2.5% other races. The shift will continue so that the projected population in the year 2050 will be 24.4% Hispanic, 14.6% black, 8% Asian, and 5.3% other races! This means that by year 2050, the U.S. population will be majority people of color.

Even as these diverse populations continue to increase, we still have a limited knowledge about ethnic skin. Evidence-based data about structural and functional differences (if any) in the skin of people of color is lacking. It is of utmost importance that these population groups be studied further and in greater detail so that disease response and treatment may be elucidated. Cultural competency is likewise important when treating these patients. In many skin of color patients, we are seeing delayed treatment for various skin diseases, including worsening of prognosis for melanomas.

It is because of the aforementioned reasons that a textbook, such as this one, on skin of color is an important and welcomed addition to the medical literature. An understanding of diseases that occur commonly in skin of color populations, their presentation, clinical features, diagnostic criteria, and treatment are essential for all dermatologists. As important is an understanding of the cultural habits, practices, and beliefs of diverse ethnic groups, which this text also offers.

In addition to great textbooks, academic institutions and specialty societies can also make an important contribution to skin of color dermatology. The Skin of Color Society is doing just that by embarking upon the task of developing a comprehensive skin classification system for patients with skin of color. This system, designed to complement the Fitzpatrick Skin Type classification system, would provide predictive information related to a patient's response to trauma (scarring) and inflammation (dyschromias), for example.

Finally, I applaud Dr. A. Paul Kelly and Dr. Susan C. Taylor for editing this textbook, which will undoubtedly expand our understanding of dermatological problems in our patients of color.

David Rodriguez, MD
Skin of Color Society
Miami, Florida

PREFACE

Historically, mainstream dermatologic research, literature, and training had little focus on skin of color. In addition to the paucity of reliable information regarding the pathology, physiology and reactivity of more darkly hued skin, there were misconceptions based on myth, folklore, and prejudice. Fortunately, by the end of the twentieth century, new interest and attention had turned to the burgeoning field of skin of color. Textbooks first by Johnson and then by Halder and Grimes served to create a foundation upon which an understanding of ethnic skin, pigmented skins, and darker skin types have been built. Efforts by the Skin of Color Society, the Dermatology section of the National Medical Association, and the American Academy of Dermatology have also aided in advancing understanding of skin of color.

The purpose of *Dermatology for Skin of Color* is to provide an in-depth, scientific view of all aspects of skin of color. Thus, we have created a comprehensive textbook and photographic atlas written by dozens of nationally and internationally recognized experts in the field. It is intended as both a textbook and as a reference guide for all physicians, especially dermatologists, medical students, dermatology residents and physician extenders. It contains chapters on the structure, function, biology, and the myriad of diseases occurring in patients of color as well as cosmetic issues. In addition, *Dermatology for Skin of Color* provides a rich understanding of the cultural habits, practices, beliefs, and use of alternative medicine by patients of diverse backgrounds. It concludes with a section on comparative dermatology from Africa, Asia, and Latin America and a spectacular atlas of skin of color dermatology.

As our population grows increasingly multiracial, multicultural, as well as multiethnic, dermatologists will be challenged with the task of recognizing how darker skin differs from lighter skin, what is normal versus pathological, which treatments have the highest efficacy and lowest morbidity, and how to interact with patients in a culturally competent manner. It is our hope that this book will serve as an invaluable tool to help dermatologists and the larger medical community meet those challenges.

A. Paul Kelly, MD
Susan C. Taylor, MD

ACKNOWLEDGMENTS

To paraphrase a popular idiom, "It takes a village to create a dermatologist." The village for me has great depth and breadth and consists of mentors. Some of them I directly trained under at Penn, Harvard, and Columbia. Others I have had the pleasure of observing and learning from at scientific meetings and through their writing. Still others I interact with currently and are always stimulating my thoughts, ideas, and passion regarding skin of color. Dr. Vincent DeLeo, a real leader in dermatology, not only sparked my interest in skin of color but has nurtured it for the past 15 years. Dr. A. Paul Kelly, a leader in dermatology with extraordinary knowledge, insight, and vision, has been a guiding force. A profound thank you to the remainder of my village, past, present, and future.

Skin of Color Center:

Vincert DeLeo
Andrew Alexis
Nanette Silverberg
Jeffery Weinberg
Richard Mizuguchi
Maritza Perez
Fran Cook-Bolden (emerita)
Elana Jones (emerita)

Skin of Color Society:

Andrew Alexis
Cheryl M. Burgess
Valerie Callender
Pearl Grimes
Aditya Gupta
Rebat Halder
Victoria Holloway
A. Paul Kelly
Henry Lim
Harvey Liu
Amit Pandya
Marta Rendon
David Rodriguez
Richard Scher
Miguel Sanchez (emeritus)
Vincent DeLeo (emeritus)

Pigmentary Disorders Academy:

Jean-Paul Ortonne
James Nordlund
Pearl Grimes
Amit Pandya
Marta Rendon
Doris Hexsel
Mauro Picardo
Tania Cestari
Ivonne Arellano-Mendoza
Sungbin Im
Mark Berneburg
Wiete Westerhof
Joyce Lim
Harvey Lui
Henry Chan

The Skin of Color Textbook Family: Beverly Baker-Kelly, A. Paul Kelly, Anne Sydor, Sarah Granlund and Sandhya Joshi.

My Family: Ethel Taylor, Charles Taylor, Flora Taylor, Kemel Dawkins, Morgan Dawkins, Madison Dawkins.

—Susan

Drs. Kenney, Livingood and McDonald are the professors most responsible for my dermatology sojourn. Dr. John A. Kenney, Jr. my professor of dermatology at Howard University, College of Medicine, was the first person to stimulate my interest in skin diseases. As a vibrant lecturer and enthusiastic clinician, he not only influenced me to become a dermatologist, but also similarly influenced six other of my medical school classmates ("the Magnificent Seven") to choose dermatology as a career. Through his expertise, persistence and dedication, dermatologists and other physicians have become aware of the nuances unique to skin of color and implications for treatment. Dr. Kenney's efforts have led to the recognition of specialized treatment of dermatologic diseases in skin of color.

Dr. Clarence S. Livingood, and the dermatology staff at Henry Ford Hospital, provided me with a superb dermatology residency program, with a special emphasis on quality patient care. Dr. Livingood's example of hard work, commitment, dedication and excellent patient rapport were the ingredients that have not only helped me to survive in academic dermatology but have also helped me to persevere in the preparation of this textbook.

My two years with Dr. Charles J. McDonald at Brown University School of Medicine was a perfect "dermatologic finishing school". Dr. McDonald was responsible for my developing administrative and teaching skills and broadening my horizons in skin diseases related to medical disorders. He also nurtured my interest in skin diseases in skin of color, and planted the seed for me to undertake the writing of a textbook on this subject. My heartfelt thanks to these teachers: Drs. Kenney, Livingood and McDonald.

In addition, special thanks goes to Aban H. Kapadia for her indispensible word-processing and cataloging of the chapters; and to Patricia Elmore and Altona Johns-Anderson for their professional and steady editing of select chapters. Lastly, special thanks are in order for Dr. Yvonne Knight for allowing us to use many of the clinical photographs that appear herein.

Thanks to my mother, Amanda Walker Kelly, and father, Joseph Paul Kelly, MD, who always encouraged me to do the best job possible, no matter my profession or endeavor. Thanks are in order for my many colleagues, especially the members of the Section on Dermatology of the National Medical Association, who donated photos for the textbook, encouraged me to complete this textbook and gave me therapeutic pearls on treating skin disorders in skin of color.

From the bottom of my heart, I thank my daughters, Traci Allyce Kelly and Kara Gisele Kelly, who allowed me sustained seclusion while I developed my areas of expertise in skin of color.

And to my wife of forty-two years, Attorney and Professor Beverly Baker-Kelly, who unswervingly supported me throughout each phase of the production of this book. She is to be credited with the idea for the Atlas portion of the book due to her longstanding legal work, vision and commitment to internationalism.

Last, but not least, appreciation goes to my co-editor, Dr. Susan C. Taylor, who conceived of the idea of this textbook on dermatology for skin of color and who gave me the great privilege of being her co-editor.

Dermatology for Skin of Color

SECTION 1

Definitions, Epidemiology and Cultural Considerations

CHAPTER 1

Skin of Color: A Historical Perspective

A. Paul Kelly

Key Points

- Myth and religion provided the earliest explanations of skin color.
- Most early rational explanations ascribed skin color to climate.
- Nineteenth century pseudoscientific theories often supported the polygenist school, i.e, separate origins of the races.
- Darwin ended the polygenist argument and led to theories of skin color based on evolution.
- Pseudoscientific misinformation, based on faulty or undocumented evidence, justified early twentieth-century socio-political prejudices and is often still considered fact.
- Modern research has led to the Vitamin D-sunlight and camouflage theories, and an understanding of the biological process that produces skin color.

Skin of color is a subject that throughout history has been shrouded in mystery, misconception, mystique, and misunderstanding. Since antiquity,[1] people have sought answers to questions such as where skin color comes from, what was the color of the first humans, and why humans developed different skin colors.

MYTHS ABOUT SKIN OF COLOR

One of the earliest explanations for skin color of humans was proposed by the ancient Greek writers. According to their mythology, Phaeton, the son of Helios, the sun-god, persuaded his father to let him drive the sun chariot for a day. Because of his inexperience and inability to control the fiery steeds, Phaeton drove the chariot too near the earth in certain lands, burning the people black, and too far from the earth in other regions, causing he people to turn pale and cold.[2] The early Greeks, probably had brown skin tones that were midway between black and white skin pigment.

According to an early African myth, early humans quarreled over the first ox slaughtered for food. The color of their descendants thus was determined by the distribution of the meat. Those who ate the liver had black children, those who took the lungs and blood had red children, and those who ate the intestines had white children.[3]

A North American Indian legend claims that both blacks and whites were created before God had sufficient time to master his skin-coloring technique. In baking the first human, God cooked him too long, and he emerged black. The white person also was a culinary failure because he was not baked long enough and consequently turned out pale-skinned. It was only with the third attempt that God was able to produce the properly baked, golden brown Indian.[4,5]

RELIGIOUS EXPLANATIONS FOR SKIN OF COLOR

Every religion seems to have its own doctrine on the origin of skin of color, especially black verses white. One of the most widely cited versions is that the biblical Ham and his descendants became black because he was cursed by Noah. Actually, there is no mention in Genesis of the descendants of Ham or of his son Canaan being black; this belief seems to originate in the Talmud, Midrash Rabbah, and other rabbinical writings from the second to the fifth centuries A.D. as interpretations of Genesis 9:20-27.[6]

There are several versions of this story. The most popular version is that Noah forbade all the people and animals on the ark to have sexual intercourse. Ham disobeyed this order and was cursed by being turned black and became the ancestor of all black people.[7]

Another version is that while Noah was drunk and lying naked on the ground, spilling his semen, Ham laughed at him. Noah's other sons, walking backwards in order not to observe their father's nakedness, covered Noah with a garment. Noah punished Ham by having the curse fall on his son Canaan. The descendants of Ham, through Canaan, therefore, have dark skin because Ham observed his father's nakedness, they have "misshapen" lips because Ham spoke to his brothers about Noah's condition, and they have curly hair because Ham twisted his head around to observe his father's nakedness.[8]

Still another version of the story is that Ham was cursed with blackness because he resented the fact that his father desired to have a fourth son. To prevent the birth of a rival heir, Ham is said to have castrated his father.[7]

The Midrash Rabbah, Genesis-Noah, Chapter 37, gives yet a different version. It states that in the quarrel between Ham and Noah, Noah said, "You have prevented me from doing something in the dark, i.e., sexual intercourse; therefore, your seed will be ugly and dark-skinned,"[6] thus giving rise to another commonly held rationale for black skin.

The "curse of Ham" had been used by some members of Abrahamic religions to justify racism and the enslavement of people of black African ancestry, who were believed to be descendants of Ham. They were often called Hamites and were believed to have descended through Canaan or his older brothers. This racist theory was widely held during the eighteenth to twentieth centuries but largely has been abandoned since the mid-twentieth century by even the most conservative theologians.[9]

In the story of Cain and Abel, Cain slew Abel because of jealousy over God's favor. He became an outcast, but in order to protect Cain from vengeful hands, God placed a protecting mark on him. The brand he bore has associated Cain and his kind with evil. Many who wanted to prove that black people were inferior claimed that Cain's protecting mark was blackness.[9]

Some black ministers, on the other hand, have viewed the story of Cain and Abel in a different light. According to their interpretation, Cain was originally black when he killed Abel, and when God shouted at him in the Garden, he turned white from fright, and his features shrank up.[10]

Another biblical teaching is that white skin is the result of leprosy. The ancestor of whites, they say, was Gehazi, servant of Elisha, who was cursed with leprosy for having solicited money from Naaman (II Kings, 5:21).[11]

The Mormon prophet Joseph Smith claimed that the "Lamanites," a white people, were changed to black by God for their sins. The book of Mormons, II

Nephri, verses 21–23, reads: "And he caused the cursing to come upon them, yet, even a sore cursing because of this inequity. For behold they had hardened their hearts against him that they had become like flint; wherefore as they were white and exceedingly fair and delightsome that they might not be enticing unto my people, the lord God did cause a skin of blackness to come upon them."[12]

EUROPEAN THOUGHT ON SKIN OF COLOR

In 1520, Paracelsus, a Swiss physician, declared that the children of Adam occupied only a small part of the earth. He also held that black people and other nonwhite people had a wholly separate origin. "God could not endure to have the rest of the world empty so by his admirable wisdom filled the world with other men." Likewise, Isaac de la Peyrere, a French Protestant, in a book published in 1655 argued that there had been two separate creations of humans. In the first chapter of Genesis, a man and a woman are given domain over every living thing, but not until the second chapter is anything said of the creation of Adam and Eve. Cain chose his wife from the earlier race when he was cast off by his own people for the murder of Abel. Peyrere believed that it was from the pre-Adamite race that the natives of Africa, Asia, and the New World were descended.[13]

Leonardo da Vinci was convinced that humankind was really unified and that physical difference among races could be explained by environment. He thought that people born in hot countries were black because they found the cool, dark nights refreshing and did much of their work at that time, thus becoming dark. Likewise, the people of northern climates were white because they worked during the day.[14]

John Friedrich Blumenbach, (1752–1840), a professor of medicine at the University of Gottingen, made a lifelong study of racial differences. It was he who coined the word *Caucasian* to describe the white race. The word is based on a single skull in Blumenbach's collection that came from the Caucasus Mountain Region of Russia. Blumenbach thought that the differences in human color were produced by a combination of climate and other factors. Although he had no solution to the question of race and color, he speculated that the blackness in Negroes might be caused by a tendency in the tropics for carbon to be imbedded in the skin. Carbon on contact with oxygen would darken. He also postulated there might be some connection between the blackness that white women sometimes develop during pregnancy and the blackness that Negroes develop permanently.[15]

In 1837, Viroy disagreed that climate and external factors had any effect on skin color, having observed that newborn black children are of a reddish or yellowish color with a brownish hue to some parts of their bodies, such as the circles around the nails of the fingers and toes and genital organs. A week after birth, their skin darkens, either in a cold or a warm climate, whether exposed to the sunlight or kept in a dark place. Therefore, Viroy concluded, since blackness seemed to be hereditary in all countries and in all generations, external causes must have little, if any, effect on the determination of skin color.[16]

Dr. Johann Meckle, and other eighteenth- and nineteenth-century anatomists, thought that the complexion of Negroes was caused by color contained in the cortical part of the brain. It was his opinion that nerves emerging from the brain medulla oblongata convey a black color to all the body, including the skin.[17]

AMERICAN TREATISES ON RACE AND SKIN COLOR

One of the first American treatises on race and skin color was by the Reverend Samuel Stanhope Smith (1751–1819), a Presbyterian minister and professor of moral philosophy at the College of New Jersey (now Princeton) and later its president. His "Essay on the Causes of the Variety of Complexion and Figure" attributed color mainly to climate. He maintained that dark skin might well be considered one universal freckle. "As one moved towards the tropics one would find successively darker shades of skin." He believed that, in time, the dark color would become hereditary.[18]

What seemed to be a dramatic confirmation of Smith's theory on the influence of climate on human skin color was the case of Henry Moss. Born a slave in Virginia, Moss fought in the Revolutionary War and then moved to the North. After many years there, he developed white spots on his body (probably vitiligo) and in three years had become almost completely white. In 1796 he was exhibited in Philadelphia as a scientific curiosity. Dr. Smith, of course, claimed Moss was living proof that the human species is a single unit and that Negroes would, in time, change their complexion to white in a northern climate. Smith noted that "wherever there were vents in the thin clothes that covered Moss there were generally seen the largest spots of black," proof that the sun was the determinant of a dark color.[18]

He thought that if Negroes were perfectly free, enjoyed property, and were admitted to a liberal participation of the society, rank, and privileges of their masters, they would change much faster their African peculiarities of skin, large lips, and large noses.[18]

Benjamin Rush (1745–1813), a founding father of the United States and an eminent physician of the late eighteenth century, also was fascinated by the case of Henry Moss. He based his argument on "scientific findings" that being black was a heredity illness, which he referred to as "negroidism." In an address to the American Philosophical Society, Rush said that the only evidence of a "cure" occurred when the skin color turned white. Rush drew the conclusion that "blackness was a mild form of a noncontiguous disease." He stated that "the black Color as it is called in Negroes is derived from Leprosy, but Moss was, for some reason, undergoing a cure induced by nature itself and was thus reverting to his natural white color."[19,20]

PSEUDOSCIENTIFIC THEORIES OF SKIN COLOR

Many pseudoscientific theories of race and skin color abounded in the nineteenth century. Various arguments seemed to support one or the other of the two main camps: the monogenist or polygenist school of thought. The leader of the polygenist school was Dr. Samuel Morton (1799–1851), a famous physician and researcher in natural history. According to Morton, the key to the separate origin of races was found in hybrids, or mulattoes. Since Linneaus, the test of species in natural history had been the ability of two organisms to produce fertile offspring. It was Morton's opinion that mulatto women bore children only with great difficulty, and if these women mated only with other mulattoes, their children are less fertile, so the progeny would eventually die out. From his conviction that "half-breeds" cannot propagate themselves indefinitely, Morton concluded that blacks and whites are not varieties of a single race but entirely different species.[21,22]

In the nineteenth century, the theory of maternal impression resurfaced, an earlier explanation for why white women have black babies and black women have white ones. The theory is attributed to Hippocrates, who saved the honor of a princess accused of adultery because she bore a black baby by saying that the princess, while in intercourse with her husband, saw a picture of a Negro cohabitating with a white woman.[23]

The Midrash Rabbah, a collection of ancient Jewish legends, supports the theory of maternal impression: "The Ethiopian wife presents her black husband with a light colored child. The husband tells the rabbi that the child is not his. The rabbi asks whether there was a picture of a man in the room at the moment of intercourse, being told there was, inquires whether it was white or black. When told it was white, the rabbi answered, "This accounts for the color of your son."[24]

Hardlicka, in the early nineteenth century, believed that the pure strains of the colored races will not show a red mark on the skin when the fingernails are drawn over the chest with pressure. However, if there is any intermixture with whites, the lines will show as fairly broad red marks, and the flush will be of some duration, both features being more marked the more white blood present in the individual examined.[25]

DARWIN'S THEORY OF EVOLUTION

Charles Darwin's (1809–1882) theory of evolution ended the monogenist-polygenist controversy over race. Darwin left no doubt that all human races belong to the same species. He wrote: "Although the existing races of man [*sic*] differ in many respects as in color, hair, shape of the skull, proportions of the body, etc., if their whole structure is taken into consideration they are found to resemble each other closely in a multitude of points. Many of these are so unimportant or of so singular a nature that it is extremely improbable that they should have been independently acquired by aboriginally distinct species or races."[26]

One evolutionary concept of race and color was advanced by Robert Chambers, an Edinburgh publisher and amateur scientist, who in 1844 anonymously published "Vestiges of the Natural History of Creation." He argues that man [*sic*] began as Negro, passed through Malay, Indian, and Mongolian phases, and finally emerged as Caucasian. The nonwhite people were thus simply a representation of the development of the highest, the Caucasian.[27]

An oft-quoted early-twentieth-century opinion on the origin of skin of color was that of Brace. He believed that early humans lived in the tropics and exchanged his anthropoidean fur coat for an improved sweat gland system that allowed him to run down game in the heat of the day. The loss of body hair thus exposed the early hominoids to the dangers of skin cancer and the need for protection from ultraviolet radiation damage led to the development of black skin. Successful and extensive human occupation of the north temperate zones, as a permanent habitat, did not occur until the last glaciation, 70,000 years ago. While the previous glaciations had forced people to areas closer to the equator, by the end of the third interglacial movement, they had developed technology for the cold further north, where large game abounded. There, the adaptive significance of melanin was substantially reduced, with the inevitable result that mutations detrimental to melanin production allowed people with nonblack skin to survive and multiply.[28]

PSEUDOSCIENTIFIC DATA ON SKIN OF COLOR

Controversy still abounds when one discusses the scientific data documenting the anatomic and/or physiologic differences between black skin and white skin. One of the main reasons for this controversy was the undocumented evidence published by "experts" on the subject, such as Neidelman's article, "Abnormalities of Pigmentation in the Negro," in which the introductory paragraph includes the sentence "the skin of persons of the Negro race differs from that of members of the white race not only in structure and physiology but in its reaction to trauma and infection."[29]

An early-twentieth-century publication by Fox is one of the classics on the difference between Negro (black) and white skin. Fox made such statements as "the skin of the Negro, especially the dermis, is thicker than that of the white. This is also true of the subcutaneous tissues, as exemplified by the characteristic thick lips of the Negro."[30,31]

Fox's statements were probably influenced by the monumental publication of Matas in 1896. Matas made the following statements about Negro skin: "The greater thickness of the whole skin is [a] generally conceded characteristic of the Negro"; "the glandular cutaneous system is more highly developed in the Negro than in the white; and "the Negro has excess activity of the sebaceous glands."[32]

Although Matas and scientists of his day did not have the luxury of the modern investigative tools, they were able to determine that the chemical composition of pigment in blacks is identical with that in whites. "This melanin of the Negro differs from that of the white in quantity and general distribution rather than in quality."[32]

Unfortunately, Matas, as did other eminent scientists of that era, used pseudoscientific data to advance, justify, and defend some of the prejudicial sociopolitical doctrines of the day. Examples of how erroneous cutaneous data were used in a direct or indirect fashion to propagate some of these beliefs are the follwoing: "It is well known that the blacker the Negro the healthier and stronger he is"; "any diminution in color of the pure race, outside of albinism, is a mark of feebleness or ill health;" "physiological baldness is one of the rarest phenomena, even in the oldest of seniors"; "the Negro is not esthetic and a mere cosmetic complaint would not appeal to his intelligence requiring a therapeutic approach."[33,34]

Not only in skin, but also, according to Balloch, "the Negro differs from the Caucasian anatomically, physiologically and pathologically."[35] He carried his erroneous clinical observations further by stating that "the dominant physiologic peculiarity of the Negro is the lessened sensibility of the nervous system, the Negro bears surgical operations remarkably well: he seldom suffers from shock, and wounds of all kind heal with quickness, and that is certainly delightful to the surgeon."[35] Unfortunately, much of this misinformation has been disseminated throughout the scientific literature, and some still is regarded as fact rather than fiction.

MODERN SCIENTIFIC THEORIES

The most widely accepted modern-day explanation of skin of color is the vitamin D–sunlight theory. It assumed that the first humans lived in a very warm climate, such as that found in Africa. Only those with dark skin were protected from the damaging effects of ultraviolet light; those with lighter skin were less successful and not chosen as mates, and so, after thousands of years, essentially vanished.[36]

Early humans, however, were hunters, and as nearby game was depleted, they followed their prey into cooler areas. There the dark skin, which had protected them from ultraviolet rays, now screened out too much of the sun's light, resulting in lower synthesis of too little vitamin D. Insufficient amounts of vitamin D in infants would have resulted in bowed legs, knock knees, scoliosis, and other manifestations of rickets and similar ossification defects in older children. Women deprived of adequate vitamin D during puberty, pregnancy, and lactation were predisposed to osteomalacia. On the other hand, people with lighter skin would thrive away from the equator because excessive amounts of vitamin D often lead to kidney stones and other metastatic calcifications in infants.[37]

When humans moved north of the Mediterranean Sea and latitude 40°N, where the winter sun is less than 20 degrees above the horizon and most of the needed ultraviolet light is removed from the powerful filtering action of the atmosphere, their more deeply pigmented infants must have been especially likely to develop the grossly bent legs and twisted spines characteristic of rickets, crippling their ability to hunt game as adults and making them undesirable as mates.[38] The realization that infants born in the spring and summer had fewer growth defects may have led to the popularity of June weddings.

Another argument for the vitamin D–sunlight theory is that most infants, of all races, have lighter skin at birth than they gradually develop as they mature,[39] paralleling the declining need for vitamin D.

A notable exception to the correlation between latitude and skin color is the Inuits. While having medium brown skin and enduring long, dark Arctic winters, they remain completely free of rickets.[38] A plausible explanation is that their diet contains large quantities of vitamin D, in the form of fish oil and meat, making it unnecessary to have light skin to prevent rickets.

The vitamin D–sunlight theory seems to offer a better explanation of color than the initial early sunlight and heat theories, especially since studies by Weiner and colleagues show that black Yoruba skin reflects only 24% of the incident light, whereas untanned European skin reflects as much as 64%.[39] Therefore, one would expect that the heat-absorbing black skin would be found in the cold northern climates and the reflective white skin near the equator. Also, according to Loomis, ultraviolet regulation rather than heat regulation explains why Caucasians are white in the winter and pigmented in the summer.[36,40]

Morrison, however, takes the opposite view. According to him, prehumans slept without the benefit of fire or clothing, although presumably living in the tropical and subtropical regions of Africa, where nighttime temperatures are often below 20°C. The critical environmental temperature for humans is 27–29°C; at lower temperatures, deep body temperature falls during the night, and this defect must be corrected before the next night. Thus, having melanin to absorb sunlight would aid survival by permitting rapid restoration of body temperature and obviating the need for additional food. The heat-absorption theory also might explain the phenomenon of immediate pigment darkening in darker-skinned people on exposure to sunlight. This obviously would accelerate the absorption of heat.[41]

Morrison also vividly summarized the camouflage theory of skin color, which posits that humans developed in a forest environment, as evidenced by the anatomy and physiology of vision. First, the spectral sensitivity for photopic vision in humans peaks at the 550 nm range, closely corresponding with the spectral composition of light on a forest floor, which is yellow-green with a fairly narrow peak close to the 500-nm range. On the other hand, under an open sky, the sunlight spectrum peaks at between 400 and 700 nm. Second, color discrimination in humans correlates well with the special composition of light in a forest.

Third, the fovea in the human retina provides equal visual sensitivity in vertical and horizontal planes, necessary in the forest, where there is no visual horizontal plane and predators may lurk above and around.[41] Grassland animals, on the other hand, have a visual streak across the retina which provides maximal visual sensitivity in a horizontal plane, giving them panoramic vision. Finally, exposure to bright sunlight for more than a day results in a 50–90% reduction in retinal sensitivity to the visible component of sunlight that can last for more than a week. Humans are obviously not adapted to living in sunlight under an open sky.[41]

In a forest world, dark skin would be advantageous for survival. White skin reflects two to three times more light than black skin, and since we see objects by light reflected from them, a person with light skin would be seen more easily by predators.[41]

While there has been much philosophical, religious, and scientific speculation on the cause of skin of color, the light and electron microscopes have provided us with the answer to what we observe clinically. Szabo[42,43] has demonstrated that melanocytes are symmetrically distributed and do not differ significantly in size, shape, or population density in the various races. The skin of the forehead, cheek, and genital areas contain over 2000 melanocytes per square millimeter, whereas the skin of the trunk has less than 1000 melanocytes per square millimeter, variations that impart the clinical differences in skin color. Also, we know that melanin pigmentation results from the melanin present in melanocytes versus to keratinocytes. Since the ratio of keratinocytes to melanocytes in the epidermis is 36:1, it must be the amount of melanin present in keratinocytes that it is the essential factor in determining of skin color. According to Fitzpatrick and Quevedo,[44] pigmentation of the skin is related to four biologic processes:

1. Formation of melanosomes in melanocytes
2. Melanization of melanosomes in melanocytes
3. Secretion of melanosomes into keratinocytes with and without degradation in lysosomal-like granules
4. Transportation of melanosomes by keratinocytes to the epidermal surface

Step 1 is essentially the same in all races. Blacks, with almost all stage IV melanosomes, have more melanization of their melanosomes than whites, who have mostly stage II and III melanosomes. In melanocytes of all races, the melanosomes are discrete particles, but in the keratinocytes of Caucasoids, Mongoloids, and American Indians, melanosomes are aggregated into groups of two to eight surrounded by a membrane. Mitchell,[45] on the other hand, found that melanosomes in the keratinocytes of Negroes and Australian aboriginals are larger and not aggregated but are found in single bodies. These are the ultramicroscopic differences that impart the clinical differences in the color of people's skin.

Let us hope that our long history of dividing people into social classes based on skin color is nearing an end, and that people of the twenty-first century acknowledge that we are all members of the same family.

At the same time, the real differences between dark and light skin too often have gone unrecognized, resulting in incorrect treatment. The following chapters will examine those differences and their implications for dermatologists.

REFERENCES

1. Khaldun I. *The Muqaddimah: An Introduction to History.* Translated from the Arabic by Franz Rosenthal, Vol I. Princeton, NJ, Princeton University Press, 1996, pp 34-36.
2. Watts AE. *The Metamorphosis of Ovid.* Berkeley, University of California Press, 1954, pp 24-35.
3. Werner A. *African Mythology on the Mythology of All Races,* Vol VII. Cannon J, MacCulloch D (eds). Boston, Cooper Squire Publishers, 1964, p 150.
4. Brown DM. *Indian Fireside Tales.* Madison, WI, Wisconsin Folklore Society Booklet, 1947, pp 3-4.
5. Swanton JR. *Myths and Tales of the Southeastern Indians.* Washington, DC, Smithsonian Institution Bureau of American Ethnology. Bulletin 88, 1919, p 74.
6. Freedman H, Simon S. *Midrash Rabbah, Genesis,* Vol III. London, Soncino Press, 1929, pp 213, 674.
7. Goldberg DM. *The Curse of Ham, Race And Slavery in Early Judaism, Christianity and Islam: Jews, Christians, and Muslims from the Ancient to the Modern World.* Princeton, NJ, Princeton University Press, 2003, pp 154-160.
8. Schwartz RM. *The Curse of Cain: The Violent Legacy of Monotheism.* Chicago, University of Chicago Press, 1997, pp 226-236.
9. Haynes SR. *Noah's Curse: The Biblical Justification of American Slavery.* Oxford, UK, Oxford University Press, 2002, pp 56-87.
10. Rogers JA. *Sex and Race,* Vol III. New York, Helga M Rogers, 1944, pp 316-317.
11. Blank W,. Gehazi. The Church of God Daily Bible Study, A Ministry of God's Word, *www.keyway.ca,* p 1.
12. Smith J. *The Book of Mormon.* Salt Lake City, UT, The Church of Jesus Christ of Latter-Day Saints, 1921, p 61.
13. Campbell A. *White Attitudes Toward Black People.* Ann Arbor, MI, Institute for Social Research, 1971, pp 12-14.
14. Oxford World's Classics. *The Lives of Artists.* Oxford, UK, Oxford University Press, 1998, p 186.
15. Bendyshe MA. *The Anthropological Treaties of Johann Friedrich Blumenbach.* London, Longman, Rogers and Green, 1865, pp 210, 221.
16. Viroy JJ. *Nature History of the Negro Race.* Extracted from the French Edition by Guenebault LJ, Beile B. New York, Babcock & Co., 1837, pp 22-23.
17. Meckle J. *Deutsche Archiv Fir Die Physiologie, Bonn,* Vol 2, pp 287-1875.
18. Zilversmith A (ed). An essay on the causes of the variety of complexion and the figure, in Smith SS (ed), *The Human Species,* 1810. *William and Mary Quarterly* 1966;23(3):506.
19. Rush B. *The Autobiography of Benjamin Rush: "Travels through Life" Together with his Commonplace Book for 1789-1813.* Indianapolis, IN, Bobbs-Merrill, 1812, p 78.
20. Brodsky A. *Benjamin Rush: Patriot and Physician.* New York: Truman Talley Books/St Martin's Press, 2004, pp 102-105.
21. Smith CH. *The Natural History of the Human Species.* Edinburgh, 1848, p 160.
22. Bondeson J. *A Cabinet of Medical Curiosities.* Ithaca, NY, Cornell University Press, 1897, p 146.
23. Zonta M. *A Hebrew Translation of Hippocrates' De Superfoetatione: Historical Introduction and Critical Edition.* Bloomington, Indiana University Press, 2003, pp 97-102.
24. Ginzberg L. *The Legend of the Jews,* Vol 5. Philadelphia, Jewish Publication Society of American, 1925, pp 56, 169-170.
25. Hardlicka A. Anthropometry. *Am J Phys Anthropol* 1919;2:17.
26. Darwin C. *On the Origin of Species by Means of Natural Selection and the Preservation of Favored Races in the Struggle for Life.* London, John Murry, 1859, p 203.
27. Chambers R. *Vestiges of the Natural History of Creation.* London, George Rutledge and Sons, 1844, pp 226-228.
28. Brace CL. *The Stages of Human Evolution,* 3rd ed. Englewood, NJ, Prentice-Hall, 1987, pp 75, 104-105.
29. Niedelman ML. Abnormalities of pigmentation in the Negro. *Arch Dermatol Syphyllol* 1945;51:123.
30. Fox H. Observations on skin diseases in the american negro. *J Cut Dis* 1908;26:67.
31. Rogers JA. Nature *Knows No Color-Line: Research into the Negro Ancestry in the White Race.* New York, Helga M. Rogers, 1952, p 21.
32. Matas R. The surgical peculiarities of the Negro. *Transact Am Surg Assoc* 1896; 14:483.
33. Stanton W. Leopard spots, in *Scientific Attitudes Towards Race in America, 1815-1859.* Chicago, University of Chicago Press, 1960, pp 5-6.
34. Montellane BR, Ortiz. Melanin, Afrocentricity, and pseudoscience. *Yearbook of Physical Anthropology* 1993;36: 33-58.
35. Balloch EA. The relative frequency of fibroid processes in the dark skinner races. *Am J Epidemiol* 1989;79:340-349.
36. Loomis WF. Skin pigment regulation of vitamin-D biosynthesis in man. *Science* 1967;157:501-506.
37. Kirchweger G. The biology of skin color: Black and white—the evolution of race was as simple as the politics of race is complex. *Discover* 2001;22:78.
38. Thomas WA. Health of a carnivorous race: A study of the Eskimo. *JAMA* 2007;88:1559.
39. Weiner JS, Harrison GA, Singer R, et al. Skin color in southern Africans. *Hum Biol* 1964;36:294-307.
40. Quevedo WC, Fitzpatrick TB, Pathak MA, Jimbow K. Light and skin color, in Pathak MA, Harber LC, Seiji M, Kukita A (eds), *Sunlight and Man: Normal and Abnormal Photobiologic Responses.* Consulting editor TB Fitzpatrick. Tokyo, University of Tokyo Press, 1974, pp 165-194.
41. Morrison WL. What is the function of melanin? *Arch Dermatol* 1985;121: 1160-1163.
42. Szabo G. Quantitative histological investigations on the melanocyte system of the human epidermis, in Gordon M (ed), *Pigment Cell Biology.* New York, Academic Press, 1959, pp 99-125.
43. Szabo G, Gerald IB, Pathak MA, Fitzpatrick TB. Racial differences in the fate of melanosomes. *Nature* 1969;222: 1081-1082.
44. Fitzpatrick TB, Quevedo WC, Szabo G, Seiji M. Biology of the melanin pigmentary system, in Fitzpatrick TB et al (eds), *Dermatology in General Medicine.* New York, McGraw-Hill, 1971, pp 117-146.
45. Mitchell RE. The skin of the Australian Aborigine: A light and electromicroscopical study. *Austral J Dermatol* 1968;9: 314-328.

CHAPTER 2

Defining Skin of Color

Susan C. Taylor
Pamela Summers

Key Points

- The term skin of color identifies individuals of racial groups with darker skin than Caucasians, such as Asians, Africans, Native Americans, and Pacific Islanders.
- Patients with skin of color often have distinctive cutaneous characteristics, disorders, and reaction patterns, as well as diverse cultural practices affecting skin care.
- There is a diversity of skin hues, cutaneous diseases, and responses to cutaneous stimuli within each racial or ethnic group.
- The rapid increase of the population with skin of color requires dermatologists and other physicians to have textbooks focusing on their distinct cutaneous disorders, reaction patterns, and cultural practices.

HOW DO WE DEFINE *SKIN OF COLOR*? (Table 2-1)

The term *skin of color* identifies individuals of particular racial and ethnic groups who share similar cutaneous characteristics and disorders, as well as reaction patterns to those disorders and other cutaneous stimuli. In general, these individuals have darker skin hues.

TABLE 2-1
Defining Skin of Color

- How do we define *skin of color*?
- Who are individuals with *skin of color*?
- Why is it useful to define individuals as having *skin of color*?
- Is there a need for a textbook on *skin of color*?

The term also may be used to bring together patients, clinicians, and scientists interested in the treatment and investigation of disorders that occur in these individuals.

WHO ARE INDIVIDUALS WITH *SKIN OF COLOR* AND FROM WHERE DID THEY ORIGINATE?

Individuals with *skin of color* have darker skin hues than those individuals with white skin. Where did these individuals originate from? A set of unique event polymorphisms associated with the nonrecombining portion of the Y chromosome has provided evidence of a common African heritage for all humankind.[1] Mitochondrial DNA analysis likewise has determined that all the women in the world descended from three African women, identified as L1, L2, and L3.[2] Descendants of L1 and L2 populated Africa, whereas descendants of L3 migrated to and populated the remaining continents. Presumably, these African ancestors had darker skin hues, or *skin of color*.

Underhill and colleagues analyzed DNA from 1062 men from 21 populations and demonstrated 131 unique haplotypes.[1] These haplotypes were used to trace the microevolutionary trajectory of global modern human genetic diversification (Table 2-2). Early humans first populated Africa, then Southeast Asia and Japan, Australia, New Guinea, and Central Asia, and finally, the remainder of the continents.

As early humankind migrated into and populated the six continents, they provided the basis for the modern-day concept of racial groups. Races are groups of people identified or defined by the continent from which they derived. Again, genomics supports this concept of race. Rosenberg demonstrated that it is possible to cluster persons into population groups based on geographic origin (continent) with high statistical accuracy.[3] Likewise, Stephens demonstrated, based on single-nucleotide polymorphisms or their corresponding haplotypes, some degree of classification of humans according to continent.[4] Selectively neutral, nonexpressed genes from populations from Africa, Eurasia, East Asia, Oceania, and America correspond with self-reported population ancestry or the concept of racial classifications (for an alternate view of racial classifications, see Chapter 3). The U.S. Census Bureau recognizes five racial groups or categories[5] (Table 2-3).

TABLE 2-2
Migration, Colonization, and Differential Survival of Populations of Humans

- Groups I and II: Africans (Khoisan, Bantu, Pygmy, Sudanese, Ethiopia, and Mali)
- Group III and IV: Africans, Southeast Asians/Japanese
- Group V: Australians, New Guineans, Southeast Asians, Japanese, and Central Asians
- Groups VI–X: Migration across the remainder of the world (except sub-Saharan Africa)

From Underhill PA. The phylogeography of Y-chromosome binary haplotypes and the origins of modern human populations. *Ann Hum Genet* 2001;65:43–62. Used with permission.

TABLE 2-3
Five Catagories for Race (U.S. Census 2000)

- American Indian or Alaska Native
  - Native Americans, Eskimos, Aleuts
- Asian
  - Filipino, Chinese, Japanese, Korean, Vietnamese, Thai, Malaysian, Laotian, Hmog, Indian, Pakistani
- Black
  - African, African Caribbean, African American
- Native Hawaiian or other Pacific Islanders
- White

When referring to individuals with darker skin hues, or *skin of color*, the first five U.S. Census–defined races as listed in Table 2-3 would be included. It is important to note that there is a diversity of skin hues, cutaneous diseases, and responses to cutaneous stimuli in individuals within each racial group. The Asian population reflects this intraracial diversity in that Southeast Asians and South Asians are, in general, of darker skin hues than the East Asian population (Table 2-4).

Individuals with skin of color are also defined by ethnic group. An *ethnic group* is a group of people who share a common culture, language, religion, history, and other source of group identification. In the United States, the largest and the fastest-growing ethnic group is Hispanics or Latinos[6] (Table 2-5). This group is also a diverse one, with people hailing from many counties and from different racial groups. An individual of Hispanic or Latino ethnicity may be

TABLE 2-4
Subdivisions of Asian Populations

- East Asians (Chinese, Japanese, Koreans)
- Southeast Asians (Indonesians, Malaysians, Singaporeans, Thais, Cambodians, Vietnamese)
- South Asians (Bangladeshis, Indians, Pakistanis, Sri Lankans)

either white or black. Furthermore, some Hispanics or Latinos are of mixed ancestry, having Caucasian and Native Indian heritage (Meztisos) or African and European heritage (Mulattos).

As early humankind, who presumably had skin of color, migrated across the continents, differences in skin color, craniofacial features, and hair texture and color developed. The differences displayed in the appearance of various racial groups are felt to be due to environmental, dietary, and adaptive factors. Recently, Lamason identified the *SLC24A5* gene, localized to the melanosome, which determines skin pigmentation.[7] West Africans with the normal form of *SLC24A5* have brown skin, whereas European whites have a modified form of the gene. The modified form accounts for fewer and smaller melanosomes and hence white skin. This gene, however, does not play a role in determining skin tones in Asian people, which probably are determined by yet another gene.

WHY IS IT USEFUL TO IDENTIFY AND HIGHLIGHT INDIVIDUALS WITH SKIN OF COLOR?

The total number of individuals in the United States with *skin of color* was approximately 85 million in the year 2000.[5] These individuals resided in major metropolitan areas as well as throughout the heartland of America. In the United States as well as in many nations around the globe, the non-Caucasian *skin of color* population is expanding rapidly. The

TABLE 2-5
Hispanic or Latino Ethnic Group (U.S. Census 2000)

- Mexican
- Cuban
- Puerto Rican
- Central American
- South American
- Other Spanish descent

TABLE 2-6
U.S. Census Population Projections for 2050 (% of population)

- American Indian or Alaska Native 0.9%
- Asians 8.2%
- Blacks 13.6%
- Native Hawaiian or other Pacific Islanders
- Whites 52.8%
- Hispanics 24.5%

U.S. Census Bureau projections for the year 2050 are that this population will approximately equal the non-Hispanic white population[8] (Table 2-6). The changing face of America, as well as the remainder of the globe, highlights the importance of understanding this population. Their population growth, coupled with the ease of international travel and immigration into the United States, will cause dermatologists to be faced with the challenge of diagnosing and treating skin diseases in racially and ethnically diverse populations.

IS THERE A NEED FOR A TEXTBOOK ON SKIN OF COLOR?

Individuals with *skin of color* have distinctive cutaneous disorders and reaction patterns to disorders as well as to cutaneous stimuli. Additionally, they have diverse cultural practices and habits. Often they will rely on alternative medicine, including botanicals or herbs. This textbook on *skin of color* is designed to educate dermatology students, residents, attending physicians, and their extenders about *skin of color*.

WHAT ARE SOME OF THE CUTANEOUS DISORDERS THAT OCCUR IN INDIVIDUALS WITH *SKIN OF COLOR*?

Individuals with skin of color include a wide array of individuals from several racial and ethnic groups. Unfortunately, data regarding the epidemiology of cutaneous diseases in individuals with skin of color are limited (see Chapter 3). Insight into diseases in various populations is often based on health care service utilization data such as retrospective private and clinic practice surveys, as well as dermatologists' published reports of their personal experience.[9,10] Although these data are useful, they are limited by several factors, including the location of the practice, patient demographics, patient access to health care, patient customs and practices, the genetics of the ethnic population, and the time period of the study. In the United States, the largest surveys have been conducted by the National Center for Health Statistics, which conducts the National Ambulatory Care Survey (NAMCS).[11] In this survey, samples of a nationally representative group of visits to the offices of non–federally employed physicians in the United States are obtained. The NAMCS provides the primary diagnosis for dermatologists by race and ethnicity. The data for the years 1993–2002 are found in Tables 2-7 through 2-12.

Asian Populations

Cutaneous diseases in Asian populations vary according to the country of ancestry of the individuals as well as their skin type. The NAMCS for Asians living in the United States reveals the

TABLE 2-7
Race = White Only

DIAGNOSIS	COUNT	PERCENT
Other acne	33,707,252	11.8013
Actinic keratosis	25,021,822	8.7605
Viral warts, unspecified	14,335,002	5.0189
Unspecified cause	13,360,224	4.6776
Malignant neoplasm of skin, site unspecified	12,653,888	4.4303
Benign neoplasm of skin, site unspecified	11,903,783	4.1677
Other psoriasis	8,375,894	2.9325
Acne	7,716,844	2.7018
Other seborrheic keratosis	7,521,141	2.6332
Rosacea	6,675,758	2.3373
Sebaceous cyst	5,980,310	2.0938
Actinic keratoses	5,943,607	2.0809
Eczema	4,037,590	1.4136

(continued)

TABLE 2-7 (Continued)
Race = White Only

Diagnosis	Count	Percent
Seborrheic dermatitis, unspecified	2,997,293	1.0494
Benign neoplasm of skin	2,635,862	0.9228
Psoriasis	2,568,689	0.8993
Melanoma	2,526,437	0.8845
Other atopic dermatitis and related cutaneous disorders	2,316,606	0.8111
Unspecified disorder of skin and subcutaneous tissue	2,149,858	0.7527
Malignant neoplasm of skin of other and unspecified parts of face	2,095,519	0.7337
Other dyschromia	2,087,079	0.7307
Keratoderma, acquired	2,049,281	0.7175
Actinic keratosis	1,957,429	0.6853
Personal history of other malignant neoplasms	1,736,431	0.6079
Inflamed seborrheic keratosis	1,708,400	0.5981
Other specified disorders of skin	1,678,580	0.5877
Other specified viral warts	1,662,858	0.5822
Alopecia, unspecified	1,590,687	0.5569
Other specified diseases of hair and hair follicles	1,568,961	0.5493
Unspecified hypertrophic and atrophic conditions of skin	1,558,806	0.5458

frequency of cutaneous disorders not to be dissimilar from that reported in populations from Singapore[11,12] (Tables 2-13 and 2-14). Acne and eczematous dermatoses occur frequently in this population, as they do in the general population.

Certain pigmentary disorders appear to occur frequently in Asian populations. Melasma is reportedly a common pigmentary disorder.[13] The frequency of melasma has been reported to range from 0.25–4.0% in several Southeast Asian populations (Table 2-15).

There are several disorders that either occur almost exclusively in Asian populations or are very common in this racial group.[14] Several of the disorders are either pigmentary in nature or related to cultural practices. The pigmentary disorders, namely, Hori's nevus, nevus of Ota, nevus of Ito, and Mongolian spots, all represent dermal melanosis. Of the cultural practices, alternative medicine is often practiced in Asian culture, resulting in self-inflicted skin abnormalities. These practices can be misdiagnosed as child abuse when their results are seen in children. Knowledge of these disorders and practices is important to dermatologists (Table 2-16).

Within the Asian population, there are differences in cutaneous diseases that occur in adults and children. Data regarding pediatric populations from Singapore, India, Hong Kong, and Thailand have been reported[15–18] (Tables 2-17 through 2-20). Eczema is a common disease in all the Asian pediatric populations. Likewise, a number of cutaneous infections ranging from bacterial to fungal and viral occur commonly in the pediatric populations.

Black Populations

The black population in the United States, as well in other countries, also represents a diverse population. These individuals are African, African American, African Caribbean, African European, and of mixed races. Cutaneous disease patterns have been studied in several different countries that have predominant or sizable black populations. These include, in

TABLE 2-8
Race = Black/African American Only

Diagnosis	Count	Percent
Other acne	2,576,186	15.6627
Unspecified cause	1,654,334	10.0580
Seborrheic dermatitis, unspecified	756,789	4.6011
Other atopic dermatitis and related conditions	756,417	4.5989
Acne	632,753	3.8470
Other psoriasis	356,465	2.1672
Alopecia, unspecified	351,811	2.1389
Noncodable diagnosis/insuff info for coding	350,140	2.1288
Keloid scar	343,986	2.0914
Viral warts, unspecified	339,162	2.0620
Alopecia areata	299,681	1.8220
Sebaceous cyst	293,260	1.7830
Dermatophytosis of scalp and beard	282,261	1.7161
Other specified disorders of skin	261,082	1.5873
Benign neoplasm of skin, site unspecified	251,438	1.5287
Pityriasis versicolor	245,344	1.4916
Rosacea	237,140	1.4418
Dyschromia, unspecified	237,025	1.4411
Contact dermatitis due to other specified agent	221,906	1.3491
Keratoderma, acquired	180,373	1.0966
Dyshidrosis	177,590	1.0797
Other dyschromia	175,988	1.0700
Other specified diseases of hair and hair follicles	173,421	1.0544
Dermatophytosis of unspecified site	149,217	0.9072
Lichen planus	142,704	0.8676
Actinic keratosis	133,445	0.8113
Dermatophytosis of nail	133,253	0.8102
X-ray of facial bones	128,616	0.7820
Psoriasis	110,516	0.6719
Malignant neoplasm of skin, site unspecified	109,573	0.6662

TABLE 2-9
Race = Asian Only

Diagnosis	Count	Percent
Other acne	1,489,170	15.0628
Unspecified cause	1,325,556	13.4079
Benign neoplasm of skin, site unspecified	478,422	4.8392
Other atopic dermatitis and related conditions	387,744	3.9220
Other psoriasis	325,440	3.2918
Viral warts, unspecified	255,134	2.5807
Other seborrheic keratosis	228,917	2.3155
Urticaria, unspecified	197,914	2.0019
Acne	186,549	1.8869
Sebaceous cyst	170,833	1.7280
Keratoderma, acquired	170,496	1.7246
Actinic keratosis	163,628	1.6551
Lichenification and lichen simplex chronicus	151,121	1.5286
Keloid scar	148,219	1.4992
Puerperal infection	129,051	1.3053
Rash and other nonspecific skin eruption	128,402	1.2988
Seborrheic dermatitis, unspecified	126,764	1.2822
Blank (no data given)	125,269	1.2671
Other specified diseases of hair and hair follicles	123,244	1.2466
Other dyschromia	122,882	1.2429
Alopecia, unspecified	116,155	1.1749
Rosacea	115,689	1.1702
Examination following other treatment	102,898	1.0408
Eczema	91,356	0.9241
Psoriasis	91,064	0.9211
Other specified disorders of skin	88,976	0.9000
Dermatophytosis of feet	85,127	0.8611
Dyschromia, unspecified	83,029	0.8398
Unspecified disorder of skin and subcutaneous tissues	73,065	0.7390
Other specified anomalies of skin	72,496	0.7333

TABLE 2-10
Race = Native Hawaiian/Other Pacific Islander Only

Diagnosis	Count	Percent
Other acne	178,576	16.3957
Other seborrheic keratosis	94,703	8.6950
Acne	77,774	7.1407
Viral warts, unspecified	49,735	4.5664
Sebaceous cyst	43,198	3.9662
Other atopic dermatitis and related conditions	41,874	3.8446
Dermatophytosis of nail	38,112	3.4992
Malignant neoplasm of skin of other and unspecified parts of face	35,926	3.2985
Unspecified cause	35,338	3.2445
Lichenification and lichen simplex chronicus	31,478	2.8901
Other dyschromia	27,157	2.4934
Dermatophytosis of feet	26,316	2.4162
Other specified diseases of nail	25,032	2.2983
Unspecified pruritic disorder	25,032	2.2983
Dyshidrosis	22,627	2.0775
Unspecified hypertrophic and atrophic conditions of skin	21,751	1.9970
Melanoma	20,105	1.8459
Alopecia areata	20,105	1.8459

(continued)

TABLE 2-10 (Continued)
Race = Native Hawaiian/Other Pacific Islander Only

Diagnosis	Count	Percent
Other and unspecified mycoses	20,105	1.8459
70630	18,977	1.7423
Other psoriasis	18,774	1.7237
Eczema	17,442	1.6014
Scabies	17,356	1.5935
Pruritus of genital organs	15,210	1.3965
Rosacea	14,318	1.3146
Keloid scar	13,700	1.2578
Malignant neoplasm of skin of ear and external auditory canal	12,922	1.1864
Benign neoplasm of skin, site unspecified	12,704	1.1664
Herpes simplex without mention of complication	12,704	1.1664
Malignant neoplasm, other w/o specific cancer type	12,704	1.1664

addition to the United States, the United Kingdom and the Caribbean countries of Jamaica and Guadeloupe[19–22] (Tables 2-21 through 2-24).

There are differences in the dermatologic disorders occurring in children compared with adult blacks.[19,23] Bacterial, fungal, and viral infections occur commonly in the black pediatric population (Tables 2-25 and 2-26). Acne vulgaris and eczema occur in both U.S. and U.K. black populations with increased frequency.

TABLE 2-12
Ethnic = Hispanic or Latino

Diagnosis	Count	Percent
Other acne	1,648,305	14.2357
Unspecified cause	807,133	6.9709
Acne	579,366	5.0037
Other psoriasis	549,461	4.7455
Viral warts, unspecified	423,396	3.6567
Sebaceous cyst	315,229	2.7225
Psoriasis	313,307	2.7059
Actinic keratosis	299,493	2.5866
Benign neoplasm of skin, site unspecified	223,646	1.9315
Alopecia areata	200,309	1.7300
Lichenification and lichen simplex chronicus	188,752	1.6302
Eczema	182,724	1.5781
Rosacea	179,618	1.5513
Seborrheic dermatitis, unspecified	175,900	1.5192
Actinic keratosis	168,949	1.4591
Malignant neoplasm of skin, site unspecified	140,114	1.2101
Other dyschromia	135,991	1.1745
Other atopic dermatitis and related conditions	135,889	1.1736
Puerperal infection	134,581	1.1623
Other specified diseases of hair and hair follicles	133,374	1.1519
Molluscum contagiosum	130,127	1.1239
Alopecia, unspecified	128,648	1.1111
Dyshidrosis	109,869	0.9489
Other specified erythematous conditions	105,174	0.9083
Benign neoplasm of skin	96,243	0.8312
Dermatophytosis of nail	91,706	0.7920
Unspecified disorder of skin and subcutaneous tissues	90,996	0.7859
Other specified viral warts	87,526	0.7559
Other specified disorders of skin	81,662	0.7053
Unspecified hypertrophic and atrophic conditions of skin	77,158	0.6664

TABLE 2-11
Race = American Indian/Alaska Native Only

Diagnosis	Count	Percent
Viral warts, unspecified	44,339	52.7299
Rosacea	23,610	28.0781
Scabies	16,138	19.1920

TABLE 2-13
Pattern of Skin Disease in the United States in the Asian population

Acne (15.1%)
Benign neoplasm of the skin (4.8%)
Atopic dermatitis/eczema (3.9%)
Psoriasis (3.3%)
Verruca (2.6%)
Seborrheic keratosis (2.3%)
Urticaria (2.0%)
Sebaceous cyst (1.7%)
Keratoderma (1.7%)
Actinic keratosis (1.7%)
Lichenification/lichen simplex chronicus (1.5%)
Other

From National Ambulatory/Health Care Survey; available at *www.cdc.gov/nchs/about/major/ahcd.ahcd1.html.*

TABLE 2-14
Pattern of Skin Disease at the National Skin Center in Singapore

Chinese 77.2%; Indian 9.9%; Malay 7.6%; Other 5.3%
Dermatitis (34.1%)
Acne (10.9%)
Viral infections (5.7%)
Fungal infection (5.4%)
Urticaria (4.7%)
Contact dermatitis (4.7%)
Psoriasis (3.3%)
Bacterial infection (3%)
Alopecia (2.4%)
Nonvenomous insect bite (2.5%)
Postinflammatory pigmentation (1.9%)

From Chua-ty G, Goh CL, Koh SL. Pattern of skin diseases at the National Skin Center (Singapore) from 1989–1090. *Int J Dermatol* 1992;31:555–559.

TABLE 2-15
Pigmentary Disorders in Asian Populations: Melasma

0.25–2.62%	Thailand (Suvanprakorn)
0.98%	Indonesia (Pusponegoro)
3.05%	Thailand (Kotrajaras)
4%	Malaysia (Hussein)

From Sivayathorn A. Melasma in Orientals. *Clin Drug Invest* 1995;10:34–40. Used with permission.

TABLE 2-16
Common/Exclusive Cutaneous Disorders in Asian Populations

Mongolian spots
Nevus of Ota
Nevus of Ito
Hori's nevus
Kawasaki disease
Primary cutaneous amyloidosis (lichen, macula, anosacral)
Kikuchi-Fujimoto disease
Lipodystrophia centrifugalis abdominalis infantilis
Conditions as a result of alternative medicine (e.g., cupping, coin-rubbing, and moxibustion)

From Lee CS, Lim HW. Cutaneous disease in Asians. *Dermatol Clin* 2003;21:669–677.

TABLE 2-17
Skin Diseases Among Children in a Referral Skin Clinic in Singapore

Chinese 70.8%; Indian 11.1%; Malay 12.6%; Other 5.5%
Ages 1–15 years
Eczema (49.3%)
Viral infection (6.5%)
Pigmentation (5.5%)
Bacterial infections (4.9%)
Insect bites (4.8%)
Parasitic infection (3.8%)
Urticaria (3.8%)
Acne vulgaris (3.1%)
Fungal infection (2.5%)
Alopecia (1.8%)
Psoriasis (1.1%)

From Goh CL, Akarapanth R. Epidemiology of skin disease among children in a referral skin clinic in Singapore. *Pedriatr Dermatol* 2004;11:125–128. Used with permission.

TABLE 2-18
Pediatric Skin Disease in India, 12,586 Children, 50.5% Male, Ages 6–14 Years

Skin conditions (38.8%)
Infections (11.4%)
Pityriasis alba (8.4%)
Dermatitis/eczema (5.2%)
Infestations (5.0%)
Disorders of pigmentation (2.6%)
Keratinization disorders (1.3%)
Nevi/hamartomas (1.1%)

From Dogra S, Kumar B. Epidemiology of skin diseases in school children: A study from northern India. *Pediatr Dermatol* 2003;20: 470–473.

TABLE 2-19
Pediatric Skin Disease in Hong Kong, Prince Wales Hospital, 331 Chinese Children, 50% Male, Age Younger than 18 Years

Eczema (33%)
Nevi (20%)
Viral warts (6%)
Vitiligo/hypopigmentation (5%)
Tinea (3%)
Urticaria (3%)
Acne vulgaris (2%)
Neurofibromatosis (2%)
Molluscum contagiosum (2%)
Keratosis pilaris (1%)
Folliculitis/impetigo/cellulitis (1%)

From Kon KL, Leung TF, Wong Y, et al. Skin diseases in Chinese children at a pediatric dermatology center. *Pediatr Dermatol* 2004;21: 109–112.

TABLE 2-20
Pediatric Skin Disease in Thailand, Siriraj Hospital, 2361 Children, 50% Male, Age Younger than 13 Years

Eczema (41.2%)
Skin infections (21.9%)
Pigmentary disorders (7.0%)
Hypersensitivity diseases (4.1%)
Scabies (4.1%)
Vitiligo (4.1%)
Tinea capitis (3.31%)
Alopecia areata (2.4%)
Papular urticaria (2.2%)

From Wisuthsarewong W, Vivavan S. Analysis of skin diseases in a referral pediatric dermatology clinic in Thailand. *J Med Assoc Thai* 2000;83:999–1004. Used with permission.

TABLE 2-21
Most Common Dermatoses of Black Private Patients Compared with Thos of White Private Patients in the Same Geographic Location

Dermatosis	Black	White
Acne vulgaris	27.7%	29.5%
Eczema	20.3%	10.7%
Pigmentary disorders (excluding vitiligo)	9%	1.7%
Seborrhea dermatitis	6.5%	1.8%
Alopecia	5.3%	—
Fungal infections	4.3%	1.1%
Contact dermatitis	4.2%	2.2%
Warts	3.1%	8.4%
Tinea versicolor	2.4%	0.2%
Keloids	2.2%	—
Pityriasis rosea	2.1%	—
Urticaria	2%	1.2%
Benign tumors	2%	7.3%

From Halder RM et al. Incidence of common dermatoses in a predominately black dermatology practice. *Cutis* 1983;32: 388–390.

Latino or Hispanic Populations

There is sparse information regarding disorders that occur in individuals of Latino or Hispanic ethnicity. Sanchez reported commonly occurring disorders in Latino patients in both a private practice and a clinic-based setting in the United States[24] (Tables 2-27 and 2-28). The inflammatory disorders acne vulgaris and eczema occurred commonly in both populations, as well as the pigmentary disorders hyperpigmentation and melasma.

TABLE 2-22
Most Common Cutaneous Diseases in Black Adult Patients in Southeast London, England

Acne (13.7%)
Acne keloidalis, nuchae and scalp folliculitis (13.7%)
Eczema (20.3%)
Psoriasis (4.8%)
Keloid scars (4.1%)
Pityriasis versicolor (3.8%)
Postinflammatory hyperpigmentation (3.4%)
Alopecia areata (3.1%)
Dermatofibroma (2.7%)
Urticaria (1.7%)
Pityriasis rosea (1.7%)
Lichen simplex (1.7%)

From Child FJ, Fuller LC, Higgins EM, et al. A study of the spectrum of skin disease occurring in a black population in southeast London. *Br J Dermatol* 1999;141:512–517. Used with permission.

TABLE 2-23
Most Common Cutaneous Diseases in 1000 Black Patients, Kingston, Jamaica

Acne (29.21%)
Seborrheic dermatitis (22.02%)
Pigmentary disorders (16.41%)
Atopic eczema (6.1%)
Keratosis pilaris (2.18%)
Tinea infections (2.18%)
Hirsuitism (1.89%)
Folliculitis keloidalis (1.74%)
Viral warts (1.67%)
Dermatosis papulosa nigra (1.59%)
Confluent and reticulated papillomatosis (1.45%)
Alopecia areata (1.23%)

From Dunwell P, Rose A. Study of the skin disease spectrum occurring in an Afro-Caribbean population. *Int J Dermatol* 2003;42:287–289. Used with permission.

TABLE 2-24
Most Common Cutaneous Diseases in 5000 Black Patients, Guadeloupe

Acne (19.5%)
Superficial mycosis (13.1%)
Eczema (11.1%)
Seborrheic dermatitis (6%)
Pigmentary disorders (4.4%)
Pityriasis alba (3.8%)
Pyoderma (3.6%)
Prurigo (3.2%)
Alopecia (3.2%)
Verruca (2%)

From Mahe A, Mancel E. Dermatological practice in Guadeloupe (French West Indies). *Clin Exp Dermatol* 1999;24:358–360. Used with permission.

TABLE 2-25
Racial Comparisons Among the Six Most Frequent Pediatric Cutaneous Diseases

Dermatosis	Black	White
Atopic dermatitis	73.4%	26.6%
Impetigo	84.6%	15.4%
Tinea capitis	90%	10%
Acne vulgaris	49.3%	50.7%
Verruca vulgaris	37.4%	62.6%
Seborrhea dermatitis	73.2%	26.8%

From Schachner L, Ling NS, Press A. A statistical analysis of a pediatric dermatology clinic. *Pediatr Dermatol* 1983;1b:157–164. Used with permission.

TABLE 2-26
Most Common Cutaneous Diseases in Black Pediatric Patients in Southeast London, England

Atopic eczema (36.5%)
Tines capitis (26.5%)
Pityriasis alba (3.7%)
Viral warts (3.7%)
Keloid scars (2.6%)
Molluscum (2.1%)
Alopecia areata (2.1%)

From Child FJ, Fuller LC, Higgins EM, et al. A study of the spectrum of skin disease occurring in a Black Population in southeast London. *Br. J Dermatol. 1999;*141:512-517. Used with permission.

TABLE 2-27
Dermatologic Diagnosis in 1000 Latino Patients Treated in a Dermatology Private Practice

Acne vulgaris (20.7%)
Eczema/contact dermatitis (19.3%)
Photoaging (16.8%)
Tinea and onychomycosis (9.9%)
Facial melasma (8.2%)
Condyloma/warts (7.1%)
Hyperpigmentation (6%)
Seborrheic keratosis (4.5%)
Acrochordons (4.2%)
Seborrheic dermatitis (3.2%)
Alopecia (2.3%)
Psoriasis (0.8%)

From Sanchez MR. Cutaneous diseases in Latinos. *Dermatol Clin* 2003;21:689–697. Used with permission.

TABLE 2-28
Dermatologic Diagnosis in 2000 Latino Patients Treated in a Hospital Clinic

Eczema/contact dermatitis (20.1%)
Condyloma/warts (17.5%)
Acne vulgaris (12.3%)
Tinea and onychomycosis (9.3%)
Pyoderma (8.8%)
Hyperpigmentation (7.5%)
Seborrheic dermatitis (7.2%)
Psoriasis (5.5%)
Facial melasma (4.1%)
Pruritus (2.3%)
Drug eruptions (1.9%)
Acrochordons (1.1%)

From Sanchez MR. Cutaneous diseases in Latinos. *Dermatol Clin* 2003;21: 689–697. Used with permission.

SUMMARY

The rapid increase in the *skin of color* population worldwide, coupled with their distinct cutaneous disorders, reaction patterns, and cultural habits and practices, makes textbooks highlighting *skin of color* important and necessary for dermatology students, residents, physicians, and physician extenders. This textbook will provide both a quick reference guide and an in-depth view of all aspects of *skin of color.*

REFERENCES

1. Underhill PA, Passarino G, Lin AA, et al. The phylogeography of Y chromosome binary haplotypes and the origins of modern human population. *Ann Hum Genet* 2001;65:43-62.
2. Brown MD, Hosseini SH, Torroni A, et al. MtDNA haplogroup X: An ancient link between Europe/western Asia and North America? *Am J Hum Genet* 1998;63: 1852-1861.
3. Rosenberg NA. Genetic structure of human populations. *Science* 2003;300: 1877.
4. Stephens JC. Hlotype variation and linkage disequilibrium in 313 human genes. *Science* 2001;293:489-493.
5. US Census Bureau. Population Statistics 2000; available at *www.census.gov/population/pop-profile/dynamic/RACEHO.pdf.*
6. US Census Bureau. Population Growth; available at *www.census.gov/Press-Release/www/releases/archives/population/001720.html.*
7. Lamason RL. *SLC24A5*, a putative cation exchanger, affects pigmentation in zebrafish and humans. *Science* 2005;310: 1782-1786.
8. US Census Bureau. Population Projections; available at *www.census.gov/ipc/www/usinterimproj/natprojtab01a.pdf.*
9. Taylor SC. Epidemiology of skin diseases in ethnic population. *Dermatol Clin* 2002; 21:601-607.
10. Taylor SC. Epidemiology of skin diseases in people of color. *Cutis* 2003;71:271-275.
11. National Center for Health Statistics. Ambulatory Health Care Data; available at *www.cdc.gov/nchs/about/major/ahcd/sampnam.htm.*
12. Chua-ty G, Goh CL, Koh SL. Pattern of skin diseases at the National Skin Center (Singapore) from 1989–1990. *Int J Dermatol* 1992;31:555-559.
13. Sivayathorn A. Melasma in Orientals. *Clin Drug Invest* 1995;10:34-63.
14. Lee CS, Lim HW. Cutaneous disease in Asians. *Dermatol Clin* 2003;21:669-677.
15. Goh CL, Akarapanth R. Epidemiology of skin disease among children in a referral skin clinic in Singapore. *Pedriatr Dermatol* 2004;11:125-128.
16. Dogra S, Kumar B. Epidemiology of skin diseases in school children: A study from northern India. *Pediatr Dermatol* 2003;20: 470-473.
17. Kon KL, Leung TF, Wong Y, et al. Skin diseases in Chinese children at a pediatric dermatology center. *Pediatr Dermatol* 2004;21:109-112.

18. Wisuthsarewong W, Vivavan S. Analysis of skin diseases in a referral pediatric dermatology clinic in Thailand. *J Med Assoc Thai* 2000;83:999-1004.
19. Halder RM, Grimes PE, Mclaurin CI, et al. Incidence of common dermatoses in a predominately black dermatology practice. *Cutis* 1983;32:388-390.
20. Child FJ, Fuller LC, Higgins EM, et al. A study of the spectrum of skin disease occurring in a black population in southeast London. *Br J Dermatol* 1999;141:512-517.
21. Dunwell P, Rose A. Study of the skin disease spectrum occurring in an Afro-Caribbean population. *Int J Dermatol* 2003;42:287-289.
22. Mahe A, Mancel E. Dermatological practice in Guadeloupe (French West Indies). *Clin Exp Dermatol* 1999;24:358-360.
23. Schachner L, Ling NS, Press S. A statistical analysis of a pediatric dermatology clinic. *Pediatr Dermatol* 1983;1:157-164.
24. Sanchez MR. Cutaneous diseases in Latinos. *Dermatol Clin* 2003;21:689-697.

CHAPTER 3

Epidemiology of Cutaneous Diseases

Michael Bigby

Key Points

- The epidemiology of cutaneous disease can be expressed using the four standard measurements of mortality, incidence, prevalence, and utilization of health care services.
- Commonly used racial classification systems lack biologic validity, are inherently racist, and can be misleading.
- The incidence and mortality of melanoma are lower in people with skin of color.
- Data indicate that different ethnic groups seek treatment for different dermatologic disorders.
- Establishing rapport and communication is more important in health care than pigeonholing patients into racial categories.

THE EPIDEMIOLOGY OF CUTANEOUS DISEASE

Cutaneous (skin) diseases are very common. They can cause morbidity and have a significant impact on quality of life. With a few notable exceptions (e.g., melanoma, toxic epidermal necrolysis, cutaneous T-cell lymphoma, and autoimmune bullous diseases), deaths from skin diseases are uncommon. This chapter will review the data on the descriptive epidemiology of cutaneous disease in people of color employing four commonly used measures: mortality, incidence, prevalence, and utilization of health care services.

Mortality is the number of deaths from a specific disease occurring in a population in a defined period of time. The *incidence* of a disease is the number of new cases occurring in a population in a defined period of time. Incidence and mortality are commonly expressed as number of cases or deaths per 100,000 people per year, respectively. Accurate incidence and mortality data can be obtained only if cases or deaths are reliably identified and reported. Reporting of death and the cause of death is mandatory in the United States. Therefore, fairly accurate estimates of mortality rates for skin diseases are available. In the United States, accurate incidence data for skin diseases are available only for a few diseases, including melanoma, nonmelanoma skin cancer, Kaposi sarcoma, and cutaneous T-cell lymphoma. The *prevalence* of a disease is the number of cases in a population at a given time. It is a snapshot of the frequency at which a disease is present in a given population at a given time. Prevalence is best determined by performing a randomized survey of the population. *Health care service utilization* can be measured by determining the number of visits to physicians in a defined period of time for specific reasons (e.g., diagnoses or complaints). Such information can be obtained from data collected for other purposes (e.g., billing records or drug dispensing), or it can be obtained specifically to study resource utilization. To understand the data on the epidemiology of skin diseases in people of color, however, the problems of the racial classification of human populations must be addressed.

RACIAL CLASSIFICATION SYSTEMS LACK BIOLOGIC VALIDITY AND ARE INHERENTLY RACIST

For an alternate view of racial classifications, see Chapter 2. The first scientific attempt to classify human populations into races was written by Carolus Linnaeus in 1735.[1] He divided the races into four groups that were described as follows: white (Europeans), "acute, gentle, inventive"; red (Americans), "obstinate, merry, free"; dark (Asians), "stiff, haughty, avaricious"; and black (Africans), "phlegmatic, indolent, negligent." The dictionary definition of Caucasian is "the 'white' races of man."[2] However, it was Johann Blumenbach who introduced the term *Caucasian* into the medical lexicon in 1795.[3] He divided the races into five groups (i.e., Caucasian, Mongolian, Ethiopian, American, and Malayan) and described Caucasians as a beautiful people who derive their name from Mount Caucasus," the Caucasus Mountain Range in the southwestern Soviet Union between the Black and Caspian seas. These people were in fact not all "white," and this idea actually was derived from Jean Chardin (1643–1713), a French explorer who had traveled to Mount Caucasus and described the people.[3] As noted by Holubar, "When saying Caucasian, we should be aware of the historical origin of this term, of the fact that it is a misnomer, of the time when it entered scientific literature and what we may understand it to mean (and what not)."[3]

Who is "black" in America? It is also important to remember that race in America is a pervasive political and social construct. The designation of who is black is a product of our nation's history and has been used to separate those with rights (whites) from those who could be sold as property (blacks) and later for varying degrees of discrimination. It is a pervasive idea that is accepted legally and in the medical community that any person with any discernible feature of being black *is* black. This practice (known as the "one drop [of black blood] rule") makes a mockery of the notion that racial classification can be of genetic or biologic usefulness.[4] Until recently, black, white, and other were the only racial groups recognized in the American Census.[5] Recognizing the inadequacy of the data-collection system and the significant change in the demographics of the American population, the Census now classifies people into larger groups (e.g., black, white, Asian or Pacific Islander, American Indian, Eskimo or Aleut, and other), with the additional category of Hispanic (any of whom also can choose to be of one of the aforementioned racial groups).[5] Census 2000 included 63 racial categories.[6] This system clearly makes as little sense genetically or biologically as its predecessors.

Modern genetic analyses have been used to separate people into genetically determined groups. Based on polymorphisms in mitochondrial DNA or in the Y chromosome, modern humans appeared first in East Africa about 44,000 years ago. Using polymorphisms in the Y chromosome, Underhill was able to divide human populations into 21 distinct groups that roughly corresponded to the regions in the world where they are located.[7] Similar results are obtained using polymorphisms in mitochondrial DNA.[8] Based on 100 Alu polymorphisms examined in 565 people, four distinct groups were identified [two sub-Saharan African groups (Mbuti Pygmies, other), Europeans, and East Asians].[9] Based on 375 short tandem repeats examined in 1000 people from 52 ethnic groups, five distinct groups were identified (sub-

Saharan Africans, Europeans and Asians west of the Himalayas, East Asians, New Guineans, and Melanesians).[9] If a large enough number of polymorphism are studied (e.g., thousands), even smaller divisions of populations sharing genetic similarity can be made (e.g., Chinese and Japanese or Hispanics, African Americans, and European Americans).[10]

It is important to remember, however, that even using modern genetic techniques to attempt to divide populations into distinct groups based on the frequency of genes expressed, the genetic variation within groups is greater than the variation between them. The average nucleotide diversity between two randomly chosen people is about 1 in 1000 to 1 in 500, or 0.2 to 3 million base pairs.[10] The nucleotide diversity between a human and a chimpanzee is about 1 in 100. Most human genetic variance is within population variance (85–90%), with only 10–15% represented by between-population variance.[10]

The implicit assumption made in identifying a person's race in clinical medicine is that it (racial group identification) imparts useful genetic and therefore biologic information about the person. Unfortunately, often it does not.[11,12] For example, recent attention has been paid to differences in responsiveness between African Americans and European Americans to angiotensin-converting enzyme (ACE) inhibitors. A meta-analysis revealed that the mean difference in systolic blood pressure (BP) reduction between African Americans and European Americans was 4.6 mm Hg.[10] The standard deviation of the change was 12 and 14 mm Hg in African Americans and European Americans, respectively, indicating that the group's responses overlapped considerably and that a large number of African Americans will have significant diastolic blood pressure reduction using ACE inhibitors.

At its worse, identifying a person's race in clinical medicine can be destructive or completely misleading. Thus the diagnosis of rosacea is often not considered in black patients because of the mistaken (or at least unsubstantiated) belief that rosacea is uncommon in this group.[12,13] A "black" patient with pityriasis rosea is more likely to be thought to have secondary syphilis (and have an RPR drawn) than a "white" patient, even though the need for serologic testing in patients with a typical herald patch and rash is doubtful.[12,14] Therapeutic assumptions based on racial classification also abound. Many physicians are reluctant to use topical retinoids in "blacks" for fear of postinflammatory hyperpigmentation despite a randomized, controlled clinical trial indicating that tretinoin is beneficial in reducing hyperpigmentation in dark patients with acne.[12,15]

TABLE 3-1
Melanoma Deaths by "Race," United States, 2001

Group	No. of Deaths	Rate	Age-Adjusted Rate
All	7542	2.6	2.7
White	7403	3.2	3.0
Black	104	0.3	0.4
Other race	35	0.3	0.4
Hispanic	145	0.4	0.8
Non-Hispanic	7387	3.0	2.8
Non-Hispanic white	7250	3.7	3.2
Non-Hispanic black	102	0.3	0.4

Source: www.cdc.gov/nchs/data/nvsr/nvsr52/nvsr52_03.pdf.

EPIDEMIOLOGY OF CUTANEOUS DISEASES IN PEOPLE OF COLOR

Mortality

Skin diseases were estimated to cause 10,710 deaths in 2006, with melanoma (7910) and nonepithelial skin cancer (2800) accounting for these deaths.[16] Melanoma caused 7542 deaths in 2001, a death rate of 2.6 per 100,000 based on the population data from the 2000 Census.[17] There were 7403, 104, and 35 deaths from melanoma among "whites," "blacks," and all "others," respectively. The corresponding death rates were 3.2, 0.3, and 0.3 per 100,000, respectively. There were 145 deaths among Hispanics, a death rate of 0.4 (Table 3-1).

Incidence

Fairly accurate estimates of the incidence of some skin cancers (i.e., melanoma, Kaposi sarcoma, and cutaneous T-cell lymphoma) are available based on data from national cancer registries (Table 3-2). Estimates are also available for several reportable diseases that have cutaneous manifestations (e.g., syphilis, leprosy, and measles) based on reports to health departments.[17] Underreporting is a potential problem with all these data. The incidence of melanoma is significantly lower in people of color.

Prevalence

The only systematically collected data on the prevalence of skin diseases in the general population in the United States was collected as part of the National Health and Nutrition Examination Survey (NHANES).[18] Whereas 75% of participants actually were examined as part of this survey and more than 20,000 Americans aged 1–74 years were examined, the survey has three major weaknesses that limit its usefulness for determining the prevalence of disease in people of color. First, the data were collected more than 20 years ago (1971–1974), and the results do not reflect the demographics of today's population and may not reflect disease prevalence of today. Second, the only "race" categories were black, white, and other. Third, the "race" of the population was "marked by observation." *The interviewers were instructed to assume that the race of all related persons was the same as the respondent unless otherwise learned. The race categories were "white," "black," or "other." If the appropriate category could not be marked by observation, then race was asked. Interviewers were instructed to record persons who responded with something other than white or black, such as Japanese,*

TABLE 3-2
Age-Adjusted Incidence of Selected Diseases in 2001 (per 100,000)

	Incidence by Group				
Disease	White	Black	American Indian/Alaskan Native	Asian or Pacific Islander	Hispanic
Melanoma	21.1529	0.7269	2.0250	1.4075	4.2616
Kaposi sarcoma	0.7490	1.8456	0.7436	0.3230	1.0206
Non-Hodgkin lymphoma	19.5748	14.1301	9.0716	14.5608	15.3868

Source: www.cancer.org/downloads/STT/CAFF2006PWSecured.pdf.

TABLE 3-3
Prevalence of Skin Disease: NHANES

Skin condition	Number of Cases	Prevalence by Race: All	Whitee*	Negro**	Other***
Dermatophytosis	1227	0.059	0.057	0.067	0.094
Acne vulgaris	1198	0.058	0.059	0.054	0.068
Seborrheic dermatitis	436	0.021	0.022	0.017	0.009
Atopic dermatitis	337	0.016	0.015	0.017	0.056
Psoriasis	145	0.007	0.008	0.002	0.000
Icthyosis/keratosis	120	0.006	0.005	0.007	0.000
Vitiligo	95	0.005	0.004	0.006	0.000
Verruca vulgaris	91	0.004	0.005	0.002	0.004
Folliculitis	70	0.003	0.004	0.002	0.000
Herpes simplex	61	0.003	0.004	0.001	0.000

* N = 16351
** N = 4163
*** N = 235
Source: National Health and Nutrition Examination Survey (NHANES), *www.cdc.gov/nchs/data/nhanes/nhanesi/4151.pdf.*

TABLE 3-4
Most Common Skin Diseases, United States

	Black	White
Acne	28	30 (1)
Atopic dermatitis	20	11 (2)
Pigmentary disorders	9.0	1.7 (7)
Seborrheic dermatitis	6.5	1.8 (8)
Alopecias	5.3	—
Dermatophytosis	4.3	1.1 (17)
Contact dermatitis	3.1	2.2 (8)
Warts	3.1	8.4 (3)
Pityriasis versicolor	2.4	0.2
Keloids	2.2	—

Source: From Halder RM, Grimes PE, McLaurin CI, et al. Incidence of common dermatoses in a predominately black dermatology practice. *Cutis* 1983;32:388–390. Used with permission.

Chinese, American Indian, Korean, Hindu, Eskimo, etc., as "other" and to include Mexicans, Puerto Ricans, and other persons of Latin American descent in the "white" category unless definitely black, American Indian, or of other nonwhite race.[18]

These limitations notwithstanding, nearly a third of those examined had at least one skin lesion warranting a physician visit. The most common skin diseases were disease of the sebaceous glands (acne), dermatophytosis, tumors, seborrheic dermatitis, atopic dermatitis, contact dermatitis, and icthyosis/keratoses (Table 3-3).

Utilization of Health Care Resources

Several studies have been published that measured the reasons that people of color seek dermatologic care[19–24] (Tables 3-4 through 3-8). In several instances, the frequencies of visits for different disorders were compared in different ethnic groups in the same locale. Halder and colleagues compared the reasons for visits to a predominantly black practice and a predominantly white practice in the Washington, DC, area.[19] Pigmentary disorders, seborrheic dermatitis, dermatophytosis, alopecia, pityriasis versicolor, and keloids were disorders prompting visits by black patients (see Table 3-4). Child and colleagues compared the reasons for visits to a single practice in London by black, white, and Asian patients (see Table 3-5).[20] The population in the surrounding community was roughly 50% black, 40% white, and 10% Asian. Therefore, if the prevalence of disease was the same in each group and each group was motivated to seek dermatologic care for similar reasons, you would expect that for each diagnosis, 50%, 40%, and 10% of the patients would be black, white, or Asian. The overwhelming majority of visits for acne keloidalis were by blacks. A disproportional high percentage of visits for atopic dermatitis, alopecia areata, and keloids were by Asians. A disproportional high percentage of visits for hyperpigmentation were by Asians and blacks. A disproportional high percentage of visits for psoriasis were by whites. The most common reasons for dermatologic consultations have been studied among black adults in the United Kingdom[18] (see Table 3-6). What is most striking about these data (see Tables 3-4 through 3-6) is that the lists are so similar.

The most common reasons for dermatologic consultations have been studied in children in Singapore and Kuwait[19,20] (see Tables 3-7 and 3-8). What is most striking about these data is that the lists are so similar. The high proportion of visits for atopic dermatitis, especially in the Singaporean study, and the proportion of visits for alopecia areata in Kuwait stand out.

The reasons for visits to a dermatologist cannot be taken as a proxy for the

TABLE 3-5
Comparison by Ethnic Group, United Kingdom

Disorder	Black	White	Asian
Acne	51	41	8
Acne keloidalis	95	5	0
Atopic dermatitis	32	50	18
Psoriasis	7.5	82	11
Keloids	60	8.5	32
Pityriasis versicolor	48	35	17
Hyperpigmentation	73	9	18
Alopecia areata	29	48	24
Dermatofibroma	13	75	13
Urticaria	32	53	15
Sarcoidosis[a]	100	0	0
Lupus[a]	47	41	12
Traction[a]	100	0	0
Pigmentation nail/sole[a]	100	0	0

[a]Few patents seen.
Source: From Child FJ, Fuller LC, Higgins EM, et al. A study of the spectrum of skin disease occurring in a black population in southeast London. *Br J Dermatol* 1999;141:512–527. Used with permission.

TABLE 3-6
Most Common Skin Diseases in Black Adults, United Kingdom

Disorder	Frequency (%)
Acne	14
Acne keloidalis/folliculitis	14
Atopic dermatitis	9.6
Psoriasis	4.8
Keloids	4.1
Pityriasis versicolor	3.8
Hyperpigmentation	3.4
Alopecia areata	3.1
Dermatofibroma	2.7
Urticaria	1.7

Source: From Child FJ, Fuller LC, Higgins EM, et al. A study of the spectrum of skin disease occurring in a black population in southeast London. *Br J Dermatol* 1999;141:512–517. Used with permission.

TABLE 3-8
Most Common Skin Diseases in Children, Kuwait

Disorder	Frequency (%)
Atopic dermatitis	31
Warts	13
Alopecia areata	6.7
Pityriasis alba	5.2
Psoriasis	4.0
Diaper dermatitis	4.0
Molluscum	3.1
Seborrheic dermatitis	3.0
Impetigo	3.0
Scabies	3.0

N = 10,000. 96% Arab.
Source: From Nanda A, Al-Hasawi F, Alsaleh QA. A prospective survey of pediatric dermatology clinic patients in Kuwait: An analysis of 10,000 cases. *Pediatr Dermatol* 1999;16:6–11. Used with permission.

prevalence of disease in different ethnic groups. Many other factors, such as severity, impact on quality of life, availability and cost of care, and competing concerns, play a role in why and when patients seek medical attention.

WHAT DO "THEY" WANT ANYWAY?

In caring for patients, establishing communication is far more important than pigeonholing them into racial categories. Effective communication between doctor and patients, a skill not emphasized in medical education programs, is essential for patient satisfaction and optimal patient care. In many teaching hospitals, the doctor is commonly white and middle class, and the patient, "of color" and indigent. Ethnic differences, even in the absence of social class differences, may have a negative impact on the quality of the doctor-patient relationship. Levy reviewed the impact of racism on health care delivery and made recommendations to enhance the relationship between doctors and patients[23] (Table 3-9). His recommendations are even more germane given the increasing diversity of populations of patients and medical care providers in all countries.

TABLE 3-7
Most Common Skin Diseases in Children, Asia

Disorder	Frequency (%)
Atopic dermatitis	49
Viral infection	6.5
Bacterial infection	4.9
Insect bites	4.8
Pigmentation	5.5
Parasitic infection	3.8
Urticaria	3.8
Acne	3.1
Fungal infection	2.5
Alopecia	1.8
Psoriasis	1.1

N = 9273. 69% Chinese, 13% Malay, 12% Indian, 5.4% other.
Source: From Chua-ty G, Goh CL, Koh SL. Pattern of skin diseases at the National Skin Center (Singapore) from 1989–1090. *Int J Dermatol* 1992;31:555–559. Used with permission.

TABLE 3-9
Caring for Patients from Different Cultures

Be courteous.
Understand missed or late appointments.
Self-awareness.
Avoid stereotyping and labeling.
Understand "maladaptive" behavior.
Be aware of patient's distrust.
Be aware of your and patient's energy.
Learn patient's experience.
Learn patient's attribution.

Source: From Levy DR. White doctors and black patients. *Pediatrics* 1985;75:639–643. Used with permission.

REFERENCES

1. Jon Morro, *www-personal.umich.edu/~jonmorro/ race.html.*
2. *http://dictionary.reference.com/search?q= Caucasian.*
3. Holubar K. What is a Caucasian? *J Invest Dermatol* 1996;106:800.
4. Davis FJ. *Who Is Black.* University Park, PA, Pennyslvania State University Press, 1991.
5. *www.census.gov/population/www/documentation/twps0029/twps0029.html.*
6. *www.census.gov/prod/2001pubs/mso01icdp.pdf.*
7. Underhill PA, Shen P, Lin AA, et al. Y chromosome sequence variation and the history of human populations. *Nat Genet* 2000;26:358-361.
8. Jorde LB, Watkins WS, Bamshad MJ, et al. The distribution of human genetic diversity: A comparison of mitochondrial, autosomal, and Y-chromosome data. *Am J Hum Genet* 2000;66:979-988.
9. Bamshad M, Olson S. Does race exist. *Scientific American,* December 2003.
10. Jorde LB, Wooding SP. Genetic variation, classification and "race." *Nat Genet* 2004; 36:S28-33.
11. Witzig R. The medicalization of race: Scientific legitimization of a flawed social construct. *Ann Intern Med* 1996; 125:675-679.
12. Bigby M, Thaler D. Describing patients' "race" in clinical presentations should be abandoned. *J Am Acad Dermatol* 2006;54: 1074-1076.
13. Rosen T, Stone MS. Acne rosacea in blacks. *J Am Acad Dermatol* 1987;17: 70-73.
14. Horn T, Kazakis A. Pityriasis rosea and the need for a serologic test for syphilis. *Cutis* 1987;39:81-82.
15. Bulengo-Ransby SM, Griffiths CE, Kimbrough-Green CK, et al. Topical tretinoin (retinoic acid) therapy for hyperpigmented lesions caused by inflammation of the skin in black patients. *N Engl J Med* 1993;328: 1438-1443.
16. *www.cancer.org/downloads/STT/CAFF2006 PWSecured.pdf.*
17. *www.cdc.gov/nchs/data/nvsr/nvsr52/nvsr52_03.pdf.*
18. *www.cdc.gov/nchs/data/nhanes/nhanesi/4151.pdf.*
19. Halder RM, Grimes PE, McLaurin CI, et al. Incidence of common dermatoses in a predominately black dermatology practice. *Cutis* 1983;32:388-390.
20. Child FJ, Fuller LC, Higgins EM, et al. A study of the spectrum of skin disease occurring in a black population in southeast London. *Br J Dermatol* 1999;141: 512-527.
21. Chua-ty G, Goh CL, Koh SL. Pattern of skin diseases at the National Skin Center (Singapore) from 1989-1990. *Int J Dermatol* 1992;31:555-559.
22. Nanda A, Al-Hasawi F, Alsaleh QA. A prospective survey of pediatric dermatology clinic patients in Kuwait: An analysis of 10,000 cases. *Pediatr Dermatol* 1999;16: 6-11.
23. Levy DR. White doctors and black patients: Influence of race on the doctor-patient relationship. *Pediatrics* 1985;75: 639-643.

CHAPTER 4

Multicultural Competence in Dermatologic Practice

Flora N. Taylor

Key Points

- Limited treatment time and lack of understanding too often causes multiculturally competent care to be sidelined.
- To empathize with the patient's cultural issues, the physician should explore his or her background, using tools provided in this chapter.
- Intake procedures should incorporate cultural assessment, and provision be made for the language needs of patients.
- Multiculturally competent care can improve patient outcomes.

The skills associated with providing multiculturally competent health care have reached greater appreciation in the health care community than ever before. Unfortunately, many health care professionals still fail to provide multiculturally competent health care to their patients. For a variety of reasons, including limited treatment time and ignorance, the value of providing multiculturally competent health care may be sidelined in the service of quicker patient visits. Physicians may complain that they do not have enough time to focus on anything beyond the patient's presenting illness. The approach described in this chapter attempts to help practitioners identify how valuable the multicultural context is and how it actually can help physicians provide better medical care to their patients. One very important intermediate step along the way to connecting with the multicultural aspects of patients' identities is to learn to value one's own multicultural parts. Toward this end, this chapter begins with exercises that clinicians can do to improve their personal understanding of just how important a patient's multicultural identity may be to him or her.

A LOOK WITHIN

One might wonder if it is necessary to look within at one's own multicultural identities in order to be more available to the multicultural identities of our patients. This is very much the case. The development of empathy requires the capacity to feel what others feel. With respect to identity, it is notoriously difficult and very well documented how more empowered groups lose touch with or perhaps never grasp an understanding of those who are less powerful. For a variety of reasons, possibly including self-protection, it takes more effort to empathize with others than to ignore them. Hence, in this case, physicians may find it easier, and certainly less time-consuming, to ignore the multicultural identities of their patients, but in no way does this serve the doctor-patient relationship well.

Patients, though they may be reluctant to state it, feel their doctor's interest in them or the lack thereof keenly. Sometimes patients will keep such an observation private, for fear of creating an even greater distance from the doctor. Other patients may just choose to see another physician or continue with an unsatisfactory rapport and limit visits to absolute emergencies. A much healthier alternative is for the care provider to acknowledge and even explore his or her own identities more broadly. This allows the caregiver to appreciate the value of multiple identities in clients. The client can feel that he or she is seen as a whole person and not only as the carrier of a particular disease constellation, lesion, etc. The patient and the physician in this scenario can form a deeper working pair (or trio if extended family need be involved), and from that, a greater health benefit can develop. Toward this end, please take a moment to complete the questions found in Table 4-1 that are designed for the health care provider's multicultural growth.

TABLE 4-1
Self-Quiz for Physicians

1. Do you know your maternal and paternal ethnic/racial designation(s)? What are they? Do they affect the way you think about your identity?
2. Have you ever considered how your cultural background might shape the way in which you respond to the health care system when seeking medical services?
3. Can you recall stories about how your family has responded to the health care system (e.g., refusals to seek treatment because of "old-fashioned" fears, blanket reverence toward all doctors, blanket distrust of health care providers as a group, or acceptance of health care providers of a certain gender, race, or organizational affiliation only)?
4. With which cultural groups do you associate yourself? In answering this question, do you consider regional affiliation, religion, gender, or sexual orientation? These, too, are considered to be culture-loaded designations.

Take a moment to think about what may have surprised you in your answers to the self-quiz. Have you thought about these issues before? Are you a person who tends to give a great deal of meaning to multicultural issues? Are you a person who tends to give little attention to the multicultural aspects of other people? What might happen if you discuss (in turn) these questions and answers with those you work with most closely?

The self-quiz is designed to help the practitioner develop greater multicultural empathy for patients by providing a basis for understanding how the multicultural identities of the physician may interact with the multicultural identities of the patient. Exacerbated by the economic pressure that managed care may add, doctors treat their patients as quickly as possible and all too easily lose touch with this part of the patient's personhood. It is also easy to assume that if a patient looks or talks like you that he or she automatically feels understood on a cultural level by you or that you are providing culturally competent health care simply by being, presumably, of the same cultural group. Neither may be true. Similarly, if a patient does not look like you, then practitioners, rightly or not, may not assume that the same cultural background exists. They may cast a more careful eye to be sure that communication is smooth and accurate, but quite often they may ignore any possible cultural differences and treat the lesion, ache, pain, etc., assuming that this will be sufficient and is, after all, that for which the patient has come. Are patients well served by physicians and other health care providers working from such an assumption?

So what is the point? How does culture relate to providing health care? The premise of this chapter is that "although largely unconscious, cultural patterns have a powerful influence on [the perception of] health and illness."[1] If culture affects the way that one sees the world, then it also will affect the way one sees health and illness. The practitioner who appreciates the influence multicultural memberships has on the patient's receptivity to treatment is better positioned to reach the patient, formulate a strong working alliance with him or her, and elicit the patient's cooperation in his or her own treatment.

DEFINING OUR TERMS

Perhaps some definitions of the concepts used in the chapter will help the reader with what may appear to be amorphous terminology. What exactly is meant by the terms *culture, multicultural, multicultural competence,* and *multiculturally competent health care*? *Culture* is a commonly used term, but one that is not so easily defined. Much of the reason for this is the broadness of the term. It is used to refer to periods of time (e.g., *Culture Shock,* the culture of the 1980s, etc.), regional distinctions, ethnic/racial distinctions, religious distinctions, and even workplace distinctions (e.g., the corporate culture). By the term *of the same culture,* I am referring to people who associate themselves with each other according to many possible dimensions. For example, regional boundaries suggest some cultural affiliations, (e.g., national boundaries or subnational: southern, eastern, or midwestern) or the culture of the suburbs, etc. Thus culture, often immediately interpreted as racial or ethnically based subgroupings visually identifiable by dress, food, music, language, and the like, alternatively can be "loaded" with region, religion, political affiliation, economic class, etc. The essential factors are that group members acknowledge the affiliation, and that customs, beliefs, and world view are, in part, shaped by the affiliation.[2,3]

Hidalgo (1993) parses the term *culture* into three levels: concrete, behavioral, and symbolic.[3] At the concrete level, she refers to what differentiates groups *that can be seen,* such as food, dress, and music. These elements might be thought of as the fun aspects of culture. At the behavioral level, she refers to *what people do* that differentiates them, such as how (and what) we speak and how we construct family, gender, and other social roles. Therefore, while less visible per se than what food we eat, this level of culture could be said to describe who provides for, buys, prepares, eats, and cleans up the food. At the third or symbolic level, even less visible than the preceding two levels, Hidalgo isolates how individuals within a group *define themselves,* for example, through religion, world view, spirituality, customs, etc. Continuing with food as the unifying example, the symbolic application would be why we do or do not eat certain foods and how eating (or not) certain foods helps to define who we are.

How is this helpful to the practitioner? Awareness on the part of the health care provider of the concrete level of culture helps patients to feel that they are *seen* by their doctor. Awareness of the second, or behavioral, level of culture helps doctors to understand how their patient fits into a social system that likely affects the patient's health. For example, whose role(s) is it to bring children to seek medical care? Whose role in the family is such that illness in that person cannot be tolerated? Awareness of the third, or symbolic, level on the part of the health care provider suggests a broader understanding of the world and the way in which this patient and the patient's affiliations fit into that world. For example, in the excellent nonfiction film, *Worlds Apart,* a Western doctor allows herself to understand and accept a Laotian mother's hesitation about allowing heart surgery for her daughter based on the maternal grandmother's fear that the child will become too scarred to enter into the afterlife.[4] In this way, the potential for continued care is kept aloft rather than shut down in a rush of intolerance, impatience, and misunderstanding.

Multiculturalism is a term that came into prominence in the early 1980s and had its initial introduction in the early 1960s through the discipline of education.[5] Not exclusive to but certainly included among the leaders were the Canadians in the journey to create multicultural classrooms. Concretely, this meant having posters and other audiovisual materials that reflected the backgrounds of the children learning in that classroom. Behaviorally, it meant recruiting and admitting students who represent the broad spectrum of humanity. Symbolically, it meant integrating those differences, religious, racial, socioeconomic, etc., into the school's or university's fabric (e.g., the school calendar, the teachers and professors' training, etc.) in such a way that the success of a multicultural student body could be supported.

The definition of *multiculturalism,* which in its simplicity seeks to encompass most of the others is, "The doctrine that several different cultures (rather than one national culture) can coexist peacefully and equitably in a single country."[6] *Multicultural* does not refer exclusively to, though it does include, ethnic and racial groupings. Multiculturalism represents a departure from these designations to a more encompassing view of others. "Multiculturalism, in an absolute sense, recognizes the broad scope of dimensions of race, ethnicity, language, sexual orientation, gender, age, disability, class status, education, religious/spiritual orientation, and other cultural dimensions."[2] Multiculturalism may be thought of as a theoretical container that allows more space for people's identities. This includes hearing and respecting the ways in which individuals choose to be identified. Multiculturalism also avoids having one culture dominate a setting. For example, in a multicultural classroom, the readings, the material, the posters, the children, and the teachers will represent some combination of cultures so that all cultures feel their value reflected.

What is the reader's level of awareness of his or her multicultural thumbprint? One way to answer this question is to complete a sociogram. Figure 4-1 is a template for a sociogram. It is offered to help the reader think about his or her multicultural self. The circle in the center of the diagram represents the reader. The spokes of the wheel represent branches of the reader's identity, for example, level of education, religion, religiosity, regional background, sexual orientation, marital status, parenthood status, race, occupation, ethnicity, socioeconomic status, gender, etc. *Please take five minutes to create your own sociogram.* Use the aspects of identity that hold the most meaning for you. If you like, you may add spokes to the wheel. Once you have completed the sociogram, consider these follow-up questions:

1. Was completing the sociogram familiar? Unfamiliar? Comfortable? Uncomfortable? Pleasant? Unpleasant?
2. Did you have more difficulty with certain aspects of identity than with others? How so?
3. Who in your life would know what you have identified on your sociogram without being told?

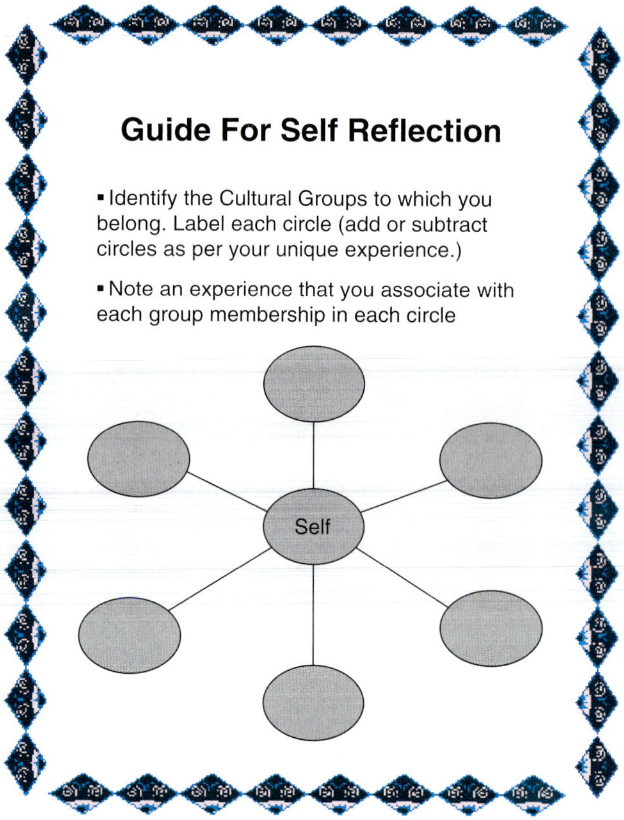

▲ **FIGURE 4-1**

4. Each of your patients has a sociogram that describes important parts of him or her. Can you imagine how recognition of this fact (with or without knowing the details) might allow you to connect more fully with your patients?

One step beyond considering how awareness of multiculturalism in individuals can be helpful to patients is to consider the issue in an institutional context. If, for example, the professional and administrative staff of a large practice has an appreciation for and an understanding of the importance of multicultural factors in patient care, that office is on its way to developing multicultural competence. "Cultural competence can be defined as a combination of knowledge, clinical skills, and behaviors that lead to positive outcomes of patient care with culturally diverse populations."[7] This includes providing "services that are respectful of and responsive to the health beliefs, practices, and cultural and linguistic needs of diverse patient populations."[1]

Kleinman offers the following list of cultural assessment questions (Table 4-2) that practitioners may choose to include in their intake procedures in order to collect more culturally sensitive information.[7,8] The questions could be asked by a medical assistant if the physician feels that there is insufficient time in his or her clinical interview. In this case, the interviewer must be trained in identifying and quickly and reliably communicating to the physician key information so that the physician can then make use of the information in an initial assessment.

Once your intake procedures integrate more fully the multicultural identities of your patients, you will have additional information. This may enable you to consider your patient base as a whole and thereby find interesting and informative patterns. The questions in Table 4-3 are designed to help you elicit your clientele's cultural fingerprint(s).

Can you identify patterns that describe the patients you tend to treat, or do you see more of a random scatter in terms of clientele? In either case, there are implications for multicultural com-

TABLE 4-2
Possible Cultural Assessment Questions to Incorporate in Intake Procedure

Cultural Assessment Questions

1. Where were you born?
2. If you were born outside the United States, how long have you lived in this country?
3. Who are the people you depend on the most for help (family members, friends, community services, church, etc.)?
4. Are there people who depend on you for care? Who are they? What kind of care do you provide?
5. What languages do you speak?
6. Can you read and write in those languages?
7. What is the first thing you do when you feel ill?
8. Do you ever see a native healer or other type of practitioner when you don't feel well?
9. What does that person do for you?
10. Do you ever take any herbs or medicines that are commonly used in your native country or cultural group?
11. What are they, and what do you take them for?
12. What foods do you generally eat? How many times a day do you eat?
13. How do you spend your day?
14. How did you get here today?
15. Do you generally have to arrange for transportation when you have appointments?

Tools to Elicit Health Beliefs

1. What do you call your problem? What name does it have?
2. What do you think caused your problem?
3. Why do you think it started when it did?
4. What does your sickness do to you? How does it work?
5. How severe is it? Will it have a short or long course?
6. What do you fear most about your disorder?
7. What are the chief problems that your sickness has caused for you?
8. What kind of treatment do you think you should receive? What are the most important results you hope to receive from treatment?

(continued)

TABLE 4-2 (Continued)
Possible Cultural Assessment Questions to Incorporate in Intake Procedure

Further Questions to Consider

1. Do individuals in this culture feel comfortable answering questions?
2. Does the patient or family perceive a provider asking questions as a lack of knowledge?
3. Who should be told about the illness?
4. Does the family need a consensus, or can one person make decisions?
5. Does the patient feel uncomfortable owing to the gender of the provider?
6. Does more medicine mean more illness to the patient?
7. Does no medication mean healthy?
8. Does the patient prefer to feel the symptoms or mask them?
9. Does the patient prefer *one* solution or choices of treatment?
10. Does the patient want to hear about risks?

petence in your office. If, for example, you work in West Philadelphia, Pennsylvania, where a large Hmong community of recent immigrants and their first- and second-generation children reside, you may need access to a professional translator. You may need to read about Hmong medical decision-making practices and hierarchies. You may need to understand the role of the traditional healer. You may need to provide forms, resource pamphlets, and the like in multiple languages. For this as well as other scenarios, the physician may find it useful to consider the practice issues outlined in Table 4-4.

TABLE 4-3
Who is your patient base?

Take a moment to consider your patient base.

- Do you treat more women than men?
- More Caucasians than Asians?
- Hispanics than African Americans?
- West Indians than African Americans?
- Caucasians of northern versus southern European decent?
- Is there an enclave of ethnic immigrants that your practice serves?
- Do you serve more first-, second-, or third-generation immigrants?
- High-, middle-, or lower-income-bracket clients?
- Rural, urban, or suburban dwellers?
- Those who speak English as a first language?
- Those who speak English as a second language or perhaps no English at all?
- Extremely religious versus not at all religious?
- What religions?
- Older, middle-age, or younger clients?
- Do you serve gay clients who are out?
- Closeted?
- Which groups of patients do you serve that are not culturally described by the preceding questions?

CONCLUSION

In the popular film, *My Big Fat Greek Wedding*, the bride's father carries around a bottle of Windex, always ready to spray into submission any cut, bite, scrape, scratch, itch, etc. that may need tending. As amusing as it may be, it offers a precious example of how the perception of illness can be influenced by culture. This chapter has provided information about how to provide multiculturally competent medical care to patients. This includes several exercises that physicians can do to raise their awareness of the multicultural aspects of their identities. The premise for this chapter is the belief that by becoming multiculturally aware, clinicians can in fact provide more comprehensive and therefore superior care to patients, who, in turn, will be more cooperative with the physician in their care and who will likely post better outcomes. If there were just one improvement health care providers could implement that would take relatively little effort but reap a huge benefit, it would be to learn to pronounce each patient's name fully and correctly the very first time you meet.[5] At the very least, a patient has a right to expect that his or her identity, as represented in his first and last name, will be respected by his or her doctor. Whatever stumbling and repetition may be required to accomplish this task is small payment for the benefits reaped. In the end, not only is the multicultural approach a winning approach, but it is also increasingly the only viable approach as world demographic patterns continue to change in their current directions.

TABLE 4-4
Is your office culturally sensitive?

- Do you provide magazines, posters, signs, and other reading material in languages that all or most of your patients can understand?
- Do you provide or have access to a translator, especially a professional one, when clients need one (and not only when they ask for one)?
- Is your receptionist trained to skillfully and sensitively handle patients who can neither read nor write English or perhaps any language?
- Do you provide resource information relevant to the life issues of clients who sit in your waiting room?
- Do you know enough about your patients' cultures to be able to ask pertinent questions about how their culture and their perception of their illness may interface?
- If your medical assistant flags a multicultural item on intake, do you feel sufficiently comfortable to discuss it with your patient?
- Do you include one or two multicultural questions in your own face-to-face interview of the patient that elevates the importance of those questions in the patient's perception of what you find noteworthy?
- Would you consider having a consultant visit your office anonymously to assess its multicultural competence without informing staff?

REFERENCES

1. West Virginia University Center on Aging. Culturally competent health care. Available at *www.hsc.wvu.edu/coa/;* retrieved March 6, 2004.
2. American Psychological Association Online Public Interest. Guidelines on multicultural education, training, research, practice, and organizational change for psychologists, 2002. Available at *www.apa.org/pi/multiculturalguideleines/definitions.html;* retrieved March 6, 2004.
3. Hidalgo N. Multicultural teacher introspection, in Perry T, Fraser J (eds), *Freedom's Plow: Teaching in the Multicultural Classroom.* New York: Routledge, 1993.
4. Grainger-Monsen M, Haslett J. World's apart: A four-part series on cross-cultural health care, *Justine Christena's Story* (motion picture), 2003. Available from Fanlight Productions, 4196 Washington Street, Boston, MA 02131.
5. Gorski P, Covert B. Defining multicultural education. Multicultural pavilion: Working definitions, 2000. Available at *www.edchange.org/mulitcultural/initial.html;*retrieved March 2004.

6. Dimopoulos K, Siolas A. The industrial and modern city: The rise of the multicultural metropolis. National Technical University of Athens, Greece. Available at *www.opencontent.gr/imtiie/pdf/dimopoulos.pdf*; retrieved January 2004.
7. Hall GH. Culturally competent patient care: A guide for providers and their staff. Institute for Health Professions Education, 2001. Available at *www.azdes.gov/dcyf/cmdpe/reports/www.azdes.gov/dcyf/cmdpe/reports/*.
8. Kleinman AA. Patients and healers in the context of culture, in Institute for Health Professions Education, *Culturally Competent Patient Care: A Guide for Providers and Their Staff*. The Regents of the University of California, 1981. Available at *www.de.state.az.us/dcyf/ cmdpe/reports/Cultural%20Competence%20Guide1.pdf*; retrieved April 2, 2004.

CHAPTER 5

Impact of Cultural Beliefs on Health Care

Marta I. Rendon
Jorge I. Gaviria

Key Points

- Physicians need to understand the attitudes, beliefs, values, and traditional healing practices of the ethnic groups they treat.
- Genetic, environmental, ethnic, and socioeconomic factors play complex roles in disease.
- Minority Americans typically receive poorer health care than whites.
- Increased awareness of racial and cultural differences has begun a trend to more egalitarian health care delivery.

More than 5000 distinct ethnic groups exist in the world today. As people migrate to the United States and other developed countries in search of jobs, they bring along a broad collection of customs and cultural beliefs. In its relatively short existence, the United States has become a melting pot of colors and cultures. In 1998, only 28% of the U.S. population was comprised of ethnic and racial minorities. By 2030, this figure is expected to reach 40%.[1] In many metropolitan areas, cultural diversification has become the norm. Miami, for example, has the largest foreign-born population of any city in the world and is home to blacks, Cubans, Central Americans, South Americans, Europeans, and people born in the Caribbean. New York and Los Angeles also have large foreign-born populations.[2] Even traditionally homogeneous cities are seeing a dramatic influx of immigrants that is changing their demographic profiles.

Little has been published in the dermatologic literature on how cultural influences affect health care practices or physician–patient relationships. This chapter will attempt to shed light on this issue. One thing is for certain: As physicians, our cultural backgrounds influence how we communicate with patients and how patients respond to us. In order to deliver the best possible care, we must understand culturally driven health-related behaviors and adapt our practices to accommodate them. Failure to do so may result in noncompliance or potentially harmful interactions between folk remedies and prescription medications, as well as missed opportunities for prevention.[3]

To the benefit of physicians and patients alike, things have changed dramatically since the 1970s, when the dominant model of illness was strictly biomedical. No room was left for the cultural, behavioral, psychological or social dimensions of illness. Fortunately, it is generally accepted today that the social sciences can be used to bridge the gap between clinical medicine and specific ethnic or cultural groups, and biopsychosocial models are now being incorporated in medical school curricula, research, and teaching.

THE PROBLEM OF DEFINING ETHNIC GROUPS

Just who comprises a specific ethnic group can be difficult to define. *African American* implies family origin in Africa. The first black Africans were brought to the New World by Spanish conquistadors and slave traders in the sixteenth century. The first colonies were located in northern South American countries such as Colombia and Venezuela and in the Caribbean countries of Cuba, Dominican Republic, Jamaica, Haiti, the Antilles, and Puerto Rico. Shortly thereafter, slaves were introduced to the English colonies in what is today the United States. Contemporary African Americans represent a mixture of Africans, European Caucasians, and Native Americans.

Many native English-speaking blacks in the United States consider themselves African Americans, whereas blacks from Spanish- or French-speaking heritage tend to identify with their country of origin rather than Africa and prefer to be known as a descendant of that country—for example, Cuban American or Haitian American—rather than an African American.

Hispanic means "of Spanish descent." Natives of Spain, however, view the term to be derogatory. Although *Hispanic* is used widely in reference to people born in Central and South America, the term *Latino* is preferred. In this chapter we will use *Latino* in reference to people from the Caribbean Islands, Central America, and South America.

Asian American refers to people of Asian heritage. Asian Americans are the second fastest growing population after Latinos and the most ethnically diverse minority group in the United States. In Census terminology, *Asian* is used to designate heritage from all countries lying between Europe and the Pacific Ocean. In common practice, however, it describes people from countries lying west of the Middle East.

As a note, *Indian* means "from India." Christopher Columbus incorrectly called Native Americans Indians because he thought he had landed in India. The correct term for indigenous people to the continental United States is *Native American;* in Alaska, it is Alaska Native; in Canada, it is Canadian Native or Canadian Aboriginal; in South America, it is Colombian, Peruvian, Bolivian, or Brazilian Native.

The conventional practice of clustering ethnic groups into the three broad minority categories mentioned earlier plus white (Caucasian) risks perpetuating outdated stereotypes. Calling all Asians "Chinese" or all blacks "African Americans" results in the inclusion of people from very different cultures and socioeconomic strata with little in common. A white from the Dominican Republic living in the United States may have nothing in common with a black Dominican or a Mexican, even though they all speak Spanish. A black Haitian may have no common ground with a black Jamaican, an Ethiopian, or a black Cuban.

It behooves every physician to be aware of the differences between various cultures and to treat patients in a manner that reflects an understanding of their unique cultural characteristics.[4] Respect is key. An open mind is essential in understanding how patients' beliefs affect their health and how they will respond to treatment suggestions. Patients bring their cultural and ideological beliefs with them when they seek health care. These beliefs may challenge what you believe to be the best for them. Cultural insensitivity or disrespect result in noncompliance or ineffective physician–patient relationship. Understanding and respecting cultural beliefs are critical to gaining a patient's trust and respect and in establishing a relationship that ultimately will benefit the patient.

COMMUNICATION AND LANGUAGE BARRIERS

Communication presents one of the biggest challenges faced by physicians and other health care workers. Language barriers, the real meaning of certain words, the use of telephones, and how much information is given and by whom are all issues in the forefront. Interpreters are not always accessible and some groups—for example, South Asians (those from Afghanistan, Bangladesh, Bhutan, India, Nepal, Pakistan, and Sri Lanka) and those from China, Hong Kong, Korea, and Vietnam—prefer same-sex physicians, nurses, and translators. Some patients are uncomfortable discussing sexual matters, sexually transmitted diseases, or illegal drug use. Minorities like Latinos or Middle eastern people are embarrassed to discuss personal and sexual matters with their physicians. Mental illness for Latinos is a "taboo" a strong social prohibition, and they do not want to deal with mental illness in close family members. Others are reluctant to use the telephone, preferring face-to-face discussions. African Americans and Latinos are less likely than whites to find antidepressant medications acceptable.[5]

When English is a second language, communicating complex medical information can be a challenge. Some Asian languages, for example, that spoken by the Hmong of Laos, lack medical terms, making direct translation impossible. Language barriers in health care present a challenge that needs cultural competent providers. This obviously can lead to serious misunderstandings.[6] To help reduce the impact of communication barriers, multilingual resources and high-quality, carefully verified translations of necessary information should be used by health care providers who treat substantial numbers of patients from particular backgrounds.

ATTITUDES, BELIEFS, AND PERCEPTIONS

It is important to become familiar with the traditional healing techniques and preferences used by various ethnic groups in order to integrate these practices into individual health care plans. A good place to start is the report on policies and strategies regarding traditional medicine released by the World Health Organization (WHO).[7] In addition, the National Center for Complementary and Alternative Medicine (NCCAM), a division of the National Institutes of Health, offers meetings, workshops, and financial support for clinical trials designed to increase understanding of the alternative and complementary medicines used in the United States.[8]

African Americans

Four centuries of black history in America have produced a population with very specific needs, marked differences in cultural beliefs, and socioeconomic disparities that affect their health care. Two questions that arise from studies of health care in U.S. blacks and that can be extrapolated to some Asian and Latin ethnic groups are, Why do they receive poorer quality health care than whites? and Why do they suffer from some diseases more often than whites?

African Americans suffer disproportonally from diseases such as hypertension, diabetes, and peripheral vascular disease[9], yet cultural factors may play a role in the lower number of referrals for surgery.[10] Food plays an important role in every Caribbean, Central American, and South American country, and poor dietary habits and cultural practices may well account for their propensity toward diabetes, hypertension, and obesity.[11] Substantial delays exist in the period between the diagnosis and treatment of breast cancer in African-American women versus white women ages 20–54, but the exact contribution of cultural beliefs, diet, and genetics is unclear.[12]

Asian Americans

Asians tend to view health care providers with respect and authority. Asian patients may not ask questions because questions are considered disrespectful. Patient information is usually discussed with the family, not the patient. Most South Asian patients are not accustomed to being informed of every detail of their diagnosis, especially negative ones. The family acts like a buffer to filter out what the patient should be told and not be told.

Those who follow Buddhist or Confucian doctrines tend to view illness as a natural way of life. Symptoms may be seen as bad luck, misfortune, and the result of karma or payback for something done in the past. They also may view health as a balance between complementary energies, such as cold and hot, and traditional treatments often are preferred over Western medications.

Bracelets, beads, and other symbolic jewelry are sacred for some Hindus, Muslims, and Sikhs and cannot be removed without family permission to do so. In addition, observant Sikhs do not cut their hair. When hair must be cut or jewelry removed for surgery, physicians are advised to discuss the dilemma with a family member or the religious leader of that particular faith.

Latin Americans

Latinos who have recently arrived in the United States and Latinos born in the United States share similar values, languages, and health care beliefs. Although they share a common language in Spanish, marked differences in socioeconomic status among their countries of origin and very different cultures create strong differences between Latinos of Caribbean, Central American, and South American origin.

In the 1970s and early 1980s, Latino immigrants primarily came from lower socioeconomic classes. Lower socioeconomic class generally is accompanied by lack of medical insurance and a tendency toward noncompliance with physicians' recommendations. Starting in the 1990s, the United States began experiencing a wave of educated middle- and upper-class businesspeople leaving South America to escape political instability.

Alternative treatment is a way of life. In one survey, 17% of Latinos initially sought health care from a folk healer, 32% used a health care professional, and the remainder opted for self-treatment.[13] Latinos tend not to have regular health care and are twice as likely to use emergency room services as the general population.[14] Lower socioeconomic Latinos are not accustomed to use medical care routinely. Some of them do not have access to adequate health care due to either lack of insurance or lack of knowledge of how to get access to the health care system. Therefore, medical issues are left untreated and eventually they will end up in a emergency room for acute care. A survey of Puerto Rican patients suffering from hypertension revealed that 21% relied solely on herbal preparations or tea as the sole treatment for their disease. Although Puerto Rico has been a U.S. territory for more than 100 years, lack of education, the absence of health care policies, and different cultural beliefs regarding medical treatments continue to interfere with proper medical treatment.[15]

When populations turn to traditional healers for help, remedies may include psychotropic compounds, herbs, roots, stones, and seeds. Some of these remedies may have no scientific rationale and may even cause harm. Physicians should be reminded to ask about the use of home remedies and folk medicines in order to avoid adverse reactions that might occur when they are combined with prescription drugs.[16]

RELIGION AND HEALTH

Among city-dwelling Latinos, the use of *curanderos* is very common, particularly when the illness or disease is believed to have a supernatural cause. *Curanderos* are traditional healers believed to get power from God. *Sobadores* (masseuses) and *yerbateros* (herbalists) are also traditional healers.

One example of a supernatural power believed to cause disease is the *mal de ojo,* or "evil eye," which is essentially a curse: a superstitious believe that somebody creates harm just by looking at you or saying something about the future. It is believed a cure can be obtained by placing an egg over the body and then placing it in a bowl under the pillow overnight. If the egg is cooked in the morning, the curse has been removed. It is also believed that placing red and white seeds in a colorful wristband on a child's wrist within the first hours of life affords some protection from the evil eye.

Although not a popular practice, *brujeria* (witchcraft) plays an important role in some cultures. A hex (*hechizo* or *maldicion*) can be placed on someone by a black witch (*bruja*) or another person who knows witchcraft. Symptoms vary, but the cure involves Catholic prayers, herbs, massages, chili powder, medicinal enemas, showering with spices and vegetables, and making crosses with water and olive oil.

Santeria (also called *Candomble, Quimbanda,* and *Umbanda* in Brazil), is an Afro-Cuban religious tradition derived from traditional beliefs of the people from Nigeria. This religious practice is similar to Voodoo. This practice is common to the people of the Caribbean, Brazil and other countries in Central and South America. *Santeria* comes from the Spanish word *santo,* meaning "saint." Practitioners are called *santeros.* Although slaves brought to the Caribbean Islands and Central and South America from Africa were converted to Catholicism, they preserved some of their traditions, fusing their beliefs and rituals with elements of Catholicism. Today, any city with a large Latino population has many *santeros* as well as Catholics because many people practice both.

In cities such as Miami, New York, and Los Angeles, *botanicals* are a fundamental part of some subsets of Latino society. Botanicals are places where the *Santeria* paraphernalia can be found. The practice of *Santeria* and the use of recommended products from botanicals may replace physician advice and treatment or be used concomitantly with physician-prescribed medications.

Voodoo comes from an African word for "spirit." Slaves from Nigeria brought the religion with them to the New World. Although it was suppressed by colonial governments, it survived through underground societies. More than 60 million people practice Voodoo primarily in Haiti, the Dominican Republic, Ghana, Togo, and in the southern United States (Florida and Louisiana). Followers believe that each person has a soul composed of two guardian angels that work together and offer protection.[17–19] Voodoo priests and priestess treat every ailment from AIDS and cancer to lovesickness, sometimes recommending working in tandem with Western physicians and sometimes interfering with a physician's recommendations.

GENETIC RESPONSE TO DISEASE

Environmental conditions, ethnic differences, genetic factors, and socioeconomic status play a complex role in the presence of disease.[20] Although the incidence of cancer has decreased in the Asian, black, and Latino populations, mortality rates are higher than those for whites.[21] Cigarette smoking and obesity are prevalent in the Latino population and may play a role in the fact that they suffer a higher incidence of cancer and other diseases related to these lifestyle factors. This being said, the age-adjusted death rates for cancer, heart disease, and stroke are lower for Latinos than for African Americans or whites.[22]

Genetic factors found in different populations can affect response to certain medications, and polymorphisms can cause differences in drug levels by the absence or presence of drug-catabolizing enzymes. For example, Asians are also known to be rapid metabolizers of codeine and suffer more adverse effects. The Chinese are more sensitive to morphine's emetic effect and less sensitive to respiratory depression and hypotension. They also require less heparin and warfarin than whites to produce the same effects.

One area where racial differences are already well recognized is in the management of hypertension. Changes in hypertension treatments are necessary to accommodate a different response by the renin-angiotensin system in people of African and Caribbean origin. The Joint National Committee on Prevention, Detection, Evaluation, and Treatment of High Blood Pressure advises low doses of thiazide diuretics as first-line treatment in black patients but angiotensin-converting enzyme (ACE) inhibitors or beta-blockers in young white patients and ACE inhibitors for white patients over age 50. Asians metabolize propanolol faster than African Americans, whites, and Latinos and, in general, achieve better hypertension control with calcium antagonists, diuretics, and beta-blockers.[23]

Genetics plays only a small part in ethnic differences in health. Cultural and environmental factors play a more influential role on health than genetics.

AN UNEQUAL HEALTH CARE DELIVERY SYSTEM

Minority Americans do not fare as well as the white majority in the U.S. health care system. Even after adjustments for insurance status and income, racial and ethnic minorities tend to have less access to health care and receive lower-quality health care than nonminorities.

In an analysis of 150,391 visits by Medicare patients to 4300 primary care doctors, researchers from Memorial Sloan-Kettering Center and the Center for Studying Health System Change verified this inequality. African American and white patients were treated by different doctors. Physicians who treated black patients were less qualified academically. Doctors in the study who cared for blacks were less likely to be board certified in a specialized area of medicine than doctors treating white patients (77.4% versus 86.1%). These noncertified doctors were less likely to diagnose conditions and more likely simply to treat symptoms. About 2% of visits by black patients were made to doctors who said they could not consistently provide high-quality care, high-quality diagnostic imaging, high-quality ancillary services, or nonemergency hospital admission compared with 19% of visits by whites.

When asked specifically if they were able to provide access to high-quality care for all their patients, 27.8% of the primary care physicians responded negatively compared with 19.3% of physicians treating white patients. They also answered that they were unable to always provide access to high-quality specialty services (overall: 24% versus 17.9%; diagnostic imaging: 24.4% versus 16.6%; nonemergency hospital admissions: 48.5% versus. 37.0%; and quality ancillary services: 36.6% versus. 27.7%).[24] This type of discrimination is not a consequence of intentional malpractice but the result of a greater proportion of African Americans, Caribbean Americans, and Latinos living in poorer neighborhoods with fewer high-quality clinics and well-paid physicians.[25] Also, minorities are less represented in the health care professions.

The American College of Physicians has identified specific disparities affecting racial and ethnic minorities in the U.S. health care system. Addressing these important issues are the following: continued research, increasing access to quality health care, patient care, provider issues, societal concern, and systems that deliver health care.[26]

DISCUSSION

As physicians, we must make a serious effort to understand the beliefs, cultures, expectations, perceptions, and realities of the patients we serve. We cannot do this alone. Cultural sensitivity training must start in medical school. Fortunately, medical schools are beginning to teach medical students and residents about the presentation of common skin conditions in populations with different backgrounds.

The University of Washington has a Cross-Cultural Health Care Program (CCHCP) that helps underserved communities interact with the health system. The University of California, San Francisco, started a cultural competence initiative in 1999 with a collection of resources for physicians and the public. Their goal is to motivate medical professionals and the public to create behavioral and institutional changes that respect the multiple cultures of their patients. Baylor College of Medicine has an ethnocultural introduction program that promotes communication issues with patients from different ethnic, racial, and religious backgrounds. George Washington University Medical Center offers interdisciplinary student community patient education services in their curricula. The Community College of San Francisco has a health care interpreter certification program.

Even the U.S. government is finally getting into the act. The Department of Health and Human Services' Healthy People 20 20 initiative has made the reduction of racial disparities a national health priority."[27]

In some ways, the focus on cultural differences has been beneficial, resulting in the creation of a wide variety of resources designed to better know and understand our communities. Yet insufficient resources are available to overcome the provider bias, and insufficient research has been conducted on the impact of race on health care.

One of the most challenging factors in raising cultural sensitivity is the origin of medical students. There continues to be a disproportionate representation of whites in medical schools. African Americans and Latinos produce a smaller number of physicians, regardless of socioeconomic class. Black and Hispanic physicians play an important role in caring for poor people and members of minority groups.[28]

Increased awareness of cultural differences has started a trend toward more egalitarian health care delivery. For example, articles have been published in the field of dermatology on skin of color in response to a growing interest in African Americans, Asian Americans, and Latinos.[29–34] The increasing importance of minority groups has led to the creation of societies such as the Skin of Color Society, whose primary purpose is the understanding of skin diseases, further research, and education in people with skin color other than white.

LOOKING AHEAD

There is a wealth of evidence that ethnic and racial disparities exist in our health care system. However, there is still a big contrariety between this nation's democratic principles and egalitarian commitments and the realities of its racial policies and practices that needs to be quantified in order to improve the quality of health care and reduce racial disparities.[35–36]

More ethnographic studies need to be conducted to determine the perspectives and beliefs of specific groups and how these influence the experience of people from different cultures seeking Western medical care. Most published studies are biased and lack a cultural understanding of ethnic minorities. Data should not originate solely from the medical establishment; there is a great need to explore the cultural competence of physicians from patients' point of view.

In designing a prospective study to evaluate the impact of cultural beliefs on health care in Asian Americans, African Americans, and Latinos, core variables that will reflect economic, geographic, and social diversity should be applied. Comparative approaches should be used to focus on the diverse manifestations of disease among different ethnic groups, aiming to incorporate the cultural aspects of illness into the clinical arena. Studies must go beyond epidemiology to explain the factors that give rise to our data and to help us better understand how cultural beliefs affect the delivery of medical care to African Americans, Asian Americans, and Latinos.

It is a reality that physicians will continue to encounter a higher number of patients with backgrounds different from their own. In response, physicians must learn to conduct a comprehensive cultural assessment on every patient. Only by evaluating a patient's cultural, ethnic, and racial background will they be able to understand the impact of genetic and cultural variables in response to medications and compliance with treatment and prevention suggestions.

REFERENCES

1. US Department of Commerce, Bureau of Census. Resident population, 1980 to 1989 and projections, 1999 to 2050, in *Statistical Abstracts of the United States: National Data Book,* 119th ed. Washington, US Government Printing Office, 1999, Table 19.
2. United Nations Development Program, *http://hdr.undp.org/reports/globa1/2004.*
3. Brach C, Fraser I. Can cultural competency reduce racial and ethnic health disparities? A review and conceptual model. *Med Care Rees Rev* 2000;57:18-217S.
4. Cross T, Bazron B, Dennis K, Isaacs M. *Toward a Culturally Competent System of Care,* Vol 1. Washington, Georgetown University Press, 1989.
5. Cooper LA. The acceptability of treatment for depression among African-American, Hispanic, and white primary care patients. *Med Care* 2003;41:479-490.
6. Johnson SK. Hmong health beliefs and experiences in the Western health care system. *J Transcult Nurs* 2002;13:126-132.
7. World Health Organization Unit on Traditional Medicine. *Legal Status of*

Traditional Medicine and Complementary/ Alternative Medicine. Geneva, WHO Unit on Traditional Medicine, 2002:43-48.

8. National Center for Complementary and Alternative Health. Program Announcements 2002; available at *http://NCCAM.nih.gov/announcements/PA /Index.htm#active.*
9. Selvin E, Erlinger TP. Prevalence of and risk factors for peripheral arterial disease in the United States: Results from the National Health and Nutrition Examination Survey, 1999-2000. *Circulation* 2004;110:738-743.
10. Haitchcock B, Velanovitch V. Comparison of antireflux surgery among ethnicity. *J Natl Med Assoc* 2004;96:535-541.
11. Sharma S, Cruickhank JK. Cultural differences in assessing dietary intake and providing relevant dietary information to British, African-Caribbean populations. *J Hum Nutr Diet* 2001;146: 449-456.
12. Gwyn K, Bondy ML, Cohen DS, et al. Racial differences in diagnosis, treatment, and clinical delays in a population-based study of patients with newly diagnosed breast carcinoma. *Cancer* 2004; 100:1595-1604.
13. World Health Organization. *Legal Status of Traditional Medicine and Complementary/ Alternative Medicine.* Geneva, WHO Unit on Traditional Medicine, 2002.
14. Diaz VA, Jr. Cultural factors in preventive care: Latinos. Primary Care 2002;29(3): 503-517,viii.
15. Vergara C, Martin AM, Wang F, Horowitz S. Awareness about factors that affect the management of hypertension in Puerto Rican patients. *Conn Med* 2004;68:269-276.
16. Boyd EL, Taylor SD, Shimp LA, Semler CR. An assessment of home remedy use by African Americans. *J Natl Med Assoc* 2000;92:341-353.
17. West African Dohomean Vodoun: Historical Background. Available at *www. mamiwata.com/historyl.html.*
18. The Vodoun Page, *http://members.aol.com/ racine125/index.html.*
19. Sponsors of the National African Religion Congress (NARC World). Le Peristyle Haitian Sanctuary. Available at *http:// leperistylehaitiansanctuary.com.*
20. Cooper RS. Race, genes, and health: New wine in old bottles? *Int J Epidemiol* 2003;32:23-25.
21. Glanz K, Croyle RT, Chollette VY, et al. Cancer-related health disparities in women. *Am J Public Health* 2003;93:292-298.
22. http://cdc.gov/omhd/About/PDFs/ omhdpresentation.pdf
23. Pearce N, Foliaki S, Sporle A, et al. Genetics, race, ethnicity, and health. *Br Med J* 2004;328:1070-1072.
24. Bach PB, Pham HH, Schrag D, et al. Primary care physicians who treat blacks and whites. *N Engl J Med* 2004;351: 575-584.
25. Epstein AM. Health care in America: Still too separate, not yet equal. *N Engl J Med* 2004;351:603-605.
26. Racial and ethnic disparities in health care. A position paper of the American College of Physicians. *Ann Intern Med.* 2004;141:226-232.
27 Healthy People 2010. What are its goals? Conference ed. Washington, D.C.: Department of Health and Human Services, 2003. http://www.healthypeople. gov/About/goals.htm.
28. Komaromy M, Grumbach K, Drake M. et al. The role of Black and Hispanic physicians in providing health care for underserved populations. *N Engl J Med.* 1996; 334:1305-1310.
29. Halder RM. Ethnic skin diseases. *Dermatol Clin* 2003;21(4);595-768.
30. Taylor SC. Understanding skin of color. *J Acad Dermatol* 2002,46(S2):41-124.
31. Rendon MI, Ciocca GR, Gaviria J. The challenge of diagnosing melasma in Hispanic populations. Poster 576. AAD Meeting, San Francisco, CA, 2003.
32. Rendon MI, Melasma and Post inflammatory Hyperpigmentation. *Cosmet Dermatol* 2003;16(S3):9-17.
33. Rendon MI. Del Rosso JQ. Current assessment of melasma in hispanic populations: Focus on approaches to management and quality of life issues. Poster. Summer AAD, New York, NY, 2004.
34. Rendon MI, Benitez, AL, Gaviria JI. Telangiectatic Melasma: A New Entity? *Cosmet Dermatol* 2007;20(1):17-21.
35. Van Ryn M, Fu SS. Paved with good intentions: Do public health and human service providers contribute to racial/ ethnic disparities in health? *Am J Public Health* 2003;93(2):247-255.
36. Geiger HJ. Race and health care—an American dilemma. *N Engl J Med* 1996;335(11):815-816.

RECOMMENDED READINGS

Geiger HJ. Race and health care: An American dilemma. *N Engl JMed* 1996;335:815-816.

Halder RM. Ethnic skin diseases. *Dermatol Clin* 2003;21:595-768.

Healthy People 2010. What Are Its Goals? Washington, Department of Health and Human Services, 2003. Available at *www. healthypeople.gov/About/goals.htm.1*

Komaromy M, Grumbach K, Drake M, et al. The role of black and Hispanic physicians in providing health care for underserved populations. *N Engl JMed* 1996; 334:1305-1310.

Kudzma EC. Cultural competence: Cardiovascular medications. *Prog Cardiovsc Nurs* 2001;16:152-160.

Racial and ethnic disparities in health care: A position paper of the American College of Physicians. *Ann Intern Med* 2004;141: 226-232.

Rendon MI, Ciocca GR, Gaviria J. The challenge of diagnosing melasma in Hispanic populations. Poster, AAD Meeting, San Francisco, CA, 2003.

Rendon MI. Melasma and postinflammatory hyperpigmentation. *J Cosmet Dermatol* 2003;16:9-17S.

Rendon MI, Del Rosso JQ. Current assessment of melasma in hispanic populations: Focus on approaches to management and quality of life issues. Poster, AAD Summer Meeting, New York, 2004.

Rendon, MI. Benitez, AL, Gaviria JI. Telangiectatic Melasma: A New Entity? *Cosmet Dermatol* 2007;20(1):17-21.

Taylor SC. Understanding skin of color. *J Acad Dermatol* 2002,46:41-124S.

Van Ryn M, Fu SS. Paved with good intentions: Do public health and human service providers contribute to racial/ethnic disparities in health? *Am J Public Health* 2003;93:247-255.

CHAPTER 6

Impact of Cultural Beliefs in Health Care in Blacks: Afro-Caribbean Culture, Traditions, Habits, and Practices

Fran E. Cook-Bolden
Jocelyne Papacharalambous

Key Points

- The use of folk remedies is associated with lack of access to health care owing to shortage of doctors, language or cultural barriers, socioeconomic status, or distrust of doctors, and is unrelated to level of education.
- Traditional practitioners believe that illness is caused by divine punishment, environmental hazards, or impaired social relationships, and can be cured only by carefully following the prescribed plan of the master (God).
- Black folk medicine incorporates African and Native American beliefs and practices, and elements of spiritualism, religion, Voodoo, and astrology.
- Folk practitioners include conjurers, psychics, prophets, herbalists, magic vendors, and divine healers.
- Dermatologists must be aware of cultural beliefs and taboos in order to recognize remedies that may be harmful or interact with prescription drugs.

The ethnic and cultural diversity of the American population has grown throughout history. Established American groups assumed that new immigrants would become incorporated into existing cultural patterns, the so-called melting-pot theory. This assimilation model has been recognized as neither a good description of what has happened nor a likely predictor of what may happen as our population continues to change rapidly. Culture, traditions, habits, and practices, as well as barriers to communication, in American society are now more varied than ever—hence the need in medicine to develop appropriate cultural competencies to serve the diverse American population.

Historically, use of folk remedies has been associated with a lack of access to health care owing to a shortage of doctors, language or cultural barriers, socioeconomic status, or mistrust of doctors. However, researchers have found no relationship between the use of home or folk remedies and level of education attained. These findings suggest that folk remedy use is not necessarily attributable to restricted access to medical care and poverty but rather represents the impact of tradition that is handed down by the elders of the specific culture. The strong influence of culture and tradition further supports the fact that cultural competence is a key to serving the diverse population in the United States.[1] This competence is necessary for treating the full gamut of disease processes but is even more important when treating diseases that are unique to or are found more commonly in specific ethnic populations. To this end, we must be aware of the belief systems, traditions, and customs of our patients' cultures. These traditions and belief systems often affect the success or failure of the treatment of the disease process.[2]

CULTURAL COMPETENCE AND ETHNOSENSITIVITY

There is sizable literature from social, behavioral, and health sciences that promotes a philosophy of cross-cultural competence to which all medical professionals working with multicultural groups should subscribe. *Cultural competence* is defined by Campinha-Bacote as "a process for effectively working within the cultural context of an individual or community from a diverse cultural or ethnic background."[3] She proposes a culturally competent model of health care that encompasses four levels: cultural awareness, cultural knowledge, cultural skill, and cultural encounter.

Ethnocentrism is a concept that often plays a part in confusing an already difficult situation when working with ethnically diverse individuals or cultural groups.[4,5] It is an individual's assumption that his or her way of believing and behaving is the most preferable and correct one. Often the physician is unaware of his or her own ethnocentric behavior and that it can lead to dysfunctional treatment encounters. For example, the physician may directly or indirectly discount or ignore a patient's cultural orientation and belief system, considering them unimportant, incorrect, or in conflict with the physician's own perceptions or worldview of how best to treat the patient's health problem or issue. This can leave the patient feeling angry, frustrated, and uncooperative.

Of equal importance is the awareness that whereas the physician may be caught in his or her own ethnocentric dance, so too may the culturally diverse patient the physician is serving. The patient may view the physician as foreign, ignorant of illness or disease causality, or uneducated regarding proper social customs, forms of address, and nonverbal behaviors deemed appropriate by the patient for dealing directly or indirectly with his or her health problem or concern.[6,7]

Ethnosensitivity is the process of becoming more sensitive and respecting of cross-cultural differences. Borkan and Neher describe a developmental model of ethnosensitivity that can be used to help train physicians to improve their cross-cultural communication and practice skills.[8] Their model proposes a seven-stage developmental range that can be used to access a health care provider's ethnosensitivity. These stages consist of

1. Fear or mistrust of different cultural groups
2. Denial of cultural differences
3. Feelings of superiority over other cultural groups
4. Minimization of cultural differences
5. Cultural relativism (acceptance and respect for differences)
6. Empathy
7. Cultural integration

During the final stage, the practitioner becomes a multicultural person able to relate well to different cultural groups.

THE AFRICAN-AMERICAN CULTURE AND ILLNESS

Explaining the Cause of Illness

In African-American culture, illness often has been attributed to one of two major categories: the natural or the unnatural. This categorization may affect the methods that traditional health practitioners use to treat or cure an illness. Historically, the majority of traditional practitioners and followers believed that illness could be cured only if special care was taken to follow the prescribed plan of the master (God). Therefore, causes of illness generally fell into three domains: divine punishment, environmental hazards, and impaired social relationships.[9] Within the natural category, illnesses were defined as being caused by stress; drinking or eating too much; discord among friends or neighbors; impurities in air, food, or water; cold air or winds; improper eating habits or diets; weakness; and lack of moderation in daily activities and other related factors. Natural illnesses could occur at any time and often were viewed as a punishment from God visited directly on the person or his or her children. Thus disorders such as mental retardation, seizures, deformities, severe eczema, disorders of keratinization, and even severe breakouts of acne in adulthood were viewed as demonstrations that innocent children suffer the consequences of their parents' misdeeds or sins.

Unnatural illnesses are caused by evil influences that may have been induced by witchcraft and do not respond to self-treatment or remedies administered by friends, relatives, practitioners, or the usual traditional or Western treatment modalities. In this situation, a Voodoo practitioner is required to manipulate the spirits or demons and remove the spell, curse, or hex.

AFRICAN-AMERICAN ETHNOMEDICINE

Ethnomedicine among blacks emerged within the context of North American slavery. The term refers to practices and knowledge that existed before the arrival of modern conventional medicine that were used to promote, maintain, and restore health and well-being. Worldwide, people developed unique indigenous healing traditions adapted and defined by their culture, beliefs, and environment that satisfied the health needs of communities over centuries. Because many folk beliefs about health and illness exhibit close similarities and parallels cross-culturally, it is often difficult to differentiate the concepts and practices in the ethnomedicine of blacks that are of African origin from those that are of Indian-American or even European origin. In African-American communities, the use of folk healers and folk remedies continues to be carried on in place of or in a complementary manner with Western treatment modalities. Lassiter observes that beliefs about health and health practices vary widely and are highly dependent on the degree of adherence to traditional ideas, geographic locale, education, scientific orientation, and socioeconomic status.[10] She also observes that most African Americans retain a holistic philosophy of health and perceive the mind and body as inseparable, with balance and harmony in one's life central to maintaining health.

Typology of Black Folk Healers

The typology of black folk healers constructed by Baer has two axes. The first is the institutional affiliation of the healer and the extensiveness of his or her practice.[7] If the healer operates as an individual or is affiliated with some sort of occult supply store, either as the owner, as an employee, or as someone who rents office space therein, Baer refers to the healer as an *independent healer*. Baer further explains that if a healer is affiliated with a religious group, he or she will be referred to as a *cultic healer*. Independent healers function exclusively or almost exclusively in private settings; cultic healers may practice in both pubic and private settings.

The second axis recognizes the extensiveness of a healer's practice, whether it tends to be broad or generalized in scope, dealing with a wide variety of illnesses and conditions, or it tends to be limited, focusing on specific disorders or problems. However, such distinction may not always be clear-cut in the case of a particular therapist. Baer intersected the two axes and developed four categories of healers: (1) independent generalists, (2) independent specialists, (3) cultic generalists, and (4) cultic specialists.[11]

INDEPENDENT GENERALISTS The central character in ethnomedicine among blacks traditionally has been the conjurer, who also has been referred to as a *rootworker*. However, many African Americans used the term *roots* to refer to folk doctoring with herbs and prescriptions. The most important functions of the traditional conjurer were to cure persons who had been "conjured," "crossed," or "hexed" and to place a direct spell or counterspell on clients' enemies. Conjurers also concerned themselves with a wide variety of other conditions ranging from organic ailments to problems of everyday life. In an attempt to solve their clients' problems, conjurers prescribed a variety of remedies, such as perfumes, oils, seeds, powders, roots, pictures of Catholic saints, candles, medals, and readings from the Bible or the Sixth and Seventh Books of Moses.

After the turn of the twentieth century, as blacks migrated to the cities of both the North and the South, conjurers became incorporated and transformed into new forms such as spiritualistic readers; psychics and prophets then began to predominate. They often became associated with churches or in some cases assumed the title of minister (which protected them from possible legal repercussions, especially if they were not licensed as psychologists or ministers). In reality, though, they also functioned as independent healers who were willing to treat a wide array of problems and concerns. In contrast to the original conjurers and rootworkers, who made extensive use of roots and herbs in an attempt to gain control over the forces of the universe, spiritualists tended to have limited knowledge of the use of these substances and were more likely to use them in the form of baths and teas.

INDEPENDENT SPECIALISTS The best-known independent specialists are herbalists. They are specialists in the application of various medicinal plants and other remedies for common ailments. Although herbalists are found most commonly in rural areas, herbalists' shops also can be found in urban areas.

Female neighborhood practitioners are closely related to herbalists and are basically local consultants on common ailments. These practitioners do not have office hours or dispense medicines but only advise clients on how to treat ordinary illnesses. They rarely receive monetary compensation for their services but sometimes will accept an expression of gratitude or a gift of food. There is also the neighborhood prophetess, who works out of her home with clients on an individual basis. Clients are neighbors who usually are seeking assistance for various emotional, personal, and domestic problems. Prayer, prophecy, and counseling are the primary techniques used by these particular healers.

An important source of advice for some blacks in their quest for health, love, economic success, and interpersonal power is the magic vendors. In contrast to other healers, magic vendors view themselves primarily as businesspeople or employees of a commercial enterprise that specializes in the sale of occult articles. Magic vendors, especially those who are employees rather than owners of candle stores, are involved primarily in giving customers advice as to which occult items might help them solve a particular problem. Magic vendors have sold specific aids, such as soap, incense, lotions, aerosol sprays, candles, and oils, for the purposes of keeping away evil spirits, bringing luck at Bingo games or the races, and keeping spouses at home. Webb reported that some of these seemingly primitive remedies are successful because of the psychotherapeutic quality of such medicines to heal or destroy, as in Voodoo deaths.[12] Some supermarkets and drug stores in urban areas stock a variety of occult items. While usually no explicit reference to Voodoo is made on the articles sold in these stores, there is little doubt that many of them are paraphernalia associated with this tradition.

CULTIC GENERALISTS Religion, as a group ceremonial activity, and medicine are intertwined in most sociocultural systems. Therefore, it should be no surprise that healing activities are part and parcel of various black religious groups in the United States. This kind of black folk healer works within the context of the highly syncretistic spiritual movement, which essentially combines elements from spiritualism, black Protestantism, Roman Catholicism, Voodoo (or its diluted form of Hoodoo), and other esoteric systems, such as New Thought, Islam, Judaism, and/or astrology.[13] Spiritual prophets profess to possess a gift from the spirit, which enables them to prophesize and heal. Although they generally treat various physical ailments, spiritual prophets tend to focus on a wide variety of socioeconomic and psychosocial problems that particularly poor blacks but also middle-class and working-class blacks, as well as some whites, encounter in everyday life.[13,14]

CULTIC SPECIALISTS Many healers functioning within religious congregations tend to focus on a somewhat narrower range of problems than the cult generalists. In addition to prophets or advisors, for example, spiritual churches have members, often referred to as *divine healers,* who claim to have the gift of healing (but note that they lack the gift of prophecy). These divine healers appear to function in a capacity not greatly unlike that of many evangelistic faith healers in fundamentalist Protestant congregations, particularly of the Holiness, Pentecostal, and some of the Baptist varieties. There are many remedies that are believed to have the ability to treat calamities caused by evil influences, and these include food, medicine, antidotes, healing, and prayer proposed to God by a medium with unusual powers.[9] Other cures and treatments include external aids such as magic and visible protection in the form of prayer cards, charms, and asafetida bags. Guillory reports that folk remedies include eating garlic for hypertension, drinking teas made from herbs for colds, applying tallow to the chest and covering it with a cloth for colds, pouring kerosene into cuts as a disinfectant, and wearing garlic around the neck to keep from catching disease.[15] Use of vinegar, Epson salts, Ben-Gay, and copper wire or bracelets for arthritis, horehound tea or buttermilk for diabetes, and tea made of rabbit tobacco and pine top for asthma is common. Dermatologists should acquaint themselves with the cultural beliefs and practices of African Americans and determine which may be beneficial or potentially hazardous and sensitively replace dangerous practices with alternatives, when possible.

IMPACT AND APPLICATIONS OF AFRO-CARIBBEAN TRADITIONS, BELIEFS, AND PRACTICES IN DERMATOLOGY

Many of today's beliefs, habits, and practices in the black community are strongly steeped in the tradition and culture of our ancestors. Many of these historical practices are strongly influenced by African and Caribbean traditions, hence the designation of *Afro-Caribbean.* They also may represent a mixture of other cultures. There has been a trend toward what is considered more "natural" practices, and these are considered to result in less harm. Over the years, the actual benefits of many of these practices have been confirmed through evidence-based medicine, whereas many others have either not been evaluated or are found to have no proof of benefit, possibly resulting in deleterious effects and delaying the implementation of effective treatment.

When taking a look at the numerous practices that remain a part of today's culture, we find that much attention is placed on the hair, especially in the female population. Both beauty and community acceptance have long been at the core of many of the practices; however, the impact of health, well-being, and quality of life is also key. It is often helpful to separate those which have intentional effects on the hair and skin from those which have secondary or nonintentional results.

Practices Involving the Hair and Scalp

Practices involving the hair and scalp that encompass beauty and acceptance but also the need to easily manage and care for skin and hair date back to our African ancestors. They include hair styles and adornments, the use of tools to achieve these styles, and the application of various hair care products to aid in management (Table 6-1). While many of the practices can be beneficial and certainly are appealing, they also can result in permanent damage to the scalp and resulting hair loss.

Practices Involving the Skin

Practices involving the skin are also steeped in adornment in the form of tribal tattoos and other forms of labeling and identification. Today these practices are continued, but to a lesser extent, and more often represent a form of adornment than health aide. Application of topical products to the skin is often used to promote skin health, but such products are still often used to treat other unrelated illnesses of the body and the "soul" (see Table 6-1).

CONCLUSION

There is a growing popularity of cosmetic and minimally invasive procedures among African Americans, as well as a significant increase in the access to and use of specialized care of the hair and skin. Blacks have become the biggest consumers of beauty products in the United States, spending at least $20 billion a year.[16] Blacks account for nearly 5 percent of the 87 million cosmetic procedures.[16,17,18] As the numbers grow, physicians will have to adapt to their clientele in terms of the cultural taboos they will have to overcome.[19,20] Dermatologists and plastic surgeons will have to determine when the remedies are beneficial, neutral, or harmful and incorporate beneficial and neutral remedies into the plan of care and consider potential drug interactions.

TABLE 6-1
Afro-Caribbean Cultural Pratices, Traditions, and Beliefs

Practice/Tradition	Belief	Negative Effect	Other
Diseases and Concerns of the Hair			
1. Pomade use in hair	Assist in styling and manageability, straightening hair	Folliculitis or other occlusive syndrome	
2. Styling hair with weaving, braiding	Cultural and self-acceptance, ease of styling hair	Traction alopecia	Today, widely practiced in many cultures
3. Use of hot combs and chemical straighteners	Same as 1 and 2	Traumatic alopecia	
4. Limiting hair washing to once a week	Avoidance of dry hair shaft ("You will dry your hair out.")	Likely none; maybe, seborrheic dermatitis	Simplifies grooming processes for those with heat or chemically straigntened styles
5. Do not wash hair in the winter or cold season	Avoidance of cold ("You will catch cold if you wash your hair when its cold.")	Seborrheic dermatitis	
6. Cutting your hair on a full moon will allow it to grow more, coconut oil, Castor oil, other greases, and pomades	Promotes hair growth (oils used in Caribbean tradition)	Folliculitis	
7. The more the perm (chemical relaxer) burns, the straighter the hair becomes	Promotes optimal hair straightening	Chemical burns, traumatic alopecia	
8. Cutting hair with dirty clippers	Causes acne keloidalis	Impetigo, delay in treatment	
Other Dermatologic Diseases and Conditions			
9. Praying away or "talking away" of warts	Treatment or removal of warts	Delay in treatment, possible spread	Brought to the Sea Islands by German immigrants
10. Application of calamine lotion, oatmeal paste on skin or oatmeal bath, cornmeal and water, baking soda with Vaseline, lemon juice, flour scorched in a skillet, olive oil, warm sardine grease, hot tea, stay in the house and wait it out	Treatment for chicken pox	Secondary infection, delay in treatment	Olive oil thought to keep skin from drying out and scarring; prospect of going blind from sunlight
11. "Blowing in the mouth" by someone who never saw the father, a man whose mother died during birth, a woman whose father died before birth, a man who never saw his father, someone white	Treatment for oral candidiasis (thrush)	Spread of infectious particles, delay in treatment	
12. Butter, flush with cold water, application of ice, application of scorched flour, mullein juice, Vaseline, cocoa butter, Clorox and water wash, mustard, toothpaste, soda and syrup paste, mayonnaise, lard, sulfur poultice strapped to burn, pack with ashes from a fireplace or wood stove, pack with black soot from the chimney, pour baking soda in water, let settle to bottom, scoop out baking soda with clean white rag and place on the burn.	Treatment for burns	Delay in healing, secondary infection, contact dermatitis, delay in treatment	
13. Urine (a pregnant woman's first morning urine, from a baby's diaper, one's own, applied directly or as a bath	Treatment of ringworm, "rashes," acne breakouts	Contact dermatitis, spread of infectious particles, delay in treatment	
14. Fatback or salted pork to dry up boils and bring them to a head, scriffin (a membrane that lines the inside of an egg shell), egg white,	Treatment of furuncle	Contact dermatitis, worsening of or prolonging disease process, delay in treatment	

(continued)

TABLE 6-1 (Continued)
Afro-Caribbean Cultural Pratices, Traditions, and Beliefs

Practice/Tradition	Belief	Negative Effect	Other
white potato, warm compresses, sulfur poultice, eat raisins, Epson salts in a hot-water bath, sterilize a needle by burning it and open it up, tie off the boil with a string, and put a cloth with mullein juice over it to bring it to a head, put paper in a bottle and light it so that it fills with smoke and let the smoke out over the boil to bring to a head, cross a fork over the boil in the shape of the cross three times and say, "In Jesus' name" (then the boil goes away in three days)			
15. Watkins salve, caliber pinks pills, Asorbin Jr., tinactin, Adam powder, Curdeure ointment with sulfur, baking soda, oatmeal paste, walnut husks, castor oil, application of one's own urine with a rag	Treatment of ringworm	Delay in treatment, spread of disease	
16. Cocoa butter, Shea butter, Vaseline	Treatment for dry skin (xerosis)		Shown beneficial for xerosis and ashy dermatosis
17. Vicks VapoRub on acne pimple	Treatment for acne	Worsens acne	
18. Cocoa butter	Treatment for stretch marks, uneven skin tone, dry skin		
19. Liver spots	Name given to idiopathic guttate hypomelanosis		
20. Intentional wounding and patterened scarring of skin	Cultural and traditional ritual in western Africa and other cultures	Scar and keloid formation	
21. Henna and other tattoos	Decorative at weddings and other celebrations in African culture and various ethnic groups	Contact dermatitis, scarring	Today, still prevalent across many ethnic groups as a form of self-expression
Treatment of Unrelated Diseases with Possible Secondary Dermatologic Effects			
22. Asafetida worn in a bag around the neck (also can be taken internally)	Treatment for colic	Irritant or allergic contact dermatitis, delay in treatment	
23. Vanilla flavoring and red liniment, yank the tooth, then lay an aspirin on the socket, paste from cloves and vanilla, vanilla drops, drops of clove oil, kerosene, or cinnamon, fill hole in tooth with lemon extract, perfume, salt heated in a spoon to burn and kill the nerve endings	Treatment for toothache	Irritant or allergic contact dermatitis, delay in treatment	
24. Castor oil and a warm compress on the chest	Treatment for tuberculosis (TB)	Irritant or allergic contact dermatitis, delay in treatment	
25. Heat, liniment rub, and heating pad, apply brown paper bag soaked in boiled vinegar with or without being wrapped in a cloth, mixture of kerosene, vinegar, and pepper, a dime on a copper chain around the ankle, wear a copper bracelet, a copper wire around the wrist or ankle, WD-40 (a mechanical lubricant), rub on camphor in Varsaw, rub on chips of Octagon soap in alcohol	Treatment of arthritis	Erythema ab igne, burn, irritant or allergic contact dermatitis, delay in treatment	

As the world around us becomes increasingly diverse, it is ever more important that practitioners embrace ethnosensitivity and cultural competence. Being able to relate well to people of all cultures will result in the best possible patient care.

REFERENCES

1. Spectrum of Skin of Color, in Program and Abstracts of the 64th Annual Meeting of the American Academy of Dermatology, San Francisco, CA, Symposium 346, March 3–7, 2006.
2. Parks Fayth M. The role of African American folk beliefs in the modern therapeutic process. *Clin Psychol* 2003;10:456.
3. Campinha-Bacote J. Cultural competence in psychiatric mental health nursing: A conceptual model. *Nurs Clin North Am* 1994;29:1-8.
4. Spector RE. *Cultural Diversity in Health and Illness,* 3rd ed. Norwalk, CT, Appleton & Lange, 1991.
5. US Department of Health and Human Services, Centers for Disease Control and Prevention, National Center for Health Statistics. *Complementary and Alternative Medicine Use Among Adults: United States, 2002.* No 343. Atlanta, CDC, May 27, 2004.
6. Jack L Jr, Harrison IE, Airhihenbuwa CO. Ethnicity and the health belief systems, in Matielly AC (ed), *The Multicultural Challenge in Health Education*. Santa Cruz, CA, ETR Associates, 1994.
7. Huff RM, Kline MV. *Promoting Health in Multicultural Population: A Handbook for Practitioners*. Thousand Oaks, CA, Sage Publications, 1998.
8. Borkan JM, Neher JO. A developmental model of ethnosensitivity in family practice training. *Family Med* 1991;23:212-217.
9. Snow LE. Folk medical beliefs and their implications for care of patients. *Ann Intern Med* 1974;81:82-96.
10. Lassiter SM. *Multicultural Clients: A Professional Handbook for Health Care Providers and Social Works*. Westport, CT, Greenwood, 1995.
11. Baer Hans A. Toward a systematic typology of black folk healers. *Phylon* 1982;43: 327-343.
12. Webb JY. Louisiana Voodoo and superstitions related to health. *HSMHA Health Reps* 1971;86:291-301.
13. Baer Hans A. Prophets and advisors in black spiritual churches: Therapy, palliative, or opiate? *Culture Med Psychiatry* 1981;5:145-170.
14. Haskins J. *Voodoo and Hoodoo: The Craft as Revealed by Traditional Practitioners.* New York: Scarborough House, 1990.
15. Guillory J. Ethnic perspectives of cancer nursing: The black American. *Oncol Nurs Forum* 1987;14:66-69.
16. American Academy of Facial Plastic and Reconstructive Surgery. Membership Survey: Trends in Facial Plastic Surgery, 2005. February 2006.
17. Magazine Publishers of American. African-American Market Profile; available at *www.magazine.org;* retrieved in July 2006 and February 2008.
18. Humphreys JM. The multicultural economy 2004, in *America's Minority Buying Power Guide,* Vol 64. Atlanta, University of Georgia, Selig Center for Economic Growth, 2004, pp 2-4.
19. US Census Bureau News, US Department of Commerce Population Division, Washington, August 2004.
20. McKinnon J. The Black Population in the United States, March 2002. Washington, US Census Bureau, Current Population Reports, Series P20-541.

CHAPTER 7

Asian Cultural Habits and Practices

Richard S. Mizuguchi

Key Points

- Traditional Chinese medicine (TCM) employs herbs, dietary therapy, massage, and acupuncture.
- Herbal remedies are often effective but may cause allergic reactions and side effects, including dermatitis.
- Traditional Asian practices of cupping, coining, and moxibustion can cause bruises and lesions sometimes mistaken for physical abuse, but distinguishable by their circular appearance.
- Physicians should realize that TCM is not quackery; many therapies are currently used in Western hospitals, and some have shown efficacy in double-blind studies.

Why is it important for dermatologists to be familiar with the cultural habits and practices of the Asian population? According to the 2000 Census report, the Asian and Pacific Island population currently represents about 4.4% of the U.S. population but is projected to increase to more than five times the current size to 41 million by the year 2050. The Asian population then would represent 10.3% of the U.S. population.[1] Since Asians represent a fast-growing segment of the population, dermatologists should become familiar with the treatment of Asian skin and also have a rudimentary knowledge of some of their more common cultural practices.

The Asian population has a steep tradition in alternative medicine. Asian immigrants, like other immigrants and refugees who settle in the United States, tend to visit physicians in their local communities. Therefore, many of the cultural practices go unnoticed in health care centers outside the Asian community. A study of a Vietnamese refugee community in San Diego showed that even after settling in the United States, most Vietnamese preferred both Vietnamese entertainment and Vietnamese health services. Both new and old refugees continued to use traditional health practices, such as coining, steam inhalation, and acupuncture.[2] However, in emergencies or when patients move outside their communities and are forced to seek treatment from dermatologists, the dermatologist should be aware of the side effects of traditional Asian treatments. In the current milieu of alternative medicine, Asian as well as non-Asian patients may present with side effects, including contact allergic and irritant dermatitis, to Asian remedies. This chapter will review some of the more common cultural habits and practices, including traditional Chinese medicine, acupuncture, and the practices of *chope* and coining. Finally, like most communities, there are also myths and misconceptions within the Asian community. Many Asians seek "natural remedies," believing that they don't have any side effects. However, as this chapter will illustrate, this is not always the case, and some of the side effects may be more serious than those of Western medicine.

TRADITIONAL CHINESE MEDICINE (TCM)

Traditional Chinese medicine (TCM) is an alternative method of therapy practiced throughout China and East Asia by millions of people. Since the dawn of time, alternative medicine has been the fundamental method used by humans to treat diseases and to preserve their health. It is used by those who live where there are no physicians. Even where physicians are readily available, many people still prefer the holistic approach to medicine. Typically, TCM refers to the medical practice of using herbs, dietary therapy, massage, and acupuncture. The use of medicinal herbs combined specifically for each individual patient is stressed. Shen Nung's herbal book, dated 2700 BC, is considered the oldest Chinese medical book and contains details of more than 300 plants.

Among the Asian population, TCM is a very popular mode for treating systemic as well as dermatologic diseases. A survey in the United States between 1990 and 1997 showed that 8.6% of people used TCM for the treatment of dermatologic problems.[3] This popularity, which extends beyond the Asian population, is based on the misconception that alternative therapies are safe and cost less then Western medicine. Patients who are increasingly frustrated by modern medicine also tend to seek alternative medical therapy. In the United States, alternative therapy in 1990 generated expenditures estimated at around $14 billion, which doubled by 1997.[4] Because of the increasing popularity of TCM, it is important to address the safety of TCM.

Herbal treatments are becoming increasingly popular and are often used for dermatologic conditions. Despite the misconception that TCM has no adverse effects owing to its "natural" composition, possible adverse effects such as hepatotoxicity have occurred. The most common adverse reactions with topical TCM are contact and irritant dermatitis. Topical TCM is often adulterated with balsam of Peru, and the North American standard patch tray now includes allergens such as tea tree oil and ylang-ylang, also found in TCM.

Many dermatologists are still unaware of the existence of placebo-controlled studies involving TCM. Sheehan and colleagues, working in conjunction with Chinese herbalist Luo in London, England, conducted one of the first placebo-controlled, double-blind study involving atopic dermatitis.[5] Therapeutic agents including *Potentilla chinensis, Tribulus terrestris, Rehmannia glutinosa, Lophatherum gracile, Clematis armandii, Ledebouriella saseloides, Dictamnus dasycarpus, Paeonia lactiflora, Schizonepeta tenuifolia,* and *Glyccyrrhiza glabrae* were compared with placebo herbs that had no known efficacy for the treatment of atopic dermatitis. The results revealed that erythema was decreased by 91.4% with the active herbs compared with 10.6% with the placebo herbs. Safety was demonstrated, and liver function tests, renal function tests, and complete blood cell counts were stable during the study period.

Furocoumarins are found in many Chinese herbal medicines used in the treatment of psoriasis. Several studies have been conducted with herbal medicine such as *Radix Angelicae dahuriace* and have demonstrated efficacy in conjunction with ultraviolet A (UV-A) radiation.[6] The difference in the efficacy between psoralen plus ultraviolet A (PUVA) and *Radix Angelicae dahuricae* UV-A was not statistically significant. There was an increase in dizziness and nausea. However, a similar herb, *Radix Angelicae pubescentis,* although equally successful in the treatment of psoriasis, showed increased lens changes.[7] As seen here, without specific knowledge of the side-effect profile, the side effects may warrant a more conventional therapy with close medical supervision even though the herb may be effective therapeutically.

As the previously mentioned studies demonstrate, there is a real possibility that TCM has efficacy beyond a simple placebo effect. However, associated adverse effects may occur that can be fatal. A 66-year-old woman developed Stevens-Johnson syndrome after drinking a health drink containing ophiopongonis tuber.[8] She tested positive in drug lymphocyte stimulation and on a rechallenge with 1/1000 the original dose.

TOPICAL TRADITIONAL MEDICINE

The use of traditional medicated oils and ointments is increasing the United States. It is important to note that brand names are just brand names and do not indicate the ingredients in the TCM. For example, Tiger Balm and 3-Snake Oil do not contain any materials from these two animals (Figure 7-1). One of the frequent arguments of patients using topical TCM is the absence of topical corticosteroids. However, the most common and prevalent adulterants in herbal creams are indeed corticosteroids.[9–15] More alarmingly, oral formulations also have been found to contain corticosteroids.[16–18] In a large-scale study from Taiwan, 2609 samples of traditional Chinese remedies were analyzed, and 24% of them were found to contain corticosteriods, some with significant amounts of clobetasol propionate.[19] In a study from London, 8 of 11 creams analyzed contained dexamethasone at concentrations inappropriate for use on the face or by children.[20] Vena and colleagues reported the presence of triamcinolone acetonide in a phytocosmetic cream marketed in Europe as a skin care cosmetic product.[21,22] Unfortunately, unaware of the potential adverse effects of these and other products, both adults and infants may use them for long periods of time.

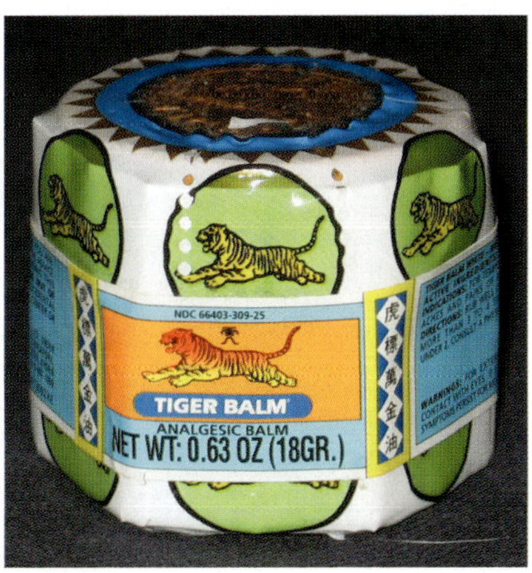

▲ **FIGURE 7-1** Tiger Balm.

TABLE 7-1
Rare Side Effects Other than Allergic Reactions or Contact Dermatitis

INGREDIENT	ADVERSE REACTION	REFERENCE
Arnica extracts, paprika	Sweet's syndrome	40,41
Arsenic	Arsenic dermatoses	42–44
Garlic	Urticaria, angioedema	45
Kakkon-to	Fixed drug eruption	46
Kombucha tea	Pellagra	47
Mercury	Mercury poisoning	26
Piperaceae	Contact leukomelanosis	48

Herbal remedies frequently cause allergic reactions.[23] The list of reported reactions in the medical literature is too extensive to be reviewed here. Some of the more common ingredients will be discussed below, and other rare adverse effects are listed in the Table 7-1. Essential oils used topically for aromatherapy and in herbal creams have been responsible for photosensitization.[24] Bergamot has been implicated in some cases because it contains 5-methosypsoralen. St John's Wort, a best-selling herbal antidepressant, has photosensitivity as an adverse effect as well.[25] This may be significant in patients beginning phototherapy for dermatologic conditions. Contamination of oral herbal preparations has been reported, resulting in arsenic and mercury poisoning.[26] In a patient presenting with either arsenical dermatoses or mercury poisoning, a detailed history of TCM use may elucidate the cause of intoxication.

As these studies indicate, some herbal medications have been demonstrated to improve dermatologic conditions in placebo-controlled studies. Dermatologists should be aware that herbal treatments are by no means free of dermatologic adverse effects. It is important to realize that many TCM remedies have the potential to cause allergic contact dermatitis or photosensitization. A patch test or photo–patch test may be necessary to determine the offending herb.

ACUPUNCTURE

Acupuncture is an ancient system of healing developed over thousands of years as a part of the traditional medicine of China, Japan, and other Eastern countries. The earliest records of acupuncture date back over 4700 years ago. It was described by Huang Ti Nei Ching Wen in *The Yellow Emperor's Classic of Internal Medicine,* which is considered the authoritative early Chinese medical book.[27] Today, there are over 3 million practitioners worldwide.

The practice of acupuncture is thought to have begun with the discovery that the stimulation of specific areas on the skin affects the functioning of certain organs of the body. Acupuncture uses fine needles to stimulate the body's own healing process through the body lines of energy or the vital energy (*Qi*). The *Qi* is thought to flow through channels know as *meridians* (i.e., wood, water, metal fire, and earth). When the free flow of this energy is obstructed, a symptom appears. The aim of acupunture is to remove these obstructions, thus allowing the energy to flow freely. This is done by the insertion of fine needles into acupuncture meridian points just beneath the skin (Figure 7-2). Magnets are also used on the same acupunture meridian points. Magnets most commonly are placed with tape or a bandage, as shown in Figure 7-3. Acupuncture is used in a number of dermatologic conditions, such as atopic dermatitis, urticaria, and psoriasis.[28]

Some cultural practices, including moxibustion, cupping, and coining, are important for physicians to understand because they may mimic physical abuse. However, the lesions usually are transient, although there are reported cases of permanent scarring from moxibustion.[29,30] Moxibustion, cupping, and coining will be discussed below.

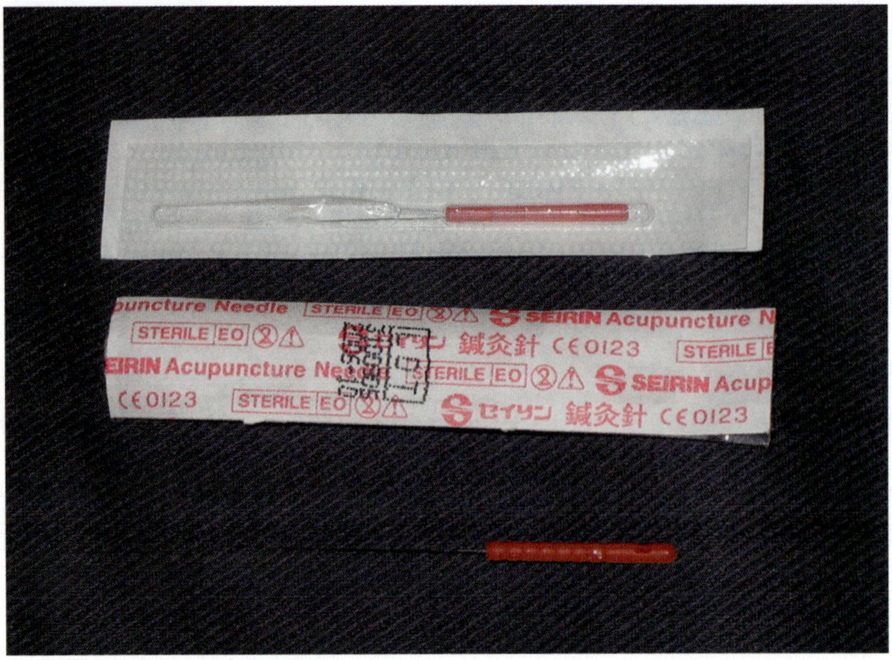

▲ **FIGURE 7-2** Commonly used acupuncture needles.

MOXIBUSTION

Moxibustion is a procedure practiced most commonly in Southeast Asia, almost exclusively by the Mien.[39] *Moxibustion* is a word derived from the words *moxa* and *combustion. Moxa* is an herb derived from the plant mugwort, or *Artemisia vulgaris.* It is felt that this herb, when burned on acupuncture points, can restore the flow of *Qi.* The procedure consists of heat application with use of the herb *moxa* on acupuncture points.

Similar to acupuncture, moxibustion is used to treat a variety of ailments, such as anemia, chronic stasis, acute lymphangitis, and immune suppression.[31] *Moxa* can be used either directly or indirectly. In direct use, *moxa* is simply placed on the skin and is lighted with an incense stick. The burning *moxa* then is pinched out or taken away by the therapist before it burns down completely to the skin. In indirect use, the burning *moxa* is placed at the head of an inserted acupuncture needle. Japanese acupuncturists tend to prefer the direct method, and Chinese acupuncturists prefer the indirect method. Patients often report a rush of warmth throughout their body during the treatment.

The moxibustion techniques require a great deal of training for a therapist to master. The lesions may mimic physical abuse, as in cupping and coining,[32] because permanent burn scars can occur from improper use.[33] Physicians unfamiliar with these practices may suspect abuse, especially if a woman or a child presents with cutaneous lesions resulting from this traditional health practice. Misdiagnosis could lead to grave consequences; for example, in one case, a false accusation of child abuse resulted in the suicide of a Vietnamese father.[34]

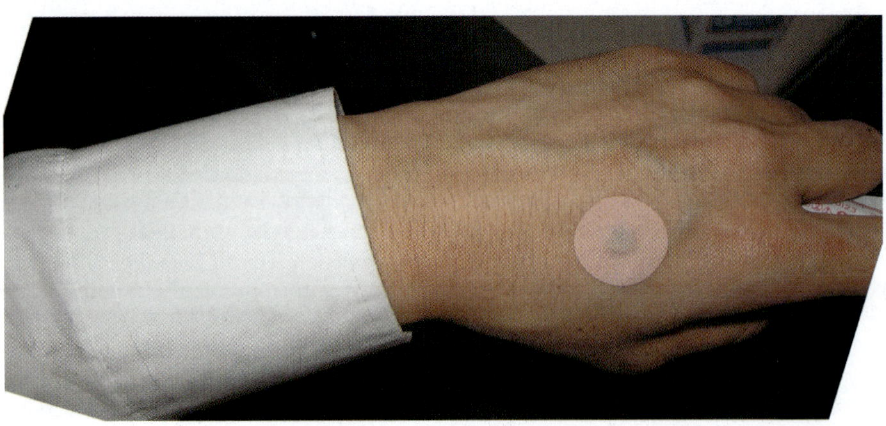

▲ **FIGURE 7-3** Magnet applied to skin.

CHOPE

Chope is a Southeast Asian (Cambodian or Vietnamese) custom used in the treatment of chest infections, muscular pain, headaches, arthritis, and other forms of pain. It consists of placing a lighted candle on the patient's forehead, either directly on the skin or on a coin. The coin is expected to catch the drippings of hot wax.

CUPPING

In cupping, a bottle is placed over the candle and coin with the bottle lip in direct contact with the skin. As the candle consumes the oxygen, a vacuum is produced. This vacuum is intended to draw out the "fire wind" (pain). With this procedure, blood is drawn to the surface of the skin by the suction of the glass vessel on the skin. The cups are placed on areas in need of treatment, such as the chest, back, buttocks, chin, and dorsum of the foot. The cups are left on the specific areas of the skin until they stick by negative pressure. They are then removed, leaving raised red patches that represent superficial skin inflammation. The lesions produced by cupping are round or annular as a consequence of both suction and the mild burn caused by the heated bottle before the lack of oxygen extinguishes the flame (Figure 7-4). This is thought to reduce inflammation in deeper adjacent organs. Both pain and infection are thought to be alleviated by the effect of counterirritation.

COINING

Coining is a Vietnamese practice used commonly to treat a variety of illnesses, including febrile illnesses, headaches, myalgia, and malaise. This folk remedy is also known as *cao gio.* Coining is the process of applying hot mentholated oil or Tiger Balm to the chest and back. The edge of a coin is rubbed over the spine and ribs, producing linear petechiae and ecchymoses.[35] When found in Vietnamese children, lesions produced by coining have been misdiagnosed as child abuse, and legal actions have been brought against the parents. Fortunately, physicians acquainted with this practice testified that coining was not a form of child abuse but a form of therapy.[36]

The most common complications of coining have been minor burns. There is an isolated report of a 45-year-old woman who caught fire during a coining

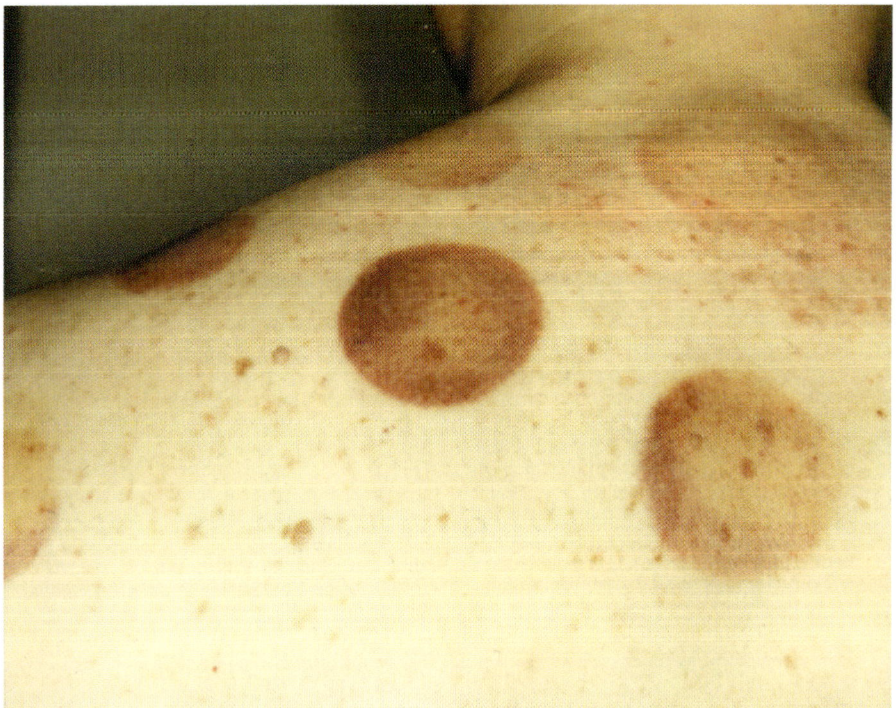

▲ **FIGURE 7-4** Bruises on the back of an Asian male as a result of cupping.

treatment and sustained full-thickness burns requiring admission to a burn unit.[37] There was one report of coning or brain stem compression secondary to the practice of coining, and this seems to be an idiosyncratic reaction.[38] Since many Vietnamese Americans and other Southeast Asians living in the United States fear criticism from their physicians for practicing coining, the true incidence is not known. It is probably much higher than appreciated. In a survey of a clinic in Washington, coining was the most commonly used practice among the Cambodians (70%), Chinese (35%) and Lao (10%).[39]

Another Asian healing practice, pinching, uses the same principle as coining. In this case, pressure is applied by pinching the skin between the thumb and index finger to the point of producing a contusion.

CONCLUSION

In conclusion, the fast-growing Asians population has diverse cultural customs and practices. Additionally, their cultural practices and habits are being adapted by many non-Asians for the treatment of medical illnesses. It is important for clinicians to be knowledgeable of these cultural practices and habits. This is especially true in those practicing in urban areas, which have higher immigrant populations.

There are many myths regarding TCM. It is important to realize that TCM is not quackery. Many of the therapies are currently being used even in Western hospitals, such as acupuncture for the treatment of stress and aches. Some therapies have shown efficacy in double-blind studies. However, like most over-the-counter and prescription medications, both topical and oral herbal medications have shown to cause significant side effects, particularly allergic contact dermatitis and photosensitization.

Finally, it is important to be aware of practices such as *chope,* coining, and moxibustion that have been misconstrued as spousal or child abuse. A basic understanding of the various Asian cultural habits and practices hopefully will facilitate communication and understanding of various signs and symptoms during a clinical examination.

REFERENCES

1. United States Census Bureau 2000.
2. Ries AL, Picchi MA, Nguyen LH, et al. Asthma in a Vietnamese refugee population. *Am J Respir Crit Care Med* 1997;155:1895-1901.
3. Eisenberg D, David RB, Ettner SL, et al. Trends in alternative medicine use in the United States, 1990-1997. *JAMA* 1998;280:1569-1575.
4. Eisenberg DM, Kassler RC, Foster C, et al. Unconventional medicine in the United States: Prevalence, costs, and patterns of use. *N Engl J Med* 1993;328:246-252.
5. Sheehan MP, Rustin M, Atherton DJ, et al. Efficacy of traditional Chinese herbal therapy in adult atopic dermatitis. *Lancet* 1992;340:13-17.
6. Zhang GW, Wang HJ, Zhou YH, et al. Treatment of psoriasis by photochemotherpy: A comparison between the photosensitizing capsule of *Angleica dahurica* and 8-MOP. *Natl Med J China* 1983;63:16-19.
7. Li FQ, Fang FY, Li SH. A long-term follow-up of 58 cases of psoriasis treated with traditional Chinese medicine, *Angelica dahuricae* and long wave ultraviolet. *Chin J Phys Ther* 1984;7:154-155.
8. Mochitomi Y, Inoue A, Kawabata H, et al. Stevens-Johnson syndrome caused by a health drink containing ophiopogonis tuber. *J Dermatol* 1998;25:662-665.
9. Ahmed S, Riaz M. Quatitation of corticosteroids as common adulterants in local drugs by HPLC. *Chromatographica* 1991;31:67-70.
10. Wood B, Wishart J. Potent topical steroid in a Chinese herbal cream. *NZ Med J* 1997;110:420-421.
11. Ernst E. Adverse effects of herbal drugs in dermatology. *Br J Dermatol* 2000;143:923-929.
12. Allen BR, Parkinson R. Chinese herbs for eczema. *Lancet* 1990;336:177.
13. O'Driscoll J, Burden AD, Kingston TP. Potent topical steroid obtained from a Chinese herbalist. *Br J Dermatol* 1992;127:543-544.
14. Graham-Brown RAC, Bourke JF, Bumphrey G. Chinese herbal remedies may contain steroids. *Br Med J* 1994;308:473.
15. Hughes JR, Higgins EM, Pembroke AC. Dexamethasone masquerading as a Chinese herbal. *Be J Dermatol* 1994;130:261.
16. Van der Stricht BI, Parvais OE, Vanhaelen-Fastre RJ, et al. Safer use of traditional remedies: Remedies may contain cocktail of active drugs. *Br Med J* 1994;308:1162.
17. Morice A. Adulteration of homeopathic remedies. *Lancet* 1987;324:62.
18. Josepht AM, Biggs T, Garr M, et al. Stealth steroids. *N Engl J Med* 1991;324:62.
19. Huang WF, Wen KC, Hsiao ML. Adulteration by synthetic therapeutic substances of traditional Chines medicine in Taiwan. *J Clin Pharmacol* 1997;37:334-350.
20. Keane FM, Munn SE, du Vivier AWP, et al. Analysis of Chinese herbal creams prescribed for dermatological conditions. *Br Med J* 1999;318:563-567.
21. Vena GA, Cassno N, Mastrolonardo M, et al. Management of inflammatory dermatoses with a cosmetic preparation containing antioxidant/anti-inflammatory agents. *J Ital Dermatol Venerol* 1998;133:373-380.
22. Bircher AJ, Hauri U, Niederer M, et al. Stealth triamcinolone acetonide in a phytocosmetic cream. *Br J Dermatol* 2002;146:524-540.
23. Mantyranta T, Haahtela T. Luonnolaakeiden aiheuttamat allergiset reaktiot. *Duodecim* 1993;109:301-308.
24. Cocks H, Wilson D. Letter. *Burns* 1998;24:82.

25. Stevinson C, Ernst E. Safety of hypericum in patients with depression. *CNS Drugs* 1999;11:125-132.
26. Ernst E, de Smet PAGM. Risks associated with complementary therapies, in Dukes MNG (ed), *Meyler's Side Effects to Drugs,* 13th ed. Amsterdam, Elsevier, 1996.
27. Veith I. *The Yellow Emperor's Classic of Internal Medicine,* Vol 18. Berkeley, University of California Press, 1984, pp 56-78.
28. Chen CJ, Yu HS. Acupuncture treatment of urticaria. *Arch Dermatol* 1998;134: 1397-1399.
29. Crutchfield CE III, Bisig TJ. Images in clinical medicine: Coining. *N Engl J Med* 1995;332:1552.
30. Wong, HCG, Wong JKT, Wong NYY. Signs of physical abuse or evidence of moxibustion, cupping or coining. *Can Med Assoc J* 1999;160:785-786.
31. Zhou W. Acute lymphangitis treated by moxibustion with garlic in 118 cases. *J Trad Chin Med* 2003;23:198.
32. Look KM, Look RM. Skin scraping, cupping, and moxibustion that may mimic physical abuse. *J Forens Sci* 1997;42:103-105.
33. Conde-Salazar L, Gonazlez MA, Guimarens D, Feuente C. Burns due to moxibustion. *Contact Dermatitis* 1991;25: 332-323.
34. Nong TA. "Pseudo-battered child" syndrome (letter). *JAMA* 1976;236:2288.
35. Yeatman GW, Dang VV. Cao gio (coin rubbing): Vietnamese attitudes towards health care. *JAMA* 1980;244:2748-2749.
36. Yeatman GW, Dong VV. Cao gio (coin rubbing): Vietnamese attitudes toward health care. JAMA 1980;244:2748-2749.
37. Amshel CE, Caruso DM. Vietnamese "coining": A burn case report and literature review. *J Burn Care Rehabil* 2000;21: 112-114.
38. Ponder A, Lehman L. "Coining" and "coning": An unusual complication of unconventional medicine. *Neurology* 1994;44:774-775.
39. Buchwald D, Panwala S, Hooton T. Use of traditional health practices by Southeast Asian refugees in a primary care clinic. *West J Med* 1992;156:507-511.
40. Greer JM, Rosen T, Tschen JA. Sweet's syndrome with an exogenous cause. *Cutis* 1993;51:112-114.
41. Delmonte S, Brusati C, Parodi A, Rebora A. Leukemia-related Sweet's syndrome elicited by pathergy to arnica. *Dermatology* 1998;197:195-196.
42. Kew J, Morris C, Aihie A, et al. Arsenic and mercury intoxication due to Indian ethnic remedies. *Br Med J* 1993;306: 506-507
43. Wong SS, Tan KC, Goh CL. Cutaneous manifestations of chronic arsenicism: Review of seventeen cases. *J Am Acad Dermatol* 1998;26:179-185.
44. Tay CH. Cutaneous manifestations of arsenic poisoning due to certain Chinese herbal medicine. *Austral J Dermatol* 1974; 15:121-131.
45. Asero R, Mistrello G, Toncarolo D, et al. A case of garlic allergy. *J Allergy Clin Immunol* 1998;101:427-428.
46. Fujimoto N, Tajima S. Extensive fixed drug eruption due to the Japanese herbal drug "Kakkon-to." *Br J Dermatol* 2003;149: 1292-1308.
47. Wood B, Rademaker M, Oakley A, Wallace J. Pellagra in a woman using alternative remedies. *Austral J Dermatol* 1998; 39:42-44.
48. Yuan-Li Liao, Yuh-Chiau C, Tsen-Fang T, et al. Contact leukomelanosis induced by the leaves of Piper betle L. (Pieperaceae): A clinical and histopathologic survey. *J Am Acad Dermatol* 1999; 40:538-539.

CHAPTER 8

Hispanic Skin Remedies and Practices

Miguel Sanchez

Key Points

- Most often, traditional remedies are complementary to allopathic care, and Hispanics generally have more confidence in physicians than in alternative medicine providers.
- Ancient Meso-American Indians had an elaborate and advanced system of healing based on botanical remedies.
- Traditional treatment of dermatologic disease employs a number of herbs.
- Physicians have limited knowledge of botanicals and their interactions with pharmacologic agents.
- Curandismo is a popular health care practice that integrates Christianity, folk medicine, psychology, and magic.

Paradoxically, at a time when scientific gains have resulted in impressive pharmacologic advances, folk medicine remains as popular as ever in Hispanic communities. The U.S. Census Bureau reported that over the past year, Hispanics accounted for 59% of this country's population growth, and immigration from Latin American countries accounted for 39% of the surge. Hispanic immigrants bring over the health systems and practices that have been effective throughout generations of use.[1] Nonallopathic medicine is popular in the United States, with the White House Commission on Complementary and Alternative Medicine Policy reporting use of dietary supplements by over 158 million persons and an expenditure of $17 billion annually. In fact, in one study, approximately 25% of the population uses complementary alternative therapies, and 70% of them do not tell their physicians.[2]

Unfortunately, such practices as prayer, folk healing, and *Santeria* were excluded from the study. Texan Hispanics use complementary and alternative treatments, such as massage (19.4%) and herbal remedies (12.4%), at a higher rate than national trends indicate. In a survey, 44% of Mexican American respondents had seen an alternative practitioner at least once during the past year.[3] In another, 59% of Hispanic women engaged in nonallopathic healing methods, including home remedies (38%), botanica products (9.5%), faith healing (17%), and consultations by a spiritist (3.5%), *curandero* (1.9%), or *santero* (1%).[4] An evaluation of surgical patients reported that 62% of Hispanics in the United States and 81% in Mexico admitted to herbal product use during the past year, and 58% of the former and 49% of the later rated the products as "excellent" in treating their conditions. More than 90% from each group had not shared this information with their surgeons.[5]

While dissatisfaction with modern medical care is an important reason for seeking alternative care, more often these treatments are complementary to allopathic care and a cultural custom that is passed on from generation to generation.[1,6] In addition to wide accessibility and low cost, their value is reinforced by conventionalism and tradition. In general, Hispanics believe that prescribed medications are more effective than herbs and have more confidence in physicians than in alternative medicine providers.[7] No doubt barriers to health care, including lack of insurance, poverty, low education levels, and language impediments, cause many Latinos to seek alternatives to the often inaccessible health care system and unaffordable allopathic medicines.[7] However, some complementary therapies can be expensive and may decrease compliance with medical visits and adherence to conventional therapy.[8] The medical profession has tended to attribute observed benefits from folk remedies to placebo effects, but many of these remedies have been used for thousands of years and may indeed have variable degrees of effectiveness.[9]

Traditional medicine refers to "health practices, approaches, knowledge and beliefs incorporating plant-, animal- and mineral-based medicines, spiritual therapies, manual techniques and exercises, applied singularly or in combination to treat, diagnose and prevent illnesses or maintain well-being."[10] The choice of health care practice is influenced by cultural heritage, education, health care beliefs, degree of acculturation, and socioeconomic factors. Cultural beliefs affect acceptance of health care, compliance, and therapeutic outcomes, and in order for physicians to be more effective in delivering care, an understanding of the basis and impact of cultural and religious credence and practices is essential.[10] Countries in Latin America use folk medicine to help meet some of their primary health care needs. Intrinsic to understanding the behavior toward illness and expectations for care of Latinos is the traditional concepts of health and disease. Latinos traditionally have viewed health as the absence of symptoms.[10] As a result of this point of view, the adoption of preventive care practices, such as periodic skin evaluations or the use of sunscreen, is particularly challenging.[11]

The Meso-American Indians established the first medical school on the continent 50 years before the settlement of Jamestown and had developed an elaborate and advanced system of healing with more than 5000 botanical remedies that had been evaluated and considered efficacious. Some of these are recorded in the De la Cruz-Badiano and Florentino codices. The native healers were particularly adept at treating such illnesses as edema, wounds, and podagra. Unfortunately, they had no therapy for the Western scourge variola, which exterminated much of the Aztec population. The tradition of herbalism continues to this day in folk medicine practices and in groups, such as the Kallawaya of northern Bolivia, who have a botanical formulary of more than 300 medicinal plants that are studied in training that can last up to 8 years.

Indigenous natives from Mexico and the subcontinent categorized diseases and therapies as hot or cold. Variations of this concept are practiced to this day in certain communities. Hot illnesses, such as hypertension, which was believed to be caused by *coraje* (anger), *susto* (fear), or thick blood, and diabetes, require cool remedies, whereas infections and other cold diseases require hot treatments, such as penicillin.[11] Dermatologic disease may be hot or cold depending on the perceived etiology, but it is usually treated with cold agents (e.g., bean paste and lemon juice).[11]

REMEDIOS CASEROS (HOME REMEDIES)

The most common healing products and practices used by Hispanics are *remedios caseros,* which include foods (e.g., herbal teas, lemon juice, garlic, honey, vinegar, baking soda, and onion), metal salts, and ointments.[12,13] In one study, a third of Hispanics surveyed admitted to combining complementary treatments with prescription drugs and over-the-counter medications.[14] Chest and back rubdowns with Vicks VapoRub ointment during cough or wheezing episodes is a memory nearly universally shared by Hispanics. Preparation H ointment is used to dry up chickenpox lesions. Olive oil heated with either ruda or garlic is a common treatment for earaches. Garlic cloves are rubbed on bee stings to decrease swelling. Warts are covered with thin slices of potato, and burns are topped with slivers of onion. Aloe vera salve from the cut leaf is applied to bites, burns, wounds, itchy skin, and cutaneous eruptions. Watermelon rind and vinegar soaks also alleviate pruritus, whereas bean paste cools sunburned skin.

The remedies are usually purchased at local groceries or botanicas, stores that traditionally have sold products such as candles, beaded necklaces (*elekes*), figurines of orishas and saints, ritual vessels, and scented spray solutions that purportedly protect from misfortune and restore health[15]. Concurrent with the surge in the Hispanic population in the United States, these stores are erupting in Hispanic neighborhoods and generally maintain low profiles, although some have designed Web sites to sell products through the Internet. These establishments have expanded to provide medicinal products, including fresh and dry herbs, plant sections, infused healing oils, and skin care products . The incorporation of mercury into some of these creams, used for acne and bleaching predominantly, has resulted in dangerously high mercury levels in several users. Alcohol-based products with herbs or other ingredients (*alcolados*) are sold for rubbing on skin eruptions, especially pruritic ones. These include plain alcohol, bay rum (alcohol with bay leaves and oils of lavender, rosemary, and sandalwood), *alcolado glacial* or *alcolado relampago* (alcohol, camphor, menthol, eucalyptus, and pine needle oils), *agua de Florida* (dilute alcohol with fragrances), and witch hazel, an astringent with little witch hazel. These tinctures and astringents can further irritate inflamed skin. Notably *agua Maravilla,* a popular distillate that does contain witch hazel, has no alcohol. Witch hazel has a soothing, antipruritic effect when applied to the skin as a cream, ointment, or compress. Poisonings from products with high alcohol content that lack child-resistant packaging have been reported.[16]

In my experience, botanica employees and even folk healers, frequently recommend pharmaceutical consultation for over-the-counter preparations or encourage medical evaluation. Possibly, the visibility of skin disease places too much pressure and accountability on folk medicine practitioners.[11]

HERBAL MEDICINE

Most *remedios caseros* are plants, herbs, and foods made into a potable tea; boiled into an infusion for compresses; mixed in oil and compounded into a cream, paste, liniment, or poultice; or applied directly to the skin.[12] Herbs also come in capsules, tablets, and solutions. Although the use of these remedies is widespread among all economic strata, they are particularly popular among low-income Hispanics. Physicians have limited knowledge about botanical therapies. In one study, 69% of the providers indicated that they had received no education about herbs or supplements, although 71% were asked about them by patients at least twice a month.[17] There is a commodious repository of information on herbal medicine, but most of the studies have been done in remote parts of the world without strict adherence to scientific protocol.[1]

In many Latin American and Caribbean countries, herbs are harvested locally and prescribed by folk healers and health care practitioners as part of a therapeutic plan in both rural and urban areas.[1] In Mexico and some Latin American countries, vendors (*merolicos*) sell their *remedios caseros* on streets and in markets. Studies to determine the use of alternative treatments for skin disease by Hispanics need to be performed, but surveys have evaluated the use of alternative medicine for systemic diseases in Hispanic communities. The use of herbal products was found to be very prevalent among both HIV-negative (79%) and HIV-positive (71%) Mexican Americans.[18]

Herbal products are not commonly consumed for skin disease, but they are used routinely for the prevention and relief of a variety of symptoms, including nausea or gastritis [e.g., chamomile (*manzanilla*), lemon verbena (*cedron*), and mint (*menta*)], anxiety [linden (*tilo*)], edema or arthritis [cinnamon (*canela*)], anxiety [linden (*tilo*)], and fatigue [Paraguay tea (*yerba mate*)], although some are ingested because systemic properties, such as an antibacterial effect, may benefit the disease course. On the other hand, topical botanical remedies are applied commonly as treatments for a variety of mucocutaneous diseases and symptoms, including acne, eczema, pruritus, hematomas, wounds, burns, animal bites, bacterial infections, calluses, hyperhidrosis, warts, herpes, and aphthous ulcers (Table 8-1). Use of medicinal herbs is particularly high among low-income and elderly Hispanics.[19]

Seventy-one percent of Latinos from south Florida who completed a survey reported using at least one herb in the last 12 months.[20] Women between 25 and 34 years of age are most inclined to use herbal remedies.[21] The most frequently used herbs were chamomile (58.5%), aloe vera (45.3%), linden (35.8%), and star anise (33.0%). In addition to low cost, family tradition (36%) and safety (17%) were the major reasons provided for the use of herbal remedies.[21] The actual prevalence of medicinal herbal and plant use varies according to the demographics, ethnicity, and size of the Hispanic population studied, but there is no question that it is significant[22] and was as high as 59% in a primary care clinic[23] and 77% among surveyed geriatric-aged Hispanics living in New Mexico.[19] Notably, skin problems, along with dyspepsia, upper respiratory tract infection, and anxiety, is one of the most common complaints for which these remedies are used.[20]

It is beyond the scope of this chapter to list all the botanical products used by Hispanics or discuss each herb in detail. However, a list of popular herbs for the treatment of dermatologic disease has been compiled (Table 8-2). A brief discussion of some of the drugs used follows:

- *Arnica* reportedly has anti-inflammatory activity when applied externally. This effect may be due to inhibition of the activation of the transcription factor NF-κB. Sesquiterpenoids isolated from the plant have been found to have activity against gram-positive bacteria, including methicillin-resistant *Staphylococcus aureus* (MRSA).[24] The mechanism of this antibacterial activity is unknown.[24] However, *arnica* can cause contact dermatitis. On the other hand, reports examining the effect of oral *arnica* on healing have not found significant benefit. A placebo-controlled study evaluating the effect of oral *arnica* on healing after removal of impacted wisdom teeth reported more pain and

TABLE 8-1
Dermatologic Diseases for Which Hispanics Commonly Use Plants and Herbs

Alopecia	*Cantuezo, espinosilla, romero, sangre de drago, cintul, saponaria, culantrillo,* hot paste with olive oil, *arnica* tincture and cinnamon, *aceite Moska,* aloe vera
Acne	*Acedera, coronillo, cardamomo,* 0.33% vinegar solution, *barro,* oatmeal and honey, *Aloe vera,* salt and tomato, *arcilla*
Aphthous ulcers	*Alfilerillo, capitaneja, nogal, árnica, bistorta, zarzamora, araroba, corre corre, martinia, salvia, sangre de dragon, totora, caña de azúcar*
Arthropod bites	*Llantén fresco, árnica, romero, tomillo,* salvia
Astringents	*Crameria, encino, guamuchil, limonero, morera, zarzamora, hojas de guayabo, abrojo rojo, bistorta*
Burns	*Achiote, llanten, siempreviva, tepezcohuite,* aloe vera
Blisters	*Zavila, adormidera, llanten, caroba, bardana, lapacho, verónica, cola de caballo, balsamo, cuachalalate, rnica, ceibo, guayabo, guaco, hierba del alacrán, mangle, nogal, mora, tlalchichonole, toloache*
Callouses	Avocado, olive oil
Deodorant allergy	*Alumbre piedra* powder, infusion of orange peel and *cola de caballo*
Ecchymosis	Vitamin E, *cuachalalate, bija*
Eczema	*Fumaria, lipocodio, ñapindá, quina quina*
Furunculosis	*Fenogreco, levadura de cerveza, palán palán*
Herpes	*Bardana, celidueña, dulcamara, mangle, nogal, ortiga, zarzaparrilla, milhombres, calaguala, caroba, centaurea mayor, cola de caballo, charrúa*
Hyperhidrosis	*Yemas de pino* in boiled water soaks, diluted formaldehyde, *kava kava* tea
Pigmentation, melasma	Coco, *azucena, Aloe vera, porotos, escrofularia acuática, fumaria oficinal, dulcamara*
Pruritus	Parsley, watercress, celery, cucumber, cornstarch
Psoriasis	*Yuca, yezgo, verdolaga, tragacanto, onagra, olivo, acedera, agrimonia, alerce, ámbar, aralia, escoba amarga, ginkgo, hibisco*
Scabies	*Ajo, altramuz, codo de fraile, chilillo, estramonio, jicama, hierba mora, hediondilla, romero, tabaco, fumaria, quina quina, ruda, verbena*
Seborrheic dermatitis of scalp	*Cauba, fumaria morada, ortiga, tabaco, tilausia, Aloe vera, encorvada, tola tola, topasaire, toronjil, pipí*
Syphilis	*Calancapatli, cáscara amarga, guayacán, guacima, maguey, palo mulato, pegarropa, sinicuiche, tepopote, zarzaparrilla. bardana, palo mulato, arnica, zarzaparrilla, diente de león*
Tinea	*Jicama, hierba, dulcamara, golondrina levadura de cerveza, Aloe vera, ajenjo, dulcamara*
Ulcers	*Cancerina, cuachalalate, arnica, malulanten, mispatle, sinicuiche, tabachin, tlalchichinole, zavela, hiedra terrestre, fenogreco, yerba mate, artemisa, marrubio, milenrama, hipérico, caléndula, consuelda, cola de caballo, romero, llantén,* dilute vinegar solution (for infected ulcers)
Urticaria	*Barbasco, sanalotodo, yerba larca, efedra, apazote, malva, achicoria, lentejil, ortiga, pegarropa*
Varicella	*Saúco, lino, ambay, vara de pastor*
Varicose veins	*Agrimonia, roble, avellano, cipres, llantén, col salicaria, castano de India, consuelda, cola de caballo*
Warts	*Aloe vera, higuera,* garlic

swelling in the *arnica*-treated group. A double-blind, placebo-controlled, randomized trial of oral *arnica* after total hysterectomy found no significant improvement in the rates of pain and infection. Allergic contact dermatitis is a potential complication.[24]

- *Echinacea* is a North American plant that is, nevertheless, popular among Hispanics as an antimicrobial agent. Previous to the introduction of sulfa drugs, Echinacea tincture was a widely available agent for treatment of infections. It can be applied to the skin or ingested in extract or capsules. There is evidence that its polysaccharides, such as inulin, and alkymides increase the function of T cells and increase natural killer activity, but the herb can worsen autoimmune diseases and decrease the effectiveness of immunosuppressants, including systemic corticosteroids.[25] It promotes wound healing, and its anti-inflammatory action can be valuable in the healing of burns, insect bites, ulcers, psoriasis, acne, and eczema.
- *Passion flower* (which is often combined with valerian root) has a sedating effect and can produce oversedation if taken with tranquilizers.[26]
- *Bromelain,* a proteolytic enzyme from the pineapple plant, inhibits production of proinflammatory prostaglandins while inducing the synthesis of anti-inflammatory prostaglandins.[25] It also reduces capillary permeability. In some studies, the agent reduced surgical pain and swelling and accelerated healing. It is ingested orally or applied topically.
- *Curcumin,* an extract of the Southeast Asian plant *tumeric* is a potent antioxidant and anti-inflammatory agent that inhibits leukotriene formation, prevents platelet aggregation, and stabilizes neutrophilic lysosomal membranes.[25]
- The latex or sap of *Sangre de Drago,* an Amazon tree, contains the phenanthrene alkaloid taspine, which has been shown to have activity against human oral epidermoid carcinoma and anti-inflammatory activity.[27] Applied topically, the sap relieves burning and pain.
- *Calendula,* derived from the marigold plant, contains flavonoids and saponins that have anti-inflammatory and antiseptic activities.[26]
- *Lemon* or *lime juice* is applied topically to relieve the inflammation and symptoms of arthropod bites and sunburn, to treat bacterial or viral skin infections, to relieve pruritus, to even out skin pigmentation, and to loosen scales on the scalp. However, it can irritate eczematous dermatitis and prevent improvement despite treatment.[25]
- *Gordolobo* contains flavonoids, glycosides, polyacethylenic compounds, terpenes, and sesquiterpene lactones. As a tea or ointment, it is used for varicella and skin bacterial infections, and as a poultice, it is used for hemorrhoids. Reports of lethal hepatotoxicity have resulted from use of a mistaken species of the genus *Senecio.*

TABLE 8-2
Selected Herbs and Plants Used by Hispanics

Abuta	*Abuta* (*Cissampelos pareira*)	Analgesic and anti-inflammatory, snakebites
Apazote de zorro	*Anamu* (*Petiveria alliacea*)	Hives, dermatophytosis, bacterial abscesses
Apazote (yerba de Santa Maria)	Wormseed (*Chenopodium abrosioides*)	Urticaria, tinea
Achiote (annatto)	*Achiote* (*Bixa orellana*)	Burns, antiseptic cicatrizant, inflammatory skin diseases
Acahua	*Amica* (*Heterotheca inuloides*)	Wounds, hematoma, and bruising prevention, inflammatory skin diseases
Acahuete	Montezuma cypress (*Taxodium mucronatum*)	Wounds
Ajo	Garlic (*Allium sativum*)	Bacterial infections
Balsam tolu and balsam of Peru	*Myroxylon balsamum*	Pruritus, scabies, bacterial infection, tinea, chronic eczema
Bardana	Burdock (*Arctium lappa*)	Antibacterial, antifungal, acne, seborrhea, diaper rash, eczema, urticaria
Berro	Watercress (*Nasturtium* sp.)	Stomatitis, gingivitis
Boldo	Boldo (*Peumus boldo*)	Melasma, wounds
Bromelaína	Bromelain (*Ananas comusus*)	Postoperative wounds
Brusca	Bucher's broom (*Ruscus aculeatus*)	Psoriasis
Cardosanto	Holy thistle (*Carbenia benedicta*)	Carbuncles, eczema
Cebada	Barley (*Hordeum vulgare*)	Weeping and pustular dermatitis
Chaparral	Chaparral (*Larrea divericata*)	Tinea
Cola de caballo	*Equisetum arvense*	Edema, wounds, hemorrhoids
Corteza del sauce (salicilin)	Willow bark (*Silix alba*)	Pruritus, pain
Consuelda	Confrey (*Symphytum officinale*)	Wounds
Contrayerba	*Asclepias sestosa*	Varicella, erysipelas, snake bites, wounds
Cuachalate	*Amphipterygium adstingens*	Wound astringent, insect bites, acne
Culandrillo	*Avevea* (*Adiantum capillus-veneris*)	Alopecia, infections
Curcumin	Tumeric extract (*Vurcuma longa*)	Inflammatory skin diseases
Dulcamara	Bittersweet (*Solanum dulcamara*)	Inflammatory skin diseases, arthritis
Equinacea	Echinacea (*Echinacea purpurea*)	Wound healing, burns, furuncles, acne, skin ulcers, inflammatory skin diseases
Espinillo	*Espinillo* (*Acacia caven*)	Suppurative skin lesions
Flor de sauco	Mexican elder (*Sambucus mexicana*)	Scalp seborrheic dermatitis, hair loss
Gobernadora	*Chaparral* (*Larrea tridentate*)	Arthritis (poultice), cancer, veneral disease, analgesic
Gordolobo	Everlasting (*Gnaphalium* sp.)	Varicella, hemorrhoids
Guayaba	Guava (*Psidium guajava*)	Scabies, vesicles, acne, astringent
Guayacan, amapa	Yellow *poui* (*Tabebuia chrysantha*)	Syphilis, tuberculosis
Hamamelis	Witch hazel (*Hamamelis virginiana*)	Pruritus, astringent, eczema
Hierba Luisa, cidron	*Verbena olarosa* (*Aloysia triphylla*)	Skin eruptions
Hiedra terrestre	Ground ivy (*Glechoma hederacea*)	Suppurative skin disease
Higuerilla	Castor oil tree (*Ricinus communis*)	Wounds, inflammation
Majorama	Marjoram (*Oréganum marjorama*)	Antiaging, antiviral, stimulates circulation
Malva	Mallow (*Malva neglecta*)	Suppurative lesions, dry skin
Manzanilla	Chamomile (*Anthemis nobilis*)	Inflammatory skin diseases (eczema)
Mastuerzo	*Capuchina* (*Tropaeolum majus*)	Antibiotic, skin pigmentation
Mercadela (maravilla)	*Calendula* (*Calendula officinalis*)	Wounds tinea, candidiasis, antiseptic, skin diseases (eczema), sunburn
Milenrama	Yarrow (*Achillea millefolium*)	Astringent, chronic eczema, pruritus
Morro (Jicara)	Calabash tree (*Crescentia cujete*)	Antibacterial
Neem	*Neem* (*Azadirachta indica*)	Eczema, tinea, bacterial skin infections
Noche buena	Poinsettia (*Euphorbia pulcherrima*)	Warts, wounds, folliculitis
Nogal	*Nuez de Castilla* (*Juglans regia*)	Inflammatory diseases of the skin and eyes, abrasions, hair loss
Nopal	Prickly pear cactus (*Opuntia* sp.)	Burns, cuts, insect bites, oozing eruptions, sunburn
Nuez moscada	Mace (*Myristica fragrans*)	Used in cosmetic creams
Onagra	Primrose (*Oenothera biennis*)	Eczema, skin aging
Oregano	*Oregano Europeo* (*Origanum vulgare*) and *Oregano Mexicano* (*Lippia berlandieri*)	Acne, dermatitis
Pasionara	Passion flower (*Passiflora* sp.)	Anxiety, vascular disease
Pastorcita	*Damiana* (*Tumera diffusa*)	Chickenpox
Pensamiento	*Violeta* (*Viola tricolor*)	Eczema, urticaria, acne, psoriasis, furunculosis

(continued)

TABLE 8-2 (Continued)
Selected Herbs and Plants Used by Hispanics

Poleo	Pennyroyal (*Mentha pulegium*)	Insect repellent
Propoleo (Propolis)	Bee glue	Acne, tinea, wounds, antibacterial, psoriasis
Romero	Rosemary (*Rosmarinus officinalis*)	Seborrheic dermatitis, alopecia, skin disinfectant
Ruda	*Ruda* (*Ruta chalepensis*)	Insect repellent, antibiotic, inflammatory and vascular diseases
Sage	*Salvia Europea* (*Salvia officinalis*)	Seborrheic dermatitis, wound antiseptic
Salvia de bolita	Mexican sage	Hyperhidrosis
Sangre de drago	*Croton lechleri*	Inflammatiory diseases, acne, insect bites, viral infections, wounds
Santa Maria	*Feverfew* (*Tanacetum parthenium*)	Insect repellent, arthritis, fever
Saponaria	Bouncingbet (*Saponaria officionalis*)	Scalp psoriasis, eczema, acne, furuncles
Taloache	Jimson weed (*Datura innoxia*)	Wounds, hemorrhoids, pustular eruptions
Tepescohuite	Mimosa (*Mimosa tenuiflora*)	Burns, wounds, acne, psoriasis
Tronadora	Trumpet flowers (*Tecoma stans*)	Chickenpox
Tomillo	Thyme (*Thymus vulgaris*)	Seborrheic dermatitis, skin eruptions
Ulnaria	Meadowsweet (*Filipendula ulnaria*)	Edema, astringent, cellulitis, wounds
Una de gato	*Uncaria tomentosa*	Wounds, inflammatory skin diseases
Virreina	Quinine bark (*Cinchone officionalis*)	Eczema
Yerba buena	Peppermint (*Mentha piperita*)	Dyspepsia, colic
Yerba de la negrita	Scarlet globe mallow (*Sphaeralcea coccinea*)	Wounds, hemorrhoids, damaged hair
Zábila	Aloe vera	Wounds, burns, striae, acne, herpes, psoriasis, radiation dermatitis, eczema, lichen planus
Zarzaparilla	Sarsaparilla (*Smilax ornate*)	Acne, syphilis

- *Rosemary oil* is used widely for scaly scalp conditions. It has antimicrobial properties but can be irritating to the skin and mucous membranes and may cause allergic and photosensitive reactions. It also can exacerbate seizures, even when used topically over large areas. Both rosemary and sage cheilitis have been reported.[28] Rosemary should not be taken by pregnant women because it can stimulate the uterus. A number of other herbs have antimicrobial activity. In one study, oregano oil had the highest bacterial inhibitory activity, followed by coriander and basil extracts. Anise oil inhibited the growth of molds but not bacteria.[29]

Although there are a few published studies, the potential interactions of plants and herbs with pharmacologic agents remains poorly understood. However, adverse reactions from chemical interactions, direct toxicity, and systemic or topical hypersensitivity do occur. Phytophotodermatitis caused by furocoumarin chemicals is seen after rubbing lime or lemon on the skin or contact with other plants (e.g., ruta or parsley) followed by exposure to the ultraviolet A (UV-A) spectrum of sunlight. Within a few hours, vesicles and bullae form on the exposed areas, which may heal with long-standing hyperpigmentation.[30] Allergic contact dermatitis is particularly common from plants in the Compositae family, which contain sesquiterpene lactones. The typical presentation is a chronic eczematous eruption rather than an acute vesicular dermatitis. Among agents that can cause contact urticaria are balsam of Peru, benzoic acid, cinnamic alcohol, cinnamic aldehyde, and sorbic acid.

Other nonbotanical remedies can cause serious illnesses. Hypersensitivity reactions may develop after use of Penesol cream, which contains penicillin and sulfa, in persons with allergy to these antibiotics. A cluster of nine children with elevated levels of mercury was reported from a bottle removed from a supplier of *santeria* artifacts.[31] Toxic levels of mercury have been found in women who use mercury-containing creams (e.g., Crema Santa, Crema de Belleza-Manning, and Miss Key Crema Blanqueadora) and soaps (e.g., Jabon Germicida) as treatment for melasma and acne.[32] Lead poisoning has been reported from salts given for *empacho* (gastroenteritis).[33] Acute, lethal poisoning from an abnormally high dose of oil of chenopodium recommended by a *curandera* has been described.[34]

CURANDERISMO

Curanderismo is a practice that integrates Christian religious concepts, folk medicine, psychotherapy, rituals, and magic. As many as 90% of Latinos do not seek care from a *curandero* initially but obtain their remedies from a hierarchy of lay healers. The first consultant is usually an elderly family member or experienced neighbor. Depending on the condition or the complexity of the symptoms, the case may be referred to a *yerbero* (herbalist), *partera* (midwive), or *sobador* (massage therapist).[1,22] If the disease is complicated or preternatural, the person is treated by a *curandera(o)* (a lay practitioner with special training and spiritual gifts for healing). Folk illnesses have strong psychological and spiritual influences, and religious practices, personal confidence in the remedies, and familial commitment are required for treatments to be effective. Among the most common of these illnesses are *empacho* (gastroenteritis), *mal de ojo* (evil eye), *susto* (fright), *caida de mollera* (fallen fontanel), and *mal puesto* (sorcery).[35] Some of these folk illnesses occur primarily in children, so it is not surprising that one study found that 20% of Mexican-American mothers had taken their children to *curanderos* for treatment.[36] Much of the *curandero*'s practice involves prayers, meditation, baths, and botanical products, including hallucinogenic plants. In order to impress and promote therapeutic trust, they also may employ magic as part of the service.[1]

Recently, there has been the emergence of bilingual nurse-*curanderas* who integrate nursing and allopathic health care with traditional folk medicine.[37] Participation of folk healers may be beneficial when religious and emotional factors are influencing a patient's prognosis. In one instance, the "hex casting" by a *curandero* was considered to be valuable and complementary to dermatologic treatment in improving an exfoliative dermatitis believed by the patient to have been caused by a curse.[38] A survey of 405 Hispanic subjects conducted in the primary and urgent care clinics at a public city hospital (Denver Health Medical Center) revealed that 29.1% had sought health care from a *curandero* at some time in their lives. Those who had been to a *curandero* were poorer and had lower levels of formal education.[37]

Santeria (*Regla Lucumi*) is a syncretic religion brought by West African slaves that combines elements of West African religious practices with Christian cultural elements. It is particularly popular among Cubans, Puerto Ricans, and Dominicans. Forbidden to pray to their *orishas,* the divinities that interact with humans by controlling nature, the slaves designated Catholic saints as symbols of these folk deities to fool plantation owners into believing that they were devoutly practicing the Catholic religion.[39] The rites involve animal sacrifice, hypnotic drum music, energetic dancing, and trances in order to communicate with and obtain the assistance of ancestors and deities. *Santeria* provides a way to control harmful supernatural forces and reduce stress.

Espiritismo (spiritism) or *espiritualismo* (spiritualism) are often used synonymously because many *espiritistas* dabble in *Santeria.* These terms denote not a religion but a form of folk healing that stresses that dead spirits can harm people, resulting in symptoms and disease for which special protection is required and consultation with an *espiritista* may be necessary. A study of HIV-infected Puerto Ricans treated in a medical clinic found that two-thirds of respondents (31% were born in the United States) engaged in either folk healing or *Santeria*. Most believed in good and evil spirits that controlled their infection.[40]

Espiritualidad (spirituality), in contrast, refers to deep piety and religious fervor that results in intense veneration of God and saints in order to achieve intercession and favors. It is a common practice for Hispanics to keep crucifixes, religious pictures, and even personal altars in their homes. The spectrum of this form of religiosity ranges widely. At one end, people observe religious services and pray mainly at times of stress or "bargaining" for health restoration, whereas at the other, these practices consume several hours of their daily schedule. These believers invariably consider illness as a punishment for past sins or transgression that can only be alleviated through atonement achieved by prayers and personal sacrifice. Prayer nodules can form from extended sessions of kneeling during prayer. Calluses between the first and second fingertips of the dominant hand may be seen from rubbing rosary beads. The rosary consists of prayers repeated in sequence and can be regarded as a form of meditation in which the prayers serve as the repetitive mantra. *Fatalismo* refers to the belief that divine providence governs the world and that unfortunate events are intentional, need to be accepted, and are unavoidable. This passive reaction to negative situations reduces the sense of personal failure, guilt, and despair that often is the outcome of such tragic events. In one survey, 35% of people living in this country prayed for health concerns (75% of these for wellness and 22% for specific medical conditions).[41] More than half (54%) of Hispanic children with chronic asthma pray for health, with rubs (53%) and massage (45%) being the other two most common methods of alternative medicine used.[42] Thirty-six percent of depressed Hispanics reported counseling by a religious priest or minister (17% had taken herbal remedies, and 5% had visited a *curandero*).[43] The majority of Mexican-American diabetics interviewed in one study indicated that prayer influences health by reducing stress and bringing healing power to medicines.[44]

CONCLUSION

As Hispanics acclimate and acculturate, they become acquainted with and tend to embrace the health care practices of their new country.[45] However, studies show that there are strong attachments to traditional cultural customs at least in early generations. Hispanics appear to combine allopathic medicine with some folk remedies routinely and effortlessly. Considering the tenets underlying Eastern medicine, an attraction to certain alternative and complementary treatments, such as acupuncture, is not surprising, but this modality may have limited value in skin disease. Expectedly, the use of folk remedies, prayer, and massage will remain at the forefront of alternative and complementary therapies in Hispanic communities. Considering potential adverse effects or interactions with pharmacologic drugs and the possibility of interference or more relaxed compliance with the prescribed regimen, it is important for physicians to be aware of their popularity and to encourage discussion of their use with their patients.

REFERENCES

1. Balick MJ, Kronenberg F, Ososki AL, et al. Medicinal plants used by Latino healers for women's health conditions in New York City. *Econ Bot* 2000;54:344-357.
2. Eisenberg DM, Kessler RC, Foster C, et al. Unconventional medicine in the United States: Prevalence, costs, and patterns of use. *N Engl J Med* 1993;328:246-252.
3. Keegan L. Use of alternative therapies among Mexican Americans in the Texas Rio Grande Valley. *J Holist Nurs* 1996; 14:277-294.
4. Laws MD, Carballeira N. Use of nonallopathic healing methods by Latina women at midlife. *Am J Public Health* 2003;93:524-525.
5. Rivera JO, Chaudhuri K, Gonzalez-Stuart A, et al. Herbal product use by Hispanic surgical patients. *Am Surg* 2005; 71:71-76.
6. Eisenberg DM, Davis RB, Ettner SL, et al. Trends in complementary medicine use in the United States, 1990-1997: Results of a follow-up survey. *JAMA* 1998;280: 1569-1575.
7. Astin JA. Why patients use alternative medicines. *JAMA* 1998;279:1548-1553.
8. Mikhail N, Wali S, Ziment I. Use of alternative medicine among Hispanics. *J Altern Compl Med* 2004;10:851-859.
9. Ramus-Remus C, Gamez-Nava JL, Gonzalez-Lopez L, et al. Use of alternative therapies by patients with rheumatic disease in Guadalajara, Mexico: Prevalence, beliefs, and expectations. Arthritis Res 1998;1:411-418.
10. *Traditional medicine*. World Health Organization Fact Sheet No 134. Geneva, WHO, 2003, pp 1-2.
11. Moy JA, McKinley-Grant L, Sanchez MR. Cultural aspects in the treatment of patients with skin disease. *Dermatol Clin* 2003;21:733-742.
12. Trotter RT II. Remedios caseros: Mexican American home remedies and community health problems. *Soc Sci Med* 1981; 15B:107-114.
13. Burge SK, Albright TL. Use of complementary and alternative medicine among

family practice patients in South Texas. *Am J Public Health* 2002;92:1614-1616.
14. Marsh WW, Hentges K. Mexican folk remedies and conventional medical care. *Am Fam Phys* 1988;37:257-262.
15. Gomez-Beloz A, Chavez N. The botanica as a culturally appropriate health care option for Latinos. *J Altern Compl Med* 2001;7:537-546.
16. Mull DS, Agran PF, Winn DG, Anderson CL. Household poisoning exposure among children of Mexican-born mothers: An ethnographic study. *West J Med* 1999;171:16-19.
17. Planta M, Gundersen B, Petitt JC. Prevalence of the use of herbal products in a low-income population. *Fam Med* 2000;32:252-257.
18. Rivera JO, Gonzalez-Stuart A, Ortiz M, et al. Herbal product use in non-HIV and HIV-positive Hispanic patients. *J Natl Med Assoc* 2005;97:1686-1691.
19. Dole EJ, Rhyne RL, Zeilmann CA, et al. The influence of ethnicity on use of herbal remedies in elderly Hispanics and non-Hispanic whites. *J Am Pharm Assoc* 2000:40:349-351
20. Ortiz BI, Clauson KA. Use of herbs and herbal products by Hispanics in South Florida. *J Am Pharm Assoc* 2006;46:161-167.
21. Laws MB, Carballeira N. Use of nonallopathic healing methods by Latina women at midlife. *Am J Public Health* 2003;93:524-525.
22. Rivera JO , Ortiz M, Lawson ME, Verma KM. Evaluation of the use of complementary and alternative medicine in the largest United States-Mexico border city. *Pharmacotherapy* 2002;22:256-264.
23. Plotkin SR, Post R. Folk remedy use in the inner city. *South Med J* 1999;92:795-798.
24. Ernst E, Pittler MH. Efficacy of homeopathic arnica: A systematic review of placebo-controlled clinical trials. *Arch Surg* 1998;133:1187-1190.
25. Graff J, Sanchez, MR. Alternative and complementary medicines in dermatology, in Freedberg IM, Sanchez MR (eds), *Current Dermatologic Diagnosis and Treatment.* Philadelphia, Lippincott Williams & Walkins, 2001, pp 222-223.
26. Graf J. Herbal anti-inflammatory agents for skin disease (letter). *Skin Ther* 2000; 5:2-5.
27. Jones K. Review of sangre de drago (*Croton lechleri*): A South American tree sap in the treatment of diarrhea, inflammation, insect bites, viral infections, and wounds—Traditional uses to clinical research. *J Altern Compl Med* 2003;9: 877-896.
28. Guin JD. Rosemary cheilits: One to remember. *Contact Dermatitis* 2000;45:63.
29. Elgayyar M, Draughon FA, Golden DA, Mount JR. Antimicrobial activity of essential oils from plants against selected pathogenic and saprophytic microorganisms. *J Food Prot* 2001;64:1019-1024.
30. Naafs B. Allergic skin reactions in the tropics. *Clin Dermatol* 2006;24:158-167.
31. Alison Newby C, Riley DM, Leal-Almeraz TO. A cluster of pediatric metallic mercury exposure cases treated with meso-2,3-dimercaptosuccinic acid (DMSA). *Environ Health Perspect* 2000;108: 575-577.
32. Alison Newby C, Riley DM, Leal-Almeraz TO. Mercury use and exposure among *Santeria* practitioners: Religious versus folk practice in northern New Jersey, USA. *Ethnogr Health* 2006;11: 287-306.
33. Baer RD, Garcia de Alba J, Leal RM, et al. Mexican use of lead in the treatment of empacho: Community, clinic, and longitudinal patterns. *Soc Sci Med* 1998;47: 1263-1266.
34. Montoya-Cabrera MA, Escalante-Galindo P, Meckes-Fisher M, et al. Fatal poisoning caused by oil of epazote, *Chenopodium graveolens. Gac Med Mex* 1996;132:433-437.
35. Trotter RT. Curanderismo: A picture of Mexican-American folk healing. *J Altern Compl Med.* 2001;7:29-31.
36. Risser AL, Mazur LJ. Use of folk remedies in a Hispanic population. *Arch Pediatr Adolesc Med* 1995;149:978-981.
37. Padilla R, Gomez V, Biggerstaff SL, Mehler PS. Use of curanderismo in a public health care system. *Arch Intern Med* 2001;161:1336-1340.
38. Garcia RL. "Witch doctor": A hexing case of dermatitis. *Cutis* 1977;19:103-105.
39. Sandoval MS. Santeria. *J Fla Med Assoc* 1983;70:620-628.
40. Suarez M, Raffaelli M, O'Leary A. Use of folk healing practices by HIV-infected Hispanics living in the United States. *AIDS Care* 1996;8:683-690.
41. McCaffrey AM, Eisenberg DM, Legedza AT, et al. Prayer for health concerns: Results of a national survey on prevalence and patterns of use. *Arch Intern Med* 2004;26;164:858-862.
42. Braganza S, Ozuah PO, Sharif I. The use of complementary therapies in inner-city asthmatic children. *J Asthma* 2003;40: 823-827.
43. Sleath BL, Williams JW Jr. Hispanic ethnicity, language, and depression: Physician-patient communication and patient use of alternative treatments. *Int J Psychol Med* 2004;34:235-246.
44. Hunt LM, Arar NH, Akana LL. Herbs, prayer and insulin: Use of medical and alternative treatments by a group of Mexican-American diabetes patients. *J Fam Prac* 2000;49:216-223.
45. Mackenzie ER, Taylor L, Bloom BS, et al. Ethnic minority use of complementary and alternative medicine (CAM): A national probability survey of CAM utilizers. *Altern Ther Health Med* 2003;9: 50-56.

CHAPTER 9

African-American Skin Remedies and Folk Healing Practices

Elena Jones
Jeanine Downie

Key Points

- Many African-Americans rely on folk healing for skin, hair, and nail disorders and concerns.
- The history of skin remedies likely harkens back to their Native American and African ancestors.
- Topical skin remedies are most often derived from plants, herbs, foods, and other natural elements.
- Modern science has provided evidence of the efficacy of some of these remedies.

African-American culture has been rich in the use of skin remedies and folk healing (Table 9-1). Many remedies adapted by African-Americans most likely originated from their African and Native American ancestors. Native Americans are known to have recognized and used plants, grasses, and herbs for healing. Early settlers held Native American healers in high regard. In 1650, one Dutch explorer wrote, "The Indians know how to cure very dangerous and perilous wounds and sores by roots, leaves and other little things. . . . Among all the discoveries of America by the French and Spaniards, I wonder why none of them was so kind to the world as to have kept a catalog of the illnesses they found the natives able to cure."[1] Examples of natural remedies derived from Africa include the use by Cleopatra of milk baths to promote healthy skin and the use of aloe vera for skin infections.

Skin remedies and folk healing continue to be used by many in the African-American community to this day (Table 9-2). Many of these skin remedies are discussed and listed in this chapter. The list, which is compiled in alphabetical order, was obtained by surveying patients, families, and associates of the authors as well as reviewing existing literature. This chapter represents only a fraction of the vast number of natural remedies that exist. Practical applications of some of the folk remedies have been included to allow for a better understanding of practices that are still being used by African-American patients.

TABLE 9-3
Cutaneous Treatment with *Aloe vera*

- Acne
- Burns
- Cutaneous bacterial and fungal infections
- Dry skin
- Eczema
- Frost bite
- Insect bites
- Poison ivy
- Seborrheic dermatitis
- Ulcers

ALOE VERA[2–4]

Aloe vera, also known as *lily of the dessert,* was first used by Ancient Egyptians to treat skin infections and to lubricate the skin. Containing mucopolysaccarides, amino acids, enzymes, and various minerals, *Aloe vera* has demonstrated steroid, antibiotic, and antiviral properties. It has been used historically in the African-American community to treat a variety of cutaneous disorders from burns to eczema (Table 9-3).

AVOCADO[5]

Avocados are replete in vitamin A, vitamin B, natural oil, and protein. They are higher in protein than many other fruits and have been used to treat acne in the

TABLE 9-1
Historic African-American Remedies and Folk Healing[4]

Boiled grass (Costa Rica): elixir used to treat colds and acne
Cement (South Africa): to treat foot fungus
Cigarette ash paste: to clear sinuses and help allergies
Cinnamon and nutmeg: to freshen breath and used topically to remove moles
Chocolate: used topically as an aphrodisiac
Crisco (Mexico): to treat nipple eczema and mastitis
Salt: used as a scrub around the eyes to remove stys and chalazions
Tobacco: used in bathwater to treat insect bites, poison ivy, and eczema
Turpentine: to treat eczema, insect bites, and psoriasis
Watermelon juice: to remove facial and body hair

TABLE 9-2
A Snapshot of Home Remedies Often Practiced by African-Americans[1,4]

Air drying cuts better for healing
Alcohol to dry out darkly colored necks, dark pimples, and razor bumps
Baby powder to lengthen eyelashes, dry oily hair, to stop itching; to kill fleas, ticks, and bed bugs
Ben Gay to firm a sagging chest and treat cellulite
Carrots boiled and applied topically to protect skin from sunburn
Castor oil to clear skin, cleanse the colon, condition and moisturize hair; taken orally to harden nails
Chamomile to highlight hair color, heal wounds, and treat skin infections
Cod liver oil taken orally to strengthen and grow hair and nails
Gelatin taken orally in foods or as a pill to strengthens nails
Hemp (Panama) to draw out pus and infection
Ketchup to treat acne, cysts, and nail fungus
Milk of magnesia as a facial mask to treat acne and smooth texture of the skin
Octagon soap for black neck discoloration, acne, athletes' foot, and body odor
Oregano (crushed) to treat a toothache and joint pain and to grow hair
Preparation H to decrease undereye puffiness and to treat cuticle swelling and throbbing leg veins
Smelling salts to treat acne, eczema, dandruff, and psoriasis when used topically
Sulfur to cure pus-filled shingles
Thyme (crushed) to improve brittle hair and to add shine to hair and nails
Tree bark brewed in water to treat corns and calluses of the feet
Urine (from babies) to clear fungus and treat acne

form of a facial mask. They are also commonly used as a skin moisturizer and hair conditioner.

BAKING SODA[3]

Baking soda (sodium bicarbonate) is a gentle alkaline powder with a myriad of uses. It has been used for more than 75 years as a deodorant and mouthwash, as well as to treat burns, foot odor, and eczema and as a skin exfoliant.

BEER[5]

Beer, a popular alcoholic beverage, has been used as a setting lotion and hair rinse. It is felt that the proteins, carbohydrates, and sugars in beer work synergistically to thicken hair.

BLACK COHOSH[6,7]

Black cohosh (*Micifuga racemes*) was used by the Algoquin Indians to treat gynecologic illnesses in the 1870s. It is also known as *bugbane* because it repels insects. Native Americans believed that it could relieve the discomfort of scarlet fever, smallpox, and arthritis.

BURDOCK[1]

Burdock (*Articum*) is an herb that is purported to have significant antifungal, antibacterial, and anticancer properties. Burdock has been used by Chinese and Native Americans for at least a century. It is used to cool and soothe inflamed skin in such conditions as acne, eczema, and psoriasis.

CALENDULA[2,7]

Calendula, also known as *marigold,* is an herb that has been used to treat inflammatory processes of the skin, including acne, eczema, and psoriasis. It is also used as an antiseptic for burns, scars, and wounds. Native Americans have used calendula for years for its antifungal properties and its ability to treat athlete's foot.

CAPSICUM[4,7]

Capsicum is a genus of plants from the nightshade family (Solanaceae). The fruit of most species of *Capsicum* contains capsaicin, the component responsible for the pungent effects of red pepper. When used topically, it is felt to relieve the itch of chickenpox and the pain of herpes zoster and treat psoriasis. It is also felt to be effective in stopping minor bleeding.

TABLE 9-4
Oily Skin Mask[9]

- 1 tablespoon witch hazel
- 1 teaspoon bentonite or alternate facial clay
- 1 mashed strawberry
- 2 drops cypress essential oil
- 2 drops lemon essential oil

Strawberries, cypress oil, and lemon oil essential oils help to decrease activity of oil glands.

CLAY[8,9]

Clay has been used medicinally since biblical days. This natural substance from the earth has been used topically to dry acne and reduce swelling. Clay also has been used as a means to "draw out impurities" from infections such as stasis dermatitis. Clay masks are used commonly to benefit facial skin (Table 9-4).

COCOA BUTTER[6]

Cocoa butter is a creamy, fatty wax that is obtained from the seeds of the cocoa plant. It has been used to make skin softer, to treat stretch marks, and to fade dark marks, particularly on elbows and knees. Topically, it is also used to soothe sunburn and friction-induced blisters.

DANDELION[3,7]

Dandelion is used as an antiseptic herbal remedy for sores, wounds, and oral inflammation. Topically, slices of dandelion are used to treat canker sores. Nails infected with fungus have been soaked in dandelion water.

EMU OIL[8]

This unique oil is derived from a relative of the ostrich. Rich in essential fatty acids, emu oil is used as an emollient moisturizer in cosmetic and skin-care products. It is used to treat dry skin conditions, including eczema, psoriasis, and xerosis.

GARLIC[2,3]

Raw garlic is believed to be a potent therapeutic food with antibiotic, antifungal, antiparasitic, and antiviral activity. Used externally for eye infections, including chalazions, its high levels of thiamine allows it to be used as an insect repellent. Garlic also contains germanium, which is an antioxidant that aids with wound healing.

GOLDENSEAL[2,3]

Goldenseal is one of America's most popular herbs. It contains berberine, which is a natural substance with antibacterial, antifungal, and antiparasitic properties. Goldenseal has been used by Native Americans, who discovered its medicinal properties and used it as an antiseptic to treat wounds. Goldenseal also has used to treat yeast infections, canker sores, athlete's foot, ringworm, and eczema.

GRAPEFRUIT SEED EXTRACT[5]

Grapefruit seed extract is considered a natural antibiotic as well an antifungal and antiviral agent. It has been used to treat candidal yeast infections, infected cuts, mild parasitic infections, staphyloccal infections, nail fungus, ringworm, warts, dandruff, and gingivitis.

GRAPESEED OIL[5]

Grapeseed oil is a light, hypoallergenic, unscented oil that has various hair applications. It has been used as a hair-styling oil and a hair conditioner, and it is believed to enhance hair growth.

HORSE CHESTNUT[5]

Horse chestnut seeds have been used traditionally for varicose veins and phlebitis. People who bruise easily also have found a use for horse chestnut seeds. Topically, it has been used as a skin brightener and to prevent lymphedema and to treat leg ulcers and hemorrhoids. It also been noted to relieve pain.

HYDROGEN PEROXIDE[9]

Hydrogen peroxide is a very popular therapeutic chemical compound that has myriad uses, including to unplug earwax, lighten hair on the body, and as an antiseptic for minor bruises, cuts, and burns. Additionally, it is believed to have antifungal activity and has been used to treat yeast infections and as a mouthwash.

IODINE[5]

Iodine is a mineral that has antibiotic-like actions and is necessary for skin, nail, and hair health. Iodine is unique in its ability to aid wound healing when used both topically and orally.

JOJOBA OIL[1,9]

Jojoba oil (*Simondsia chinensis*) is a plant that is found in the southern regions of Arizona and California. Jojoba seeds contain approximately 50% oil, and they are added to soaps for moisturization and to shampoos for conditioning. Jojopba also was used by Native Americans to treat burns, bruises, cuts, and sores. It is also reputed to treat hair loss.

LAVENDER[3,7]

Lavender is a violet-blue flower that has been used to calm and soothe skin inflammation for decades. It is used specifically to treat conditions such as eczema and psoriasis, which are felt to be worsened by stress.

LEMON[3,7]

This popular citrus fruit acts as a natural bleaching agent. It has been used to lighten age spots, freckles, and hair. As a soak, lemons are used to remove the top layer of dead skin cells, which help to even skin tone. It is specifically used to treat dark elbows and knees.

LICORICE[4,7]

Licorice is derived from the root of *Glycyrrhiza glabra*. It has been used topically for canker sores, eczema, herpes, and ulcers.

MAYONNAISE[5,9]

Mayonnaise is a dressing made from oil, eggs, and vinegar or lemon juice that is often an ingredient in natural beauty treatments used by African-Americans. The oil and eggs are used for their ability to moisturize skin. Egg whites tend to act as an astringent and can be drying, whereas yolks are a major source of lecithin, a natural emollient. The function of the vinegar or lemon juice is to help to restore the skin's natural acid pH. Mayonnaise is used as a moisturizer for dry skin or as a conditioner for hair. A mayonnaise hair conditioner is used frequently to treat dry hair and hair that has been damaged by too much sun or blow drying. After shampooing, mayonnaise is massaged into the hair, left on for 15 minutes or more to allow the ingredients to penetrate, and then rinsed out. Weekly mayonnaise conditioning treatments are felt to restore moisture and radiance to hair (Table 9-5).

TABLE 9-5
Common Mayonnaise-Based Hair Treatments[5,9]

Mayonnaise Hair Treatment
- Use approximately ¼ cup of mayonnaise (less or more depending on length of hair).
- Apply mayonnaise treatment to clean, damp hair.
- Wrap hair with plastic wrap to hold in heat and open up the hair follicles for deep conditioning.
- Leave on for at least 15 minutes.
- Rinse thoroughly with cool water.

For dry hair:
- Combine 2 tablespoons coconut oil with ¼ cup each of pureed banana and avocado and ¼ cup of mayonnaise.

For normal hair:
- Combine 2 tablespoons of olive oil with 1 egg and ¼ cup each of mayonnaise and yogurt.

For oily hair:
- Add only 1–2 teaspoons of lemon juice to the product for normal hair. (*Beware:* Lemon juice can bleach hair.)

MILK[2,9]

Milk, which is rich in protein, natural fat, and lactic acid, is used as a natural cleanser and beautifier. In addition to cleansing and detoxifying the skin, it is known to leave skin soft, smooth, and well hydrated. The use of milk baths dates back to ancient Egypt, where they were purportedly used by Cleopatra (Table 9-6). Other natural cleansers used by African-Americans include sour cream and plain yogurt.

TABLE 9-6
Milk Bath Treatment[2,9]

Combine ¼ cup dry nonfat milk powder with ¼ cup dry buttermilk powder and 1 tablespoon cornstarch. Pour ¼ cup of mixture into full tub of warm water.

MINERAL OIL[3,5,6]

Mineral oil is an ingredient widely used in cosmetics that is stable and does not spoil over time. It is used frequently as a skin emollient. Mineral oil consists of refined liquid hydrocarbons derived from petroleum. Petroleum jelly (Vaseline) is the solid form of this oil. Vaseline is used widely by the African-American population for a variety of purposes. Its primary use is as a topical emollient for the skin and dry or chapped lips, hands, and feet. It also has been used on the hair as a hair pomade or moisturizer. Use on the hair or faces of children and young adults has resulted in pomade acne.

MINT[4,7]

Mint leaves have many medicinal uses in the African-American community, from soothing indigestion to serving as a natural astringent or insect repellent. Mint is rich in iron and menthol and is felt to energize and help to raise metabolism. The menthol is believed to help tighten the skin pores. Pennyroyal (*Mentha puleguim*), a member of the mint family, is used as an insect repellant. Its leaves are crushed, and the liquid is applied to exposed skin. Hanging dried pennyroyal plants in the home is also believed to repel insects.

NETTLE (*URTICA DIOCA*)[4,7]

Nettles are plants with a high mineral content. The leaves and roots have many medicinal uses, including the treatment of rashes, dandruff, and hay fever. Nettles also have been used as an astringent. Nettle leaves combined equally with horsetail, johnny-up, and lavender has been brewed into a tea and employed as a leave-in herbal dandruff treatment.

OATS (*AVENA SAVITA*)[2,8,10]

Oatmeal was used for skin health and beauty as early as 2000 BC in Arabia and Egypt to soothe and protect dry or itchy, inflamed skin. Oatmeal is a grain that has been used as an effective and popular nonsoap cleanser. This nontoxic, soothing grain is rich in protein, potassium, iron, phosphates, magnesium, and silicon. It is gentle and mild and is used by people with all African-American skin types. It is especially useful in baths for individuals with eczema-prone skin or other dry, itchy, or sensitive skin conditions (Table 9-7).

TABLE 9-7
Oatmeal Bath[2,8]

To make an oatmeal bath:
• Take 1 cup of edible oats and put them in a handkerchief or cheesecloth.
• Tie it over the faucet, and let the water run through it.
• Soak in the tub for 20–30 minutes.
• Immediately apply a moisturizer to damp skin,
Warning: When getting out of the tub, oatmeal can make skin and tub very slippery.

OLIVE OIL[4,9]

Olive oil has been used as a good, inexpensive basic moisturizer by African-Americans. It is used for seborrheic dermatitis, xerosis, and calluses. Pure olive oil has been applied to scalps of infants with cradle-cap or seborrheic dermatitis, left on for about 15 minutes, and washed off. The emolliency of the natural oil can help to lift the adherent flakes.

ONION[4,7]

Onion, a close botanical cousin to garlic, has been used to help heal burns, soothe insect stings, and fight infections. An old folk remedy is to cut a slice of white onion and tape it over an insect sting for 1 hour (after removing the insect stinger). Although it is unclear how the onion actually works, its moist and cooling properties are soothing.

PAPAYA (*CARICA PAPAYA*)[5,9]

Papaya is a tropical fruit that is known for its digestive properties, as well as its dermatologic properties. Papaya contains papain, a proteolytic enzyme, with unripe papayas having the highest content of papain. Papaya is a skin softener and antiaging cream (Table 9-8). Fresh papaya is also used to help soothe jellyfish stings.

TABLE 9-8
Antiaging Papaya Peel

Two tablespoons of crushed unripe papaya mixed with 1 tablespoon of dry oatmeal can be used as a peel to help reduce the appearance of fine lines.

PLANTAIN (*PLANTAGO IANCEOLATA*)[3,4]

Plaintain, another tropical fruit, has been used to stop infections and inflammation. Topically, it has been used to treat wounds, burns, and bites. Fresh leaves can be crushed and the juices applied directly to a burn as a soothing lotion. It also has been used to treat urinary and respiratory tract infections.

PUMICE[9]

Pumice stones are light, porous bits of volcanic lava used to remove dead skin and calluses from the feet, knees, elbows, and hands. They are used frequently by African-American women.

ROSEMARY (*ROSEMARY OFFICINALIS*)[4,7]

Rosemary is used often for hair and scalp disorders. The three essential oils associated with healthy hair are rosemary, lavender, and sandalwood. Rosemary is thought to stimulate hair growth (Table 9-9). In addition, the potent essential oils in rosemary are felt to help control overproduction of scalp oil. Rosemary leaves are used to make a strong tea that can be used as a rinse for oily hair and to highlight brunette hair color.

TEA TREE OIL (*MELALEUCA ALTERNIFOLIA*)[1,4,9]

Tea trees have been used as medicinal plants for thousands of years by Australian aboriginals. It is the oil found within the leaves that has antibacterial, antifungal, and antiviral properties. The volatile oil from the leaves and small branches of the tree contains terpinen-4-ol, a skin antiseptic and anti-inflammatory agent. Another component, cineol, present in small yet varying amounts depending on the quality of the oil, can act as a skin irritant and cause a rhuslike dermatitis.

Tea tree oil is used for a variety of purposes by African-Americans, including as a treatment for acne (Table 9-10). In fact, a 5% tea tree oil gel is felt to be as effective as 5% benzoyl peroxide against acne. While the tea tree oil gel is slower to take effect, it is much less drying to the skin.

Tea tree oil is also used to treat a variety of fungal disorders, including foot, nail, and groin fungus. A combination of equal parts of olive oil and tea tree oil or *Aloe vera* gel and tea tree oil applied twice daily has been used as a fungicidal (Table 9-11). For maximum benefit, tea tree oil must be applied for 6–8 weeks.

Because of its antibacterial effects, tea tree oil is also believed to be effective for abscesses and furuncles. When applied topically as a cream or diluted in water, it helps to drain purulent discharge.

TABLE 9-9
Natural Alternatives for Hair Loss[4,6]

Saw palmetto (*Serenoa repens*)
320–400 mg daily of an 85% liposterolic extract
Biotin
2000–3000 mg daily
Methylsulfonylmethane
3000 mg daily
Silica
500 mg twice daily
Rosemary essential oil
3–5 drops per 1 ounce of shampoo daily

TABLE 9-10
Natural Alternatives for Acne[9,10]

Essential fatty acids
1–2 tablespoons of flaxseed oil, daily for 6 weeks
3–5 g of fish oil daily for 6 weeks
Zinc
50 mg twice daily with meals for 3 months, then reduce to 50 mg daily (take in conjunction with 3–5 mg copper for 3 months)
Zinc works to reduce the buildup of dihydrotestosterone (DHT) and promote skin healing
Burdock root
300–500 mg daily
Tea tree oil
Apply 5% solution twice daily

TABLE 9-11
Natural Alternatives for Tinea Pedis[8,9]

Tea tree oil
Apply daily for 6–8 weeks
Oregano oil
500 mg three times daily with meals, or tincture also can be applied topically
Garlic
500–1000 mg twice daily
Echinacea and goldenseal
500 mg three times daily or apply 2–4 mL of tincture three times

TOMATO[5,8]

Tomatoes have astringent properties that aid in skin exfoliation and cleansing. They are useful for comedones and oily skin. In addition, tomato juice can be used as a hair rinse to help remove odors, such as smoke, from hair.

VINEGAR (ACETIC ACID)[2,9]

Vinegars have a high acid content; therefore, they are useful as antibacterial, antiyeast, and antifungal agents. Vinegar eardrops used after swimming help to prevent swimmer's ear by creating an acidic environment that retards bacterial overgrowth. Vinegar soaks can be used for nails and intertriginous areas to prevent and diminish the colonization of yeast and fungal species. Finally, vinegar is used to remove alkaline residues from skin and hair.

VITAMIN E (TOCOPHEROL)[2,6]

Vitamin E is found in vegetable oils, seeds (e.g., sunflower), nuts, brown rice, and whole grains. Applied topically, vitamin E is used by African-Americans to improve skin tone and texture, as well as to help with unsightly scars. A contact dermatitis can result.

WATERCRESS (*NASTURTIUM OFFICINALE*)[3]

Watercress is a plant that grows in shallow creeks or along the edges of slow-moving rivers, ponds, and lakes throughout the United States, Mexico, and most of Canada. It is exceptionally nutritious with significant amounts of vitamins A, C, and E, along with minerals such as calcium, magnesium, iron, and copper. Native Americans used watercress to treat myriad disorders, including upper respiratory infections, gallstones, acne, eczema, and tinea infections. The juice was applied to the scalp in an attempt to prevent hair loss. Today, watercress is made into a tea and used as an astringent for acne or as a soothing bath for eczema.

WITCH HAZEL[2,8]

Witch hazel, derived from the shrub *Hamamelis virginiana,* has been used to treat itchy, inflamed skin. The shrub's bark and leaves have been used as a local anesthetic and astringent. It is used commonly by African-Americans as a toner because the large quantities of tannins contained in witch hazel cause the skin to tighten, remove excess surface oil, and decrease bacteria on acne-prone skin.

YOGURT[6,9]

Plain yogurt is rich in protein, calcium, and vitamins. It has skin-softening qualities, making it a soothing cleanser that is absorbed easily. It can be an excellent mask for all skin types. The lactobacilli in yogurt have been used to control vaginal yeast infections.

CONCLUSION

Traditionally, the use of plants, herbs, and other natural elements has been at the center of healing in African-American culture. These natural remedies often proved to be far less expensive and, at time, equally effective as "modern medicine." We have reviewed the more common remedies used by many African-American patients.

REFERENCES

1. Shimer P. *Healing Secrets of the Native Americans.* New York, Black Dog & Leventhal Publishers, 2004.
2. Gaeddert A. *Healing Skin Disorders: Natural Treatments for Dermatological Conditions.* Berkeley, CA, North Atlantic Books, 2003.
3. Page L. *Healthy Healing: A Guide to Self-Healing for Everyone.* Berkeley, CA, Healthy Healing, 2004.
4. Dole EJ, Rhyne RL, Zeilmann CA, Skipper BJ, McCabe ML, Dog TL. The influence of ethnicity on the use of herbal remedies. *J Am Pharm Assoc* 2000; 40:359-365.
5. Prevention Health Books (eds). *The Doctor's Book of Home Remedies.* New York, Bantam Dell, 2002.
6. Gaston Hughes M, Porter G. *Prime Time: The African American Woman's Guide to Midlife Health and Wellness.* New York, Ballantine Publishing Group, 2001.
7. Prevention Health Books (eds). *The Doctor's Book of Herbal Home Remedies.* New York, Rodale, 2000.
8. Balch J. *Prescription for Natural Cures.* Hoboken, NJ, Wiley, 2004.
9. Cox J. *Natural Beauty at Home.* New York, Holt, 2002.
10. Baumann LS. Cosmeceutical critique: Oatmeal. *Skin & Allergy News,* November 2004, p 44.

CHAPTER 10

Homeopathic Medicine and Spiritualism: African-American Voodoo and Healing Remedies

Wilbert C. Jordan

Key Points

- Voodoo in the United States is rooted in both African religion and Christianity.
- Therapy is provided by three characters with distinct roles: the "old lady," the spiritualist, and the hougan (priest).
- Animals figure importantly in Voodoo, especially the chicken and snake.
- Rituals and spells are integral parts of the tradition.
- The moaning style of singing derives from Voodoo ceremonies and is the root of the "blue note."

Voodoo is a form of religion based on a belief in "things," many more powerful and sacred than human themselves. Although Voodoo can be found as the sole religion in parts of Haiti and Africa, in the United States it functions symbiotically with Christianity.

Voodoo, like any religion, affords explanations for unanswered mysteries and provides a means of dealing with them. It is African in origin, but in the United States it has developed into many forms with varying degrees of similarity to one another and to the African model.

This chapter will discuss Voodoo primarily as it exists in the United States, but it will also show its derivation from the classical African forms. The focus will be on its influence as an unorthodox form of medical practice.

FROM AFRICA TO AMERICA

Voodoo functions to serve the needs of a people. Its laws, taboos, medicines, and rituals were derived and established for the perpetuation of a given group, clan, or tribe. It was so much "of the people" that the dehumanization of American slavery did not erase it from their minds.

Slavery destroyed many aspects of black culture by systematically separating the family and by placing together members from tribes with different languages in order to prevent communication. This resulted in the breakdown of the African family system in America; however, remnants of the former culture survived. American Voodoo's, kinship with African Voodoo parallels that of black American music with African music. In music, what remained was the common denominator of all African music, the *chant–response*. In fact, the oldest pure black American music, the spirituals and the moaning hymns, are both based primarily on the chant– response. Likewise, in Voodoo, the specifics became lost, but the structure common to all Africans remained and was adapted to the needs of the new environment that black faced.

THE BASIC ELEMENTS OF VOODOO

Black folk medicine has three principal characters:

1. The "old lady," "granny," or "Ms Markus," who is well versed in herbs and functions as the local consultant for common ailments. She is also well versed in child rearing and usually has raised several children of her own and grandchildren as well.
2. The spiritualist, the predominant and most heterogeneous character today.
3. The oldest character, and in many ways the most powerful, the Voodoo priest, or hougan.

Each of these characters has important and different roles that are deeply established in the traditions of black American culture.

The Old Lady

Ms Inoshe (pronounced "I-no-she") is an example of an old lady in a rural southern town. She does not have office hours; people come to her home at any time. Most of her clients are young mothers who seek help with raising children or treating their illnesses. Unlike the priest, priestess, or spiritualist, she does not dispense medicines, only gives instructions. On rare occasions; she may be compensated with money, however, most likely she will receive only a "thank you" or food products in exchange for her advice. She is typically found in the more rural South.

Occasionally, when she is unfamiliar with a problem the old lady consults a priest or priestess or refers the patient to him or her. She eliminates from the priest's practice patients who only need advice about medications. This system makes it possible for others to learn of folk remedies and how to make them so that the next generation may be educated in folk medicine.

The institution of the old lady is unique. Many are mothers who have successfully raised children through hardship and poverty, with little assistance from the traditional medical community.

Perhaps their success in child raising despite obstacles has led to their selection as paraprofessionals, so to speak, in folk medicine. There is no certification or recertification; their credentials come from word of mouth.

The Spiritualist

Spiritualists serve an important function in black culture. Black-oriented radio and newspapers routinely carry advertisements promising "to solve all personal problems, to heal incurable diseases, to solve financial anxieties, to give 'hot numbers.'" Many radio stations play tapes of persons bearing witness to the powers of a given spiritualist, telling how their troubled lives have improved since meeting him or her. Integration and technology have affected them because a majority are in urban areas. Historically, their primary form of advertisement was in the black-oriented newspapers, such as the *Chicago Defender, Pittsburgh Courier,* or *Amsterdam News.* Today, in addition, they use a wide range of other means, including radio, circulars, cards, and the Internet, as well as word of mouth.

Presently, this group stands as the predominant, the most urban, and the most heterogeneous of the three characters in black folk medicine. The major differences in the United States between the Voodoo priest and the spiritualist are as follows:

- Spiritualists are "called" to their profession. Many of them claim to have received a gift from God or to have been specifically chosen by Him. The relationship to the traditional black church and its influence is apparent. In fact, many spiritualists are former Christian ministers who were "called" and ordained (but not formally trained) in the Christian church before becoming spiritualists. Many spiritualists perform both functions simultaneously.

- All spiritualists have their basis in Christianity.
- Spiritualists are not trained in the art of Voodoo beyond the level of knowledge of the old lady. Many spiritualists once functioned as old ladies.
- Spiritualists are primarily urban (although some are found in rural areas), whereas Voodoo priests are overwhelmingly rural-based. Although many spiritualists once functioned as old ladies, not all spiritualists are women; the ratio of males to females is approximately 1:1.

Figure 10-1 shows a woman who functioned as a spiritualist and a Voodoo priestess.

Haiti is regarded as the ultimate base of Voodoo knowledge and its powers. In the United States, Louisiana and Georgia are the states where folk medicines and its are most often found. Among the most famous mythical personalities in black culture is the group known as the *Famous Seven Sisters of New Orleans,* whose legendary powers in Voodoo were unsurpassed. Louisiana is considered to be where Voodoo began in this country, with Georgia the state of its second birth. Old ladies, spiritualists, and hougans who were born in Louisiana or Georgia, or who have traveled extensively in those states, or Haiti, are thought to possess greater power than others of their kind. Consequently, many spiritualists advertise themselves as having traveled to Haiti, Louisiana, or Georgia and as being related to well-known Voodoo practitioners there. Phrases such as *Georgia mojo, Louisiana mojo,* and *Louisiana conja* are well known in black America.

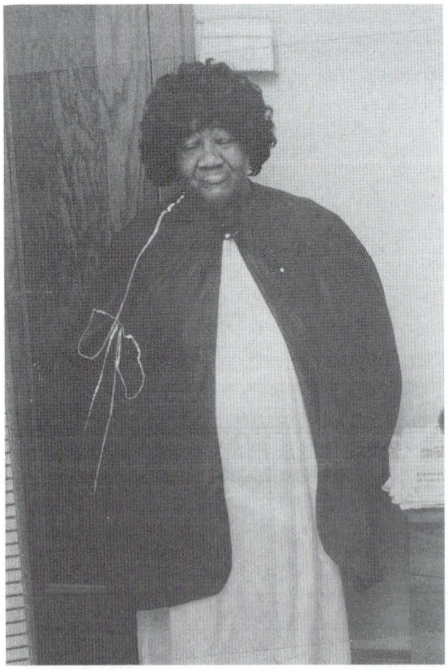

▲ **FIGURE 10-1** Bishop Sam Ella Jordan, spiritualist. She was well known on the south side of Chicago and later moved to Los Angeles. Her clientele was nationwide.

The titles of spiritualists are drawn from religion: mother, father, reverend, prophet, or bishop, all proclaiming to heal. Most of their clientele are poor, uneducated, and devoutly religious. As in the case of the Voodoo priest, most of the spiritualist is clients seek help with an unsteady romance, financial problems, or "treasure hunting," or they complain of being pursued by ghosts.

Many clients have physical illnesses that require medical attention, for which the spiritualist provides a substitute. Certain spiritualists sell (gambling) numbers and are overt confidence; others serve in a capacity similar to that of a trained psychiatrist, listening and offering advice to the chronically anxiety-laden or neurotic patient. Spiritualists deal with the fears and neuroses of their patients by helping them to cope better with their lives. The first requirement is the patient's devout trust in the spiritualist. The client must believe that the spiritualist has a special ability to communicate with the lord. Later, a long-standing relationship evolves through visits or correspondence. Patients in rural areas where there is no Voodoo activity communicate with practitioners by mail; frequently complete psychotherapy is conducted by mail.

What is important to appreciate is that the more disconnected the black patient is from mainstream society, the greater is the chance he or she will seek help from a spiritualist. This is someone who can be trusted. Distrust of the mainstream system remains problematic in many segments of the black community. Many patients who live in rural areas where there is no Voodoo activity communicate with Voodoo practitioners by mail; frequently complete psychotherapy is conducted by mail.

Spiritualists must know their patients well. Few, if any, keep files or records; they rely primarily on memory. Spiritualists may be found in any American city where a sizable black population exists.

The Hougan (Priest)

The relationship of the hougan, or Voodoo priest, with the ruling body of a given African society parallels that of the Pope or the Archbishop of Canterbury with the governments of Italy and England in the past.

Training consists of learning the philosophy of elders, as well as the techniques of dealing with people and their problems. It involves recognizing the importance of various herbs, their actions, and their side effects. The functions of Voodoo priests combine those of many professions, including judicial, medical, psychosocial, and legal. Therefore, training is more extensive than one might imagine. The new priest must be well equipped with the skills to deal with family and personal problems as they exist in his society to handle illnesses or other medical concerns, and interpret signs as good or bad omens. Figure 10-2 shows a voodoo priest in his office with a patient.

In any given generation of priests and priestesses, however, a priest is usually respected as being stronger than a priest. The origin of this tradition of successors to the priesthood is unclear, but it is commonly observed among Voodoo practitioners in the mid-South.

Naming of babies is rarely done now, but was a unique practice in the rural South in the late 1800s and early 1900s. When a mother felt her daughter was going to be pretty and might face

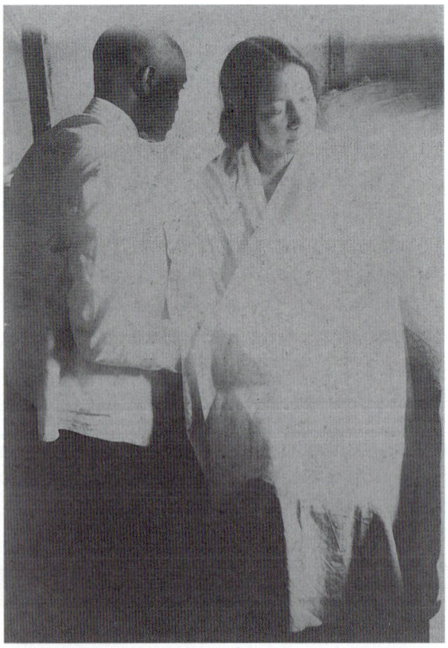

▲ **FIGURE 10-2** Dr. William Jordan of Wheatley, Arkansas, a Voodoo priest, in his office with a patient who had neurotic complaints about a growth in the abdomen.

molestation, by white men, the priest would give the babies protective names. Names had predictive value. For instance, Bertha, Bessie, and Beulah were typically the "Butt sisters." Being overweight was the best protection against sexual molestation by white men in small southern towns before the 1950s. Ironically, many black women named Bertha, Bessie, and Beulah are well endowed with adipose tissue.

ANIMALS AND VOODOO

A beautiful aspect of African culture is its relation to animals. The dances parallel the motions of certain animals. Priests rely heavily on animals in determining which herbs to use. In treating an illness, the priest imitates the symptoms of the affected person; recalls which animal(s) displays the same symptoms, especially their more subtle aspects, and what they mean; and relies on the same herbs that the animal would use. If the priest has never seen the symptoms in an animal, he imagines the symptoms in an animal that has been studied extremely well. For these reasons, it is important for Voodoo priests to have a thorough knowledge of animal habits.

For example, if a patient presents with a complaint of intractable diarrhea, the priest, drawing on a deep familiarity with animal habits, tells him which herbs to use. For example, since it is common for dogs with diarrhea to eat wild grass, many priests prescribe wild grass either eaten or taken with tea, as the treatment.

In Voodoo, one does not think in terms of gods, but spirits such as power, good, and evil. The two most important spirits are good and evil, power, usually representative by fire can merge with either of them. Evil is represented by the snake, and one's ability to handle the snake implies ability to overpower evil and control it. Good is represented by the chicken; biting its head off and drinking the blood represents one's ability to master and contain good. Some ceremonies, when a client is thought to be possessed of evil, involve having the subject drink blood from the chicken in hopes that the power from that good will overcome the power of the evil possessing him and drive it out.

Other animals are used in black American Voodoo, but not in ceremonies. It is the responsibility of the priest or priestess to become familiar with other animals in order to role-play their habits and personalities.

The Chicken

In the United States, the animal most commonly studied by Voodoo practitioners is the chicken, followed by the dog and the cat. The chicken symbolizes the ability of human beings to overcome their weaknesses. Drinking the blood from a freshly killed chicken imparts self-awareness, a feeling of being in control of one's own destiny.

The Snake

The snake is the animal most identified with Voodoo and its priests, but while its function is distinct from that of other animals the association is a Western phenomenon and not part of classical African Voodoo. The role of the snake reflects the Christian influence on Voodoo, including Haitian Voodoo in the United States, it is used to show the priest's power over evil and representing the "serpent" described in the Bible. In the black American vernacular, the snake and evil are synonymous. In America, the most commonly used snake is the diamondback rattler, usually a tamed or one with its poison sacs removed. The copperhead moccasin is also used; however, use of the coral snake or the cottonmouth moccasin is unknown to this author. Some priests use snake venom as the base for facial dyes (Table 10-1).

Priests do not carry snakes with them routinely; however, in certain religious ceremonies and programs, priests display their powers by demonstrating their power over the serpent. The fact that the priest is not bitten by the snake during a ceremony is obviously awesome to the spectators. Bishop James, a priest in Kansas City, would collect venom from his snake in the presence of an audience. Occasionally, he would allow the snake to strike him. A few priests claim to be immune to snake bites, especially rattlesnake bites, presumably through slow desensitization. Whether such claims to immunity are accurate has not been investigated.

THE SPELL

When a person (the aggressor) seeks to have a spell cast on another person (the victim), the act is known as *seeking a hex or controlling, or conjuring*. The victim may not be aware of the act. The hex enables the aggressor to control, relate to, or deal

TABLE 10-1
Dyes for Cosmetic and Domestic Purposes

Color	Ingredients and Preparation	Uses
Red	Flowers from poinsettia plant are boiled in small amount of water until water turns dark red; flowers are then strained off and solution is cooled.	1. The concentrated dark red solution is added to 1 Tbsp boiled snake venom; this is added to 1 cup of clay dirt, and the mixture is used as red paint for face during ceremonies. 2. The boiled dark-red solution is added to fresh water, and clothing is soaked for dying.
Brown	Birch bark is left in water until it turns brown; also used are walnut bark and persimmon bark with small piece of charcoal.	Same as above.
Yellow	Persimmon bark, tin, and sunflower leaves are boiled in water.	Same as above.
Blue	The entire indigo plant is boiled in water, and the water is strained off when it appears black; this is concentrated blue dye.	Same as above.
Black	Pieces of scrap iron are boiled slowly for 2–3 hours, then vigorously; water is strained off.	Same as above.
Green	Hickory bark is boiled until it appears black; water is strained off; 1 part hickory bark water is mixed with 1 part indigo water. Concentrated green dye results.	Same as above.

with the victim better though the victim may not be aware of the hex.

A hex, when performed by a priest may take place in a congregational setting or with the aggressor albine. When it is performed by a priest, the hex is completed, the priest and the aggressor cease communication. This type of hex is administered independently of the victim. No form of powder, material, body part, or instrument is exchanged between the aggressor and the priest, nor are any of the victim's possessions involved.

When the hex is completed, the priest and the aggressor separate and have no further communication. The priest may have remaining procedures to accomplish, or he may feel that the verbal communication between himself and the aggressor was sufficient psychotherapy to enable the aggressor to control the problem with the victim.

The victim may be the active party seeking help for having had a spell put on him; that is, he may want protection from a spell or may desire to have a spell broken. The help that the "conjured" victim receives may be given an object, clothing, hair particles, fingernails, or a bag of some sort by the priest to retain or to spread around his surroundings or the surroundings of the aggressor, provided that the aggressor's identity is known. The victim may furnish the priest with articles belonging to the aggressor or body parts such as hair, fingernails, or toenails of the aggressor, or alternatives, the priest may give the victim a bag of "conja" to spray, spread, clump, etc. on a particular possession of the aggressor. The victim may be instructed to place the conja on his or her clothing, around his or her door, across his or her sidewalk, etc. Conja is given to help protect a person and is not used for aggressive acts.

It is forbidden for the victim to visit the same priest as the aggressor, nor can the same priest knowingly serve both. It does happen, however, that a priest unknowingly serves both the aggressor and the victim since it is very common not to refer to persons by name.Thus a victim will talk about the aggressor at length and perhaps over several visits, describing the person in every way and giving the sex, mentioning his or her name; the aggressor does the same in regard to the victim. In fact, many priests forbid the use of names by their clientele. This means that the client must be able to describe the other party in great detail. The description allows the priest to visualize the other party, but more important, it enables the client to develop a detailed and extensive dialogue with the priest. In describing the other party in detail, the client makes clear his or her feelings about him or her, and the priest concentrates on these feelings.

This strict separation of the interaction of the priest with the victim and with the aggressor is not practiced by spiritualists, who may give the aggressor as well as the victim a "bag." This is an important factor in distinguishing a classical Voodoo priest, of whom there are only a few remaining in America, from a spiritualist.

CEREMONIES AND RITUALS

In black American Voodoo, there are several well-defined occasions for rituals or ceremonies. These are not traditional in nature; the priest is free to outline the ritual or state what is necessary for a particular ceremony. The Christian influence is obvious. Most ceremonies consist of three acts, with each act relating to one part of the Trinity. Ceremonies and rituals most common in black American Voodoo are listed in Table 10-2.

The most impressive and important of all rituals in Voodoo is the *reading of bones*. Bones are used as a means of communicating with an individual's subconscious (see Figures 10-3 through 10-5 for patterns and explanations). The ritual is performed with only the patient present, and occasionally is preceded by a testimony of the patient's faith in the priest. The type of patient who receives a reading is usually one who would be diagnosed in psychiatric language as having a character disorder; however, some neurotics are also read. The priest decides that a reading is necessary. The reading follows a defined pattern. The priest spreads a cloth over a table or kneels with the patient on the floor with or without a cloth. The priest asks the patient to think of an object, something specifying the number of sides the object is to have usually based on a statement the patient has made in the preceding conversation with the priest; for example, a love triangle equals a three-sided object or a dream of 10 coffins equals a 10-sided object). After visualizing the requested object, the patient is asked to draw the figure on the cloth or the floor, usually with white chalk but occasionally with powder or flour. The patient receives the bones in a container, most likely a turtle's shell or a human skull. He or she is first instructed to pick each bone up individually, while the priest explains what it represents. All the bones are placed either back into the container or on a certain spot on the table or floor. The Priest then instructs the patient to arrange the bones in any order either on the chalk lines or inside the drawing, but never both. For each topic chosen, the procedure is repeated an undefined number of times as the priest interprets to the patient what the patterns express. The patterns are always interpreted with the patient alone.

Many mothers take their infants to a priest to have a "lucky" or "healthy" number bestowed on them. Customarily, the number is derived from a combination of birth factors, especially a characteristic that makes the infant unique, positively or negatively. For example, a child who was born on the same day as a death in the family may be given that date as a healthy number, provided the death occurred after the birth. If the death occurred before the birth, however, the date may be considered a bad sign and that number may be given to the child as his or her "number to be aware of" or an "unlucky number."

On occasion, the priest also examines the placenta, and depending whether the umbilical cord is inserted in the center or on the periphery, may make predictions about the infant's health.

Treasure hunting, the most challenging of ceremonies is rooted in the rural

TABLE 10-2
Voodoo Ceremonies and Rituals

Ceremonies	Rituals
Recognition of son or daughter into priesthood	Treasure hunting
Challenge of a candidate's right to priesthood	Reading of bones
Removal of curses	Interpretation of birth signs
Placing of hexes (sometimes resulting in Voodoo death)	
Communicating with the dead	
Driving out evil spirits from a "possessed" person, that is a psychotic; usually unsuccessful	

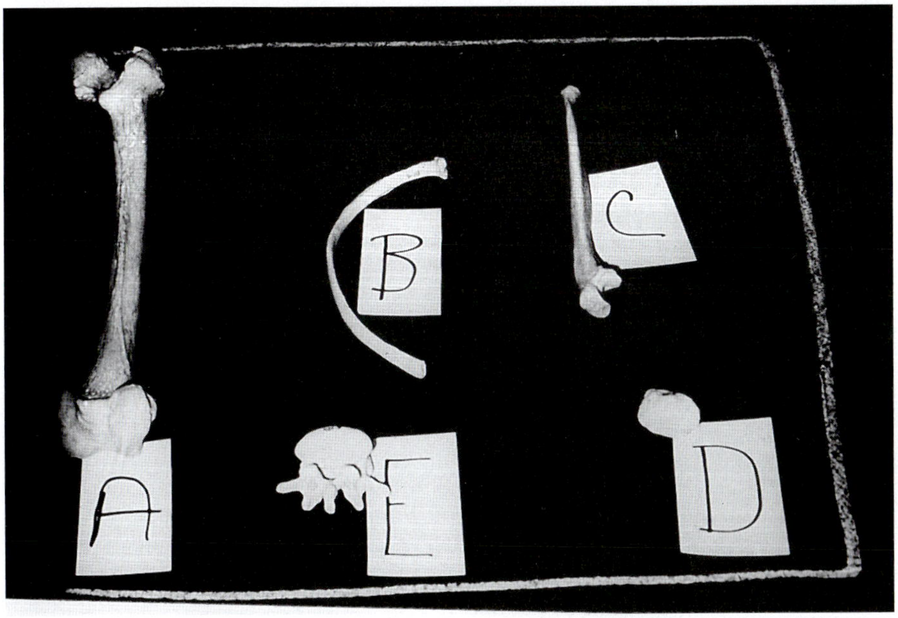

▲ **FIGURE 10-3** Reading of bones. *A.* The femur, representing (1) a strong character, (2) the patient, (3) a dominating parent, (4) father, (5) male character. *B.* A rib, representing (1) a woman, (2) the patient's wife. *C.* The tibia, humerus, ulna, or radius; any of these can represent (1) a female, (2) a dependent character separate from the patient, (3) weak character, male or female. *D.* The patella, representing children, male or female. *E.* A vertebra, representing children, male or female.

South. This has its basis in the rural South. It is rarely practiced today, but in the 1930s through 1960s it was a successful priest/priestess' primary source of income. At that time, many blacks did not put their money in banks because there were instances and rumors of instances where white bankers claimed money was never deposited. In small southern towns there was little a black person could do about it. Therefore, many put their money in a different kind of bank, a river bank. That people often buried their money creek or river. It was easy to remember the hiding place and to instruct others, but often it was on someone else's a white man's property, and so had to be dug up at night. Consequently, when a "depositor" died, the heirs usually came in the dark night to dig it up. Fearing spirits and the landowner's shot gun, they would hire a priest to lead the party across some field to where the deceased person had left instructions that the money was buried. The priest's function was to keep the spirits at bay and allow the dig to go quietly. There are tales of hands coming out of the ground, trains approaching where there were no tracks, and the sound of big truck and ferocious dogs barking.

The treasure hunt ceremonies involved moaning. It was also a way to condition the group to think the same thing or feel the same sensations, this inducing mass hypnosis.

MUSIC

Although music is an integral part of Voodoo, the role of music in ceremonies and rituals differs somewhat from its role in the traditional black church. Most of the songs are derived from slavery and are related to death, earthly fear, or the need for help. The song used most has been "The Day Is Past and Gone." This song, the most definitive statement pertaining to death in all of black music, is sung in the a cappella quartet style. All songs in black American Voodoo are sung a cappella in a moaning style. Other songs include "Life's Evening Sun," "Hush, Somebody's Calling My Name," "Somebody Touched Me," and "Hold to God's Unchanging Hand."

Moaning is an incomplete artform. The best example is to ask a person over age 50 about his or her mother's or grandmother's moan. It was easy to tell if she was moaning about a son who was away from home, debt, or marital problems, but not about the stock exchange. The point is that moans varied according to the issues, but the issues were always the day-to-day problems of rural blacks. The great early gospel singers were known for their ability to moan. A study was done once with gospel great Bessie Griffith had her moan in a gospel concert until the audience went into a frenzy. She was asked on one occasion to moan about problems in the home, another time about kids gone astray, and a third about having too much debt and not knowing how to pay. When the members of the audience were asked what had been on their minds when they did shout, remarkably, they mentioned the same themes about which Bessie Griffith had moaned.

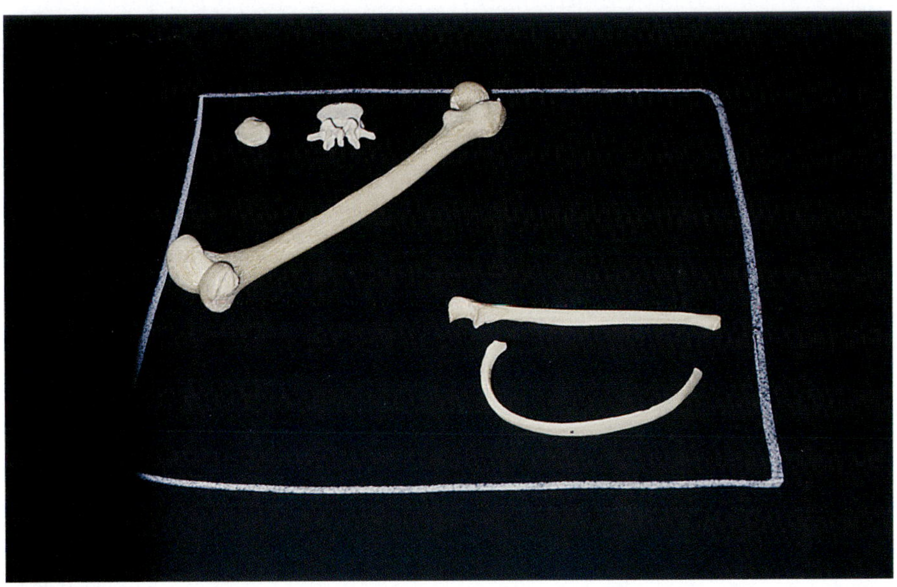

▲ **FIGURE 10-4** This pattern can imply that the patient (a man) is romantically involved with a woman other than his wife. Placement of bones representing the children (patella and vertebra); above the femur indicates the patient's concern for his children. Placement of the rib below the bone representing the other woman and implies less love for the wife than for the other woman.

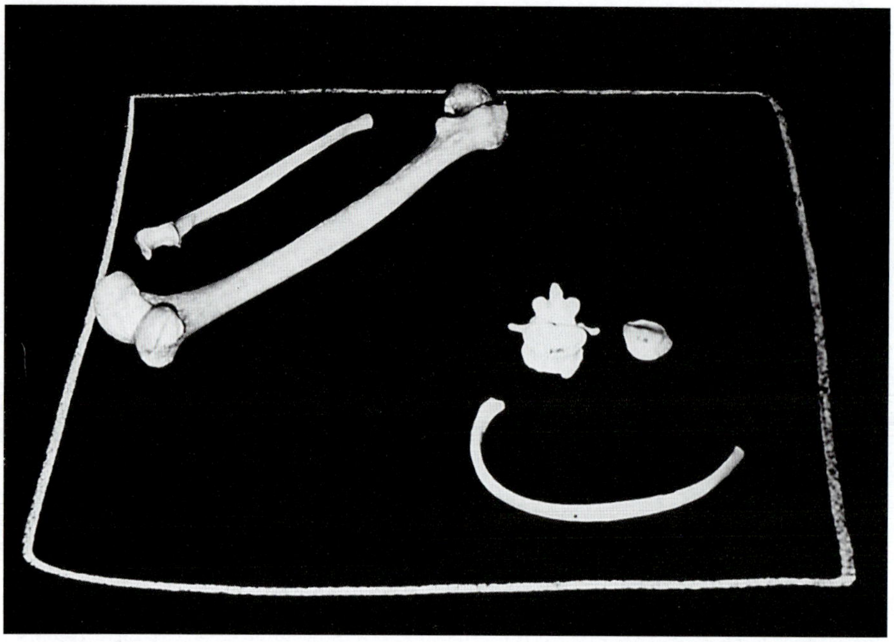

▲ **FIGURE 10-5** In this pattern, the patient has placed the other woman above himself and again has put the wife in the lowest position, below the children. This pattern implies real attraction to the other woman.

There was no way of communicating during slavery. It is the root of that (blue note) or note bending. There are no notes for moaning: It cannot be scripted. You can rhyme nearly any line. In Voodoo, the Priest often introduces moaning, this most often with treasure hunting, to induce mass hypnosis.

Only priest, and only the most powerful ones, used hypnosis, never spiritualist or old lady. Their style was different from what is regarded today as hypnosis. Their goal was to control the individual. It often came out of a challenge between priests. Whoever was successful in hypnotizing the other first had an upper hand. Usually a posthypnotic suggestive act or statement was left, making it easier to accomplish the act again. There were no ties or close calls. In a challenge ceremony, only one priest came out the clear victor. The other was not a loser, but close to a slave or zombie. In other words, the winner controlled the loser. The black American definition of zombie is related to hypnosis.

The *zombie* in black American Voodoo is a person whose will has been broken. In Voodoo, the human is seen as having a conscious and unconscious personality, or consciousness A and B. Consciousness B is what we call our subconscious, but in Voodoo, it is really conscious and aware of everything we do. It is thought that if one is hypnotized and level, consciousness A is made to sleep, and now consciousness B will be active. If consciousness B feels that consciousness A has done evil or horrible things to its body, it may not wish to go back. Sometimes it is felt that it wills itself to die, that is, the voodoo death. Alternatively, an experienced priest can put consciousness A to rest and allow consciousness B to be the conscious form, which means a new level, consciousness C, is created as what we would be calling the subconscious. There are always two conscious levels. To be complete, the priest can put consciousness B to rest and allow consciousness C to be the first level, or what we would call the conscious. This means that a new subconscious would be created, or consciousness D. This person, with a conscious C and subconscious D, basically would be unaware of his or her past life. It would be for the priest to hold them, or control them. This is a zombie.

DISCUSSION AND CONCLUSIONS

It is important to understand that all positive accomplishments of Voodoo priests or spiritualists tend to reinforce their position and power. However, their importance as mystic possessors of supernatural powers is most often magnified.

Studies dealing with black American folk medicine are scarce, and many of the existing few are inadequately organized, but the literature is sufficient to point out the significance of this form of medicine. A study printed in *Mental Hygiene*[1] examined the practices of eight African-American healers in Georgia. The author used two black undergraduate students as interviewers. Both were native-born Georgians, one a political science major and the other a sociology major. The two students interviewed 8 practitioners and 25 patients. The results of the study indicated that (1) five of the eight practitioners reported that they had learned their art from a member of their family, (2) practitioners gave as reasons for being in the practice that they had been called by God, that they had a supernatural gift, and that they had a desire to help people, and (3) the range of years in practice was 34 to 75, and the average age of those beginning in practice was 19 years. No mention in this article was made of whether the practitioners interviewed were priests or spiritualists or simply old ladies, nor was sufficient information given for the reader to decide. Most important, the article did not enter into the details of the doctor–patient relationship, the rituals and ceremonies involved, or the community's relation to the practitioners.

A better study appears in the November 1972 issue of *Medical Opinion*.[2] The author's discussion of "rootwork," as he calls it, is an excellent case study of a 37-year-old black man unsuccessfully treated at the psychiatric unit of the University of Connecticut–McCook Hospital in Hartford until the aid of a "rootworker" was included.

A case report of a patient who had a questionable death by hex is presented in Harvey and Bordley's textbook, *Differential Diagnosis*.[3] An excellent review of cases of Voodoo death can be found in the *American Anthropologist*.[4] Several cases of death apparently caused by spells, hexes, and fears are presented, again raising questions about the power of one's emotions over one's constitution and life. To eliminate doubt, one should participate in Voodoo ceremonies, such as treasure hunting and communicating with the dead; the powers of group emotion and mass hypnosis soon become obvious. Sizable questions are still unanswered in this area; perhaps Voodoo will provide the road to understanding them.

The Voodoo priest, the spiritualist, and the old lady are true professionals in the black community; the millions of blacks using their services and the millions who have survived because of them establish their reality and legitimacy. With origins that revert to southern rural traditions, Voodoo medicine is now serving many in

TABLE 10-3
Dermatologic Medications and Substances Used by Voodoo Practitioners*

Illness	Remedy	Ingredients, Preparation	How Given
1. Herpes simplex	Ear wax		Applied as a cream to affected areas
2. Acne	Juice from honey suckle plant	Juice from honeysuckle plant (usually 1 tsp) added to butter, grease, or face cream	Applied as regular face cream qhs
3. Acne	Oyster, crayfish, or crab oil	Any of these crustaceae are boiled in small amount of water; oil is taken off the top	Applied as cream qhs
4. Sunburn	Poplar tea	Leaves and buds of poplar boiled in water	Applied over affected area prn
5. Dandruff	Honey shampoo		Hair is washed with water; then honey is rubbed in, and scalp is massaged
6. Short hair	Dandruff	Dandruff from someone with long hair	Scalp massaged after dandruff has been sprinkled over it; repeated nightly
7. Ringworm	Axle grease	Axle grease taken from the wheel of a wagon	Applied over scalp; not massaged
8. Eczema or hives	Dandelion lotion	Root of dandelion plant boiled in water; 1 cup mixed with ½ cup of root of dandelion plant, allowed to soak over 24 h in alcohol or kerosene	Applied prn or qhs
9. Eczema or hives	Snake oil	Oil from the skin of the snake	Rubbed over affected area qhs
10. Underarm odor	Flour		Used as underarm talcum
11. Underarm odor	Baking soda		Used as underarm talcum
12. Gonorrhea (in men)	Stale bread	Stale bread beginning to smell of mold	5 pieces eaten qd for a week
13. Syphilis	Molded bread	Molded bread soaked in tea or milk	A bowlful eaten qd for a week
14. Gonorrhea (in women)	Stale bread	Stale bread smelling of mold; a pot sterilized with boiling water; pour off some of the water, leaving half a pot of water to cool; when the water has cooled, add the stale bread and let it soak; after an afternoon of soaking, strain the water into a second sterilized pot; this water, now strained, is used as a douche	Bread is eaten for a week,and douche is done every night until pain goes away
15. Acne (thought due due to lack of orgasm)	Sexual intercourse or masturbation		
16. Warts		On day 1, patient eats several oranges and lemons with salt; he or she then takes the urine of that afternoon or the following day (while still on orange-lemon regimen)	Urine is applied weekly to wart
17. Syphilis	Egg mold	Put white of a chicken's egg into pot; add to this the mold from bread; mix	Applied as salve to chancre
18. "Bad complexion"	Honey water	1 cup honey or 1 cup water boiled with honeysuckle flowers (unopened) in it; add either to pot of sterilized water	Face is washed with solution every morning and qhs
19. Skin burn	Blueberry root salve	Roots of blueberry plant boiled as a tea; ¼ cup is added to ½ cup lard, petroleum jelly, or butter and mixed	Applied to burned area
20. Skin burn	Blackberry root salve	Same as for item 19	Applied to burned area
21. Impetigo	Peach wine mold	In fermenting peaches, allow mold to set in	The wine is drunk

(continued)

TABLE 10-3 (Continued)
Dermatologic Medications and Substances Used by Voodoo Practitioners*

Illness	Remedy	Ingredients, Preparation	How Given
22. Impetigo	Bread mold	Mold from bread mixed with small amount of petroleum jelly	Mixture is applied to affected areas
23. Pruritus	Tulip tree bark tea	Bark of tulip tree boiled as a tea	Drunk prn
24. Pruritus	Popular bark tea	Same as in item 23	Same as in item 23
25. Itching of face		½ cup honey and ½ cup vinegar added to rinse wate	Patient washes face with soap, then rinses with solution by taking deep breath and placing face in pan as long as possible
26. Onychomycosis		To a pan of hot water, add 1 cup alcohol and some "detoxified" cottonmouth moccasin poison (detoxified by putting in a jar and placing the jar in a pot of boiling water for 5 min)	Feet are bathed every night
27. Bad skin	Ant butter	1 tsp sugar mixed with level teaspoon butter; allow to draw ants; mash this mixture up until ants are blended with butter and sugar	1 tsp eaten with meals; butter applied to face at bedtime
28. Bedsore		1 part baking soda; 1 part flour; ¼ part salt	Applied over affected area
29. Bed sore	Moss butter	One packed cup fresh moss from flowing spring water, beaten up in butter until thoroughly mixed	Applied over affected area
30. Chickenpox	Sassafras tea		Drunk tid and qhs
31. Measles	Sassafras tea		Drunk tid and qhs
32. Acne	Lemon and petroleum jelly	½ cup petroleum jelly; add the juice from two lemons and mix	Applied generously qhs

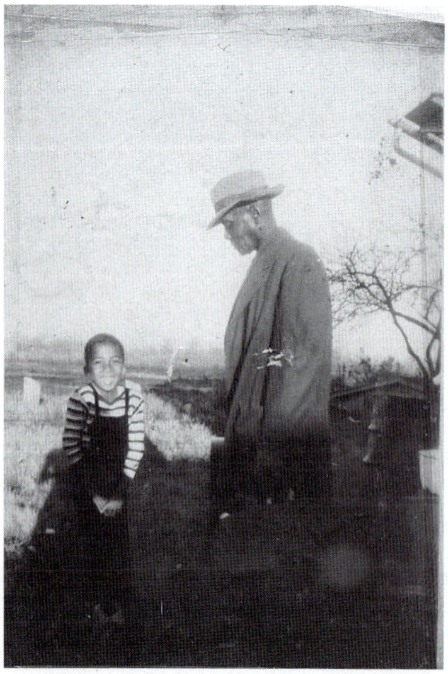

▲ **FIGURE 10-6** Dr. William Jordan is shown with his son, the author, Dr. Wilbert Jordan.

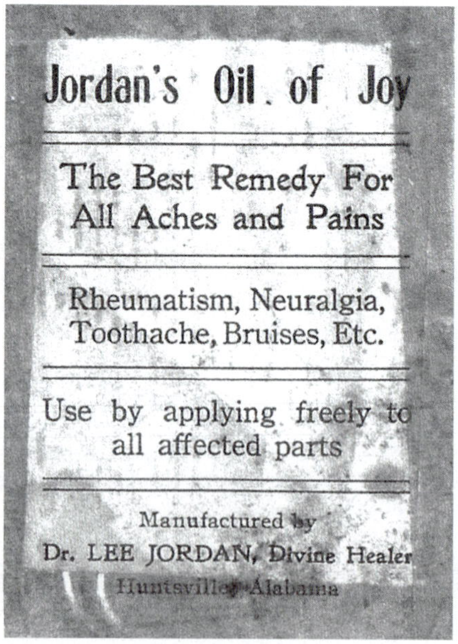

▲ **FIGURE 10-7** Advertisement for an analgesic preparation used by Dr. Lee Jordan, 1870–1912. Bottled in 4- and 8-oounce sizes (or in larger amounts in jars), it was sold throughout the Southeast from Louisiana and Arkansas to Georgia and South Carolina and north to Tennessee.

the urban environment, and as with all forms of the healing art, it must be continually reexamined.

It must be recognized that there are situations where a black patient may be better served by a priest or a spiritualist than by a medical doctor. At times, the physician must suppress his or her ego for the patient's sake when spiritualists or priests are consulted.

Table 10-3 contains a list of some medicines and remedies used by Voodoo practitioners. Figure 10-6 shows Dr. William Jordan with his son, the author, Dr. Wilbert Jordan, and Figure 10-7 shows an advertisement for a famous remedy.

I wish to express my thanks to Mrs. Annie Mae Jordan, Mrs. Helen Brown, and Bishop Sam Ella James for their help and cooperation.

REFERENCES

1. Start H. Kindling of hope in the disadvantaged: A study of the Afro-American healer, *Ment Hyg* 1971;55.
2. Wintrobe RW. Hexes, roots, snake eggs? MD vs occult. *Med Opinion* 1972;1.
3. Harvey, Bordley. *Differential Diagnosis.* Philadelphia. Saunders, 1970, pp 237-244.
4. Cannon WB. Voodoo death. *Am Anthropol* 1942;44.

CHAPTER 11

Psychiatric Aspects of Skin of Color

Curley L. Bonds

Key Points

- Skin color is the major contributor to race consciousness and prejudice, with psychological implications for the individual that are often overlooked.
- Dermatologic conditions are frequently linked to psychiatric disorders such as anxiety, depression, and social phobia.
- Medications for skin imperfections sometimes induce depression or suicidal thoughts.
- Skin abnormalities often should be evaluated to determine if they represent an underlying psychiatric disorder.
- Some psychotropic medications are associated with a wide range of skin lesions that can be serious or even life-threatening.
- Skin bleaching, tattooing, and branding are culturally-specific forms of self-mutilation in people with skin of color.
- Shared management and close collaboration among clinicians treating individuals with psycho-cutaneous disorders are important for the best outcome.

Skin color, texture, and tone are among the first things that we notice about a person. In a culture where appearances and first impressions dominate interpersonal interactions, it is appropriate that we consider the role that the skin plays in psychological health. While race is largely a sociopolitical concept, skin color is perhaps the single largest contributor to race consciousness, whereas other, less prominent physical characteristics play a secondary role.

For centuries, social inequalities have been linked to race and, as a result, to the characteristics of one's skin. The institution of slavery for African Americans was predicated in large part on the ability to distinguish one group of individuals from another based on the color of their skin.

However, other examples of bias based on skin tone and color exist throughout the globe and across most cultures. Brazilians identify social classifications along lines of skin color rather than racial ancestry.[1] In fact, Brazilian Portuguese has more than 30 words to describe various skin colorations.

In preapartheid South Africa, elaborate social classification schemas were developed based on skin tone and other racial features. For health care providers, is it essential to recognize the interrelationships between colored skin and mental health.

Research has demonstrated that cultural stereotypes exist based on skin-tone bias. This is true for both whites and minorities. An illustration of this fact comes from a historic rhyme popular among African-Americans in the mid-1900s: "If you're white, you're all right; if you're yellow, you're mellow; if you're brown, stick around; if you're black, get back."[2]

In *The Future of Race,* Henry Louis Gates, Jr., described being subjected to the "paper bag principle" during a social event that he encountered at Yale in the late 1960s. The party involved a traditional discriminatory practice that illustrates skin tone bias in the southern United States. People darker than a brown paper bag placed on the door of the party were denied entry.[3]

While empirical evidence about relative advantages of lighter or darker skin is limited, several examples in the literature demonstrate that many people attribute positive personality characteristics to lighter-skinned individuals and negative traits to those with darker skin.[4–9]

The observed preferences for lighter skin extend to members of various ethnic groups as well as to majority individuals. Discrimination based on skin tone within an ethnic group is referred to as *colorism* and can be associated with profoundly negative social and interpersonal consequences including low self-esteem and discrimination.

Keith and Herring studied African-Americans and skin-tone variance and demonstrated that higher occupational prestige, educational achievement, and family income were linked to lighter skin tones.[10] The long-term psychological implications of coping with the effects of skin-tone bias are poorly understood but should be considered when working to provide mental health interventions.

From early embryonic development, the ectoderm and neuroectoderm are connected and remain so throughout life. As a result, a strong association between dermatologic and psychiatric disorders exists. Up to a third of dermatologic conditions coexist with psychiatric disorders. A number of psychiatric, behavioral, and medical presentations have unique presentations in skin of color. A few examples will be presented in this chapter, but the list is by no means exhaustive.

PSYCHIATRIC DISORDERS WITH DERMATOLOGIC SYMPTOMS

Body Dysmorphic Disorder

Body dysmorphic disorder (BDD) is a somatoform spectrum illness characterized by a preoccupation with an imagined bodily defect (Table 11-1). Patients initially may present to primary care physicians or dermatologists with concerns about their skin. The psychopathology is the perception that a flaw or imperfection exists in the skin. The patient may be convinced that the coloring of their skin is abnormal or that his or her skin's elasticity is amiss. The patient also may perceive imagined imperfections such as scars, acne, moles, or cellulite. The focus of attention is frequently the face. Freud's Wolfman was excessively concerned about his nose and is the classic example of BDD.

BDD occurs in 10–14% of dermatology patients and 1% of the general population. Women are affected more commonly than men. The age of onset is between 15 and 20 years. Sixty percent have concurrent comorbid depression,

TABLE 11-1
Diagnostic Criteria for Body Dysmporphic Disorder (DSM-IV-TR)

A. Preoccupation with an imagined defect in appearance. If a slight physical anomaly is present, the person's concern is markedly excessive.
B. The preoccupation causes clinically significant distress or impairment in social, occupational, or other important areas of functioning.
C. The preoccupation is not better accounted for by another mental disorder (e.g., dissatisfaction with body shape and size in anorexia nervosa).

Source: From *Diagnostic and Stastical Manual of Mental Disorders,* 4th ed, text revision (DSM-IV-TR). Washington, American Psychiatric Association Press, 2000.

and the lifetime risk of depression in BDD patients is 80%. About a third of patients suffer from social phobia, usually because they are fearful of others seeing their defects. Treatment with selective serotonin reuptake inhibitors (SSRIs) helps to reduce the intensity of symptoms in about 50% of patients. Surgical, dermatologic, and other medical interventions should be avoided because they typically worsen the patient's condition. Cognitive behavioral psychotherapy also has been shown to reduce the impairment caused by symptoms.

Mood and Anxiety Disorders

Skin lesions and disfigurement resulting from dermatologic conditions may have a profound impact on psychological functioning. Visible scars and depigmented or hyperpigmented patches of skin often become the focus of depressive thoughts in those who are prone to mood disorders. Social anxiety and reclusive behavior may result from severe disfigurement. The stress of living with chronic acne, warts, herpes, or psoriasis may trigger feelings of shame, depression, rage, and hopelessness.

Cultural stigma associated with mental health treatment means that patients of color are much more likely to consult a dermatologist or primary care provider, hoping that treatment of the perceived skin lesion may improve their sense of well-being. Patients who experience permanent visible scarring, such as those with keloids (Figure 11-1) or cystic acne, should be questioned about psychosocial functioning and mood symptoms during the clinical interview. Assessing the seriousness of depressive symptoms is important for these patients so that appropriate treatment can be initiated. Depression as a clinical syndrome requires the presence of at least five of nine cardinal symptoms, including

1. Depressed mood
2. Sleep disturbance (hyposomnia or hypersomnia)
3. Appetite disturbance (increased or anorexia)
4. Decreased interest in usual activities
5. Poor energy (or restless energy)
6. Problems with concentration
7. Guilty thoughts
8. Psychomotor slowing or agitation
9. Suicidal thoughts (or recurrent death-themed fantasies)

Depressed individuals also may report low self-worth and feelings of hopelessness and helplessness. The presence of these symptoms in the absence of clearly precipitating changes in psychosocial circumstances is suggestive of a major depressive episode. Psychosis may complicate severe depression. The psychosis may take the form of delusional thoughts, including somatic delusions focused on skin abnormalities.

While some skin conditions certainly may cause depression and anxiety, there exist psychophysiologic disorders in which the dermatologic condition is precipitated or aggravated by stress.[11] The list includes atopic dermatitis, *acne excoriée des jeune filles*, hyperhidrosis, urticaria, seborrheic dermatitis, rosacea, and pruritus. In most cases, treatment of the comorbid psychological distress helps the skin condition to improve.

It is important to note that several medications used to treat dermatologic conditions may induce depression as a side effect. The most common offenders include isotretinoin, interferon, prednisone, and other steroids. In February 1998, Roche laboratories issued a letter to all physicians warning of the increased risk of depression with isotretinoin (Accutane):

> Psychiatric disorders: Accutane may cause depression, psychosis and, rarely, suicidal ideation, suicide attempts and suicide. Discontinuation of Accutane therapy may be insufficient; further evaluation may be necessary. No mechanism of action has been established for these events.

The product labeling now states that discontinuation of therapy in some patients resulted in a reduction in depression but that depression recurred when the drug was reinstituted. Clinicians should be cautious in using this agent, especially in patients who have a history of depression.

In many cases, the medication-induced depression is severe and may lead to suicidal thoughts or plans. This level of depression is considered a psychiatric emergency, and the inciting drug should be stopped or tapered immediately and the patient referred for a full psychiatric assessment.

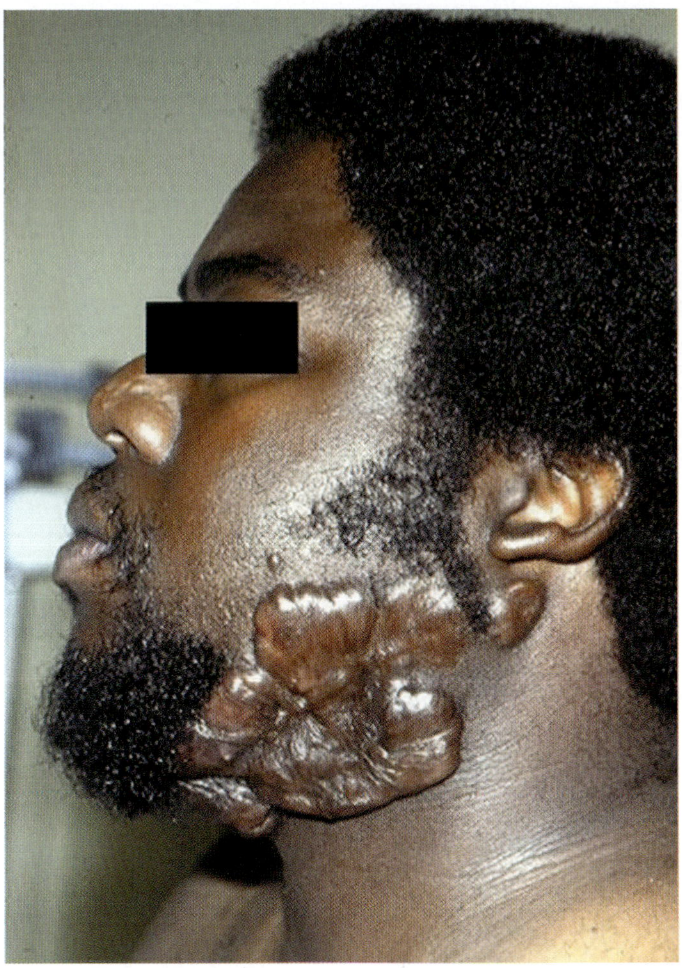

▲ **FIGURE 11-1** Keloid. Profile shot showing large keloid on chin and neck area.

TABLE 11-2
Diagnostic Criteria for Trichotillomania

A. Recurrent pulling out of one's hair resulting in noticeable hair loss.
B. An increasing sense of tension immediately before pulling out the hair or when attempting to resist the behavior.
C. Pleasure, gratification, or relief when pulling out the hair.
D. The disturbance is not better accounted for by another mental disorder and is not due to a general medical condition (e.g., a dermatologic condition).
E. The disturbance causes clinically significant distress or impairment in social, occupational, or other important areas of functioning.

Source: From *Diagnostic and Stastical Manual of Mental Disorders,* 4th ed, text revision (DSM-IV-TR). Washington, American Psychiatric Association Press, 2000.

Trichotillomania

Trichotillomania is an impulse-control disorder characterized by recurrent hair pulling resulting in visible hair loss (Table 11-2). Patients often report an increase in anxiety or tension prior to the pulling out of hair that is resolved by the act. Attempts to resist the behavior result in escalating anxiety and tension, making the behavior difficult to resist. Symptoms usually worsen when the individual is under stress. However, some individuals pull or twist their hair in an absent-minded, distracted fashion when they are bored or inactive. The scalp is most commonly affected. However, the hairs of eyebrows, eyelashes, the pubic area, the extremities, and the trunk also may become targets.[12] In about a quarter of patients, the onset is linked to some stressful event. Diagnostic criteria include a sense of pleasure, gratification, or relief when hair pulling occurs. The activity of hair pulling must cause clinically significant distress or impairment in social, occupational, or other important areas of functioning.

While the condition may be benign, effective treatments usually involve co-management by a psychiatrist and dermatologist. Psychopharmacologic options include clomipramine (a serotonergic tricyclic antidepressant), SSRIs, lithium, and naltrexone. Antipsychotic agents, particularly pimozide (Orap) or the newer atypical neuroleptics, may be useful to augment the effects of serotonergic drugs. Nonpharmacologic psychiatric interventions that have shown some success include hypnosis, relaxation training, biofeedback, and behavior therapy. Recently, Lee and colleagues described a novel dermatologic approach to trichotillomania in a case report of laser hair removal as a treatment option.[13] The patient's illness involved hairs on the legs only, so the ability to generalize this approach to other patients is limited.

Pathologic skin picking is related to trichotillomania, but it also has been linked to obsessive-compulsive and body dysmorphic disorders. Patients with the condition may spend minutes to hours of each day picking. Individuals with BDD may specifically focus their picking behaviors on areas of skin that they feel are abnormal. Eventually, the picking itself leads to scarring, which then can intensify the attention paid to the area, creating a vicious cycle of inspection, picking, and tissue damage. Multiple medications have been studied. Unfortunately, most trials have been open label and limited in size. Drug interventions showing the greatest effectiveness are similar to those used to treat trichotillomania: SSRIs and tricyclic antidepressants, dual noradrenergic and serotonin reuptake inhibitors, and lamotrigine.

PSYCHOGENIC SKIN DISORDERS

Delusions of Parasitosis

Delusions are firm and fixed beliefs that can occur in a variety of forms. Classic paranoid delusions involve thoughts that someone is following, watching, or monitoring the individual, usually with malicious intent. Other delusional disorders may involve grandiose, jealous, erotic, or somatic themes. Delusions of parasitosis are classified as somatic type and consist of the belief that parasites are living beneath the skin. This condition should be distinguished from *formication,* the sensation of bugs crawling beneath the skin, which is frequently experienced during cocaine withdrawal.

MORGELLON SYNDROME

A condition related to delusions of parasitosis is Morgellon syndrome. In addition to the sensations of insect-like creatures crawling beneath the skin, Morgellon patients also experience debilitating fatigue, cognitive dysfunction, and fiber-like filaments, granules, or crystals beneath the skin that can be extracted from their lesions. This disorder has gained a strong following of self-proclaimed sufferers who have developed support groups and proposed diagnostic criteria. Patients usually present to dermatologists for care. Individuals may bring in "samples" of the alleged offending organism wrapped in paper tissue or cellophane wrap. They may spend an inordinate amount of time scratching, picking, and surveying their epidermis in efforts to locate parasites or other organisms thought to be responsible for their infestation. Pimozide (Orap) traditionally has been the "gold standard" of treatment, but newer atypical antipsychotics also should be considered and may be better tolerated.

Published studies about psychiatric interventions for this disorder are sparse because affected individuals often reject psychiatric diagnoses or care. The best approach to the patient is to avoid excessive biopsies and manipulations of skin to prove or disprove the existence of invaders. The clinician should provide support and reassure the individual that he or she is aware of the distress that the alleged parasites cause despite their origins. Patients sometimes can be convinced to take medications if they learn that they may increase their ability to cope with what appears to be a medically unsolvable situation.

DERMATOLOGIC AND MEDICAL DIAGNOSES

Dermatitis Artefacta and Other Self-Inflicted Lesions

A great number of dermatologic conditions have unique psychological components when they occur in pigmented skin. *Dermatitis artefacta* is the deliberate production of skin wounds to resolve an unconscious psychological conflict or emotional need. It is considered to be a factitious disorder because the patient is aware of his or her behavior but denies responsibility for the lesions. Although rare overall, some forms of *dermatitis artefacta* are worth mentioning here because of cultural factors that may place people of color at increased risk for them. In the clinical assessment, looking for a life-altering event or trauma is important because the onset of self-inflicted skin injury frequently follows an emotional disturbance.[14]

Self-Mutilation

The incidence of *self-mutilating* or *cutting behaviors* appears to be increasing. This is particularly true among adolescents, in whom awareness of this behavior is

TABLE 11-3
Diagnostic Criteria for Borderline Personality Disorder

A pervasive pattern of instability of interpersonal relationships, self-image, and affects and marked impulsivity beginning by early adulthood and present in a variety of contexts, as indicated by five (or more) of the following:

1. Frantic efforts to avoid real or imagined abandonment. *Note:* Do not include suicidal or self-mutilating behavior covered in criterion 5.
2. A pattern of unstable and intense interpersonal relationships characterized by alternating between extremes of idealization and devaluation.
3. Identity disturbance: markedly and persistently unstable self-image of sense of self.
4. Impulsivity in at least two areas that are potentially self-damaging (e.g., spending, sex, substance abuse, reckless driving, and binge eating). *Note:* Do not include suicidal or self-mutilating behavior covered in criterion 5.
5. Recurrent suicidal behaviors, gestures, or threats or self-mutilating behavior.
6. Affective instability owing to a marked reactivity of mood (e.g., intense episodic dysphoria, irritability, or anxiety usually lasting a few hours and only rarely more than a few days).
7. Chronic feelings of emptiness.
8. Inappropriate, intense anger or difficulty controlling anger (e.g., frequent displays of temper, constant anger, and recurrent physical fights).
9. Transient, stress-related paranoid ideation or severe dissociative symptoms.

Source: From *Diagnostic and Stastical Manual of Mental Disorders,* 4th ed, text revision (DSM-IV-TR). Washington, American Psychiatric Association Press, 2000.

increasing. Self-mutilation may be associated with personality disorders and in fact is an essential feature listed in the diagnostic criteria for borderline personality disorder (Table 11-3).

Usually the individual cuts, pierces, or picks at his or her skin in efforts to replace psychic pain with physical pain. Patients often report an increase in mental tension or anxiety prior to an episode of self-mutilation. This tension may be released after the act of cutting, resulting in a powerful but temporary sense of well-being and calmness. Patients may go to great lengths to disguise marks or place them only on private skin so that the behavior is not easily detected.

The highest-risk group for self-mutilation remains young white women; however, in jail and prison settings, inmates often engage in self-injury in efforts to gain attention and medical or mental health treatment. In emergency departments, roughly 50% of patients who self-mutilate have a psychiatric diagnosis.[15] When a patient presents for medical care of a self-inflicted wound, the clinician should seize the opportunity to screen for psychiatric illness and to offer a referral for mental health services when appropriate. In some native Africans and aboriginal tribes, ritual mutilation may be a culturally sanctioned practice and therefore not considered to be psychopathologic.

Tattooing

Over the past two decades, social norms have shifted and moved tattoos into the mainstream. Earlier literature linked tattooing to antisocial and other unstable personality traits. The popularity of tattooing renders these perspectives dated and obsolete today. An online poll conducted in 2003 by Harris Interactive showed that 16% of American adults had at least one tattoo. The numbers increased for those between the ages of 25 and 29 to 36%. Themes and images present in tattoos can give the clinician insight into how the individual views himself or herself and his or her relationship with the world around him or her. Gang affiliations are often memorialized with tattoos. This, of course, creates problems when the individual opts to make a lifestyle change because these semipermanent markers serve as a reminder of past affiliations and behaviors. Self-inflicted tattoos, common among teens and inmates, can have specialized meanings. For instance, in Mexican gangs and prison culture, a teardrop tattoo worn on the face usually indicates that the individual has committed murder at some time. The symbol is intended to intimidate viewers and warn them that the tattooed individual is dangerous and powerful. In Filipino culture, a tattoo of a question mark anywhere on the body indicates membership in the notoriously violent and dangerous *Bahala Na Gang* (BNG, or "Come What May"). Understanding the meaning behind tattoos requires knowledge of local and regional codes that may change over time.

In other settings, impulsive, intoxicated individuals may wake up from a night on the town during which a tattoo was obtained and live to regret their decision to be tattooed. Only about 17% of Americans in the same poll previously quoted expressed regret about their tattoos. The risk factors most commonly sited for regret include being a Republican, living in the South, and having a person's name in the tattoo. Fortunately, laser technology has made tattoo removal possible. However, the effectiveness of the equipment on darker skin and the cost can be prohibitive for many minority patients. However, the importance of erasing distinctive gang tattoos from visible skin should not be underestimated in the full psychosocial rehabilitation of patients who aspire to move beyond past life choices.

Branding

Some African-American fraternity brothers use self-inflicted wounds caused by branding to indicate a sense of group identity and belonging. This controversial rite of passage for inductees to black Greek letter organizations creates unpredictable results. Some brand wounds heal with neatly raised scars outlining an emblem or symbol; in other cases, careful cleansing creates a flat scar (Figure 11-2). Some individuals intentionally pick at scabs that form on the wound in hopes of creating a keloid. In a psychological context, the history of using branding among plantation owners to mark slaves as property is difficult to overlook. One interpretation of an individual's independent decision to undergo branding is that he is advertising his ability to make choices for himself.[16] Generally, self-inflicted branding does not represent a psychiatric symptom but rather a form of self-expression.[17] Ironically, branding can be viewed by disapproving outsiders as a form of identification with a historical aggressor because pain is inherent to the process of branding. Branding also may be used in some tribal cultures as a form of therapeutic healing.[18] The complications of branding that may require medical attention include infections, transmission of blood-borne pathogens, allergic reactions, and injury related to a third-degree burn.

Skin Bleaching

The desire to have lighter skin leads some individuals with skin of color to extreme measures. Skin bleaching

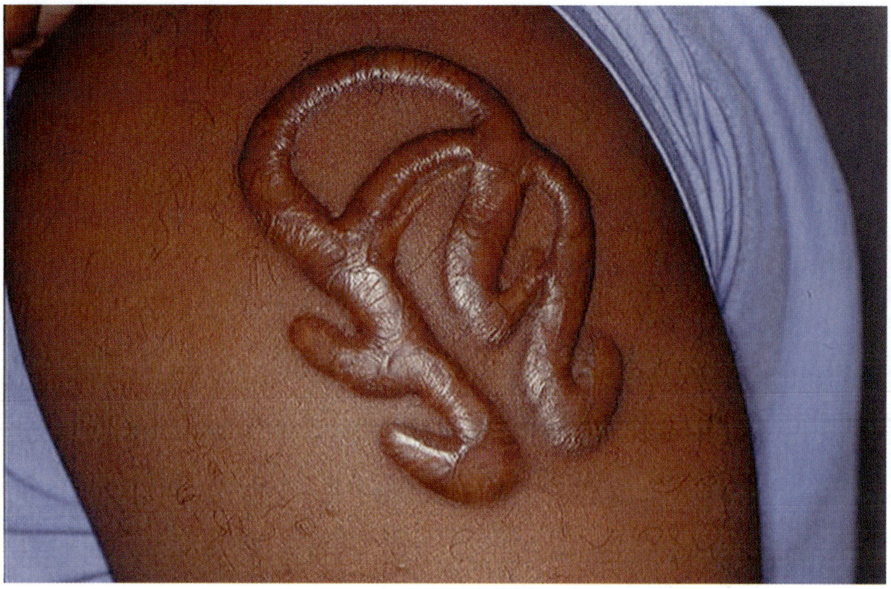

▲ **FIGURE 11-2** Fraternity branding. Bicep showing Greek letter brand.

agents are aggressively marketed to Asian consumers, who sometime will go to great lengths to lighten their complexions. The psychological motivation among Asians as well as others with darker skin is the rationale that lighter skin is associated with greater wealth, education, and upper-class status. Many of the commercially available products are poorly regulated and contain hydroquinone in dangerous quantities.

VITILIGO

Vitiligo results in a marked loss of skin pigmentation, which is more easily noticeable in individuals with a naturally dark skin color (Figure 11-3). Individuals with this autoimmune depigmenting disorder can experience extreme shame and depression related to the seemingly uncontrollable and unpredictable course of the disease. Retreat from society because of "anticipated rejection" is common, especially in children, who can be subjected to extremely hurtful and humiliating comments.[19] Michael Jackson's public disclosure that he has vitiligo during a 1993 interview with Oprah Winfrey resulted in greater public awareness of the illness. Prior to this, even he was the victim of many unkind comments from critics who saw his progressive depigmentation, along with facial plastic surgery, as an attempt to transform himself into a Caucasian.

PSYCHOTROPIC MEDICATIONS AND DERMATOLOGIC PROBLEMS

Mood Stabilizers

Lithium remains a mainstay for treatment of bipolar disorder. It is an excellent mood stabilizer that has the reputation of decreasing the risk of completed suicides in depressed patients. In addition, it may be used in lower doses to augment antidepressants. It also may cause or worsen acne and psoriasis and should be avoided in patients with these preexisting conditions because compliance may be adversely affected. Male patients are at greater risk than female patients.[19] Gupta and colleagues reported a case of lithium-induced hidradenitis suppurativa and also found that other cutaneous side effects of lithium include folliculitis, alopecia, and a maculopapular/macular eruption.[21] Hair also may lose its curl or wave. Lithium-related cutaneous lesions are also slower to respond to conventional therapy while the patient continues to receive lithium.[21]

Anticonvulsant Mood Stabilizers

Lamotrogine is an anticonvulsant mood stabilizer that is also indicated by the Food and Drug Administration (FDA) for treatment of major depression.[22] The primary dermatologic concern with this medication is that it may cause Stevens-Johnson syndrome, or toxic epidermal necroylsis. The incidence is low, and the syndrome is usually prevented when proper dosing guidelines are followed. Serious rashes from lamotrigine are usually confluent and located on the face, neck, soles, and palms. The rash may be manifested by

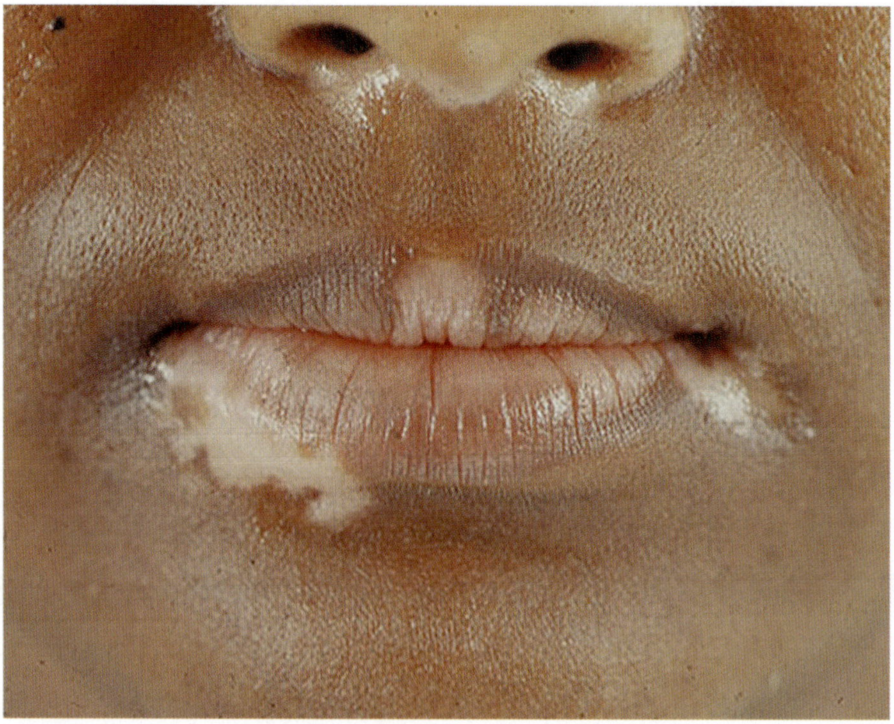

▲ **FIGURE 11-3** Vitiligo. Lips with surrounding patches of hypopigmentation.

a purpuric or hemorrhagic appearance and may be associated with fever, malaise, pharyngitis, anorexia, or lymphadenopathy.[23] The patient should stop the drug immediately and seek emergency medical attention. Critical care in an intensive care unit setting is usually warranted. The risk of rash increases exponentially when valproic acid is coadministered with lamotrigine. Thus, when the two drugs are used simultaneously, the initial dose and rate of dose escalation of lamotrigine should be adjusted accordingly. Calabrese published a thorough review of lamotrigine-related rashes, including a detailed discussion of clinical management.[24]

Other anticonvulsant mood stabilizers include valproic acid and carbamazepine. Carbamazepine is much more likely to cause rashes, but most of these are benign. Oxcarbamazepine (Trileptal) is a newer alternative to carbamazepine and appears to cause fewer rashes. About 75% of patients who develop rash with carbamazepine will tolerate oxcarbamazepine.[25] Valproate is known to interfere with liver function and may cause elevated clotting times. Visible bruises may be the first warning that liver function has been adversely affected. Valproate is also known to cause alopecia. This can be addressed by administering a multivitamin containing zinc and selenium.[26]

Other classes of psychotropic medications are also associated with multiple dermatologic diagnoses. Table 11-4 provides an outline of the cutaneous side effects attributed to other psychopharmacologic agents.

TABLE 11-4
Cutaneous Side Effects of Psychiatric Drugs

Antipsychotics	Blue-gray discoloration of skin Photosensitivity Lupus-like syndrome Erythematous maculopapular rash Contact dermatitis Seborrheic dermatitis SJS/erythema multiforme Purpura Urticaria Palmar erythema
Anxiolytics	Exacerbation of porphyria Fixed drug eruption Hyperpigmentation Bullous lesions Maculopapular rash Photosensitivity Urticaria Erythema multiforme Erythema nodosum
Antidepressants	Maculopapular, pustular rash Urticaria Petechiae Photosensitivity Vasculitis Leukonychia Acne Alopecia Erythema multiforme Pustular psoriasis
Anticonvulsants	Maculopapular rash Hypersensitivyt reactions Exfoliative dermatitis Systemic lupus erythematosus Alopecia Erythema multiforme/SJS/TEN Urticaria Hair color changes Scleroderma Vasculitis
Lithium	Psoriasiform lesions Acneiform lesions Vaginal and other mucosal ulcerations Hidradenitis suppurativa Follicular hyperkeratosis Exacerbation of Darier's disease Lichenoid stomatitis Erythematous maculopapular rash Hair loss Increased growth of warts Geographic tongue

Abbreviations: SJS = Stevens-Johnson syndrome; TEN = toxic epidermal necrolysis
Source: From Jafferany M. Psychodermatology: A guide to understanding common psychocutaneous disorders. *Primary Care Companion J Clin Psychiatry* 2007;9:203–211.

CONCLUSION

The interrelationships between psychological and dermatologic disorders are complex. Treating these conditions in patients of color presents the clinician with added challenges. The best approach to psychocutaneous disorders involves shared management between medical and mental health professionals working toward agreed-on treatment goals. The overall health status of all patients can be improved if psychological factors are considered during the treatment of dermatologic disorders.

ACKNOWLEDGMENT

Special thanks to Michelle O. Clark, M.D. (reviewer).

REFERENCES

1. Telles E. *Race in Another America: The Significance of Skin color in Brazil.* Princeton, NJ, Princeton University Press, 2004.
2. Brown KT. Consequences of skin tone bias for African-Americans: Resource attainment and psychological/social. *Afr Am Res Perspect* 1998;4:1–9.
3. Gates HL. *The Future of Race.* New York, Vintage Books, 1997.

4. Seeman M. Skin color values in three all-Negro school classes. *Am Sociol Review* 1946;11:315–321.
5. Porter CP. Social reasons for skin tone preferences of black school-age children. *Am J Orthopsychiatry* 1991;61:8149–154.
6. Goering JM. Changing perceptions and evaluations of physical characteristics among blacks. *Phylon* 1971;33:231–241.
7. Robinson TL, Ward JV. African-American adolescents and skin color. *J Black Psychology* 1995;21:256–274.
8. Bond S, Cash FT. Black beauty: Skin color and body images among African-American college women. *J Negro Ed* 1992;46:76–88.
9. Hall RE. Bias among African-Americans regarding skin color: Implications for social work practice. *Res Social Work Prac* 1992;2:479–486.
10. Keith VM, Herring C. Skin tone and stratification in the black community. *Am J Sociol* 1991;97:760–778.
11. Jafferany M. Psychodermatology: A guide to understanding common psychocutaneous disorders. *Primary Care Companion J Clin Psychiatry* 2007;9:203–211.
12. Hautmann G, Hercogova J, Torello L. Trichotillomania. *J Am Acad Dermatol* 2003;45: 807–826.
13. Lee SJ, Park SG, Kang JM, et al. Laser hair removal as an option for treatment of trichotillomania: A case report. *Eur Acad Dermatol Venereal* 2006;21:1413–1450.
14. Fabish W. Psychiatric aspects of dermatitis artefacta. *Br J Dermatol* 1980;102: 29–34.
15. Olfson M, Gameroff MJ, Marcus SC, et al. Emergency treatment of young people following deliberate self-harm. *Arch Gen Psychiatr* 2005;62:1122–1128.
16. Posey SM. Burning messages: Interpreting African-American fraternity brands and their bearers. *Voices* 2004;30: 3–4.
17. Karamanoukian R, Ukatu C, Lee E, et al. Aesthetic skin branding: A novel form of body art with adverse clinical sequela. *J Burn Care Res* 2006;27:108–110.
18. Kumar S, Kumar PR. Skin branding. *J Postgrad Med* 2004;50:204.
19. Parsand D, Prasand S, Kumarasing W. *Psychosocial Implications of Pigmentary Disorders in Asia.* Singapore, PanAmerican Society for Pigment Cell Research Commentary, 2006.
20. Chan H, Wing Y, Su R. A control study of the cutaneous side effects of chronic lithium therapy. *J Affect Disord* 2000;57: 107–113.
21. Gupta AK, Knowles SR, Gupta MA, et al. Lithium therapy associated with hidradenitis suppurativa: Case report and a review of the dermatologic side effects of lithium. *J Am Acad Dermatol* 2004;32:382–386.
22. Lamictal (prescribing information), in *Physicians' Desk Reference,* 59th ed. Montvale, NJ, Medical Economics Company, 2005.
23. Guberman A, Besag F, Brodie M, et al. Lamotrigine-associated rash: Risk/benefit considerations in adults and children. *Epilepsia* 1999;40:985–991.
24. Calabrese JR, Sullivan JR, Bowden CL, et al. Rash in multicenter trials of lamotrigine in mood disorders: Clinical relevance and management. *J Clin Psychiatr* 2002; 63:1012–1019.
25. Ketter TA, Wang PW, Post RM. Carbamazepine and oxcarbazepine, in Schatzberg AF, Nemeroff CB (eds), *Essentials of Clinical Psychopharmacology*. Washington, American Psychiatric Publishing, 2006.
26. Hurd RW, Van Rinsvelt HA, Wilder BJ, et al. Selenium, zinc, and copper changes with valproic acid: Possible relations to drug side effects. *Neurology* 1984;34: 1393–1395.

American Psychiatric Association. *Diagnostic and Stastical Manual of Mental Disorders,* 4th ed., text revision. Washington, American Psychiatric Association Press, 2000.

SECTION 2

Structure, Function, and Biology

CHAPTER 12

The Structure and Function of Skin of Color

Sonia Badreshia-Bansal
Susan C. Taylor

TABLE 12-1
Population Distribution by Race/Ethnicity[1,2]

YEAR	NON-HISPANIC WHITE	AFRICAN AMERICAN	ALL OTHER
2000	69.1%	12.3%	18.6%
2005	67.1%	12.5%	20.4%
2010	64.8%	12.7%	22.5%
2015	62.8%	12.9%	24.3%
2020	60.8%	13.1%	26.1%

Source: Modified version of Census Bureau middle-series projections.

Key Points

- It has been predicted that the international population will constitute a majority in the United States in the twenty-first century.
- There is a dearth of medical knowledge on racial and ethnic differences in skin of color.
- Epidermal differences include stratum corneum structure, lipid content, and melanin dispersion.
- Dermal differences include varied structural organization and concentration of dermal components.
- Although few definitive conclusions can be made with sparse research, biologic differences do exist.
- These biologic differences in skin structure and function account for lower rates of skin cancers and less pronounced photoaging but also increased incidence of keloids and a variety of pigmentary disorders.

The latest Census figures forecast an increasing ethnically diverse population in America. Demand for health care services by individuals with skin of color is increasing as these groups grow. Higher birth rates among racial and ethnically diverse groups, as well as immigration, suggest that this trend will continue. Table 12-1 exhibits the current and projected distribution of the population across three diverse groups.[1] As this trend continues into the twenty-first century, the rapidly expanding skin of color population will become the majority and constitute most of the American and global health care frontier. Although the current U.S. population is still predominately Caucasian, minority populations are growing 12 times faster than the white population. In the next 25 years, there will be a 50% growth in ethnically and racially diverse populations.

Racial and ethnic populations are currently unevenly distributed geographically within the United States. Their proportions vary substantially by state, with disproportionate numbers in major metropolitan areas. If health care utilization patterns and physician productivity patterns remain constant over time, an increasing amount of total patient care hours will be spent by individuals who have skin of color[1] (Figure 12-1). In 2020, physicians will be spending approximately 14% of patient care hours with African-Americans and 26% of hours with patients of other racial and ethnically diverse groups. Although the racial and ethnic composition of the physician workforce varies substantially by specialty, it is composed predominantly of Caucasians. This highlights the need to educate all physicians, especially dermatologists, regarding the differences between the structure and function of ethnic skin[2] (Table 12-2 and Figure 12-2).

Several studies that will be discussed have conflicting data regarding racial differences.[3] The few studies that have been cited in the literature lack a standard approach in study design and include small patient populations. Therefore, few definitive conclusions can be made.

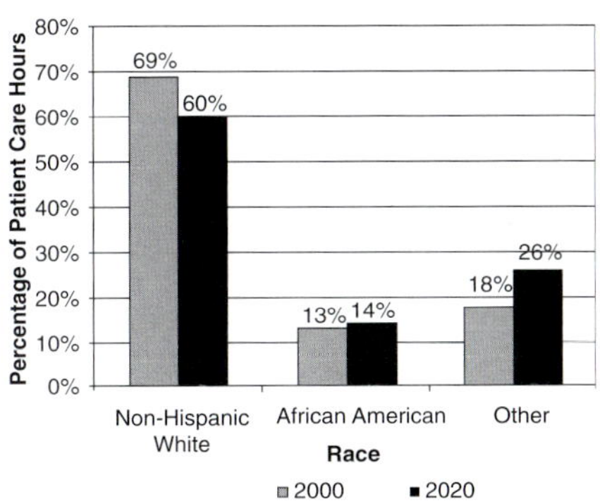

▲ **FIGURE 12-1** Distribution of total patient care hours by patient race: total active physicians in patient care.[1]

STRATUM CORNEUM

Structure and Function

The stratum corneum forms the interface between the external environment and the body and influences barrier function and subsequently the potential for irritant reactions. The primary function of the stratum corneum is to prevent evaporative water loss from the aqueous interior cell layers. The stratum corneum also protects against mechanical insults, foreign chemicals, microorganisms, and ultraviolet light.

The stratum corneum consists of a two-compartment system, termed *bricks and mortar,* that is composed of polyhedral corneocytes surrounded by a matrix of lipid-enriched membranes. The corneocytes are filled with keratin filaments and osmotically active small molecules, including filaggrin. The corneocyte cytosol is encased by a chemically resistant, flexible cell envelope. Lipids in the intercellular spaces of the stratum corneum provide the permeability barrier of the skin. The main lipids comprising the barrier are ceramides, cholesterol, and long-chain saturated fatty acids. The intercellular lipids of the stratum corneum are organized into elaborate multilamellar structures. In a variety of pathologic conditions, the lipid composition and organization are altered, leading to a reduced capacity to hold water and increased transepidermal water loss (TEWL).

Structural Differences

Attention has been focused on the thickness, density, and compactness of the stratum corneum when comparing skin of color with white skin. The thickness of the stratum corneum in white and black skin is generally thought to be similar.[4] A comparative study investigating the number of tape strips required to completely remove the stratum corneum

TABLE 12-2
Percent Distribution of Physicians by Race and Ethnicity in 1999[3]

Specialty	Non-Hispanic White	African American	Hispanic	Asian	Other	American Indian /Alaskan Native
Total MDs	75.4	3.6	4.9	12.6	3.5	0.1
Aerospace medicine	91.1	2.1	3.4	2.1	1.3	0.0
Allergy and immunology	79.0	1.4	3.7	12.2	3.6	0.1
Anesthesiology	71.5	3.4	4.2	16.9	4.1	0.1
Cardiovascular disease	71.1	2.4	4.9	15.2	6.2	0.1
Child psychiatry	73.5	4.8	7.0	10.2	4.3	0.2
Colon/rectal surgery	81.6	1.8	5.1	9.8	1.7	0.0
Dermatology	**87.4**	**2.5**	**2.7**	**5.9**	**1.4**	**0.0**
Diagnostic radiology	80.2	2.0	3.5	11.5	2.7	0.1
Emergency medicine	82.4	4.1	4.2	7.3	1.8	0.1
Family practice	79.2	4.1	5.4	8.8	2.3	0.2
Forensic pathology	82.2	3.7	4.7	8.3	0.7	0.3
Gastroenterology	71.5	3.1	4.8	14.8	5.8	0.0
General practice	75.5	2.2	7.9	13.6	0.7	0.0
General preventive medicine	82.1	6.3	3.5	6.6	1.4	0.1
General surgery	78.3	3.4	4.6	10.9	2.7	0.1
Internal medicine	67.0	4.1	5.1	17.9	5.8	0.1
Medical genetics	84.6	1.9	3.4	8.0	2.2	0.0
Neurology	72.8	1.9	5.2	14.1	5.9	0.0
Neurologic surgery	82.7	2.5	3.9	7.8	3.1	0.1
Nuclear medicine	71.0	2.0	5.7	16.8	4.4	0.0
Obstetrics/gynecology	77.2	6.2	5.3	9.3	2.0	0.1
Occupational medicine	88.6	2.9	3.0	4.6	0.9	0.1
Ophthalmology	84.6	2.2	2.9	7.9	2.4	0.1
Orthopedic surgery	88.7	2.4	2.4	4.7	1.7	0.1
Otolaryngology	84.3	2.0	3.2	8.7	1.7	0.0
Pathology, anatomic/clinical	74.5	1.9	4.9	15.5	3.3	0.0
Pediatrics	68.6	4.8	6.7	15.7	4.0	0.1
Pediatric cardiology	75.7	2.0	5.6	11.5	5.0	0.1
Physical medicine/ rehababilitation	65.2	4.4	6.2	20.6	3.7	0.1
Plastic surgery	84.8	1.8	3.6	7.5	2.3	0.0
Psychiatry	75.0	3.2	5.6	12.7	3.4	0.1
Pulmonary diseases	75.7	2.6	5.2	12.3	4.2	0.1
Radiology	85.7	1.4	2.2	8.8	1.7	0.0
Radiation oncology	73.5	2.7	3.2	17.4	3.2	0.0
Thoracic surgery	67.2	4.2	5.6	10.5	12.2	0.3
Urologic surgery	82.7	2.8	3.5	8.7	2.2	0.1
Other	88.2	2.0	3.4	5.5	0.9	0.0

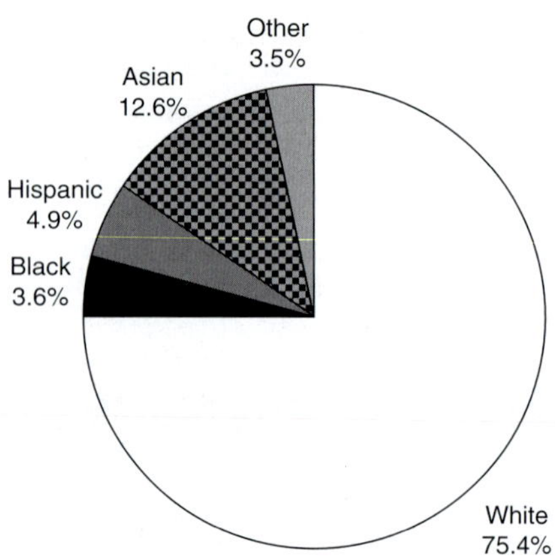

▲ **FIGURE 12-2** Race distribution of the physician workforce, 1999.[3]

(a measure of the number of layers of the stratum corneum) demonstrated a greater variability in tape strippings in black subjects compared with white subjects. Black subjects required a higher number of tape strippings than white subjects.[4–7] The degree of pigmentation had no correlation with the number of cell layers observed in a few studies.[4,8] Microscopic differences also included greater average stratum corneum layers in black skin compared with white skin. This led to the conclusion that since thickness was equal in both groups, the stratum corneum in black skin must be more cohesive and compact.[4]

This observation was confirmed when comparing skin phototypes V and VI with phototypes II and III.[7] The darker skin phototypes required more tape strippings to disrupt the epidermal barrier. This led to the conclusion that more cornified compact cell layers in dark skin could display superior epidermal barrier function and faster recovery from barrier damage. No differences were found between white skin and Asian skin. Hence the differences were demonstrated to be related to skin phototype instead of race.

Another recent study of a small number of patients confirmed equal stratum corneum thickness with greater cohesiveness and intercellular lipid content in blacks compared with whites.[9] In one experiment, the composition of lipids was found to vary, with the lowest ceramide level found in blacks, followed by whites, Hispanics, and Asians.[10] Ceramide levels were inversely correlated with TEWL and directly related to water content.

In examining corneocyte surface area, there appears to be inconsistent data. A comparative study among African-Americans, white Americans, and Asians of Chinese descent showed no difference in corneocyte surface area, but there was increased spontaneous corneocyte desquamation in the black group, which was attributed to a difference in the composition of the lipids of the stratum corneum.[11] This contrasts with another study that found a greater desquamation index of corneocytes of the cheeks and foreheads of white subjects compared with black subjects.[12]

In contrast to these observations, one study reported a trend toward a thicker stratum corneum in black skin compared with white skin.[13] However, these finding have not been substantiated using standard methodologies.

Functional Differences

The barrier properties of the skin depend on an intact stratum corneum, among several other factors.[14] Skin permeability is related to the thickness of the epidermis and density of cutaneous appendages, thus allowing penetration into the capillary system in the dermis.[15–17] Studies of racial and ethnic differences in percutaneous absorption have demonstrated conflicting results. Small study populations do not allow for unequivocal results. When investigating black versus white skin by several methodologies, including evaluation of vasodilatation or laser Doppler velocimetry (LDV) in response to percutaneous absorption of methyl-nicotinate, there was no difference in absorption.[18,19] However, one study did demonstrate greater LDV output in both black and Asian skin versus white skin.[20]

Skin irritation is another controversial area where multiple poorly designed studies offer conflicting results. Methodologic flaws include studies relying on investigator observation of erythema induced by various chemicals as a primary endpoint in pigmented skin.[4,21–24] As a result, this subjective assessment led these researchers to conclude that black subjects were less susceptible to irritants than white subjects. Irritation was inversely proportional to skin color, so white or lightly complected subjects were most susceptible to irritation.[25,26] Also, interindividual variability to irritants can be a confounding variable leading to inaccurate conclusions.

Instead of using the subjective measurement of erythema, more recent studies relied on TEWL and other objective measures of irritancy.[27–34] However, these studies have their own flaws. These studies used occluded topical sodium lauryl sulfate (SLS) in normal skin but also in pretreated skin that removed the stratum corneum and in preoccluded skin that increased water content. Clinical relevance is questioned when the normal skin model is not used. The irritant effect of SLS was secondary to disruption in stratum corneum integrity that used objective measurements, including TEWL (evaporimetry), capacitance (water content), and LDV (microcirculation). These studies concluded that black subjects (1) display a stronger skin irritant reaction, (2) have more sensitive skin, and (3) display less erythema, blood vessel reactivity, and cutaneous blood flow than white subjects. They also concluded that Hispanic subjects showed (1) strong irritant reaction similar to black subjects, (2) strong irritant reactions when injured, and (3) similar erythematous reactions when compared with white subjects.

However, these conclusions are based only on an altered preoccluded skin model. A compromised skin barrier undoubtedly will result in increased susceptibility to irritants. However, for the untreated normal skin model, there were no significant differences in stratum corneum integrity. Therefore, the conclusions noted earlier would better substantiated if these values were observed in an untreated skin model.[3]

Another comparative study of skin complexion among fair-skinned Chinese, darker-skinned Malaysians, and dark-skinned Indians found no difference in irritation indices measured by TEWL to 2% SLS.[32] However, a follow-up study in black, white, and Asian subjects evaluating only TEWL and LDV without exposure to irritants or chemicals that disrupt the stratum corneum showed an increase in baseline TEWL in Asian and black subjects. This led to the conclusion that black and Asian subjects have a more compromised barrier function that would likely be more susceptible to irritants.[33] Higher TEWL at higher temperatures in black cadaveric skin was observed in another study.[30] However, some studies have found no apparent difference.[34,35] A more recent study evaluating irritant contact dermatitis using confocal histopathology in vivo interestingly demonstrated more severe reactions in white forearm skin, which was characterized by parakeratosis, spongiosis, perivascular inflammatory infiltrate, and microvesicle formation.[36] In addition, when comparing reactions to 2% and 4% SLS, white skin had a greater mean increases in TEWL after exposure to 4% SLS than did black skin. These results support the theory that those with black skin are more resistant to irritants.

EPIDERMIS

Structure and Function

Melanocytes are an important component of the epidermis that displays differences in structure among the various racial and ethnic groups. Derived from neural crest cell precursors, melanocytes migrate through the mesenchyme into the basal layer of the epidermis, the hair matrix and the outer root sheath of hair follicles, epithelia of various mucous membranes, leptomeninges, the cochlea in the inner ear, and the uveal tract of the eye. Immunohistochemical staining reveals that primitive melanocytes first appear diffusely throughout the dermis of the head and neck region during the eighth week of fetal life.[37] Melanocytes are identified in the epidermis as early as day 50 of gestation, and by 120 days, melanosomes are recognizable by electron microscopy.[38] At the end of gestation, active dermal melanocytes disappear presumably owing to programmed cell death. The arborization of melanocytes among 30–40 neighboring keratinocytes occurs during development with subsequent transfer of melanosomes into the keratinocytes.[39] This relationship of cells is termed the *epidermal-melanin unit.* One known function of melanin is to provide the skin with natural protection from the effects of daily ultraviolet radiation.

Structural Differences

Pigment cell biology has determined that the number of melanocytes is constant among races.[40,41] However, the activity of melanocytes does vary among the races, as well as from one individual to another and among different anatomic regions of the body.[42] Pigmentation of the skin depends on an orderly transfer of melanosomes from melanocytes to keratinocytes. The amount, density, and distribution of melanin within the melanosome, as determined by melanocyte activity, are the primary determinants of the variability of human skin color.[37,40–49] Differences in melanosome size, density, and aggregation correlate closely with skin color. Figure 12-3 illustrates these differences in various skin hues. For example, early stage I or II melanosomes, seen in fair-skinned individuals, are small, clustered in groups or aggregations and are degraded more quickly in the stratum spinosum. This is in contrast to late stage IV melanosomes, seen in darker-skinned individuals, which are larger, individually dispersed and degraded more slowly, and remain in the stratum corneum longer. In general, dark-skinned black subjects tend to have larger, nonaggregated, dense, and more oval melanosomes than subjects with white skin. Although skin of color contains melanosomes that tend to be larger and nonaggregated, this is not absolute. The size and distribution of melanosomes within ethnic groups vary with skin hues and skin phototypes. For example, black individuals with lighter skin tones have a unique combination of single, large as well as small, aggregated melanosomes.[44] Similar variability also occurs in white and Asian subjects of darker and lighter hues.

Melanosomal distribution throughout the epidermis has racial variability. In black skin, melanosomes are distributed throughout the entire epidermis, which is in contrast to unexposed fair white skin, in which melanosomes are confined to the stratum basale and absent in the upper epidermal layers.[46,50] Sun exposure can play an important role in melanosomal distribution and groupings. The distribution of melanosomes

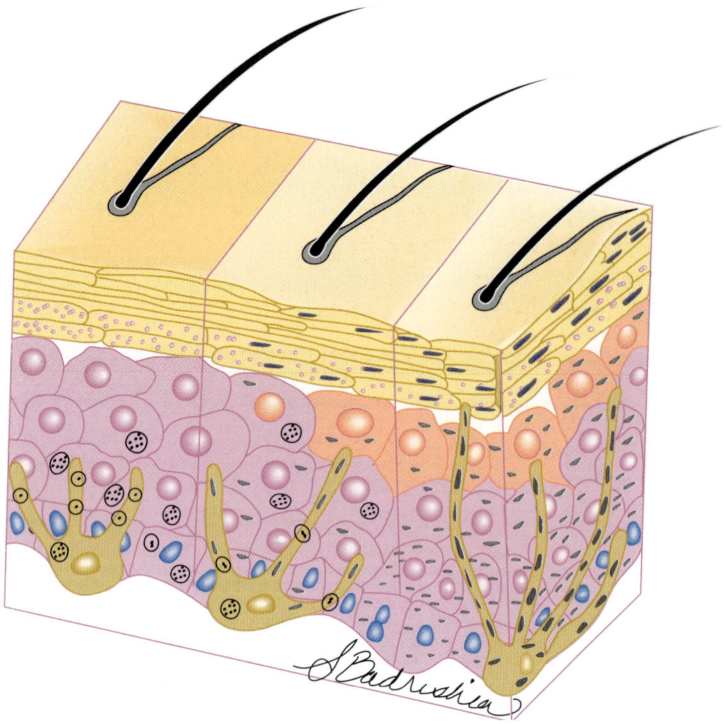

▲ **FIGURE 12-3** Schematic representation illustrating differences in melanosome organization in dark skin, tan skin, and light skin.

in sun-exposed, deeply tanned skin was noted to be similar to the distribution of melanosomes black skin.[46,47] A study in deeply tanned Thai patients showed that melanosomes in these subjects tended to have dense clusters in the basal layer with distribution throughout the epidermis and heavy pigmentation in the stratum corneum.[51]

There appears to be a size requirement that dictates melanosomal aggregation in a membrane. Melanosomes in fair skin are smaller than 0.35 μm and can group into a membrane-bound unit called a *phagosome*.[42,47] However, melanosomes in dark skin are larger than 0.35 μm and therefore cannot be complexed and aggregated physically. As expected, total melanin content has been found to be greater in darker skin than in lighter skin, as determined through melanocyte cultures.[44]

Functional Differences

The amount, density, and distribution of melanin that correlates with human skin color have substantial benefits for photoprotection and the incidence of skin cancer. It has been established that melanin confers protection from ultraviolet (UV) light.[47,48,52] In skin of color, the higher number of nonaggregated stage IV melanosomes absorb more UV light than the aggregated, smaller melanosomes in fair-skinned white patients.[52] Skin color rather than stratum corneum thickness is responsible for differences in skin color reflectance measurements, as demonstrated by the similarities between albino Africans and European whites.[53] Darkly pigmented black skin had average minimal erythema doses (MEDs) 15–33 times greater than white skin, depending on skin tone.[47,52] The melanin pigment in black skin is considered a neutral-density filter, reducing all wavelengths of light equally.[52] A similar trend occurs in other populations with skin of color. In a study of Asian skin, Japanese women demonstrated that greater melanin content, as evidenced by darker complexion, reacted less severely to the sun.[54]

Although melanin in pigmented skin confers protection from UV radiation, pigmented skin is not immune from damage. Individuals with this skin type have the ability to experience significant photodamage, including atypia, atrophy, collagen and elastin damage, and hyperpigmentation.[50,51] A study of Thai women found that melanin is not an efficient absorber of UV light of longer wavelengths, including UVA and infrared rays.[51] Furthermore, melanin also can be photoreactive with the production of damaging oxygen free radicals.[55]

Variability in melanin protection correlates with differences in extrinsic and intrinsic aging among racial and ethnic groups. In general, there is a marked difference in atrophy and cell cytology between black and white skin, with blacks displaying fewer changes.[46] Chronologic aging in black subjects does occur with more pronounced changes, such as epidermal thinning, effaced rete ridges, and dyskeratosis occurring in older individuals [50] This parallels findings in a study performed on Thai subjects over age 50 with heavy sun exposure, who were noted to have greater disordered differentiation and atrophy.[51] Table 12-3 summarizes the substantiated evidence discussed earlier regarding differences in the epidermal structure and function of the various ethnic groups.

TABLE 12-3
Comparison of the Epidermis Across the Top Three Racial Groups[3,75]

	White	Black	Asians
Stratum corneum thickness	Equal	Equal	
Stratum corneocyte size	Equal	Equal	
Stratum corneum layers	Less	More	
Stratum corneum lipids	Low	High	
Ceramide concentration	High	Low	High
Vitamin D production	High	Low	
Minimal erythema dose	Low	High	
Photodamage	High	Minimal	
Melanin	Low	High	Intermediate
Melanosomes	Small, aggregated	Large, dispersed	Mixed

DERMIS

Structure and Function

The dermis is a highly vascular structure made up of several components, including collagen, elastin, and ground substance, as well as various glands. The cells of the dermis are derived from primitive mesenchymal cells, including fibroblasts, which produce collagen, elastin, and the matrix, and several specialized cells, including histiocytes, mastocytes, lymphocytes, plasma cells, and eosinophils.

Eccrine sweat glands, a key part of the body's thermoregulatory system, form in the fourth month of gestation from a downward budding of the epidermis. The coiled secretory portion is located in the reticular dermis, which then spirals upward onto the skin's surface, forming the acrosyringium, the excretory portion of the duct that secretes hypotonic saline. There are an estimated 2–5 million eccrine ducts located throughout the skin, with the densest population present in the axillae, palms, soles, and forehead, where they are under sympathetic cholinergic control.[56]

Apocrine glands are phylogentic remnants of the mammalian sexual scent gland and function very similar to the eccrine ducts.[56] These glands are outgrowths of the pilosebaceous unit, and they deposit their contents into the infundibulum of hair follicles. Apocrine glands are densely populated in the axillae, perineum, areolae, and external auditory canal. They become active just before puberty, generating odorless sweat by decapitation secretion that develops an odor after interacting with the skin's bacteria. Apocrine sweat glands are innervated by sympathetic adrenergic nerve fibers.

Sebaceous glands comprise the third gland found in the dermis, and they produce sebum, which consists of various lipids, including squalene, cholesterol, cholesterol esters, wax esters, and triglycerides, that transcend the follicular canal to the skin surface. These lipids function as the skin's natural moisturizer.

Structural and Functional Differences

The existence of well-documented racial and ethnic differences in the quantity, structure, and function of the eccrine sweat glands is not confirmed.[3] Most of the literature suggests no significant differences. Because of the premise that races evolved as a result of environmental selection, it is plausible that differences in sweat glands between races exists owing to adaptation to hot, humid climates versus colder climates. It is unclear whether these differences would be based on genetics or strictly environmental adaptations.

The literature does not support difference in the number of eccrine glands between black and white skin.[57,58] However, a racial differential in the functional activity of eccrine sweat glands has been noted. Higher sweating rates by white subjects during physical labor[59] or by cholinergic stimulation by pilocarpine tests[60,61] has been identified compared with either black Africans or Asian Indians. The sodium content in sweat showed a lower concentration in black Africans, suggesting a more efficient electrolyte conservation system.[62] Electrophysiologic studies showed higher skin resistance and therefore greater eccrine gland activity in black subjects compared with white subjects.[63–66] Interestingly, in Hispanic and Spanish subjects, gland activity was between black and white eccrine gland activity.[63] This would suggest that skin color correlates with eccrine activity and that darker individuals have higher skin resistance than fair-skinned individuals.

There are limited and less than optimal studies in the literature regarding racial differences in apocrine glands.[3] Three early studies with a small study design concluded that black subjects had larger apocrine glands[67] in greater numbers[67,68] and with more turbid secretions.[69] However, the small study design and lack of investigator-blinded assessment preclude definitive conclusions.

An apoeccrine gland, also called a *mixed sweat gland,* develops at puberty from an eccrine gland that underwent apocrinization in the axilla, perineum, and nasal skin.[70] The secretory rate in an apoeccrine gland is 10 times more than that in an eccrine gland. Although there is great interindividual variation, one study found a greater number in black versus white facial skin.[46,71] The significance of this finding is unclear.

Racial differences in sebaceous gland size and activity have been suggested. However, there are limited studies that seem contradictory owing to a lack of well-controlled protocols, methodologic flaws, and small study populations. The literature suggests that black subjects tend to have higher sebum levels and larger glands than white subjects.[72,73] However, another study found a trend toward increased sebum production on the foreheads of black versus white men, although it did not reach statistical significance. The opposite finding was true when comparing black and white females. In a more recent study, there was no statistical difference when measuring sebum excretion among white, black, and Asian patients.[74] Finally, an Asian study using Japanese women demonstrated a positive correlation between the amount of skin surface lipids and darker pigmentation.[54]

Although there are no differences in caliper-assisted skin thickness encompassing both epidermis and dermis, there may be differences at the cellular level between dermis of black and white individuals.[75] Fibroblasts in black female facial skin were larger, binucleate or multinucleated, and of greater quantity than in white female facial skin.[46] There was greater interindividual variability in white subjects compared with blacks. Collagen fiber bundles in black skin were smaller, more closely stacked, and ran more parallel with more collagen fibrils and glycoprotein fragments in the interstices versus larger more sparse fiber fragments in white skin. Fibroblast hyperreactivity is the result of the interaction among mast cells, cytokines, and fibroblasts. Number and size of mast cells are constant between the two racial groups.[46] However, there are greater and larger macrophages in the papillary dermis, along with a decrease in collagenase, in black skin. This may explain in part the propensity for keloid formation in black individuals. Tables 12-4 and 12-5 summarize these findings and their implications for clinical disease in ethnic skin.

TABLE 12-4
Comparison of Dermal Structure Between Black and White Skin[3,75]

	White	Black
Dermis	Thin and less compact	Thick and compact
Papillary and reticular layer	More distinct	Less distinct
Collagen fiber bundles	Large	Small, close stacking
Fiber fragments	Sparse	Prominent and numerous
Melanophages	Few	Numerous and larger
Lymphatic vessels	Moderate, dilated	Dilated empty channels
Fibroblasts	Few	Numerous, large, binucleated and multinucleated
Elastic fibers	Several, elastosis	Few, elastosis uncommon
Superficial blood vessel	Sparse to moderate	Numerous, mostly dilated
Glycoprotein	Variable	Numerous in the dermis

TABLE 12-5
Therapeutic Implications of Key Biologic Differences in Skin of Color[3]

Biologic Factor	Therapeutic Implications
Epidermis	
Increased melanin content	Lower rates of skin cancer
Increased melanosome dispersion	Less pronounced photoaging
	Pigmentation disorders owing to both biologic predispositions and cultural practices
Dermis	
Multinucleated and larger fibroblasts	Greater incidence of keloids

REFERENCES

1. US Department of Health and Human Services, Health Resources and Services Administration. Changing Racial and Ethnic Composition of the Population, 2003. Available at *http://bhpr.hrsa.gov/healthworkforce/reports/changingdemo/composition.htm.*
2. Pasko T, Seidman B (eds). *Physician Characteristics and Distribution in the US, 2001–2002.* Washington, American Medical Association Press, 2001.
3. Taylor SC. Skin of color: Biology, structure, function, and implications for dermatologic disease. *J Am Acad Dermatol* 2002;46:S41–62.
4. Weigand DA, Haygood C, Gaylor JR. Cell layers and density of Negro and Caucasian stratum corneum. *J Invest Dermatol* 1974;62: 563–568.
5. Freeman RG, Cockerell FG, Armstrong J, et al. Sunlight as a factor influencing the thickness of epidermis. *J Invest Dermatol* 1962;39:295–297.
6. Thomson ML. Relative efficiency of pigment and horny layer thickness in protecting the skin of Europeans and Africans against solar ultraviolet radiation. *J Physiol (Lond)* 1955;127: 236–238.
7. Reed JT, Ghadially R, Elias PM. Effect of race, gender, and skin type on epidermal permeability barrier function. *J Invest Dermatol* 1994; 102:537.
8. Berardesca E, Rigol J, Leveque JL. In vivo biophysical differences in races. *Dermatologica* 1991; 182:89–93.
9. La Ruche G, Cesarini JP. Histology and physiology of black skin. *Ann Dermatol Venereol* 1992;119:567–574.
10. Sugino K, Imokawa G, Maibach HI. Ethnic difference of stratum corneum lipid in relation to stratum corneum function. *J Invest Dermatol* 1993;100: 597.
11. Corcuff P, Lotte C, Rougier A, et al. Racial differences in corneocytes. *Acta Derm Venereol* 1991;71: 146–148.
12. Warrier AG, Kligman AM, Harper RA, et al. A comparison of black and white skin using noninvasive methods. *J Soc Cosmet Chem* 1996;47: 229–240.
13. Johnson BL Jr. Differences in skin type, in Johnson BL Jr, Moy RL, White GM (eds), *Ethnic Skin: Medical and Surgical.* St Louis, MO, Mosby, 1998, pp 3–5.
14. Bereson PA, Burch GE. Studies of diffusion through dead human skin. *Am J Trop Med Hyg* 1971;31:842.
15. Malkinson FD, Gehlman L. Factors affecting percutaneous absorption, in Drill VA, Lazar P (eds), *Cutaneous Toxicology.* New York, Academic Press, 1977.
16. Scheuplein RJ, Blank IH. Permeability of the skin. *Physiol Rev* 1971;51:702.
17. Marzulli FN. Barriers to skin penetration. *J Invest Dermatol* 1962;39:387.
18. Wickrema-Sinha, Wickrema-Sinha AJ, Shaw SR, Weber DJ. Percutaneous absorption and excretion of tritium-labeled diflorasone diacetate: A new topical corticosteroid in the rat, monkey and man. *J Invest Dermatol* 1978;7: 372–377.
19. Guy RH, Tur E, Bjerke S, et al. Are there age and racial differences to methyl nicotinate-induced vasodilatation in human skin? *J Am Acad Dermatol* 1985;12:1001–1006.
20. Gean CJ, Tur E, Maibach HI, et al. Cutaneous responses to topical methyl bicofinate in black, Oriental and Caucasian subjects. *Arch Dermatol Res* 1989;281:95–98.
21. Marshall EK, Lynch V, Smith HV. Variation in susceptibility of the skin to dichloroethylsulfide. *J Pharmacol Exp Ther* 1919;12: 291–301.
22. Schwartz L, Tulipan L, Birmingham DJ. *Occupational Diseases of the Skin.* Philadelphia, Lea & Febiger, 1939.
23. Shelley WB. Newer understanding of ecology in dermatology, in Rees RB (ed), *Dermatosis Due to Environmental and Physical Factors.* Springfield, IL, Charles C. Thomas, 1962, p 12.
24. Frosch RJ, Kligman AM. The chamber scarification test for assessing irritancy of topically applied substances, in Drill VA, Lazar P (eds), *Cutaneous Toxicology.* New York: Academic Press, 1977, p 150.
25. Marshall J, Heyl T. Skin diseases in western Cape Province. *S Afr Med J* 1963;37:1308.
26. Marshall J. New skin diseases in Africa. *Trans St Johns Hosp Dermatol Soc* 1970;56: 3–10.
27. Berardesca E, Maibach HI. Racial differences in sodium lauryl sulfate–induced cutaneous irritation: Black and white. *Contact Dermatitis* 1988;18:65–70.
28. Berardesca E, Maibach HI. Sodium-lauryl-sulphate–induced cutaneous irritation comparison of white and hispanic subjects. *Contact Dermatitis* 1988;19:136–140.
29. Berardesca E. Racial differences in skin function. *Acta Derm Venereol.* 1994;185:44–46.
30. Wilson D, Berardesca E, Maibach HI. In vivo transepidermal water loss: Differences between black and white skin. *Br J Dermatol* 1988;119: 647–652.
31. Berardesca E, Maibach HI. Sensitive and ethnic skin: A need for special skin care agent? *Dermatol Clin* 1991;9:89–92.
32. Goh CL, Chia SE. Skin irritability to sodium-lauryl sulphate: As measured by skin water vapor loss—by sex and race. *Clin Exp Dermatol* 1988;13:16–19.
33. Kompaore F, Marty JP, Dupont C. In vivo evaluation of the stratum corneum barrier function in blacks, Caucasians and Asians with two non-invasive methods. *Skin Pharmacol* 1993;6:200–207.
34. DeLuca R, Balestrieri A, Dinle Y. Measurement of cutaneous evaporation: 6. Cutaneous water loss in the people of Somalia. *Boll Soc Ital Biol Sper* 1983;59: 1499–1501.
35. Pinnagoda J, Tupker RA, Agner T, et al. Guidelines for transepidermal water loss (TEWL) measurement. *Contact Dermatitis* 1990;22: 164–178.
36. Hicks SP, Swindells KJ, Middelkamp-Hup MA, et al. Confocal histopathology of irritant contact dermatitis in vivo and the impact of skin color (black vs white). *J Am Acad Dermatol* 2003;48: 727–734.
37. Bolognia JL, Orlow SJ. Melanocyte biology, in Bolognia JL, Jorizzo JL, Rapini RP (eds), *Dermatology.* St Louis, MO, Mosby, 2003, p 935.
38. Holbrook KA, Underwood RA, Vogel AM, et al. The appearance, density, and distribution of melanocytes in human embryonic and fetal skin revealed by the anti-melanoma monoclonal antibody, HMB-45. *Anat Embrol* 1989;180:443–455.
39. Jimbow K, Quevedo WC Jr, Fitzpatrick TB, et al. Some aspects of melanin biology: 1950–1975. *J Invest Dermatol* 1976;67:72–89.
40. Szabo G. Mitochondria and other cytoplasmic inclusions, in Gordon M (ed), *Pigment Cell Biology.* New York, Academic Press, 1959.
41. Starkco RS, Pinkus S. Quantitative and qualitative data on the pigment cell of adult human epidermis. *J Invest Dermatol* 1957;28:33.
42. Toda K, Pathak MA, Parrish JA, et al. Alteration of racial differences in melanosome distribution in human epidermis after exposure to ultraviolet light. *Nat New Biol* 1972;236: 143–144.
43. Johnson BL Jr. Differences in skin type, in Johnson BL Jr, Moy RL, White GM (eds), *Ethnic Skin: Medical and Surgical.* St Louis, MO, Mosby, 1998, pp 3–5.
44. Masson P. Pigment cells in man, in Miner RW, Gordon M (eds), *The Biology of Melanosomes,* Vol IV. New York, New York Academy of Sciences, 1948, pp 10–17.
45. Szabo G, Gerald AB, Pathak MA, et al. Racial differences in the fate of melanosomes in humane epidermis. *Nature* 1969;222:1081–1082.
46. Montagna W, Carlisle K. The architecture of black and white facial skin. *J Am Acad Dermatol* 1991;24:929–937.
47. Olson RL, Gaylor J, Everett MA. Skin color, melanin, and erythema. *Arch Dermatol* 1973;108: 541–544.
48. Mitchell R. The skin of the Australian Aborigines: A light and electron micro-

scopical study. *Australas J Dermatol* 1968; 9:314.
49. Smit NM, Kolb RM, Lentjes EM, et al. Variations in melanin formation by cultured melanocytes from different skin types. *Arch Dermatol Res* 1998;290: 342–349.
50. Herzberg AJ, Dinehart SM. Chronologic aging in black skin. *Am J Dermatopathol* 1989;11: 319 328.
51. Kotrajaras R, Kligman AM. The effect of topical tretinoin on photodamaged facial skin: The Thai experience. *Br J Dermatol* 1993;129:302–309.
52. Kaidbey KH, Agin PP, Sayre RM, et al. Photoprotection by melanin: A comparison of black and Caucasian skin. *J Am Acad Dermatol* 1979;1:249–260.
53. Thomson, ML. Relative efficiency of pigment and horny layer thickness in protecting the skin of Europeans and Africans against solar ultraviolet radiation. *J Physiol* 1955;127:236–238.
54. Abe T, Arai S, Mimura K, et al. Studies of physiological factors affecting skin susceptibility to ultraviolet light irradiation and irritants. *J Dermatol* 1983;10:531–537.
55. Hill HZ, Li W, Xin P, et al. Melanin: A two-edged sword? *Pigment Cell Res* 1997;10: 158–161.
56. Hurley HJ. Diseases of the eccrine sweat glands, in Bolognia JL, Jorizzo JL, Rapini RP (eds), *Dermatology.* St Louis, MO, Mosby, 2003, p 567.
57. Johnson LG, Landon MM. Eccrine sweat gland activity and racial differences in resting skin conductance. *Psychophysiology* 1965;1:322–329.
58. Montagna W, Parakkal PF. *The Structure and Function of Skin,* 3rd ed. New York, Academic Press, 1974.
59. Robinson S, Dill D, Wilson J, et al. Adaptation of white men and Negroes to prolonged work in humid heat. *Am J Trop Med* 1941;21:261–287.
60. McCance RA, Purohit G. Ethnic differences in response to the sweat glands to pilocarpine. *Nature* 1969;221:378–379.
61. McCance RA, Rutishauser IH, Knight HC. Response to sweat glands to pilocarpine in the Bantu of Uganda. *Lancet* 1968;1:663–665.
62. Calhoun DA, Oparil S. Racial differences in the pathogenesis of hypertension. *Am J Med Sci* 1995;310:S86–90.
63. Homma H. On apocrine sweat glands in white and Negro men and women. *Bull Johns Hopkins Hosp* 1956;38:365.
64. Johnson LC, CorahNL. Racial differences in skin resistance. *Science* 1960;139: 766–767.
65. James CL, Worland J, Stern JA. Skin potential and barometer responsiveness of black and white children. *Psychophysiology* 1976;13: 523–527.
66. Juniper K Jr, Blanton DA, Dykman RA. Skin resistance, sweat-gland counts, salivary flow, and gastric secretion: Age, race, and sex differences, and intercorrelations. *Psychophysiology* 1967;4:216–222.
67. Schiefferdecker P. Dsaael be (vollkomin Mitt). *Zoologica* 1922;27:1–154.
68. Homma H. On apocrine sweat glands in white and Negro men and women. *Bull Johns Hopkins Hosp* 1926;38:365.
69. Hurley HJ, Shelley WB. The physiology and pharmacology of the apocrine sweat gland, in *The Human Apocrine Sweat Gland in Health and Disease.* Springfield, IL, Charles C Thomas, 1960.
70. Ito T. Morphological connections of human apocrine and eccrine sweat glands: Occurrence of the so-called "mixed sweat glands"—A review. *Okajimas Folia Anat Jpn* 1988;65: 315–316.
71. Goldsmith LA. Biology of eccrine and apocrine sweat glands, in Freedberg IM, Eisen AZ, Wolff K, et al (eds), *Fitzpatrick's Dermatology in General Medicine,* Vol 1. New York, McGraw-Hill, 1999.
72. Kligman AM, Shelley, WB. An investigation of the biology of the sebaceous gland. *J Invest Dermatol* 1958;30:99–125.
73. Champion RH, Gillman T, Rook AJ, et al. *An Introduction to the Biology of the Skin.* Philadelphia, FA Davis, 1970, p 418.
74. Abedeen SK, Gonzales M, Judodihardjo H, et al. Racial variation in sebum excretion rate (abstract 559), in *Program and Abstracts of the 58th Annual Meeting of the American Academy of Dermatology,* San Francisco, CA, March 10–15, 2000.
75. Whitmore SE, Sago NJ. Caliper-measured skin thickness is similar in white and black women. *J Am Acad Dermatol* 2000;42:76-9, 2000.
76. Richards GM, Oresajo CO, Halder RM. Structure and function of ethnic skin and hair. *Dermatol Clin* 2003;21:595–600.

CHAPTER 13

Nuances in Skin of Color

A. Paul Kelly

Key Points

- Visual observation can be more useful than sophisticated technology in distinguishing abnormalities from common nuances of skin of color.
- *Futcher's lines*, abrupt color demarcations on the flexor surface of the upper arm, are common among adults with skin of color, although rare in infants.
- In children, hair lines, characterized by an abrupt linear demarcation between the darker, lateral, lanugo hair–containing area of the arm and the medial nonhairy area, occur in a similar pattern as Futcher's lines.
- Forearm and thigh lines, less common than *Futcher's lines* and often hard to distinguish, are seldom mentioned in the literature.
- Linea nigra and linea alba demarcations of the trunk are common among black patients.
- Palmar and plantar hyperpigmentation not found in infants becomes more common in older patients.
- Black infants frequently have localized areas of hyperpigmentation.
- Hyperpigmentation of the oral mucosa and sclera, while common in adults, is not found in young children, although infants often have a lip discoloration that disappears quickly.
- Melanonychia striata, common in older adults, is rare in young children, suggesting trauma as the usual cause, although melanoma must be considered.
- Idiopathic guttate hypomelanosis, characterized by hypopigmented patches primarily on the anterior leg, is more common in older patients.
- Mongolian spots present in Native American, Asian, and African-American infants may not appear in the classic lumbosacral region but rather on the hip.

Skin, our largest organ, is a window of human biology and pathology. Yet too often clinical observation is undervalued on the assumption that it will add nothing to information obtained by light or electron microscopy, immunofluorescent techniques, and other more sophisticated investigative approaches. This chapter focuses on visual observation of several skin nuances of individuals of color, particularly blacks. Many such nuances have not been described previously or were called abnormal, even though they were common to a large percentage of people with darker skin

Although Neidelman's article entitled, "Abnormalities of the Negro," was published over 60 years ago,[1] and Kelly[2] and Johnson[3] have since better defined these norms, confusion remains as to what is normal and abnormal when evaluating skin of color. This chapter will clearly elucidate and discuss cutaneous variants in skin of color.

PIGMENTARY DEMARCATION LINES

Futcher's lines were described by Futcher[4] as an abrupt linear demarcation on the flexor surface of the upper arm; the medial side was lighter in color than the lateral side. However, in 1913, Matsumoto[5] was the first to report this finding. Other Japanese authors also described this demarcation line, and their findings were summarized by Ito, who reported that it was present in 43% of the Japanese and 10 times more often in females.[6] Maruya, cited by Miura,[7] screened more than 1300 Japanese and found the line in 39% of females and 23% of males. Vollum observed it in 26% of Jamaican children ages 1–11, but unlike the Japanese reports, there was no male/female difference.[8] James and colleagues described six types of pigmentary demarcation lines,[9] of which type A lines corresponded to the classic Futcher's lines. They found a 44% incidence of type A lines, with a higher incidence in female patients. Selmanowitz and Krivo reported that 37% of 100 black patients had this type of pigmentary demarcation on the arm, with an approximately equal sex ratio.[10]

In order to localize Futcher's lines anatomically they were divided into quadrants. The upper outer surface was quadrant 1, counted clockwise on the left arm and counterclockwise on the right arm. Most of the demarcations were in quadrant 1. The next most common was quadrant 2, where the line was more proximal and often continued for a short distance along the posterior auxiliary fold (Figure 13-1).

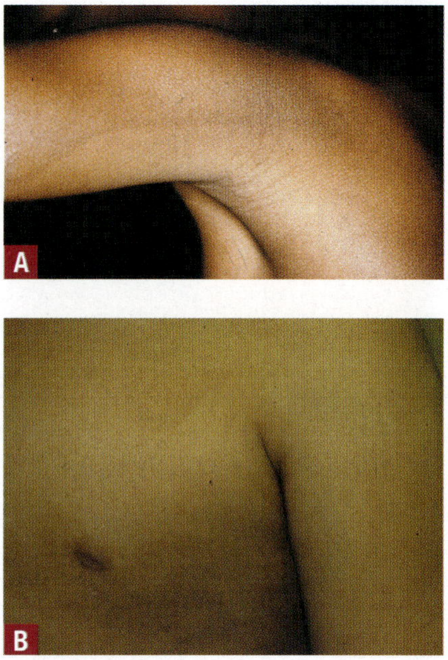

▲ **FIGURE 13-1** **A** and **B** *Futcher's lines.* Four quadrants on left/right arm; quadrant 1 shows the most demarcation.

Studies performed at King Drew Medical Center (KDMC) indicate that more than 50% of the black patients examined had this abrupt color change bilaterally and fewer than 10% unilaterally.[2] There was no correlation of unilateral lesions with the dominant hand or body build. There was no significant variation in the frequency of these lines in males and females, except in senior citizens, in whom demarcation lines were found in 20% fewer males. Futcher's demarcation lines averaged approximately 10 cm in length. There was no correlation of these lines with skin color. Anatomically, Futcher's lines follow no definite muscle, nerve, or blood vessel, although they have been associated with the biceps muscle, division of the C8 and T1, and the course of the cephalic vein, respectively.[4]

Black infants seldom demonstrated Futcher's lines. Most, however, displayed a *hair line,* in a similar pattern as Futcher's lines, that is characterized by an abrupt linear demarcation between the darker, lateral, lanugo hair–containing area of the arm and the medial nonhairy area (Figure 13-2). Once the long lanugo hairs were no longer present, classic Futcher's lines became visible. Since there was a definite hair line in approximately the same percentage of infants as Futcher's lines in adults, a possible explanation for the lines is that the larger or more numerous hair follicles impart a darker color to the skin. This is further illustrated by the often abrupt

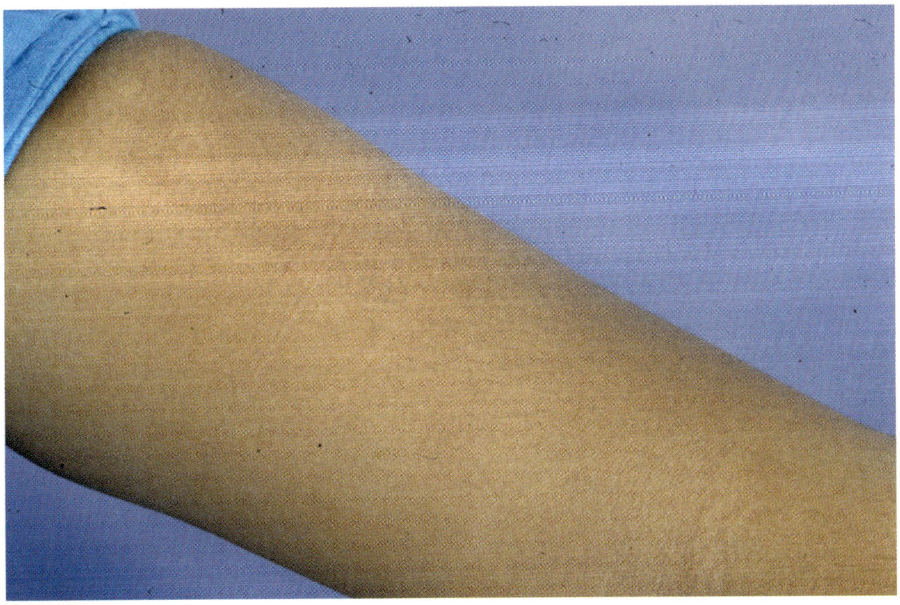

▲ **FIGURE 13-2** Black infant showing a hair line similar to a Futchers line, Laungo/medial lighter non-hairy area.

demarcation between the dark sideburn areas in infants and the lighter brown skin anterior and posterior to this future hair-bearing area (Figure 13-3).

A hair line appeared on the first quadrant of the arm in 50% of the KDMC black infants, and 80% of these had a concomitant line extending from the upper back, above the axillae, and down the proximal third of quadrant 2 of the arm[2] (see Figure 13-2). This divided the arm into two separate colors without the blending that is usually observed on the dorsal (exterior) aspect of the arm in children and adults. Since this demarcation is usually on the ventral surface of the arm on the one side, it should not represent Voigt's lines separating the ventral from the dorsal aspect of the body, as discussed by Matsumoto[5] and Wasserman.[11]

Forearm lines, a color demarcation on the medial aspect of the forearm, were present in 60% of males and 75% of females in the KDMC study[2] (Figure 13-4). More than 50% of males had only one forearm involved, and this was usually on the dominant side. A few of these demarcations seemed to be continuations of Futcher's lines, although most had no connection. No mention was made of this demarcation by James and colleagues.[9] This may be due to the fact that although the incidence is high, the lines are often hard to discern.

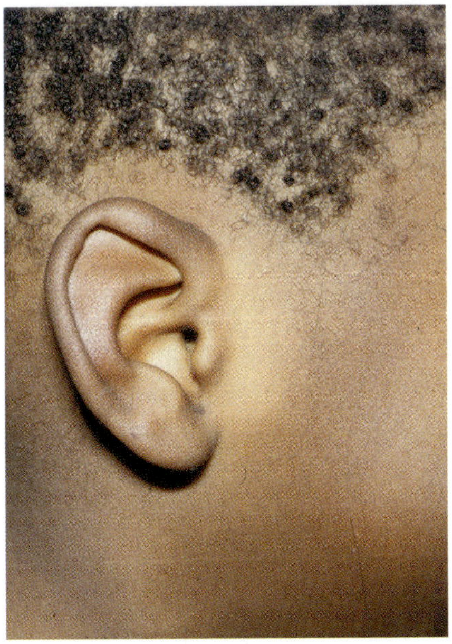

▲ **FIGURE 13-3** Black infant showing an abrupt demarcation between the dark sideburn area and the lighter brown anterior and posterior.

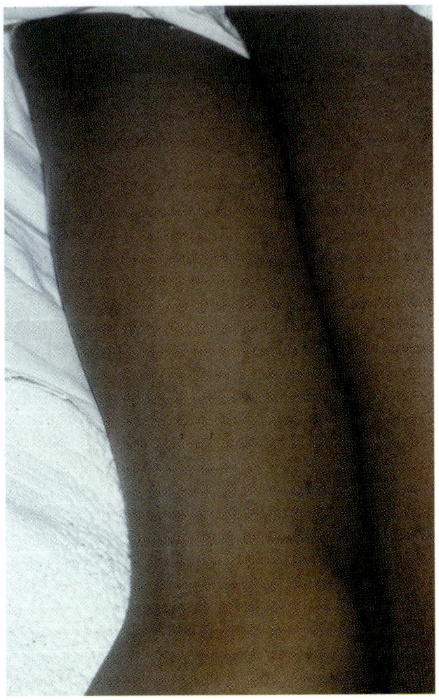

▲ **FIGURE 13-4** Thigh line.

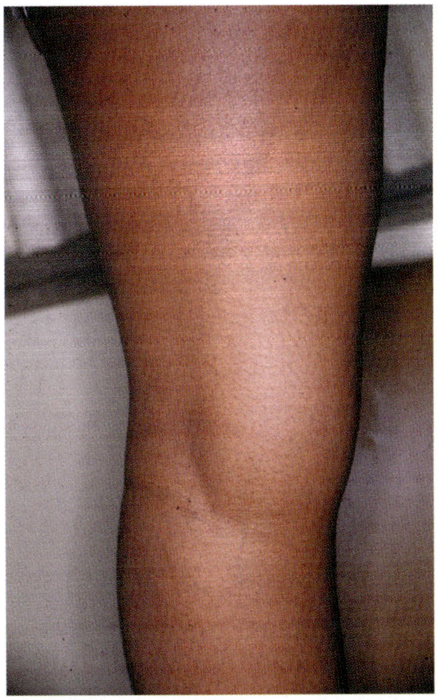

▲ **FIGURE 13-5** Thigh demarcation.

Thigh lines (James type B lines[9]) were present in approximately one-quarter of black males and females examined, and two-thirds of those examined had concomitant Futcher's lines[2] (Figures 13-5). They are most often present on the posteriomedial aspect of the thigh. Thigh lines seemed to follow the area innervated by the anterior femoral cutaneous nerve (I 1, 2, 3) medially and the posterior femoral cutaneous nerve (S 1, 2, 3) laterally. Some people with thigh lines had extensions across the popliteal area onto the calf, sometimes extending to the medial aspect of the ankle. Although the incidence in males and females was the same, more females had bilateral thigh demarcations.

This *leg demarcation line* was either not reported or seldom mentioned in previous articles on skin lines. It may be an extension of the thigh line, and sometimes it is the only demarcation on the lower extremity. The most likely reason that these leg and thigh lines have seldom been described by other investigators and are considered a rarity is the phenomenon of "ashyness." When dark skin is dry, especially in cold weather, it seems to be covered with grayish branlike scales, termed *ashy.* The legs are especially prone to ashyness, which most likely masks most linear demarcations. Since the leg demarcation is not as vivid as that of the arm, wiping the leg with a wet cloth or applying an emollient cream or an oil preparation before examining the leg for lines is imperative. The leg demarcations usually extended from the popliteal fossa to the medial ankle, being most prominent above the calf. There was no difference in the incidence according to age, gender, or body build, with the exception of infants, who had questionable hair line demarcations on the thighs and legs. Hair lines on their lower extremities occurred in approximately the same configurations and frequency (30%) as in adults with true lower extremity linear cutaneous demarcations.

James and colleagues reported two women who developed lower extremity linear demarcations (James type B lines) during pregnancy. Fourteen percent of their black mothers claimed that they first noted these lines during pregnancy.[12] Fulk also supported this observation.[13]

MIDTRUNK DEMARCATIONS

Cutaneous linea nigra and linea alba are interesting skin markings in blacks. Two-thirds of all black patients examined at KDMC had *linea nigra,* a dark line extending from the suprapubic area to the umbilicus.[2] There was no variation based on age or gender. This demarcation ranged from 1–14 cm in length and from 1–8 mm in width. Usually it extended from the umbilicus to the suprapubic area, although 20% of patients had the line extending to a supraumbilical location (Figures 13-6). The longest line was 9 cm above the umbilicus. There were no subjects in whom the linea nigra was located only in a supraumbilical position.

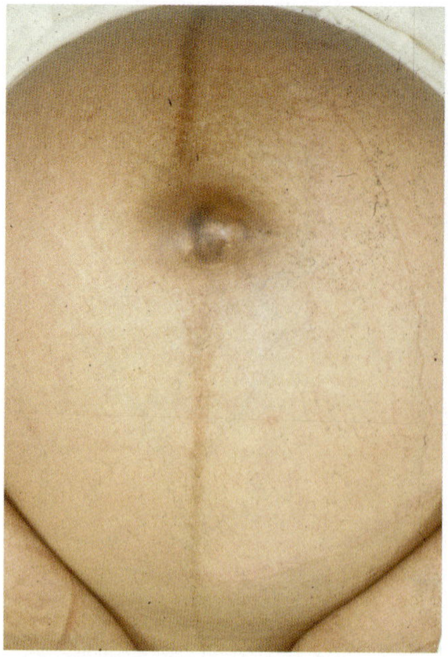

▲ **FIGURE 13-6** Linea nigra—a dark line extending from the suprapubic area to the umbilicus; no variations in age or gender.

Cutaneous *linea alba,* also termed *midline hypopigmentation,* is a vertical hypopigmented demarcation in or near the midsaggital line that may begin on one side of the trunk, cross the midline, and continue in a vertical direction on the opposite side (Figure 13-7). Niedelman mentioned but did not elaborate on this line.[1] Selmanowitz and Krivo found a linea alba in 43% of black males and 33% of black females.[14] In contrast, the KDMC evaluations showed a greater than 60% occurrence in both sexes, with a slightly higher incidence in males. Linea alba appeared anywhere from the dorsal aspect of the manubrium to the umbilicus. However, none extended below the umbilicus. Size ranged from 2 mm to 2 cm in diameter and from 4–25 cm in length. Linea alba corresponds to the type C lines that James and colleagues found in 36% of their black patients (44% male, 20% female).[9] Others found these lines in approximately 40% of their black patients, with a slight male predominance.[14,15]

It is unknown why the upper half of the anterior trunk would have a hypopigmented ventral midline demarcation and the lower anterior trunk a hyperpigmented demarcation. One plausible explanation is that melanocytes, migrating in a dorsal to ventral direction from the neutral crest origin, do not always complete their journey in the upper, wider chest region and come together to the point of supersaturation on the lower abdominal area owing to its smaller girth. Color, gender, and body build did not seem to have any influence on the presence or absence of these ventral linear color demarcations.

A broad area of midback vertical hypopigmentation (James type D lines[9]) was found in 3 of 50 infants and 5 of 100 adults. The lines are often hard to discern, and the incidence is not sufficient to be considered common in blacks.

Bilateral hypopigmented macules (James type E lines) were found in 12% of the KDMC patients, with a slight male predominance.[9] Selmanowitz and Krivo found a 16% incidence, with male patients having twice the incidence of females,[14] whereas James and colleagues reported a 13% incidence with an equal sex ratio.[9] Since these are not linear demarcations but bilateral hypopigmented macules, it is sometimes difficult to differentiate the changes from postinflammatory hypopigmentation or pityriasis alba.

Futcher also described a midchest demarcation,[16] and we have also seen it in an occasional patient at KDMC (Figure 13-8). The frequency of the

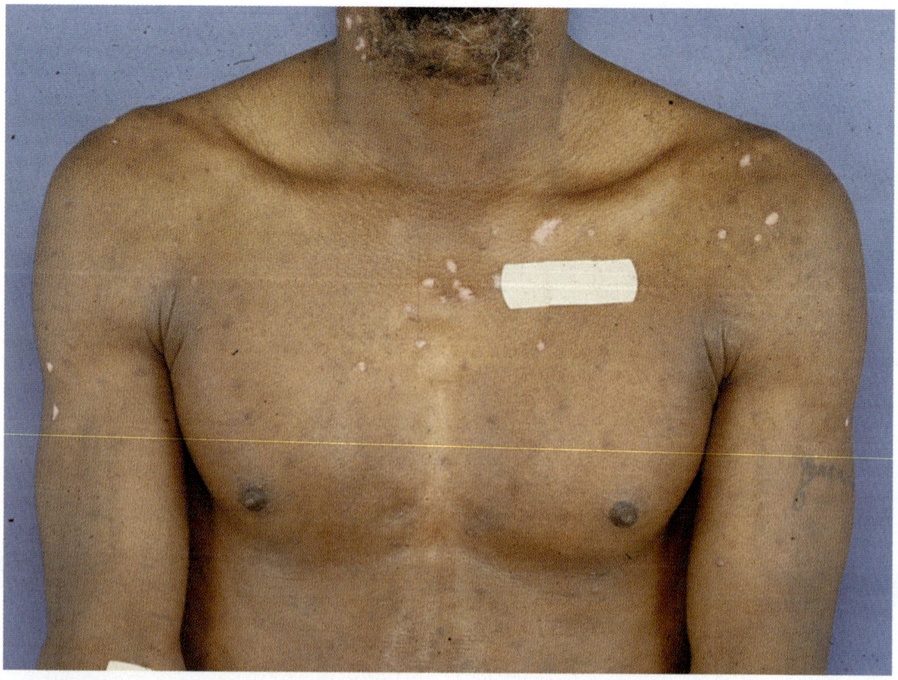

▲ **FIGURE 13-7** Cutaneous linea alba, vertical hypopigmentation in or near the midsaggital line. It often starts on one side, crosses the midline, and then moves down the opposite side.

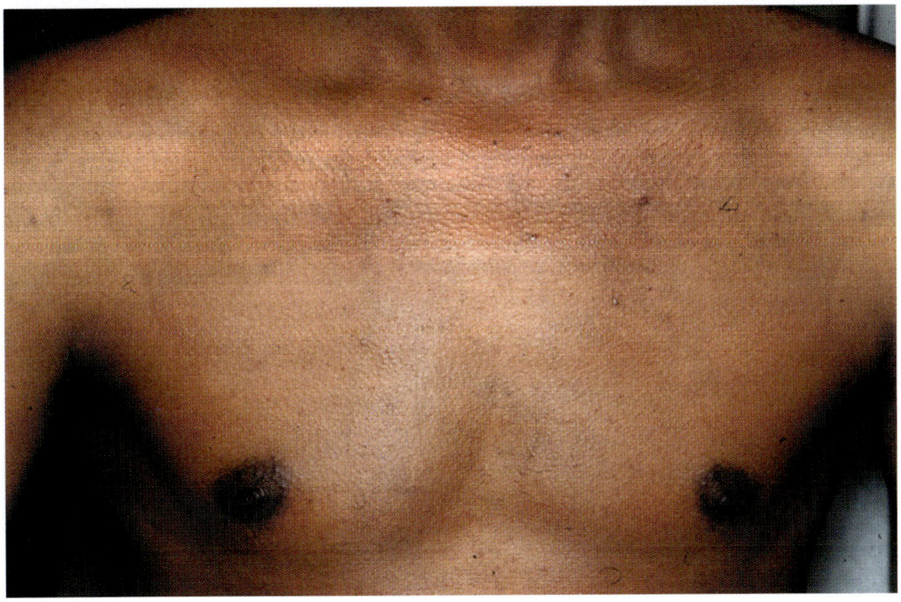

▲ **FIGURE 13-8** Futcher midchest demarcation.

demarcation makes it difficult to determine if there is any association with age, gender, body type, skin color, or disease.

PALMAR AND PLANTAR HYPERPIGMENTATION

Palmar and plantar hyperpigmentation is a common finding in blacks. A study at KDMC revealed that hyperpigmented macules and patches of the palms were present in 35% of black adults examined and in more than 50% of those over age 50 but absent in black infants (Figure 13-9 A-D). The youngest patient in the KDMC study demonstrating palmar hyperpigmentation was 4 years old. None of the black infants examined had plantar hyperpigmentation, whereas it was present in more than 70% of blacks over age 50. Since hyperpigmentation of neither the palms nor the soles is present at birth, trauma leading to postinflammatory changes may be the precipitating factor. Going barefooted as a child did not seem to explain with any predictability the presence or absence of plantar hyperpigmentation.

PUNCTATE KERATOSIS OF PALMAR CREASES

Darker skin of color patients often develop keratotic plugs in their palmar and finger creases. When the plugs are removed, shallow pits are left (Figure 13-9A and B). Some patients have sole involvement but only to a lesser degree. Atopy and manual labor are associated with this skin abnormality, but the exact cause is unknown. Therapy is usually not needed; however, if the plugs become painful, a daily use of 40% Urea cream usually provides a successful therapy.

LOCALIZED HYPERPIGMENTATION IN INFANTS

Black infants have localized areas of hyperpigmentation. This phenomenon is not mentioned in any dermatology textbooks, including the *Atlas of Black Dermatology*.[17] The usual areas of involvement are the helix of the ears, lips, fingernail and toenail matrix areas, penis, scrotum, vulva, nipples, umbilicus, axillae, and anal orifice (Figure 13-10). Between 60% and 85% of all black infants have these localized areas of darkness. There was no correlation with skin color, gender, or body build. Finger, toe, nail matrix, nipple, penis, scrotum, and vulvar hyperpigmentation seems to persist for the duration of one's life, whereas earlobe and axillary hyperpigmentation seems to disappear during the first year of life, whether the infant is exposed to sunlight or not. The rest of the skin seems to get darker, and the dark areas seem to get somewhat lighter.

It is difficult to explain why the ears (with 1400 ± 80 melanocytes per square

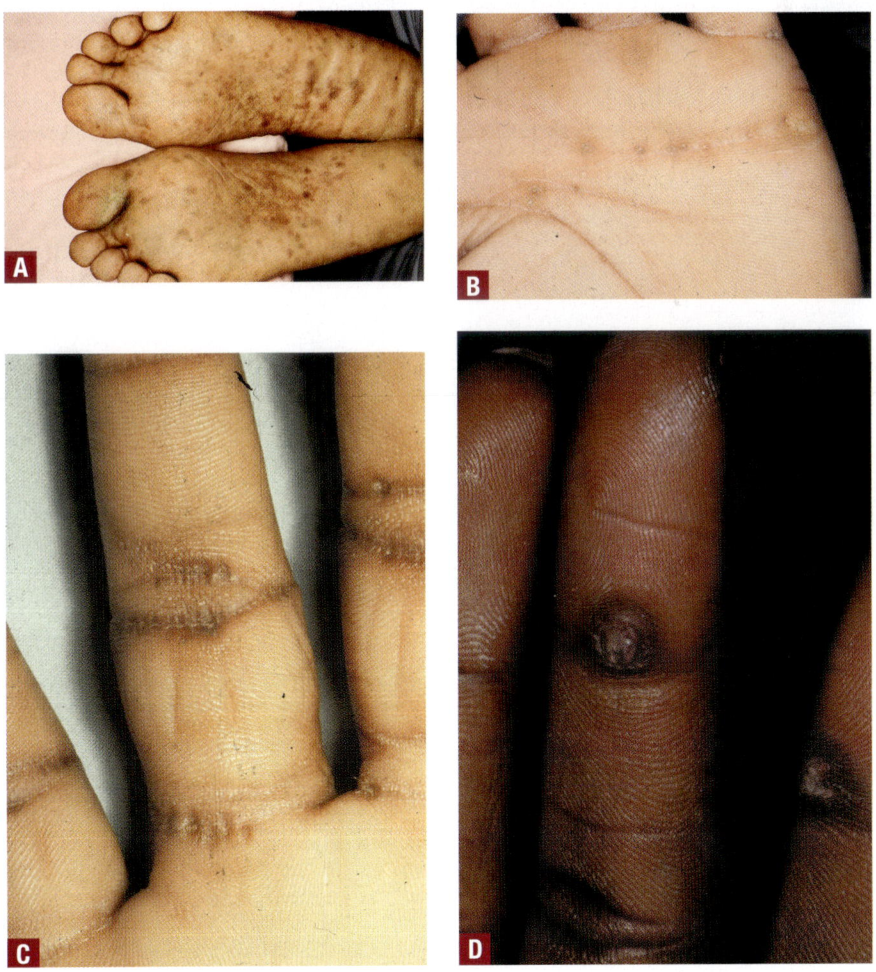

▲ **FIGURE 13-9** **A** Hyperpigmentation of souls, adults over age 50. **B, C and D** Punctate Keratosis of Palmar Creases.

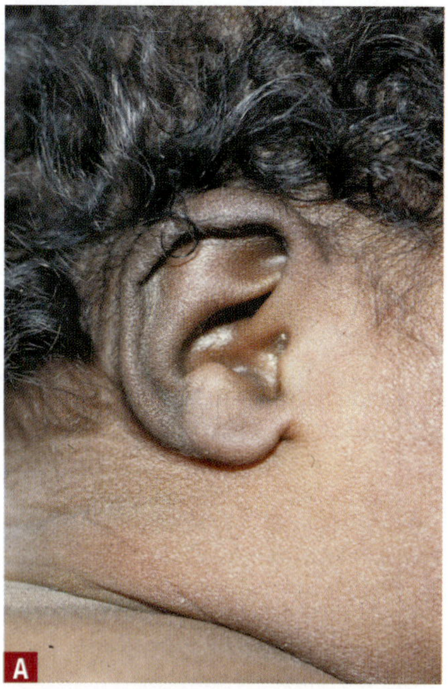

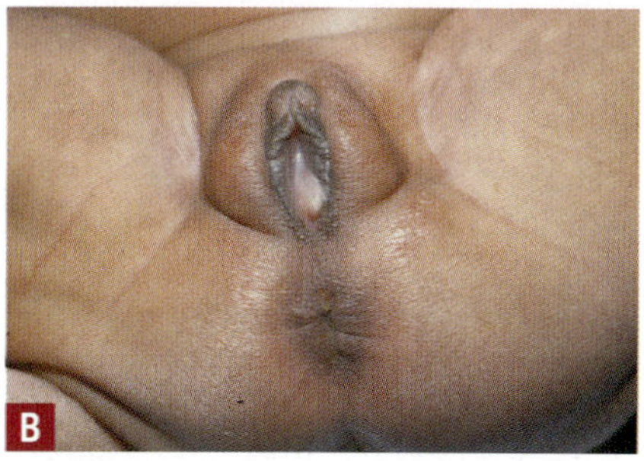

▲ **FIGURE 13-10** **A** and **B** Hyperpigmentation of ears (a) and genitourinary (b) region in infants.

millimeter) and not the cheeks (with 2310 ± 150 melanocytes per square millimeter)[18] are darker at birth. In black culture, these dark areas are often used to predict the ultimate skin color of the baby, that is, the color he or she will have as an adult.

MUCOUS MEMBRANE HYPERPIGMENTATION

Oral mucous membrane hyperpigmentation is common in black adults, infants, and children. (Figure 13-11). Hyperpigmentation of the lips is common in older blacks; however, in the KDMC study we found a deep grayish to violaceous, dry discoloration of the lips, especially the upper lip, in 60% of infants examined. It seemed to start at the lower or inner aspect of the free margin of the lips and progress inward approximately 5–7 mm. The discoloration clears within a few weeks of life without residual cutaneous markings.

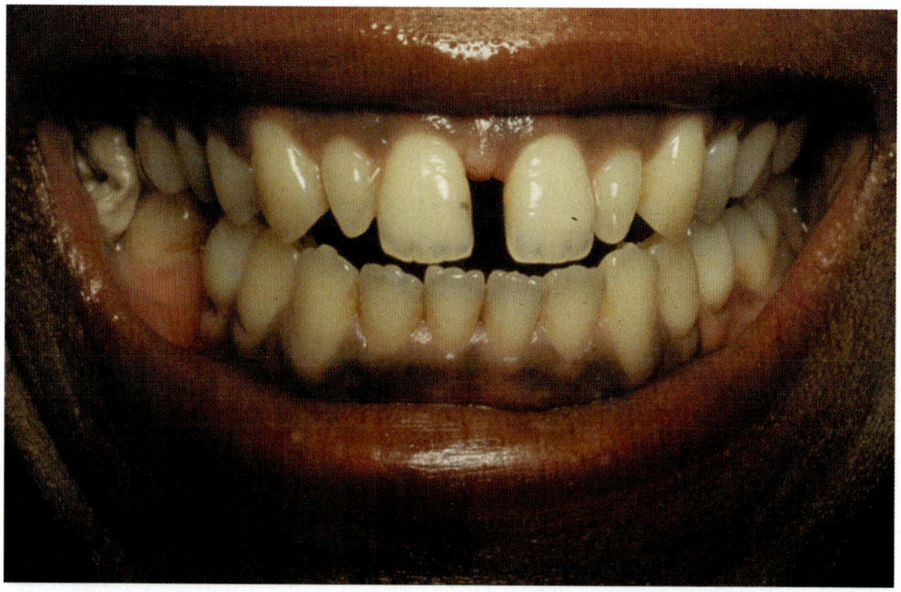

▲ **FIGURE 13-11** Mucous membrane hyperpigmentation, gums, adult over age 65.

Search of the dental, otolaryngology, and dermatology literature failed to reveal any mention of this nuance. One possible explanation is lip sucking in uteri.

Hyperpigmentation of the gums appeared in 25% of infants, and fewer than 10% had hyperpigmentation of the buccal mucosa. The severity and frequency of oral pigmentation seem to increase with age. Almost 80% of blacks over age 65 will have some type of oral mucous membrane hyperpigmentation, with the gums and lips being the areas most commonly involved.

An absence of scleral pigmentation was noted in all the black infants and children younger than 5 years of age. Scleral (actually the overlying conjunctiva) pigmentation seems to start in that portion of the conjunctiva exposed to sunlight and other elements, such as wind, heat, cold, and airborne particles. Over 80% of the black adults examined at KDMC had conjunctival pigmentation. Brown discoloration was the most common, but reddish brown, red, and yellowish brown discolorations also were noticed. Males had a higher incidence than females, suggesting that environmental exposure may be a contributing factor.

MELANONYCHIA STRIATA

Between 50% and 90% of black senior citizens have at least one fingernail with a vertical linear streak (i.e., longitudinal melanoychia, or melanoychia striate) (Figures 13-12). The youngest patient with melanonychia striata identified at KDMC was 6 years of age, but it is found primarily in adults. This suggests trauma, either acute or chronic, as the etiologic agent, especially since the thumb and/or index finger were involved most often. There seems to be no association of melanonychia with any systemic diseases; however, melanoma must be ruled out. Involvement of one nail with a width of 6 mm or more and variegation in color are features of longitudinal melanonychia secondary to malignant melanoma.

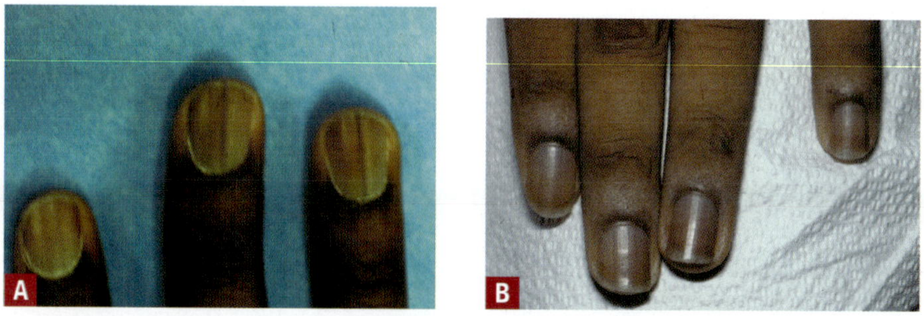

▲ **FIGURE 13-12** **A** and **B** Nail streaks, black senior citizens.

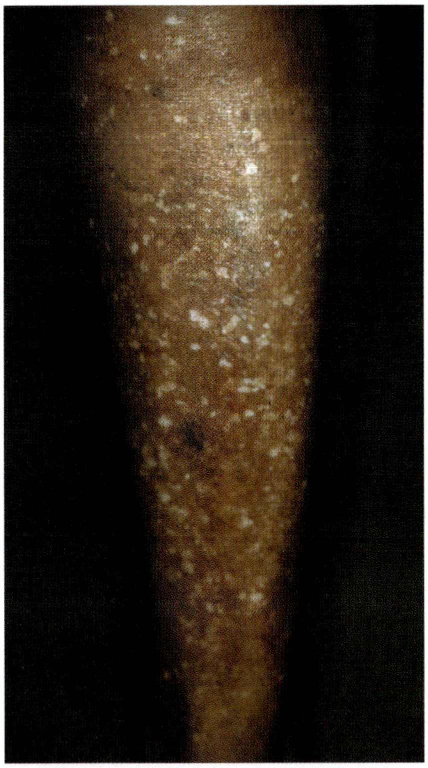

▲ **FIGURE 13-13** Idiopathic guttate hypomelanosis, lesions yellow-brown, asymptomatic hypopolymacules or patches primarily on anterior legs, senior citizens, females.

IDIOPATHIC GUTTATE HYPOMELANOSIS

Idiopathic guttate hypomelanosis is an overt pigmentary nuance in blacks. Although present in whites, it is often difficult to discern.[19] In individuals with very dark skin, the initial lesions are often yellow-brown in color. It is characterized by asymptomatic, hypopigmented, polygonal macules or patches (1–20 mm in diameter with an average diameter of 4 mm) primarily affecting the anterior legs.

The incidence varies according to age. It is present in more than 90% of black senior citizens, with the legs, thighs, abdomen, arms, and back involved in decreasing order (Figure 13-13). It appears to begin earlier in females and is rare in children and young adults.[20] Patients with idiopathic guttate hypomelanosis do not have an increased susceptibility to other pigmentary disorders.

CIRCUMSCRIBED DERMAL MELANOCYTOSIS (MONGOLIAN SPOTS)

Circumscribed dermal melanocytosis, originally termed *Mongolian spots*, consists of dark blue-gray macules and patches present at birth. They occur in 98% of African-American infants, 90% of Native American infants, 81% of Asian-American infants, 40–70% of Hispanic infants, and 10% of Caucasian infants. The color of the lesions is uniform, and there is no grossly visible change in the epidermis.

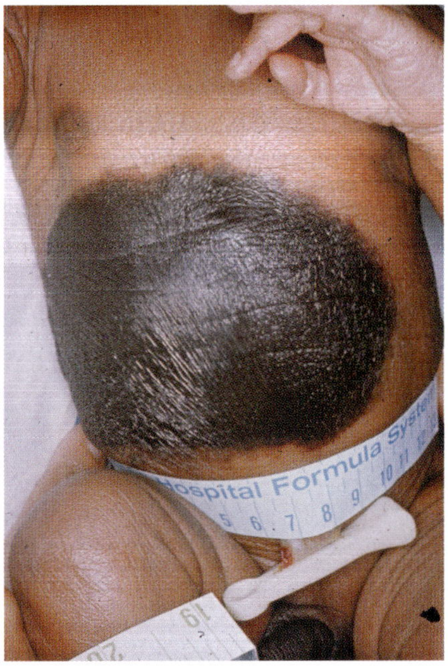

▲ **FIGURE 13-14** **Large** Mongolian spot on the abdomen.

Circumscribed dermal melanocytosis is a perfect example of how clinical observation has led to erroneous assumptions before cause and incidence are delineated. Erwin Balz, a German professor of internal medicine, was teaching in Tokyo in the early 1930s when he observed blue spots on the buttocks of Japanese children and named them "Mongolian spots," thinking them a characteristic of Mongolians.[21] When Adachi found the same spot in a white child, he insisted that it should be called a "child spot" instead. Initially, the Japanese believed that the spot was caused by bleeding in the fetus.[22] It is now known that the Monoglian spot is caused by the arrest of melanocytes in the dermis as they migrate from the neural crest to the epidermis during the eleventh to the fourteenth week of gestation.[21,22]

The KDMC studies demonstrated that the frequency of Mongolian spots was approximately the same in black babies with skin colors ranging from very fair to very dark.[2] They were most noticeable in medium-brown infants and often difficult to detect in very dark babies. In 18% of the cases, the Mongolian spots were not in the classic lumbosacral area; approximately half of these were located on the hips (Figure 13-14). The maximum number of lesions present in any infant was seven. Our 92% incidence is similar to that reported by other authors.[22]

CONCLUSION

There are many skin nuances in individuals of color that are not readily recognized by physicians or are mistaken for abnormalities. As physicians continue to treat a growing population of patients of color, it is important to recognize skin lesions that are variants of normal. Patients then can be reassured that the lesion is indeed normal, and potentially unnecessary procedures may be avoided.

REFERENCES

1. Niedelman ML. Abnormalities of pigmentation in the Negro. *Arch Dermatol Syphilol (Berl)* 1945;51:1-9.
2. Kelly AP. *Nuances of black skin: Study performed at King Drew Medical Center (KDMC)*. Presented at the NMA Section on Dermatology, New Orleans, LA, 1974.
3. Johnson S. The black skin: Norms and abnorms. *Cutis* 1978;22:332-336.
4. Futcher PH. A peculiarity of pigmentation of the upper arm of Negros. *Science* 1938;88:570-571.
5. Matsumoto S. Ube rein eigentumliche. Pigmentaverteilung an der Voigtschen Liniean (Beitrag zur kenntnis der Voigtschen Grenzen). *Arch Dermatol Syphilol (Berl)* 1913;118:157-164.
6. Ito K. The peculiar demarcation of pigmentation along the so-called Voigt's lines among the Japanese. *Dermatol Int* 1965;4:45-47.
7. Miura O. On the demarcation lines of pigmentation observed among Japanese on inner sides of their extremities and on the anterior and posterior sides of their medial regions. *Tohoku J Exp Ed* 1951;54: 135-140.
8. Vollum DI. Skin markings in Negro children from the West Indies. *Br J Dermatol* 1972;86:260.
9. James WD, Carter JM, Rodman OG. Pigmentation demarcation lines: A population survey. *J Am Acad Dermatol* 1987;16: 584-590.
10. Selmanowitz VJ, Krivo JM. Pigmentary demarcation lines. *Br J Dermatol* 1975;93: 371-377.
11. Wasserman HP. Peculiar pigment division along Voigt's line in an European and in a Xhosa woman. *Dermatologica* 1967;135: 461-464.
12. James WD, Meltzer MC, Guill MA, et al. Pigmentary demarcation lines associated with pregnancy. *J Am Acad Dermatol* 1984;11:438-440.

13. Fulk CS. Primary disorders of hyperpigmentation. *J Am Acam Dermatol* 1984;10:1-16.
14. Selmanowitz J, Krivo JM. Hypopigmented markings in Negroes. *Int J Dermatol* 1973;12:229-235.
15. Kisch B, Nasuhoglu A. A mediosternal depigmentation line in Negroes. *Exp Med Surg* 1953;11:265-267.
16. Futcher PH. The distribution of pigmentation on the arm and thorax of man. *Bull Johns Hopkins Hosp* 1940;67:372-373.
17. Rosen T, Martin S. *Atlas of Black Dermatology.* Boston, Little, Brown, 1981.
18. Fitzpatrick T, Szabo G. The melanocyte cytology and cytochemistry. *J Invest Dermatol* 1959;32:197-209.
19. Whitehead WJ, Moyer DG, Vander Plueg DE. Idiopathci guttate hypomelanosis. *Arch Dermatol* 1966;94:279-281.
20. Treadwell PA. Dermatoses in newborns. *Am Fam Physician* 1997;56:443-450.
21. Muraoka K. On the Mongolian spot in the Japanese. *Acta Anat Jpn* 1931;3:1371-1390.
22. Kikuchi I. What is a Mongolian spot? *Int J Dermatol* 1982;21:131-133, 1982; and Brennemann J. The sacral or so-called "Mongolian" pigment spots of earliest infancy and childhood, with especial references to their occurrence in the American Negro. *Am Anthropol* 1907;9:12-30.

CHAPTER 14

Skin Lesions: Normal and Pathologic

Sharona Yashar
Jennifer Haley

TABLE 14-1
Pigmentary Demarcation Lines (PDLs)

Type	Location	Pigment
A	Anterolateral upper arms, pectoral area	Hyperpigmented
B	Posteromedial aspect of lower legs	Hyperpigmented
C	Vertical line in presternal area	Hypopigmented
D	Posteromedial area of spine	Hyperpigmented
E	Chest from midthird of clavicle to periareolar skin	Hypopigmented
D	Straight of curved convex line on the face	Hyperpigmented

Key Points

- Pigmentary demarcation lines are normal boundaries of the skin that represent a transition between levels of melanin pigment in the skin corresponding to dermatomal innervation.
- Longitudinal melanonychia is a normal pattern of nail pigmentation seen in patients with skin of color that must be differentiated from benign and malignany melanocytic proliferations and extraneous pigment deposition.
- The gingiva of people with darker skin is often pigmented as well.
- Erythema dyschromicum perstans can be seen more often in people with skin of color.
- Lability of pigment in this population causes dramatic changes in skin color after inflammatory processes of the skin.
- Many common dermatologic conditions manifest with follicular or papular lesions in dark-skinned individuals.
- Keloidal scarring is common in patients with skin of color.

NORMAL VARIATIONS IN SKIN OF COLOR

There are a number of skin lesions that are part of the normal variant in people with skin of color. Since the non-Caucasian population of the United States and abroad is increasing,[1,2] knowledge of normal variations in skin is crucial in evaluating and treating dermatology patients with skin of color. Historically, lack of recognition of benign variations in dark skin has led to unnecessary treatment and potentially poor results. These lesions fall into pigmentary and nonpigmentary categories.[3]

PIGMENTARY VARIANTS

Pigmentary Demarcation Lines

Pigmentary demarcation lines are normal boundaries of the skin that represent a transition between darker and lighter melanin pigment distribution corresponding to dermatomal innervation of the skin by spinal nerves. There are six types of pigmentary demarcation lines[4] (Table 14-1). In one study, 79% of African-American women and 75% of men had at least one pigmentary demarcation line. These lines may be present at birth, arise later in life, or occur during pregnancy.[5]

Type A, also termed *Voigt's* (*Futcher's*) *lines*, are sharply demarcated, frequently bilateral lines of pigmentation found at the anterolateral junction of the upper arms (Figure 14-1). The change from darker to lighter pigment occurs at the junction of the extensor to flexor surface of the arm. Type B lines occur at the posteromedial aspect of the lower legs and often arise during pregnancy.[6] Up to 14% of black women present with type B lines during pregnancy.[5] Other pigmentary demarcation lines occur on the spine, chest and legs (Figure 14-2), and face.[7] Type E demarcation lines are also referred to as *midline hypopigmentation*. Midline hypopigmentation occurs over the anterior aspect of the central and midsternal chest and consists of hypopigmented linear or oval macules. There may be an autosomal dominant inheritance pattern of this condition.[3] The differential diagnosis includes ash leaf macules of tuberous sclerosis, postinflammatory hypopigmentation, idiopathic guttate hypomelanosis, vitiligo, seborrheic dermatitis, and tinea versicolor.[8]

The etiology of pigmentary demarcation lines is unclear. Genetic and hormonal influences have been proposed for type B pigmentary demarcation lines. Compression of peripheral nerves between S1 and S2 by the pregnant uterus also may be a factor.[9] Although reported in Caucasian people, pigmentary demarcation lines are rare compared with darker-skinned individuals. Skin biopsy shows increased pigmentation in the basal keratinocytes of the epidermis

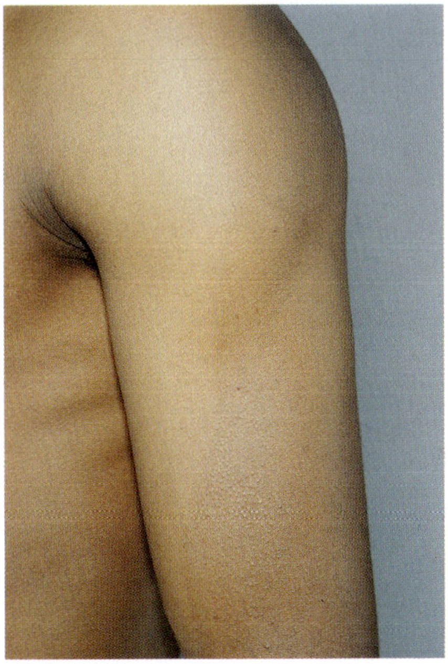

▲ **FIGURE 14-1** Futcher's line of demarcation on the arm.

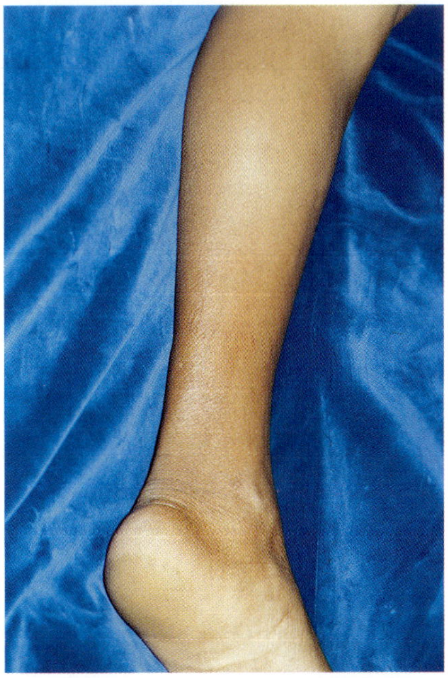

▲ **FIGURE 14-2** Demarcation line on the posteromedial aspect of the lower leg.

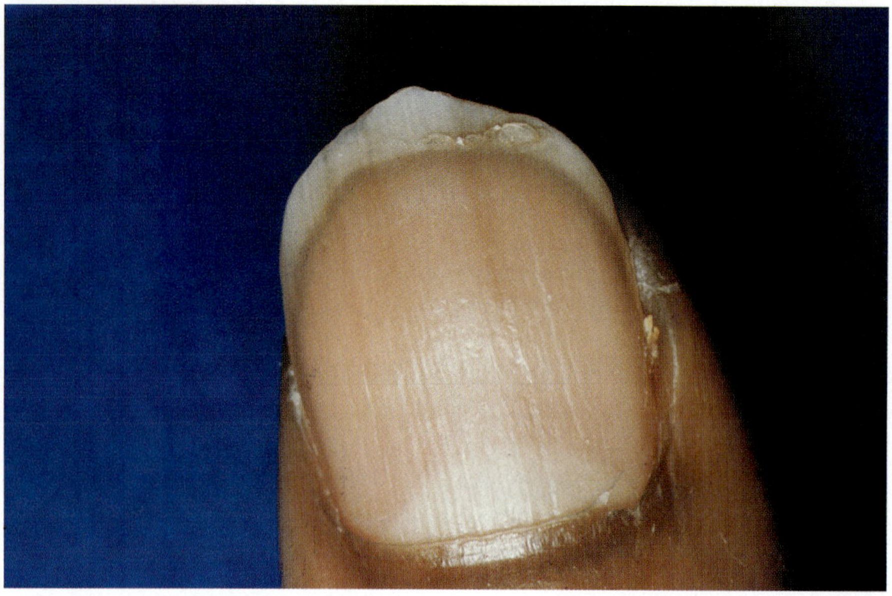

▲ **FIGURE 14-3** Longitudinal melanonychia.

without an inflammatory infiltrate or increase in melanocytes.[6]

Pigmentary demarcation lines represent a change in the amount of melanin pigment in the skin and should be differentiated from the rare condition of acquired dermal melanocytosis, in which there is an increase in melanocytes in the dermis. These lesions appear as blue-gray patches on the face, trunk, or extremities and may appear during pregnancy.[10]

Nail Pigmentation

Another frequent pigmentary variant in skin of color is nail pigmentation (longitudinal melanonychia) (Figure 14-3). Longitudinal bands of brown pigment often occur as an acquired condition in pigmented skin, and there is often a history of trauma. Over 50% of African-Americans over age 50 have at least one nail involved. The degree of nail pigmentation is increased in patients with darker skin. Histologically, there is increased melanin in the matrix and nail plate. The differential diagnosis includes melanocytic nevus, melanoma, and pigmentation owing to infection, drugs, chemicals, or postradiation changes. Malignant longitudinal melanonychia is usually wider than 5 mm.[11] Recently, dermoscopy has become an increasingly helpful tool in the diagnosis of nail pigment. A grayish background and thin, regular gray lines are common characteristics in ethnic-type nail pigmentation,[12] whereas longitudinal black lines of subungual melanoma tend to be irregular in color, spacing, thickness, and parallelism.

Oral Pigmentation

Oral pigmentation is seen commonly on the gingivae, hard palate, buccal mucosa, and tongue of people of darker skin and varies in color from light brown to blue discoloration[13] (Figure 14-4). The prevalence of oral pigmentation in black Brazilian children was 93.2% compared with 12.5% in white Brazilian children.[14] This physiologic pigmentation is due to greater melanocytic activity rather than a greater number of melanocytes.[15] The gingiva is the most common intraoral site of pigment.[16] Lesions appear as a bilateral, well-demarcated, ribbon-like dark brown band that usually spares the marginal gingiva, an important feature that helps to distinguish them from other pathologic causes of pigmentation, such as Addison disease.[17] In contrast, pigmentation of the buccal mucosa, hard palate, lips, and tongue may appear as less well-demarcated brown patches. In contrast to nail pigmentation, the association between the frequency of oral mucosal pigmentation and darker skin pigment is not as clear. Some observers have suggested that the degree of pigmentation may be partly related to mechanical, chemical, and physical stimulation, which can increase melanin production.[18,19]

The differential diagnosis for oral mucosal pigmentation is broad. Oral pigmentation has been classified as endogenous or exogenous, localized or generalized, melanin-based or non-melanin-based, and benign or malignant (Table 14-2). One always must distinguish the normal variation of oral pigmentation from melanoma, melanocytic nevi, postinflammatory changes, contact dermatitis, smoker's melanosis, secondary syphilis, and drug or heavy metal ingestion. Physiologic oral pigmentation usually appears in infancy and darkens with puberty.[17] Systemic disease or exogenous influence must be suspected when pigmentation develops or darkens rapidly in adulthood.[17] Melanoma in the oral cavity is rare and has a poor prognosis.[20] Peutz-Jegher syndrome is a genetic disorder defined by intestinal hamartomas and mucocutaneous pigmentation. Oral pigmented lesions are

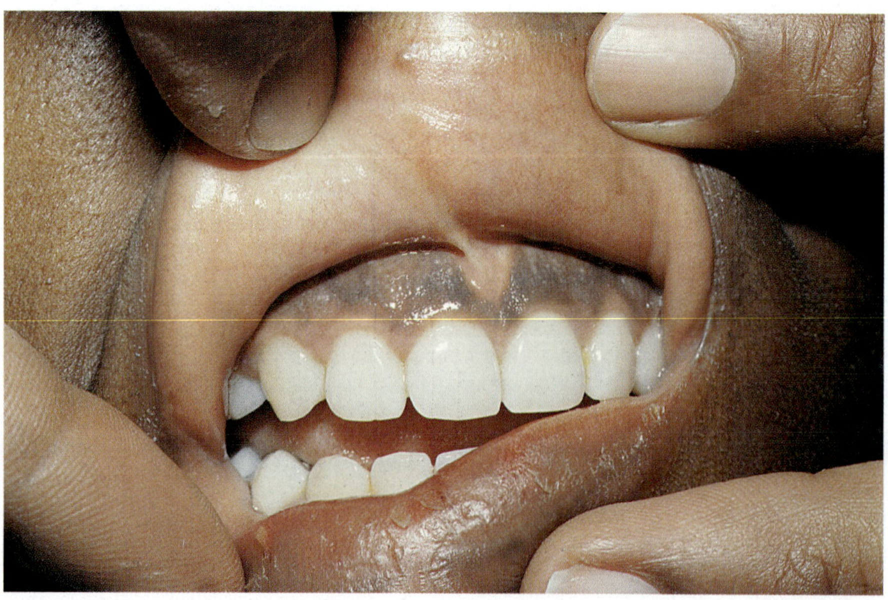

▲ **FIGURE 14-4** Oral pigmentation involving the gingival.

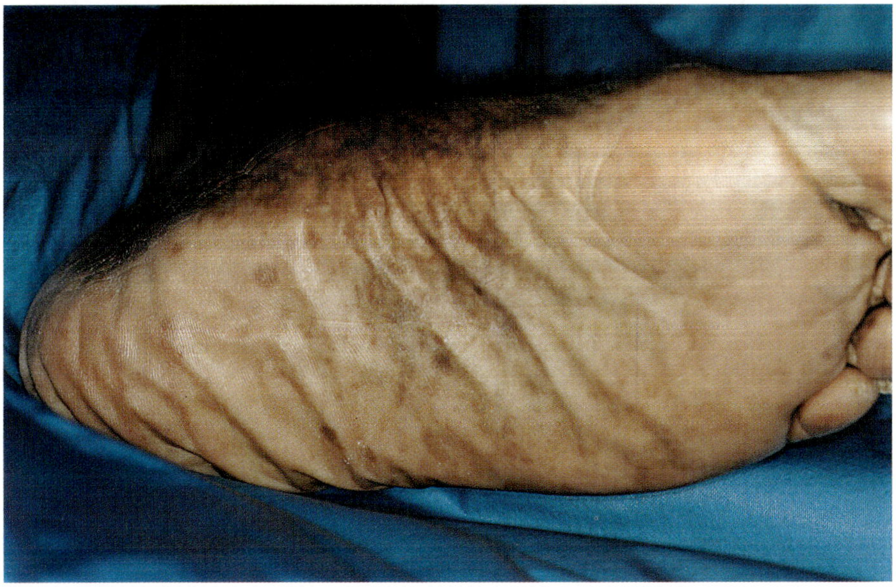

▲ **FIGURE 14-5** Plantar hyperpigmented macules.

usually found on the lower lip and buccal mucosa and rarely on the upper lip, tongue, palate, and gingiva.[18] Smoker's melanosis is directly related to tobacco use and represents a benign focal pigmentation of the oral mucosa.[21,22] Lesions present as multiple brown pigmented macules less than 1 cm in diameter at the attached labial anterior gingival and interdental papillae of the mandible.[18] Antimalarial agent—induced oral pigmentation is characterized as slate gray in color.

Palmar and Plantar Hyperpigmented Macules

Hyperpigmented macules on the palms and soles are another normal pigmentary variant in people with skin of color. These lesions vary in size and shape and may be sharp or ill-defined with a reticulated appearance[3] (Figure 14-5). They must be distinguished from similar-appearing lesions of secondary syphilis, tinea nigra, nevi, and melanoma.

NONPIGMENTARY VARIANTS

Punctate Keratoses of the Palms and Soles

Most often occurring in the creases of the palms and soles, punctate keratoses are 1- to 5-mm depressed comedo-like keratinous plugs (Figure 14-6A and 14-6B). There have been reports that this is an acquired condition as a result of repetitive trauma. However, autosomal dominant inheritance has been seen. Punctate keratoses are a benign normal variant seen most often in black patients. A personal or family history of atopy has been reported in up to 80% of patients with keratosis palmaris et plantaris.[2] Histologically, these pits show hyperkeratosis and parakeratosis overlying a pyknotic, vacuolated epidermis and some spongiosis in the basal layer, and occlusion of glands may be present. Keratosis palmaris et plantaris must be differentiated from the palmar pits of nevoid basal cell carcinoma syndrome, in which lesions tend to spare the creases, and from perforating disorders such as Kyrle disease, in which keratotic papules with central plugs are seen on the extremities.

Oral Leukoedema

Leukoedema is a benign, pearly, whitish gray, nonkeratotic lesion of the buccal mucosa that is present as a normal variant in many people of color. It may develop at any age and is usually asymptomatic.[23] Leukoedema is seen in as

TABLE 14-2
Classification of Oral Pigmentation

Localized pigmentation
Amalgam tattoo
Graphite tattoo
Nevus
Melanotic macule
Melanoacanthoma
Kaposi sarcoma
Epithelioid oligomatosis
Verruciform xanthoma
Melanoma
Generalized pigmentation
Genetic
Physiologic (ethnic)
Peutz-Jegher syndrome
Laugier-Hunziker syndrome
Spotty pigmentation
Carney syndrome
Leopard syndrome
Lentiginosis profuse
Hemochromatosis
Neurofibromatosis
Wilson disease
Endocrine
Addison disease
Albright syndrome
Acanthosis nigricans
Pregnancy
Hyperthyroidism
Drugs
Antimalarials
Antimicrobials
Minocycline
Amiodarone
Clorpromazine
Zidovudine
Ketoconazole
Methyldopa
Busulfan
Menthol
Contraceptive pills
Other
Smoking
Heavy metals
HIV
Nutritional deficiency
Benign vascular tumors

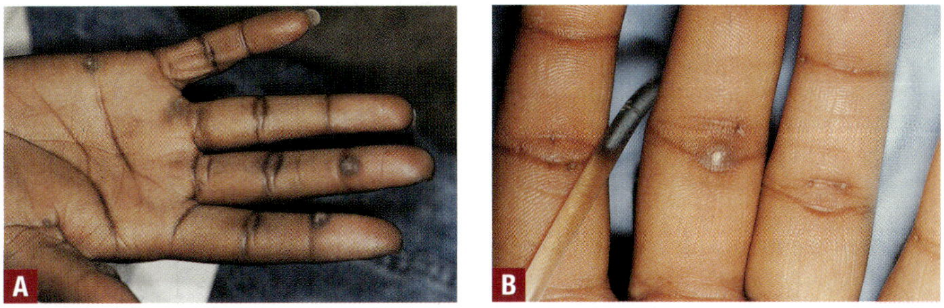

▲ **FIGURE 14-6** A and B Punctate keratoses palms and fingers.

TABLE 14-3
Common Skin Conditions Reported in Black, Hispanic, and Arab Groups in the United States

Blacks[a]		Hispanics[b]		Arabs[c]	
Acne	27.7%	Acne	20.7%	Acne	37.7%
Eczematous dermatitis	23.4%	Eczematous dermatitis	19.3%	Eczematous dermatitis	25.5%
Pigmentary disorders	9.0%	Photoaging	16.8%	Fungal infection	20.0%
Seborrheic dermatitis	6.5%	Tinea/onychomycosis	9.9%	Condyloma/warts	20.0%
Alopecia	5.3%	Melasma	8.2%	Melasma	14.5%
Fungal infections	4.3%	Condyloma/warts	7.1%	Keloid	10.7%
Condyloma/warts	2.4%	Hyperpigmentation	6%	Psoriasis	4.7%
Tinea versicolor	2.2%	Seborrheic keratosis	4.5%	Vitiligo	2.0%
Keloids	2.1%	Acrochordon	4.2%		
Pityriasis rosea	2.0%	Seborrheic dermatitis	3.2%		
Urticaria	2.0%	Alopecia	2.3%		
		Psoriasis	0.8%		

[a]From Halder RM, Roberts CI, Nootheti PK. Cutaneous diseases in the black races. *Dermatol Clin* 2003;21:679–687, ix.
[b]From Sanchez MR. Cutaneous diseases in Latinos. *Dermatol Clin* 2003;21:689–697.
[c]El-Essawi D, et al. A survey of skin disease and skin-related issues in Arab Americans. *J Am Acad Dermatol* 2007.

many as 90% of adult blacks and, although less prominent, in half the Caucasian population.[24] Tobacco smoking and chewing may enhance the whiteness and size of the lesions. Leukoedema is characterized histologically by intracellular edema and vacuolated epithelial cells with some pyknosis.[25] The epithelium is hyperplastic with elongated rete ridges. Treatment for leukoedema is unnecessary, and there is no malignant potential. The differential diagnosis includes white sponge nevus, frictional keratosis, smokeless tobacco keratosis, and Witkop syndrome (scalp hair normal to thin, hypodontia of secondary teeth, normal sweating, and prolonged retention of primary teeth).

Pearly Penile Papules

Pearly penile papules are benign, dome-shaped papules found on the corona of the glans penis. They vary in size (ranging from 1–2 mm in width and up to 4 mm in length), color (pink, white, yellowish, or translucent), and shape (dome, acuminate, or annular). In most cases, they are asymptomatic and are found incidentally. A higher incidence has been reported in blacks and in uncircumcised men.[26–28] Histologically, pearly penile papules resemble angiofibromas with prominent orthokeratosis, hypergranulosis, ectatic capillaries and venules, and stellate fibroblasts with dermal fibrosis.[29] No treatment is necessary, but ablative methods such as cryotherapy and CO_2 laser have been tried with equivocal results.[30,31]

COMMON SKIN DISORDERS SEEN PREDOMINANTLY IN DARKER SKIN

There have been several reports of the rates of common skin disorders in pigmented skin. Table 14-3 shows the common skin diagnoses seen in black, Hispanic, and Arab-American populations in the United States.[32–34] The most common skin disorders seen in skin of color include acne and eczematous dermatitis.

Acne lesions in people with skin of color include papules, pustules, comedones, and numerous acne hyperpigmented macules and a high percentage of keloidal scarring (up to 54.1%) (Figure 14-7).[35] Halder showed that comedonal lesions biopsied from African-American females showed marked inflammation, including polymorphonuclear leukocytes, in contrast to comedonal lesions in white skin, which did not show significant inflammation. This may account for why acne in darker skin commonly results in postinflammatory hyperpigmentation.[36]

Melasma is another very frequent and distressing disorder that occurs in people with skin of color.[37] Hormonal causes, ultraviolet (UV) radiation, and

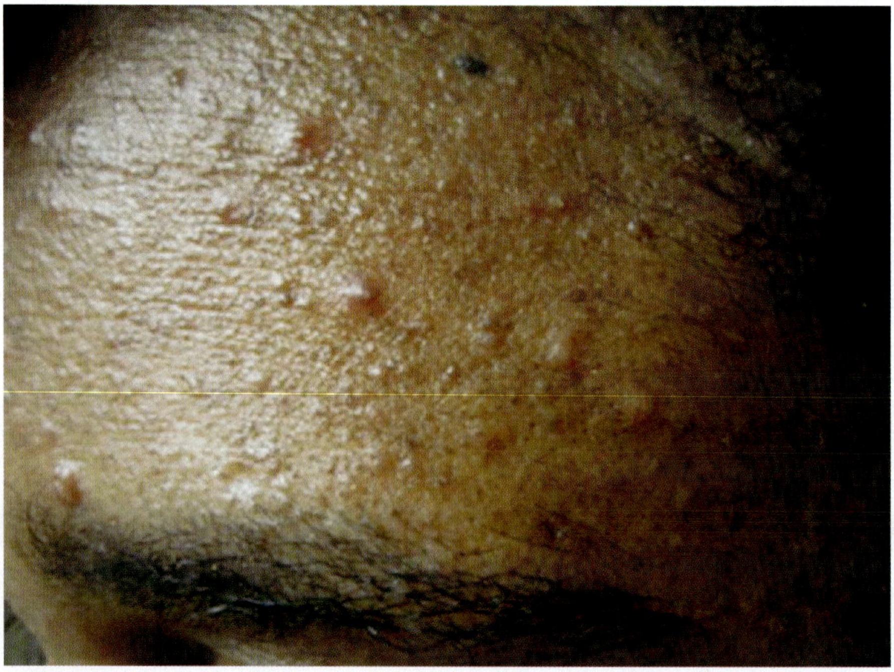

▲ **FIGURE 14-7** Acne vulgaris.

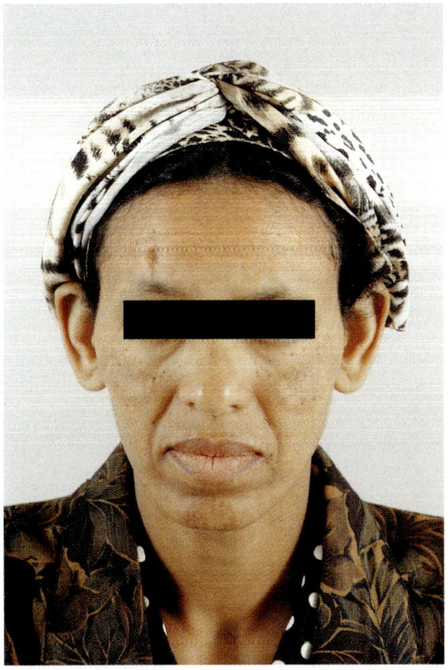

▲ **FIGURE 14-8** Facial melasma

lability of melanocytes may be influential etiologic factors (Figure 14-8).[38]

In addition to common skin disorders seen in all skin types, there are several dermatoses that are far more frequent in darker skin. One well-known example is the high prevalence of actinic prurigo seen in Native Americans and the Mestizo population in Latin America.[39] Actinic prurigo is an idiopathic photodermatosis that affects the sun-exposed skin, resulting in erythematous papules, nodules, and lichenified plaques secondary to chronic pruritus.[40] Its onset is usually in childhood, and there is a 2–4:1 ratio of females to males affected.[41,42] Early-onset lesions usually affect the lower lip. Conjunctivitis and pterygium formation also have been reported.[43] The differential diagnosis for actinic prurigo includes polymorphous light eruption, atopic dermatitis with photosensitivity, and chronic actinic dermatitis.

Histopathologic characteristics of actinic prurigo have been elucidated recently and include hyperkeratosis, ortho- or parakeratosis, regular acanthosis, and a dense lymphocytic inflammatory infiltrate in the superficial dermis. There is usually a lack of deep inflammatory infiltrate, periadnexal involvement, and solar elastosis. The dense lymphoplasmacytic infiltrate may be lichenoid or form follicles or germinal centers. In addition, numerous eosinophils are usually present. It has been proposed that the prevalence of actinic prurigo in certain ethnic groups is a reflection of certain genetic predisposition. There are several reports of human leukocyte antigen (HLA) associations with actinic prurigo, including HLA-A24 and HLA-Cw4 in Cree Indians from Saskatchewan, Canada,[44] HLA-Cw4 in Chimila Indians from Colombia,[45] and HLA-DR4, HLA-A28, and HLA-B39 in Mexicans.[46]

Erythema dyschromicum perstans (ashy dermatosis) is a rare, idiopathic skin condition that appears in the first few decades of life and consists of asymptomatic blue-gray patches of varying size over the trunk, extremities, and neck, with early lesions reported to have an advancing erythematous border.[33] This disease is common in people with dark skin, particularly in women of Asian or Latin descent.[47,48] The differential diagnosis includes lichen planus, idiopathic eruptive macular pigmentation, fixed drug eruptions, mastocytosis, macular amyloidosis, and postinflammatory hyperpigmentation.[49]

The histopathologic findings from the active border include increased pigmentation of the basal layer of the epidermis, vacuolar alteration of the basement membrane, and a mild perivascular lymphohistiocytic infiltrate with melanophages. A range of predisposing factors for erythema dyschromicum perstans has been revealed, including ingestion of ammonium nitrate,[50] nematode-induced intestinal parasitosis,[51] use of oral contrast media,[52] and contact with chemicals such as the pesticide chlorothalonil[53] and cobalt.[54] Although the exact immunologic basis of erythema dyschromicum perstans has not been elucidated, a recent study performed in the Mexican population pointed to a higher association of HLA-DR4 (DRB1*0407) in this condition.[55]

CUTANEOUS REACTION PATTERNS IN SKIN OF COLOR

Both hereditary and environmental factors contribute to the appearance and incidence of certain dermatoses in skin of color. Hereditary factors likely include pigmentary differences, as well as other, yet to be identified key differences in immunology. Environmental factors that are important in altering skin disease include nutrition, emotions, socioeconomic status, hygiene, and occupation. In addition to the unequal prevalence of certain dermatologic and systemic disorders in individuals with dark skin, there is also a predisposition to develop atypical reaction patterns to common dermatoses. Some cutaneous reaction patterns seen more commonly in skin of color include: follicular, annular, papular, granulomatous, keloidal, fibromatous, and ulcerative patterns.[8]

Lability of Pigment

Pigmentary disorders are a significant concern in individuals with Fitzpatrick skin types 4–6. The lability of pigmentation in this population causes dramatic change in skin color after inflammatory or bullous diseases characterized by postinflammatory hypopigmentation or hyperpigmentation (Figure 14-9).[34] Although the exact mechanism of postinflammatory pigment change is not known, the normal release of inflammatory mediators and cytokines from inflammatory cells has specific effects on melanocyte biology.[56] Leukotriene B_4, prostaglandins D_2 and E_2, endothelins, interleukins 1 and 6, and tumor necrosis factor alpha have been shown to increase melanogenesis, whereas leukotriene C_4 may decrease melanogenesis and also cause movement of melanocytes.[57] Postinflammatory pigment change is often more dramatic in dark skin, and lesions may persist for an extended period of time than similar inflammatory conditions in lighter skin (Fitzpatrick skin types 1–3).

Follicular and Papular Reactions

There is a tendency to develop follicular or papular reactions to many common dermatoses in dark-skinned individuals. This may be a result of yet unknown factors that cause an affinity for the pilar apparatus (Figure 14-10). Follicular tinea versicolor, papular pityriasis rosea, papular lichen planus, and follicular eczema are seen more often in black individuals. Disseminate and recurrent

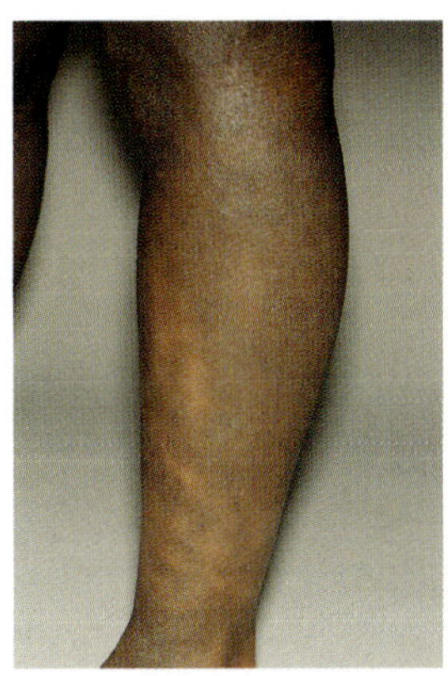

▲ **FIGURE 14-9** Post inflammatory hypopigmentation and hyperpigmentation on the leg.

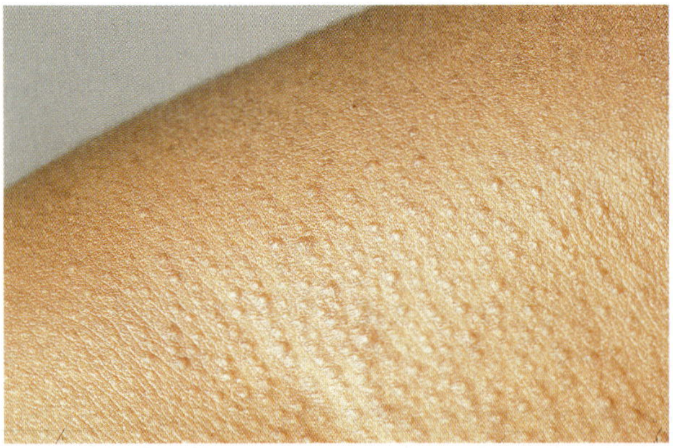

▲ **FIGURE 14-10** Follicular Accentuation in Atopic Dermatitis.

infundibulofolliculitis is a variant of follicular eczema that presents as recurrent, pruritic follicular-based papules on the neck, trunk, and proximal extremities. Black adults tend to develop a papular variant of lichen simplex chronicus.[58] Sarcoidosis may be papular, lichenoid, or verrucous. Secondary syphilis may be pruritic and present in a papular or follicular distribution.[1] Dermatosis papulosa nigra, histologically identical to seborrheic keratosis, presents as small 1- to 5-mm papular lesions on the face of up to 70% of black individuals.[59]

Vesiculobullous Diseases

Bullous lichen planus,[60,61] papulovesicular pityriasis rosea,[62] and bullous secondary syphilis have been reported in patients with skin of color. In addition, acropustulosis of infancy, transient neonatal pustular melanosis, and erythema toxicum neonatorum have a tendency to occur more commonly in black children.[63]

Granulomatous Lesions

There is a propensity to develop granulomatous reactions in dermatoses in skin of color. Sarcoidosis has been reported more commonly in black individuals. In a recent study, the risk of sarcoidosis among the African-American population is three to four times greater than among Caucasians in the United States. Familial clustering also was found, indicating a certain genetic susceptibility. Familial sarcoidosis is more frequent among African-Americans (17%) than among Caucasians (6%). Sarcoidosis may present as hypopigmented or hyperpigmented, papular, nodular, plaquelike and ichthyosiform lesions.[64] Secondary syphilis,[65] rosacea, and seborrheic dermatitis may become granulomatous as well.[8]

Keloidal Reactions

Keloid scarring occurs in all races but has been reported to occur more frequently in skin of color. It has been reported to arise from 3–18 times more often in black persons than in white persons[66,67] and to be more common in the Chinese population in Asia.[68] Although not fully understood, keloidal scarring occurs through the interaction between fibroblasts and cytokines that serve to aid the production of excessive collagen and inhibit the degradation of the extracellular matrix components.[69] Studies show that fibroblasts are larger and binucleated or multinucleated in the skin of black persons.[70] Several etiologic factors for keloids have been proposed, including: trauma, infection, abnormal metabolism of melanocyte-stimulating hormone, physiologic hyperactivity of the pituitary gland (e.g., during puberty and pregnancy), genetic and familial disorders, malnutrition, and theories suggesting an immunologic basis for keloid formation.[71–76] However, the exact mechanism through which there is a higher incidence of keloidal scarring in darker-skinned individuals is still not known.

REFERENCES

1. Abell E, Marks R, Jones EW. Secondary syphilis: clinico-pathological review. *Br J Dermatol* 1975;93:53-61.
2. Anderson WA, Elam MD, Lambert WC. Keratosis punctata and atopy: Report of 31 cases with a prospective study of prevalence. *Arch Dermatol* 1984;120:884-890.
3. Henderson AL. Skin variations in blacks. *Cutis* 1983;32:376-377.
4. Amichai B, Grunwald MH. Pigmentary demarcation lines of pregnancy. *Eur J Obstet Gynecol Reprod Biol* 2006; 239-240.
5. James WD, Carter JM, Rodman OG. Pigmentary demarcation lines: A population survey. *J Am Acad Dermatol* 1987;16:584-590.
6. Bonci A, Patrizi A. Pigmentary demarcation lines in pregnancy. *Arch Dermatol* 2002;138:127-128.
7. Malakar S, Dhar S. Pigmentary demarcation lines over the face. *Dermatology* 2000;200:85-86.
8. McLaurin CI. Cutaneous reaction patterns in blacks. *Dermatol Clin* 1988;6:353-362.
9. Ozawa H, Rokugo M, Aoyama H. Pigmentary demarcation lines of pregnancy with erythema. *Dermatology* 1993;187:134-136.
10. Rubin AI, Laborde SV, Stiller MJ. Acquired dermal melanocytosis: Appearance during pregnancy. *J Am Acad Dermatol* 2001;45:609-613.
11. Haneke E, Baran R. Longitudinal melanonychia. *Dermatol Surg* 2001;27:580-584.
12. Ronger S, Touzet S, Ligeron C, et al. Dermoscopic examination of nail pigmentation. *Arch Dermatol* 2002;138:1327-1333.
13. Gaeta GM, Satriano RA, Baroni A. Oral pigmented lesions. *Clin Dermatol* 2002;20:286-288.
14. Eleuterio D. [Clinical study of intraoral physiologic melanin pigmentation in children selected from three distinct ethnic groups: White, yellow and Negro.] *Rev Fac Farm Odontol Araraquara* 1969;3:19-47.
15. Kauzman A, Pavone M, Blanas N, et al. Pigmented lesions of the oral cavity: Review, differential diagnosis, and case presentations. *J Can Dent Assoc* 2004;70:682-683.
16. Ozbayrak S, Dumlu A, Ercalik-Yalcinkaya S. Treatment of melanin-pigmented gingiva and oral mucosa by CO_2 laser. *Oral Surg Oral Med Oral Pathol Oral Radiol Endod* 2000;90:14-15.
17. Eisen D. Disorders of pigmentation in the oral cavity. *Clin Dermatol* 2000;18:579-587.
18. Cicek Y, Ertas U. The normal and pathological pigmentation of oral mucous membrane: A review. *J Contemp Dent Pract* 2003;4:76-86.
19. Dummett C. Clinical observation on pigment variations in healthy oral tissues in the Negro. *J Dent Res* 1945;24:7-13.
20. Gloster HM Jr, Neal K. Skin cancer in skin of color. *J Am Acad Dermatol* 2006;55:741-760.
21. Dummett CO. Oral tissue color changes, part I. *Quintessence Int Dent Dig* 1979;10:39-45.
22. Araki S, Murata K, Ushio K, et al. Dose-response relationship between tobacco consumption and melanin pigmentation in the attached gingiva. *Arch Environ Health* 1983;38: 375-378.
23. Martin JL. Leukoedema: An epidemiological study in whites and African-Americans. *J Tenn Dent Assoc* 1997;77:18-21.
24. Bouquot JE. Common oral lesions found during a mass screening examination. *J Am Dent Assoc* 1986;112:50-57.
25. Martin JL. Leukoedema: A review of the literature. *J Natl Med Assoc* 1992;84:938-940.
26. Rehbein HM. Pearly penile papules: Incidence. *Cutis* 1977;19:54-57.
27. Glicksman JM, Freeman RG. Pearly penile papules: A statistical study of incidence. *Arch Dermatol* 1966;93:56-59.
28. Neinstein LS, Goldenring J. Pink pearly papules: An epidemiologic study. *J Pediatr* 1984;105:594-595.

29. Agrawal SK, Bhattacharya SN, Singh N. Pearly penile papules: A review. *Int J Dermatol* 2004;43:199-201.
30. McKinlay JR, Graham BS, Ross EV. The clinical superiority of continuous exposure versus short-pulsed carbon dioxide laser exposures for the treatment of pearly penile papules. *Dermatol Surg* 1999;25:124-126.
31. El Essawi J, Hammad A, Lim H. A survey of skin disease and skin-related issues in Arab Americans. *J Am Acad of Dermatol* 2007;56:933-938.
32. El-Essawi J, Hammad A, Lim H. A survey of skin disease and skin-related issues in Arab Americans. *J Am Acad Dermatol* 2007;56:933-938.
33. Sanchez MR. Cutaneous diseases in Latinos. *Dermatol Clin* 2003;21:689-697.
34. Halder RM, Roberts CI, Nootheti PK. Cutaneous diseases in the black races. *Dermatol Clin* 2003;21:679-687, ix.
35. Taylor SC, Fran Cook-Bolden F, Rahman Z, et al. Acne vulgaris in skin of color. *J Am Acad Dermatol* 2002;46:S98-106.
36. Halder RM, Brooks HL, Callender VD. Acne in ethnic skin. *Dermatol Clin* 2003; 21:609-615, vii.
37. Grimes PE, Stockton T. Pigmentary disorders in blacks. *Dermatol Clin* 1988;6:271-281.
38. Grimes PE. Melasma: Etiologic and therapeutic considerations. *Arch Dermatol* 1995;131:1453-1457.
39. Cornelison RL Jr. Cutaneous diseases in Native Americans. *Dermatol Clin* 2003; 21:699-702.
40. Zuloaga-Salcedo S, Castillo-Vazquez M, Vega-Memije E, et al. Class I and class II major histocompatibility complex genes in Mexican patients with actinic prurigo. *Br J Dermatol* 2007;1074-1075.
41. Lane PR, Hogan DJ, Martel MJ, et al. Actinic prurigo: Clinical features and prognosis. *J Am Acad Dermatol* 1992;26: 683-692.
42. Birt AR, Davis RA. Hereditary polymorphic light eruption of American Indians. *Int J Dermatol* 1975;14:105-111.
43. Fletcher DC, Romanchuk KG, Lane PR. Conjunctivitis and pterygium associated with the American Indian type of polymorphous light eruption. *Can J Ophthalmol* 1988;23:30-33.
44. Sheridan DP, Lane PR, Irvine J, et al. HLA typing in actinic prurigo. *J Am Acad Dermatol* 1990;22: 1019-1023.
45. Bernal JE, Duran de Rueda MM, Ordonez CP, et al. Actinic prurigo among the Chimila Indians in Colombia: HLA studies. *J Am Acad Dermatol* 1990;22:1049-1051.
46. Hojyo-Tomoka T, Granados J, Vargas-Alarcon G, et al. Further evidence of the role of HLA-DR4 in the genetic susceptibility to actinic prurigo. *J Am Acad Dermatol* 1997;36: 935-937.
47. Convit J, Piquero-Martin J, Perez RM. Erythema dyschromicum perstans. *Int J Dermatol* 1989;28:168-169.
48. Novick NL, Phelps R. Erythema dyschromicum perstans. *Int J Dermatol* 1985;24:630-633.
49. Pandya AG, Guevara IL. Disorders of hyperpigmentation. *Dermatol Clin* 2000;18:91-98, ix.
50. Jablonska S. Ingestion of ammonium nitrate as a possible cause of erythema dyschromicum perstans (ashy dermatosis). *Dermatologica* 1975;150:287-291.
51. Stevenson JR, Miura M. Erythema dyschromicum perstans (ashy dermatosis). *Arch Dermatol* 1966;94:196-199.
52. Lambert WC, Schwartz RA, Hamilton GB. Erythema dyschromicum perstans. *Cutis* 1986;37:42-44.
53. Penagos H, Jimenez V, Fallas V, et al. Chlorothalonil, a possible cause of erythema dyschromicum perstans (ashy dermatitis). *Contact Dermatitis* 1996;35: 214-218.
54. Zenorola P, Bisceglia M, Lomuto M. Ashy dermatosis associated with cobalt allergy. *Contact Dermatitis* 1994;31: 53-54.
55. Correa MC, Vega Memije E, Vargas-Alarcón, G. HLA-DR association with the genetic susceptibility to develop ashy dermatosis in Mexican Mestizo patients. *J Am Acad Dermatol* 2007;56: 617-620.
56. Morelli JG, Norris DA. Influence of inflammatory mediators and cytokines on human melanocyte function. *J Invest Dermatol* 1993;100:191S-195.
57. Morelli JG, Kincannon J, Yohn JJ, et al. Leukotriene C_4 and TGF-α are stimulators of human melanocyte migration in vitro. *J Invest Dermatol* 1992;98:290-295.
58. Brauner G. Cutaneous diseases in the black races, in Demis DJ, Dobson RL, McGuire J (eds), *Dermatology*. 1975, pp 1704-1733.
59. Grimes PE, Arora S, Minus HR, et al. Dermatosis papulosa nigra. *Cutis* 1983: 32:385-386, 392.
60. Huang C, Chen S, Liu Z, et al. Familial bullous lichen planus (FBLP): Pedigree analysis and clinical characteristics. *J Cutan Med Surg* 2005;9:217-222.
61. Mora RG, Nesbitt LT Jr, Brantley JB. Lichen planus pemphigoides: Clinical and immunofluorescent findings in four cases. *J Am Acad Dermatol* 1983;8:331-336.
62. Miranda SB, Lupi O, Lucas E. Vesicular pityriasis rosea: Response to erythromycin treatment. *J Eur Acad Dermatol Venereol* 2004;18:622-625.
63. Laude TA. Approach to dermatologic disorders in black children. *Semin Dermatol* 1995;14:15-20.
64. Griffiths CE, Leonard JN, Walker MM. Acquired ichthyosis and sarcoidosis. *Clin Exp Dermatol* 1986;11:296-298.
65. Green KM, Heilman E. Secondary syphilis presenting as a palisading granuloma. *J Am Acad Dermatol* 1985;12:957-960.
66. Shaffer JJ, Taylor SC, Cook-Bolden F. Keloidal scars: A review with a critical look at therapeutic options. *J Am Acad Dermatol* 2002;46:S63-97.
67. Louw L. Keloids in rural black South Africans, part 1: General overview and essential fatty acid hypotheses for keloid formation and prevention. *Prostaglandins Leukot Essent Fatty Acids* 2000;63:237-245.
68. Alhady SM, Sivanantharajah K. Keloids in various races: A review of 175 cases. *Plast Reconstr Surg* 1969;44:564-566.
69. Louw L. The keloid phenomenon: Progress toward a solution. *Clin Anat* 2007;20:3-14.
70. Montagna W, Carlisle K. The architecture of black and white facial skin. *J Am Acad Dermatol* 1991;24:929-937.
71. Murray JC, Pollack SV, Pinnell SR. Keloids: A review. *J Am Acad Dermatol* 1981;4:461-470.
72. Chait LA, Kadwa MA. Hypertrophic scars and keloids: Cause and management—Current concepts. *S Afr J Surg* 1988;26:95-98.
73. Lawrence WT. In search of the optimal treatment of keloids: Report of a series and a review of the literature. *Ann Plast Surg* 1991;27:164-178.
74. Tritto M, Kanat IO. Management of keloids and hypertrophic scars. *J Am Podiatr Med Assoc* 1991;81:601-605.
75. Darzi MA, Chowdri NA, Kaul SK, et al. Evaluation of various methods of treating keloids and hypertrophic scars: A 10-year follow-up study. *Br J Plast Surg* 1992;45:374-379.
76. Tuan TL, Nichter LS. The molecular basis of keloid and hypertrophic scar formation. *Mol Med Today* 1998;4:19-24.

CHAPTER 15

Histology

Jennifer Haley
Chandra Smart

Key Points

- The skin consists of three main layers that all contain different cell types.
- The epidermis contains four layers: stratum corneum, stratum granulosum, stratum spinosum, and stratum basale.
- The dermis contains the skin appendages, blood vessels, and nerves, as well a mixture of cells including fibroblasts, dendritic cells, and mast cells.
- The subcutis consists predominately of mature adipose tissue separated by fibrous bands.
- The racial differences in pigmentation are due to the number, size, and aggregation of melanosomes in the melanocytes and adjacent keratinocytes.
- The stratum corneum in African Americans is more compact when compared with that of Caucasians.
- African Americans have a wider distribution of apocrine glands and a greater amount of apocrine secretions when compared with Caucasians.
- African Americans have more lipid content in their hair owing to higher amounts of sebum production than Caucasians.
- African Americans have differences in hair pattern, elastic fiber and melanosome distribution, total hair density, and ultrastructure of the hair when compared with other races.
- African Americans have a greater number of fibroblasts and more compact collagen bundles in the dermis than other ethnic groups.

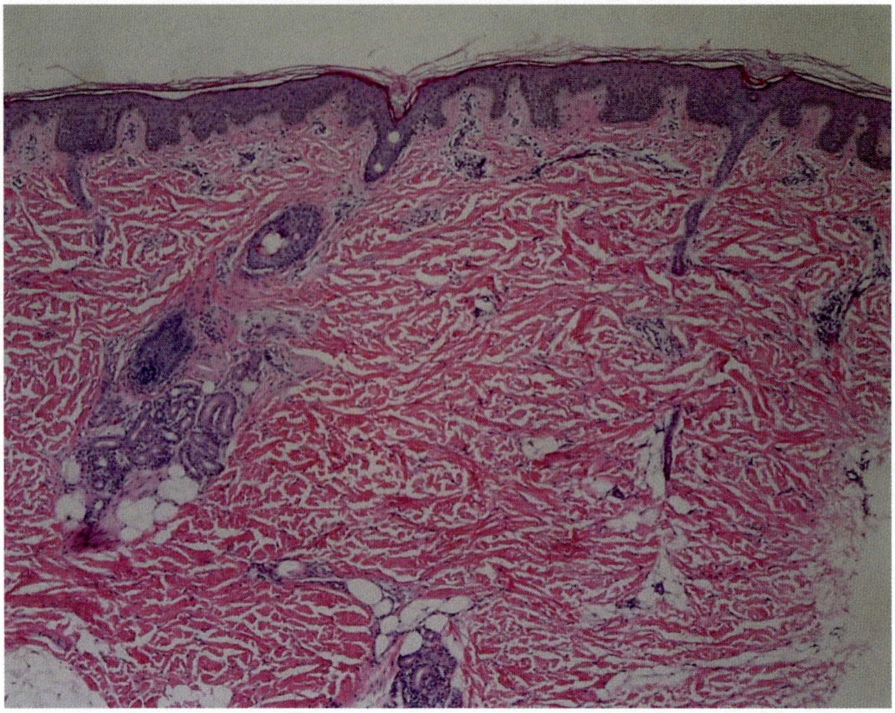

▲ **FIGURE 15-1** Normal skin. There are three anatomic layers of the skin: epidermis, dermis, and subcutis. Epidermal appendages include pilosebaceous units and eccrine glands.

NORMAL SKIN PHYSIOLOGY

The skin is the largest organ in the body. It serves as a protective barrier, is integral in thermal regulation, is an important sensory organ, and plays an important role in immunologic function. The skin is divided into three main anatomic layers: epidermis, dermis, and subcutis (Figure 15-1). Epidermal appendages include pilosebaceous units and eccrine glands.

Epidermis

The epidermis derives from the ectoderm and is the most superficial layer of the skin. It is composed of several layers: stratum corneum, stratum granulosum, stratum spinosum, and stratum basale. The stratum spinosum and stratum basale together are sometimes referred to as the *malpighian layer.*

STRATUM BASALE The stratum basale, or basal cell layer, is composed of proliferating stem cells separated from the dermis by a thin basement membrane composed of type IV collagen.[1] In histologic sections, these cells are seen as a single layer above the basement membrane.[1] The daughter cells differentiate and undergo keratinization as they migrate upward toward the surface of the skin. This process of regeneration takes place every 28–40 days.

STRATUM SPINOSUM The stratum spinosum lies above the basal cell layer. This layer is composed of several layers of keratinocytes. These cells differentiate from basal cells and accumulate keratin as they approach the surface of the epidermis. Desmosomes, or cell adhesion molecules, are responsible for the "spiny" appearance of this layer and hence its name.

STRATUM GRANULOSUM In the granular layer, cells continue to accumulate keratin and basophilic keratohyaline granules. These granules, coupled with the desmosomes, help to form a waterproof barrier, protecting the body from excessive water loss. They also serve as promoters for aggregation of keratin filaments in the cornified layer via the protein filaggrin.[1]

STRATUM CORNEUM The stratum corneum is the thickest of the epidermal layers. Cells are anucleate, flattened, and filled with keratin. As cells migrate up to this layer, it is thought that rupture of lysosomal membranes releases enzymes that eventually cause cell death. These dead cells then take on the characteristic flattened, eosinophilic morphology and eventually shed from the surface of the skin.[1]

Epidermal Cell Types

The subdivisions of the epidermis are the cornified layer, the spinous layer, and the granular cell layer. The dermis is divided into the papillary dermis and the wider, deeper reticular dermis (Figure 15-2).

KERATINOCYTES Keratinocytes constitute the major cell population of the epidermis, accounting for approximately 80% of all cells.[2] They are subclassified by their location in the epidermis (see above).

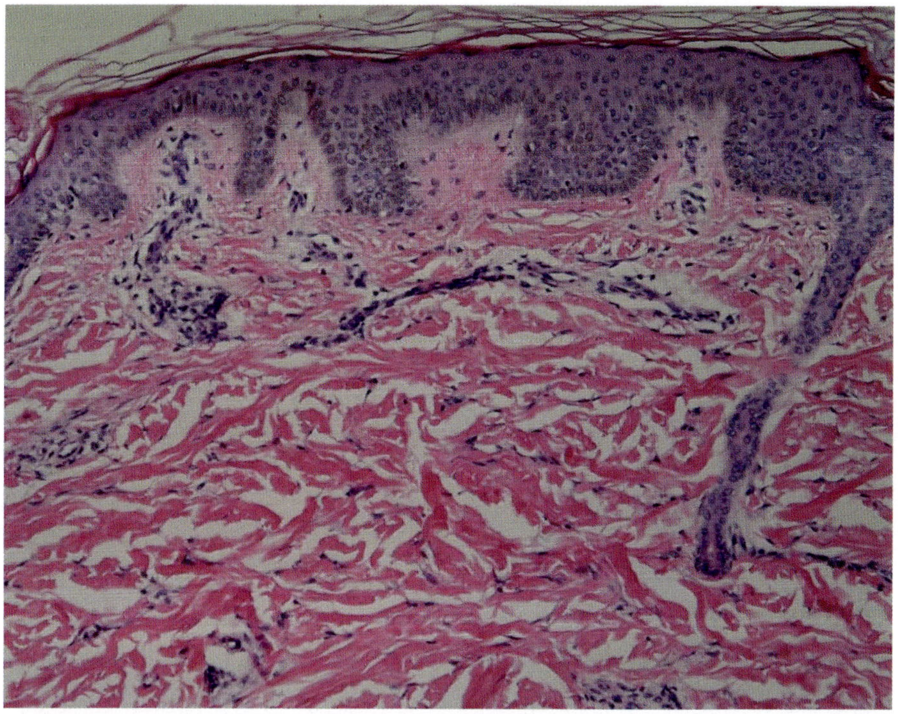

▲ **FIGURE 15-2** Normal skin. The subdivisions of the epidermis are the cornified layer, the spinous layer, and the granular cell layer. The dermis is divided into the papillary dermis and the wider, deeper reticular dermis.

MELANOCYTES Melanocytes are derived from neural crest cells and migrate to the epidermis during the first 3 months of development. Melanocytes are located in the basal layer of the skin and contain melanosomes. Melanosomes are the cellular organelles where the synthesis of melanin takes place via the enzyme tyrosinase. This enzyme is responsible for converting tyrosine into dopa, one of the key steps in melanin production.[3] Developing melanosomes containing melanin are transferred to neighboring basal and hair follicular cells via phagocytosis of the dendritic tips of melanocytes by surrounding keratinocytes. Melanin can either be yellow to reddish-brown (pheomelanin) or brown to black (eumelanin).[1] The most important function of melanin is to protect against the effects of nonionizing ultraviolet (UV) irradiation.[1] The number of melanocytes in normal skin is constant in all races, with a ratio of one melanocyte per every 4–10 keratinocytes.[1]

LANGERHANS' CELLS Langerhans' cells are derived from precursor cells in the bone marrow and serve as the antigen-presenting cells integral to immune surveillance in the skin. They are normally located in the middle to upper part of the epidermis.[1] These dendritic cells process and present antigens to helper T cells and are related in function to tissue macrophages, forming an important immunologic barrier of the skin.

MERKEL CELLS

Merkel cells are thought to be responsible for mediating tactile sensation.[1] They are located predominately in the basal layer of the epidermis and are found in increased concentration in the glabrous skin of the digits, lips, and oral cavity. Their site of origin is debatable, with some authors postulating a neural crest origin and others favoring differentiation from adjacent keratinocytes.[1]

Melanocytes appear as cuboidal cells with clear cytoplasm along the basal layer. Langerhans cells may resemble melanocytes with hemotoxylin and eosin stain but are located in the middle to upper dermis (Figure 15-3).

Dermis

The dermis is derived from the mesoderm and serves as the connective tissue support structure for the skin. It contains the blood vessels, nerves, and cutaneous appendages. The dermis consists of two layers: papillary dermis and reticular dermis. The papillary dermis is composed of loosely arranged type I and III collagen fibers, elastin fibers, abundant ground substance, capillaries of superficial plexuses, and fibroblasts.[1] It is named after the dermal papillae, or protrusions of dermal connective tissue, that indent the base of the epidermis. The reticular dermis is composed of predominately type I collagen, forming layers that are thick, densely packed, and arranged parallel to the epidermis. The cellular makeup of the reticular dermis includes fibroblasts, dendritic cells, macrophages, and mast cells.[1]

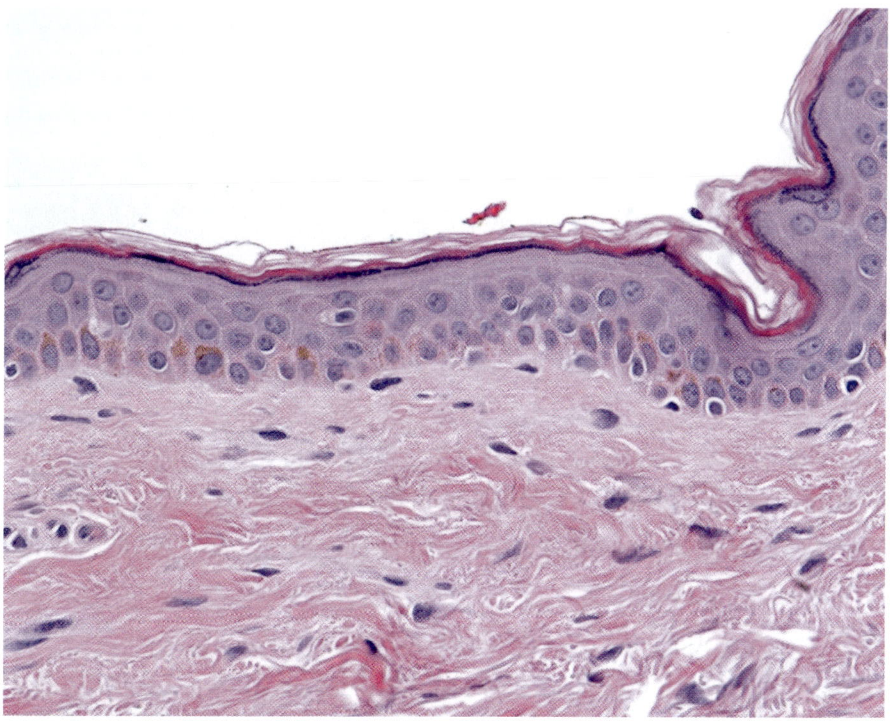

▲ **FIGURE 15-3** Pigmented skin. Melanocytes appear as cuboidal cells with clear cytoplasm along the basal layer. Langerhans cells may resemble melanocytes with hemotoxylin and eosin stain but are located in the middle to upper dermis.

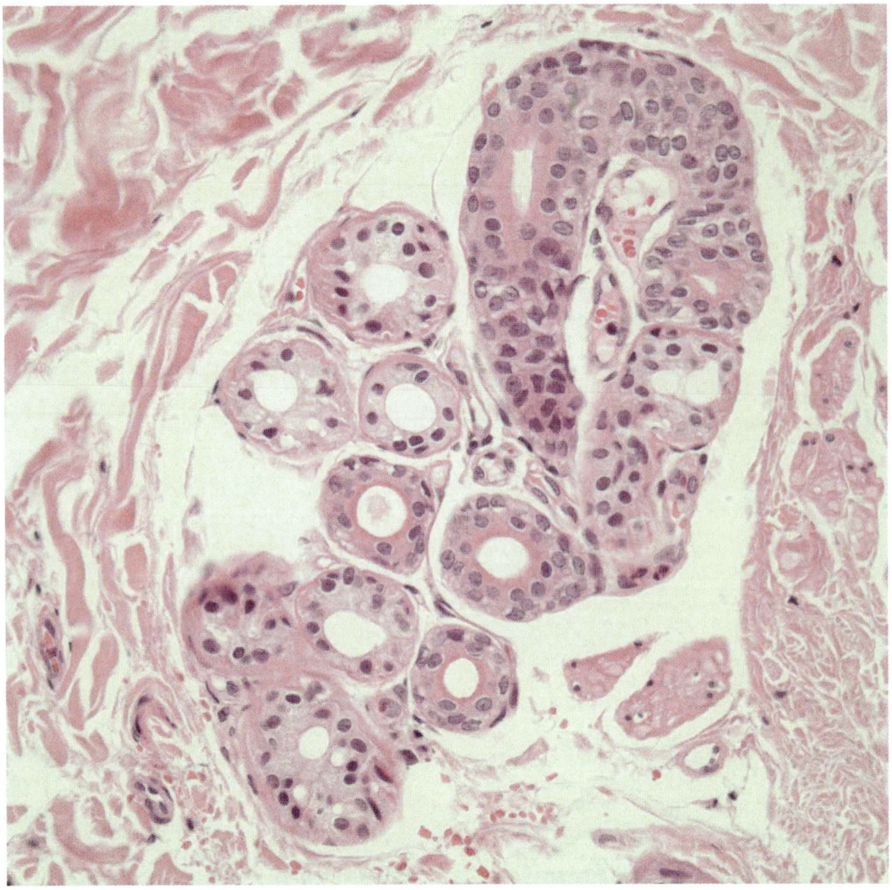

▲ **FIGURE 15-4** Normal eccrine gland.

Subcutis

The subcutis is arranged into lobules of mature adipocytes separated by fibrous connective tissue septa. The thickness of the subcutis varies with gender, nutritional status of the individual, and anatomic location.[2]

Skin Appendages

ECCRINE GLANDS These glands are the true sweat glands, important in regulating temperature. The eccrine gland is composed of a secretory coil (pictured) which leads into a coiled proximal duct and then a straight duct which eventually passes through the epidermis (Figure 15-4). They are found predominately in the palms, soles, forehead, and axillae. Eccrine glands produce an isotonic to hypertonic secretion that is modified by the ducts to emerge on the skin surface as sweat.[2] This is especially useful for people who engage in physical activity or live in hot climates.

APOCRINE GLANDS These glands are found primarily in the axillae, groin, eyelids, and ears, as well as in the mammary and perineal regions.[3] The function of these glands is not well understood, but they are known to cause body odor when their secretions are excreted onto the skin owing to the presence of bacteria that colonize the skin surface.

PILOSEBACEOUS UNIT
The pilosebaceous unit is composed of the hair follicle, hair shaft, arrector pili, and sebaceous glands (Figure 15-5). The hair follicle is divided into three main segments: the infundibulum, the isthmus, and the inferior segment, or hair bulb.[1] Hair follicles are associated with sebaceous glands, which are present everywhere except on the palms and soles. The sebaceous glands are holocrine glands that secrete oily, lipid-rich secretions composed predominately of disintegrated cells into the hair follicle.[1] The arrector pili are composed of bundles of smooth muscle fibers that are controlled by the autonomic nervous system.[2]

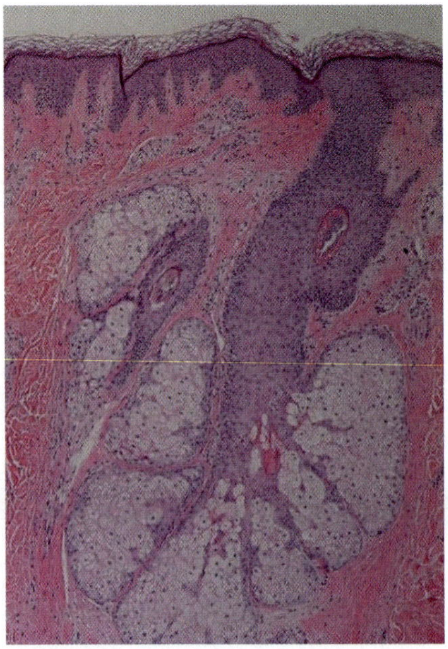

▲ **FIGURE 15-5** Pilosebaceous unit.

SKIN PHYSIOLOGY IN SKIN OF COLOR

Pigmentation

One of the most striking differences in skin of color is the varying degree of pigmentation seen in this population. As stated earlier, melanocytes are responsible for producing the cutaneous pigment melanin, but there are no racial differences in the number of melanocytes present in skin.[3] The racial and ethnic differences in pigmentation are mainly due to the number, size, and aggregation of melanosomes within the melanocyte and the keratinocyte.[3] People of color, particularly African-Americans, tend to have large, nonaggregated melanosomes that absorb and scatter more energy, providing higher photoprotection in pigmented skin.[4] The number of melanocytes in normal skin is constant. The number and shape of melanosomes account for differences in skin color (Figure 15-6).

Epidermis

STRATUM CORNEUM The average stratum corneum thickness is similar between African-Americans and Caucasians, but the stratum corneum was found to be more compact in African-Americans. Studies have been performed demonstrating that removal of the stratum corneum in African-American skin requires more cellophane tape strips than removal in Caucasian skin.[5] This finding may be a reflection of the greater intercellular cohesion present in African-American skin. The spontaneous desquamation rate of the stratum corneum in African-Americans is 2.5 times greater than that seen in Caucasians and Asians, which may account for the increased frequency of xerosis seen clinically in African-Americans.[4]

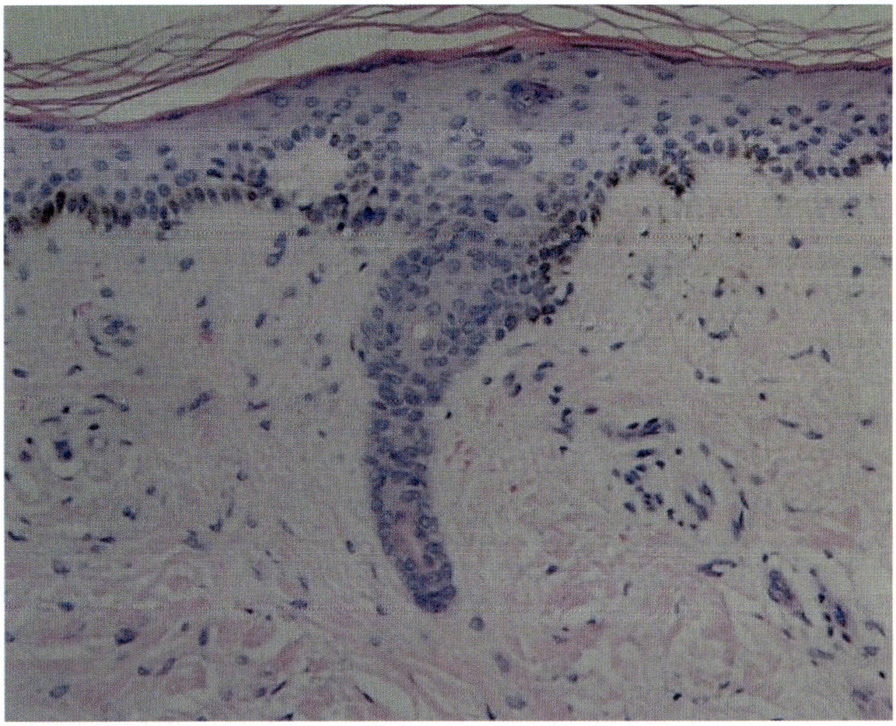

▲ **FIGURE 15-6** Pigmented skin at low power. The number of melanocytes in normal skin is constant. The number and shape of melanosomes account for differences in skin color.

Skin Appendages

ECCRINE SWEAT GLANDS There are few differences in the number of eccrine sweat glands between races, but some functional differences are of note. One such difference was an increased sweating rate in Caucasians compared with black Africans.[1] Furthermore, black Africans had a lower concentration of salt in their sweat than Caucasians.[3]

APOCRINE SWEAT GLANDS As stated earlier, the function of apocrine sweat glands is poorly understood, but African-Americans have a greater distribution of secretion as reported in one limited study.[3]

SEBACEOUS GLANDS African-Americans have more lipid content in their hair owing to higher sebum production, and one study showed that African-Americans have larger sebaceous glands.[3]

HAIR FOLLICLES There are distinctive differences in the hair follicles of African-Americans when compared with other races. These differences consist of hair pattern, elastic fiber and melanosome distribution, total hair density, and ultrastructure of the hair. Four hair patterns have been noted: straight, wavy, helical, and spiral with spiral being the most largely represented in African-Americans.[3] The follicles on the scalp and the hair are curved, but there are no discernible differences in the thickness of the cuticle and shape and size of scale and cortical cells between the hair of African-Americans and Caucasians.[3] African-Americans have fewer elastic fibers anchoring the hair follicles to the dermis. Melanosomes are distributed in both the outer root sheath and the bulb of vellus hairs. African-Americans have more heavily pigmented hair owing to the presence of larger melanin granules. The ultrastructure of African-American hair tends to be altered such that it has a tendency to form knots, longitudinal fissures, and splits along the hair shaft.

Dermis

The major differences in the dermis of African-Americans are present within its cellular components. African-Americans have an increased quantity and larger fibroblasts that are either binucleated or multinucleated.[3] In addition, the collagen bundles present in the dermis of African-Americans are smaller, more closely stacked, and run in a pattern parallel to the epidermis. Microscopic examination of African-American skin reveals that the mast cells present in the dermis contain larger intracellular granules.[5]

REFERENCES

1. Sternberg, SS. *Histology for Pathologists,* 2nd ed. Philadelphia, Lippincott Williams & Wilkins, 1997, pp 25-43.
2. Hood AF, Kwan TH, Mihm MC, et al. *Primer of Dermatopathology,* 3rd ed. Philadelphia, Lippincott Williams & Wilkins, 2002, pp 3-15.
3. Taylor SC. Skin of color: Biology, structure, function, and implications for dermatologic disease. *J Am Acad Dermatol* 2002; 46:S44.
4. Berardesca W, Maibach H. Racial differences in skin pathophysiology. *J Am Acad Dermatol* 1996;34:667-672.
5. Wesley NO, Maibach HI. Racial (ethnic) differences in skin properities: The objective data. *Am J Clin Dermatol* 2003; 4:843-860.

CHAPTER 16

Genetics of Skin Diseases

Saundrett G. Arrindell
Shirley B. Russell

Key Points

- Differences in the incidence and prevalence of disease in different racial and ethnic populations provide evidence for a genetic contribution to the etiology of a disorder.
- Familial clustering of disease and more frequent concordance of disease in monozygotic than dizygotic twins provide further support for a genetic component.
- Genome-wide linkage and gene association studies provide evidence for involvement of genes at specific chromosomal regions.
- Systemic lupus erythematosus (SLE), vitiligo, systemic sclerosis (SSc), sarcoidosis, and keloids are genetically complex, with multiple genetic loci and environmental triggers conferring risk for the disease and its severity.
- Autoimmune diseases, including SLE, SSc, sarcoidosis, and vitiligo, share susceptibility loci at human chromosomal region 6p21, which contains the genes of the major histocompatibility complex (MHC).
- Genome-wide linkage studies of autoimmune diseases have identified at least 30 chromosomal regions of overlap for different autoimmune diseases, suggesting shared susceptibility loci for these clinically related disorders.
- In addition to shared genetic susceptibilities, some gene differences are observed mainly within a single disorder, within a single racial or ethnic group, or within a group of patients with similar clinical symptoms.
- To better identify the roles of specific genes in different populations, genetic studies are being refined by analyzing results from different racial and ethnic groups separately, by using subsets of patients with similar clinical symptoms, and by using ordered subset analysis (OSA) to obtain evidence for gene interaction (epistasis) between different genetic loci.

There is much evidence that supports a genetic contribution to human disease. Differences in incidence and prevalence in different racial and ethnic populations provide strong suggestive evidence for a genetic contribution to the etiology of a disorder. Although socioeconomic, behavioral, and environmental factors confound the identification and contribution of genetic factors, dissimilar frequencies of rare alleles and polymorphisms that associate with disease in different racial and ethnic groups support a role of genetic factors. Gene admixture makes assignment of individuals to a single group complicated. However, recent studies in multiple populations have provided estimates of the degree of admixture of genes among different groups, from which the expected distribution of genes in an individual may be predicted more accurately[1–3] (Table 16-1). While optimal diagnosis and treatment of disease will require identification of the complete spectrum of at-risk genotypes in single individuals, characterization of the genetic contributions to disease occurrence and severity in racial and ethnic populations can provide, when used judiciously, important diagnostic and prognostic information for clinicians. Familial clustering of disease and more frequent concordance of disease in monozygotic than dizygotic twins provide further support for a genetic component. Twin studies depend on the fact that monozygotic twins have virtually identical genomes (except for somatic mutations and contributions from mitochondrial inheritance), whereas dizygotic twins share, on average, only 50% of their genes. If both members of pairs of monozygotic twins develop a disease (concordance) more often than both members of dizygotic twins, a genetic contribution to the disease is supported. Concordance of significantly less than 100% in monozygotic twin pairs is evidence for the contribution of both genetic and environmental factors.

Differences in occurrence of a disease in different populations and evidence from twin studies and familial clustering of a disease provide strong support for a genetic predisposition. However, great strides in clarifying the genetic contribution to disease in recent years have been facilitated by the sequencing of the human genome. Technological advances in molecular biology needed for genome-wide linkage studies, characterization of small differences within genes, and testing of associations between particular gene variations and disease have facilitated understanding. The genome contains 3 billion base pairs and an estimated 30,000 genes. The human genome sequence is essentially the same (>99.9%) in all people. Genetic diversity between individuals is attributable to the remaining 0.1%. A small variation in one's DNA sequence, such as a single-nucleotide

TABLE 16-1
Admixture Estimates for Different Populations[1]

		Population Contribution Assessed by Structure (%)			
Sample Examined	N	European	African	Asian	Amerindian
European American					
Chicago	39	98.4	0.4	0.7	0.5
Baltimore	39	97.5	0.4	0.9	1.3
African American					
Chicago	18	18.4	80.6	0.7	0.3
Pittsburgh	23	18.3	80.6	0.6	0.5
Baltimore	45	15.9	83.2	0.5	0.5
North Carolina	23	18.8	79.6	0.5	1.1
African					
Senegal	46	2.8	95	1.6	0.6
Ghana	33	0.1	99.8	0.1	0.1
Cameroon	20	0.1	99.8	0.1	0.1
Botswana	21	1.2	98.4	0.3	0.1
Chinese					
Cantonese	40	0.2	0.1	98.9	0.8
Amerindian					
Mexican Zapotec	29	4.3	0.3	0.5	94.8

change in a rare mutation or a single-nucleotide polymorphism (SNP), can be critical in determining whether an individual has a genetic predisposition to a disease and its severity. The human genome has been shown to have at least 10 million SNPs. Genetic mapping of SNPs has made it possible to trace the migration of the human species, affording a window into the multifaceted genetic makeup of different populations.

The role of a genetic component in dermatologic diseases has been evident anecdotally for centuries. Many skin diseases were observed more commonly in certain families, and several hereditary syndromes were noted to have characteristic cutaneous manifestations. Ongoing research and discovery of genes, gene loci, and gene mutations are serving to define the complex molecular interactions that result in a particular skin disorder or syndrome.

Most, if not all, disorders discussed here, notably systemic lupus erythematosus (SLE), vitiligo, systemic sclerosis (SSc), sarcoidosis, and keloids, are genetically complex, with multiple genetic loci as well as environmental triggers conferring risk for the disease and its severity. Even where an autosomal dominant pattern of inheritance has been observed in some families, reduced penetrance supports contributions by more than one gene, and variable expression within the same individual supports a role for environmental factors. Involvement of different genes in the etiology of a disease (i.e., locus heterogeneity) has been suggested by clinical heterogeneity in disease presentation and confirmed by genetic linkage to different chromosomal regions in different families and in different racial and ethnic groups. This complexity has made it difficult to replicate linkage studies, even within the same racial or ethnic group. However, the rapidly expanding capacity to identify genes and environmental factors that contribute to differential disease prevalence and severity in different individuals and populations will provide the basis for more rational approaches to diagnosis, prevention, and treatment.

Autoimmune diseases, including but not limited to SLE, SSc, vitiligo, and sarcoidosis, arise from interactions between multiple genetic and environmental factors. Genome-wide linkage studies of autoimmune diseases have identified at least 30 chromosomal regions of overlap for different autoimmune diseases, suggesting shared susceptibility loci for these clinically related disorders[4] (Table 16-2). Many autoimmune diseases share susceptibility loci on the short arm of chromosome 6 (Figure 16-1) at 6p21.3 (Figure 16-2). This chromosomal region contains the genes of the major histocompatibility complex (MHC), including the highly polymorphic class I human leukocyte antigen (HLA) genes (B, C, and A), class II HLA genes (DR, DQ, and DP), genes in the class II region that code for components of the proteasome, and class III HLA genes (cytokines and complement proteins). Patterns of inheritance seen in some familial cases indicate a predisposition to autoimmune disease development rather than to a specific autoimmune disease.[5] The occurrence of different types of autoimmune diseases within a pedigree may be determined by additional genetic loci and environmental influences. Recently, microarray studies have identified clusters of genes that are differentially expressed in multiple autoimmune diseases, many of which are located in chromosomal regions that contain susceptibility loci for autoimmune disease.[6] This convergence of genetic linkage and differences in gene expression at linked loci provides a strong basis for exploring the clinical significance of gene differences in different diseases and populations.

SYSTEMIC LUPUS ERYTHEMATOSUS

Systemic lupus erythematosus (SLE) is a multisystem autoimmune disorder characterized by the deposition of autoantibodies leading to tissue injury in multiple organs, including but not limited to the skin, heart, kidneys, brain, lungs, and joints. The etiology of SLE is multifactorial. Genetic and nongenetic factors, such as environmental and hormonal influences, affect disease expression, activity, severity, and outcome. Evidence supporting a genetic predisposition to SLE is strong but complex.[7,8] The overall prevalence of SLE is estimated at 1 in 2000. Ninety percent of cases occur in women, mainly in childbearing ages, suggesting a hormonal influence.[9,10] Increased prevalence in certain ethnic populations and within families supports a genetic component. African-Americans, Asians, and Hispanics have an increased incidence, estimated at 1 in 1000 African-American women versus 1 in 4000 Caucasian- American women. Both prevalence and phenotype are strongly affected by ethnicity. African-Americans and Hispanics experience more active, aggressive disease that occurs at a younger age.[11] Genetic admixture underscores the observation that Hispanic SLE patients of Mexican and Central American ancestry have more severe disease than mainland Puerto Rican patients, although mainland Puerto Ricans have more cutaneous manifestations.[3] Familial aggregation and a high monozygotic-to-dizygotic-twin concordance ratio support a genetic component. The monozygotic-to-dizygotic-twin concordance ratio has been estimated at 10, with a monozygotic twin concordance rate of 24–58% and a dizygotic twin concordance rate of 2–5%, similar to that of nontwin siblings.[12,13] The risk for a sibling is 20- to 40-fold higher than the risk for an unrelated person in the general population.[14]

Candidate gene association analysis and genome-wide linkage studies have been used to detect multiple susceptibility genes and loci for SLE. Genome-wide linkage analyses[8,12,15–22] and targeted genome scans[23–29] using cohorts of SLE multiplex families (two or more affected individuals) of multiple ethnicities have detected chromosomal regions that show evidence of linkage to SLE. Chromosomal regions with significant linkage to SLE are shown in Table 16-2.

Candidate gene association analysis has implicated the MHC genes *HLA-DR2* and *HLA-DR3* located at chromosome 6p21, interleukin 1 at 2q14, human Fc-γ low-affinity receptors *FcGR2A* and *FcGR3A* at 1q23, and deficiency of complement components C4 and C2 at 6 p21, C1q at 1p36, and C1r/s at 12p13 in increased risk of disease development.[8,13,25,30–36] Individuals with a hereditary deficiency of C1q develop SLE at a young age with severe photosensitivity rash without respect to gender or ethnicity. In addition, a strong risk of developing rheumatic disease occurs in greater than 90% of patients with deficient C1q, 75% with deficient C4, and 10% with deficient C2. A hereditary deficiency of complement component C4A denoted a risk for SLE development in almost all ethnic groups evaluated. Variation in gene copy number has been recognized recently as a heritable source of susceptibility to complex genetic diseases. In this regard, low *FcGR3B* copy number has been associated with increased risk for autoimmune glomerulonephritis in a subset of SLE patients.[37] Reduced copy number of C4 has been shown to be a risk factor for and increased copy number has been shown to be protective against SLE in European Americans.[38] A risk haplotype in the upstream region of the tumor

TABLE 16-2
Susceptibility Loci for Autoimmune Disorders

Chromosome	Autoimmunity	Systemic Lupus Erythematosus	Vitiligo	Systemic Sclerosis	Sarcoidosis
1	1p21-22	1p36.11	1p13	1p 36.2	1p22
	1p31	1q23	1p31-p32	1q31-q32	
	1q24-25	1q 25-q31	1p36		
	1q42	1q41-q42			
2	2q32-36	2q33	2p16.3	2q25	2p25
		2q34-q35		2q31	
		2q312q35-q37			
3	3q21	3p24		3	3p14-11
					3p21
4	4q28	4p16-p15.2	4q13-q21	4q27	
5	5p11	5p13-p15		5q31.3-q32	5q11
	5p15	5q21-q22		5q36	5q35
	5q31-33	5q36			
6	6p12-q11	6p11-p21	6p21-p22	6p21	6p21-22
	6q27	6p21.3	6q24-q25		
		6q25-p27	7	7q22.1	
7	7p15-22				
	7q31		7q11-q21		
		7q32			7q36
8	8q22	8q21.11	8		
			8p21		
9	9p22				9q33
					9q34
10	10p12	10q22.3	10q11.2-q21	10q12	
		10q23-q24			
11	11p13-p15	11p13-p15.5		11	11p15
		11q14		11q13.1	
12	12p13	12q24	12q12-q14		
13		13q32			
14	14q31-32	14q21-q23	14q12-q13		
15	15q11			15q21.1	
	15q26				
16	16q12-21	16q12		16p12.1-p11.2	
17	17p13	17p13	17p13	17p13	
	17q22	17q21		17q21-q23	
18		18q21			
		18q23			
19	19p13	19p13		19	
	19q13	19q13.1		19q13.1	
20	20p11	20p13-p11			
	20q13				20q13
21	21q22			21	
22	22q12-13	22q13.1-13,31	22q11.2-q12		
X	Xp11				Xq

Sources: Chromosomal regions listed are found in references cited in text and Locuslink at *www.ncbi.nlm.gov/LocusLink*.

necrosis factor (TNF) superfamily gene *TNSF4* at chromosome 1q25 that causes increased expression of the gene has been associated with increased risk for SLE.[39]

Some gene associations have been identified mainly in specific ethnic groups. An association with the programmed cell death 1 (*PD-1*) allele (2q37 linkage) is seen in people of European descent but not in African-American families. A *PD-1* association in Spanish cases of lupus was found.[40–42] A study of SLE patients stratified for discoid lupus manifestations revealed linkage at 11p13 in African-American families.[43] SLE susceptibility linkage at 12q24 was observed mainly in Hispanic and European families.[21] An important SLE susceptibility gene, *SLEH1* at 11q14, was found in African-Americans when pedigrees were stratified by the presence of antinucleolar autoantibodies[44] or hemolytic anemia.[45] When pedigrees were stratified for renal disease, three SLE susceptibility loci were identified: *SLEN1* at 10q22.3 in Caucasians and *SLEN2* at 2q34-35 and *SLEN3* at 11p15.5 in African-Americans.[46,47]

Overlap of SLE susceptibility loci with other autoimmune diseases is evident[7,8] (see Table 16-2). Candidate genes for multiple autoimmune diseases have been observed at chromosomal regions 1p13 (*P2PN22*), 2q37 (*PDCD1*), 2q33 (*CTLA4*), and 16q12 (*NOD2/CARD150*).

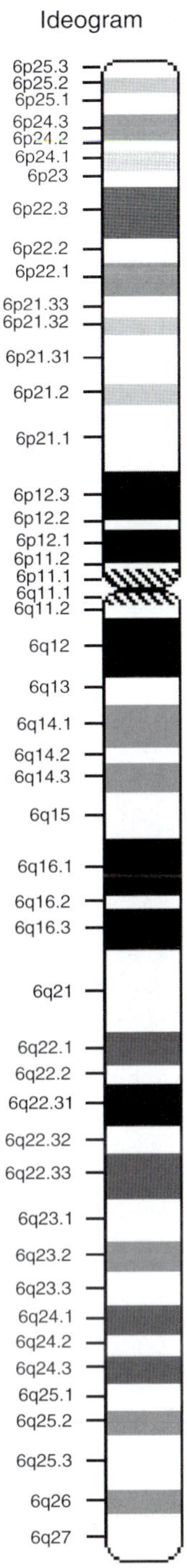

▲ **FIGURE 16-1** Ideogram of chromosome 6 (NCBI MapView). Many autoimmune diseases share susceptibility loci on the short arm of human chromosome 6 at region p21.3.

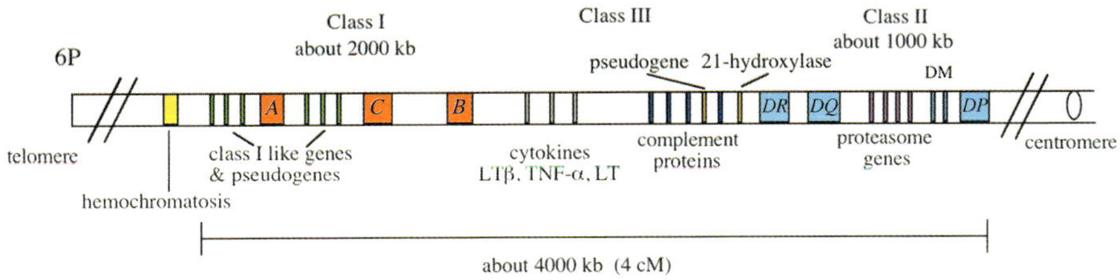

▲ **FIGURE 16-2** Major histocompatibility locus. Chromosomal region 6p21.3 contains the highly polymorphic class I human leukocyte antigen (HLA) genes (*B*, *C*, and *A*), class II HLA genes (*DR*, *DQ*, and *DP*), genes in the class II region that code for components of the proteasome, and class III HLA genes (cytokines and complement proteins).

For example, cytotoxic T-lymphocyte antigen 4 (*CTLA-4*) polymorphisms at chromosomal region 2q33 have been implicated in several types of autoimmunity, suggesting a role for *CTLA-4* as a general susceptibility gene for autoimmune diseases, including SLE.[48–50] Chromosomal regions 10q22.3, 2q34-q35, and 11p15.5 are seen in SLE with an increased risk for lupus nephritis,[46] 17p13 in SLE associated with vitiligo,[51] 11q14 in SLE associated with hemolytic anemia,[45] and 1q41 with thyroid-lupus autoantigen.[52]

Gene association studies also have provided direct evidence for the involvement of specific pathways in the pathogenesis of SLE. For example, the expression of many interferon (IFN)–inducible genes is increased in the peripheral blood of SLE patients. Evidence that the IFN pathway plays a causal role in SLE has been provided by findings that several different functional variants of the gene for IFN regulatory factor 5 confer susceptibility for or protection against SLE.[53]

The identification of genes for SLE, as well as for other genetically complex diseases, is in a dynamic state, with many findings not replicated in subsequent studies. The failure to replicate is due to a number of factors. These include (1) different genes cause the same disease in different racial and ethnic populations, (2) different genes cause different forms of disease characterized by different clinical features, and (3) interactions between genes at different loci (i.e., epistasis) may influence whether a particular gene causes susceptibility to the disease. As indicated earlier, to address these issues, an increasing number of gene linkage and gene association studies are taking genetic heterogeneity and gene interactions into account by analyzing results from different racial and ethnic groups separately, by examining the role of specific genes in subsets of patients with a similar set of symptoms, or recently, by using ordered subset analysis (OSA) to obtain evidence for gene interaction (epistasis) between loci in two different chromosomal regions.[54]

VITILIGO

Vitiligo is a disorder of pigmentation characterized by the destruction of melanocytes owing to a complex pathogenesis of genetic susceptibility, autoimmune destruction, biochemical defects, and environmental factors. Phenotypic variance is evident in the different clinical expressions of vitiligo, such as focal, vulgaris (generalized), universal, segmental, acrofacial, and mucosal. Vitiligo affects 0.1–2.0% of various populations.[55,56] In a survey of 2624 vitiligo probands (83% Caucasian) from North America and the United Kingdom, the frequency in males and females was equal. The prevalence of vitiligo was reported to be 0.19% in the Chinese Han people, the ethnic group representing greater than 90% of the Chinese population. An evaluation of 2247 probands revealed that the age of onset with the highest prevalence was 10–14 years compared with a later age of onset of 20–24 years in U.S. females. Distribution between males and females was equal. First-degree relatives had a 3- to 13-fold higher relative risk of developing vitiligo; the risk was two to four times higher for second-degree relatives.[57] A prevalence of 0.34% was seen in the French West Indies (Isle of Martinique), where 96% of the population is of African-European descent (black Caribbean). The prevalence among relatives was 7%, and the age of onset was much later (31 years).[58] A study of 357 Nigerian vitiligo patients showed a male:female ratio of 1:1.3, onset in the second and third decades of life, and a family history in 18% of probands.[59] The prevalence of vitiligo in the United States has been estimated at 1%. Studies in other countries have reported a prevalence of 0.38% in Denmark, 1.13% in Surat, India, and 0.45% in Calcutta.[60]

Progress in defining the genetic component has depended on clearly defining the disorder. Consequently, most studies have focused on generalized vitiligo. Strong evidence for genetic factors in the pathogenesis of generalized vitiligo comes from studies of patients' close relatives.[61] Among Caucasians, the frequency in probands' siblings was 6.1%, approximately 18 times the population frequency, and 20% of probands had at least one affected first-degree relative, highly suggestive of a genetic component.

There is a similar risk of generalized vitiligo in other first-degree relatives: 7.1% in Caucasians, 6.1% in Indo-Pakistanis, and 4.8% in Hispanics. A lower risk is seen in more distant relatives. Also, among Caucasians, the mean age of onset is 21.5 years in patients from families in which multiple family members are affected[62] but is 24.2 years in unselected (mainly sporadic) patients. Earlier disease onset in familial cases and a lower risk of disease with increased genetic distance from an affected family member are commonly observed features of polygenic disorders.[63] However, while there is strong evidence for genetic factors in the pathogenesis of vitiligo, the concordance of vitiligo in monozygotic twins was only 23%, suggesting additional nongenetic triggers.[63]

The association of vitiligo with other autoimmune diseases is well documented. In 23% of patients with generalized vitiligo there was an increase in the frequency of six autoimmune disorders in probands and their first-degree relatives: vitiligo, autoimmune thyroid disease, pernicious anemia, Addison disease, SLE, and inflammatory bowel disease.[63] Additionally, associations with diabetes mellitus and alopecia areata have been documented.[64] A combination of gene linkage and gene association studies have found susceptibility loci for vitiligo at chromosomal regions 1p31 [*AIS1* (autoimmune susceptibility 1)], 1p13 (*PTPN22*), 6p21.3 (*HLA-DRB-1, HLA-DRB4,* and *HLA-DQB-1*), chromosome 7 (*AIS2*), chromosome 8 (*AIS3*), and 17p13 [*SLEV1* (*NALP1*)].[61,65–69] *NALP1* encodes a key regulator of the immune system that activates the IL-1β and possibly other inflammatory pathways.[70] Linkage to *AIS1, AIS2,* and *NALP1* is theorized to predispose to vitiligo associated with susceptibility to autoimmune diseases, whereas linkage at *AIS3* is not noted for that association.[69] While many of these linkage results have been confirmed in Caucasian populations, different linkage results have been obtained in Chinese families, suggesting that different genes may be involved in the pathogenesis of vitiligo in different populations.[61]

SYSTEMIC SCLEROSIS

Systemic sclerosis (SSc) is a chronic systemic fibrotic disease. Although the defining characteristics of SSc are thickening of the skin and peripheral vascular abnormalities, the clinical phenotype varies from limited cutaneous involvement and Raynaud phenomenon to diffuse and life-threatening fibrosis of skin and visceral organs and very severe vascular abnormalities.

Three types of evidence support a genetic component in the pathogenesis of SSc. The first is variation in disease prevalence and incidence among ethnic and racial groups. Prevalence and severity are significantly higher in African-Americans than in Caucasians.[71] An Oklahoma Choctaw Indian population has the highest reported prevalence owing, it is believed, to a founder effect.[72] The ancestry of the SSc patients in this population was traced to five founding families in the eighteenth century.[73,74] Second, SSc occurs significantly more frequently in families, a positive family history being the strongest risk factor for the disease.[75] Third, candidate polymorphisms and rare mutations have been identified that show a positive association with the disease, including genes for the class II HLA loci (6p21), tumor necrosis factor α (12p13), interleukin 4 receptor α (16p12.1-p11.2), IL-8 receptor 2 (2q35), topoisomerase 1 (20q12), transforming growth factor (TGFβ) (19q13.1), and connective tissue growth factor (CTGF) (6q23-27).[76–79] Several susceptibility loci, including fibrillin (15q21) and *SPARC* (secreted protein, acidic and rich in cysteine) (5q31-33), were observed in the Oklahoma Choctaw Indian population referred to earlier.[76] The combination of genetic association and gene linkage studies for regions of systemic sclerosis susceptibility indicates that the disorder is multifactorial, with a number of genetic loci contributing to SSc (see Table 16-2), and is consistent with the view that some autoimmune rheumatic disorders share genetic determinants. Although there have been no reported differences in disease concordance between monozygotic and dizygotic twins, concordance for antinuclear and anticytoplasmic antibodies was significantly higher in monozygotic than in dizygotic twins (90% versus 40%).[80–82]

In addition to differences in disease prevalence in different racial and ethnic groups, certain clinical phenotypes may be unequally distributed. African-Americans and Hispanics have a higher frequency of diffuse disease than European Americans.[83,84] In addition, there appears to be a higher prevalence of SSc renal crisis among African-Americans, characterized by abrupt onset of severe uncontrolled hypertension and rapidly progressive oliguric renal failure with high renin levels.[85] A significantly lower proportion of Caucasians has diffuse skin involvement, digital pits and ulcers, and hypopigmentation/hyperpigmentation. A higher proportion has facial telangiectasia. Hypothyroidism is diagnosed more frequently in whites than in non-white Hispanics and appears to be absent in African-Americans.[83]

At least some of these clinical differences may be attributed to differences in the type of autoantibodies produced.[86] Patients with SSc express a number of autoantibodies to nuclear antigens, each with its own clinical associations. These include anticentromere antibodies (ACAs), antitopoisomerase 1 (Scl-70), RNA polymerase I and III (RNAPI and -III), and antinucleolar antibodies (AnoAs). Each SSc patient typically produces only one of these antibody types.[76,77,87] There is strong evidence from twin studies and from associations with MHC genes that the types of autoantibodies produced in SSc are influenced by hereditary factors. The types produced also vary in different racial and ethnic groups.[86] ACAs occur most frequently in Caucasians, with significantly lower frequency in Hispanic, African-American, and Thai patients. They are strongly associated with limited cutaneous SSc, with a higher risk for calcinosis and ischemic digital loss and with a lower frequency of interstitial pulmonary fibrosis. Patients who are ACA-positive have a lower mortality than those who are positive for antitopoisomerase 1 antibodies or AnoAs. Antitopoisomerase 1 antibodies that are unique to SSc occur at higher frequency in Mexican-American, African-American, Native American, Thai, and Japanese patients.[88] Antitopoisomerase 1 antibodies are associated with fibrosing alveolitis but not with scleroderma renal crisis. African-American and Japanese patients with SSc had a significantly lower survival rate than Caucasian individuals with antitopoisomerase 1 antibodies. This may be explained by a higher frequency of progressive pulmonary interstitial fibrosis in these two groups.[89] A particular class of AnoA, antifibrillarin/anti-U3RNP, is found with higher frequency in SSc patients of African descent than in Caucasians and is associated with diffuse skin involvement, gastrointestinal dysmotility, myositis, pulmonary hypertension, cardiac involvement, and renal disease.[78,83,86,90,91] Another group of AnoAs, antiRNAP antibodies, is associated with diffuse cutaneous involvement and renal crisis.[76] Overproduction of the nucleolar protein fibrillarin has been reported in fibroblasts from scleroderma patients,[87] and decreased fibrillarin level has been shown to result in decreased collagen secretion.[92] Thus overproduction of fibrillarin may play a role in the very severe fibrosis seen in some scleroderma patients. Associations have been shown between particular class II MHC alleles and the type of autoantibodies made.[76] These findings, along with the results of twin studies, support a genetic influence on which class of autoantibodies will be produced. Since the autoantibody class produced appears to correlate with some of the phenotypic variability, further characterization of the genetic basis and functional significance of differences in autoantibody production and the distribution of relevant alleles in different individuals and populations may help to identify, prevent, and treat different forms of scleroderma.

SARCOIDOSIS

Sarcoidosis is an autoimmune systemic granulomatous disease associated with an accumulation of CD4-negative T cells.[93] Although its etiology has not been determined, hypothetical causative agents include infectious organisms and noninfectious environmental agents, including metals and organic and inorganic dusts, and autoantigens.[94,95] Pulmonary involvement occurs in most cases, but any organ system may be involved, most commonly the skin, eye, heart, liver, and nervous system. In addition to heterogeneous manifestations, the disease lacks a precise definition, and clinical overlap with other diseases and insensitive and nonspecific diagnostic tests lead to misclassification.

A genetic component in the pathogenesis of sarcoidosis is supported by (1) variation in disease prevalence and incidence among ethnic and racial groups, (2) an adjusted annual incidence approximately threefold higher among African-Americans than among Caucasian Americans and the greater likelihood that the disease is chronic and fatal in African-Americans,[96] (3) the greater likelihood that relatives of individuals with sarcoidosis will have the disease,[76,97] (4) the appearance of familial clustering in different populations,[98] and (5) gene linkage and gene association studies.[99]

Candidate genes for this multifactorial disorder include loci that influence immune regulation, T-cell function, antigen presentation or recognition, and polymorphisms in class I and II HLA loci and genes for immunoregulatory cytokines, growth factors, and angiotensin-converting enzyme.[76,100] Of particular note are polymorphisms in the HLA class 2 genes located in the MHC and mutations in the butyrophilin-like gene (*BTNL2*) at human chromosome region 6p21-22.[96,99–101] These polymorphisms appear to be susceptibility markers not only for sarcoidosis but also for a particular clinical phenotype. Studies of HLA *DRB1* alleles have shown that HLA *DRB1-1101* is a risk factor for sarcoidosis in African-American and Caucasian populations. Significant differences have been observed in the distribution of HLA class II alleles between African-Americans and Caucasians. The HLA *DRB1*1501* allele increases risk in Caucasians but is protective in African-Americans.[102] Other allelic forms are associated with different clinical phenotypes, including eye and bone marrow involvement in African-Americans and hypercalcemia in Caucasians.[102]

Two genome scans for linkage have been reported, one in German families[103] and the other in African-Americans.[104] Several linkage peaks were seen in the German study, with the highest signal at 6p21 and other peaks of interest at chromosome locations 1p22, 3p21, 7q36, 9q33, and on the long arm of the X chromosome. In the African-American study, linkage was detected at 2p25, 5q11, 5q35, 9q34, 11p15, 20q13, and 3p14-11. Further studies are in progress to determine whether these peaks can be confirmed and whether differences in the German and African-American populations can be attributed to different genetic bases for sarcoidosis in the two populations.[99] Also, as in the case of SLE, sarcoidosis has a great deal of phenotypic heterogeneity that may reflect underlying genetic heterogeneity, and searching for genes linked to particular clinical phenotypes may simplify the identification of relevant genes.[105]

While the evidence for a genetic component is strong, family members may share common exposures. Sarcoidosis shares many features with chronic beryllium disease, which is known to have an occupational origin in genetically predisposed individuals. Recent studies have indicated that specific polymorphisms in HLA class II genes may interact with environmental exposures in determining susceptibility to sarcoidosis.[106]

KELOIDS

Keloids are benign collagenous tumors of the dermis that form during a prolonged wound-healing process.[107,108] The genetic predisposition to form keloids is found predominantly in people of African and Asian descent. A prolonged period of fibroblast proliferation and an elevated rate of collagen synthesis relative to normal wound healing characterize keloid formation. The key alteration(s) responsible for the pathologic processes resulting in keloid formation has not been identified, and there is no satisfactory treatment for this disorder. Keloid formation is one of a group of fibroproliferative diseases characterized by an exaggerated response to injury that occur at higher frequency or with more severe manifestations in people of African ancestry. These diseases include hypertension,[109] nephrosclerosis,[110] scleroderma,[71] sarcoidosis,[93] asthma,[111] and uterine fibroma.[112] We[113,114] and others[109,110,115] have suggested that a common etiopathology may operate in these diseases and that common genetic factors may account for their unusual racial distribution.

While most cases of keloid formation occur sporadically, suggesting nongenetic or genetically complex mechanisms of inheritance, familial patterns have been observed. A strong genetic component for keloid formation is supported by the occurrence of keloids at different frequencies in different racial and ethnic populations. Keloids have been estimated to occur in approximately 1 in 30 African-Americans and approximately 1 in 625 of the overall U.S. population.[116] In a study of 14 pedigrees with familial keloids, the inheritance pattern was consistent with an autosomal dominant trait with incomplete penetrance and variable expression.[117] Earlier reports provided evidence for both autosomal dominant[118] and autosomal recessive inheritance.[119] Locus heterogeneity appears likely. In one family, linkage was detected at a region on human chromosome 14q22-q23,[120] whereas in two others, linkage to chromosomes 2q23 and 7p11 was shown.[107] All three families exhibited autosomal dominant inheritance. A microarray study indicating altered expression of multiple genes at or close to these regions in keloid fibroblasts suggested candidate genes for further study.[113] In pedigrees supporting autosomal dominant inheritance, reduced penetrance suggests genetic complexity involving contributions of other susceptibility loci.

Although some cases of keloid formation may be due to somatic mutation,[121] multiple keloids in the same individual and evidence for a multicellular origin of keloids[122–124] argue against somatic mutation as the primary event and suggest that an environmental factor present during wound healing triggers abnormal gene expression in genetically susceptible individuals.

REFERENCES

1. Smith MW, Patterson N, Lautenberger JA, et al. A high-density admixture map for disease gene discovery in African-Americans. *Am J Hum Genet* 2004;74(5):1001-1013.
2. Parra EJ, Marcini A, Akey J, et al. Estimating African-American admixture proportions by use of population-specific alleles. *Am J Hum Genet* 1998;63(6):1839-1851.
3. Vila LM, Alarcon GS, McGwin G Jr, et al. Early clinical manifestations, disease activity and damage of systemic lupus erythematosus among two distinct US Hispanic subpopulations. *Rheumatology (Oxford)* 2004;43(3):358-363.
4. Becker KG. The common genetic hypothesis of autoimmune/inflammatory disease. *Curr Opin Allergy Clin Immunol* 2001;1(5):399-405.
5. Shamim EA, Miller FW, Familial autoimmunity and the idiopathic inflammatory myopathies. *Curr Rheumatol Rep* 2000;2(3):201-211.
6. Aune TM, Parker JS, Maas K, et al. Co-localization of differentially expressed genes and shared susceptibility loci in human autoimmunity. *Genet Epidemiol* 2004;27(2):162-172.
7. Rhodes B, Vyse TJ, General aspects of the genetics of SLE. *Autoimmunity* 2007;40(8):550-559.
8. Wong M, Tsao BP, Current topics in human SLE genetics. *Springer Semin Immunopathol* 2006;28(2):97-107.
9. Hochberg MC. The epidemiology of sysemic lupus erythematosus. In: Wallace DJ, Hahn BH, Quismorio FP, eds. *Dubois' lupus erythematosus*. Baltimore, MD: Williams and Wilkins; 1997:49-65.
10. Rus VHA. Systemic lupus erythematosus. In: Silman AJHM, ed. *Epidemiology of Rheumatic Diseases*. Oxford University Press; 2001:123-140.
11. Uribe AG, McGwin G Jr, Reveille JD, et al. What have we learned from a 10-year experience with the LUMINA (Lupus in Minorities; Nature vs. nurture) cohort? Where are we heading? *Autoimmun Rev* 2004;3(4):321-329.
12. Cantor RM, Yuan J, Napier S, et al. Systemic lupus erythematosus genome scan: support for linkage at 1q23, 2q33, 16q12-13, and 17q21-23 and novel evidence at 3p24, 10q23-24, 13q32, and 18q22-23. *Arthritis Rheum* 2004;50(10):3203-3210.
13. Shen N, Tsao BP. Current advances in the human lupus genetics. *Curr Rheumatol Rep* 2004;6(5):391-398.
14. Wandstrat A, Wakeland E. The genetics of complex autoimmune diseases: non-MHC susceptibility genes. *Nat Immunol* 2001;2(9):802-809.
15. Gaffney PM, Kearns GM, Shark KB, et al. A genome-wide search for susceptibility genes in human systemic lupus erythematosus sib-pair families. *Proc Natl Acad Sci U S A* 1998;95(25):14875-14879.
16. Moser KL, Neas BR, Salmon JE, et al. Genome scan of human systemic lupus erythematosus: evidence for linkage on chromosome 1q in African-American pedigrees. *Proc Natl Acad Sci U S A* 1998;95(25):14869-14874.
17. Gaffney PM, Ortmann WA, Selby SA, et al. Genome screening in human systemic lupus erythematosus: results from a second Minnesota cohort and combined analyses of 187 sib-pair families. *Am J Hum Genet* 2000;66(2):547-556.
18. Gray-McGuire C, Moser KL, Gaffney PM, et al. Genome scan of human systemic lupus erythematosus by regression modeling: evidence of linkage and epistasis at 4p16-15.2. *Am J Hum Genet* 2000;67(6):1460-1469.
19. Lindqvist AK, Steinsson K, Johanneson B, et al. A susceptibility locus for human systemic lupus erythematosus (hSLE1) on chromosome 2q. *J Autoimmun* 2000;14(2):169-178.
20. Shai R, Quismorio FP Jr, Li L, et al. Genome-wide screen for systemic lupus erythematosus susceptibility genes in multiplex families. *Hum Mol Genet* 1999;8(4):639-644.
21. Nath SK, Quintero-Del-Rio AI, Kilpatrick J, et al. Linkage at 12q24 with systemic lupus erythematosus (SLE) is established and confirmed in Hispanic and European American families. *Am J Hum Genet* 2004;74(1):73-82.
22. Koskenmies S, Lahermo P, Julkunen H, et al. Linkage mapping of systemic lupus erythematosus (SLE) in Finnish families multiply affected by SLE. *J Med Genet* 2004;41(1):e2-e5.
23. Tsao BP, Cantor RM, Grossman JM, et al. PARP alleles within the linked chromosomal region are associated with systemic lupus erythematosus. *J Clin Invest* 1999;103(8):1135-1140.
24. Tsao BP, Cantor RM, Kalunian KC, et al. Evidence for linkage of a candidate chromosome 1 region to human systemic lupus erythematosus. *J Clin Invest* 1997;99(4):725-731.
25. Moser KL, Gray-McGuire C, Kelly J, et al. Confirmation of genetic linkage between human systemic lupus erythematosus and chromosome 1q41. *Arthritis Rheum* 1999;42(9):1902-1907.
26. Criswell LA, Moser KL, Gaffney PM, et al. PARP alleles and SLE: failure to confirm association with disease susceptibility. *J Clin Invest* 2000;105(11):1501-1502.
27. Graham RR, Langefeld CD, Gaffney PM, et al. Genetic linkage and transmission disequilibrium of marker haplotypes at chromosome 1q41 in human systemic lupus erythematosus. *Arthritis Res* 2001;3(5):299-305.
28. Magnusson V, Lindqvist AK, Castillejo-Lopez C, et al. Fine mapping of the SLEB2 locus involved in susceptibility to systemic lupus erythematosus. *Genomics* 2000;70(3):307-314.
29. Johanneson B, Lima G, J von Salome, et al. A major susceptibility locus for systemic lupus erythemathosus maps to chromosome 1q31. *Am J Hum Genet* 2002;71(5):1060-1071.
30. Nath SK, Kilpatrick J, Harley JB, Genetics of human systemic lupus erythematosus: the emerging picture. *Curr Opin Immunol* 2004;16(6):794-800.
31. Graham RR, Ortmann WA, Langefeld CD, et al. Visualizing human leukocyte antigen class II risk haplotypes in human systemic lupus erythematosus. *Am J Hum Genet* 2002;71(3):543-553.
32. Magnusson V, Johanneson B, Lima G, et al. Both risk alleles for FcgammaRIIA and FcgammaRIIIA are susceptibility factors for SLE: a unifying hypothesis. *Genes Immun* 2004;5(2):130-137.
33. Ghebrehiwet B, Peerschke EI. Role of C1q and C1q receptors in the pathogenesis of systemic lupus erythematosus. *Curr Dir Autoimmun* 2004;7:87-97.
34. Manderson AP, Botto M, Walport MJ. The role of complement in the development of systemic lupus erythematosus. *Annu Rev Immunol* 2004;22:431-456.
35. Slingsby JH, Norsworthy P, Pearce G, et al. Homozygous hereditary C1q deficiency and systemic lupus erythematosus. A new family and the molecular basis of C1q deficiency in three families. *Arthritis Rheum* 1996;39(4):663-670.
36. Haywood ME, Hogarth MB, Slingsby JH, et al. Identification of intervals on chromosomes 1, 3, and 13 linked to the development of lupus in BXSB mice. *Arthritis Rheum* 2000;43(2):349-355.
37. Fanciulli M, Norsworthy PJ, Petretto E, et al. FCGR3B copy number variation is associated with susceptibility to systemic, but not organ-specific, autoimmunity. *Nat Genet* 2007;39(6):721-723.
38. Yang Y, Chung EK, Wu YL, et al. Gene copy-number variation and associated polymorphisms of complement component C4 in human systemic lupus erythematosus (SLE): low copy number is a risk factor for and high copy number is a protective factor against SLE susceptibility in European Americans. *Am J Hum Genet* 2007;80(6):1037-1054.
39. Graham DS, Graham RR, Manku H, et al. Polymorphism at the TNF superfamily gene TNFSF4 confers susceptibility to systemic lupus erythematosus. *Nat Genet* 2008;40(1):83-89.
40. Prokunina L, Castillejo-Lopez C, Oberg F, et al. A regulatory polymorphism in PDCD1 is associated with susceptibility to systemic lupus erythematosus in humans. *Nat Genet* 2002;32(4):666-669.
41. Ferreiros-Vidal I, Gomez-Reino JJ, Barros F, et al. Association of PDCD1 with susceptibility to systemic lupus erythematosus: evidence of population-specific effects. *Arthritis Rheum* 2004;50(8):2590-2597.
42. Prokunina L, Padyukov L, Bennet A, et al. Association of the PD-1.3A allele of the PDCD1 gene in patients with rheumatoid arthritis negative for rheumatoid factor and the shared epitope. *Arthritis Rheum* 2004;50(6):1770-1773.
43. Nath SK, Namjou B, Kilpatrick J, et al. A candidate region on 11p13 for systemic lupus erythematosus: a linkage identified in African-American families.

J Investig Dermatol Symp Proc 2004; 9(1):64-67.
44. Sawalha AH, Namjou B, Nath SK, et al. Genetic linkage of systemic lupus erythematosus with chromosome 11q14 (SLEH1) in African-American families stratified by a nucleolar antinuclear antibody pattern. *Genes Immun* 2002; 3(suppl 1):S31-S34.
45. Kelly JA, Thompson K, Kilpatrick J, et al. Evidence for a susceptibility gene (SLEH1) on chromosome 11q14 for systemic lupus erythematosus (SLE) families with hemolytic anemia. *Proc Natl Acad Sci U S A* 2002;99(18):11766-11771.
46. Quintero-Del-Rio AI, Kelly JA, Kilpatrick J, et al. The genetics of systemic lupus erythematosus stratified by renal disease: linkage at 10q22.3 (SLEN1), 2q34-35 (SLEN2), and 11p15.6 (SLEN3). *Genes Immun* 2002;3(suppl 1):S57-S62.
47. Quintero-del-Rio AI, Kelly JA, Garriott CP, et al. SLEN2 (2q34-35) and SLEN1 (10q22.3) replication in systemic lupus erythematosus stratified by nephritis. *Am J Hum Genet* 2004;75(2):346-348.
48. Hudson LL, Rocca K, Song YW, et al. CTLA-4 gene polymorphisms in systemic lupus erythematosus: a highly significant association with a determinant in the promoter region. *Hum Genet* 2002;111(4-5):452-455.
49. Fernandez-Blanco L, Perez-Pampin E, Gomez-Reino JJ, et al. A CTLA-4 polymorphism associated with susceptibility to systemic lupus erythematosus. *Arthritis Rheum* 2004;50(1):328-329.
50. Liu MF, Wang CR, Lin LC, et al. CTLA-4 gene polymorphism in promoter and exon-1 regions in Chinese patients with systemic lupus erythematosus. *Lupus* 2001;10(9):647-649.
51. Nath SK, Kelly JA, Namjou B, et al. Evidence for a susceptibility gene, SLEV1, on chromosome 17p13 in families with vitiligo-related systemic lupus erythematosus. *Am J Hum Genet* 2001;69(6):1401-1406.
52. Online Mendelian Inheritance in Man, OMIM (TM). McKusick-Nathans Institute of Genetic Medicine, Johns Hopkins University (Baltimore, MD) and National Center for Biotechnology Information, National Library of Medicine (Bethesda, MD), World Wide Web URL: http://www.ncbi.nlm.nih.gov/omim/
53. Graham RR, Kyogoku C, Sigurdsson S, et al. Three functional variants of IFN regulatory factor 5 (IRF5) define risk and protective haplotypes for human lupus. *Proc Natl Acad Sci U S A* 2007;104(16): 6758-6763.
54. Gaffney PM, Langefeld CD, Graham RR, et al. Fine-mapping chromosome 20 in 230 systemic lupus erythematosus sib pair and multiplex families: evidence for genetic epistasis with chromosome 16q12. *Am J Hum Genet* 2006;78(5):747-758.
55. Hann S, Nordlund JJ. In: Hann SK, ed. *Vitiligo: A monograph on the Basic and Clinical Science.* Oxford, England: Blackwell Science; 2000.
56. Bolognia J, Nordlund JJ, Ortonne J-P. Vitiligo vulgaris, In: Nordlund J, Boissy RE, Hearing VJ, King RA, Ortonne J-P, eds. *The Pigmentary System.* New York, NY: Oxford University Press; 1998.
57. Zhang XJ, Liu JB, Gui JP, et al. Characteristics of genetic epidemiology and genetic models for vitiligo. *J Am Acad Dermatol* 2004;51(3):383-390.
58. Boisseau-Garsaud AM, Garsaud P, Cales-Quist D, et al. Epidemiology of vitiligo in the French West Indies (Isle of Martinique). *Int J Dermatol* 2000;39(1): 18-20.
59. Onunu AN, Kubeyinje EP. Vitiligo in the Nigerian African: a study of 351 patients in Benin City, Nigeria. *Int J Dermatol* 2003;42(10):800-802.
60. Kovacs SO. Vitiligo. *J Am Acad Dermatol* 1998;38(5)(Pt 1):6476-66; quiz 667-668.
61. Spritz RA. The genetics of generalized vitiligo and associated autoimmune diseases. *Pigment Cell Res* 2007;20(4):271-278.
62. Laberge G, Mailloux CM, Gowan K, et al. Early disease onset and increased risk of other autoimmune diseases in familial generalized vitiligo. *Pigment Cell Res* 2005;18(4):300-305.
63. Alkhateeb A, Fain PR, Thody A, et al. Epidemiology of vitiligo and associated autoimmune diseases in Caucasian probands and their families. *Pigment Cell Res* 2003;16(3):208-214.
64. Grimes PE, Halder RM, Jones C, et al. Autoantibodies and their clinical significance in a black vitiligo population. *Arch Dermatol* 1983;119(4):300-303.
65. Fain PR, Gowan K, LaBerge GS, et al. A genomewide screen for generalized vitiligo: confirmation of AIS1 on chromosome 1p31 and evidence for additional susceptibility loci. *Am J Hum Genet* 2003;72(6):1560-1564.
66. Dunston GM, Halder RM. Vitiligo is associated with HLA-DR4 in black patients. A preliminary report. *Arch Dermatol* 1990;126(1):56-60.
67. Arcos-Burgos M, Parodi E, Salgar M, et al. Vitiligo: complex segregation and linkage disequilibrium analyses with respect to microsatellite loci spanning the HLA. *Hum Genet* 2002;110(4):334-342.
68. Orozco-Topete R, Cordova-Lopez J, Yamamoto-Furusho JK, et al. HLA-DRB1 *04 is associated with the genetic susceptibility to develop vitiligo in Mexican patients with autoimmune thyroid disease. *J Am Acad Dermatol* 2005;52(1):182-183.
69. Spritz RA, Gowan K, Bennett DC, et al. Novel vitiligo susceptibility loci on chromosomes 7 (AIS2) and 8 (AIS3), confirmation of SLEV1 on chromosome 17, and their roles in an autoimmune diathesis. *Am J Hum Genet* 2004;74(1): 188-191.
70. Bruey JM, Bruey-Sedano N, Luciano F, et al. Bcl-2 and Bcl-XL regulate proinflammatory caspase-1 activation by interaction with NALP1. *Cell* 2007; 129(1):45-56.
71. Mayes MD, Lacey JV Jr, Beebe-Dimmer J, et al. Prevalence, incidence, survival, and disease characteristics of systemic sclerosis in a large US population. *Arthritis Rheum* 2003;48(8):2246-2255.
72. Zhou X, Tan FK, Wang N, et al. Genome-wide association study for regions of systemic sclerosis susceptibility in a Choctaw Indian population with high disease prevalence. *Arthritis Rheum* 2003;48(9):2585-2592.
73. Harley JB, Neas BR. Oklahoma Choctaw and systemic sclerosis: the founder effect and genetic susceptibility. *Arthritis Rheum* 1998;41(10):1725-1728.
74. Tan FK, Stivers DN, Foster MW, et al. Association of microsatellite markers near the fibrillin 1 gene on human chromosome 15q with scleroderma in a Native American population. *Arthritis Rheum* 1998;41(10):1729-1737.
75. Arnett FC, Cho M, Chatterjee S, et al. Familial occurrence frequencies and relative risks for systemic sclerosis (scleroderma) in three United States cohorts. *Arthritis Rheum* 2001;44(6):1359-1362.
76. du Bois RM. The genetic predisposition to interstitial lung disease. Proceedings and Abstracts of the 44th Annual Thomas Petty Aspen Lung Conference: Pulmonary Genetics, Genomics, Gene Therapy. *Chest* 2002;121:1S-110S.
77. Sato H, Lagan AL, Alexopoulou C, et al. The TNF-863A allele strongly associates with anticentromere antibody positivity in scleroderma. *Arthritis Rheum* 2004;50(2):558-564.
78. Johnson RW, Tew MB, Arnett FC. The genetics of systemic sclerosis. *Curr Rheumatol Rep* 2002;4(2):99-107.
79. Fonseca C, Lindahl GE, Ponticos M, et al. A polymorphism in the CTGF promoter region associated with systemic sclerosis. *N Engl J Med* 2007;357(12): 1210-1220.
80. Feghali-Bostwick CA. Genetics and proteomics in scleroderma. *Curr Rheumatol Rep* 2005;7(2):129-134.
81. Assassi S, Arnett FC, Reveille JD, et al. Clinical, immunologic, and genetic features of familial systemic sclerosis. *Arthritis Rheum* 2007;56(6):2031-2037.
82. Mayes MD, Trojanowska M. Genetic factors in systemic sclerosis. *Arthritis Res Ther* 2007;9(suppl 2):S5.
83. Reveille JD, Fischbach M, McNearney T, et al. Systemic sclerosis in 3 US ethnic groups: a comparison of clinical, sociodemographic, serologic, and immunogenetic determinants. *Semin Arthritis Rheum* 2001;30(5):332-346.
84. Mayes MD. Scleroderma epidemiology. *Rheum Dis Clin North Am* 2003;29(2): 239-254.
85. Prisant LM, Loebl DH, Mulloy LL. Scleroderma renal crisis. *J Clin Hypertens (Greenwich)* 2003;5(2):168-170, 176.
86. Cepeda EJ, Reveille JD. Autoantibodies in systemic sclerosis and fibrosing syndromes: clinical indications and relevance. *Curr Opin Rheumatol* 2004;16(6): 723-732.
87. Zhou X, Tan FK, Xiong M, et al. Systemic sclerosis (scleroderma): specific autoantigen genes are selectively overexpressed in scleroderma fibroblasts. *J Immunol* 2001;167(12):7126-7133.
88. Arnett FC. HLA and autoimmunity in scleroderma (systemic sclerosis). *Int Rev Immunol* 1995;12(2-4):107-128.
89. Kuwana M, Kaburaki J, Arnett FC, et al. Influence of ethnic background on clinical and serologic features in patients with systemic sclerosis and anti-DNA topoisomerase I antibody. *Arthritis Rheum* 1999;42(3):465-474.
90. Tormey VJ, Bunn CC, Denton CP, et al. Anti-fibrillarin antibodies in systemic

sclerosis. *Rheumatology (Oxford)* 2001; 40(10):1157-1162.
91. Arnett FC, Reveille JD, Goldstein R, et al. Autoantibodies to fibrillarin in systemic sclerosis (scleroderma). An immunogenetic, serologic, and clinical analysis. *Arthritis Rheum* 1996;39(7): 1151-1160.
92. Lefevre F, Garnotel R, Georges N, et al. Modulation of collagen metabolism by the nucleolar protein fibrillarin. *Exp Cell Res* 2001;271(1):84-93.
93. Rybicki BA, Maliarik MJ, Major M, et al. Epidemiology, demographics, and genetics of sarcoidosis. *Semin Respir Infect* 1998;13(3):166-173.
94. Moller DR. Etiology of sarcoidosis. *Clin Chest Med* 1997;18(4):695-706.
95. Moller DR, Chen ES. What causes sarcoidosis? *Curr Opin Pulm Med.* 2002;8(5):429-434.
96. Iannuzzi MC, Rybicki BA, Teirstein AS. Sarcoidosis. *N Engl J Med* 2007;357(21): 2153-2165.
97. Rybicki BA, Iannuzzi MC, Frederick MM, et al. Familial aggregation of sarcoidosis. A case-control etiologic study of sarcoidosis (ACCESS). *Am J Respir Crit Care Med* 2001;164(11):2085-2091.
98. Rybicki BA, Kirkey KL, Major M, et al. Familial risk ratio of sarcoidosis in African-American sibs and parents. *Am J Epidemiol* 2001;153(2):188-193.
99. Iannuzzi MC, Rybicki BA. Genetics of sarcoidosis: candidate genes and genome scans. *Proc Am Thorac Soc* 2007;4(1): 108-116.
100. Rybicki BA, Walewski JL, Maliarik MJ, et al. The BTNL2 gene and sarcoidosis susceptibility in African-Americans and Whites. *Am J Hum Genet* 2005;77(3):491-499.
101. Valentonyte R, Hampe J, Huse K, et al. Sarcoidosis is associated with a truncating splice site mutation in BTNL2. *Nat Genet* 2005;37(4):357-364.
102. Rossman MD, Thompson B, Frederick M, et al. HLA-DRB1*1101: a significant risk factor for sarcoidosis in blacks and whites. *Am J Hum Genet* 2003;73(4):720-735.
103. Schurmann M, Reichel P, Muller-Myhsok B, et al. Results from a genome-wide search for predisposing genes in sarcoidosis. *Am J Respir Crit Care Med* 2001;164(5):840-846.
104. Iannuzzi MC, Iyengar SK, Gray-McGuire C, et al. Genome-wide search for sarcoidosis susceptibility genes in African-Americans. *Genes Immun* 2005; 6(6):509-518.
105. Rybicki BA, Sinha R, Iyengar S, et al. Genetic linkage analysis of sarcoidosis phenotypes: the sarcoidosis genetic analysis (SAGA) study. *Genes Immun* 2007;8(5):379-386.
106. Iannuzzi MC, Maliarik MJ, Poisson LM, et al. Sarcoidosis susceptibility and resistance HLA-DQB1 alleles in African-Americans. *Am J Respir Crit Care Med* 2003;167(9):1225-1231.
107. Marneros AG, Norris JE, Watanabe S, et al. Genome scans provide evidence for keloid susceptibility Loci on chromosomes 2q23 and 7p11. *J Invest Dermatol* 2004;122(5):1126-1132.
108. Niessen FB, Spauwen PH, Schalkwijk J, et al. On the nature of hypertrophic scars and keloids: a review. *Plast Reconstr Surg* 1999;104(5):1435-1458.
109. Dustan HP. Does keloid pathogenesis hold the key to understanding black/white differences in hypertension severity? *Hypertension* 1995;26(6)(Pt 1): 858-862.
110. August P, Suthanthiran M. Transforming growth factor beta and progression of renal disease. *Kidney Int Suppl* 2003;87: S99-S104.
111. Nickel R, Beck LA, Stellato C, et al. Chemokines and allergic disease. *J Allergy Clin Immunol* 1999;104(4)(Pt 1):723-742.
112. Flake GP, Andersen J, Dixon D. Etiology and pathogenesis of uterine leiomyomas: a review. *Environ Health Perspect* 2003;111(8):1037-1054.
113. Smith JC, Boone BE, Opalenik SR, et al. Gene Profiling of Keloid Fibroblasts Shows Altered Expression in Multiple Fibrosis-Associated Pathways. *J Invest Dermatol* 2008;128:1298-1310.
114. Russell SB, Trupin JS, Myers JC, et al. Differential glucocorticoid regulation of collagen mRNAs in human dermal fibroblasts. Keloid-derived and fetal fibroblasts are refractory to down-regulation. *J Biol Chem* 1989;264(23): 13730-13735.
115. Catherino WH, Leppert PC, Stenmark MH, et al. Reduced dermatopontin expression is a molecular link between uterine leiomyomas and keloids. *Genes Chromosomes Cancer* 2004;40(3): 204-217.
116. Barrett J. Keloid. In: Bergsma D, ed. *Birth Defect Compendium.* Baltimore, MD: Williams and Wilkens Company; 1973:553.
117. Marneros AG, Norris JE, Olsen BR, et al. Clinical genetics of familial keloids. *Arch Dermatol* 2001;137(11):1429-1434.
118. Bloom D. Heredity of keloids. *N Y State Med J* 1956;56:511-519.
119. Omo-Dare P. Genetic studies on keloid. *J Natl Med Assoc* 1975;67(6):428-432.
120. Davis KD, Garcia M, Phillips JA III, et al. Detection of a critical interval for a familial keloid locus on chromosome 14q22-q23 in an African-American pedigree. *Am J Hum Gen* 2000;67:A21.
121. Saed GM, Ladin D, Olson J, et al. Analysis of p53 gene mutations in keloids using polymerase chain reaction-based single-strand conformational polymorphism and DNA sequencing. *Arch Dermatol* 1998;134(8):963-967.
122. Chevray PM, Manson PN. Keloid scars are formed by polyclonal fibroblasts. *Ann Plast Surg* 2004;52(6):605-608.
123. Moulton-Levy P, Jackson CE, Levy HG, et al. Multiple cell origin of traumatically induced keloids. *J Am Acad Dermatol* 1984;10(6):986-988.
124. Trupin JS, Williams JM, Hammons J, et al. Multicellular origin of keloids. In: *Fifth International Conference on Birth Defects.* Montreal, QC: Elsevier; 1977.

CHAPTER 17

Biology of Hair Follicle

Candrice R. Heath
Amy J. McMichael

Key Points

- Embryologic development of hair follicles is the same for all races, with the important exception of the distribution of melanin along the hair follicle of individuals of African descent.
- The shapes of hair follicles and the hair shaft differ based on ethnicity.
- The amino acid structure of hair is consistent across all ethnic groups.
- Textured hair of individuals of African descent is more susceptible to breakage (lower tensile strength) than Asian or Caucasian hair.
- As measured by the number of hair follicles in a 4-mm punch biopsy specimen, Asian and textured African hair is less dense than Caucasian hair.
- Textured African hair swells less than either Asian or Caucasian hair when in contact with water and has a decreased moisture content.
- Despite being wet or dry, more energy (joules) is required to comb textured African hair than is required to comb Caucasian hair.

Studies regarding the biology of hair and hair follicles have focused on Caucasian, Asian, and textured African hair, but the world's population encompasses people of a multitude of backgrounds, which results in the existence of multiple hair types. De La Miettrie and colleagues gathered samples from 1442 people from 18 countries and identified eight hair types based on hair shape. They suggest that identifying hair based solely on race results in a simplification of the hair types found in the world. The danger of oversimplification is reflected in the large and diverse continent of Africa, which contains people with many hair textures that vary with their region of origin.[1] Straight hair, which can be found in people from northern Africa, is unlike the tightly coiled hair textures of people from sub-Saharan Africa.[2] Nevertheless, for the purposes of nomenclature, the designation *textured African hair* will refer to the tightly coiled hair of individuals who herald from sub-Saharan Africa, which is synonymous with unprocessed African-American or Black hair.

EMBRYOGENESIS OF THE HAIR FOLLICLE

Embryos of all racial and ethnic groups are formed from three germ layers: the endoderm, mesoderm, and ectoderm. Skin, hair, and nails arise primarily from the ectoderm.[3] Hair follicles form as the result of unique neuroectodermal and mesodermal interactions.[3,4] Hair follicle formation occurs only during the fetal stage, and therefore, hair follicles do not regenerate during adult life.[5]

Embryologically, hair follicle formation is triggered by dermal fibroblasts that cause the aggregation of cells in the overlying basal layer of the epidermis. Subsequently, the basal cells lengthen, divide, and recede into the dermis.[6] Beneath this early follicle, the dermal papilla is formed. As a consequence of the dermal papilla's upward pressure on the early follicle, basal stem cells within the matrix are stimulated to divide more rapidly and eventually produce cells that will differentiate into the hair shaft.[6,7]

Hair shafts receive pigment from the melanocytes interlaced among the matrix cells. The fibroblasts within the dermal papilla may dictate the number of matrix cells and size of the hair.[7] The hair follicle elongates, and the concave-shaped inferior portion encloses the dermal papilla. Each hair follicle grows at an oblique angle to the epidermis. Two swellings form at the posterior portion of the follicle, and they serve as the sebaceous gland and the attachment site for the arrector pilli muscle.[8] Ultimately, there are approximately 5 million hair follicles on the entire body, with 80,000–150,000 follicles located on the scalp.[9–11]

The shape of the hair follicle contributes to the cross-sectional structure of the hair shaft. A curved, helically shaped follicle produces tightly curled African hair, whereas linear Asian hair follicles give rise to straight hair.[12] Additionally, the hair follicles of African-Americans are reportedly anchored to the dermis by fewer elastic fibers than Caucasian follicles.[13]

Differences in ethnic follicular size and density on the forehead, back, thorax, upper arms, forearms, thighs, and calves of 10 Caucasians, 10 African-Americans, and 10 Asians have been reported. The most dense follicular area was reportedly the forehead of Caucasians (292 follicles/cm^2), followed by African-Americans (189 follicles/cm^2) and then Asians (138 follicles/cm^2). No significant ethnic differences were found in the number of upper arm follicles. In order to obtain representative numbers of follicles from each body site, several samples were taken from each site. The intersite averages for each body area were calculated and then compared with distant sites. Asian follicular orifice intersite diameters were uniform, whereas the Caucasian subjects had wide variations in intersite measurements. In African-American and Caucasian subjects, the smallest follicular orifices were found on the forehead, whereas the largest were observed on the thigh and calf. Overall, the Asian follicular orifices were the smallest of the groups studied regardless of body site. In Caucasians, the highest number of follicular orifices were found on the forehead, calves, and back, whereas the highest percentage of follicular orifices was found on the forehead, upper arms, and back, respectively in African-Americans and Asians.[14]

Hair shaft diameter has been noted to differ among racial groups. Hair shaft diameter on the thighs and calves of African-American and Asian subjects was less than that of Caucasians. Variations in vellus hair follicle orifice size and distribution may prove significant in topical drug penetration.[14]

BASIC HAIR STRUCTURE

Hair follicles differentiate into three epithelial cylinders: the central shaft fiber, the middle inner root sheath, and the outer root sheath[15] (Figure 17-1). The structure of the hair shaft from individuals of African, Caucasian, and Asian descent are essentially the same.[16] The central hair shaft unit includes the cuticle, cortex, and sometimes an inner medulla.[17] However, despite the same basic hair shaft structure, some variations have been identified in the cross section, shape, and pigment content.

African hair shafts have a more flattened cross section compared with the hair shafts of Asians and Caucasians.[18] The African hair shaft appears to be as

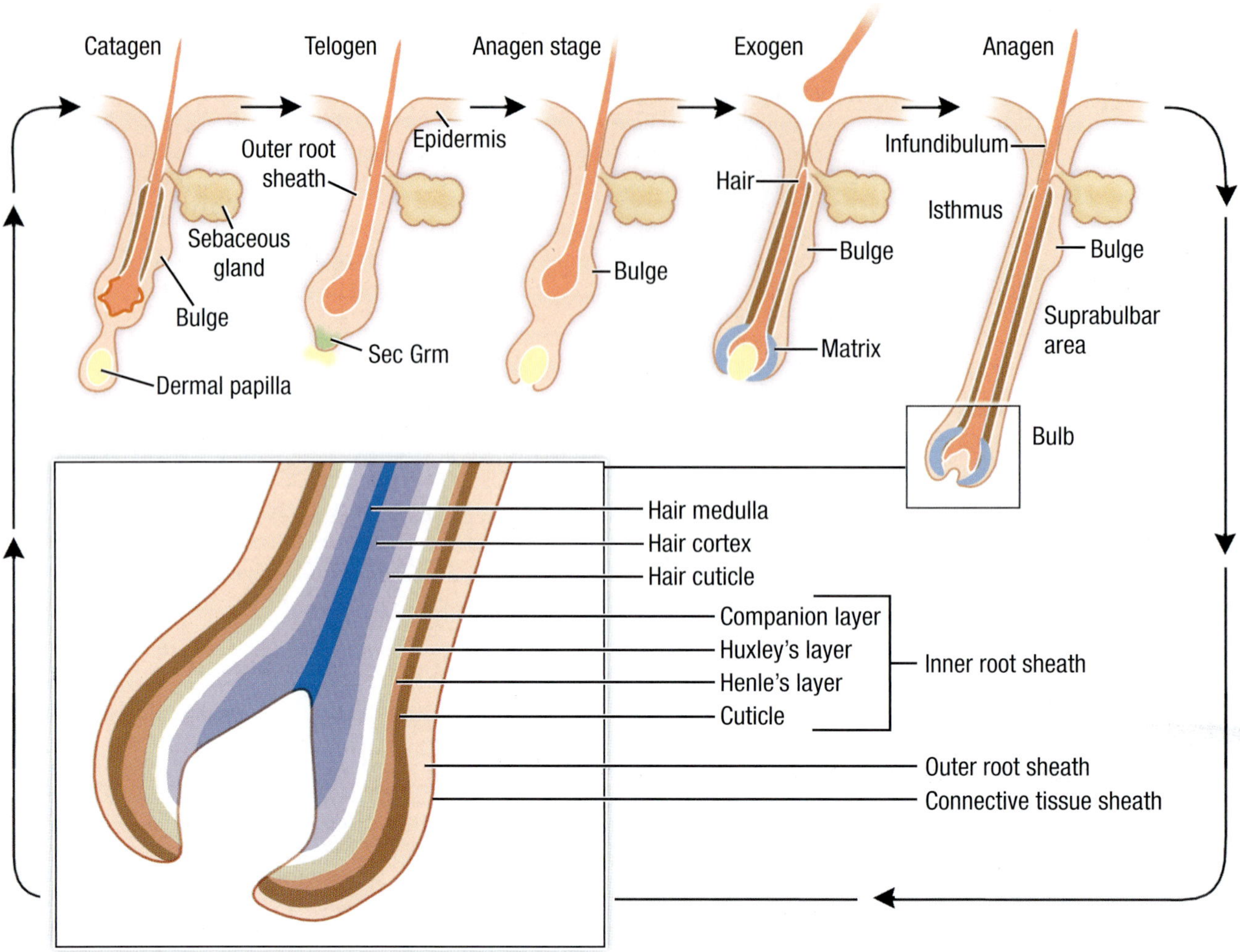

▲ **FIGURE 17-1** Hair follicle cycling and hair anatomy. (From *Fitzpatrick's Dermatology in General Medicine,* Vol 1, 7th ed. New York, McGraw-Hill, 2008, Figure 84-2.)

tightly coiled as the textured hair that emerges from it.[12,16,18] Light microscopy reveals broken and knotted African hair shafts, whereas the hair shafts of Caucasians and Asians are straight or slightly curved[16]. Furthermore, textured African hair shafts are distinct owing to the presence of melanin granules and melanosomes, which are found at deeper levels parallel to the axis of the hair shaft.[13,18]

Cuticle

Cells proliferate at the base of the follicle, migrate upward, and through protein synthesis and keratinization, transform into hair. Hair fibers are covered by a layer of overlapping flat scales called *cuticle cells,* which marginally tilt away from the hair fiber axis and contain a blend of proteins, lipids, and carbohydrates.[9,19] Scanning electron microscopy and transmission microscopy demonstrate that Asian hair cuticles have multiple cuticle layers, giving rise to a thicker, more compact cuticle layer than Caucasian hair.[20,21] In fact, Asian eyelashes reportedly have more cuticle layers with a density similar to that of Asian scalp hair.[22]

Within the cuticle cell, there are distinct layers, including the controversial epicuticle, which recently was tentatively established by transmission electron microscope as a 13-nm continuous layer found on undamaged mammalian keratin fibers.[23] The cuticle's cystine-rich A layer is positioned between the epicuticle and the exocuticle. The exocuticle has multiple cystine disulfide bonds but not nearly as many as contained within the A layer of the cuticle cell. The adjacent layer, the endocuticle, contains proteins, cellular debris, and minimal cystine.[9] Asian hair endocuticles are harder than those found in Caucasian hair.[21]

The cuticular cell membrane complex (CMC), an extremely adhesive layer, holds the cuticle cells together with its three layers, which include a central δ layer, with little protein, flanked on each side by lipid-rich β layers.[9] This CMC layer includes 18-methyleicosanoic acid (MEA), an atypical branched-chain fatty acid that is bound covalently to its protein components and to the cuticle surface.[9,24] MEA may exhibit decreased adhesion with textured African hair compared with the adhesion to Caucasian hair.[24]

Cortex

Parallel to the axis of the hair fiber lie fused spindle-like cells. These cells are packed with fine filaments into microfibrils and organized into groups to create macrofibrils. Owing to various packing methods within the macrofibrils, two arrangements, the paracortex and the orthocortex, result. Within the macrofibrils, microfibrils are immersed in a cystine matrix. In Asian, Caucasian, and textured African hair, the cystine disulfide bonds are a critical aspect of keratin stability.[9]

Inner and Outer Root Sheaths

Surrounding the central hair shaft unit (i.e., cuticle, cortex, and medulla) are the inner and outer root sheaths.[17] The outer root sheath divides this cylindrical structure from the dermis, whereas the inner root sheath guides and moves outward with the hair shaft.[15] Melanosomes are found in the outer root sheath of Black hair follicles, but melanosomes are missing from the outer root sheaths of Caucasians.[13] A portion of the outer root sheath, the bulge, is near the insertion of the arrector pili muscle. The bulge contains epithelial stem cells, which are vital to regeneration of anagen hair bulbs.[7,25] In fact, the outer root sheath, inner root sheath, hair matrix, and hair shaft emerge from stem cells within the bulge.[4]

Determination of Hair Color

Melanocytes contain melanosomes, which are transported to keratinocytes in the skin and hair via long dendritic processes. The melanosomes produce two types of melanin, which determine hair color pigment. Eumelanin produces brown to black hair, whereas pheomelanin produces yellow-blonde to red hair (3).

HAIR FOLLICLE CYCLING

Multiple growth factors and growth factor receptors are crucial for hair follicle development and cycling.[7] The main hair growth phases include the anagen, catagen, and telogen phases (see Figure 17-1). During the anagen phase, active growth occurs and may last for 2–8 years.[7,9,10] This is followed by a brief catagen rest phase for a few weeks, after which a 2- to 4-month telogen shedding phase occurs. At any point in the hair growth cycle, a percentage of the 150,000 scalp hairs are growing (85–90%), resting, or shedding.[9,10]

Hair follicles on various body areas produce hairs of different lengths. Hair length corresponds to the time spent in the anagen phase. This is evident in the comparison of the 2- to 3-month anagen phase of eyebrows compared with the 2- to 8-year scalp anagen phase.[7] If the length of time spent in the hair growth phases is altered, clinical changes may occur, including effluvium, from a shortened anagen growth phase, and hypertrichosis, from a prolonged anagen phase.[4]

Hair cycling is not synchronized.[10] However, during the late stages of fetal development, hair cycling does occur in a synchronized fashion.[3] Hair on the parietal and frontal areas of the fetal scalp is shed twice in utero.[8] The occipital scalp hairs are shed only once in utero, which may account for occipital telogen shedding during the first few weeks of life.[8] Occipital hairs may even be more susceptible to shedding owing to scalp friction from the highly recommended infant supine sleeping position, although some authors challenge sleeping position as a cause for scalp shedding in the first 3 months of life.[8,26]

HAIR TYPES

Lanugo hair, fine fetal hair, is shed in utero or during the first weeks after birth.[7] Vellus hairs are short, nonpigmented hairs, whereas terminal hairs are larger pigment-containing hairs.[4,7] The bulbs of vellus hair in Blacks contain melanosomes, in contrast to Caucasian vellus hair bulbs, which do not contain melanosomes.[13] In the setting of androgenic alopecia, a process of miniaturization occurs. Miniaturization involves large terminal hairs converting into vellus hairs. Club hairs are the ultimate product of the follicle during the telogen phase, during which 50–150 hairs may be shed daily.[7]

SKIN OF COLOR HAIR PROPERTIES

Cross Section

In cross section, Asian hair is wide and round, whereas Caucasian hair is thinner with a more elliptical shape.[27–29] Textured African hair, with its pronounced curly structure, is the most elliptical of the three most studied hair types: Asian, Caucasian, and African.[27–32] The elliptical shape of African hair resembles a flattened oval.[27] Asian hair diameter (or ellipticity) is very uniform, whereas African hair has a range of ellipticity that is speculated to be due to hair curliness.[9] The most cross-sectional variability can be found in African hair owing to frequent fiber restrictions.[27,31,32] A study of the scalps of preschool children demonstrated differences in the maximum shaft diameter in hairs from different areas, but generally, hairs from different areas of an undiseased scalp are morphologically the same.[33]

Chemical Composition

Despite differences in hair texture, the amino acid composition and distribution of cystine-rich proteins of African, Asian, and Caucasian hair is the same.[18,27,29,34] In addition, the low-sulfur proteins within the hair are identical for Caucasians, Asians, and Africans.[35] Although the sulfur-containing proteins are the same, the relationship between the low- and high-sulfur proteins varies depending on hair color.[36]

Tensile Strength

Since textured African, Asian, and Caucasian hair share the same protein structure, textured African hair is not inherently fragile from structural abnormalities, but mechanical damage is likely.[18,28] Owing to daily hair grooming practices and textured African hair's tightly coiled shape, the easily damaged hair is more prone to breakage.[18,28,29,37] Under both wet and dry conditions, textured African hair breaks more easily than Caucasian hair.[31]

Despite the larger diameter and higher tensile force required to disrupt Asian hair, Caucasian and Asian hair responds similarly during scientific strain tests. Asian and Caucasian hairs are more resistant to tensile stress, whereas African hair is more fragile and breaks in a much shorter time period.[27] Under the stress of extension, Asian hair loses cohesion between the cuticle cells (cuticle cell membrane complex) because this area absorbs the stress, thus allowing the cuticles to lift and break. In contrast, under extension stress, Caucasian hair cuticles fall off in small pieces.[21]

Effects of Hair Processing

Textured African hair can be straightened by temporary heat pressing or permanent lanthionization (relaxer) processing to relax the curl pattern of the hair.[29,37,38] The chemical bonds within hair are broken temporarily by heat and permanently by lanthionization processing with sodium hydroxide, guanine hydroxide, potassium hydroxide, sulfites, and thioglycolates[37–39] Textured African hair, susceptible to mechanical damage, may be further fractured or broken if the hair is overprocessed with chemicals or repeatedly pressed at extremely high temperatures.[40]

Hair Density and Growth Rate

Hair density, defined as the number of hair follicles in a 4-mm biopsy specimen, is higher in Caucasians than in

Blacks.[41] Reportedly, the hair density ratio of Blacks compared with Caucasians is less than 3:5, with higher ratios reported as well.[17,41] Caucasians and Asians have, on average, one follicular unit per square millimeter on the scalp, whereas Africans average 0.6 follicular units per square millimeter.[2] In Caucasians and Asians, each follicular unit produces two hairs, whereas each African follicular unit produces three hairs. Bernstein and Rassman hypothesize that low hair density, higher follicular grouping, and the tightly curled hair pattern seen in Africans may have evolved as a means of scalp cooling by protection from the sun.[42]

In a study of 4-mm punch scalp biopsies from Caucasians and African-Americans, the total numbers of terminal follicles and terminal anagen hairs were lower in the African-American specimens than in samples from Caucasians.[41] In addition, a study examining Asian 4-mm punch scalp biopsies found lower hair density than that seen in Caucasian and black hair. Much lower numbers of terminal, vellus, and total hairs were found in Asians than in Caucasians.[43] These observations are important in the interpretations of scalp biopsy specimens.[41]

Not only is the hair density lower in persons of African descent, the hair growth rate is slower than in Caucasians. Loussouarn found a growth rate of 256 ± 44 μm/day for African hair and 396 ± 55 μm/day for Caucasian hair, respectively.[44] Despite the data that textured African hair experiences daily growth, many people with textured African hair may have the same overall length of hair for long periods of time. This length threshold may be due to daily breakage of tightly coiled hair from daily hair care maintenance techniques.[2]

Water Swelling and Moisture

Textured African hair swells less with a lower radial swelling rate while in contact with water than Asian and Caucasian hair.[27] Even when the moisture content of textured African hair is compared with that of Caucasian hair using a scientific weight calculation, the content of moisture in African hair is less than that in Caucasian hair. This decreased moisture content may have a considerable role in the relative fragility of textured African hair.[31] Further study is required to explain the differences in hydration despite the same hair chemical composition.[27]

Combability and Wear

When measured in joules, the work of combing wet textured African hair is nearly 5 times that of combing wet Caucasian hair. Moreover, the work of combing dry textured African hair is 50 times greater than that of combing dry Caucasian hair (Figure 17-2). Overall, it's about 8 times more challenging to comb wet textured African hair than dry textured African hair.[31] However, other authors have explained that by and large, textured African hair is easier to comb while wet owing to a reduction in the waving pattern[9,29].

Owing to the tightly coiled springlike quality of textured African hair, the hair shafts often intertwine when the hair is combed. The more curled and intertwined the hair, the more it breaks.[18,28,29] As a result, short unprocessed hair is easier to comb than longer tresses. Depending on the degree of coiling, the hair is frequently fractured in order to remove knots. Since combing creates daily breakage, a point occurs when the amount of new growth equals the breakage, and any hair growth is difficult to appreciate.[28]

Under scanning electron microscopy, textured African, Caucasian, and Asian hair tips exhibit a loss of cuticular pattern owing to wear. A long-haired Caucasian subject demonstrated complete loss of cuticular structure owing to wear. In this study, textured African hair shafts had longitudinal fissures, shaft splitting, and knots and were fractured in contrast to the wear exhibited by Asian and Caucasian hair.[16] In another study comparing Asian and Caucasian hair, daily grooming induced cuticle removal at a faster rate in Asian hair.[21]

The similarities and differences in hair properties among various ethnic groups may dictate optimal treatment options, give insight into the pathophysiology of diseases disproportionately affecting those of a specific ethnic background, and serve as the premise for further scientific investigations.

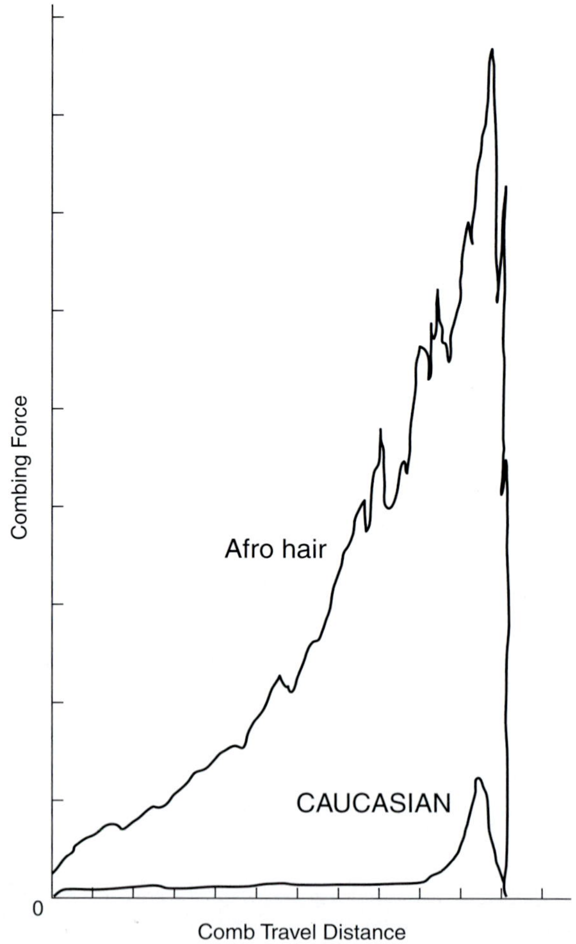

▲ **FIGURE 17-2** Dry combing of African and Caucasian hair. African hair is more difficult to comb and requires a progressive rise in the combing force to displace the individual curl entanglements. When the comb engages Caucasian hair, little effort is required to move through the hair mass, except at the tip of the tresses.

REFERENCES

1. De La Mettrie R, Saint-Leger D, Loussouarn G, et al. Shape variability and classification of human hair: A worldwide approach. *Hum Biol* 2007;79:265-281.
2. Khumalo N. African hair length: The picture is clearer. *J Am Acad Dermatol* 2006;54:886-888.
3. Furdon S, Clark D. Scalp hair characteristics in the newborn infant. *Adv Neonat Care* 2003;3:286-296.
4. Paus R, Foitzik K. In search of the "hair cycle clock": A guided tour. *Int Soc Different* 2004;72:489-511.
5. Whiting D. Diagnostic and predictive value of horizontal sections of scalp biopsy specimens in male pattern androgenic alopecia. *J Am Acad Dermatol* 1993;28:755-763.
6. Gilbert S. The epidermis and the origin of cutaneous structures, in *Developmental Biology,* 6th ed. Sunderland, MA, Sinauer Associates, 2000.
7. Paus R, Cotsarelis G. The biology of hair follicles. *N Engl J Med* 1999;341:491-497.
8. Dawber R. The embryology and development of human scalp hair. *Clin Dermatol* 1988;6:1-6.
9. Wolfram LJ. Human hair: A unique physicochemical composite. *J Am Acad Dermatol* 2003;48:S106-114.
10. Krause K, Foitzik K. Biology of the hair follicle: The basics. *Semin Cutan Med Surg* 2006;25:2-10.
11. McMichael A. Hair and scalp disorders in ethnic populations. *Dermatol Clin* 2003;21: 629-644.
12. Lindelof B, Forslind B, Hedblad M. Human hair form morphology revealed by light and scanning electron microscopy and computer aided three-dimensional reconstruction. *Arch Dermatol* 1988;124: 1359-1362.
13. Montagna W, Carlisle K. The architecture of black and white facial skin. *J Am Acad Dermatol* 1991;24:929-937.
14. Mangelsdorf S, Otberg N, Maicach H, et al. Ethnic variation in vellus hair follicle size and distribution. *Skin Pharmacol Physiol* 2006;19:159-167.
15. Stenn K, Paus R. Controls of hair follicle cycling. *Physiol Rev* 2001;81:449-494.
16. Khumalo NP, Doe PT, Dawber RPR, et al. What is normal black African hair? A light and scanning electron-microscopic study. *J Am Acad Dermatol* 2000;43: 814-820.
17. Schlake T. Determination of hair structure and shape. *Semin Cell Dev Biol* 2007;18:267-273.
18. Khumalo NP, Dawber RPR, Ferguson DJP, et al. Apparent fragility of African hair is unrelated to the cystine-rich protein distribution: A cytochemical electron microscopic study. *Exp Dermatol* 2003;14:311-314.
19. Kajiura Y, Watanabe S, Itou T, et al: Structural analysis of human hair single fibres by scanning microbeam SAXS. *J Struct Biol* 2006;155:438-444.
20. Kim BJ, Na JI, Park WS, et al. Hair cuticle differences between Asian and Caucasian females. *Int J Dermatol* 2006;45:1435-1437.
21. Takahashi T, Hayashi R, Okamoto M, et al. Morphology and properties of Asian and Caucasian hair. *J Cosmet Sci* 2006;57: 327-338.
22. Na J, Dwon O, Kim W, et al. Ethic characteristics of eyelashes: A comparative analysis in Asian and Caucasian females. *Br J Dermatol* 2006;155:1170-1176.
23. Swift JA, Smith JR. Microscopical investigations on the epicuticle of mammalian keratin fibres. *J Microsc* 2001;204:203-211.
24. Breakspear S, Smith JR, Luengo G. Effect of the covalently linked fatty acid 18-MEA on the nanotribiology of hair's outermost surface. *J Struct Biol* 2005;149:235-242.
25. Tiede S, Kloepper J, Bodo E, et al. Hair follicle stem cells: Walking the maze. *Eur J Cell Biol* 2007;86:355-376.
26. Cutrone M, Grimalt R. Transient neonatal hair loss: A common transient neonatal dermatosis. *Eur J Pediatr* 2003;164: 630-632.
27. Franbourg A, Hallegot P, Baltenneck F, et al. Current research on ethnic hair. *J Am Acad Dermatol* 2003;48:S115-119.
28. Khumalo NP. African hair morphology: Macrostructure to ultrastructure. *Int J Dermatol* 2005;44:10-12.
29. Ramos-e-Silva M. Ethnic Hair and skin: What is the state of the science? *Clin Dermatol* 2002;20:321-324.
30. Steggerda M, Seibert HC. Size and shape of head hair from six racial groups. *J Hered* 1941;20:315-318.
31. Syed AN, Kuhajda A, Ayoub H, et al. African-American hair. *Cosmet Toiletries* 1995;110:39-48.
32. Kamath YK, Hornby SB. Mechanical and fractographic behaviour of Negroid hair. *J Soc Cosmet Chem* 1984;35:21-43.
33. Bhatia R, Rao K, Rao N. Site variations in scalp hair morphology in pre-school children. *Ind J Med Res* 1980;71:890-892.
34. Gold RJM, Scriver CR. The amino acid composition of hair from different racial origins. *Clin Chim Acta* 1971;33:465-466.
35. Dekio S, Jidoi J. Hair low-sulfur protein composition does not differ electrophoretically among different races. *J Dermatol* 1988;15:393-396.
36. Nappe C, Kermicic M. Electrophoretic analysis of alkylated proteins of human hair from various ethnic groups. *J Soc Cosmet Chem* 1989;40:91-99.
37. McMichael A. Hair breakage in normal and weathered hair: Focus on the black patient. *J Invest Dermatol Symp Proc* 2007; 12:6-9.
38. Syed AN. Ethnic hair care: History, trends and formulation. *Cosmet Toiletries* 1993;108:99-107.
39. Brooks G. Treatment regimens for "styled" black hair. *Cosmet Toiletries* 1983; 98:59-68.
40. Halder R. Hair and scalp disorders in blacks. *Cutis* 1983;32:378-380.
41. Sperling LC. Hair density in African-Americans. *Arch Dermatol* 1999;135: 656-658.
42. Bernstein R, Rassman W. The aesthetics of follicular transplantation. *Dermatol Surg* 1997;23:785-799.
43. Lee H-J, Ha S-J, Lee J-H, et al. Hair counts from scalp biopsy specimens in Asians. *J Am Acad Dermatol* 2002;46:218-221.
44. Loussouarn G. African hair growth parameters. *Br J Dermatol* 2001;145: 294-297.

CHAPTER 18

Biology of Nails

Nicole DeYampert
Gisela Torres Bonilla,
Richard K. Scher

Key Points

- Nail matrix melanocytes in patients with skin of color contain mature melanosomes that produce nail plate pigmentation.
- Melanonychia in multiple nails reduces but does not eliminate the probability of melanoma more than if there is pigment in a solitary digit.
- Although melanoma of the nail unit is uncommon in people of color, acral locations, including nails, are disproportionately more frequent.
- Over 90% of melanonychias arise from the distal rather than the proximal nail matrix.
- Melanomas are more frequent in the great toe and thumb than in other digits.
- Most melanomas arising from melanonychia striata are in situ melanomas.

The nail unit is composed of the matrix, plate, bed, proximal and lateral nail folds, and hyponychium (Figure 18-1). The nail develops from an ingrowth of the epidermis into the dermis during gestational week 9, and the nail unit is fully developed at week 15 and then continues to grow throughout life. Since the nail unit lies immediately above the periostium of the distal phalanx, disorders of the nail and bone can affect each other. The shape of the distal phalangeal bone also determines the shape and transverse curvature of the nail. The nail functions to protect the distal phalanges and to increase tactile sensation. Toenails protect the distal toenail and aid in pedal biomechanics.

TABLE 18-1
Nail Embryology

	Gestational Development (week)
Digits	8
Nail	9
Primary nail field	10
Nail folds	13, 14
Nail plate	17

EMBRYOLOGY

The development of the digits, nails, and nail folds occurs early in embryonic development (Table 18-1). Individual digits are developing by the eighth week of gestation.[1] The nail develops during the ninth embryonic week from the same primitive epidermis that gives rise to hair, sweat glands, and the stratum corneum. At week 10, the primary nail field is developed. Proximal and lateral nail folds develop during weeks 13 and 14. The nail plate covers the majority of the nail bed at week 17. From week 20 to birth, the nail unit and digit grow in unison.

TABLE 18-2
Nail Matrix and Plate Formation

Dorsal matrix	Upper nail plate
Intermediate matrix	Intermediate nail plate
Ventral matrix	Lower nail plate

NAIL MATRIX

Nail matrix keratinocytes divide in the basal cell layer and keratinize in the absence of a granular layer. The site of keratinization of nail matrix onychocytes can be clearly distinguished in histologic sections as an eosinophilic area where cells show fragmentation of their nuclei and condensation of their cytoplasm. The maturation and differentiation of nail matrix keratinocytes occur along a diagonal axis that is distally oriented. Thus keratinization of the proximal nail matrix produces the dorsal nail plate, and keratinization of the distal nail matrix cells produces the intermediate plate (Table 18-2).

Cultured nail matrix keratinocytes are larger and have a greater proliferation rate than epidermal keratinocytes. At the ultastructural level, nail matrix cells contain a higher euchromatin:heterochromatin ratio and a lower nucleus:cytoplasm ratio than epidermal keratinocytes.[2] Both soft and hard keratins are produced by the nail matrix keratinocytes.[3] Soft keratins are produced by the dorsal matrix in bovine hoofs, whereas the ventral matrix produces mainly hard keratins, with a small population of keratinocytes coexpressing both hard and soft keratins. The proximal nail matrix is composed of soft keratins K10, K14, K16, K17, K1, K5, and K6. The distal matrix contains soft keratins K10, K14, K20, K1, and K5 and the hard keratin Ha1.[4]

When cultured in serum-containing medium, nail matrix cells produced an outgrowth of epithelium and a spontaneous migration phenomenon associated with a tendency to stratify in a semilunar area that resembles the architecture of the nail matrix.[2] The pluristratified

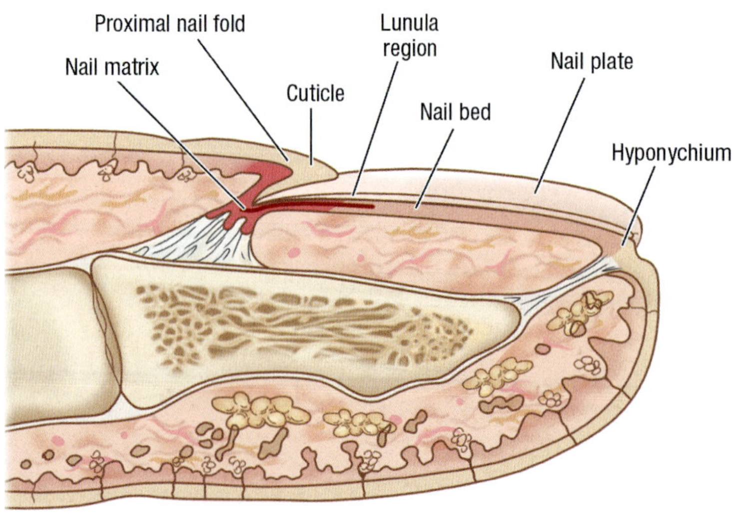

▲ **FIGURE 18-1** Basic anatomy of the nail unit.

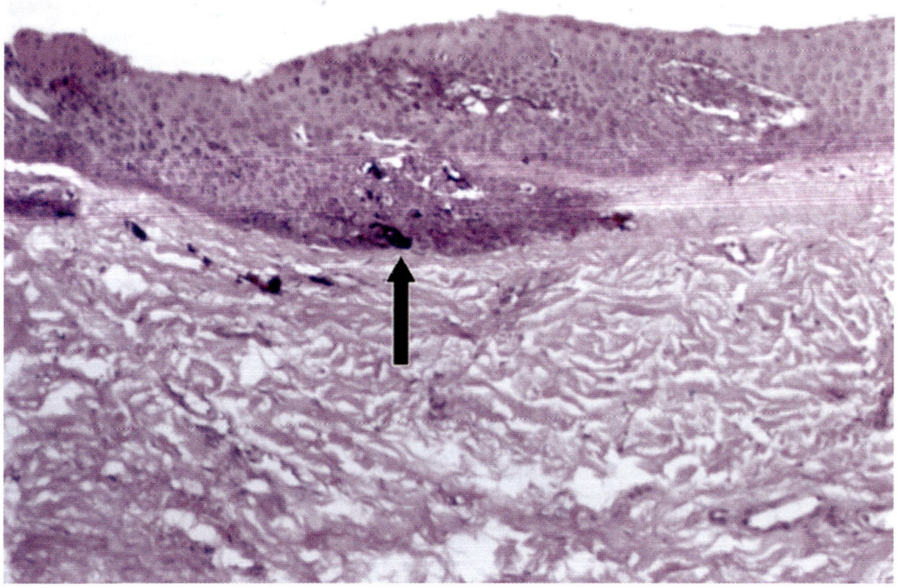

▲ **FIGURE 18-2** Histology of nail matrix biopsy with special staining for melanocytes.

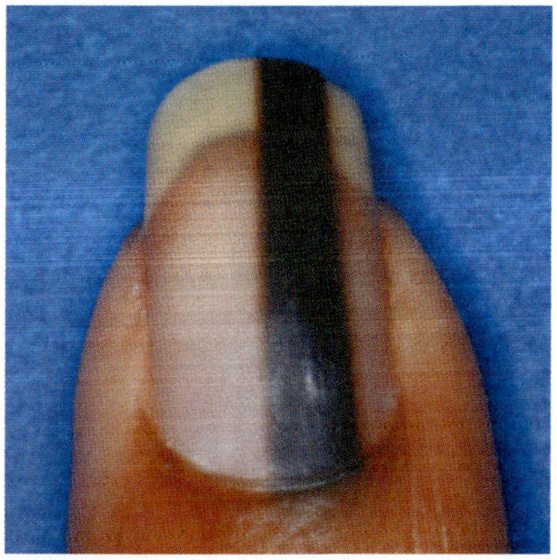

▲ **FIGURE 18-3** Photograph of a black/Latino/Asian patient with melanonychia striata.

epithelium showed characteristic markers of nail differentiation. Cultures of nail matrix cells have been a useful model to study the biology of the nails, including structure, nail disease, and effects of drugs.

MELANOCYTES

It has been demonstrated that melanocytes densely populate the nail matrix (Figure 18-2 and Table 18-3). The number of melanocytes ranges from 208–576 cell/mm^2.[5] Melanocytes are most prominent in the distal matrix. Melanocytes of the proximal matrix have been described as being in a single compartment of largely dormant cells. The distal matrix is composed of a dormant and an active component.[5] The DOPA-positive melanocytes in the distal areas are larger and more dendritic than those in proximal areas.[6] Active melanocytes in the distal matrix result in longitudinal melanonychia. A study in Japanese patients showed DOPA-staining melanocytes in the lower two to four layers of the nail matrix epithelium.[6]

There is considerable debate as to whether melanocytes are present in the nail bed. In a recent study, melanocytes were found in the nail bed when stained with TRP-1 at a density of 45 melanocytes/mm^2.[7] Nail matrix melanocytes in patients with skin of color contain mature melanonsomes that produce melanin (Table 18-4). In Japanese nails, melanocytes containing melanosomes were seen regularly in the dorsal, apical, and ventral matrices.[8] These melanocytes contained all gradations of maturing melanonsomes, the majority being an immature variety with visible longitudianal cristae and transverse striations. Transferred melanosomes were seen regularly within the keratinocytes. The melanosomes were either mature and dense or immature and half filled with dense melanin. In black nails, most of the melanonsomes were mature and dense. Transferred melanosomes also were mature.[8] The nail matrix of Caucasian patients lacks mature melanosomes but has premelanosomes, as well as stage I and stage II melanosomes. Although the Caucasian nail is not pigmented, pigmentation of the nail plate in a horizontal or longitudinal band has been reported to occur in response to an increased plasma melanocyte-stimulating hormone.[8]

Nail matrix melanocytes differ from melanocytes elsewhere in the skin in that they are located primarily in the distal matrix and suprabasal layers.[6] In the nail matrix, the melanocytes are less dense and more frequently dormant than in the epidermis.[9] Since the nail matrix is covered by the nail plate and the nail fold at the proximal areas, these melanocytes are presumed not to be stimulated by ultraviolet (UV) light. It has been postulated that this is the reason the population of DOPA-positive melanocytes is fewer in the nail matrix than in the epidermis.

Melanin in the nail plate is composed of granules derived from nail matrix melanocytes. Longitudinal melanonychia may be a benign phenomenon, particularly in black patients (Figure 18-3). Studies have reported that 77% of blacks will have melanonychia by age 20 and almost 100% by age 50.[10] A study of a Japanese population revealed a 10–20% prevalence of longitudinal melanocyhia.[11] Research also has shown that a series of 15 cases of benign melanonychia occurred secondary to an increase in the activity and number of DOPA-positive melanocytes in the

TABLE 18-3
Nail Matrix Melanocytes

Distal matrix	Longitudinal melanonychia, larger, more dendritic melanocytes
Proximal matrix	Single compartment, largely dormant melanocytes

TABLE 18-4
Nail Matrix Melanosomes

Race/Ethnicity	Percent with Melanonychia	Type of Melanosomes in Matrix
Japanese	11.4%	Immature and mature melanosomes
Blacks	77%	Mature and dense melanosomes
Whites	Rare	Premelanosomes

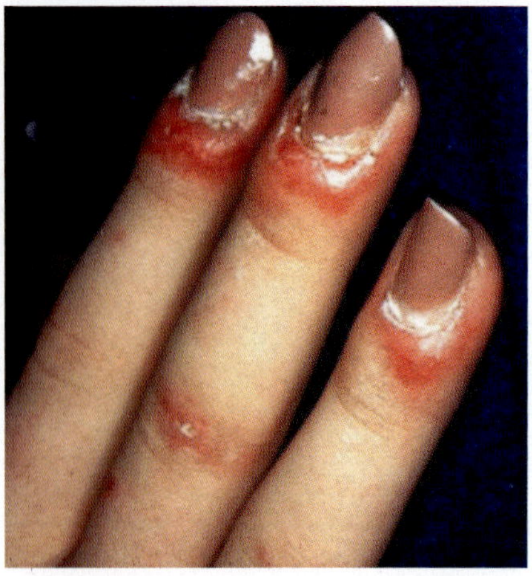

▲ **FIGURE 18-4** Photograph of a nail fold with dilated capillaries.

matrix. Unlike blacks and Japanese, in Caucasians, subungual pigmented lesions have a greater likelihood of being malignant.[12]

LANGERHAN'S CELLS/ MERKEL CELLS

Langerhan's cells are found predominantly in the suprabasal layers of the nail matrix epithelium. They are more common in the proximal rather than the distal nail matrix.[13] However, Langerhan's cells may be seen occasionally within the basal layer of the nail matrix epithelium. Merkel cells also have been demonstrated in the nail matrix. The density of Merkel cells has been shown to decrease with age because these cells are more numerous in fetal than in adult nails.[14]

LUNULA (DISTAL MATRIX)

The lunula is the convex margin of the matrix, which can be visualized through the nail plate. It is most commonly visible on the thumbs and the great toes, although the proximal nail fold may conceal the lunula. The lunula is the area where the nail plate is least adherent.

NAIL BED

The nail bed epithelium is comprised of two to five cell layers. Keratinization occurs without formation of a granular layer. Few or no melanocytes have been found in the nail bed. The nail bed epithelium is adherent to the nail plate, causing it to remain attached to the nail plate after nail avulsion. A study in 1991 revealed that the nail bed contributes one-fifth of nail thickness and mass. The ventral nail plate is formed by a horny layer produced by keratinization of the nail bed.[15] On histologic examination, the ventral portion is identified by its eosinophilic appearance. After nail avulsion, the nail bed may develop a granular layer.

HYPONYCHIUM

The epithelium of the hyponychium is equivalent to the epithelium of the volar skin, with both a granular and a thick cornified layer being present. Anatomically, it is defined as the cutaneous margin underlying the free edge of the nail, bordered distally by the distal groove at the point where the nail plate separates from the dorsal digit.

FOLDS

The dorsal portion of the proximal nail fold corresponds to the skin of the dorsal digit. The proximal nail fold contains sweat glands but lacks pilosebaceous units. It is densely innervated; thus inflammation of this area causes severe pain. The ventral portion of the nail fold continues proximally with the germinative matrix and covers approximately one-fourth of the nail plate. The border between the proximal nail fold and the nail matrix can be established histologically at the site of disappearance of the granular layer.

The horny layer of the proximal nail fold forms the eponychium, which is firmly attached to the superficial nail plate and prevents separation of the nail plate from the nail fold. The integrity of the eponychium is essential for maintaining homeostasis and minimizing the likelihood of infection.

The epithelium of the proximal nail fold contains a granular layer. Structurally, the dermis of the proximal nail fold contains superficial capillaries that are arranged in regular loops. These capillaries can provide useful information about microvascular alterations and assist in the diagnosis of connective tissue disorders[16] (Figure 18-4).

PLATE

The nail plate is composed of onychocytes, compacted keratinized epithelial cells. The plate covers both the nail bed and matrix. The nail plate is curved along both the longitudinal and transverse axes. This allows it to be embedded into the nail folds at its proximal and lateral margin, thus providing strong attachment. The curvature of the toenail is greater than that of the fingernail. The upper surface of the nail plate is smooth and may have a variable number of longitudinal ridges that increase with age.[17] The ventral surface also has longitudinal ridges that correspond to complementary grooves on the upper aspect of the nail bed. The nail plate gains thickness and density as it grows distally. A thick nail plate may imply a long intermediate matrix. This stems from the process whereby the longitudinal axis of the intermediate matrix becomes the vertical axis of the nail plate.[18] The proximal regions of matrix produce the dorsal nail plate, and the distal matrix produces the ventral nail plate.

The dorsal plate has a relatively high calcium, phospholipid, and sulphydryl group content. It has little acid phosphatase activity and is physically hard. The phospholipid content may provide some water resistance.[19] The intermediate nail plate shares a similar chemical composition as the dorsal nail plate, except that it has a high acid phosphatase activity, probably corresponding to the number of retained nuclear remnants. There are many disulfide bonds (few bound sulfhydryl groups). It also contains phospholipids and calcium. The intermediate plate cells are eosinophilic and move both upward and forward with nail growth. The nail plate has been found to have a superficial dry compartment and a deep humid one. Corneocytes of the dorsal nail plate are joined laterally by spaced deep interdigitations. The interdigitations are more frequent in the deeper parts of the nail plate.

VASCULAR SUPPLY/ INNERVATION

The nail unit has an abundant blood supply provided by four lateral digital arteries. The palmar digital arteries provide the main blood supply to the fingers. The nail fold is supplied by a superficial arcade. The distal and subungual arcades, arising from an anastomosis of the palmar arch and the dorsal nail fold, supply the subungual region. Glomus bodies contain nerve endings and arteriovenous anastomoses that regulate capillary circulation. The glomus bodies are found predominately in the dermis, with a density varying from 90–500/mm^2.[20] Their typical length is 300 μm. They are particularly important in maintaining blood supply to the periphery in cold weather. Pared digital nerves give rise to the cutaneous sensory nerves, which have a parallel course to the digital vessels. There is a very high density of nerve endings in the nail folds.

CHEMICAL PROPERTIES

The onychocytes of the nail are composed primarily of keratins. The keratins are low-sulfur filamentous proteins with a parallel orientation. Because of this orientation, the nail is more susceptible to transverse fractures. The keratins are embedded in nonkeratin proteins, which are rich in sulfur, glycine, and tyrosine. The hardness of the nail plate is secondary to the hard keratins. From 80–90% of the nail keratins are hard hairlike keratins. The soft skinlike keratins comprise the remaining 10–20%.[21]

The normal water content of the nail ranges from 7–18% compared with 15–25% in the epidermis. Most of the water is localized to the intermediate nail plate, which has been found to be 1000 times more permeable to water than the skin.[22,23] The porosity of the nail causes the nail to be readily hydrated and dehydrated. When the percentage of water decreases below 7%, the nail becomes brittle; when the water content rises above 30%, it becomes opaque and soft.[24] The nail also contains trace organic elements, including iron, zinc, and calcium. These elements do not contribute to the hardness of the nail. The total fat content of the nail plate varies from 0.1–5% in comparison with the stratum corneum, which has 10% fat content.[20] The primary lipid in the nail is cholesterol.

PHYSICAL PROPERTIES

The physical properties of the nail plate are hardness, strength, and flexibility. The presence of hard keratins and cystine-rich high-sulfur proteins determines the hardness of the nail. The strength is attributed to the curved axis in the longitudinal and transverse orientations and the firm adhesion of the onychocytes.[25] The maximum elastic stress of the nail has been found to be 420–880 kg/cm^2.[26] The flexibility is a consequence of its water content.

The ultrastructural character of the nail plate varies in each of its three layers.[22] The dorsal nail plate contains flat onychocytes with a shorter diameter perpendicular to the nail plate surface. Intermediate plate cell adhesion is provided by desmosomes and interdigitations of the cell membranes. The ventral nail plate is very thin and composed of soft keratins. The ventral nail plate provides firm attachment to the underlying nail bed.

NAIL GROWTH

Fingernails grow at 3 mm per month versus 1 mm per month for toenails, leading to a complete replacement of the fingernails in 6 months and of toenails in 12–18 months.[23] Because of this slow rate of growth, diseases of the nail matrix require a significant period of time to become apparent. The rate of nail growth is typically greatest during the second and third decades. After age 50, the rate of nail growth decreases sharply.[27] Many conditions have been associated with either increased or decreased rate of growth. Slow rate of growth is associated with fever, onychomycosis, malnutrition, and the yellow nail syndrome. Accelerated growth has been associated with pregnancy, hyperthyroidism, psoriasis, and pityriasis rubra pilaris.[28] The nail's slow rate of growth allows evaluation of pathologic events that have occurred in the past[29]. One such change is the development of Beau's lines, which are the result of a disturbance of the normal nail matrix growth.

REFERENCES

1. Lewis BL. Microscopic studies of fetal and mature nail and surrounding soft tissue. *Arch Dermatol Syph* XXXX;70: 732-744.
2. Picardo M, Tosti A, Marchese C, et al. Characterization of cultured nail matrix cells. *J Am Acad Dermatol* 1994;30:434-440.
3. Kitahara T, Ogawa H. Coexpression of keratins characteristic of skin and hair differentiation in nail cells. *J Invest Dermatol* 1993;100:171-175.
4. DeBerker D, Wojnarowsha F, Sviland L, et al. Keratin expression in the normal nail unit: Markers of regional differentiation.
5. Tosti A, Cameli N, Piraccini B, et al. Characterization of nail matrix melanocytes with anti-PEP1, anti-PEP8, TMH-1, and HMB-45 antibodies. *J Am Acad Dermatol* 1994;31:193-196.
6. Higashi N. Melanocytes of nail matrix and nail pigmentation. *Arch Dermatol* 1968;97:570-574.
7. Perrin C, Michelis JF, Pisani A, Ortonne JP. Anatomic distribution of melanocytes in normal nail unit: An immunohistochemical investigation. *Am J Dermatolpathol* 1997;19:462-467.
8. Hashimoto K. Ultrastructure of the human toenail: I. Proximal nail matrix. *J Invest Dermatol* 1971;56:235-246.
9. Higashi N, Saito T. Horizontal distribution of the dopa-positive melanocytes in the nail matrix. *J Invest Dermatol* XXXX; 53:163-165.
10. Monash S. Normal pigmentation in the nails of the Negro. *Arch Dermatol* 1932; 25:876-881.
11. Kawamura T. Pigmentation longitudinalis striata unguium and pigmentation of the nail plate in Addison's disease. *Jpn J Dermatol* 1958;68:10.
12. Baran R, Kechijian P. Longitudinal melanonychia (melanonychia striata): Diagnosis and management. *J Am Acad Dermatol* 1989;21:1165-1175.
13. DeBerker D, Angus B. Proliferative compartments in the normal nail unit. *Br J Dermatol* 1996;135:555-559.
14. Moll I, Moll R. Merkel cells in ontogenesis of human nails. *Arch Dermatol Res* 1993;285:366-371.
15. Johnson M. Nail is produced by the normal nail bed: A controversy resolved. *Br J Dermatol* 1991;125:27-29.
16. Hahn M, Heubach T, Steins A. Hemodynamics in nailfold capillaries of patients with systemic scleroderma: Synchronous measurement of capillary blood pressure and red blood cell velocity. *J Invest Dermatol* 1998;110:982-985.
17. Tosti A, Piraccini BM. Biology of nails, in Freedberg IM, Fitzpatrick TB (eds), *Fitzpatrick's Dermatology in General Medicine*, 2nd ed. New York, McGraw-Hill, 1999, pp 239-244.
18. DeBerker D, Mawhinney B, Sviland L. Quantification of regional matrix nail production. *Br J Dermatol* 1996;134:1083-1086.
19. Jarrett A, Spearman RC. The histochemistry of the human nail. *Arch Dermatol* 1989;94:652-657.
20. Dawber RPR, deBerker DAR, Baran R. Science of the nail apparatus, in Baran R, Dawber RPR, deBerker DAR (eds), *Diseases of the Nails and Their Management*. Oxford, England, Blackwell Science, 2001, pp 1-47.
21. Lynch MH, O'Guiinlum, Hardy C. Acidic and basic hair/nail ("hard") keratins: Their colocalization in the upper cortical and cuticle cells of the human hair follicle and their relationship to "soft" keratins. *J Cell Biol* 1986;103:2593-2606.
22. Jemec GBE, Serup J. Ultrasound structure of the human nail plate. *Arch Dermatol* 1989;125:643-646.
23. Spruit D. Measurement of water vapor loss through human nail in vivo. *J Invest Dermatol* 1971;56:359-361.
24. Runne U, Orfansos CE. The human nail: Structure, growth and pathologic changes. *Curr Probl Dermatol* 1981;9;102-149.
25. Finlay AY, Frost P, Keith AD. Assessment of factors influencing flexibility of human fingernail. *Br J Dermatol* 1980;10: 357-365.
26. Young RW. Strength of fingernails. *J Invest Dermatol* 1965;44:358-360.
27. Bean WB. Nail growth: 30 years observation. *Arch Intern Med* 1974;134:497-502.
28. Beau JHS. Note sur certains caracteres de semeiolgie retrospective presentes par les ongles. *Arch Gen Med* 1846; 11:447.
29. Geyer AS, Onumah N, Uyttendaele H, Scher RK. Modulation of linear nail growth to treat diseases of the nail. *J Am Acad Dermatol* 2004;50:229-234.

CHAPTER 19

Cutaneous Wound Healing

A. Paul Kelly
Elaine Bethell

Key Points

- U.S. populations of African, Asian, and Latin American origin are the fastest growing and often in poor health, putting them at risk for wound infections and pressure ulcers.
- Diversity in skin color can pose a challenge in assessing patients with wounds.
- Assessment should include patient history and examination of the wound, surrounding skin area, and the entire body.
- Assessment should consider color, temperature, moisture, and the presence of inflammation, erythema, edema, and scarring.
- Pressure ulcers are common (especially in the elderly), costly to treat, and hard to identify in darkly pigmented skin.
- Dermabrasion may not be appropriate for darkly pigmented patients.

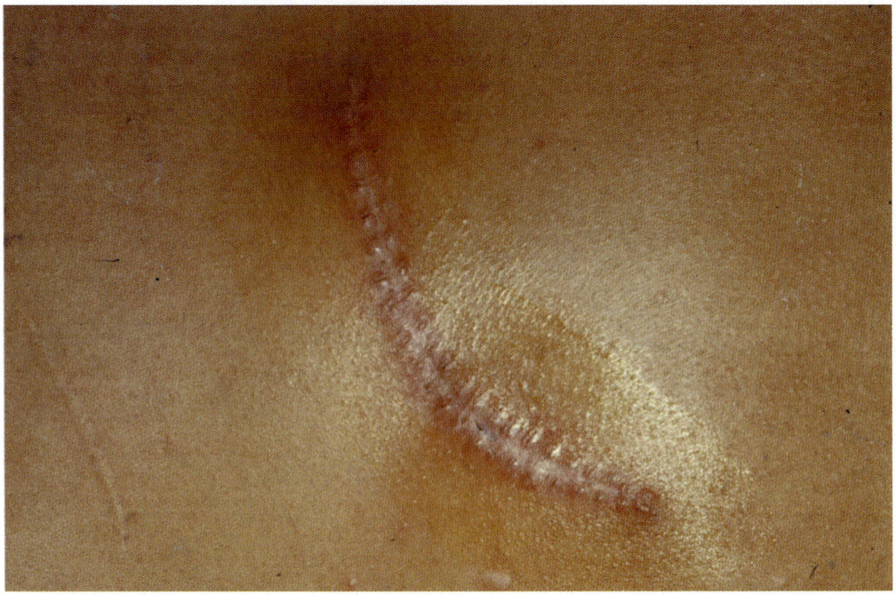

▲ **FIGURE 19-1** Incision line on lightly pigmented skin. Notice the pinkness of the postoperative site.

Diversity in skin color can pose a challenge in assessing patients with wounds. For example, the usual redness characteristic of erythema is difficult to detect in patients with darkly pigmented skin.[1,2] It is important that health care practitioners understand the differences between lightly (Figure 19-1) and darkly (Figure 19-2) pigmented skin.[3] Bennett defines darkly pigmented skin coloration as that which does not blanch when pressure is applied over a bony prominence, irrespective of the patient's race or ethnicity.[1] Failure to detect signs of inflammation or nonblanching erythema (Figure 19-3) may lead to the development of a life-threatening wound infection. This chapter focuses on wound assessment and treatment for darkly pigmented patients.

The National Institutes of Health address racial and ethnic disparities in health status and the many factors that contribute to these inequities within the United States.[4] The findings indicate that in the U.S. populations of African, Asian, and Latin American origin are the fastest growing and often in poor health,[5,6] putting them at risk for wound infections and pressure ulcers. In today's society, chronic wounds represent a major health care burden. Approximately 1–2% of people will be affected by leg ulcerations during their lifetime, and this figure likely will increase as the population ages.[7]

THE WOUND-HEALING PROCESS

A wound is a disruption of the normal anatomic structure and function of the skin[7] that may be acute or chronic.[8] Wounds can be classified using several different approaches. Wounds also may have a surgical, traumatic, neuropathic, vascular, or pressure-related etiology.[9]

Normal Wound Healing

There are three phases in normal wound healing: inflammation, proliferation, and maturation[7,10,11] (Table 19-1).

INFLAMMATION During the inflammatory phase, neutrophils and macrophages destroy bacteria and debris. In the absence of infection, the neutrophils disappear within 3 days. It is important that the immune system is healthy and there is an adequate supply of growth factors during this phase.

PROLIFERATION This phase usually begins 3 days after injury and lasts a few weeks. During this period, fibroblasts produce a collagen matrix, granulation tissue forms in the wound, and epidermal cells migrate across the surface to close the wound. Collagen deposition and remodeling contribute to the tensile strength of cutaneous wounds. Within 3 weeks of injury, tonsile strength is usually restored to 20% of normal; tensile strength never returns to normal but reaches a maximum of 70–80% of normal. Lack of adequate protein or vitamin deficiencies may impair collagen production, and necrotic tissue in the wound bed may impede formation of new epithelium.

MATURATION Maturation normally starts a week after injury and may last a year

TABLE 19-1
Three Overlapping Phases of Wound Healing

Inflammatory: Homeostasis immediately after injury platelet activation, platelet-derived growth factor activation of complement cascade. Neutrophils first inflammatory cells to respond. Macrophages attach to wound site within first 24 hours.
Proliferative Phase: Replacement of provisonal fibrin matrix with new a matrix. Angiogenesis, formation of granulation tissue, epithelization, fibroblast migration.
Remolding: Granulation tissue matures into scar, deposition of matrix materials, remolding of extracellular matrix wound closure.

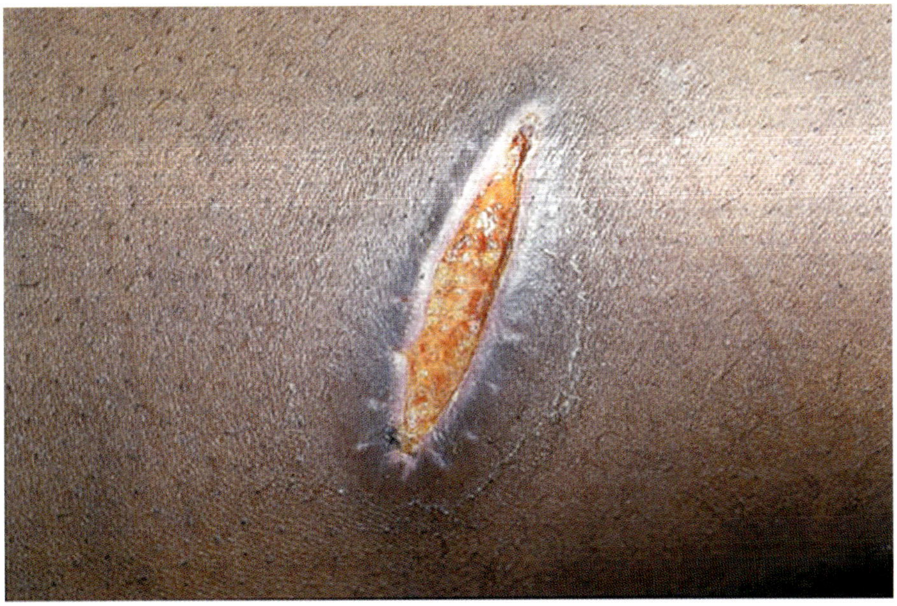

▲ **FIGURE 19-2** Type IV skin showing hyperpigmentation of the wound border. (From Knoop KJ, Stack LB, Storrow AB. *Atlas of Emergency Medicine.* New York, McGraw-Hill, 2002, p. 602.)

or more. During this phase, fibroblasts reorganize the collagen matrix and ultimately assume a myofibroblast phenotype that causes the connective tissue to become compacted and the wound to contract.

Disruption of any component of this process can delay healing. Normally, the process takes between 3 days and 2 weeks to complete.[11]

ASSESSING WOUNDS

A problem for clinicians when assessing patients with darkly pigmented skin is the lack of guidance and/or evidence. The literature primarily addresses pressure ulcers, with little on skin and wound assessment.[12] Consequently, there is no written standard for the information to include in a wound assessment, nor has any single documentation chart or tool been designated as most effective.[13]

However, as part of a comprehensive wound assessment, it is accepted practice to make a total patient assessment, including other health issues and lifestyle. It is important to know, for example, that patients have diabetes, which makes them more prone to foot and leg ulcers. The assessment and patient history should be thoroughly documented. Equally important is to document wound progress, either in writing or in pictures. This is the only way to evaluate the effectiveness of treatment interventions.[14]

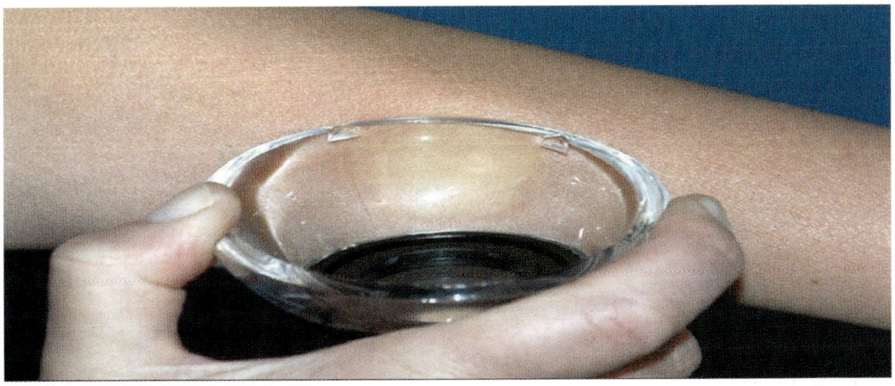

▲ **FIGURE 19-3** There is a difference in skin responses between lightly pigmented and darkly pigmented skin: A glass applied to the skin shows blanching erythema on lightly pigmented skin. In contrast, in darkly pigmented skin, the blanching is difficult to see.

WOUND EXAMINATION

A minimal wound assessment should include a thorough patient examination, etiology or wound type, and wound characteristics such as location, size, depth, exudate, and tissue type. Visually assessing the wound should determine its type, location, size, depth, exudate, and tissue type. The next step is a thorough physical examination of the wound and its surrounding skin. The skin surrounding a wound can provide valuable information for ongoing evaluations and future wound care management. When palpated, skin should quickly return to its original state. A slow return may indicate dehydration or be the effect of aging. Soft tissue may indicate an underlying infection. Tense skin may indicate lymphedema and cellulitis.[14]

It is also important to make a complete skin assessment, not just of the wound site but also of the entire body, looking for lesions, bruising, absence of hair, shiny skin, callus formation, and hypertrophic and keloid scars, which are more prevalent in darkly pigmented skin.[15] However, in dark-skinned patients, it is harder to detect signs of venous insufficiency such as hemosiderin deposits, characterized by a reddish brown color on the lower legs of lightly pigmented patients with venous ulcers, ankle flare, and *atrophie blanche*. In such cases, patient history becomes the key to diagnosis. Skin assessment also can reveal the classic signs of arterial ulcers: hair loss, weak or absent pulses, and thin, shiny, and taut skin.[14,16]

Following are some guidelines for assessment of darkly pigmented skin.

Color

Adjacent skin color can signal disruptions in circulation related to injury or infection. These can be diagnosed easily in lightly pigmented skin. Pressing on the area closes the capillaries, causing a blanching in lightly pigmented skin (see Figure 19-3); the color returns to normal when pressure is released.[1,17]

Erythema

Erythema is characteristic of many skin conditions, including pressure ulcers and allergic reactions.[17] The change in normal skin color results from dilatation of capillaries near the skin's surface and usually lasts about 2–5 days from the time of injury.

Nonblanching erythema in lightly pigmented skin is redness that does not disappear within 20 minutes of removing pressure. Nonblanching erythema

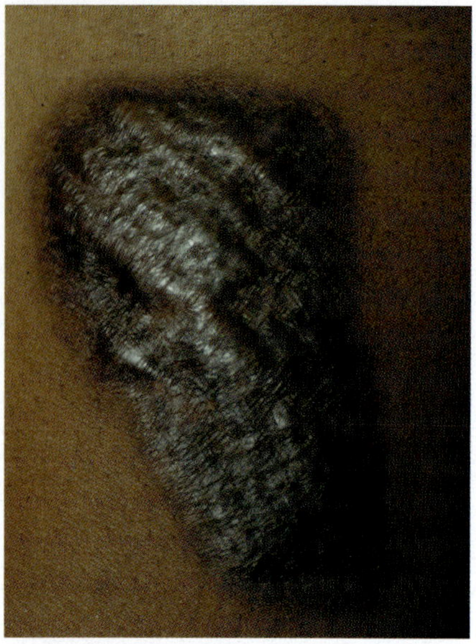

▲ **FIGURE 19-4** Postoperative keloid secondary to an excision of a cyst on darkly pigmented skin, showing a hyperpigmented border with a grayish violaceous hue.

signals erythrostasis in the capillaries and venules and hemorrhage.[2]

Erythema is more difficult to diagnose in darkly pigmented skin. Inflammation may show as a darker hue rather than redness, often a violaceous gray, indicating subcutaneous hemorrhage (Figure 19-4). Another complicating factor noted by Sussman[2] is differentiating inflammation from the darkening of the skin caused by hemosiderin staining. Hemosiderin staining usually occurs close to the wound edges, whereas injury-related color changes usually extend out a considerable distance and are accompanied by the other signs of inflammation.[18]

Sussman[2] offers the following guidelines for measuring the extent of inflammation/trauma in darkly pigmented skin:

- Use natural light or halogen light, not fluorescent light.
- Outline the margins of color change on the surrounding skin with a marking pen.
- Select a reference point for future measures.
- Calculate the area of color change (as described for all length-by-width measurements).

Inflammation

Inflammation is a normal physiologic response to tissue injury, the skin's defense against invading microbes. Signs of inflammation include erythema, heat, edema, and pain.[11]

Inflammation following a surgical incision should subside within 5 days.[12] In nonsurgical wounds, inflammation may indicate infection and a serious underlying condition. Viral inflammation may indicate herpes zoster, chickenpox, or keloids.[14]

Temperature

Skin that is warmer than usual can be a sign of inflammation or an indicator of infection or pressure damage. Warmth results from increased local blood flow and edema, followed by engorgement of surrounding vessels and tissues, resulting in warmth and redness in the area. Histologically, this is due to edema of the papillary dermis, platelet aggregation in the microcirculation,[18] and erythrocyte engorgement of the superficial blood vessels.[19]

Pale and cool skin can be a sign of poor perfusion or ischemia and may indicate the end stage of nonblanching erythema.[20,21] Increased or decreased skin temperature usually is detectable by touch.[22] Since the changes are slight, not wearing gloves is an option while assessing temperature. Flanagan[23] argues that a rise in temperature of 1–2 degrees is difficult to assess with or without gloves; most practitioners' fingers are not that sensitive. However, temperature assessment is important in patients with darkly pigmented skin because of the difficulty in observing color changes.

Edema

Shiny, taut skin or pitting impressions within 4 cm of a wound margin indicate edema, which is another sign of inflammation. Edema can be assessed by pressing the finger firmly within 4 cm of the ulcer margin, releasing, and waiting 5 seconds to look for indentations.[24] This procedure is effective regardless of the skin pigmentation.

Edema and induration occur when pressure causes the skin layers to separate, allowing interstitial fluid to accumulate.[25] Therefore, both edema and induration are good indicators of tissue damage. Parish and colleagues found that at this stage there is engorgement of capillaries and venules in the papillary dermis.[26]

In addition to being a sign of inflammation, edema also can indicate heart, liver, or kidney failure or venous insufficiency.

Moisture

Note whether skin is moist or dry. If dry, look for hyperkeratosis (flaking and scales). Also look for eczema or dermatitis, psoriasis rashes, leaking edema, or exudate. These signs may aid in diagnosing cellulitis, lymphedema, or wet gangrene.[14]

Scarring

Epithelialization is regeneration of the epidermis across the surface of a wound. As the wound migrates from its edges, the area covered with epithelium is pearly or silver and shiny. In darker-pigmented skin, the color of the epithelium will be tonally relevant to normal skin, but as with scar tissue in lighter skins, it will be different from surrounding undamaged epidermis[14] (Figure 19-5).

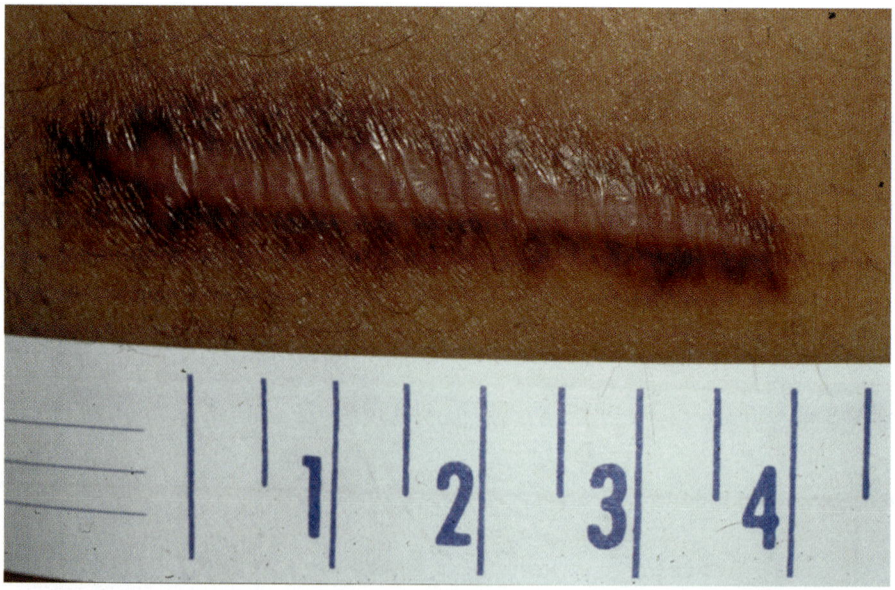

▲ **FIGURE 19-5** Four weeks after the incision, a slight hypertrophic scar has developed on the medium-color pigmented skin. The borders of the incision are hyperpigmented, and the center of the incision is hypopigmented.

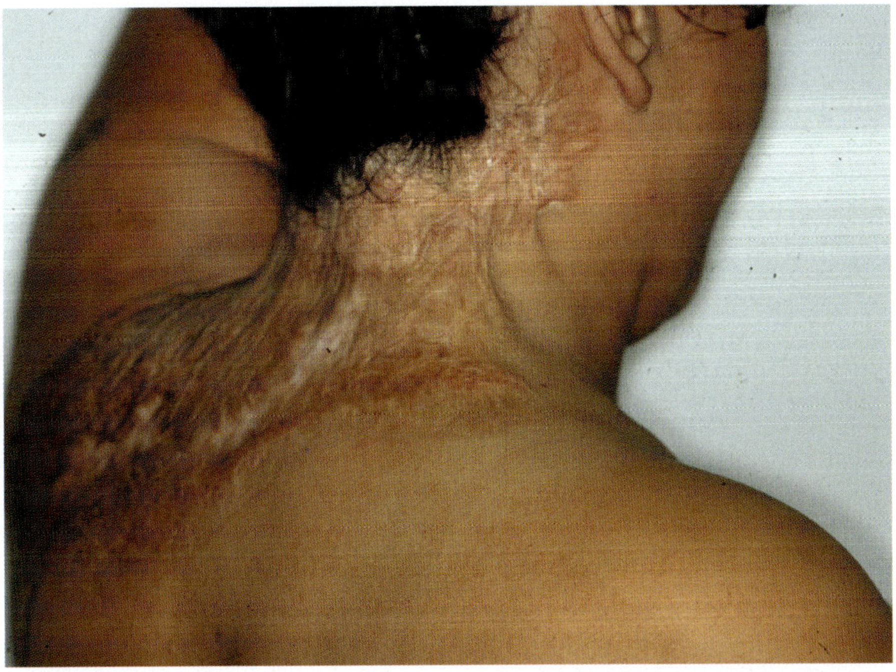

▲ **FIGURE 19-6** Hypertrophic scar secondary to a burn on the posterior neck and upper back of a Hispanic woman. Note that the wound area is both hypopigmented and hyperpigmented.

Hypertrophic and keloid scars are abnormalities associated with the maturation phase of healing. Hypertrophic scars usually regress completely in a year to 18 months. Keloids may grow larger over time and even for a lifetime in some patients[27] (Figures 19-6 and 19-7).

HYPERTROPHIC SCARS Hypertrophic scars occur directly after initial repair, tend to follow the line of the incision, and are more common in young patients. Careful placement of incisions along Langer lines (incisions are made in natural creases) and fine suture material can avoid excessive scar formation[28] (Figure 19-8).

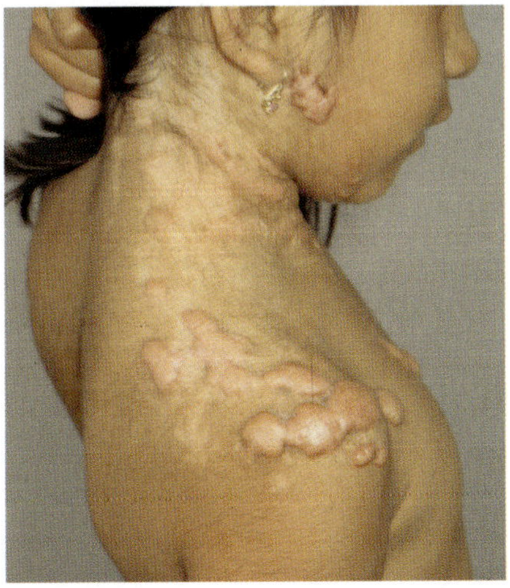

▲ **FIGURE 19-7** Scarification from a thermal burn on the posterior neck and upper back of a young Hispanic girl showing both keloids and hypertrophic scars.

KELOID SCARS Keloids result from large amounts of scar tissue around the wound site owing to an increase in collagen synthesis and decrease in collagen lysis. They are also thought to be linked to melanocyte-stimulating hormone (MSH). The role of MSH in humans is not fully understood. However, Mehendale and Martin believe that a better understanding of melanocyte responses to wounding may suggest ways to prevent posthealing pigmentary disturbances and avoid the necessity for further surgical intervention[3,29] (Figures 19-9 and 19-10).

Often keloid scars are larger than the wound itself, and even if the scar is excised, it is likely to recur. Keloid scars may occur sometime after healing and range from red to dark brown. The scars are prominent and continue to grow and spread, invading surrounding healthy tissue, whereas hypertrophic scars do not[27] (Figures 19-11 and 19-12).

Darkly pigmented skin is more likely to develop keloid scarring than lighter skin. The reasons are not fully understood. Theories include an excess of MSH, a decreased percentage of mature collagen and small increased percentages of soluble collagen, and blockage of small blood vessels resulting in lack of oxygen that contributes to keloid formation.[30] While there is no definitive theory as yet, research continues. Determining the cause should mean better prevention and treatment in the future. However, problems such as a lack of a clear cutoff of treatment, inadequate follow up of patients, and too few studies hamper the search for a cure (Figures 19-13 and 19-14).

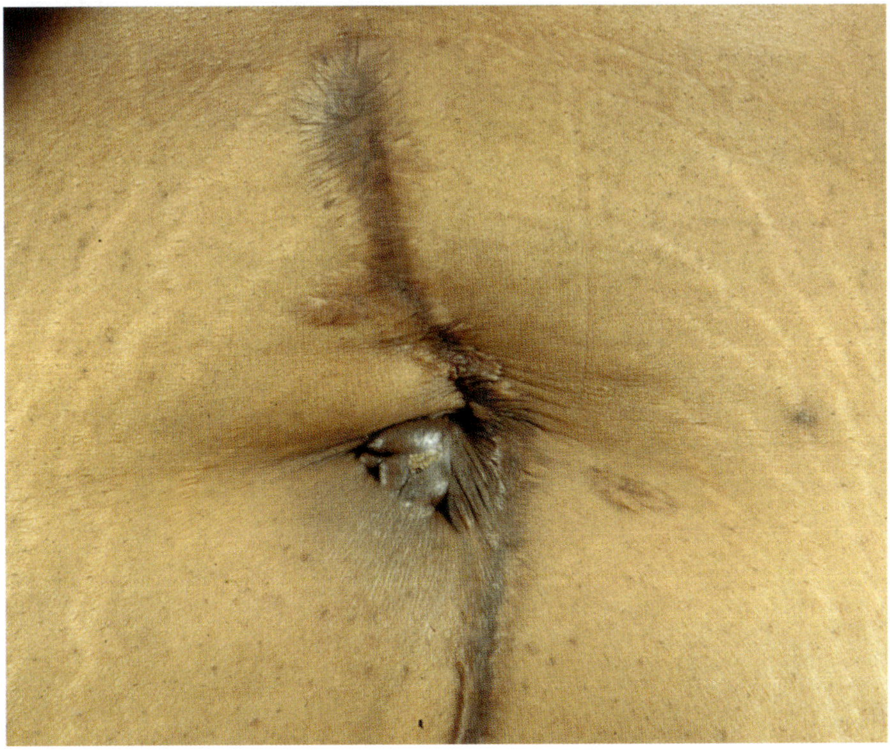

▲ **FIGURE 19-8** Hypertrophic scar of the midabdomen area secondary to abdominal surgery.

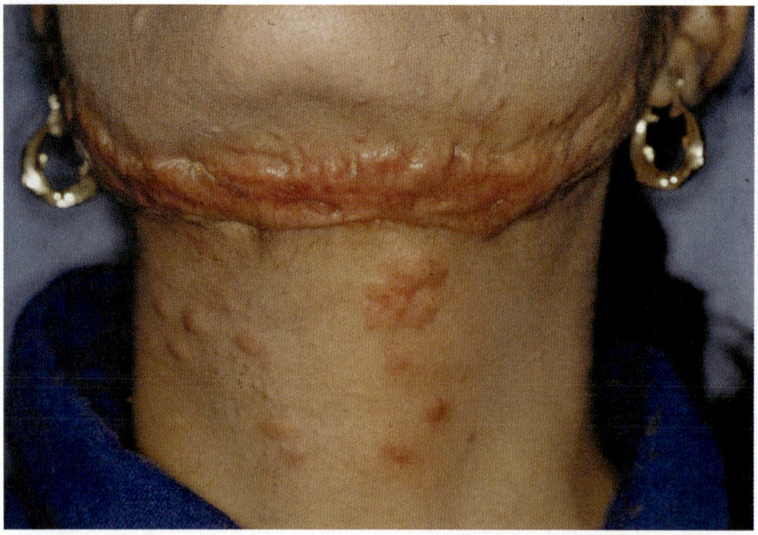

▲ **FIGURE 19-9** Ear-to-ear keloid formation secondary to an excisional surgery on a Hispanic woman.

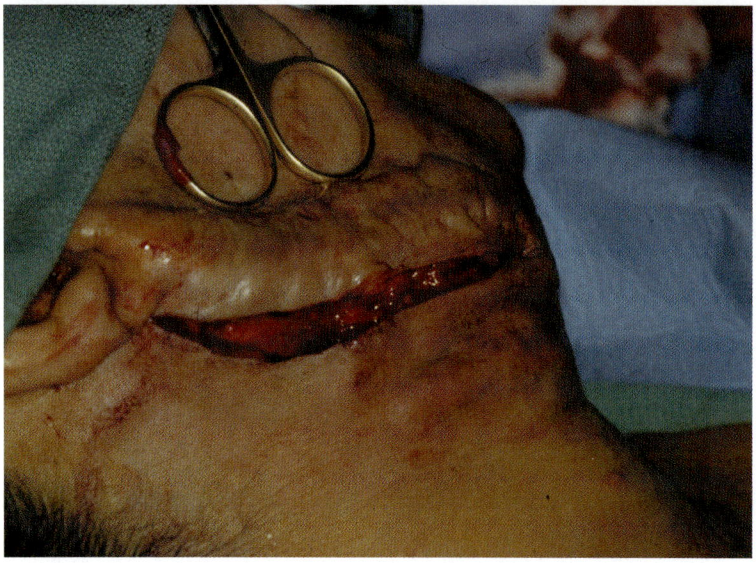

▲ **FIGURE 19-10** Keloidectomy of the patient in Figure 19-9. Patient was injected with corticosteroids at the time of excision and then every 2 weeks × 4 postoperatively to prevent recurrence.

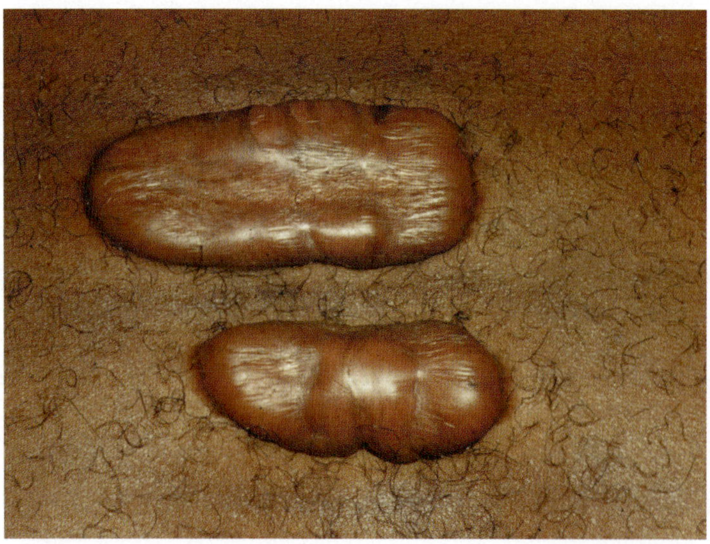

▲ **FIGURE 19-11** Horizontal keloids on the midchest area of a darkly pigmented man.

TREATMENT

Treatment varies according to the type of wound. Specific guidelines appear in other chapters. For example, see the Chapter 30 on keloids and Chapter 33 on pseudofolliculitis barbae.

Care of the skin, whether lightly or darkly pigmented, requires keeping it lubricated. Petrolatum, lanolin-based lotions, and sparing use of soaps are recommended.

PRESSURE ULCERS

Pressure ulcers are areas of localized damage to the skin and underlying tissue caused by two concurrent processes, pressure and shear, ultimately leading to tissue anoxia. They frequently occur over bony prominences and are most prevalent in elderly patients. In addition to skin, subcutaneous fat, deep fascia, muscle, and bone are involved in pressure ulcer development.

Pressure ulcers are common, and the cost of prevention and treatment is high. Estimates of costs in the United States range from $836 million in 1992 to between $1.3 billion and $2.8 billion more recently.[7]

Lyder considers nonblanching erythema a true criterion of stage 1 pressure ulcers. Nonblanching erythema signals irreversible damage, which will progress to deeper skin layers unless pressure is relieved. Failure to detect nonblanching erythema is probably why dark-skinned patients had the most severe grade 4 pressure ulcers in recent surveys. A special task force is addressing the difficulty of identifying a stage 1 pressure ulcer or nonblanching erythema in such patients.[20,23]

Stage 1 Pressure Ulcers

Bennett found that emphasizing redness in the definition of stage 1 pressure ulcers was not helpful for darkly pigmented skin.[1] Instead, the skin may be darker, taut, shiny and/or indurated, warmer, and/or painful. Lyder's definition includes coolness as well as warmth.[23] Some researchers have found a grade 1 pressure injury more likely to have a bluish tinge than reactive hyperanemia and that this signals irreversible tissue damage[19,22] (Figure 19-15).

An updated definition approved by the National Pressure Ulcer Advisory Panel (NPUAP)[21] includes temperature and purple hues, whereas the National Institute for Health and Clinical

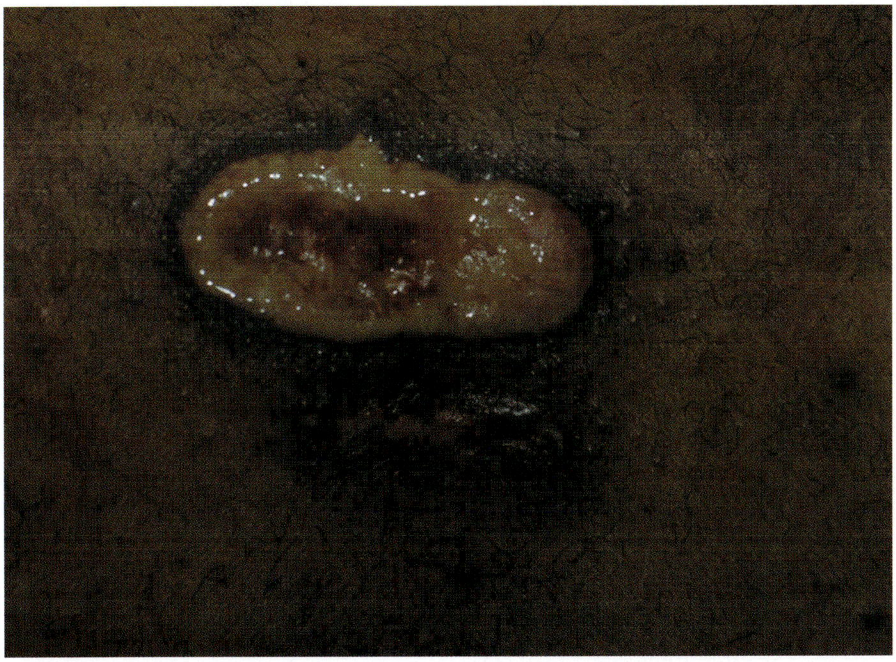

▲ **FIGURE 19-12** A 9-day postoperative examination after keloidectomy of the patient in Figure 19-11 showing rapid regrowth even with the use interlesional steroids during the surgery.

Excellence (NICE) definition emphasizes the importance of discoloration.[31]

PURPLE ULCERS Purple ulcers may be treated less seriously than they should be, especially in patients with dark skin, where they are difficult to identify. However, they signal a full-thickness skin loss; biopsy reveals hemorrhage and early gangrenous changes described as an increasing number of "purple" ulcers that are purple-red ecchymotic—caused by an effusion of blood under the skin—pale ecchymotic, or bruised. The skin may be intact or the epidermis "brushed" off, exposing a discolored area. This can rarely be reversed[32] (Figures 19-16 and 19-17).

BLANCH TEST The blanch test distinguishes between blanching (healthy skin) and nonblanching erythema (damaged skin) (see Figure 19-3). It involves gently pressing on the skin, forcing blood out of the area. In healthy tissues, color returns swiftly as blood refills the dermal capillaries. Since pressing with a finger covers the area to be observed, it is better to use a clear glass or plastic disk or both disk and thumb. Unfortunately, in patients with darkly pigmented skin, the melanin prevents seeing the evacuation and refill of blood.[33]

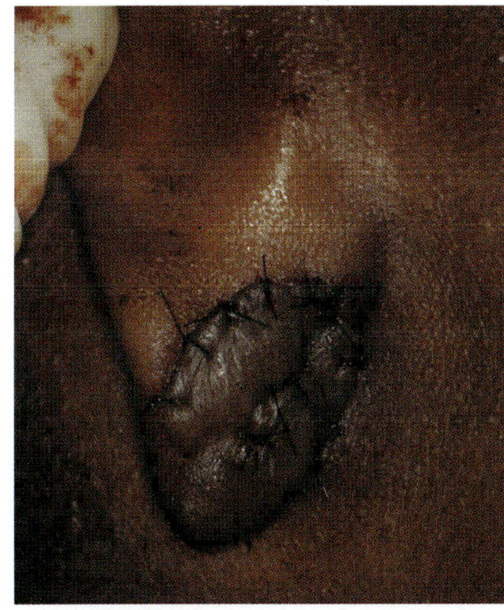

▲ **FIGURE 19-14** Primary postoperative closure of the flap from a keloidectomy in a darkly pigmented women.

PULSE OXIMETRY Noninvasive pulse oximetry is a popular method of assessing oxygenation, which is important for wound healing. However, pulse oximetry may be less reliable for darkly pigmented skin than for lighter skin.[34]

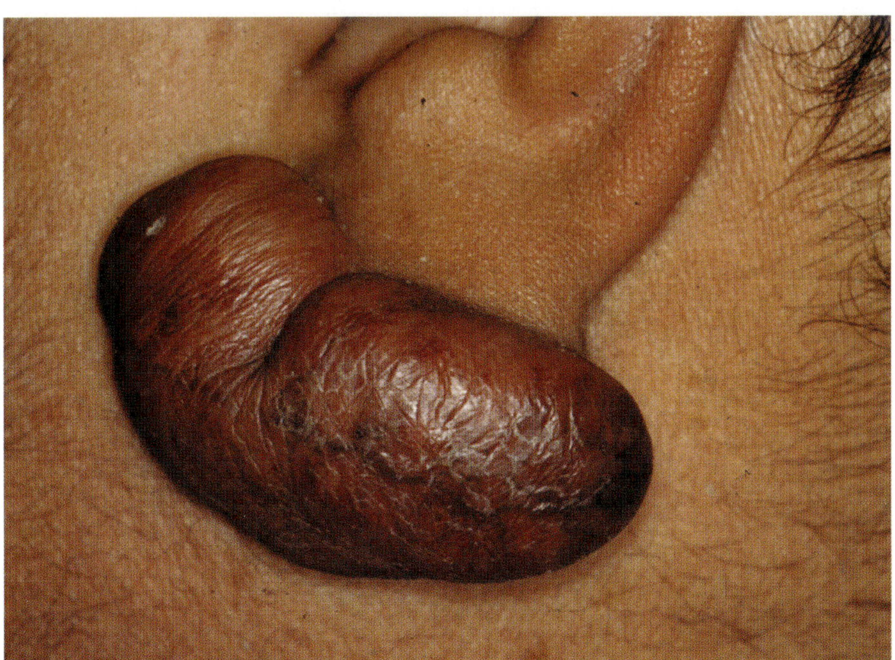

▲ **FIGURE 19-13** Keloid on the left ear.

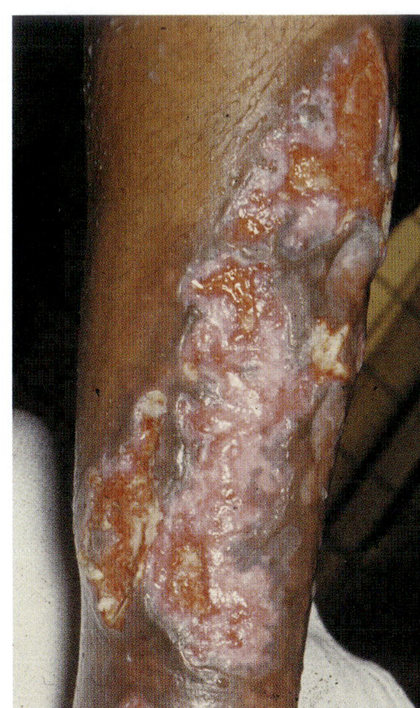

▲ **FIGURE 19-15** Stasis leg ulcer.

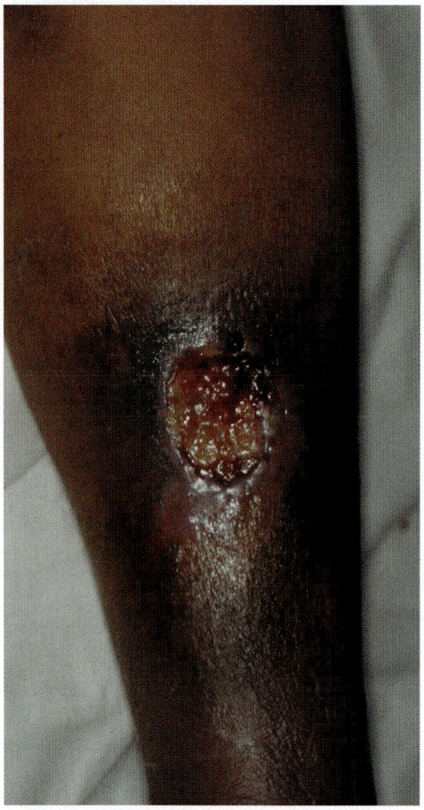

▲ **FIGURE 19-16** Purple leg ulcer.

PRESSURE ULCER RISK PREDICTION SCORES The Braden scale is the most widely used pressure ulcer assessment tool in the United States. However, Lyder and colleagues found that the Braden score significantly underpredicted the risk in black and Hispanic elders. The study also found that variables such as diet may affect the risk scores of hospitalized older blacks and Hispanics, who often refuse to eat unfamiliar foods.[23]

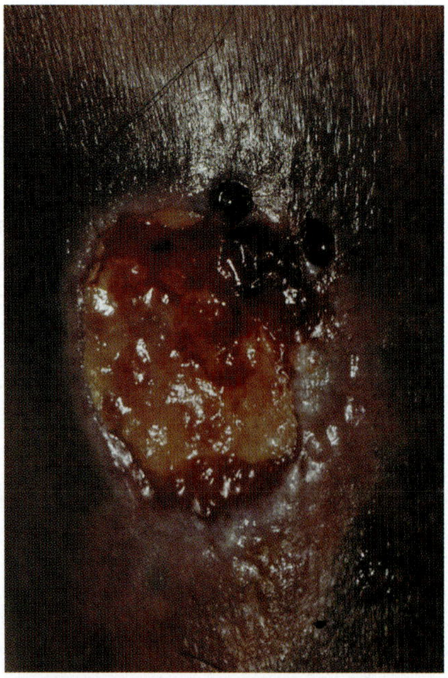

▲ **FIGURE 19-17** Purple leg ulcer.

PRESSURE ULCER RISK ASSESSMENT Few health care professionals receive the training in assessing pressure ulcer risk that the NICE (2001) guidelines called for.[35] It is particularly difficult to recognize early-stage pressure ulcers and to ascertain the extent of damage in patients with darkly pigmented skin.[36,37]

CUTANEOUS SURGERY CONSIDERATIONS

Cutaneous surgery can be divided into two categories: (1) basic surgery for removal of benign and malignant lesions and (2) cosmetic surgery, where the procedure is performed at the patient's request to enhance his or her aesthetic well-being. Sometimes the two categories overlap, as in the case of a painful keloid. The patient wants the keloid removed to eliminate both the pain and the cosmetically challenging growth.

Adverse cosmetic results secondary to cutaneous surgery usually can be avoided by taking a good preoperative history of the patient's previous response(s) to cutaneous trauma and then using this information in making operative and postoperative planning decisions. The physician also should be aware of possible psychological and/or vocational ramifications the procedure may have for the patient.

There are several basic canons that physicians should be cognizant of when performing cutaneous surgery on darkly pigmented patients and, if appropriate, explain to the patient:

- Cryosurgery that requires a freezing time of less than 20 seconds often produces hyperpigmentation that may last 6–12 months. Longer freezing may produce hypopigmentation that will last 12–18 months or longer. Liquid nitrogen, when used as a topical freezing agent prior to dermabrasion, often produces long-lasting dyschromia.
- Intralesional corticosteroid injections in strengths of more than 3 mL of triamcinolone acetonide may produce hypopigmentation that usually will remain for 6–12 months.
- Scars in darker skin, whether flat, raised, or splayed, are more often dyspigmented than similar scars in lighter skin.
- Healing is a two-dimensional process. First is primary healing, which takes place on wounds that are closed by sutures. Secondary healing involves leaving the wound open; it closes on its own without suturing (Figures 19-18 and 19-19) (see also Chapter 32).
- Skin cancer is rare in darkly pigmented skin, and if malignant melanomas develop, they are usually in acral and mucosal areas.
- Cobblestoning after hair transplants is more common in darkly pigmented patients than in lighter-skinned patients.
- Hyperpigmentation following vein sclerosing is more common in darker skin than in lighter skin.
- Depilation of unwanted hairs by electrolysis or thermolysis results in more frequent scarring and hyperpigmentation in darker skin than in lighter skin.
- When taking pre- and postoperative photographs of darkly pigmented patients, open the camera one-half to one full stop to get the same clarity of photographs that you get with lighter-skinned patients using a higher f-stop.

Most of the basic cutaneous surgical techniques are the same for darkly pigmented and lighter skin and are described in other chapters of this textbook. However, certain disorders requiring cutaneous surgery either occur more frequently in darkly pigmented patients or may require special surgical adaptations. Some of them are as follows:

- Keloids (see Chapter 30)
- Acne keloidalis (see Chapter 32)
- Hidradenitis suppurativa (see Chapter 40)
- Punch grafts for vitiligo repigmentation (see Chapter 46)
- Dermatosis papulosa nigra (see Chapter 72)
- Dermabrasion (Discussed below)

DERMABRASION

Dermabrasion may be performed with the same techniques and equipment regardless of skin color. However, before surgery, darkly pigmented patients should be informed about the possible postoperative pigmentary changes. Also, those who are known keloid or scar formers should not be dermabraded. The most common reasons for dermabrasion are for acne scarring and tattoos.

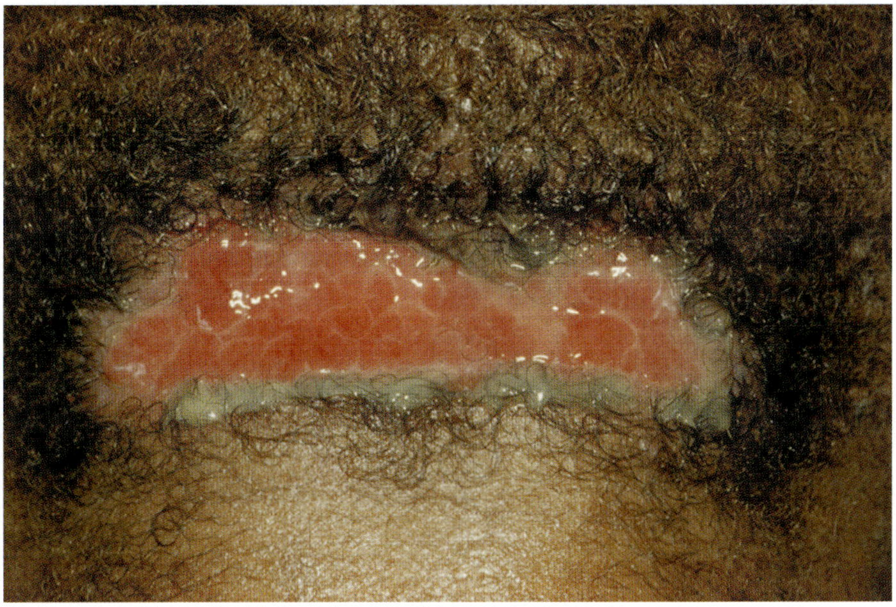

▲ **FIGURE 19-18** One week after excision of an acne keloidalis lesion of the posterior nucal area.

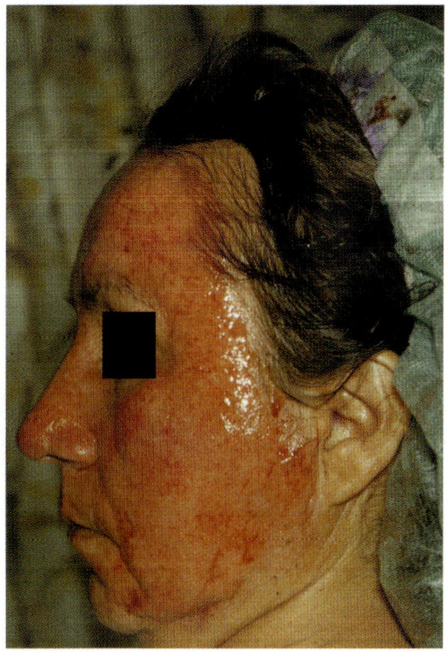

▲ **FIGURE 19-20** Dermabrasion of the face of a Hispanic woman.

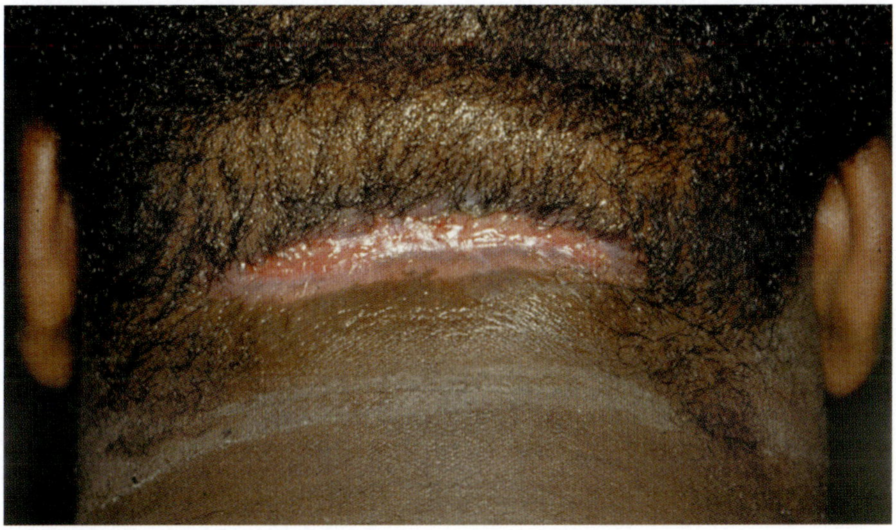

▲ **FIGURE 19-19** Three-month postoperative view of the patient in Figure 19-18. Secondary healing can be successful and can take place without scarring and having the wound splay.

Once dermabraded, the patient should avoid direct sunlight for 4 months. If not, hyperpigmentation usually develops. Twice a day use of a sunscreen after applying a hydroquinone preparation is often successful in attenuating the hyperpigmentation. Hypopigmentation is best avoided by not dermabrading too deeply. If scars develop, then the application twice a day of a class 1 or 2 topical corticosteroid and daily application of cordran tape usually will prevent further scar development; however, long-term use can produce temporary perilesional hypopigmentation and atrophy (Figure 19-20).

CONCLUSION

Medicine in general and dermatology specifically must place a greater emphasis on quality wound care for all patients, and attention needs to be focused on darkly pigmented patients as well. We emphasize that patients should not go undiagnosed because of the color of their skin. Subsequent research in education, wound healing, and pressure ulcers must include patients with darkly pigmented skin.

REFERENCES

1. Bennett MA. Report of the task force on the implications for darkly pigmented intact skin in the prediction and prevention of pressure ulcers. *Adv Wound Care* 1995;8:34-35.
2. Sussman C. Wound measurements, in Sussman C, Bates-Jensen B (eds), *Wound Care: A Collaborative Practice Manual for Physical Therapists and Nurses.* Aspen Publications, 1998, Chap 4, pp 95-96.
3. Mehendale F, Martin P. The cellular and molecular events of wound healing: Melanocytes, in Falanga V (ed), *Cutaneous Wound Healing.* London, Martin Dunitz, 2001, Chap 3, pp. 28-29.
4. National Institutes of Health. Addressing Health Disparities: The NIH Program of Action. What Are Health Disparities, 2007. Available at *http://healthdisparities.nih.gov/ware are.html.*
5. Atrash HK, Hunter MD. Health disparities in the United States: A continuing challenge, in Satcher D, Pamies R (eds), *Multicultural Medicine and Health Disparities.* New York, McGraw-Hill, 2006, Chap 1, pp 3-32.
6. Levine RS, Briggs NC, Husini BA, et al. Geographic studies of black-white mortality, in Satcher D, Pamies R (eds), *Multicultural Medicine and Health Disparities.* New York, McGraw-Hill, 2006, Chap 2, pp 33-104.
7. Fonder MA, Lazarus GS, Cowan DA, et al: Treating the chronic wound: A practical approach to the care of nonhealing wounds and wound care dressings. *J Am Acad Dermatol* 2008;58:185-206.
8. Araujo T, Kirsner RS. Atypical wounds, in Baranoski S, Ayello EA (eds), *Wound Care Essentials: Practice Principles.* Philadelphia, Lippincott Williams & Wilkins, 2003, Chap 19, pp 381-398.
9. Ayello EA, Baranoski S, Lyder CH, Cuddigan J. Pressure ulcers: Wound etiology, in Baranoski S, Ayello EA (eds),

Wound Care Essentials: Practice Principles. Philadelphia, PA: Lippincott Williams & Wilkins, 2003, Chap 13, pp 241-270.
10. Falabella AF, Falanga V. Wound healing, in Freinkel RK, Woodley DT (eds), *The Biology of the Skin.* New York, Pearl River, NY: Pantheon Publishing Group, 2001, pp 281-297.
11. Singer AJ, Clark RAF. Cutaneous Wound healing. *N Engl J Med* 1999;341: 738-746.
12. Cho M, Hunt TK. The overall clinical approach to wounds, in Falanga V (ed), *Cutaneous Wound Healing.* London, Martin Dunitz, 2001, pp 149-154.
13. Bannerjee D, Jones V, Harding KG. The overall clinical approach to chronic wounds, in Falanga V (ed), *Cutaneous Wound Healing.* London, Martin Dunitz, 2001, Chap 12, pp 165-186.
14. Baranoski S, Ayello EA. Wound assessment, in Baranoski S, Ayello EA (eds), *Wound Care Essentials: Practice Principles.* Philadelphia, Lippincott Williams & Wilkins, 2004, pp 79-90.
15. Kelly AP. Special considerations in approach to treatment and management of scars in African-Americans and other populations more at risk, in Arndt KA, Dover JS, Alam M (eds), *Scar Revision.* New York, Elsevier, 2006, Chap 7, pp 115-122.
16. Salcido RS. Finding a window into the skin. *Adv Skin Wound Care* 2002;15:100.
17. Roach LB. Assessment: Color changes in dark skin. *Nursing* 1977;77:48-51.
18. Barton A, Barton M. *The Management and Prevention of Pressure Sores.* London, Faber and Faber, 1981.
19. Witkowski J. Purple ulcers (letter). *J ET Nurs* 1993;20:132.
20. Lyder CH. Conceptualization of the stage 1 pressure ulcer. *J ET Nurs* 1991; 189:162-165.
21. National Pressure Ulcer Advisory Panel. Position Statement: Stage 1 Assessment in Darkly Pigmented Skin, 2007. Available at *www.npuap.org/positn4.html.*
22. Bliss MR. Pressure injuries: Causes and prevention. *Hosp Med* 1998;59:841-844.
23. Lyder CH. Is pressure ulcer care evidence based or evidence linked? Science of Surfaces Meeting, Warwickshire, UH, January 20-21, 2005.
24. Gardner S, Frantz R. Wound bioburden, in Baranoski S, Ayello E (eds), *Wound Care Essentials: Practice Principles.* Philadelphia, Lippincott Williams & Wilkins, 2004, pp 91-116.
25. Villa A, et al. Keloids and hypertrophic scars, in Falabella AF, Kirsner RS (eds), *Wound Healing.* Boston: Taylor & Francis, 2005, pp 623-636.
26. Parish LC, Witkowski JA, Crissey JT. Unusual aspects of the decubitus ulcer. *Decubitus* 1988;1:22-24.
27. Kelly AP. Keloids: Pathogenesis and treatment. *Cosmet Dermatol* 2003;16:29-32S.
28. Kelly AP. Medical and surgical therapies for keloids. *Dermatol Ther* 2004;17:212-218. 29.
29. Lee CP. Keloids: Their epidemiology and treatment. *Int J Dermatol* 21:9:504-505.
30. Bale S, Jones V. *Wound Care Nursing: A Patient-Centered Approach.* London, Ballière Tindall, 2000.
31. Placik OJ, Lewis VL Jr. Immunologic associations of keloids. *Surg Gynecol Obstet* 1992;175:185-193.
32. National Institute for Clinical Excellence. *Pressure Ulcer Risk Assessment and Prevention.* London: NICE, 2001.
33. Nixon J. The pathophysiology and etiology of pressure ulcers, in Morison M (ed), *The Prevention and Management of Pressure Ulcers.* St Louis, MO, Mosby, 2001, pp 17-35.
34. Matas A, Sowa MG, Taylor V, et al. Eliminating the issue of skin color in assessment of the blanch response. *Adv Skin Wound Care* 2001;14180-14188.
35. Flanagan M. Accurately assess pressure damage on patients with darkly pigmented skin. *J Wound Care* 1996;5: 454.
36. Scanlon E, Stubbs N. Pressure ulcer risk assessment in patients with darkly pigmented skin. *Profession Nurs* 2004;19: 338-341.
37. Bethell E. Assessment and prevention of pressure ulcers for patients with darkly pigmented skin. *Divers Nurs* 2003; 134-35.
38. Bethell E. Controversies in classifying and assessing grade 1 pressure ulcers. *J Wound Care* 2003;12:33-36.

CHAPTER 20

Cytokine Alterations and Cutaneous Diseases

Madeliene E. Gainers
Charles J. Dimitroff

Key Points

- Cytokines play a significant role in the immune regulatory function of skin.
- Aberrations in cytokine production can result in a number of cutaneous disorders, including vitiligo, keloids, atopic dermatitis, Behçet disease, and systemic lupus erythematosus.
- Research on cytokine dysregulation has revealed new targets for therapeutic exploitation and stimulated new directions for drug development.
- Anticytokine therapeutics or agents that dampen cytokine activity represent a promising avenue for the treatment of cutaneous disorders in persons of color.

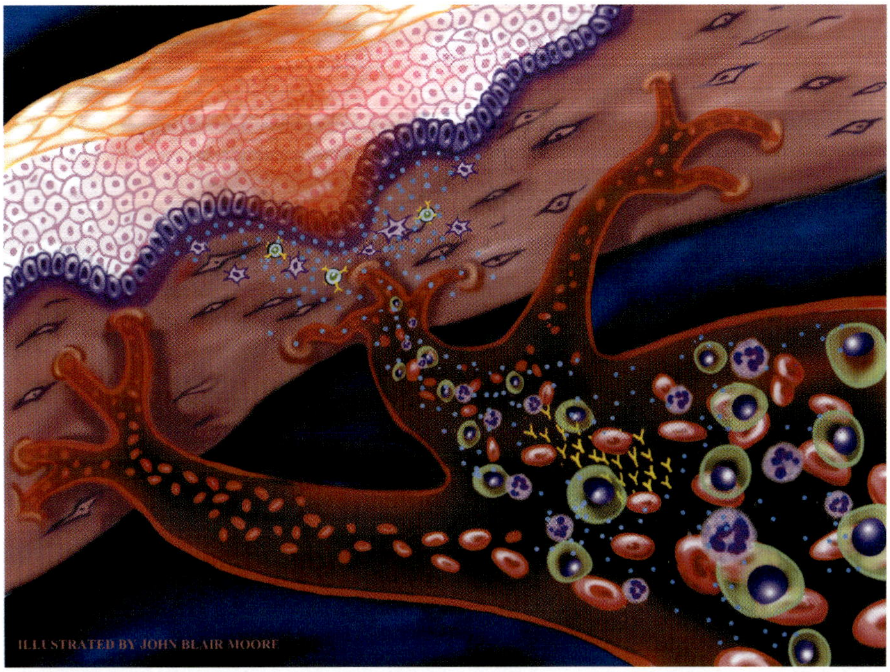

▲ **FIGURE 20-1** Cytokines coordinate cutaneous cellular activities by facilitating communication between epidermal melanocytes, keratinocytes, dermal fibroblasts, and immune cells (T cells, B cells, and antigen-presenting cells).

The response of the immune system to foreign antigen requires the coordinated activity of multiple cellular networks. This coordination is possible, in large part, owing to small secreted proteins called *cytokines* that serve as signal molecules. Cytokines are critically important in controlling cutaneous immune and inflammatory processes and ultimately affect the cellular microenvironment of the skin and dysregulation of cellular factors associated with diseases (Figure 20-1). Cytokines exhibit either autocrine (i.e., they act on the same cell that secreted it), paracrine (i.e., they act on neighboring cells), or endocrine (i.e., they act on target tissues distant from the site of cytokine secretion) activity. Table 20-1 summarizes the categories and gives examples of cytokines characteristically involved in skin diseases. On binding with its specific membrane receptor on the target cell, intracellular secondary messengers stimulate secretion of effector molecules, upregulation or downregulation of membrane proteins, and cellular proliferation. Cytokine production can involve a trimolecular complex, which consists of a major histocompatibility (MHC) class II molecule, processed antigen, and contact with a T-cell receptor and/or the proliferation/activation of an immune cell.[1–3] Immune cells involved in innate responses also elaborate cytokine secretions. This chapter will discuss recent research that explores how aberrations in cytokine production may result in cutaneous disorders associated with persons of color while focusing on the following five diseases: vitiligo, keloids, atopic dermatitis, Behçet disease, and systemic lupus erythematosus (SLE). In addition, the chapter will describe how dark skin pigmentation can be beneficial in preventing cytokine alterations on ultraviolet (UV) light exposure.

VITILIGO

Vitiligo is an acquired idiopathic skin and hair disorder characterized by absence of pigmentation with resulting well-defined white patches. The loss of pigment is caused by a destruction of melanocytes in the epidermis.[4,5] Melanocytes are cells of neural crest origin that reside in the basal layer of the epidermis and pigment skin by the production of melanin in membrane-bound organelles called *melanosomes*. The packaged melanin travels through dendrites and is distributed to and phagocytosed by keratinocytes. Melanocytes also may have other physiologically significant roles through their secretion of inflammatory substances, such as nitric oxide.[6] Vitiligo is seen worldwide among all races, affecting 0.5–1% of the population. However, dark skinned-individuals and certain ethnic groups are more likely to seek medical care for the disorder because the contrast between white lesions and darker skin can be cosmetically disfiguring and lead to social stigmatism.[4,5]

Several theories have been postulated for the complete disappearance of functional melanocytes in vitiligo lesions. These include genetic factors,[7] toxicity from melanin precursors and free radicals produced during melanin production,[8] autoimmune responses triggered by melanocyte surface antigen antibodies,[9] and melanocyte cell death caused by chemicals released from nerve endings.[5] There is even a growth factor defect hypothesis that suggests that diminished melanocyte growth is caused by inadequate secretion of mediators such as basic fibroblastic growth factor (bFGF) by neighboring cells.[5,10,11]

Other cytokines also have been implicated as having a possible role in the pathogenesis of vitiligo by altering the melanocyte microenvironment.[4,5] Stem cell factor (SCF) and endothelin (ET), which are paracrine cytokines produced

TABLE 20-1
Cytokine Definitions and Examples

	Definitions	Examples
Cytokine terms	*Cytokine*—small secreted protein that serves as a signal molecule of the immune response	IL-2 secreted by T cells on antigen stimulation
	Chemokine—chemotactic cytokine that recruits white blood cells	IL-8 produced by mononuclear cells for neutrophil recruitment
	Monokine—cytokine secreted by antigen presenting cells (monocytes)	IL-12 produced by antigen presenting dendritic cells and macrophages for stimulation of naïve T cells that results in T_H1 cell activation
	Lymphokine—cytokine derived from T cells	IL-2 secreted by T cells upon antigen stimulation
Action of Cytokines	*Autocrine*—act on the same cell	IL-2 secreted by T_H1 cells also acts on the same cells in a stimulatory capacity
	Paracrine—act on neighboring cells	IL-2 secreted by T_H1 cells acts on cytotoxic CD8+ cells in a stimulatory capacity
	Endocrine—target cells distant from cytokine secretion	IL-6 produced by monocytes, fibroblasts, and T_H cells induces fever by acting on the hypothalamus
Interleukin	Lymphokines that stimulate and regulate lymphocytes	IL-2 secreted by T cells
Interferon	Glycoproteins that block viral replication and immunomodulate cellular functions	IFN-γ secreted by T_H1 and CD8+ T cells increases MHC I and II protein synthesis on various cells and augments antigen presentation
Growth factors	Factor necessary for growth and differentiation	bFGF secreted by fibroblasts and keratinocytes stimulates melanocyte growth

Abbreviations: IL = interleukin; T = thymus; T_H = T helper; IFN = interferon; CD = cluster of differentiation; MHC = major histocompatibility complex; bFGF = basic fibroblast growth factor.

by keratinocytes that bind to receptors on melanocytes, have been identified as melanogenic cytokines that are linked to hyperpigmentation.[12–19] SCF binds to its cognate receptor KIT (transmembrane receptor tyrosine kinase) and acts via the mitogen-activated protein kinase (MAPK) pathway to stimulate microphthalmia-associated transcription factor (MITF) activation. Through MITF interaction with p300, increased pigmentation results from the activation of transcription factors for several genes, notably tyrosinase, a critical rate-limiting enzyme in the melanin synthesis pathway. Bcl2, a molecule that suppresses programmed cell death, is also activated through this pathway. Kitamura and colleagues conducted a study of 12 Japanese patients with nonsegmental vitiligo.[12] SCF and ET-1 levels were examined in lesional and nonlesional (perilesional) vitiligo epidermis. Surprisingly, their data showed that vitiliginous lesions actually have increased expression of these cytokines, suggesting that there is normal keratinocyte production of the molecules. There was, however, downregulation of c-KIT and melanocyte-specific microphthalmia-associated transcription factor (MITF-M).[12] They proposed that decreased MITF-M expression may lead to melanocyte cell death owing to the subsequent reduction of Bcl2.[12,20] Furthermore, if the SCF receptor, KIT protein, is deficient, the lack of SCF binding and resulting reduced tyrosinase expression could cause melanocyte dysfunction.[12]

In a study of 15 Caucasian patients with nonsegmental vitiligo, cytokine expression in lesional, nonlesional, and perilesional skin was investigated. Moretti and colleagues found that melanocytes were absent in lesional skin, and there was a reduction in the following keratinocyte-derived melanogenic factors: granulocyte-monocyte colony-stimulating factor (GM-CSF), SCF, and bFGF.[21,22] Furthermore, vacuolar degeneration of keratinocytes in perilesional skin of vitiligo patients was demonstrated.[21–23] This suggests that a reduction in functional keratinocytes may lead to the derangement of melanogenic factors and melanocytes. Compared with perilesional and nonlesional skin, lesional skin had increased levels of interleukin 6 (IL-6) and tumor necrosis factor α (TNF-α).[21,22] IL-6 and TNF-α are cytokines that can be produced by keratinocytes and have an inhibitory effect on melanogenesis and proliferation of melanocytes. Since TNF-α inhibits tyrosinase and tyrosinase-related protein 1,[21,22,24,25] and tyrosinase is important in the melanin synthesis pathway, melanogenesis may be compromised by elevated levels of TNF-α.

Measurement of the serum levels of various cytokines was conducted in a study of 50 Chinese patients with vitiligo.[26] They found higher serum levels of IL-6 and, in contrast with the preceding study, GM-CSF in patients with focal and generalized types of vitiligo, as well as increased IL-1β in those with generalized type compared with healthy subjects.[26]

Peripheral blood mononuclear cells were isolated from the serum of 12 vitiligo patients in Taiwan, and cytokine levels were assayed.[27] It was noted that IL-8 and, as found in similar studies described earlier, IL-6 were elevated.[27] IL-8 stimulates the recruitment of neutrophils and T cells into the skin and may help to trigger inflammation, causing melanocyte destruction.[1,27–30] IL-6 can increase the expression of intercellular adhesion molecule 1 (ICAM-1) on melanocytes[31] and may enhance leukocyte-melanocyte interactions, thus causing melanocyte death.[32] The authors proposed that activation and proliferation of B cells by IL-6 may cause autoantibody production, which could be an additional means for melanocyte cell apoptosis.[27]

In agreement with these results, data from a similar study in Taiwan demonstrated elevated levels of IL-8 secretion by melanocytes.[28] The aberrant levels of IL-8 were produced by melanocytes stimulated with IgG antibodies against melanocyte surface antigens (V-IgG) purified from 12 patients with nonsegmental vitiligo. Interestingly, IgG from healthy volunteers (N-IgG) did not stimulate enhanced IL-8 production. It was concluded that the increased IL-8 could lead to an augmented inflammatory response by T-cell infiltration, resulting in melanocyte cell destruction.[28]

In summary, to date, the cytokines implicated in the pathogenesis of vitiligo are SCF, GM-CSF, bFGF, TNF-α, IL-6, and IL-8. Owing to the diversity in patient populations, differences in detection techniques, and various sampling methods, it remains difficult to determine exactly which cytokines are responsible for vitiligo, although some key players are becoming more apparent. In all likelihood, the etiology of vitiligo may vary among patients with different presentations, otherwise known as the *convergence theory*, and can be due to several factors, such as genetics, autoimmunity, and melanocyte/nerve cell interaction, in addition to cytokine alterations.[5]

KELOIDS

Keloids are dermal fibroproliferative tumors caused by excessive accumulation of collagen usually owing to cutaneous injury, although spontaneous cases do occur. Keloids are cosmetically disfiguring lesions that extend beyond the borders of the original site of trauma. They are more prevalent among blacks, whereas Asians also may be predisposed to their development.[4,33] Enhanced transforming growth factor β [TGF-β(1 and 2)] protein expression and secretion by keloid fibroblasts are thought to play a role in the pathogenesis of the disease.[33–38] TGF-β stimulates collagen synthesis and promotes wound healing by regulating fibroblast growth, differentiation, and proliferation, as well as by inhibiting degradation of the extracellular matrix.[1,39] Therefore, this cytokine is thought to have a critical role in dermal scar formation. However, results from Bayat and colleagues, using DNA extracted from the peripheral blood cells of Caucasian keloid patients, did not demonstrate an association between TGF-β(1) polymorphisms and plasma TGF-β(1) levels and keloid development.[39] It was concluded that it is conceivable that an unknown polymorphism of the TGF-β(1) gene or another cytokine within the TGF-β regulatory system, such as TGF-β(2 and 3), could affect the development of skin fibrosis.[39]

TGF-β can also induce expression of vascular endothelial growth factor (VEGF) in cultured human keratinocytes and keloid fibroblasts.[40,41] VEGF is an angiogenic protein secreted during hypoxic states. VEGF binds and activates the tyrosine kinase receptor, resulting in vascular endothelial and smooth-muscle cell growth along with neovascularization and capillary hyperpermeability. Similar to the findings of the extra-abdominal desmoid tumor, aggressive fibromatosis, which is also characterized by excessive fibroblastic proliferation and collagenous deposition, keloids were found to have about a four-fold increase in VEGF in the stroma, in addition to TGF-β, compared to normal skin.[42] Some investigators have characterized keloids as angiogenic lesions in which the overlying hyperplastic epidermis is the source of abundant keratinocyte-derived VEGF.[43] This idea was initially controversial given that keloids are hypocellular and hypovascular with an avascular center and that there is variability in the epidermis of keloids, ranging from atrophic to hyperplastic.[44] However, multiple studies have since found an increase in VEGF and have concluded that it may contribute to keloid pathophysiology.

Evidence exists for a local state of tissue hypoxia in keloids by an increase in hypoxia-inducible factor-1α (HIF-1α).[45,46] VEGF is generated under hypoxic states, such as that which exists in the early stages of wound repair. HIF-1α activates the VEGF gene, which is an immediate downstream target.[47] This may be mediated by direct cell-cell contact between mast cells and fibroblasts and subsequent hypoxia-mediated activation of ERK 1/2 and Akt signaling pathways.[46] Activation of these pathways leads to increased HIF-1α and VEGF expression.[46] Keloids can be thought of as chronic wounds that do not heal.[45] They have been described clinically as having an erythematous, inflammatory base, a pale, raised central region, and a flattened, regressing portion. The inflammatory base, or tissue fibroplasia, is hypercellular and hypervascular and represents angiogenesis mediated by VEGF. This region mimics the early phases of wound repair.[45] The raised portion may represent altered extracellular matrix metabolism. Part of wound repair involves formation of fibrin clots and collagen deposition. However, in the case of keloids, there is an increase in antiproteolytic activities that prevent the lysis of this deposition. VEGF could induce this state, considering VEGF is increased in keloid tissues and is partly responsible for the upregulation of plasminogen activator inhibitor-1, which may also interfere with collagen degradation.[45]

An earlier study assayed cytokine production in peripheral blood mononuclear cells from black patients with keloids and black volunteers without keloids. IL-6, TNF-α, and interferon β (IFN-β) levels were higher, IL-1 and IL-2 production was similar, and IFN-α, IFN-γ, and TNF-β levels were lower in the keloid group.[48] IFN-α, IFN-β, and IFN-γ are known to inhibit collagen synthesis and fibroblast proliferation,[49] whereas IFN-γ and TNF-β also increase collagenase activity.[48–51] Abundant collagen deposition may result from a deficiency of IFN-α, IFN-γ, and TNF-β. Since both TNF-α and TNF-β stimulate collagenase function, increases in TNF-α and IFN-β may have been ineffective compensatory catabolic responses to accumulating collagen deposition.[48]

Observations of altered cytokine production contributing to keloid formation has provided insight extending beyond dermatologic diseases. Impact from keloid research reveals that effects of growth factors such as platelet-derived growth factor β (PDGF-β) and TGF-β on atherogenesis, vascular hyperplasia, and vascular smooth muscle hypertrophy also may be associated with the greater severity of hypertension and increased frequency of end-stage renal disease (ESRD) among blacks.[52]

ATOPIC DERMATITIS (ECZEMA)

Atopic dermatitis may cause profound pruritus that eventually leads to the clinical finding of lichenification secondary to scratching. It is usually associated with the allergic triad, which includes allergic rhinitis and asthma.[4] The term *atopy* refers to a hereditary predisposition to develop hypersensitive allergic reactions to various allergens, as demonstrated by a positive skin prick test and increased IgE production on allergen challenge.[53] Atopic dermatitis affects people of all races. Follicular eczema, characterized by pruritic follicular papules involving the hair follicles, is more common in African (black) and Asian children.[4] Halder and colleagues reported that eczema was common and was diagnosed almost twice as often in black patients than in white patients (20.3% versus 10.7% of patients, respectively) seen in a predominately black dermatology clinic in Washington, DC.[33,54,55] Although studies specifically examining atopic dermatitis in blacks and Asians are lacking, insight can be gained from literature concerning those with atopy or at an increased risk for atopy within the general population.

It has been documented that highly atopic children have an increased IL-4:IFN-γ ratio.[56] Highly atopic children with atopic dermatitis and plasma levels of IgE greater than 600 units/mL were compared with mildly atopic children, some of whom also had atopic dermatitis, with plasma IgE levels of less than 600 units/mL and with healthy subjects. Increased IL-4 and reduced IFN-γ levels were found by analysis of supernatants from ex vivo cultures of peripheral blood mononuclear cells.[56] Only the highly atopic group had statistically significant cytokine variations. These findings leave questions as to whether the observed differences correlate with disease severity rather than represent a correlative marker of atopy.[56] Elevated serum IgE is associated with atopic disease.[56] B-cell isotype switching from IgM to IgE, which depends on IL-4, leads to enhanced IgE levels.[1,56–58] IFN-γ, which is capable of counteracting the effect of IL-4[56,59] and of being suppressed by IL-4,[56,60] is found in reduced levels in highly atopic children with severe atopic dermatitis.[56]

Several studies have reported a deficiency in IFN-γ as a strong predictor of atopic disease. For example, a more recent study found that 2-year-old children with atopic disease had decreased levels of allergen-induced IFN-γ (specifically to house dust mite and cockroach allergen exposure) secreted by peripheral blood mononuclear cells.[61] There also was a positive correlation with increased allergen-induced IL-13 secretion (specifically to house dust mite and cat allergens) and elevated IgE early in life.[61] Since IL-13 helps to mediate antibody class switching to IgE[61] and is related to asthma etiology,[1] and since approximately 94% of children with asthma also have atopy,[62] IL-13 has been associated with atopy. Further evaluation of IL-4 and IL-13 genes revealed that specific polymorphisms are associated with atopy and atopic dermatitis in white children.[53,62]

In conclusion, atopic dermatitis appears to correlate with the selective activation of a cytokine profile related to the development of T-helper 2 (T_H2) cell phenotype. Elevations of the cytokines IL-4, IL-6, IL-10, and IL-13 lead to an increase in humoral (B-cell-mediated) immunity, increased IgE production, suppression of factors controlling T-helper 1 (T_H1) cell–mediated immunity (such as decreased IFN-γ), and eosinophilia.

BEHÇET DISEASE AND NEURO-BEHÇET SYNDROME

Behçet disease is characterized by recurrent oral aphthous ulcers along with genital aphthous ulcers, eye lesions, and cutaneous manifestations. Skin lesions often can present as punched-out ulcers, painful inflammatory nodules, pustules, or plaques. The pathogenesis is uncertain, but skin lesions may result from neutrophil accumulation in regions of immune complex–mediated vasculitis. This disease also can have neurologic manifestations such as meningoencephalitis, cranial nerve palsies, and psychosis. The prevalence is highest in Japanese, Southeast Asian, southern European, and Middle Eastern populations.[4]

IL-6 has been implicated as having a major role in the pathogenesis of neuro-Behçet syndrome. In a study involving Chinese patients, IL-6 and anticardiolipin antibodies of the IgM isotype were found to be elevated in the serum and cerebrospinal fluid (CSF) of patients with neuro-Behçet disease compared with those found in patients with noninflammatory neurologic disorders.[63] IL-6 is an important mediator of the immune and inflammatory responses and stimulates autoantibody production through its effects on B-cell differentiation and activation, indicating a potential relationship with the pathogenesis of Behçet disease.

In Korean patients with Behçet disease, an association was found between tandem repeat polymorphisms in the 3' flanking region of the IL-6 gene and the presence of the syndrome.[64] Genetic variants of the IL-6 gene have been identified in other chronic inflammatory and autoimmune diseases.

TNF-α also has been found to be overexpressed in Behçet disease. This proinflammatory molecule is thought to play a vital immunopathogenetic role in the tissue destruction and various cutaneous and central nervous system lesions.[65–69] Misumi and colleagues documented an increase in the number of cells secreting TNF-α in peripheral blood mononuclear cells from Japanese patients with active disease compared with those who had inactive disease.[70] A great deal of attention in the recent years has been focused on the effects of TNF-α and novel therapeutics for its inhibition.[70]

SYSTEMIC LUPUS ERYTHEMATOSUS

Systemic lupus erythematosus (SLE) is a polyclonal B-cell autoimmune disease affecting the vasculature and connective tissue of multiple organ systems, including the skin in 85% of patients. Cutaneous tissue injury results from immune complex (mainly autoantibody bound to DNA) deposition at the dermal-epidermal junction.[4] There is a plethora of skin lesions that SLE patients can acquire. Many patients present to a dermatologist for cutaneous manifestations, such as the butterfly-patterned rash on the face, even before a diagnosis of lupus is made and end-stage extracutaneous multisystem damage has occurred. This life-threatening disorder is most common in women (male:female ratio of 1:8) and blacks (1:250 black women versus 1:1000 white women).[4,71] Alterations in several cytokine levels have been identified and evaluated. Among them is TNF-α. Polymorphisms of TNF-α-308A and TNF-α-238, which are implicated in elevated TNF-α production, in African-American and Mexican patients, respectively, have been documented.[72,73] IL-6 also has been implicated by several groups in the pathogenesis of SLE.[74,75]

Lupus is often associated with an elevation of anti-double-stranded DNA (anti-dsDNA) antibodies, antinuclear antibodies (ANAs), anti-Smith (anti-Sm) antibodies, and anticardiolipin (aCL) antibodies. It has been reported that anti-dsDNA antibodies can interact with a cell and alter its cytokine production. Mouse monoclonal IgG anti-DNA antibody that has anti-dsDNA specificity has been shown to penetrate human peripheral blood mononuclear cells by targeting DNA or structural moieties similar to DNA that are bound to DNA receptors on cell membranes.[76] The DNA-bound IgG antibody subsequently may be internalized, making it possible for cellular activities to be altered by the antibody.[76] Data from another study demonstrated that murine monoclonal anti-DNA antibodies attached to the surfaces of cells, entered the nuclei, and stimulated the release of IL-1β, IL-8, TNF-α, and IL-10 from normal human peripheral blood mononuclear cells.[77] The significance of this effect is that IL-1β, IL-8, and TNF-α are proinflammatory cytokines that coordinate tissue destruction. Rises in IL-10 levels may alter immunologic polarity toward humoral immunity and abnormal antibody production.[77] Fc-receptor cross-linking of immune complexes with monocytes and macrophages also has been shown to induce secretion of TNF.[78]

TNF-α concentration correlates with disease activity and is thought to be the proinflammatory cytokine of central

TABLE 20-2
Cytokine Association with Cutaneous Diseases in Persons of Color

Cytokine	Source	Affected Cells	Function	Trends Noted in Studies Cited in This Chapter
IL-4	T_H2 cells	B cells T_H2 cells T_H1	• B cell growth, proliferation, and differentiation • Isotype switching (↑ IgE) • Increases T_H2 cell population • Suppresses T_H1 cell function	• ↑ Production in PBMCs from children with severe AD
IL-6	T_H cells Macrophages Keratinocytes Stromal cells	B cells Plasma cells Melanocytes Stem cells	• B cell differentiation • Causes fever • Induces acute phase protein synthesis by the liver • Enhances melanocyte ICAM-1 expression • Increases leukocyte-melanocyte interaction • May cause melanocyte cell death	• ↑ expression in vitiliginous lesions • ↑ production by cultured PBMCs of vitiligo patients • ↑ production by PBMCs of black keloid patients • ↑ levels in serum and CSF of patients with Behçet disease • ↑ levels in SLE patients
IL-8	Mononuclear cells Melanocytes Keratinocytes	Neutrophils	• Attracts neutrophils • Possibly attracts T cells	• ↑ in serum of vitiligo patients • ↑ levels implicated in SLE pathogenesis
IL-10	T_H2 cells Neutrophils Macrophages Keratinocytes	Macrophages B cells	• Inhibits dendritic cell and macrophage IL-12 production • Drives the system toward humoral immunity • Inhibits cell-mediated immunity (decreases antitumor immune action)	• No increase in black skin (SPT VI) following SSR • ↑ levels implicated in SLE pathogenesis
IL-13	T_H2 cells	B cells	• Causes asthma • May mediate antibody class switching • Increases IgE	• ↑ Production in PBMCs from atopic children on common allergen exposure
TNF-α	Macrophages Mast cells Natural Killer cells Keratinocytes CD8+ T cells T_H1 cells	Neutrophils Endothelial cells T_H cells B cells Tumor cells Melanocytes	• Activation of neutrophils • Increases synthesis of endothelial cell adhesion molecules • Enhanced lymphokine synthesis • B-cell growth • Causes endotoxin-induced septic shock • Mediates tumor necrosis • Inhibits tyrosinase and tyrosinase-related protein 1 • Interferes with melanogenesis • Stimulates collagenase activity/ collagen degradation	• ↑ expression in vitiliginous lesions • ↑ production by PBMCs of black keloid patients • ↑ secretion by PBMCs of patients with active Behçet disease • ↑ expression in SLE patients
TNF-β	T cells	Similar to TNF- α	• Binds to the same receptor as TNF-α, causing similar effects	• ↓ production by PBMCs of black keloid patients
TGF-β	T cells B cells Macrophages	T cells B cells Macrophages Neutrophils Natural Killer cells	• "Anticytokine"/inhibits the function of T cells and many other cell types • Suppression of the immune response after an infection • Stimulates wound healing • Upregulates collagen synthesis	• ↑ protein expression and secretion by keloid fibroblasts
VEGF	Smooth Muscle cells	Vascular Endothelial cells Fibroblasts Keratinocytes	• Vascular endothelial and smooth muscle cell growth	• ↑levels in keloid tissue
IFN-α	Leukocytes	Viruses Fibroblast	• Antiviral activity • Increases MHC class I • Inhibits collagen production • Inhibits rapidly dividing fibroblasts	• ↓ production by PBMCs of black keloid patients
IFN-β	Fibroblasts	Viruses Fibroblast	• Antiviral activity • Increases MHC class I • Inhibits collagen production • Inhibits rapidly dividing fibroblasts	• ↑ production by PBMCs of black keloid patients
IFN-γ	T_H1 cells CD8+ T cells	Viruses Fibroblast	• Antiviral activity • Enhances phagocytic killing	• ↓ production by PBMCs of black keloid patients

(continued)

TABLE 20-2 (Continued)
Cytokine Association with Cutaneous Diseases in Persons of Color

Cytokine	Source	Affected Cells	Function	Trends Noted in Studies Cited in This Chapter
		Macrophages Neutrophils Natural Killer cells	• Increases MHC classes I and II/enhances antigen presentation of various cells • Inhibits collagen production • Inhibits rapidly dividing fibroblasts	• ↓ Production in PBMCs from children with severe AD
GM-CSF	T cells Macrophages Keratinocytes	Granulocytes Macrophages Melanocytes	• Stimulates growth and differentiation of granulocytes, macrophages, and dendritic cells • Enhances macrophage antimicrobial activity • Melanocyte growth factor/stimulant	• ↑ serum level in Chinese vitiligo patients • ↓ expression in vitiliginous lesions of Caucasian patients
bFGF	Keratinocytes Fibroblasts	Melanocytes	• Melanocyte growth factor	• ↓ expression in vitiliginous lesions of Caucasian patients
SCF	Keratinocytes	Melanocytes	• Maintain melanocyte homeostasis and melanocyte activation	• ↑ expression in vitiliginous lesions of Japanese patients • ↓ expression in vitiliginous lesions of Caucasian patients
ET-1	Keratinocytes	Melanocytes	• Maintain melanocyte homeostasis and melanocyte activation	• ↑ expression in vitiliginous lesions of Japanese patients

Note: (1) More than one cell type can secrete the same cytokine, one cell can secrete multiple cytokines, and a cytokine can target different cell types. (2) This list may not recognize all cytokines and target cells affecting the diseases outlined here.
Abbreviations: IL = interleukin; T_H = T helper; B = bursa of Fabricius; PBMC = peripheral blood mononuclear cell; AD = atopic dermatitis; ICAM = intercellular adhesion molecule; CSF = cerebrospinal fluid; SLE = systemic lupus erythematosus; T = thymus; SPT = skin phototype; SSR = solar-simulating radiation; IgE = immunoglobulin E; TNF = tumor necrosis factor; CD = cluster of differentiation; TGF = transforming growth factor; VEGF = vascular endothelial growth factor; IFN = interferon; MHC = major histocompatibility complex; GM-CSF = granulocyte macrophage colony-stimulating factor; bFGF = basic fibroblast growth factor; SCF = stem cell factor; ET = endothelin

importance. TNF-α release by immune complex–stimulated monocytes and macrophages may help to induce other proinflammatory cytokines, such as IL-1, IL-6, IL-18, and IFN-γ.[79] TNF-α also may have an immunoregulatory role to decrease autoantibody production. Inhibiting TNF-α leads to a transient increase in IgG isotype antibody production without clinical flares of disease, however.[79–81]

Another member of the TNF family, B-cell activation factor of the TNF family (BAFF), is elevated in SLE patients. It binds to B-cell receptors to prolong their survival, and it differentiates plasma cells. Thus it may have a direct impact on serum IgG and autoantibody levels.[81]

Studies targeting the enhanced susceptibility to lupus in the black population are few. Additional research needs to be performed to determine if there are further cytokine variations that are unique to the black population that would make this group more susceptible to this devastating disease.

PHOTOPROTECTION

There is a protective value of skin of color. Darker skin pigmentation creates an increased threshold for the inflammatory response induced by ultraviolet (UV) radiation. In one study, no IL-10-positive neutrophils were found in the epidermis at 24 and 48 hours after 18,000 mJ/cm^2 of solar-simulating radiation (SSR) exposure of black subjects with skin phototype (SPT) VI. In contrast, IL-10-positive neutrophils were present in individuals with white skin of SPTs I–III after 12,000–18,000 mJ/cm^2 of SSR.[82] Since IL-10 is associated with UV-induced immunosuppression, this may explain the difference in skin cancer incidence between black and white individuals.[82] IL-10 inhibits macrophage IL-12 production, thus diminishing the activation of T_H1 cells and suppressing the antitumor effects of cell-mediated immunity,[1] which may contribute to the higher skin cancer incidence among white patients.

CONCLUSION

Owing to the limited basic science research identifying the causes of other skin and hair disorders related to persons of color, there is little known about specific cytokine alterations in several disorders. We have summarized here the association of cytokines with specific cutaneous diseases that either exhibit a predilection for expression within a particular race or are more problematic in persons of darker skin tones. Table 20-2 summarizes the activities of various cytokines associated with cutaneous manifestations when altered in persons of color. There is suspicion that cytokines may play a role to varying degrees in many other cutaneous diseases aside from those mentioned earlier. For example, they may be involved in inflammation and transfer of excess melanin to keratinocytes in the epidermis or to macrophages in the dermis, resulting in postinflammatory hyperpigmentation.[33,83] (See "Vitiligo" above for more information on melanogenic cytokines.) There remains a great deal to elucidate about the large array of cytokines that orchestrates the complex interworkings of the immune response. The potentially damaging elements of the human internal and external environments necessitate cytokine involvement for survival and self-defense. Unfortunately, owing to inherent shifts in homeostatic immune surveillance, cytokines actually may trigger the development of aberrant cellular communication within the skin, resulting in cutaneous pathologies.

Investigating the role of cytokines in dermatologic issues affecting people of color can lead to the development of potentially beneficial anticytokine therapy. For example, anti-TNF-α therapy, such as infliximab (a chimeric monoclonal antibody against TNF-α), in combination with azathioprine or methotrexate to avoid severe infusion reactions has shown promising results with rapid improvement of the inflammatory manifestations of SLE in small, open-labeled trials and single cases.[79–81,84] Randomized, controlled trials are still necessary to verify the results. Infliximab also has shown potential benefit in the treatment of Behçet disease by causing a rapid, sustained reduction in TNF-α and clinical improvement.[70] Furthermore, angiogenesis-associated cytokines that normally regulate wound healing and tumor invasion may have a significant role in the pathological mechanisms of keloid formation, maintenance, and growth. Exploitation of angiogenic targets may be beneficial to the treatment of keloids. For example, it has been demonstrated that intralesional corticosteroid treatment (i.e. dexamethasone) may lead to flattening and reduction of keloids by inhibiting endogenous VEGF expression and fibroblast proliferation via interaction with the glucocorticoid receptor pathway.[85] Owing to the promise of anticytokine therapeutics, further anticytokine therapeutic interventions need to be developed. However, more research studying cytokine dysregulation and cutaneous disease development must be addressed to stimulate new ideas and targets for therapeutic exploitation.

REFERENCES

1. Levinson W, Jawetz E. Cellular basis of the immune response, in Bernstein J (ed), *Medical Microbiology and Immunology: Examination and Board Review.* New York, Lange Medical Books/McGraw-Hill, 2002, pp 363-381.
2. Anderson W. Coordination of the immune response: Major cytokines, in *Immunology.* Madison, WI, Fence Creek Publishing, 1999, pp 71-79.
3. Decker J. Cytokines. Immunology Tutorials, Tucson, AZ, 2006; available at *microvet.arizona.edu*.
4. Fitzpatrick T. *Color Atlas and Synopsis of Clinical Dermatology: Common and Serious Diseases.* New York, McGraw-Hill, 2001.
5. Njoo MD, Westerhof W. Vitiligo: Pathogenesis and treatment. *Am J Clin Dermatol* 2001;2:167-181.
6. Tsatmali M, Ancans J, Thody AJ. Melanocyte function and its control by melanocortin peptides. *J Histochem Cytochem* 2002;50:125-133.
7. Mohr J. Vitiligo in a pair of monovular twins. *Acta Genet Stat Med* 1951;2:252-255.
8. Lerner AB. On the etiology of vitiligo and gray hair. *Am J Med* 1971;51:141-147.
9. Cui J, Arita Y, Bystryn JC. Characterization of vitiligo antigens. *Pigment Cell Res* 1995; 8:53-59.
10. Puri N, Mojamdar M, Ramaiah A. Growth defects of melanocytes in culture from vitiligo subjects are spontaneously corrected in vivo in repigmenting subjects and can be partially corrected by the addition of fibroblast-derived growth factors in vitro. *Arch Dermatol Res* 1989; 281:178-184.
11. Puri N, Mojamdar M, Ramaiah A. In vitro growth characteristics of melanocytes obtained from adult normal and vitiligo subjects. *J Invest Dermatol* 1987;88: 434-438.
12. Kitamura R, Tsukamoto K, Harada K, et al. Mechanisms underlying the dysfunction of melanocytes in vitiligo epidermis: Role of SCF/KIT protein interactions and the downstream effector, MITF-M. *J Pathol* 2004;202: 463-475.
13. Imokawa G, Yada Y, Miyagishi M. Endothelins secreted from human keratinocytes are intrinsic mitogens for human melanocytes. *J Biol Chem* 1992; 267:24675-25680.
14. Imokawa G, Miyagishi M, Yada Y. Endothelin-1 as a new melanogen: Coordinated expression of its gene and the tyrosinase gene in UVB-exposed human epidermis. *J Invest Dermatol* 1995; 105:32-37.
15. Imokawa G, Yada Y, Kimura M. Signaling mechanisms of endothelin-induced mitogenesis and melanogenesis in human melanocytes. *Biochem J* 1996;314:305-312.
16. Manaka L, Kadono S, Kawashima M. et al. The mechanism of hyperpigmentation in seborrhoeic keratosis involves the high expression of endothelin-converting enzyme-1α and TNF-α, which stimulate secretion of endothelin 1. *Br J Dermatol* 2001;145: 895-903.
17. Hachiya A, Akemi K, Atsushi O, et al. The paracrine role of stem cell factor/ c-kit signaling in the activation of human melanocytes in ultraviolet-B-induced pigmentation. *J Invest Dermatol* 2001;116: 578-586.
18. Hachiya A, Akemi K, Yoshida Y, et al. Biphasic expression of two paracrine melanogenic cytokines, stem cell factor and endothelin-1 in ultraviolet B-induced human melanogenesis. *Am J Pathol* 2004; 165:2099-2109.
19. Hattori H, Kawashima M, Ichikawa Y, et al. The epidermal stem cell factor is over-expressed in lentigo senilis: Implication for the mechanism of hyperpigmentation. *J Invest Dermatol* 2004;122:1256-1265.
20. McGill GG, Horstmann H, Widlund H, et al. Bcl2 regulation by the melanocyte master regulator Mitf modulates lineage survival and melanoma cell viability. *Cell* 2002;109: 707-718.
21. Moretti S, Spallanzain A, Amato L, et al. New insights into the pathogenesis of vitiligo: Imbalance of keratinocyte-derived cytokines. *Arch Dermatol* 2002; 138: 273-274.
22. Moretti S, Spallanzain A, Amato L, et al. Vgitiligo and epidermal microenvironment: Possible involvement of epidermal cytokines at sites of lesions. *Pigment Cell Res* 2002;15:87-92.
23. Moellmann G, Klein-Angerer S, Scollay D, et al. Extracellular granular material and degeneration of keratinocytes in the normally pigmented epidermis of patients with vitiligo. *J Invest Dermatol* 1982;79:321-330.
24. Kondo S. The roles of keratinocyte-derived cytokines in the epidermis and their possible responses to UVA-irradiation. *J Invest Dermatol Symp Proc* 1999;4: 177-183.
25. Martinez-Esparza M, Jiménez-Cervantes C, Solano F, et al. Mechanisms of melanogenesis inhibition by tumor necrosis factor-α in B16/F10 mouse melanoma cells. *Eur J Biochem* 1998;255: 139-146.
26. Tu CX, Gu JS, Lin XR. Increased interleukin-6 and granulocyte-macrophage colony stimulating factor levels in the sera of patients with non-segmental vitiligo. *J Dermatol Sci* 2003;31:73-78.
27. Yu HS, Chang KL, Yu CL, et al. Alterations in IL-6, IL-8, GM-CSF, TNF-α, and IFN-γ release by peripheral mononuclear cells in patients with active vitiligo. *J Invest Dermatol* 1997;108:527-529.
28. Li YL, Yu CL, Yu HS. IgG anti-melanocyte antibodies purified from patients with active vitiligo induce HLA-DR and intercellular adhesion molecule-1 expression and an increase in interleukin-8 release by melanocytes. *J Invest Dermatol* 2000; 115:969-973.
29. Larsen CG, Anderson AO, Appella E, et al. The neutrophil-activating protein (NAP-1) is also chemotactic for T lymphocytes. *Science* 1989;243:1464-1466.
30. Taub DD, Anver M, Oppenheim JJ, et al. T-lymphocyte recruitment by interleukin-8 (IL-8): IL-8-induced degranulation of neutrophils releases potent chemoattractants for human T lymphocytes both in vitro and in vivo. *J Clin Invest* 1996;97: 1931-1941.
31. Kirnbauer R, Charvat B, Schauer E, et al. Modulation of intercellular adhesion molecule-1 expression on human melanocytes and melanoma cells: Evidence for a regulatory role of IL-6, IL-7, TNF β, and UVB light. *J Invest Dermatol* 1992;98:320-326.
32. Morelli JG, Norris DA. Influence of inflammatory mediators and cytokines on human melanocyte function. *J Invest Dermatol* 1993;100:191-195S.
33. Burrall B. Ethnic Skin: A Spectrum of Issues, 2006, Medscape, *www.medscape.com*.
34. Lee TY, Chin GS, Kim WJ, et al. Expression of transforming growth factor beta 1, 2, and 3 proteins in keloids. *Ann Plast Surg* 1999;43:179-184.
35. Peltonen J, Hsiao LL, Jaakkola S, et al. Activation of collagen gene expression in keloids: Co-localization of type I and VI collagen and transforming growth factor-β 1 mRNA. *J Invest Dermatol* 1991;97: 240-248.
36. Babu M, Diegelmann R, Oliver N. Keloid fibroblasts exhibit an altered response to TGF-β. *J Invest Dermatol* 1992;99:650-655.
37. Bettinger DA, Yager DR, Diegelmann RF, et al. The effect of TGF-β on keloid fibroblast proliferation and collagen synthesis. *Plast Reconstr Surg* 1996;98:827-833.
38. Chin GS, Liu W, Peled Z, et al. Differential expression of transforming growth factor-β receptors I and II and activation of Smad 3 in keloid fibroblasts. *Plast Reconstr Surg* 2001;108:423-429.
39. Bayat A, Oliver B, Uli M, et al. Genetic susceptibility to keloid disease and hypertrophic scarring: Transforming growth factor β1 common polymorphisms and plasma levels. *Plast Reconstr Surg* 2003;111: 535-543.

40. Frank S, Hübner G, Breier G, et al. Regulation of Vascular Endothelial Growth Factor Expression in Cultured Keratinocytes. Implications for Normal and Impaired Wound Healing. *J Biol Chem* 1995;270:12607-12613.
41. Fujiwara M, Muragaki Y, Ooshima A. Upregulation of transforming growth factor-beta1 and vascular endothelial growth factor in cultured keloid fibroblasts: relevance to angiogenic activity. *Arch Dermatol Res* 2005;297(4):161-169.
42. Mills BG, Frausto A, Brien E. Cytokines associated with the pathophysiology of aggressive fibromatosis. *J Orthop Res* 2000;18:655-662.
43. Gira AK, Brown LF, Washington CV, Cohen C, Arbiser JL. Keloids demonstrate high-level epidermal expression of vascular endothelial growth factor. *J Am Acad Dermatol* 2004;50(6):850-853.
44. Beer TW. Keloids are not angiogenic lesions. *J Am Acad Dermatol* 2005;53(6): 1097-1098.
45. Le AD, Zhang Q, Wu Y, et al. Elevated vascular endothelial growth factor in keloids: relevance to tissue fibrosis. *Cells Tissues Organs* 2004;176(1-3): 87-94.
46. Zhang Q, Oh CK, Messadi DV, et al. Hypoxia-induced HIF-1 accumulation is augmented in a coculture of keloid fibroblast and human mast cells: involvement of ERK1/2 and PI-3K/Akt. *Exp Cell Res* 2006;312(2):145-155.
47. Forsythe JA, Jiang BH, Iyer NV, et al. Activation of vascular endothelial growth factor gene transcription by hypoxia-inducible factor 1. *Mol Cell Biol* 1996; 16(9):4604-4613.
48. McCauley RL, Chopra V, Li YY, et al. Altered cytokine production in black patients with keloids. *J Clin Immunol* 1992;12: 300-308.
49. Elias JA, Jimenez SA, Freundlich B. Recombinant gamma, alpha, and beta interferon regulation of human lung fibroblast proliferation. *Am Rev Respir Dis* 1987;135:62-65.
50. Duncan MR, Berman B. Gamma interferon is the lymphokine and beta interferon the monokine responsible for inhibition of fibroblast collagen production and late but not early fibroblast proliferation. *J Exp Med* 1985;162: 516-527.
51. Jimenez SA, Freundlich B, Rosenbloom J. Selective inhibition of human diploid fibroblast collagen synthesis by interferons. *J Clin Invest* 1984;74:1112-1116.
52. Dustan HP. Does keloid pathogenesis hold the key to understanding black/white differences in hypertension severity? *Hypertension* 1995;26:858-862.
53. He JQ, Chan-Yeung M, Becker AB, et al. Genetic variants of the IL13 and IL4 genes and atopic diseases in at-risk children. *Genes Immun* 2003;4:385-389.
54. Halder RM, Grimes PE, McLaurin CI, et al. Incidence of common dermatoses in a predominantly black dermatologic practice. *Cutis* 1983;32: 388, 390.
55. Halder RM, Nootheti PK. Ethnic skin disorders overview. *J Am Acad Dermatol* 2003;48:S143-148.
56. Tang M, Kemp A, Varigos G. IL-4 and interferon-γ production in children with atopic disease. *Clin Exp Immunol* 1993;92: 120-124.
57. Vercelli D, Jabara HH, Arai K, et al. Induction of human IgE synthesis requires interleukin 4 and T/B cell interactions involving the T cell receptor/CD3 complex and MHC class II antigens. *J Exp Med* 1989;169:1295-1307.
58. Del Prete G, Maggi E, Parronchi P, et al. IL-4 is an essential factor for the IgE synthesis induced in vitro by human T cell clones and their supernatants. *J Immunol* 1988;140: 4193-4198.
59. Pene J, Chrétien I, Rousset F, et al. Modulation of IL-4-induced human IgE production in vitro by IFN-γ and IL-5: The role of soluble CD23 (s-CD23). *J Cell Biochem* 1989;39: 253-264.
60. Vercelli D, Jabara HH, Lauener RP, et al. IL-4 inhibits the synthesis of IFN-γ and induces the synthesis of IgE in human mixed lymphocyte cultures. *J Immunol* 1990;144:570-573.
61. Contreras JP, LY Ngoc P, Gold DR, et al. Allergen-induced cytokine production, atopic disease, IgE, and wheeze in children. *J Allergy Clin Immunol* 2003;112: 1072-1077.
62. Zhu S, et al. Polymorphisms of the IL-4, TNF-α, and Fce RIβ genes and the risk of allergic disorders in at-risk infants. *Am J Respir Crit Care Med* 2000; 161:1655-1659.
63. Wang CR, Chuang CY, Chen CY. Anticardiolipin antibodies and interleukin-6 in cerebrospinal fluid and blood of Chinese patients with neuro-Behçet's syndrome. *Clin Exp Rheumatol* 1992;10: 599-602.
64. Chang HK, Jang W, Park S, et al. Association between interleukin 6 gene polymorphisms and Behçet's disease in Korean people. *Ann Rheum Dis* 2005;64: 339-340.
65. Akoglu TF, Direskeneli H, Yazici H, et al. TNF, soluble IL-2R and soluble CD-8 in Behçet's disease. *J Rheumatol* 1990;17: 1107-1108.
66. Hamzaoui K, Hamza M, Ayed K. Production of TNF-α and IL-1 in active Behçet's disease. *J Rheumatol* 1990;17: 1428-1429.
67. Mege JL, Dilsen N, Sanguedolce V, et al. Overproduction of monocyte derived tumor necrosis factor α, interleukin (IL) 6, IL-8 and increased neutrophil superoxide generation in Behçet's disease: A comparative study with familial Mediterranean fever and healthy subjects. *J Rheumatol* 1993;20: 1544-1549.
68. Sayinalp N, Ozcebe OI, Ozdemir O, et al. Cytokines in Behçet's disease. *J Rheumatol* 1996;23: 321-322.
69. Everekliogiu C, Er H, Turkoz Y, et al. Serum levels of TNF-α, sIL-2R, IL-6, and IL-8 are increased and associated with elevated lipid peroxidation in patients with Behçet's disease. *Mediat Inflamm* 2002;11:87-93.
70. Misumi M, Eri H, Mitsuhiro T, et al. Cytokine production profile in patients with Behçet's disease treated with infliximab. *Cytokine* 2003;24: 210-218.
71. Hellmann DS. Systemic Lupus Erythematosis. McGraw-Hill's Access Medicine, New York, 2006, *www.accessmedicine.com.*
72. Sullivan KE, Wooten C, Schmeckpeper BJ, et al. A promoter polymorphism of tumor necrosis factor α associated with systemic lupus erythematosus in African-Americans. *Arthritis Rheum* 1997;40: 2207-2211.
73. Zuniga J, Vargas-Alarcón G, Hernández-Pacheco G, et al. Tumor necrosis factor-α promoter polymorphisms in Mexican patients with systemic lupus erythematosus (SLE). *Genes Immun* 2001;2: 363-366.
74. Linker-Israeli M, Deans RJ, Wallace DJ, et al. Elevated levels of endogenous IL-6 in systemic lupus erythematosus: A putative role in pathogenesis. *J Immunol* 1991;147: 117-123.
75. Nagafuchi H, Suzuki N, Mizushima Y, et al. Constitutive expression of IL-6 receptors and their role in the excessive B cell function in patients with systemic lupus erythematosus. *J Immunol* 1993;151: 6525-6534.
76. Okudaira K, Yoshizawa H, Williams RC Jr. Monoclonal murine anti-DNA antibody interacts with living mononuclear cells. *Arthritis Rheum* 1987;30: 669-678.
77. Sun KH, Yu CL, Tang SJ, et al. Monoclonal anti-double-stranded DNA autoantibody stimulates the expression and release of IL-1β, IL-6, IL-8, IL-10, and TNF-α from normal human mononuclear cells involving in the lupus pathogenesis. *Immunology* 2000;99:352-360.
78. Debets JM, Van der Linden CJ, Dieteren IE, et al. Fc-receptor cross-linking induces rapid secretion of tumor necrosis factor (cachectin) by human peripheral blood monocytes. *J Immunol* 1988;141: 1197-1201.
79. Aringer M, Smolen JS. Tumour necrosis factor and other proinflammatory cytokines in systemic lupus erythematosus: A rationale for therapeutic intervention. *Lupus* 2004;13:44-47.
80. Aringer M, Graninger WB, Steiner G, et al. Safety and efficacy of tumor necrosis factor α blockade in systemic lupus erythematosus: An open-label study. *Arthritis Rheum* 2004;50:3161-3169.
81. Anolik JH, Aringer M. New treatments for SLE: Cell-depleting and anti-cytokine therapies. *Best Pract Res Clin Rheumatol* 2005;19:859-878.
82. Rijken F, Bruijnzeel PL, van Weelden H, et al. Responses of black and white skin to solar-simulating radiation: Differences in DNA photodamage, infiltrating neutrophils, proteolytic enzymes induced, keratinocyte activation, and IL-10 expression. *J Invest Dermatol* 2004;122: 1448-1455.
83. Trout CR. Disorders of hyperpigmentation, in Jorrizo J, Rapini R (eds), *Bolognia.* New York, Elsevier, 2003.
84. Segal R, Dayan M, Zinger H, et al. Suppression of experimental systemic lupus erythematosus (SLE) in mice via TNF inhibition by an anti-TNFα monoclonal antibody and by pentoxiphylline. *Lupus* 2001;10:23-31.
85. Wu WS, Wang FS, Yang KD, Huang CC, Kuo YR. Dexamethasone induction of keloid regression through effective suppression of VEGF expression and keloid fibroblast proliferation. *J Invest Dermatol* 2006;126(6):1264-1271.

CHAPTER 21

Complement System: Cellular and Molecular Biology of Inflammation

Kwame Denianke

Key Points

- Several studies have highlighted mutations in various complement components that are unique to particular ethnic groups; however, most of these studies were unable to provide a clear and sound rationale as to how these distinct abnormalities in complement manifest clinically.
- Epidemiologic and genetic studies have illustrated differences that exist between ethnic groups of various complement components. Further studies are needed to determine if there is indeed a clear link between complement, systemic lupus erythematosus (SLE), and ethnicity.

The principal physiologic functions of complement are to defend against pyogenic bacterial infections, bridge innate and adaptive immunity, and dispose of immune complexes and the products of inflammatory injury. The complement system is composed of plasma proteins that are activated by microbes and promote the destruction of microbes and inflammation.[1] It consists of three pathways: the classical, the alternative, and the lectin pathways. Although the classical pathway was discovered first, the alternative pathway is phylogenetically older. The pathways are distinct in regard to how they are initiated, but all result in the generation of enzyme complexes that are capable of cleaving the most abundant protein, C3. This results in formation of a protein complex, which lyses cells. The alternative and lectin pathways are components of innate immunity, whereas the classical pathway is a mechanism of humoral immunity.[2] Thus the complement system is critical to proper functioning of both innate and humoral immunity and contributes to the pathogenesis of disease processes, including several cutaneous diseases.

Over the past few decades, there has been a considerable amount of basic science and clinical science research on the complement system, which has contributed significantly to our understanding of the immune system as a whole. Simultaneously, epidemiologic data have been collected that have highlighted some of the ethnic differences in prevalence of complement deficiencies and complement gene mutations. It is thought that these findings also may help to explain the pathogenesis and manifestation of these diseases across ethnic boundaries.

This chapter will first review the basic science mechanisms of the complement system. Second, it will summarize some of the research that has highlighted ethnic differences in the complement system. Finally, the systemic and cutaneous manifestation of complement abnormalities will be discussed, with a special emphasis on systemic lupus erythematosus (SLE). In discussing SLE, the chapter will explore various theories focusing on genetics and ethnicity that may explain differences in prevalence and severity across different ethnic groups.

BASIC SCIENCE

Shortly after the discovery of antibodies, Jules Bordet was among the first to demonstrate the presence of complement and the integral role it plays in the immune system. He demonstrated that if fresh serum containing antibacterial antibody was added to bacteria at 37°C, the bacteria were lysed. However, if the serum was heated to 56°C or more, the lytic capacity was lost. Thus he presumed that the serum must contain a heat-labile component that *complemented* the lytic function of antibodies.[2]

Activation of complement involves a cascade that results in the generation of enzymes with proteolytic activity. The proteins and protein complexes created in this process become covalently bound to microbial cell surfaces or antibodies bound to microbes and other antigens. In fluid phase, the complement proteins are inactive and become stably active only when attached to microbes or to antibodies. Complement activation is inhibited by regulatory proteins present on normal host cells but absent on microbes. However, once activated, the cascade can proceed down one of three distinct pathways, which are illustrated in Figure 21-1 and will be discussed individually.

Classical Pathway

The classical pathway is initiated by certain isotypes of antibodies bound to antigens. Complement protein C1 binds the CH2 domain of IgG and the CH3 domains of IgM molecules that have bound antigen. Each IgFc region has a single C1q-binding site, and each C1q molecule must bind to two immunoglobulin heavy chains to be activated. This explains why only antibodies with bound antigens and not free antibodies can activate the classical pathway. Subsequently, C4 is cleaved by C1r2s2 enzyme to C4b and C4a. C4b binds to the antigenic surface and antibodies. C2 also binds to C4, resulting in cleavage of C2 and formation of a C4b2a complex (C3 convertase). C3 is cleaved by C3 convertase, creating C3a and C3b.[2] The binding of C3b to C4b2a results in the formation of C5 convertase, which ultimately leads to the late steps of complement activation, which are discussed below.

Alternative Pathway

The alternative pathway is activated on microbial surfaces in the absence of antibody. Soluble C3 in plasma undergoes slow spontaneous hydrolysis of its internal thioester bond, leading to formation of a fluid-phase C3 convertase and the generation of C3b. If the C3b is deposited on the surfaces of microbes, it binds to factor B, a serine protease, and forms the alternative pathway C3 convertase (C3bBb). The C3 convertase is stabilized by serum protein properdin. Subsequently, C5 convertase is formed, leading to the late steps of activation. Of note, the early steps of the alternative and classical pathway are homologous, with C3 in the alternative pathway being homologous to C4 in the classical pathway and factor B homologous to C2.[2]

Lectin Pathway

The lectin pathway is activated by a plasma lectin that binds to mannose residues on microbes in the absence of antibody. Mannose-binding lectin (MBL) binds to mannose residues on polysaccharides and, owing to its structural resemblance to C1q, triggers the complement system by activating the C1r–C1s enzyme complex or associating with mannose-binding protein– associated serine esterase that cleaves C4. Aside from being initiated independent of antibody,

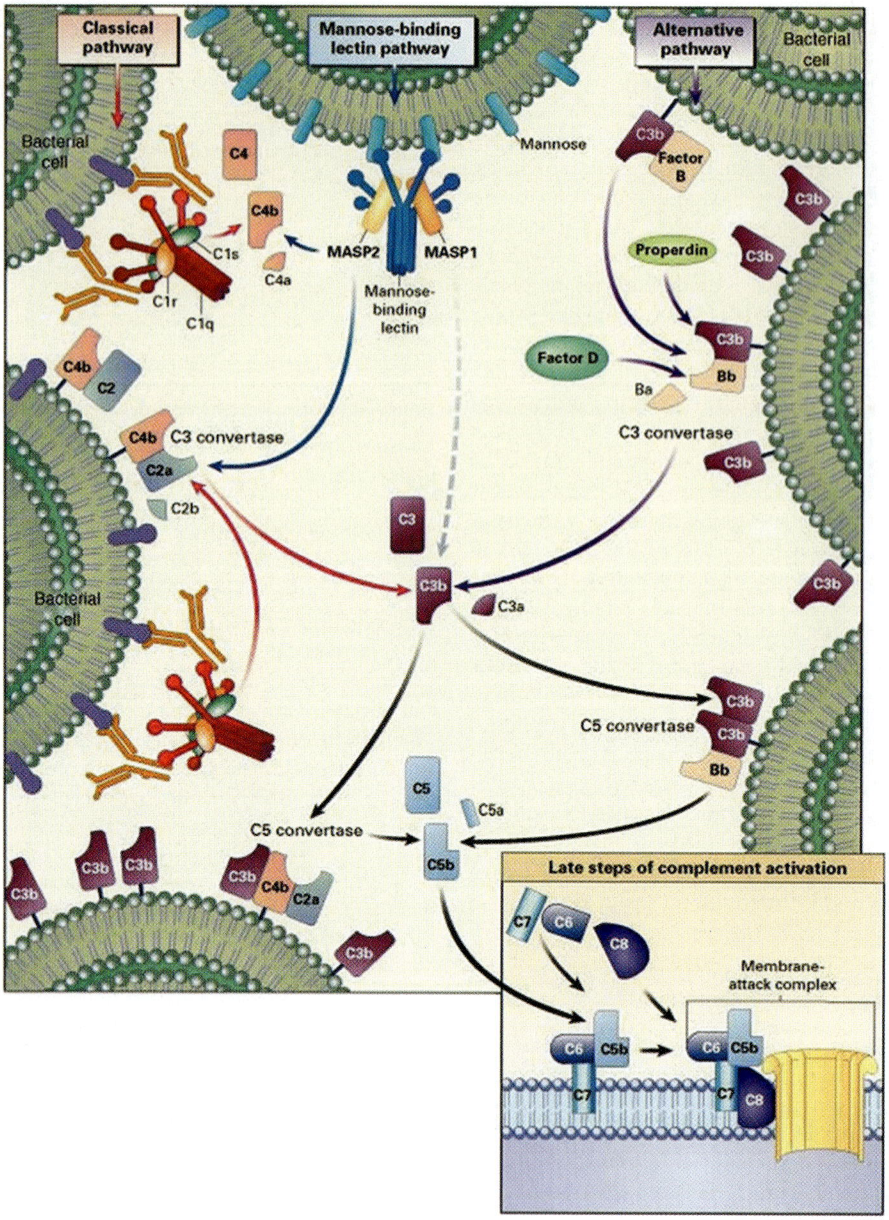

▲ **FIGURE 21-1** The three activation pathways of complement: the classical, mannose-binding lectin, and alternative pathways. The complement system is complex and comprised of three pathways that are noted to converge at the C3 cleavage point. The classical pathway is initiated by binding of the C1 complex (C1q, C1r, C1s) to antibodies bound to antigen on the surface of a bacterial cell. The mannose-binding lectin pathway is initiated by binding of the complex of mannose-binding lectin and mannose-binding lectin–associated proteases 1 and 2 (MASP1, MASP2) to mannose groups on the bacterial cell surface. The alternative pathway is initiated by the covalent binding of C3b to hydroxyl groups on cell surface carbohydrates and proteins. (From Walport MJ. Advances in immunology: Complement—First of two parts. *N Engl J Med* 2001;344(14):1058–1066, with permission.)

which is similar to the alternative pathway, the remainder of steps in the lectin pathway are identical to those of the classical pathway.[2]

Late Steps of Complement Activation

The late components of the complement system are initiated by C5 convertase generated by the early steps of the classical, alternative, and lectin pathways. Ultimately, a C5b,6,7,8 complex, also known as the *membrane attack complex* (MAC), stably inserts into the lipid bilayer of cell membranes. On binding of C9, the complex becomes activated, and pores are formed in the plasma membranes of cells, resulting in osmotic swelling and rupture of the cells. Furthermore, apoptosis is induced in nucleated cells via calcium influx.[2]

Regulation of Complement Activation

Activation of the complement cascade and the stability of active complement proteins are strictly regulated to prevent complement activation on normal host cells and to limit the duration of the response. Even when initiated on microbes or antibody-antigen complexes, degradation products may diffuse to adjacent cells and injure them. The proteolytic activity of C1r and C1s is inhibited by C1 inhibitor (C1 INH), which prevents the accumulation of enzymatically active C1r2–C1s2 in the plasma. This limits the time this complex is able to activate subsequent steps in the cascade. Deficiency of this enzyme is implicated in the autosomal dominantly inherited disease hereditary angioneurotic edema.[2]

There are several other regulators of complement activation that may contribute to the manifestation of cutaneous disease (Figure 21-2). Assembly and stability of C3 convertase can be inhibited by many regulatory proteins, such as decay-accelerating factor (DAF), type 1 complement receptor (CR1), membrane cofactor protein (MCP or CD46), and plasma protein factor H and factor I. Factor H is the dominant complement-control protein, and when it is absent, the regulation of complement activation breaks down completely.[1] Formation of the MAC is inhibited by a membrane protein called CD59, which is a glycophosphatidylinositol-linked protein expressed on many cell types. It is present on normal host cells but not microbes. There are also inhibitors present in the plasma, further ensuring that normal uninvolved cells are not involved in activation of complement and subsequent lysis. Nevertheless, the function of regulatory proteins may be overcome by increasing amounts of complement activation that may occur in the setting of immunologic disease when large amounts of antibodies are deposited on host cells.[2]

COMPLEMENT AND ETHNIC VARIABILITY

As mentioned previously, several studies have highlighted distinct mutations in various complement components that are unique to particular ethnic groups. However, most of these studies have not been able to provide a clear and sound rationale as to how these distinct abnormalities in complement manifest clinically. Nevertheless, a cursory review of these articles will follow because they may form the basis of future studies that could perhaps elucidate the pathogenesis of several disease processes. With

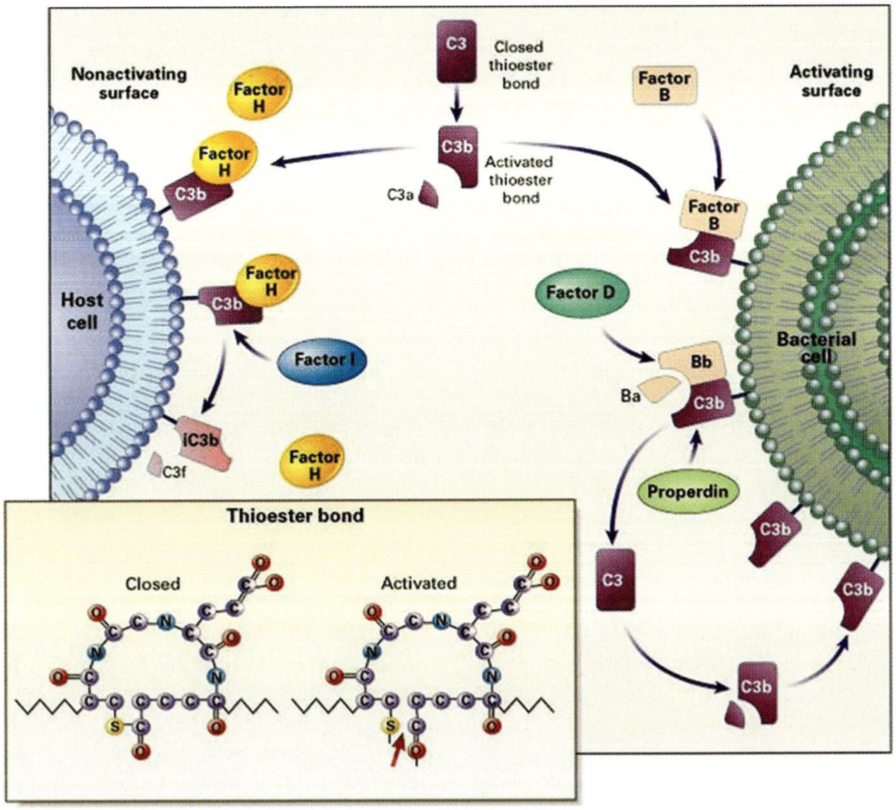

▲ **FIGURE 21-2** Regulation of the cleavage of C3 by factor H and factor I. The first product of the cleavage of C3 by C3 convertase is C3b, which has an activated internal thioester bond. This bond enables C3b to bind covalently to hydroxyl groups on nearby carbohydrates and protein-acceptor groups. If the acceptor molecule is on a host cell surface, then protective regulatory mechanisms come into play. This is illustrated by the binding of factor H to C3b, which acts as a cofactor to the serine esterase factor I. Factor I cleaves the C3 into an inactive product, iC3b, releasing a small peptide, C3f. The iC3b can no longer participate in the formation of a C3 convertase enzyme. If C3b binds covalently to a bacterium, then the enzyme precursor factor B binds to the C3b. Factor B that is bound to C3b is susceptible to cleavage and activation by the enzyme factor D. This leads to the formation of the C3 convertase enzyme C3bBb, which is stabilized by the binding of properdin. This enzyme cleaves more C3, leading to the deposition of additional C3b on the bacterium. The carbhohydrate environment of the surface on which the C3b is deposited determines the relative affinity of C3b for factor H or factor B. On host cell surface bearing polyanions such as sialic acid, factor H binds to C3b with a higher affinity than does factor B. On microbial surfaces that lack a polyanionic coating, factor B binds to C3b with a higher affinity than does factor H, leading to amplified cleavage of C3. (From Walport MJ. Advances in immunology: Complement—First of two parts. *N Engl J Med* 2001;344(14):1058–1066, with permission.)

few exceptions, most of these studies have emphasized differences in early complement components. This is not alarming because many of the systemic diseases that have been associated with complement abnormalities are found in the early steps of the cascade.

In 1977, Muff and colleagues documented that blacks have a higher frequency of the factor B allele *BF*F* than other ethnic groups.[3] These findings have been supported by other studies. Also, it has been shown and agreed on by many that C2 has the least polymorphic variability worldwide.[4] In 1992, Lipscombe and colleagues showed that Gambians in West Africa have a distinct MBP mutation compared with Europeans, Indians, Malaysians, Polynesians, and Chinese.[5] Human complement factor I (IF) allele A has been shown to have the highest frequency in the southwest Chinese Han population.[6] There is a high frequency of *C4A*Q0* and *C4B*Q0* null alleles in Telegu-speaking Hindu and Bengali-speaking Muslims in India.[7] However, despite the concordance of these studies, and others that will be discussed, the clinical significance of this genetic variability remains to be illustrated.

Based on the mechanisms of the complement cascade, many have postulated that deficiencies in the later components may serve as the basis for explaining the ethnic differences in the incidence and severity of infections, namely, *Neisseria meningitidis* and *N. gonorrhoeae*. However, many of these studies have failed to provide results with consistency. In 2000, Zhu and colleagues analyzed many of the molecular defects of early and late components across different ethnic groups. They described distinct C6 deficiency (C6D) molecular defects in African-Americans, Japanese, and the Cape colored people of South Africa. In the United States, the prevalence of C6D among African-Americans, particularly in the South, was found to be greater than that in other ethnic groups.[8] Some authors have argued that homozygous deficiency of C6 offers a selective advantage because it protects against the deleterious effects of complement activation by endotoxin in infantile gastroenteritis.[1] In a small study group, Halle and colleagues showed that C6, C8α, and C8γ deficiency is greatest in blacks, while C7 and C8B deficiency is more prevalent in Caucasians.[9] A unique nonsense mutation in the C9 gene has been found to be responsible for most C9 deficiency in Japanese patients. This gene mutation, in a paradoxical manner similar to C6 mutations described earlier, is thought to be protective because the incidence of serious meningococcal infections in complement-deficient patients is lower in comparison with normal individuals.[10]

COMPLEMENT AND DISEASE

The two primary mechanisms by which complement leads to disease are by deficiencies of the protein components and absence of regulatory components. Genetic deficiencies in the classical pathway components have been identified, with C2 being the most common. A disease that resembles SLE develops in more than 50% of patients with C2 and C4 deficiencies. It is hypothesized that defects in complement activation may lead to failure to clear circulating immune complexes. Deficiency of C3 is associated with serious pyogenic bacterial infections and a characteristic eruption.[11] Deficiencies in the alternative pathway have been associated with increased susceptibility to infection with pyogenic bacteria. Deficiencies in regulatory proteins also have been reported, the most common being C1 INH deficiency, which was mentioned earlier.

There are several cutaneous diseases in which complement clearly has been shown to have a role in the pathogenesis. This has been demonstrated in but not limited to vesiculobullous dermatoses. Paraneoplastic pemphigus, bullous pemphigoid, cicatricial pemphigoid, herpes gestations, epidermolysis bullosa acquisita, erythema multiforme, and SLE reveal C3 positivity with direct immunofluorescence.[12]

Systemic Lupus Erythematosus

It has been established by many authors that patients with active SLE exhibit hypocomplementemia.[13] However, as pointed out by Ramo-Casals and colleagues, the usefulness of low complement levels as predictors of lupus flares is controversial, with some studies finding a clear association with lupus activity and others showing no correlation.[14] Furthermore, it is widely accepted that activation of complement by immune complexes contributes to tissue injury in patients with SLE. In fact, about a third of patients have high titers of autoantibodies to C1q, which is indicative of severe disease and is associated with consumptive hypocomplementemia and lupus nephritis.[11] However, the true role that complement plays in the pathogenesis of SLE is not clearly understood, and the fact that patients with hereditary deficiencies of complement proteins of the classical pathway are in fact at increased risk for SLE seems to contradict the importance attributed to complement in this disease. Nevertheless, Nived and Sturfelt suggest that in the future, complement might be worthwhile testing in developing the American College of Rheumatology (ACR) criteria for SLE because in their study, complement was found to be the most accurate variable in the subset of patients who were negative for anti–double-stranded DNA (anti-dsDNA) antibodies, had no malar rash, but had pleurisy.[13]

Most of the literature highlights the differences in individual complement components between patients with SLE and controls within particular ethnic groups, as well as differences across ethnic groups. Homozygous deficiencies of C1q, C1r, C1s, C4, and C2 have shown to be associated with increased incidence of SLE. Also, an increased prevalence of SLE has been shown in patients with hereditary angioedema. In patients with hereditary angioedema, there is excessive cleavage of C4 and C2 by C1s, leading to an acquired C4 and C2 deficiency, which increases susceptibility to SLE.[11] Partial deficiency of C4, C4A in particular, has been shown to be a genetic risk factor for lupus in Hispanics, whites, and blacks.[15]

Two hypotheses that have been proposed to explain the association between complement deficiency and an increased incidence of SLE. The first proposes that complement determines the activation thresholds of B- and T-lymphocytes. Thus deficiency leads to incomplete maintenance of peripheral tolerance and subsequent autoimmunity. The second theory has been termed the *waste-disposal hypothesis*. This is based on the assumption that complement has inflammatory and anti-inflammatory functions. The anti-inflammatory functions are supported by its role in clearing immune complexes from the circulation and tissues. Absence of complement-dependent clearance of dying cells and immune complexes results in an increase in immunogenic self-antigens and subsequent autoantibody formation. In addition, the formation of DNA and anti-DNA immune complexes may directly induce tissue inflammation and mediate the inappropriate maturation of dendritic cells with potentially pathogenic consequences.[11]

It is also well accepted that ethnicity is a risk factor for developing SLE. Studies have reported that SLE is most common in African-American women, with a prevalence of 4 in 1000 versus 1 in 1000 in Caucasian American women.[16] Ethnicity also affects the phenotype because African-Americans have a higher frequency of nephritis, pneumonitis, and discoid lesions and a lower frequency of photosensitivity than Caucasians. Also, African-Americans tend to have an earlier age of onset and higher mortality.[17] Several investigators have explored the role that complement plays in the variable presentation of SLE in different ethnic groups. However these studies, some of which are discussed below, have failed to provide compelling arguments linking complement and ethnicity to the development of SLE. For example, Jacyk and colleagues reported that South African blacks with SLE had decreased serum complement levels compared with their white counterparts.[18] In another study, Ghaussy and colleagues showed that compared with Caucasians, Hispanics had a greater prevalence of arthritis and depressed complement levels that was statistically significant. They concluded that this indicates increased SLE disease activity and is restricted to specific domains but that "it remains to be determined if differences are genetic versus cultural versus environmental or some combination thereof."[19]

A great deal of research has centered on C4 with SLE patients from a variety of backgrounds. Hong and colleagues reported a high frequency of the C4A null allele *C4AQ0* in Caucasians, blacks, and Asians. Especially in Caucasians with SLE, there is an increased prevalence of homozygote C4 deficiency (>10%), as well as an increased frequency of heterozygote of *C4AQ0,* and about 78% of the C4A null allele was due to DR3-associated C4 gene deletion. In contrast, the C4A null allele in Asians with SLE is almost always heterozygous rather than homozygous and not an expression of the C4 gene deletion shown in Caucasians and black Americans. The *C4AQ0* allele is associated with SLE in Koreans.[20] In 1998, Reveille and colleagues showed that *C4B*2* is seen less frequently in Hispanic patients with SLE when compared with Hispanic controls without SLE ($p = 0.005$), and a similar trend has been observed in African-Americans, although it is not statistically significant ($p = 0.06$). CR1 alleles did not differ significantly between patients with SLE and Caucasian, African-American, or Hispanic controls. Given the association of *C4A*3* (most frequently observed C4 allele in all three ethnic groups) with disease activity at the time of diagnosis, it is possible that C4A null alleles are associated with a better prognosis.[21]

Although not much research has been performed assessing the role of the lectin pathway in the development of SLE, Takahashi and colleagues found an increased incidence of anti-MBL antibodies in the sera of some Japanese patients with SLE. However, it was not statistically significant when compared with Japanese controls. Thus the etiologic role of these antibodies in the development of SLE remains unclear.[22]

In summary, there have been several publications highlighting the role that complement may play in the development of SLE. Furthermore, epidemiologic and genetic studies have illustrated differences that exist between ethnic groups of various complement components. Nevertheless, further studies are needed to determine if there is indeed a clear interrelated link between complement, SLE, and ethnicity.

CONCLUSION

We have discussed the integral role that complement plays in proper functioning of the immune system. This has advanced our understanding of the pathogenesis of several systemic and cutaneous diseases. However, despite the advancements that have been made in regard to understanding the complement system, much more research is needed to establish a clear understanding of mechanisms that contribute to the development of disease. As we have discovered, several articles have highlighted ethnic and genetic differences in particular complement components. These differences may help to explain why ethnic groups are affected disproportionately by different systemic and cutaneous diseases that are influenced by complement. The best example of such a disease is SLE, which has been shown to be linked to complement deficiencies, and complement activation, which is correlated with the activity of this disease. Although the prevalence and phenotype of SLE are clearly affected by ethnicity, whether or not these differences can be explained by the genetics of complement remains to be revealed.

REFERENCES

1. Walport M. Complement: First of two parts. *N Engl J Med* 2001;344:1058-1066.
2. Abbas A, Lichtman A. Effector mechanisms of immune responses, in *Cellular and Molecular Immunology,* 5th ed. Philadelphia, Saunders, 2003, pp 326-344.
3. Muff G, Gauchel FD, Hitzeroth HW. Polymorphism of properdin factor B in South African Negroid, Indian and colored populations. *Hum Genet* 1977;33: 319-322.
4. de Massias IT, Reis A, de Almeida PT, et al. Genetic variability of the MHC class III complement proteins C2, BF, C4A and C4B in southern Brazil. *Exp Clin Immunogenet* 1994;11:192-196.
5. Lipscombe RJ, Sumiya M, Hill AV, et al. High frequencies in African and non-African populations of independent mutations in the mannose-binding protein gene. *Hum Mol Genet* 1992;1:709-715.
6. Zhang L, Stradmann-Bellinghausen B, Rittner C, et al. Genetic polymorphism of human complement factor I (C3b inactivator) in the Chinese Han population. *Exp Clin Immunogenet* 1999;16:30-32.
7. Ad'hiah A, Papiha S. Complement components C2, C3, and C4 (C4A and C4B) and BF polymorphisms in populations of the Indian subcontinent. *Hum Biol* 1996; 68:755-776.
8. Zhu Z, Atkinson TP, Hovanky KT, et al. High prevalence of complement component C6 deficiency among African-Americans in the southeastern USA. *Clin Exp Immunol* 2000;119:305-310.
9. Halle D, Elstein D, Geudalia D, et al. High prevalence of complement C7 deficiency among healthy blood donors of Moroccan Jewish ancestry. *Am J Med Genet* 2001;99: 325-327.
10. Khajoee V, Ihara K, Kira R, et al. Founder effect of the C9 *R95X* mutation in Orientals. *Hum Genet* 2003;112:244-248.
11. Walport M. Complement: Second of two parts. *N Engl J Med* 2001;344:1140-1144.
12. Cohen LM, Skopicki DK, Harrist TJ, et al. Noninfectious Vesiculobullous and Vesiculopustular Diseases. In: Elder, D et al. (eds) Lever's Histopathology of the Skin. 8th ed. Philadelphia: Lippincott-Raven; 1997; pp 209-252.
13. Nived O, Sturfelt G. ACR classification criteria for systemic lupus erythematosus: Complement components. *Lupus* 2004; 13:877-879.
14. Ramos-Casals M. Hypocomplementemia in systemic lupus erythematosus and primary antiphospholipid syndrome: Prevalence and clinical significance in 667 patients. *Lupus* 2004;777-783.
15. Moulds J, Reveille J, Arnett F. Structural polymorphisms of complement receptor 1 (CR1) in systemic lupus erythematosus (SLE) patients and normal controls of three ethnic groups. *Clin Exp Immunol* 1996;105:302-305.
16. Hochberg M. The epidemiology of systemic lupus erythematosus, in Wallace DJ, Hahn BH (eds), *Dubois' Lupus Erythematosus,* 4th ed. Philadelphia, Lea & Febiger, 1993 pp 49-57.
17. Lee L. Lupus erythematosus, in Bolognia J, Jorizzo J, Rapini R (eds), *Dermatology.* London, Elsevier, 2003 pp 601-613.
18. Jacyk W, Steenkamp K. Systemic lupus erythematosus in South African blacks: Prospective study. *Int J Dermatol* 1996;35: 707-710.
19. Ghaussy NO, Sibbitt W Jr, Bankhurst AD, et al. The effect of race on disease activity in systemic lupus erythematosus. *J Rheumatol* 2004;31: 915-919.
20. Hong GH, Kim HY, Takeuchi F, et al. Association of complement C4 and HLA-DR alleles with systemic lupus erythematosus in Koreans. *J Rheumatol* 1994;21: 442-447.
21. Reveille JD, Moulds JM, Ahn C, et al. Systemic lupus erythematosus in three ethnic groups: I. The effects of HLA class II, C4, and CR1 alleles, socioeconomic factors, and ethnicity at disease onset. LUMINA Study Group. Lupus in minority populations, nature versus nurture. *Arthritis Rheum* 1998;41:1161-1172.
22. Takahashi R, Tsutsumi A, Ohtani K, et al. Anti–mannose-binding lectin antibodies in sera of Japanese patients with systemic lupus erythemtosus. *Clin Exp Immunol* 2004;136: 585-590.

SECTION 3

Cutaneous Disorders

CHAPTER 22

Psoriasis

Amy Geng
Jason McBean
Priya Swamy Zeikus
Charles J. McDonald

Key Points

- Psoriasis occurs worldwide with differing prevalences among ethnicities; there may exist ethnic differences in the genetic predisposition to develop psoriasis.
- Higher prevalences seem to be found in Scandinavia (3–4.8%), Malaysia (4–5%), East Africa (1.25–3%), and South Africa (4–5%), and lower prevalences are seen in West Africa (0.3–0.8%), Africans-Americans (0.45–1.3%), Southeast Asians (0.4–2.3%), India and East Asians (~0.3%), and the indigenous populations of the Americas (nearly absent).
- The clinical features of psoriasis are similar across ethnicities; darker skin phototypes show a tendency toward violaceous plaques, gray scale, and postinflammatory dyspigmentation.
- Treatment of psoriasis is similar across ethnicities. Traditional medicine is not popular but is used by certain populations.

Psoriasis is a chronic inflammatory and hyperproliferative disease of the skin that presents in a number of clinical forms that are similar across ethnicities. It may be associated with mild to severe hyperproliferative skin disease and inflammatory arthritis. Onset of disease and its severity are strongly influenced by age and genetics, and may be provoked by a variety of internal and external factors such as physical injury to the skin, systemic drugs, infections, and emotional stress. The incidence of psoriasis is worldwide in distribution, but its prevalence varies by ethnicity and geography. The treatment of psoriasis varies minimally among ethnicities.

EPIDEMIOLOGY

Psoriasis appears to be most prevalent in northern European populations, particularly in Scandinavians, in whom the peak prevalence approaches 5%. In contrast, psoriasis is observed less frequently in people with darker skin phototypes. We note that in our extensive review of the dermatologic literature, there is a paucity of written reports that address psoriasis in ethnic skin. Specifically, there are very few published studies on psoriasis in Native Americans, the Andean population of South America, and the Latin American populations of North, Central, and South America. It is noteworthy that with the exception of a small group of isolated population centers in India, China, Japan, and the African continent and in African-Americans, large studies of the prevalence of psoriasis in people of color have yet to be reported. The absence of such studies makes it difficult to define with assurance the true prevalence of psoriasis among different ethnic groups. Table 22-1 summarizes the limited data available.

Data from the few studies available from the Near East and Southeast Asia show that the prevalence of psoriasis ranges from 0.5–2.3% in India, 4–5% in Malaysia, and about 0.4% in Sri Lanka.[1] In Japan, China, and the Pacific Islands, prevalence rates range from 0.05–0.3%.[2–5] On the African continent, a number of studies show that psoriasis prevalence varies widely with geographic location. In western African

TABLE 22-1
Prevalance of Psoriasis Among Ethnicities

Location or Ethnicity	Number of Patients with Skin Disease	Percent of Patients with Psoriasis	Comments
Arctic Kasach'ye[58]		12	
Jamaica[59]	1000	6	95% Afro-Caribbean 0.8% Caucasian 1.4% Indian 1.4% Chinese
Norway[60]		3–4.8	
Faroe Islands[61]		2.8	
Central Europe		1.5	
United States, overall[6,62]		1.4–4.6, 2.2	National Psoriasis Foundation
United States, Caucasian[6,7]		2.5, 2.5	National Psoriasis Foundation
United States, African-American[6,7,58]		1.3, 1.3, 0.45–0.7	National Psoriasis Foundation
South Africa[6]		4–5	
Egypt[6]		3	
Uganda[6]	3371	2.8	African black
Kenya[6]	1230	1.9	African black
Ethiopia[6]	6580	1.25	African black
Nigeria[7]	9806	0.8	
Nigeria[6]	1156	0.5	African black
Senegal[6]	45,000	0.6	Ethnicity not given
Brazil[6]	3140	0.7	35% Mestizo 25% European 40% African black
Malaysia[1]		4–5	
India[1]		0.5–2.3	
Sri Lanka[1]		0.4	
Japan[4]		0.3–1	
China[5]		0.3	
Japan, China, Pacific Islands[2–5]		0.05–0.3	
Native North American		Nearly absent	
Native South American[59]	26,000	No cases reported	
Samoa[59]		No cases reported	

countries—Nigeria, Angola, Mali, and Senegal—prevalence rates range from 0.3–0.8%, substantially below that of most European populations.[6] In northern, southern, and eastern Africa, psoriasis prevalence approaches that found in Europe, that is, 1.3–3%. Considerable discussion has centered around data showing marked similarities in psoriasis prevalence noted in African-Americans (0.7–1.4%) and that observed in western Africa.[6–10] Historically, most African-Americans trace their origins to western Africa, the center of the African slave trade. Some authors have suggested that the present-day African-American population is an amalgamation of multiple ethnic groups including Native Americans, European whites, and Africans, perhaps accounting for the slightly higher incidence of psoriasis in the African-American versus western African populations; such an assumption is speculative and must be viewed with strong caution.

ETIOLOGY AND GENETICS

For several decades, psoriasis was characterized as a disease that occurred principally as a result of epidermal cell hyperplasia and dermal inflammation. The attributed characteristics were based on the histopathologic features found in a typical psoriatic plaque and on some convincing laboratory data detailing cell cycle and cell transit time within the epidermis. The epidermis in a psoriatic plaque is hyperplastic and thickened, and there is incomplete or aberrant maturation of epidermal cells above the germinative cell area. The rapid replication of germinative cells within the epidermis is quite noticeable, and there is reduced cell transit time through the thickened epidermis. Extensive abnormalities of the cutaneous vasculature, particularly within the upper dermis, are noted, and there is an increased number of inflammatory cells, that is, lymphocytes, polymorphonuclear leukocytes, and macrophages, accumulated within the dermis and epidermis. The role of each of these cell types in disease has not been fully appreciated. Recently, it has become clear that most of the cells in the dermal cell population in psoriasis are active T cells. These cells are capable of inducing changes within dermal structures that both initiate and maintain the disease state.

Activated T cells within the cutaneous circulation are attracted to the endothelium of the cutaneous vasculature, adhere, and migrate or "traffic" through the vessel wall into the dermis. Once inside the dermis, activated T cells induce changes in keratinocytes, vascular endothelial cells, and other inflammatory cells of the dermis, including other T-lymphocytes, macrophages, and dendritic cells. The secretion of a number of proteins, or *-kines,* by these varied cell types induces changes in epidermal keratinocytes that ultimately lead to the formation and maintenance of the psoriatic lesion.

Genetic transmission of psoriasis is well documented, and considerable evidence has accumulated that susceptibility to develop psoriasis is strongly associated with certain human leukocyte antigens (HLAs), particularly HLA-A1, HLA-A2, HLA-B17, HLA-B13, HLA-B37, HLA-B39, HLA-Bw57, HLA-Cw6, HLA-Cw7, HLA-Cw11, and HLA-DR7.[11] The onset of disease at an early age is frequently associated with HLA-B13, HLA-B17, and HLA-Cw6. The frequencies of association tend to vary among different racial and ethnic groups. For example, HLA-Cw6 is felt to be the strongest risk factor in white psoriatic patients, where 50–80% have the HLA-Cw6 antigen.[12] In contrast, only 17% of Chinese patients with psoriasis carry HLA-Cw6.[13] Interestingly, however, the HLA-Cw6 allele in Chinese patients is still correlated with higher risk of psoriasis; in one study, 18.6% of Taiwanese psoriasis patients had the allele versus 6.6% of control individuals.[14,15] Among Japanese patients with psoriasis, the incidences of HLA-A1, HLA-A2, HLA-B39, HLA-Bw46, HLA-Cw1, HLA-B46, HLA-DQB1*03, HLA-DR9, HLA-Cw6, HLA-Cw7, and HLA-Cw11 are higher than in control individuals.[15–19]

In one study from northern India, HLA-Cw6 showed a very strong correlation with psoriasis.[20] In contrast, while the prevalence of psoriasis is higher in eastern Africa than in western Africa, the distribution of HLA-Cw6 in eastern Africa does not differ appreciably from that in western Africa.

Psoriatic spondyloarthritis is often associated with HLA-B27. In European whites, the prevalence of HLA-B27 in patients with psoriatic arthritis is 40–50% versus 8% in the general population. In Japan, HLA-B27 prevalence is low (<1%), and the incidence of spondyloarthropathies is also exceedingly low.[21]

CLINICAL MANIFESTATIONS

There are very few published studies that document the specific clinical features of psoriasis in ethnic populations. Based on case reports and other experiential data, psoriasis appears to present similarly across skin types. In this section we describe the general clinical manifestations of psoriasis and the available data regarding any specific ethnic variations.

The clinical onset of nonpustular psoriasis occurs during two peak age ranges. Early-onset disease peaks around the second decade, at ages 16 for females and 20 for males. Late-onset disease peaks at ages 57–60. This bimodal distribution for age of onset appears to hold true for most ethnic groups.

The primary lesion in psoriasis patients with lighter skin is a red, scaling papule that further develops into a red, scaling plaque with sharply demarcated

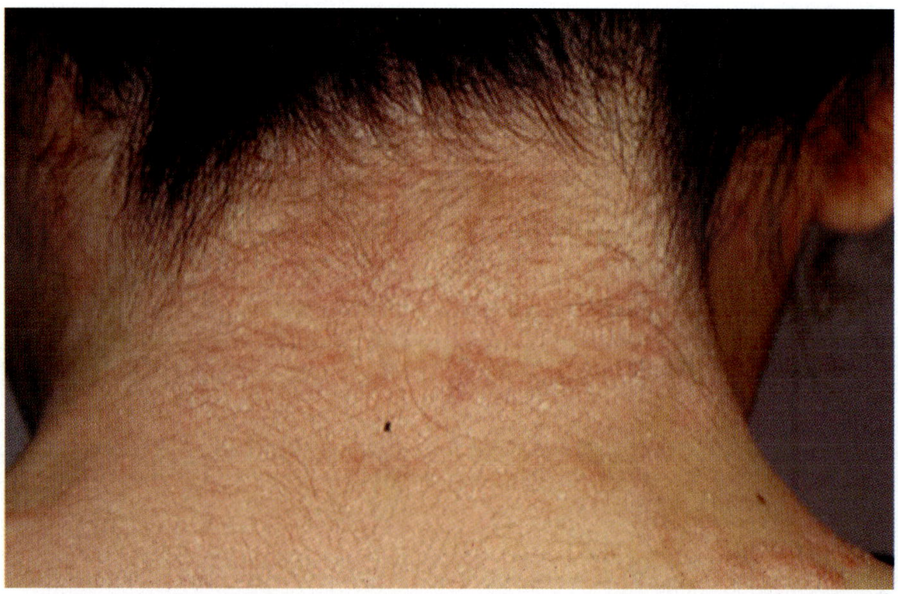

▲ **FIGURE 22-1** With lighter skin, such as that of this Hispanic patient, the primary lesions are salmon-pink plaques with silver-white scale.

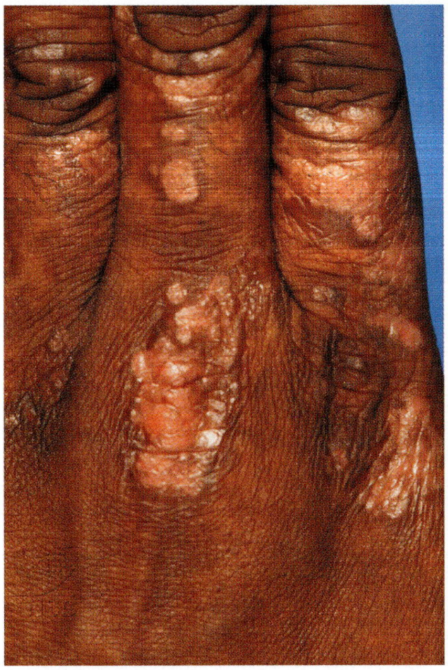

▲ **FIGURE 22-2** Chronic plaque psoriasis. Well-demarcated salmon-pink papules and plaques on the dorsum of hand and fingers of an Asian patient. Courtesy of the National Skin Centre, Singapore.

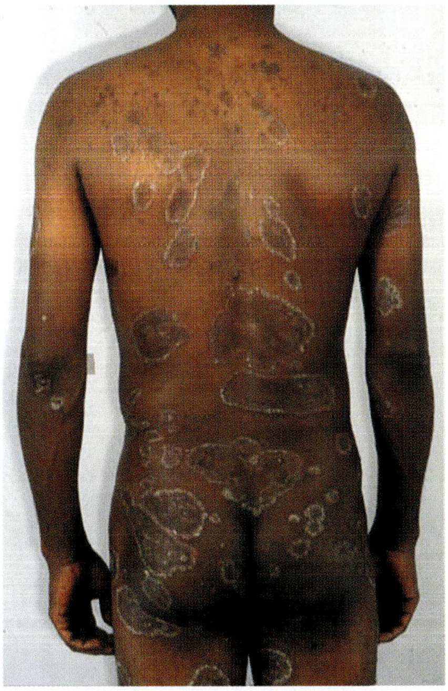

▲ **FIGURE 22-4** In patients with darker skin, such as that of this African-American patient, the papules and plaques are violaceous with gray scale.

peripheral borders (Figures 22-1 through 22-3). The scale is silvery white. Plaques are often localized to the elbows, knees, scalp, umbilicus, and intergluteal fold. In patients with dark skin, the distribution is similar, but the papules and plaques are usually violaceous with a gray scale (Figures 22-4 through 22-7). Intertriginous involvement often manifests as smooth, pink to violaceous plaques depending on underlying skin color (Figure 22-8). On the palms and soles, well-demarcated lesions with a pink to red hue may contain collections of sterile pustules and at times thick scale (Figure 22-9). Enlarging plaques may expand to encompass more than 50% of the body surface area (Figure 22-10). External trauma, including rubbing, scratching, or scrubbing of the skin, leads to long-term maintenance of the individual psoriatic plaque; this is known as the *Koebner phenomenon.*

Textbook guttate psoriasis presents with large numbers of small, red- to salmon-colored papules and plaques that may be covered with a very fine silvery scale. In darker skin with guttate psoriasis, violaceous and gray colors predominate (Figure 22-11). This type of psoriasis often occurs with an explosive or rapid onset, primarily in young patients, and its onset is frequently associated with upper respiratory infections such as viral or streptococcal pharyngitis. Guttate psoriasis is often noted as the initial episode of psoriasis.

Pustular psoriasis is characterized by the development of groups of macroscopic sterile pustules located at the periphery of stable plaques, or it may erupt spontaneously in the absence of identifiable psoriatic lesions. Generalized pustular psoriasis presents with large clusters or sheets of pustules on a fiery red base and usually represents a very serious, potentially fatal presentation of disease. High fevers, chills, and a peripheral leukocytosis accompany the acute onset of pustules. Generalized pustular psoriasis may be lethal in improperly diagnosed and treated patients. Severe cases of pustular psoriasis such as generalized pustular psoriasis are often seen in patients with extensive psoriasis who have been treated with systemic or intensive and prolonged topical corticosteroids. Pustular psoriasis of a less severe nature also may occur as a primary manifestation of palmoplantar psoriasis. The characteristic lesion may present initially on the inner sole of the foot, eventually spreading to engulf the entire foot or hand (Figure 22-12). The distinction

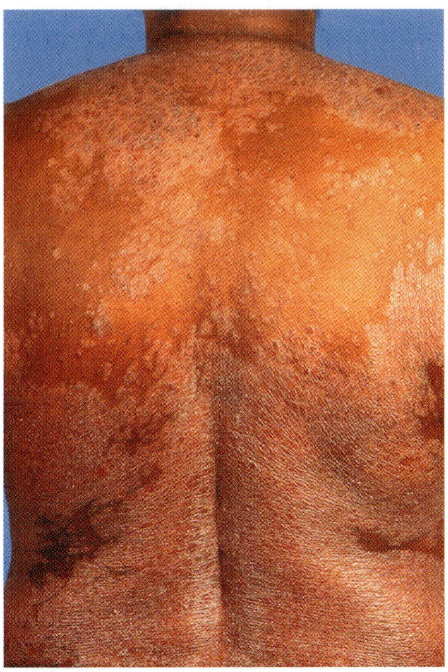

▲ **FIGURE 22-3** Chronic plaque psoriasis. Extensive well-demarcated salmon-pink scaly plaques on the back of an Asian patient. Courtesy of the National Skin Centre, Singapore.

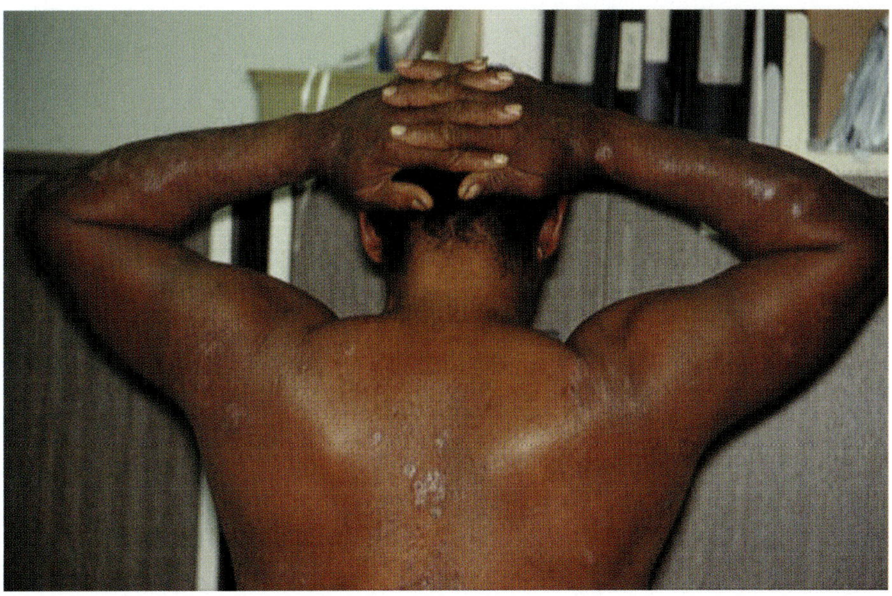

▲ **FIGURE 22-5** Well-demarcated pink to violaceous papules and plaques with scale in this African-American patient with psoriasis.

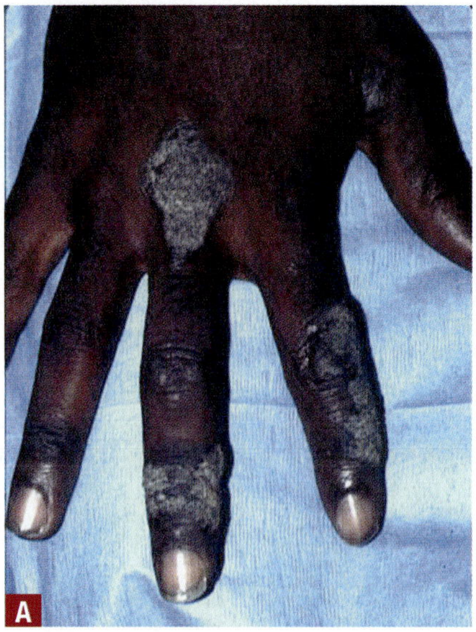

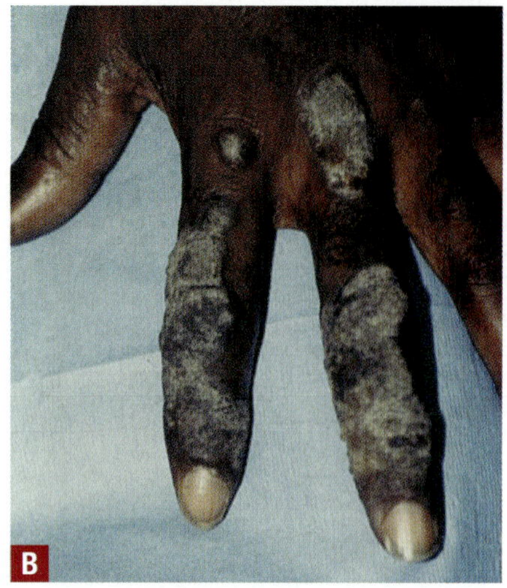

▲ **FIGURE 22-6** This African-American patient had violaceous plaques with thick, micaceous, gray scale on the dorsal fingers.

between palmoplantar pustular psoriasis and dyshidrotic eczema may be difficult to make.

Erythrodermic psoriasis may present at any time during the course of psoriasis. It manifests as diffuse, generalized redness of the skin associated with extensive scaling. The skin feels warm to touch, and body temperature control becomes quite erratic. Cutaneous blood flow increases, initiating a stream of abnormal metabolic events that result in a severely ill patient. The sudden withdrawal of long-term systemic or intensive topical corticosteroid treatment often serves as the trigger for developing erythrodermic psoriasis.

Nail changes are relatively common in psoriasis. They are quite characteristic and often diagnostic yet bear no relationship to the severity of psoriasis. Pitting of the nail is the most common finding, followed by leukonychia and longitudinal grooves and ridges. Often a reddish brown discoloration of the nail bed results in the appearance of a characteristic "oil drop" sign. Subungual hyperkeratosis also may be observed. The number of involved nails varies.

The prevalence and frequency of occurrence of psoriatic arthritis remain in dispute because the criteria for evaluating arthritis in the individual patient or large patient populations vary widely among physicians. Psoriatic arthritis, like the disease psoriasis, is believed to occur as a result of inflammation and excessive cellular proliferation. The histologic picture in affected joints of patients with psoriatic arthritis shows similar features to those found in the skin of patients with psoriasis.

Psoriatic arthritis is classified into five subgroups: (1) asymmetric oligoarticular arthritis, found in over 70% of patients with arthritis and characterized by the typical "sausage-shaped digits," (2) symmetric metacarpophalangeal joint involvement, (3) distal interphalangeal joint involvement, producing the pathognomonic "swan neck" deformity, (4) arthritis mutilans, characterized by extensive bone resorption, and (5) spondylitis or spondyloarthropathy. The age of onset peaks at about 40 years, and onset is often acute. A few cases of acute-onset psoriatic arthritis have been observed by the senior author in young female patients with a degree of severity that required long-term treatment with antineoplastic agents.

As noted previously, there are a few studies describing the clinical characteristics of psoriasis in skin of darker phototypes. In a study of 1220 psoriatic

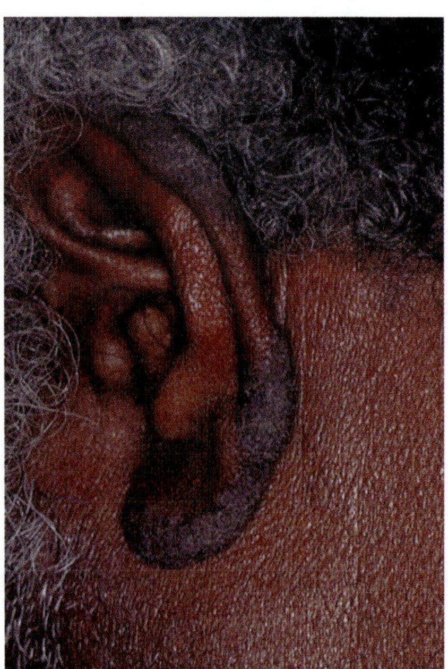

▲ **FIGURE 22-7** Well-demarcated violaceous plaques with gray scale on the helix of the ear of this African-American patient.

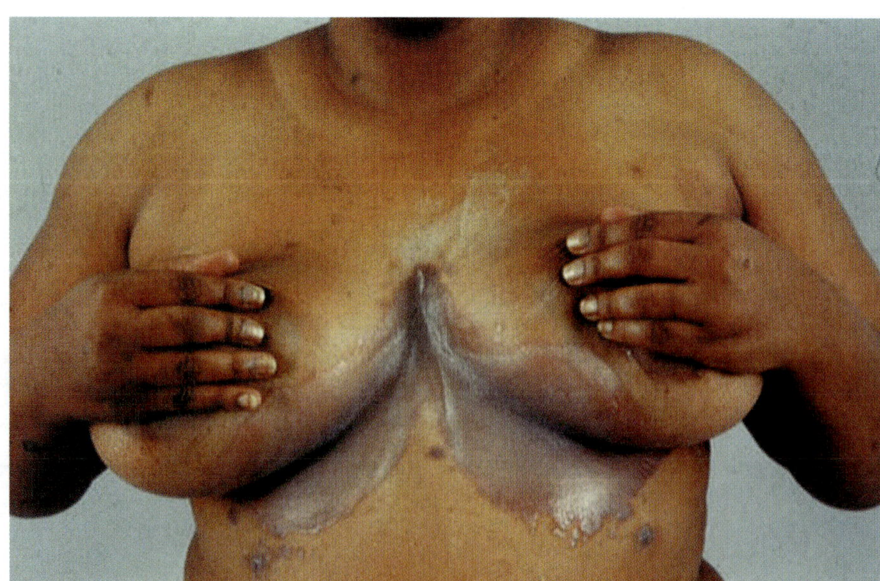

▲ **FIGURE 22-8** Intertriginous involvement manifested as smooth violaceous plaques in this African-American patient.

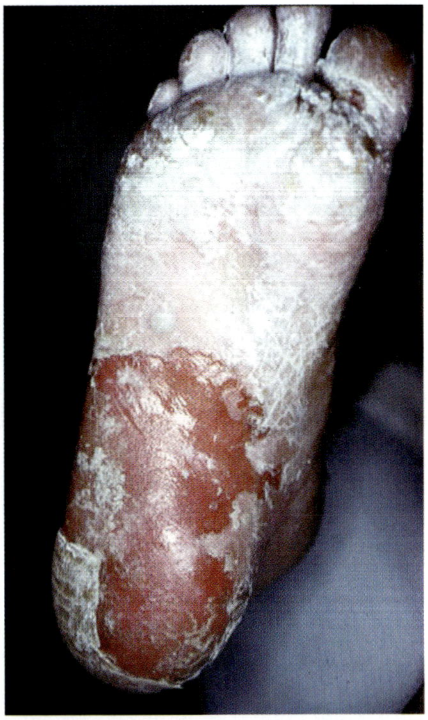

▲ **FIGURE 22-9** Plantar foot psoriasis with thick, micaceous scale in this African-American patient.

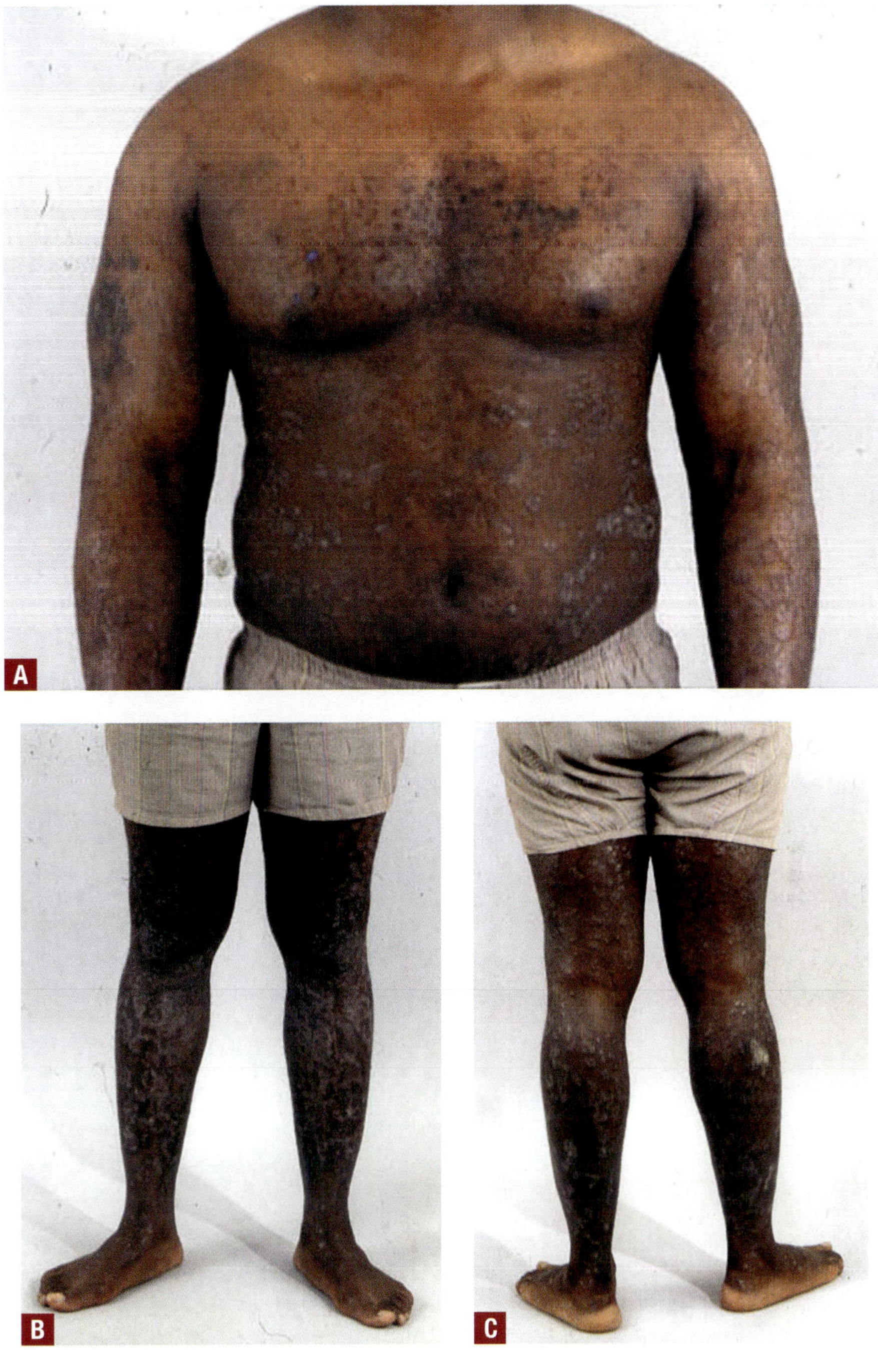

▲ **FIGURE 22-10** Enlarging plaques may expand and coalesce to encompass large body surface areas. This African-American patient had psoriasis involving the chest, arms, abdomen, back, and legs.

patients in India, 93% had plaque-type psoriasis, followed by pustular, guttate, erythrodermic, nail, flexural, and arthropathic types of psoriasis.[22] In this case series, the extent of disease in patients was mild, involving less than 25% of body surface area. Most patients described their lesions as relatively asymptomatic with minor pruritus and burning, and postinflammatory hyperpigmentation was observed more commonly than hypopigmentation. In this study, only a few of the Indian patients admitted to having cosmetic embarrassment from their skin lesions.

In a similar study from Sri Lanka, 5–10% of patients identified specific triggers of psoriasis; these included most commonly sore throat, pregnancy or parturition, and chloroquine use. Other less common precipitating factors such as chickenpox, diarrhea, alcohol use, and mental stress also were identified.[23]

Nail involvement in Indian and Sri Lankan patients varies from 14–56%, and pitting of the nail was the most commonly reported nail change. Fewer than 1% of patients had psoriasis limited to the nails.[23]

Studies from India also have described a higher incidence of palmoplantar psoriasis. Predisposing factors likely include occupational trauma from manual labor and from the practice of wearing open-toed slippers and the Indian custom of walking barefoot.[24] The prevalence of psoriatic arthritis in the Indian psoriatic population is lower (4%) than in the U.S. psoriatic population (10%). In a case-controlled study of 80 patients with psoriasis in Singapore, ethnic Indians were twice as likely to have psoriatic arthritis than ethnic Chinese patients.[25]

A survey of 28,628 Japanese patients with psoriasis revealed that the vast majority had plaque-type psoriasis vulgaris (86%), followed by guttate psoriasis (2.8%), psoriatic erythroderma (0.8%), generalized pustular psoriasis (0.9%), localized pustular psoriasis (0.5), and psoriatic arthritis (1.0%).[26] In African-American and Native American patients, there appears to be little difference in the clinical presentation of psoriasis compared with other skin phototypes; most patients seem to have classic plaque-type disease. The course of the disease has been described as "mild," with only a few reported cases of erythrodermic psoriasis.

In a 1967 study by Verhagen and colleagues of 1230 Kenyan patients, the

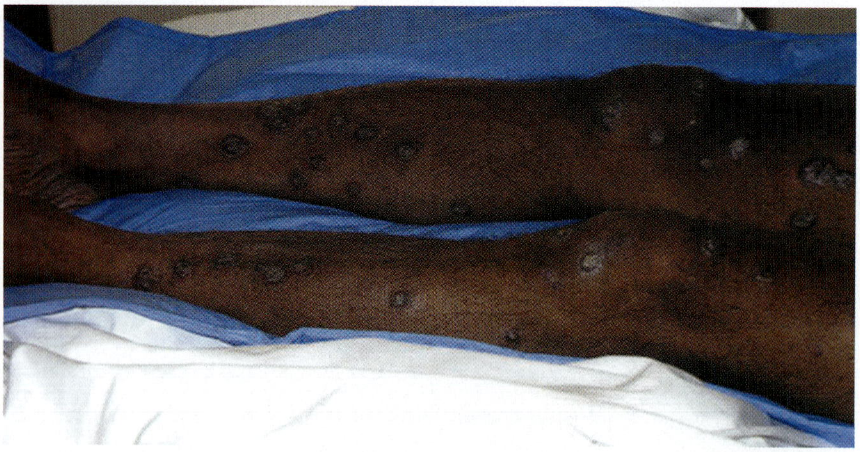

▲ **FIGURE 22-11** In darker skin with guttate psoriasis, violaceous and gray colors predominate.

prevalence of psoriasis was 2.6%. The diagnosis was established using the same criteria used in Western countries. In contrast to the hyperpigmentation seen in the Indian and Sri Lankan populations, Verhagen described "hypopigmentation as an outspoken feature in African skin" during both active disease and in residual lesions.[27]

In a series of 12 patients with hypertrophic or verrucous psoriasis, a rarely reported histologic subtype of psoriasis, the ethnicities were as follows: Caucasian (8), Hispanic (3), and African (1).[28]

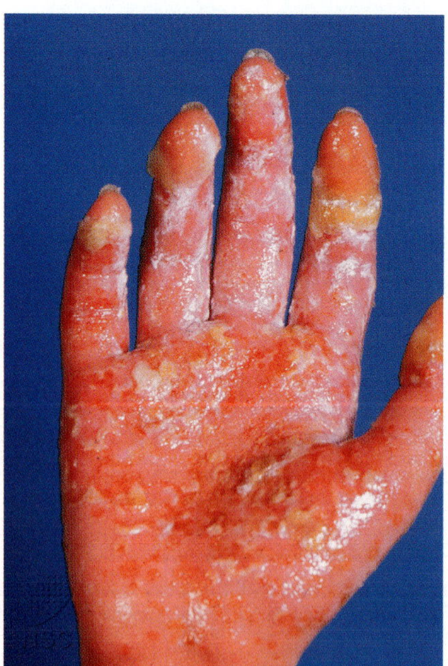

▲ **FIGURE 22-12** Pustular psoriasis may occur as a primary manifestation of palmoplantar psoriasis. In this Asian patient, the characteristic plustar and crusted erosions spread to engulf the hand and fingers. Courtsey of the National Skin Centre, Singapore.

TREATMENT OF PSORIASIS

The treatment of psoriasis seems to be similar across all ethnic populations; standard therapies include anthralins, topical and systemic glucocorticosteroids, tar, calcipotriene, topical and oral retinoids, phototherapy, and immunosuppressive medications. Newer, experimental treatments include biologic therapies and the 308-nm excimer laser. However, while standard treatments are shared worldwide, certain cultures have developed unique treatment regimens.

Complementary and alternative medicine (CAM) for psoriasis will be discussed in this section. Fifty-one percent of psoriasis patients in the United States and Great Britain have tried alternative therapies,[29,30] and in ethnic populations, the prevalence of CAM usage may be even higher.

In a study of 28,628 psoriatic patients in Japan, topical corticosteroid use was the most common treatment modality (68%). Topical vitamin D derivatives were used rarely (2.4%). Phototherapeutic regimens included use of topical psoralen and ultraviolet A (PUVA; 12%), systemic PUVA (8%), and ultraviolet B (UVB; 311-313). PUVA is contraindicated in psoriasis patients who are pregnant or lactating (0.5%). Systemic regimens included, most commonly, herbal medicine (14%), followed by etretinate (7.6%), nonsteroidal anti-inflammatory drugs (4.4%), oral corticosteroids (4.1%), methotrexate (2.8%), cyclosporine (1.6%), and other antineoplastic medications (1.4%).

Of note, phototherapy may be relatively unpopular among Asian patients owing to a cultural aversion to tanning. A tanned complexion is considered a sign of having to perform manual outdoor labor and is considered undesirable. Asian patients have been reported to complain about unwanted tanning from phototherapy,[31] and one should consider the issue of compliance when prescribing phototherapy in this ethnic population.

Several traditional Chinese herbal products have been shown to be effective in the treatment of psoriasis through anti-inflammatory and/or immunosuppressive properties, including indirubin, *Tripterygium wilfordii* Hook, and *Tripterygium hypoglaucum* Hutch. Side effects include gastrointestinal symptoms, myelosuppression, and elevated liver function tests.[32–43] *T. wilfordii* Hook was used to good effect in 638 patients with psoriatic arthritis, 16 patients with pustular psoriasis, and 5 patients with erythrodermic psoriasis.[14,44,45]

Another traditional Chinese herb, *Radix angelicae dahuricae,* has been used topically with ultraviolet A for a psoralen-like effect. *R. angelicae dahuricae* contains imperatorin, isoimperatorin, and alloimperatorin, which, like psoralens, are furocoumarins. Psoriasis clearance rates were similar between *R. angelicae dahuricae* with UVA versus PUVA, but with fewer side effects.[46–48] *R. angelicae pubescentis* also has been used successfully with UVA.[49]

Traditional Chinese medicine (TCM) usually involves the use of multiple herbs simultaneously, but there are very few studies of multiple-agent TCM treatment of psoriasis. Notably, a study of 801 patients with psoriasis found a 50–85% response rate in patients treated with a mixture of five herbs (*Rhizoma sparganii, Rhizoma zedoariae, Herba serissae, Resina boswelliae,* and *Myrrha*).[50]

Acupuncture also is used for psoriasis. In a case series of 61 patients with refractory psoriasis, 50% had complete to near-complete clearance and 33% had partial improvement with acupuncture.[51] In contrast, a Swedish study reported no difference between patients treated with TCM-indicated points and patients treated with sham points.[52] Note, however, that the use of sham points may itself have a physiologic effect and thus is not usually considered to be an adequate control.[53]

In India, the overall cost-benefit ratio of treatments becomes an important factor in treatment decisions, especially in a chronic disease like psoriasis. Coal tar is still considered to be the most useful topical agent because the cost is nearly 25 times less than that of calcipotriol.[54] Anthralin and topical steroids are also cost-effective options and are used for localized disease.[55] In extensive psoriasis, methotrexate is the drug of choice in India primarily because of its affordability and relatively few associated side effects. Hydroxyurea is used as a second-line agent for patients who are intolerant of methotrexate. Retinoids are not available, likely owing to their associated teratogenic effects.

Alternative therapeutic regimens have implemented ayurvedic or herbal therapy in treating psoriasis and psoriatic arthritis. Neem oil (from the Neem tree, *Azadirachta indixa*) has been used for treating localized plaque psoriasis primarily for its emollient properties.[56] This inexpensive oil removes scale from thickened psoriatic plaques and also functions as an anti-inflammatory agent. Its properties, like those of coal tar, are enhanced when used with ultraviolet light. Turmeric (*Curcuma longa*) is another inexpensive alternative topical agent for psoriasis. This mustard-yellow, fragrant powder is made from the stems of a ginger-root-like plant and is used most often in curry powder. Outside the kitchen, turmeric is prized for its anti-inflammatory and powerful antioxidant properties. This powder can be mixed with water or aloe vera gel to form a paste that can be applied directly to psoriatic skin lesions.[57]

Another ayurvedic therapy is the practice of *snehapanam,* in which medicated *ghee* (clarified butter) or specific herbal oils are combined and consumed by the patient over a 2-week period in increasing quantities. This process is designed to purify the blood and is thought to heal the body in conditions such as psoriasis and psoriatic arthritis.

Stress can exacerbate psoriasis and is an important factor to address especially in refractory cases of psoriasis. Complementary and alternative therapies such as TCM and ayurvedic medicine emphasize the importance of lifestyle in the management of psoriasis. Practices such as yoga, taichi, and meditation are encouraged to achieve a state of mental well-being and thus contribute holistically to the management of psoriasis.

CONCLUSION

Psoriasis occurs worldwide, but there is scant research characterizing the disease in individual ethnicities. Overall, the prevalence of psoriasis seems to be lower in certain ethnic populations, including certain populations of Africa, East Asia, India, and Samoa and indigenous populations of the Americas. Some data suggest that there may exist ethnic differences in the genetic predisposition to develop psoriasis. While clinical manifestations may differ slightly, the treatment of psoriasis seems to be similar among various populations, although certain cultures have developed unique treatment regimens, including cost-effective therapies and herbal medicine. There is a need for additional studies of psoriasis and ethnic skin.

REFERENCES

1. Raychauduri SP, Farber EM. The prevalence of psoriasis in the world. *J Eur Acad Dermatol Venerol* 2001;15:16-17.
2. Yip SY. The prevalence of psoriasis in the Mongoloid race. *J Am Acad Dermatol* 1984;10:965-968.
3. Cheng L,Zhang SZ, Xiao CY, et al. The A5.1 allele of the major histocompatibility complex class I chain-related gene A is associated with psoriasis vulgaris in Chinese. *Br J Dermatol* 2000;143:324-329.
4. Aoki T. Psoriasis in Japan. *Arch Dermatol* 1971;104:328-329.
5. Lin XR. Psoriasis in China. *J Dermatol* 1993;20:746-755.
6. Farber EM, Nall L. Psoriasis in the tropics: Epidemiologic, genetic, clinical, and therapeutic aspects. *Dermatol Clin* 1994;12: 805-816.
7. Gelfand JM, Stern RS, Nijsten T, et al. The prevalence of psoriasis in African-Americans: Results from a population-based study. *J Am Acad Dermatol* 2005;52: 23-26.
8. Jacyk WK. Psoriasis in Nigerians. *Trop Geogr Med* 1981;33:139-142.
9. Leder RO, Farber EM. The variable incidence of psoriasis in sub-Saharan Africa. *Int J Dermatol* 1997;36:911-919.
10. Gelfand JM, Stern RS, Feldman SR, et al. The prevalence of psoriasis in African-Americans: Results from a population-based study. *J Am Acad Dermatol* 2005;52: 23-26.
11. Ikaheimo I, Silvennoinen-Kassine S, Karvonen J, et al. Immunogenetic profile of psoriasis vulgaris association with haplotypes A2, B13, Cw6, DR7, DQA1*0201 and A1, B17, Cw6, DR7, DQA1*0201. *Arch Dermatol Res* 1996;288:63-67.
12. Wuepper KD, Coulter SN, Haberman A. Psoriasis vulgaris: A genetic approach. *J Invest Dermatol* 1990; 95:2-4S.
13. Cao K, Song FJ, Li HG, et al. Association between HLA antigens and families with psoriasis vulgaris. *Chin Med J* 1993;06: 132-135.
14. Tsai TF, Hu CY, Tsai WL, et al. HLA-Cw6 specificity and polymorphic residues are associated with susceptibility among Chinese psoriatics in Taiwan. *Arch Dermatol Res* 2002; 294:214-220.
15. Chang YT, Tsai SF, Lee DD, et al. A study of candidate genes for psorasis near HLA-C in Chinese patients with psoriasis. *Br J Dermatol* 2003:148:418-423.
16. Ozawa A, Miyahara M, Sugai J, et al. HLA class I and II alleles and susceptibility to generalized pustular psoriasis: Significant associations with HLA-Cw1 and HLA-DQB1*0303. *J Dermatol* 1998;25:573-581.
17. Asahina A, Kuwata S, Tokunanga K, et al. Study of aspartate at residue 9 of HLA-C molecules in Japanese patients with psoriasis vulgaris. *J Dermatol Sci* 1995;13:125-133.
18. Torii H, Nakagawa H, Ishibashi Y, et al. Genetic polymorphisms in HLA-A, -B, -C, and -DR antigens in Japanese patients with palmoplantar pustulosis. *Dermatology* 1994;188:290-292.
19. Nakagawa H, Akazaki S, Asahina A, et al. Study of HLA class I, class II, and complement genes (C2, C4A, C4B, and BF) in Japanese psoriatics and analysis of a newly found high-risk haplotype by pulsed field gel electrophoresis. *Arch Dermatol Res* 1991;283:281-284.
20. Rani R, Narayan R, Fernandez-VinMa A, et al. HLA-B and C alleles in psoriasis in patients in North India. *Tissue Antigens* 1998;51:618-622.
21. Hukuda S, Minami M, Saito T, et al. Spondyloarthropathies in Japan: Nationwide questionnaire survey performed by the Japan Ankylosing Spondylitis Society. *J Rheumatol* 2001;28: 554-559.
22. Kaur I, Handa S, Kumar B. Natural history of psoriasis: Study from the Indian subcontinent. *J Dermatol* 1997; 24:230-234.
23. Gunawardena DA, Gunawardena KA, Vasanthanathan NS, Gunawardena JA. Psoriasis in Sri Lanka: A computer analysis of 1366 cases. *Br J Dermatol* 1978;98: 85-96.
24. Kumar B, Saraswat A, Kaur I. Palmoplantar lesions in psoriasis. *Acta Dermatol Venerol* 2002;82:192-195.
25. Thumboo J, Tham SN, Tay YK. Patterns of psoriatic arthritis in Orientals. *J Rheumatol* 1997;24: 1949-1953.
26. Kawada A, Tezuka T, Nakamizo Y, et al. A survey of psoriasis patients in Japan from 1982-2001. *J Dermatol Sci* 2003;31: 59-64.
27. Verhagen ARHB, Koten JW. Psoriasis in Kenya. *Arch Dermatol* 1967;96:39-41.
28. Khalil FK, Keehn CA, Saeed S, Morgan MB. Verrucous psoriasis: A distinctive clinicopathologic variant of psoriasis. *Am J Dermatopathol* 2005;27:204-207.
29. Fleischer AB, Feldman SR, Rapp SR, et al. Alternative therapies commonly used within a population of patients with psoriasis. *Cutis* 1996;58: 216-220.
30. Clark CM, Mckay RA, Fortune DG, et al. Use of alternative treatments by patients with psoriasis. *Br J Gen Pract* 1998;48: 1873-1874.
31. Choe YB, Rim JH, Youn JI. Quantitative assessment of narrow-band UVB induced tanning during phototherapy in Korea. *Photodermatol Photoimmunol Photomed* 2002; 18:127-130.
32. Prieto JM, Recio MC, Giner RM, et al. Influence of traditional Chinese anti-inflammatory medicinal plants on leukocyte and platelet functions. *J Pharm Pharmacol* 2003;55:1275-1282.
33. Koo J, Desai R. Traditional Chinese medicine in dermatology. *Dermatol Ther* 2003; 16:98-105.
34. Wang MX, Wang HL, Lui WS, et al. Study of the therapeutic effect and pharmacological action of indirubin in treating psoriasis. *Chin J Dermatol* 1982;15: 157-160.
35. Lu YT. Treating 159 cases of psoriasis vulgaris with *pilulae Indigo naturalis compositae. Chin J Integr Tradit West Med* 1989; 9:558.

36. Yuan ZZ, Yuan X, Xu ZX. An observation on the therapeutic effect of *Indigo naturalis* in 46 cases of psoriasis. *J Tradit Chin Med* 1982; 23:43.
37. Chen LZ. Treating 23 cases of psoriasis with indirubin tablets. *J Clin Dermatol* 1981;10:157-158.
38. Ling MW, Chen DY, Zhu YX, et al. Treatment of 26 cases of psoriasis with indirubin. *J Clin Dermatol* 1982;11: 131-132.
39. Yan SF. A clinical observation of treating 43 cases of psoriasis with indirubin. *Yunnan J Tradit Chin Med* 1982;2:21.
40. Lin XR, Yang CM, Yang GL, et al. Treatment of psoriasis with meisoindigo. *J Clin Dermatol* 1989;18:29-30.
41. Yang CM, Lin XR, Yang GL, et al. A study of the treatment of psoriasis with meisindigo. *J Clin Dermatol* 1989;18: 295-297.
42. Chen NQ, Dai ZH, Wang LZ. An observation of the effectiveness of *N*-acetylindirubin in treating psoriasis. *J Clin Dermatol* 1988; 17:328.
43. Xie ZZ. Treatment of psoriasis with *pilulae Indigo naturalis compositae*. *J Tradit Chin Med* 1984;25:39-40.
44. Guan F, Wong DH. Treatment of psoriasis with *Tripterygium wilfordii* Hook. *J Clin Dermatol* 1981;10:91-93.
45. Zhang JY. Treating 148 cases of psoriasis vulgaris with *Tripterygium wilfordii* Hook. *J Clin Dermatol* 1982;11:118.
46. Zhang GW, Li SB, Wang HJ, et al. Inhibition of Chinese herb medicine, *Angelica dahurica* (Benth et Hook) and UVA synthesis of DNA of lymphocytes in vitro. *Chin J Dermatol* 1980;13:138-140.
47. Zhang GW. [Treatment of psoriasis by photochemotherapy: A comparison between the photosensitizing capsule of *Angelica dahurica* and 8-MOP.] *Zhonghua Yi Xue Za Zhi* 1983;63:16-19.
48. Shi SY, Xu S, Yian YP. A therapeutic evaluation of *Tripterygium wilfordii* Hook in the treatment of 19 cases of psoriatic arthritis. *J Clin Dermatol* 1988:17:294-296.
49. Li FQ. Cases suffering from psoriasis treated with traditional Chinese medicine *Angelicae tuhuo* and long wave ultraviolet. *Chin J Phys Ther* 1983;6:144-145.
50. Lin CH, Wang HY. Comparison of long term clinical effects of microcirculation modulation traditional drugs and ethylene diamine tetraacetylimide in the treatment of psoriasis. *J Clin Dermatol* 1988; 17:125-130.
51. Liao SJ, Liao TA. Acupuncture treatment for psoriasis: A retrospective case report. *Acupunct Electrother Res* 1992;17:195-208.
52. Jerner B, Skogh M, Vahlquist A. A controlled trial of acupuncture in psoriasis: No convincing effect. *Acta Derm Venereol* 1997;77:154-156.
53. Streitberger K, Kleinhenz J. Introducing a placebo needle into acupuncture research. *Lancet* 1998;352:364-365.
54. Sharma V, Kaur I, Kumar B. Calcipotriol versus coal tar: A prospective randomized study in stable plaque psoriasis. *Int J Dermatol* 2003;42:834-838.
55. Agarwal R, Saraswat A, Kaur I, et al. A novel liposomal formulation of dithranol in psoriasis: Preliminary results. *J Dermatol Treat* 2002;13:119-122.
56. Subapriya R, Nagini S. Medicinal properties of Neem leaves: A review. *Curr Med Chem Anticancer Agents* 2005;5:149-156.
57. Shishodia S, Sethi G, Agarwal BB. Curcumin: Getting back to the roots. *Ann NY Acad Sci* 2005;1056:206-217.
58. Farber EM, Nall ML. Epidemiology: Natural history and genetics, in Roenigk HH, Maibach HI (eds), *Psoriasis*. New York, Marcel Dekker, 1998, pp 107-158.
59. Campalani E, Barker JNWN. The clinical genetics of psoriasis. *Curr Genomics* 2005; 6:51-60.
60. Farber EM, Nall ML. Epidemiology: Natural history and genetics, in Roenigk HH, Mailbach HI. (eds), *Psoriasis*. New York, Marcel Dekker, 1991, pp 209-258.
61. Lomholt G. Prevalence of skin diseases in a population: A census study from the Faroe Islands. *Danish Med Bull* 1964;11:1-7.
62. Stern RS, Nijsten T, Feldman SR, et al. Psoriasis is common, carries a substantial burden even when not extensive, and is associated with widespread treatment dissatisfaction. *J Investig Dermatol Symp Proc* 2004;9:136-139.

CHAPTER 23

Pityriasis Rosea

Dwana R. Shabazz

Key Points

- Self-limiting papulosquamous dermatosis found worldwide without racial predilection
- Higher incidence in the spring and fall with possible viral etiology (HHV-6, HHV7)
- Violaceous- or gray-colored lesions in darker skin and salmon or rose-colored in white skin
- Association with drugs (e.g., barbiturates, metronidazole, terbinafin, isotretinoin and gold)
- Treatment with erythromycin is controversial

Pityriasis rosea (PR) is an acute, self-limiting papulosquamous dermatosis that is thought to be of viral origin. It occurs over a broad age range, most often between the ages of 10 and 35 years and rarely before age 2. Peak occurrence is during the spring and fall seasons. It usually has a classic clinical presentation and is asymptomatic and undergoes spontaneous resolution in 6–10 weeks.

PR is found worldwide without racial predilection. In an overview of disorders more commonly seen in ethnic skin, including African-Americans, Hispanics, and Asians, PR was listed as occurring in about 2% of African-Americans patient seen by dermatologists.[1]

The incidence of PR has been decreasing. This may be due to its self-limited nature, thus never coming to the attention of a physician. Furthermore, dermatologists are usually the second or third physician a patient sees for diagnosis and treatment of PR, and at that point, the patient often has cleared and wants to know the cause of the dermatosis and/or the patient has healed with postinflammatory dyspigmentation, especially hyperpigmentation (Table 23-1).

Since PR may differ clinically in those with black versus white skin, it is important to highlight clinical differences, as well as to be aware of the effects of certain treatment options on skin of color.

TABLE 23-1
General Information

- Occurs in 2% of black dermatology patients
- Onset usually between the ages of 10 and 35 years
- Spontaneous resolution in 6 to 10 weeks

PATHOGENESIS

PR is thought to be due to a virus or bacterium. Most of the literature points to a viral etiology.[2] Human herpes virus 6 (HHV-6) and human herpes virus 7 (HHV-7) are the two viruses most closely associated with PR, although this correlation is inconclusive (Table 23-2).

HHV-6 belongs to genus *Roseolavirus* and is closely homologous with HHV-7; thus HHV-7 belongs to the same genus. HHV-6 is widespread in the population and persists in hosts in a latent state in monocytes and bone marrow progenitor cells and as a chronic infection of salivary glands, which is thought to be the mode of transmission.[2] In support of the close association between the two viruses, it has been reported that infection with HHV-7 can lead to reactivation of HHV-6 from latency.[2] HHV-6 causes ballooning and induces apoptosis in uninfected CD4 T cells.[2] In addition, HHV-6 causes the enhancement of natural killer T-cell activity, suppression of peripheral blood mononuclear cell proliferation, and induction of many cytokines.[2] Approximately 95% of the human population is seropositive for HHV-6. As a result, a positive viral culture for HHV-6 does not necessarily correspond to a clinically relevant infection owing to the large number of asymptomatic carriers.

HHV-7 is also prevalent worldwide. The primary infection of HHV-7 occurs in childhood, but later than infections owing to HHV-6. HHV-7 shares its mode of infection with HHV-6 by showing latency in peripheral blood T cells and a persistent infection in the salivary glands. HHV-7 is prone to reactivation. Less is known about the pathogenecity of HHV-7, but it is thought to be the primary causative agent of PR, with HHV-6 having a close association. However, there is no definitive proof that the viruses are the pathogenesis of PR.

Both HHV 6 and HHV 7 are associated with a febrile illness and exanthem subitum (roseola infantum), which has a characteristic rash. Although a virus is not a proven cause, PR may have fever as a prodrome, a classic exanthem that resolves spontaneously and peaks in the spring and fall, thus supporting a viral etiology.

There have been reports of several drugs causing PR or rashes that look quite similar to PR. PR owing to drugs shows a more atypical pattern, has a longer course, and is more resistant to treatment. Some of the implicated drugs include arsenic, barbiturates, bismuth, captopril, clonidine, D-penicillamine, interferon-α, isotretinoin, metronidazole, gold, omeprazole, and terbinafine[3] (Table 23-3).

TABLE 23-2
Etiology

- Evidence points to a viral etiology
- Human herpes virus 6 (HHV-6) closely associated
- Human herpes virus 7 (HHV-7) also closely associated
- Peak occurrence in spring and fall supports viral origin

TABLE 23-3
Medication Induced PR

- Atypical clinical pattern
- Slower resolution
- More resistant to treatment
- Drugs include gold, arsenic, barbiturates, bismuth, captopril, terbinafine, D-penicillamine, interferon-a, metronidazole, isotretinoin, opeprazole

CLINICAL PICTURE (TABLES 23-4 AND 23-5)

Medical textbooks illustrate a classic cutaneous exanthem of salmon- or rose-colored papules and plaques in Caucasian patients with PR (Figure 23-1). However, in people with dark skin, the lesions are usually violaceous or gray in color (Figure 23-2). Following a fever and a respiratory tract infection in some patients, a herald patch ("mother patch") arises. It is seen in 50–90% of patients with PR (Figure 23-3). About 1–2 weeks later, a generalized secondary rash consisting of oval plaques with a collarette scale (the scale is on the inner border and points to the center of the lesion) develops (Figure 23-4). The secondary

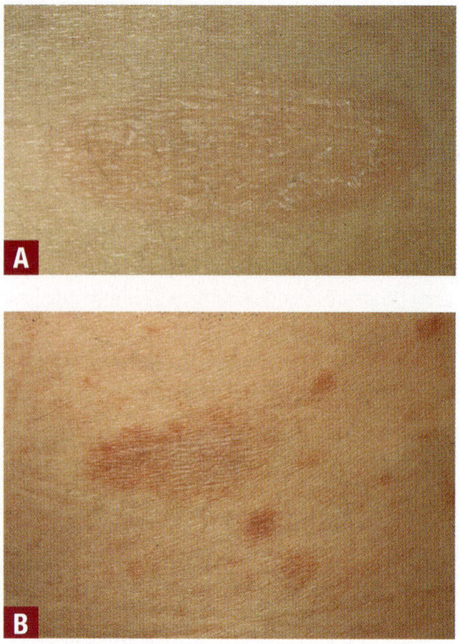

▲ **FIGURE 23-1 A.** The classic salmon-colored lesion in a Caucasian patient with PR. **B.** Rose-colored lesions in a Caucasian patient with PR.

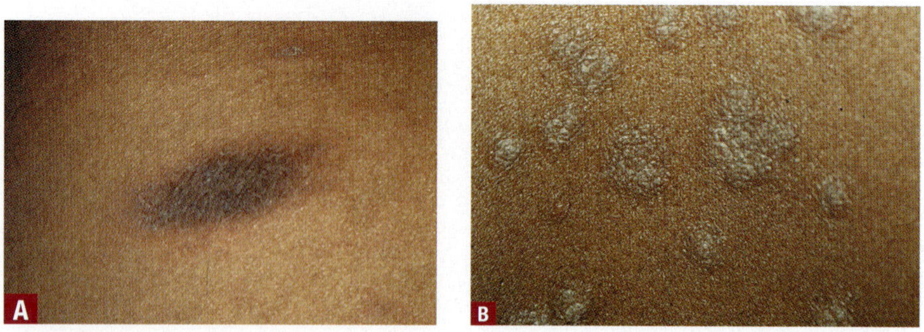

▲ **FIGURE 23-2 A.** A violaceous plaque in an African-American patient with PR. **B.** Gray plaques in an African-American man with PR.

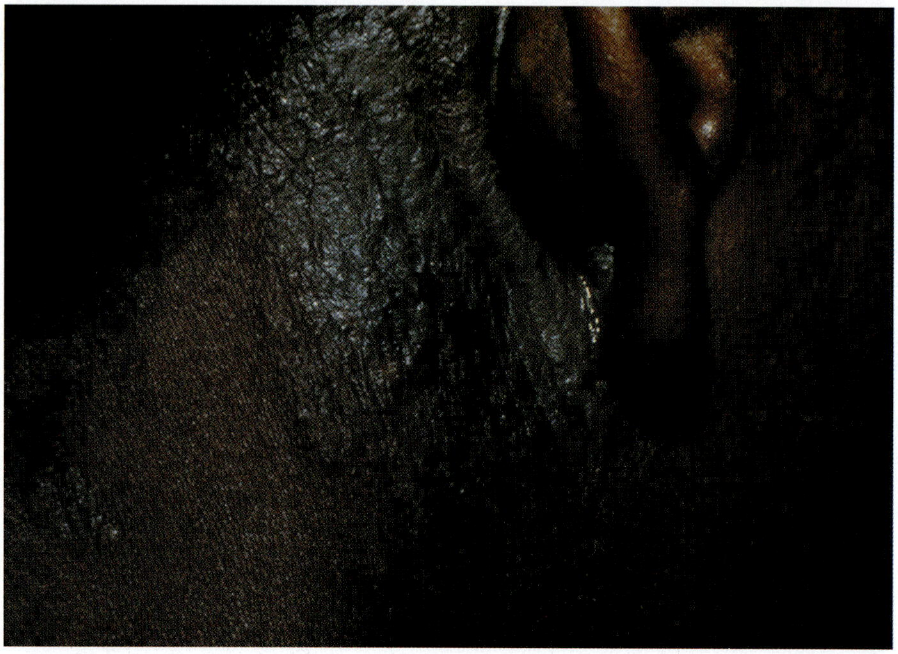

▲ **FIGURE 23-3** A violaceous herald patch of the right posterior auricular area.

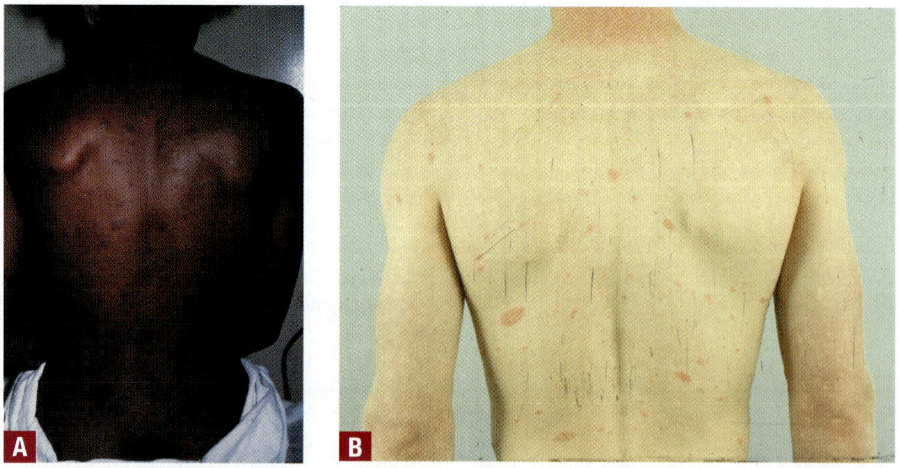

▲ **FIGURE 23-4 A.** Secondary PR rash with several residual patches with collaratte scale. **B.** Secondary lesions with several residual herald pathches in a Hispanic man. The color is a dark erythema somewhat intermediate between the rose- or salmon-colored lesion in a Caucasian and the violaceous or gray lesion seen in African-Americans.

rash develops along Langer's lines and has been characterized as occurring in a "Christmas tree" distribution on the trunk (Figure 23-5) and a "school of minnows" pattern on the flank (Figure 23-6). Sun-exposed areas are seldom involved. In African-American patients, lesions are more papular, and the papules often have small necrotic-like centers (Figure 23-7). African-American patients have more follicular accentuation (Figure 23-8), and the lesions occur in a more inverse pattern, involving the face, neck, axilla, groin, and lower abdomen[4] (Figure 23-9). African-American children are particularly predisposed to the papular variant, which is also prevalent in Hispanic children (Figure 23-10). PR can be pruritic and occurs occasionally on the palms and rarely is generalized (Figure 23-11). In a study assessing the quality of life in children with PR, the majority of the children were only minimally itchy; thus school, other daily activities, and sleep were not greatly affected.[5] PR usually resolves spontaneously in 6–10 weeks, although it occasionally may last 4–5 months. In patients with skin of color, resolution often occurs with postinflammatory hyperpigmentation, although it occasionally results in postinflammatory hypopigmentation. Rarely, the scalp, eyelids, penis, and oral mucosa may be involved.

If PR persists beyond 3 months, the diagnosis must be reconsidered. The Christmas tree distribution on the trunk can be confused with ashy dermatosis,

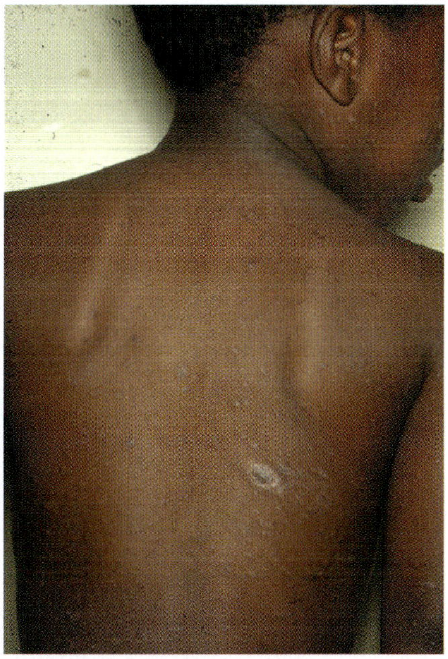

▲ **FIGURE 23-5** A Christmas tree pattern of PR lesions on the back.

other lichenoid reactions, and in the setting of human immunodeficiency virus (HIV) infection, Kaposi sarcoma. Many annular eruptions, such as pityriasis alba, nummular eczema, seborrheic dermatitis, and tinea, may resemble PR. Inverse papular PR can be difficult to distinguish from Gianotti-Crosti syndrome. Secondary syphilis may imitate papular or scaly plaque PR (Figure 23-12); thus the VDRL titer should be checked when considering PR as a diagnosis.

The herald patch may be absent or may appear as multiple lesions. The secondary lesions may be located on the extremities with little truncal involvement. Focal lesions may appear, especially in children. Oral, purpuric, vesicular, and pustular forms of PR are sometimes present in children. The palms and soles may be involved, and it may be difficult to distinguish from secondary syphilis. PR is usually diagnosed clinically. However, in some of the atypical variants, PR may be difficult to diagnose.

PATHOLOGY

The histologic findings are nonspecific. There is a decrease or absence of the granular layer, acanthosis, spongiosis, a superficial dermal infiltrate of lymphocytes, extravasated erythrocytes extending to the epidermis, and parakeratosis. The parakeratosis is often focal and in mounds. In a micropapular variant in African-American patients, there are often triangular mounds of parakeratosis that look tilted with respect to the underlying epidermis.[6] Focal spongiosis occasionally progresses to vesiculation. In older lesions, the perivascular infiltrate is often superficial and deep, with less spongiosis and more epidermal hyperplasia making it difficult to distinguish from psoriasis and lichen planus[7].

MANAGEMENT

PR is self-limiting; thus treatment is usually not necessary. When treatment is given, it is often for symptomatic relief of pruritus, for which medium-strength topical steroids and/or antihistamines are prescribed. Intramuscular or oral corticosteroids given early may help to prevent postinflammatory hyperpigmentation, especially in skin of color.[4] This usually attenuates the lesions in 2–3 weeks, but systemic corticosteroids may exacerbate PR. PR in a severe vesicular form can be treated with dapsone.

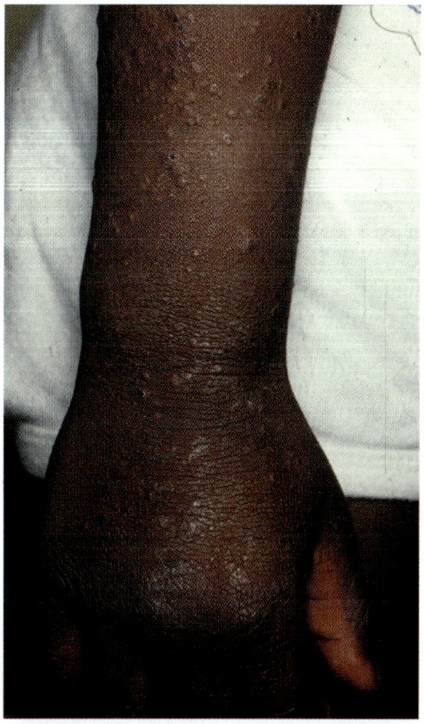

▲ **FIGURE 23-7** Papular lesions on the dorsum of the hands and forearms, many with necrotic-like centers.

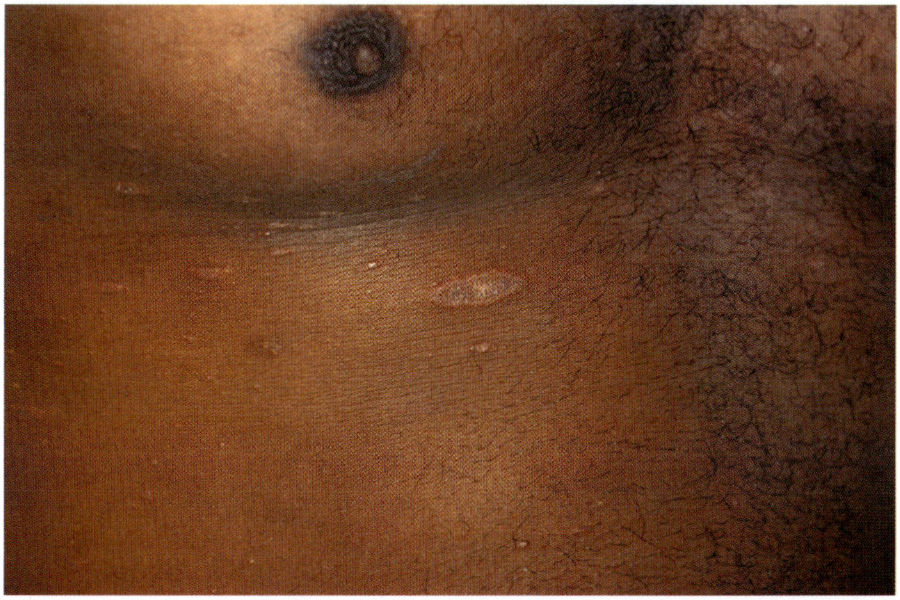

▲ **FIGURE 23-6** PR lesions appearing as a herald patch with narrow linear lesions on the flank chest (school of minnows pattern).

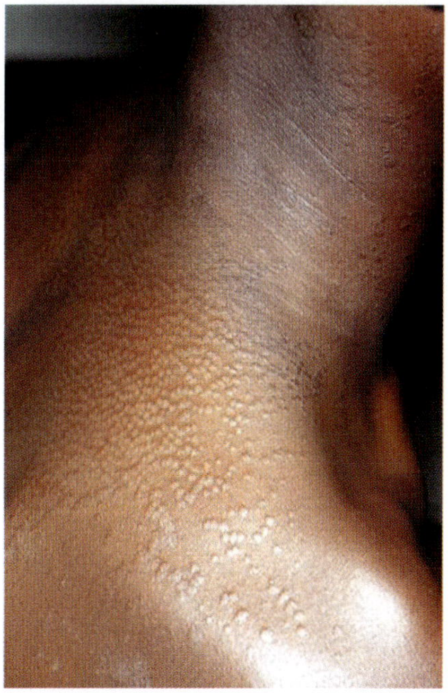

▲ **FIGURE 23-8** A male with follicular PR.

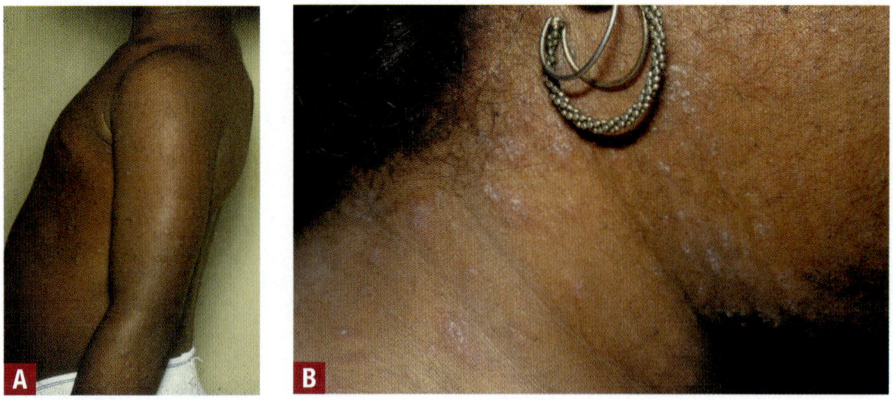

▲ **FIGURE 23-9** **A.** PR papules on the arms and chest of an African-American boy. **B.** PR lesions on the face and neck of an African-American woman.

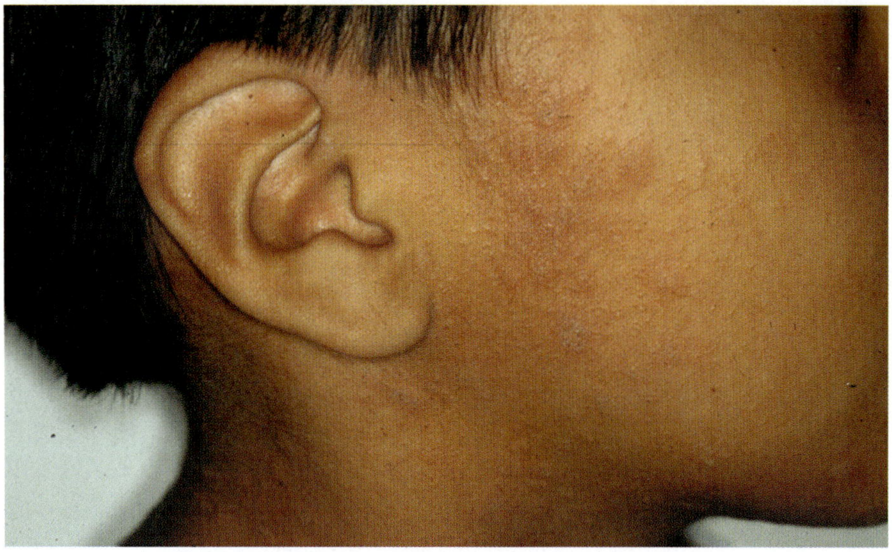

▲ **FIGURE 23-10** Erythematous papules and plaques on the face and neck of a Hispanic child.

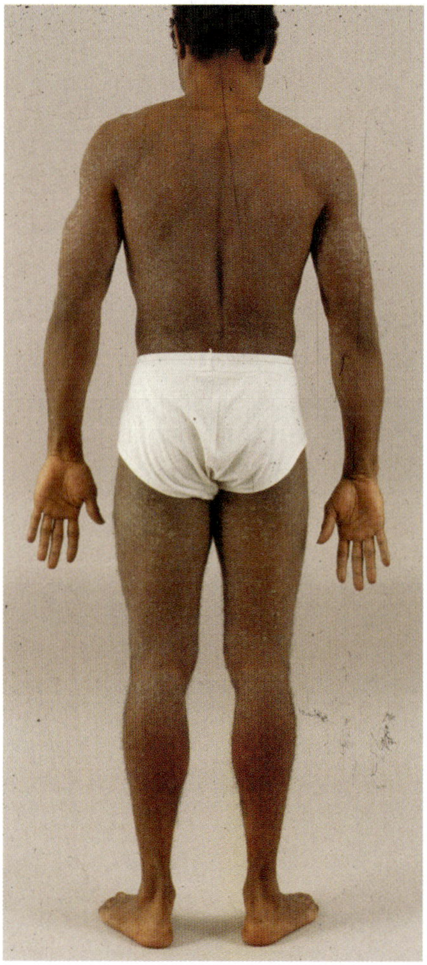

▲ **FIGURE 23-11** Generalized PR on the trunk and extremities of an African-American man.

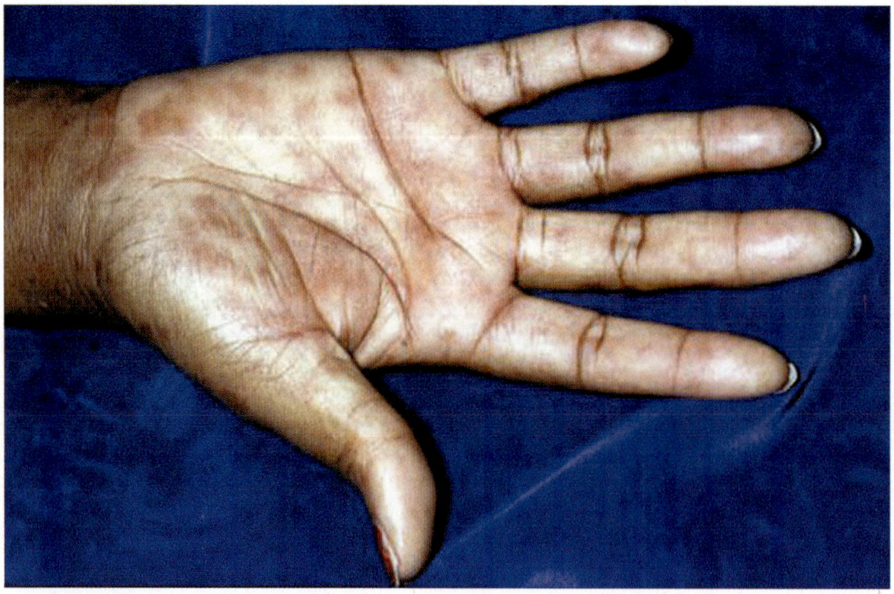

▲ **FIGURE 23-12** Palmar lesions of secondary syphilis.

TABLE 23-4
Clinical Presentation

Characteristics	White Skin	Skin of Color
Color of lesions	Rose or salmon	Gray or violaceous
Location	More on trunk	More extremity lesions
Scale	Collarette of scale	Central scale
Special features	Seldom central hyperpigmentation	Central, necrotic like, hyperpig mentation
Lesion size	More plaques central (trunk) location	More papules extremity location

Ultraviolet B radiation (UVB) has been shown to decrease the severity of the disease, but not the accompanying pruritus.[8] UVB plus a topical corticosteroid may make this mode of therapy more effective. Because UVB can cause postinflammatory hyperpigmentation, it may not be the treatment of choice for skin of color.

TABLE 23-5
Four Clinical Features of PR

1. An initial plaque (herald patch)
   - May be more than 1 day to a week before other lesions appear
   - Lasts 6–10 weeks
   - Dark skin often heals with postinflammatory hyperpigmentation
2. Characteristic individual lesions
   - Collarette scale
3. Lesions along lines of cleavage
   - "School of minnows" pattern
   - "Christmas tree" pattern
4. Papules with central necrotic-like hyperpigmentation
   - Especially on extremities in African-American children

Studies have shown that erythromycin may be effective in treating PR. In one study, 73% of the PR patients (45 total patients) treated with erythromycin, 250 mg/day, achieved complete clearance in 2 weeks,[9] whereas spontaneous remission takes at least 6 weeks. Since many organisms are sensitive to Erythromycin rather confounding factors have to be identified. As a result, erythromycin is not a definitive therapy for PR. In fact, a recent article by Rasi and colleagues found that oral erythromycin is ineffective in the treatment of PR[10] (Table 23-6).

TABLE 23-6
PR Therapy

- Self limiting = does not need treatment
- Intramuscular or oral corticosteroids
  - Use early in disease process
  - Attenuates dermatosis
- UVB and topical treatment
- Erythromycin 250 mg qid
  - Complete clearance in 2 weeks
  - Controversy exists concerning the role of erythromycin in the treatment of PR, as reported by Rasi and colleagues[10]

REFERENCES

1. Halder RM, Nootheti PK. Ethnic skin disorders overview. *J Am Acad Dermatol* 2003;48:5143-5148.
2. Araujo DT, Berman B, Weinstein A. Human herpes viruses 6 and 7. *Dermatol Clin* 2002;20:301-306.
3. Freedberg, IM. Eisen, AZ. Wolff, K. *Fitzpatrick's* (eds), *Dermatology in General Medicine,* 6th ed. New York, McGraw-Hill, 2003, pp 445-450.
4. Halder RM, Roberts CI, Nootheti PK. Cutaneous diseases in the black races. *Dermatol Clin* 2003;21:679-687.
5. Chuh AA. Quality of life in children with pityriasis rosea: A prospective case control study. *Pediatr Dermatol* 2003;20:474-478.
6. Brady SP. Parakeratosis. *J Am Acad Dermatol* 2004;50:77-84.
7. Ackerman AB. *Histologic Diagnosis of Inflammatory Skin Disease.* Philadelphia, Lea & Febiger, 1978.
8. Leenutaphong V, Jiamton S. UVB phototherapy for pityriasis rosea: A bilateral comparison study. *J Am Acad Dermatol* 1995;33:996-999.
9. Sharma PK, Yadav TP, Gautam RK, et al. Erythromycin in pityriasis rosea: A double-blind, placebo-controlled clinical trial. *J Am Acad Dermatol* 2000;42:241-244.
10. Rasi A, Tajziehchi L, Savabi-Nasab S. Oral erythromycin is ineffective in the treatment of pityriasis rosea. *J Drugs Dermatol* 2008;7:35-38.

CHAPTER 24

Lichen Planus

Khari H. Bridges

Key Points

- Lichen planus is an autoimmune inflammatory mucocutaneous condition that can affect the skin, mucosal surfaces, scalp, or nails.
- Evidence suggests that lichen planus is due to altered self-antigens on basal keratinocytes, a process that appears to be multifactorial.
- Lichen planus has a multitude of clinical variants, including some actinic variants that occur in darker skin types.
- Lichen planus is the prototypical histologic lichenoid reaction.

Lichen planus (LP) is an autoimmune inflammatory mucocutaneous condition that can affect the skin, oral mucosa, scalp, or nails. LP is often idiopathic but at times may be linked to drugs [e.g., penicillamine, gold, angiotensin-converting enzyme (ACE) inhibitors, antimalarials, and quinidine] or viral infections [especially hepatitis C virus (HCV) infection]. Topical steroids are used to treat localized LP, whereas systemic steroids and other modalities are used to treat patients with generalized LP.[1]

EPIDEMIOLOGY

LP affects from 0.22–1% of the adult population,[2] whereas oral LP (OLP) affects 1–4% of the population.[3] There is no overt racial predisposition. Incidence rates vary from 0.29% in African-Americans to 0.1–1% in East Indians.[4] Two-thirds of patients developed the disease between 30 and 60 years of age.[5] There is a slight predominance in women, although some authors have reported women being affected twice as often as men.[1,4,5] Women tend to develop the disease later in life than men (sixth versus fourth decade).[2] There may be a small genetic component to LP because 1–2% of cases are familial.[6]

OLP may be found in 50–75% of cases of cutaneous LP.[7,8] Cutaneous LP is found in 10–20% of cases of OLP. Of patients with LP of any form, 25% will have solely mucosal involvement.[8]

PATHOGENESIS

There is a growing body of evidence to suggest that LP represents a T-cell-mediated autoimmune process directed against basal keratinocytes that express altered self-antigens on their surfaces.[8] How these altered self-antigens arise appears to be multifactorial.

The role of viruses has been investigated to explain the origin of antigens in the generation of effector T cells with cytotoxic potential. HCV is one of the suspected viruses. Several case-control studies have found that HCV is more prevalent in LP populations than in controls, with numbers ranging from 4–38%.[6,9] Conversely, it has been reported that 5% of all HCV patients have LP.[6] HCV is believed to be more commonly associated with OLP than cutaneous LP. Moreover, HCV RNA has been found in 93% of OLP lesions via the polymerase chain reaction (PCR) technique.[10] Other suspected viruses include TT virus (TTV) and human herpes virus 6 (HHV-6).[11,12]

Medications also play a role in some lichenoid reactions. While any drug potentially can cause a lichenoid drug reaction, some drugs are more likely to result in this reaction than others. Beta-blockers, ACE inhibitors, nonsteroidal anti-inflammatory drugs (NSAIDs), antimalarials, quinidine, hydrochlorothiazide (HCTZ), gold, and penicillamine are the classic agents known to cause lichenoid drug eruptions. The interval to onset can be anywhere from 10 days to several years. When a lichenoid drug reaction is suspected, discontinuation of the suspected drug is recommended, if at all possible.

Contact allergens, specifically metals in dental restorations or constructions such as mercury, copper, and gold, have been linked to the induction or exacerbation of OLP. About 94% of these patients had improvement after removal of the sensitizing material.[13]

Lichenoid eruptions also have been observed in association with autoimmune liver disease, myasthenia gravis, thymoma, and ulcerative colitis.[4] LP also has been reported in association with underlying malignancy.[14]

A murine model of LP has been established by employing autoreactive T cells, which respond to self major histocompatability complex (MHC) class II antigens on macrophages and Langerhans cells. The result is induction of LP-like skin lesions with histologic changes similar to LP or lichenoid skin diseases.[15] CD8+ T cells make up a large proportion of the inflammatory infiltrate, especially in older LP lesions.[15]

After an antigen-presenting cell presents a cross-reactive antigen to an antigen-specific naive T cell, the T cell elaborates tumor necrosis factor α (TNF-α) and interferon-γ (IFN-γ), which upregulate E-selectin and subsequently intercellular adhension molecule-1 (ICAM-1) in endothelial cells, facilitating migration of T cells across the endothelium and into the dermis.[8]

IFN-γ also induces elaboration of chemokines CXCL10, CXCL9, and CXCL11, which bind to chemokine receptor 3 (CXCR3). CXCR3 has been found to be consistently expressed by the majority of CD4+ and CD8+ dermal T cells and natural killer (NK) cells and is thought to also function in the activation, recruitment, and maintenance of these effector cells.[16]

Both T_H1 and T_H2 helper subsets elaborate chemokines and cytokines in a mixed pro- and anti-inflammatory cytokine profile. The balance between these profiles determines the clinical behavior of the disease.[17]

Apoptosis of keratinocytes is likely to be effected via cross-linking of the Fas receptor expressed on the keratinocytes with the Fas ligand expressed by CD8+ T cells and possibly NK cells. An additional T-cell cytotoxic effect on keratinocytes is mediated by perforin and granzymes. IFN-γ and TNF-α, which have been shown to be present in high concentrations in LP lesions, can induce keratinocyte expression of ICAM-1, thus facilitating this latter T-cell–keratinocyte interaction.[18] IFN-γ and TNF-β also may function to enhance expression of apoptosis-associated proteins in keratinocytes.

CLINICAL FEATURES

LP is classically described as a small, polygonal, violaceous, flat-topped papules that may coalesce into plaques (Figure 24-1). There may be umbilication (Figure 24-2). The surface is shiny or transparent, with a network of fine white lines called *Wickham's striae*. Wickham's striae are usually prominent on the oral mucosa of those with darker

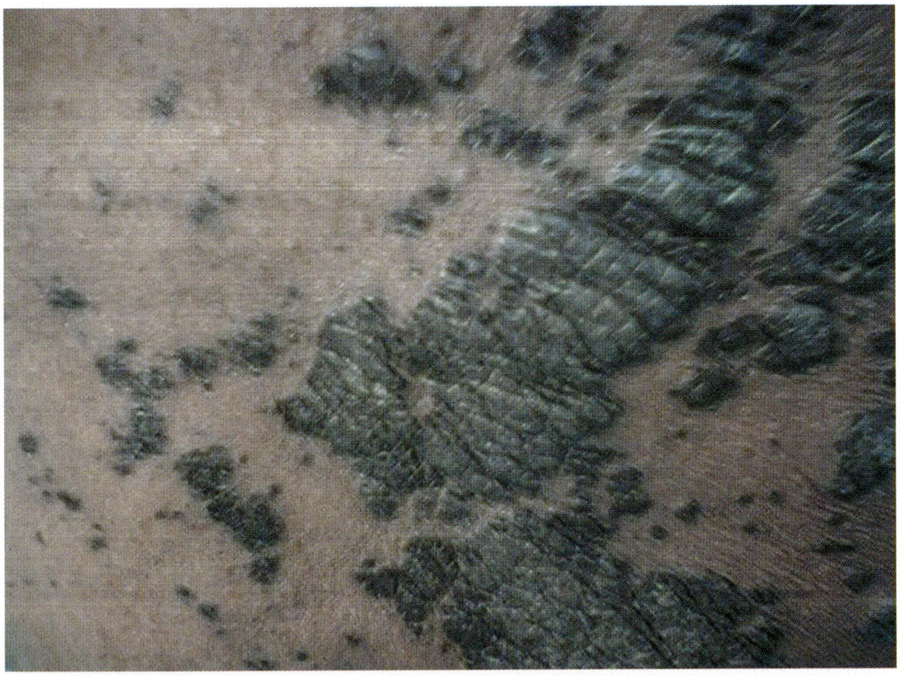

▲ **FIGURE 24-1** Polygonal, violaceous, planar papules, and plaques of lichen planus.

skin. There may be small gray-white puncta that correspond to focal thickening of the granular layer. The Koebner (isomorphic) phenomenon is commonly seen (see Figure 24-2). Most frequently involved sites are the flexor surfaces of the wrists and foreams (Figure 24-3), the dorsal surfaces of the hands, and the anterior aspect of the lower legs (Figure 24-4). The oral mucosa is affected in over half of affected patients[8] (Figure 24-5 and 24-6). Lesions begin as pinpoint papules and expand to 0.5- to 1.0-cm plaques.[6] Lesions of LP may be described using what have come to be known as "the six P's": pruritic, polygonal, planar, purple papules and plaques.[1] In skin of color, the classic purple color is often modified and may appear as black, gray, brown, or violaceous. When an exacerbation of LP occurs, it usually takes 2–16 weeks for maximal spread to occur.[19]

LP is classically an intensely pruritic condition. The itch may appear out of proportion to the amount of disease. Despite the pruritus, scratching is not a major problem because LP patients seem to experience pain when they scratch. The pruritus is spasmodic. Many patients react to the pruritus by rubbing rather than scratching, resulting in a paucity of visible excoriations.[6]

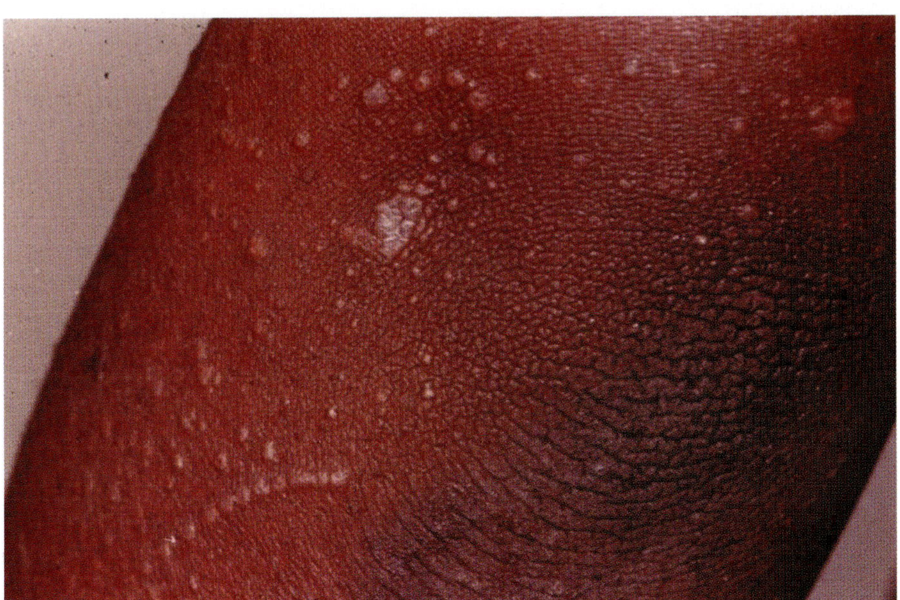

▲ **FIGURE 24-2** Lichen planus, umbilicated clinical variant, also exhibiting Koebner phenomenon.

There are many variants that deviate from this classic description. Variants include (1) acute LP, which describes eruptive lesions that occur most often on the trunk, (2) annular LP, which describes the 10% of patients who present with lesions with central inactivity or involution, (3) atrophic LP, which describes resolving lesions of LP that are classically found on the lower leg, (4) bullous LP, which describes lesions that exhibit blisters within long-standing plaques, evidenced histologically by exaggerated Max-Joseph spaces, (5) hypertrophic LP, which describes lesions that present with thick hyperkeratotic plaques (Figures 24-7 and 24-8), (6) lichen planopilaris, which describes a follicular variant of LP that can result in scarring alopecia of the scalp (there is also the Graham-Little subvariant, characterized by the clinical triad of spinous follicular lesions, mucocutaneous LP, and alopecia), (7) LP pemphigoides, which manifests as bullae in previously uninvolved skin of patients with LP and is characterized by circulating IgG autoantibodies against BPAG2 (type XVII collagen), (8) linear LP, which describes linear lesions that occur spontaneously (as opposed to by isomorphic phenomenon) along the lines of Blaschko, (9) LP–lupus erythematosus overlap syndrome, which describes patients with characteristics of both disorders, (10) nail LP, resulting in nail thinning, ridging, fissuring, or pterygium formation (Figure 24-9) (twenty-nail dystrophy represents a subvariant of nail LP), (11) oral LP, seen more commonly in women than men, which has varying morphologies, including an asymptomatic white, reticular variant (see Figure 24-6) that appears on the buccal mucosa and an erosive or bullous variants that can result in severe pain, and (12) ulcerative LP, which is seen within palmoplantar lesions of LP, consisting of bullae and permanent loss of toenails.[8] The actinic variant of LP, as well as LP pigmentosus, will be discussed later in this chapter because they have a predilection for darker-skinned individuals.

OLP occurs in approximately 50–75% of patients with cutaneous LP and is often the only affected area. Lesions can be (1) reticulate without symptoms, (2) atrophic, or (3) ulcerated and very painful, with involvement of the buccal mucosa or the gingiva.[7] The ulcerative form is the most common, occuring in

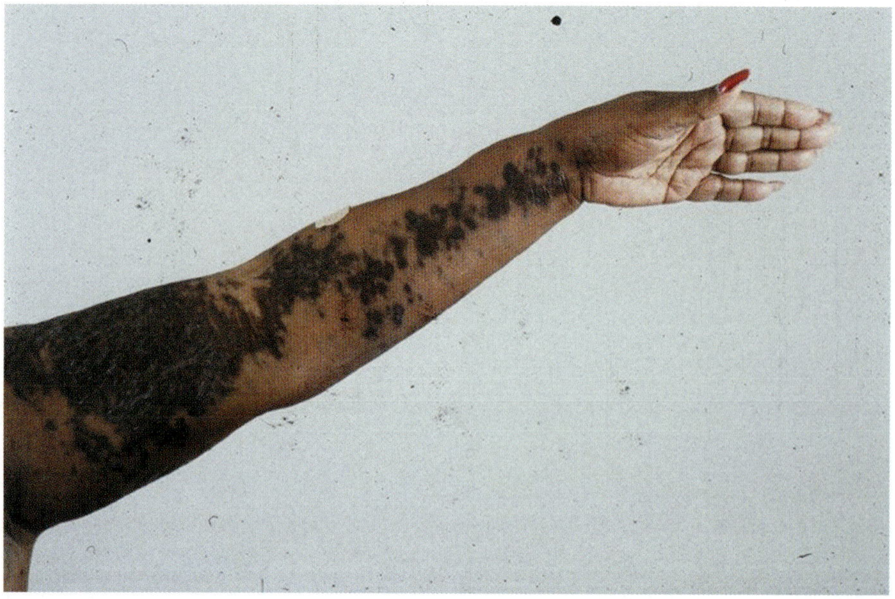

▲ **FIGURE 24-3** Lichen planus involving the flexor forearm and wrist of a dark-skinned individual.

just under half of patients with OLP. Reticulate lesions represent about a third of patients, and 20% of patients have atrophic lesions.[6] The ulcerative form also can occur in the vulvovaginal-gingival syndrome, characterized by gingival involvement in conjuction with vulvar and vaginal ulcerative lesions.[6]

Chronic ulcerative lesions, especially oral lesions, are at risk for development of squamous cell carcinoma (SCC).[8] It is important to monitor oral and genital LP for possible progression to SCC.[1] Approximately 0.5% of cutaneous LP patients will develop oral SCC, and 1% of OLP patients will develop SCC over a 3-year period. Erosive mucosal LP should be considered a premalignant condition, and the threshold to biopsy of suspicious lesions should be very low.[6]

Nail involvement occurs in approximately 10% of patients. Twenty-nail dystrophy is a variant characterized by involvement of all nails without any skin involvement.[7] Nail LP can cause multiple types of nail dystrophy, including ridging, distal splitting, thinning, subungual hyperkeratosis, pterygium formation (see Figure 24-9), and loss of the nail.[1]

Scalp involvement is called *lichen planopilaris,* and it presents as alopecia with keratotic follicular papules. It can progress to scarring alopecia if left untreated.[1] This can manifest as pseudopelade, a form of alopecia described poetically as "footprints in the snow."[19]

PATHOLOGY

The lichenoid tissue reaction is a histologic pattern characterized by hyperkeratosis, wedge-shaped hypergranulosis, "saw-toothed" acanthosis, and dyskeratotic epidermal basal cell damage (seen as Civatte/colloid/cytoid/hyaline bodies) that is associated with a massive bandlike infiltration of mononuclear cells at the dermal-epidermal junction.[1] Vacuolar damage to the basal layer can become confluent and result in small separations at the dermal-epidermal junction (Max-Joseph spaces).[8] If more than focal parakeratosis is present, LP cannot be diagnosed on histologic grounds.[20] OLP more commonly shows parakeratosis, and the epidermis is often atrophic.[8]

TREATMENT

LP is largely a self-limiting disease. Spontaneous remissions occur in the majority of patients after 1 year.[1] More

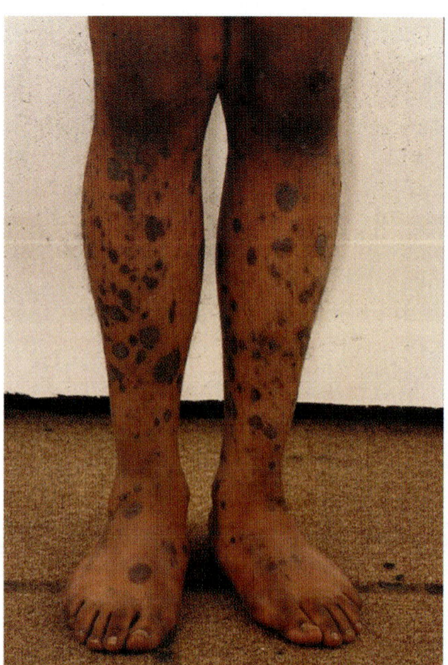

▲ **FIGURE 24-4** Lichen planus characteristically involving the anterior shins.

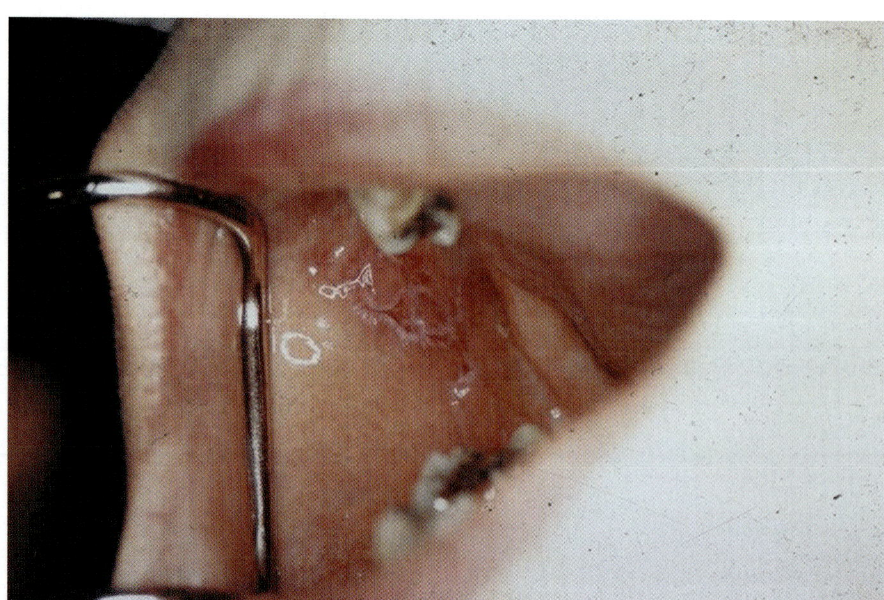

▲ **FIGURE 24-5** Oral lichen planus of the buccal mucosa.

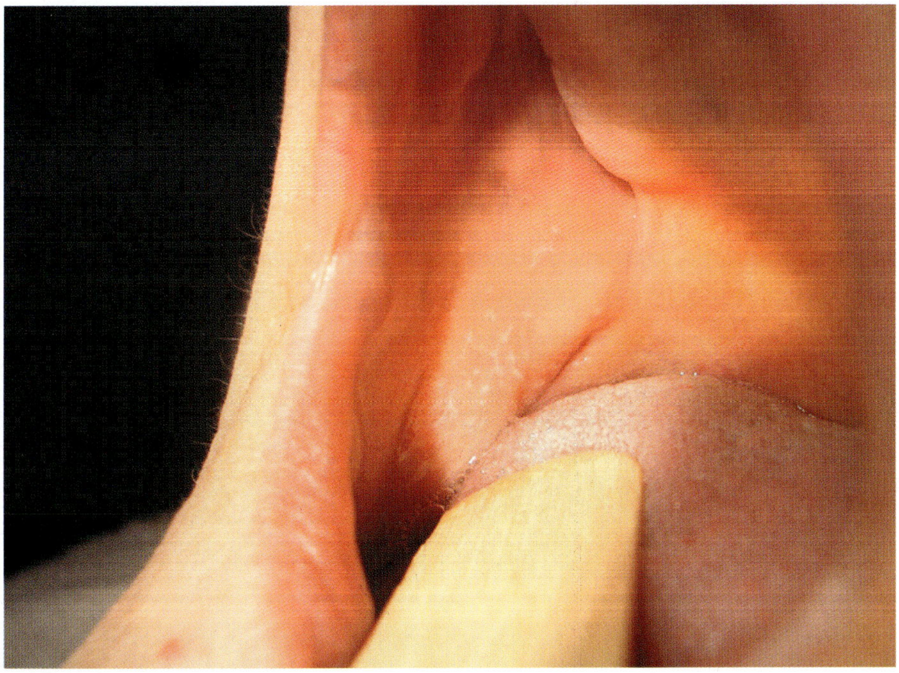

▲ **FIGURE 24-6** Oral lichen planus, reticulate variant.

specifically, more than 50% of cases will resolve within 6 months and 85% after 1 year.[19] OLP, on the other hand, lasts for an average of 5 years.[19,21] Ulcerative LP rarely resolves spontaneously.[21] Fewer than 3% of patients with OLP have spontaneous remission in an average 5-year period. Hypertrophic LP has the worst prognosis of all, lasting an average of 8 years. The duration of disease of LP variants has the following order: generalized < cutaneous < mucocutaneous < mucous < hypertrophic = lichen planopilaris.[22]

For patients who desire more rapid improvement in their condition, topical steroids are first-line therapy for localized disease. Intralesional steroids may be tried in resistant lesions or in hyperkeratotic LP. OLP can be treated with steroid mixed in Orabase, an adhesive vehicle. Systemic corticosteroids are helpful in patients with generalized involvement. Systemic steroids relieve symptoms in the short term but are not recommended for long-term therapy and are not known to affect the total duration of the disease.[1] One study has shown a reduction in median time to clearance with use of systemic steroids.[23] The usual dose of prednisone is 15–20 mg qd for 2–6 weeks, with tapering if indicated. Triamcinolone, 50–60 mg intramuscularly every 3 weeks, helps for severe LP but must be tapered gradually to prevent rebound.

Some steroid-sparing therapies are available, including acitretin, a systemic retinoid, given daily for 8 weeks at a 30-mg dose. This drug is typically reserved for men and women incapable of producing children (e.g., postmenopausal, status post tubal ligation, or hysterectomy) owing to the teratogenicity of this drug.[1] Topical tacrolimus or pimecrolims, both calcineurin inhibitors, are effective for oral and genital LP.[7,24] Low-molecular-weight heparin, 3 mg subcutaneously every week for 4–6 weeks, is reported to be very effective for skin and reticulated oral lesions owing to the immunomodulatory and antilymphoproliferative effects at low doses.[25] Psoralen with ultraviolet A (PUVA), griseofulvin, dapsone, cyclosporine, and hydroxychloroquine also have been reported anecdotally to be effective for steroid-resistant LP.[1] Griseofulvin is especially effective for erosive OLP.[2] Hydroxychloroquine, 200–400 mg qd for 6 months, has been reported to give an excellent response in OLP.[6,26] For women with the vulvovaginal syndrome, corticosteroids can be delivered in a vaginal bioadhesive glycerin-based moisturizer (Replens).[6] Cyclosporine, 1–6 mg qd, may be effective in patients with recalcitrant LP resistant to steroid and retinoid therapy. Oral antihistamines can reduce the pruritus associated with LP.[8] Recrudescence of LP occurs in approximately 15–20% of patients.[22] In skin of color, LP usually causes prominent postinflammatory hyperpigmentation on resolution of the acute disease.

The following two sections discuss variants of LP that are seen in darker-pigmented skin.

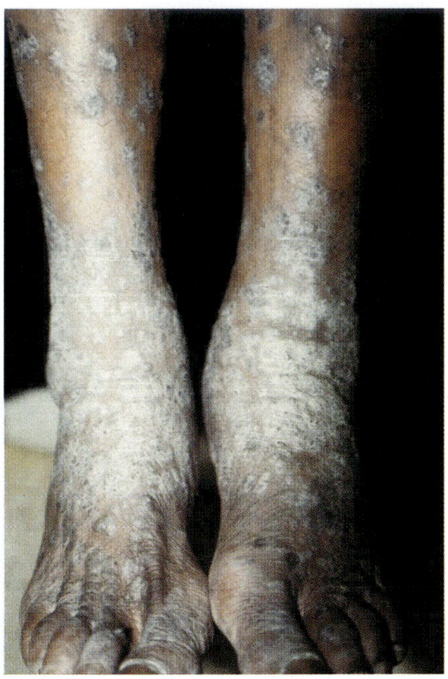

▲ **FIGURE 24-7** Hypertrophic lichen planus of the anterior shins.

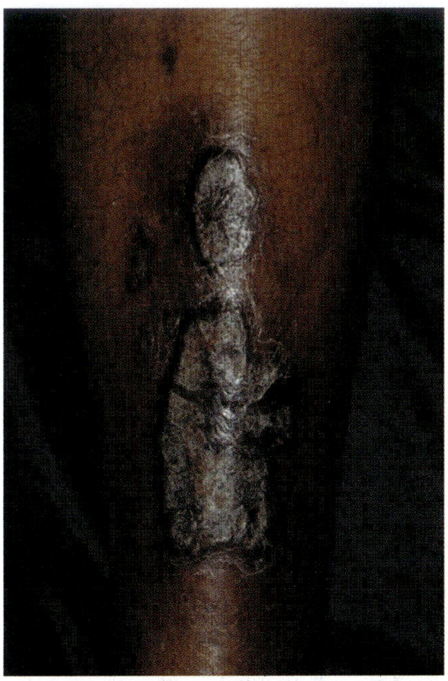

▲ **FIGURE 24-8** Hypertrophic lichen planus of the anterior shins.

LICHEN PLANUS ACTINICUS

Lichen planus actinicus (LPA), also known as *actinic LP, LP subtropicus, LP tropicus, lichenoid melanodermatitis,* and *summertime actinic lichenoid eruption,* is a photodistributed variant of LP that has a

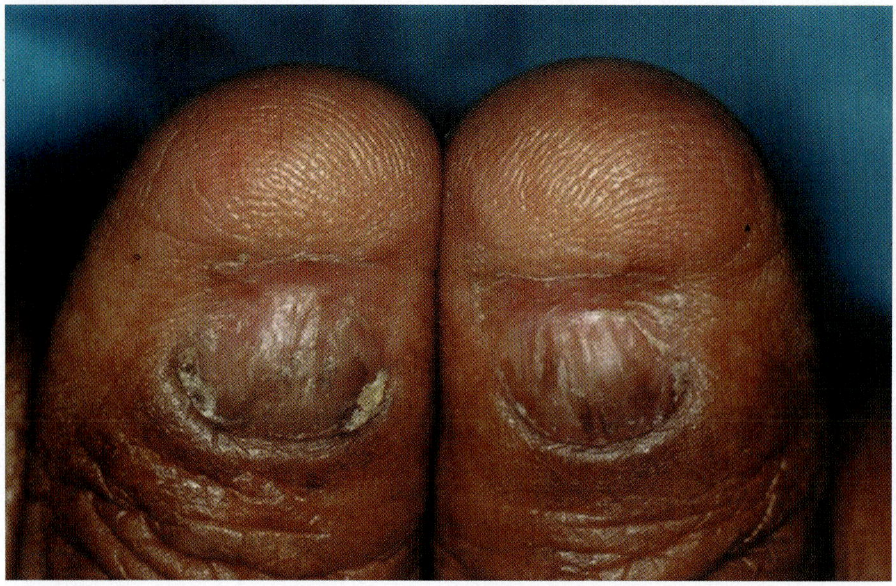

▲ **FIGURE 24-9** Pterygium formation in lichen planus involving the nails.

predilection for darker-skinned individuals, subtropical climates, and individuals of Middle Eastern, African, and Asian descent.[6,27] Sun exposure appears to be a triggering factor. Among photodistributed areas, the lateral aspect of the forehead is the most common site of presentation. There is a seasonal predilection, with most outbreaks occurring during the spring or summer with remittance during the winter months. LPA has an earlier age of onset and a longer course than classic LP. There is a female preponderance. In contrast to classic LP, pruritus, scaling, nail involvement, and Koebner reaction are frequently absent.[6,27]

Several morphologic patterns have been described: (1) annular hyperpigmented plaques (the most common type, located on dorsa of fingers and hands, with increased hyperpigmentation at the center of the plaque), (2) melasma-like patches (with hyperpigmented patches on the face and neck ranging from 5mm to 5cm), (3) dyschromic papules (2- to 3-mm papules with small central keratotic plugs found on the posterior neck and dorsa of hands), and (4) classic lichenoid papules/plaques (violaceous papules in sun-exposed areas).[27]

The histopathology of LPA is consistent with classic LP.[27] In addition, there is melanin incontinence with the presence of dermal melanin, which corresponds to the typical blue-gray hyperpigmentation.[6] There are several treatments available for LPA. Some cases remit spontaneously with sun avoidance and the use of sunblock. Some cases require more aggressive therapy with hydroxychloroquine or intralesional corticosteroids. Acitretin, used in combination with topical corticosteroids, has resulted in complete resolution of lesions without recurrence. Bismuth, grenz rays, arsenicals, and topical steroids under occlusion have been used with variable response. There are no reports of PUVA, isotretinoin, systemic corticosteroids, cyclosporine, or dapsone being successful in LPA treatment.[27]

LICHEN PLANUS PIGMENTOSUS

Lichen planus pigmentosus occurs in Latin Americans and darkly pigmented skin types. It manifests as asymptomatic dark brown macules or patches in sun-exposed areas and flexural folds. Histology reveals an atrophic epidermis, vacuolar alteration of the basal cell layer, a sparse lymphocytic lichenoid infiltrate, and pigment incontinence. This type of lichenoid dermatosis may be a case of phenotypic overlap with erythema dyschromicum perstans (ashy dermatosis).[28]

ACKNOWLEDGMENT

I would like to thank Dr. Carrie Marder for her involvement in preparing this chapter.

REFERENCES

1. Katta R. Lichen planus. *Am Fam Physician* 2000;61:3319-3324, 3327-3328; *www.aafp.org/afp/20000601/3319.html.*
2. Boyd AS, Neldner KH. Lichen planus. *J Am Acad Dermatol* 1991;25:593-619.
3. Scully C, Beyli M, Ferreiro MC, et al. Update on oral lichen planus: Etiopathogenesis and management. *Crit Rev Oral Biol Med* 1998;9:86-122.
4. Scully C, el-Kom M. Lichen planus: Review and update on pathogenesis. *J Oral Pathol* 1985;14:431-458.
5. Silverman S, Gorsky M, Luzada-Nur F. A prospective follow-up study of 570 patients with oral lichen planus: Persistence, remission, and malignant association. *Oral Surg Oral Med Oral Pathol* 1985;60:30-34.
6. Odom RB, James WD, Berger TG (eds). *Andrews' Diseases of the Skin: Clinical Dermatology,* 9th ed. Philadelphia, WB Saunders, 2000, pp 266-280.
7. Lichen Planus. DermNet NZ, September 30, 2004. New Zealand Dermatological Society, Inc. Accessed March 13, 2005 at *http://dermnetnz.org/scaly/lichen-planus.html.*
8. Shiohara T, Kano Y. Licen planus and lichenoid dermatoses, in Bolognia JL, Jorizzo JL, Rapini RP, et al (eds), *Dermatology*. London, Mosby (Elsevier), 2003, pp 175-184, 186-188.
9. Conklin RJ, Blasberg B. Oral lichen planus. *Dermatol Clin* 1987;5:663-673.
10. Nagao Y, Kameyama T, Sata M. Hepatitis C virus RNA detection in oral lichen planus tissue. *Am J Gastroenterol* 1998; 93:850.
11. Rodriguez-Inigo E, Arrieta JJ, Casqueiro M, et al. TT virus detection in oral lichen planus lesions. *J Med Virol* 2001; 64:183-189.
12. Requena L, Kutzner H, Escalonilla P, et al. Cutaneous reactions at sites of herpes zoster scars: An expanded spectrum. *Br J Dermatol* 1998;138:161-168.
13. Usman A, Kimyai-Asadi A, Stiller MJ, et al. Lichenoid eruption following hepatitis B vaccination: First North American case report. *Pediatr Dermatol* 2001;18: 123-126.
14. Helm TN, Camisa C, Liu AY, et al. Lichen planus associated with neoplasia: A cell-mediated immune response to tumor antigen? *J Am Acad Dermatol* 1994; 30:219-224.
15. Shiohara T, Moriya N, Nagashima M. Induction and control of lichenoid tissue reactions. *Springer Semin Immunopathol* 1992;13:369-385.
16. Flier J, Boorsma DM, van Beek PJ, et al. Differential expression of CXCR3 targeting chemokines CXCL10, CXCL9, and CXCL11 in different types of skin inflammation. *J Pathol* 2001;194: 398-405.
17. Simark-Mattsson C, Bergenholtz G, Jontell M, et al. Distribution of interleukin-2, -4, -10, tumour necrosis factor-alpha and transforming growth factor-beta mRNAs in oral lichen planus. *Arch Oral Biol* 1999;44:499-507.
18. Yasukawa M, Ohminami H, Arai J, et al. Granule exocytosis, and not the fas/fas ligand system, is the main pathway of cytotoxicity mediated by alloantigen-specific CD4(+) as well as CD8(+) cytotoxic T lymphocytes in humans. *Blood* 2000;95:2352-2355.
19. Chaung T, Stitle L. Lichen planus. *E-medicine,* January 12, 2005; accessed March 13, 2005 at *www.emedicine.com/DERM/topic233.htm.*

20. Prieto BG, Casal M, McNutt NS. Lichen planus-like keratosis: A clinical and histological reexamination. *Am J Surg Pathol* 1993;17:259-263.
21. Mignogna MD, Muzio LL, Russo LL, et al. Oral lichen planus: Different clinical features in HCV-positive and HCV-negative patients. *Int J Dermatol* 2000;39: 134-139.
22. Tompkins JK. Lichen planus: A statistical study of forty-one cases. *Arch Dermatol* 1955;71:515-519.
23. Cribier B, Frances C, Chosidow O. Treatment of lichen planus: An evidence-based medicine analysis of efficacy. *Arch Dermatol* 1998;134:1521-1530.
24. Rozycki TW, Rogers RS 3rd, Pittelkow MR, et al. Topical tacrolimus in the treatment of symptomatic oral lichen planus: A series of 13 patients. *J Am Acad Dermatol* 2002;46:27-34.
25. Stefanidou MP, Ioannidou DJ, Panayiotides JG, et al. Low molecular weight heparin: A novel alternative therapeutic approach for lichen planus. *Br J Dermatol* 1999;141: 1040-1045.
26. Eisen D. Hydroxychloroquine sulfate (Plaquenil) improves oral lichen planus: An open trial. *J Am Acad Dermatol* 1993; 28:609-612.
27. Meads SB, Kunishige J, Ramos-Caro FA, et al. Lichen planus actinicus. *Cutis* 2003; 72:377-381.
28. Vega ME, Waxtein L, Arenas R, et al. Ashy dermatosis versus lichen planus pigmentosus: A controversial matter. *Int J Dermatol* 1992;31:87-88.

CHAPTER 25

Lichen Nitidus

Khari H. Bridges

Key Points

- Lichen nitidus is characterized by numerous, tiny, discrete, skin-colored, uniform, pinhead-sized papules that occur in clusters.
- Histology of lichen nitidus reveals a "ball and claw" arrangement.
- There is an actinic variant of lichen nitidus that occurs predominantly in darker skin types.

EPIDEMIOLOGY

Lichen nitidus (LN) is a somewhat rare disease, and hence adequate epidemiologic data are difficult to obtain. Epidemiology, although it seems to affect blacks more than whites all studies does not show any predilection for sex, race, or age. There is a rare generalized variant of LN that has a female preponderance.[1] Rare familial cases of LN do occur.[2]

CLINICAL FEATURES

LN is characterized by asymptomatic, numerous, tiny, discrete, skin-colored, uniform, pinhead-sized papules that occur in clusters (Figure 25-1). Papules are flat-topped with a shiny surface. Papules in dark-skinned individuals tend to be hypopigmented, but sometimes they are hyperpigmented. Lesions are usually found on the flexor aspects of the upper extremities, as well as on the dorsal hands, chest, abdomen, and genitalia. Nail involvement is seen in approximately 10%; changes include pitting, rippling, ridging, fissuring, and increased longitudinal linear striations. Koebner reaction is seen in LN. Generalized LN can exhibit coalescence of the papules into plaques. Oral Lesions, Wickham striae, nail lesions, palmer lesions are somewhat rare.

PATHOLOGY

There is parakeratosis, absence or thinning of the granular layer, with epidermal atrophy. There is vacuolar change of the basal cell layer with melanin incontinence. There are hyperplastic rete ridges that surround a well-circumscribed dermal infiltrate consisting of lymphocytes, epithelioid cells, and Langerhans giant cells in a "ball and claw" arrangement. The infiltrate is typically confined to the width of two to three dermal papillae.[1,3]

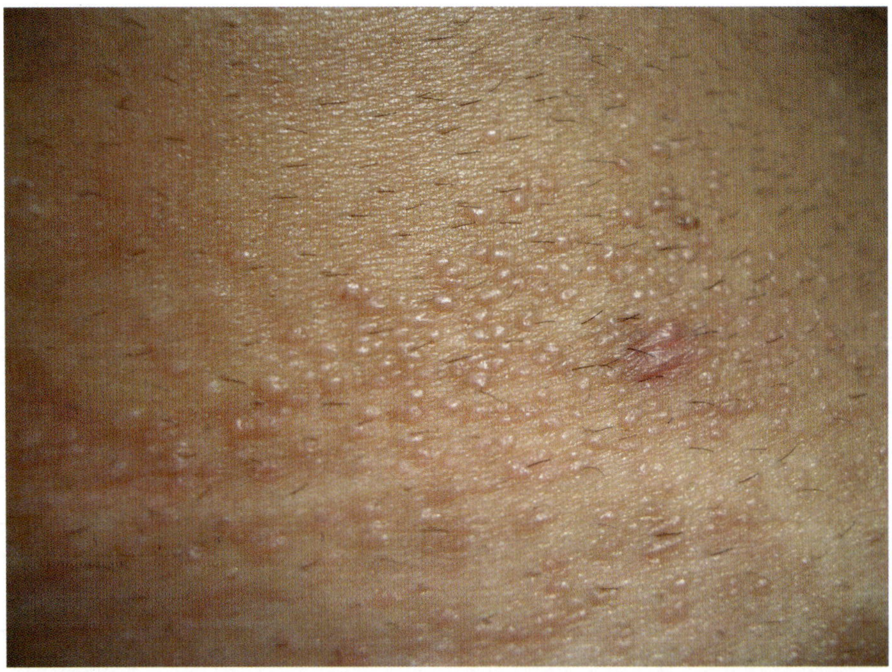

▲ **FIGURE 25-1** Discrete, skin-colored, uniform, grouped, pinhead-sized papules of lichen nitidus.

TREATMENT

Most patients experience spontaneous resolution in 1–3 years. Treatment is largely guided by symptoms. Oral antihistamines and topical steroids can relieve the pruritus sometimes associated with LN. Topical tacrolimus has proven effective anecdotally in children with LN. There are anecdotal descriptions of improvement with psoralen with ultraviolet A (PUVA), acitretin, itraconazole, and dinitrochlorobenzene (DNCB).[4,5] Low dose cyclosporin has also provided successful therapy.

ACTINIC LICHEN NITIDUS

This is a variant of LN reported in black and Middle Eastern patients, similar to actinic LP. The lesions are clinically and histologically similar to LN and occur in sun-exposed areas of the dorsal hands, extensor forearms, and posterior neck. The lesions typically respond to sun protection; topical steroids can be added for resistant lesions.[2] The majority of the patients clear spontaneously in several months to a year. In a occasional patient it may persist for a lifetime. Patients usually heal with post inflammatory pigmentary changes or scar formation.

REFERENCES

1. Shiohara T, Kano Y. Licen planus and lichenoid dermatoses, in Bolognia JL, Jorizzo JL, Rapini RP, et al. (eds), *Dermatology*. London, Mosby (Elsevier), 2003, pp 175-184, 186-188.
2. Odom RB, James WD, Berger TG (eds). *Andrews' Diseases of the Skin: Clinical Dermatology*, 9th ed. Philadelphia, WB Saunders, 2000, pp 266-280.
3. Lapins NA, Willoughby C, Helwig EB. Lichen nitidus: A study of forty-three cases. *Cutis* 1978;21:634-637.
4. Chen W, Schramm M, Zouboulis CC. Generalized lichen nitidus. *J Am Acad Dermatol* 1997;36:360-361.
5. Kano Y, Otake Y, Shiohara T. Improvement of lichen nitidus after topical dinitrochlorobenzene application. *J Am Acad Dermatol* 1998;39:305-308.

CHAPTER 26

Allergic Contact Dermatitis

Nina Desai
Vincent DeLeo

Key Points

- Environmental, cultural, occupational, genetic, individual, and racial differences are important in the study of contact dermatitis.
- The differences in skin physiology that are important to determining the relationship between race and contact dermatitis are barrier function and percutaneous absorption.
- Allergic contact dermatitis (ACD) in skin of color could be more commonly associated with lichenification and hyperpigmentation versus the vesicular, papular, erythematous response seen in Caucasians.
- Patch test interpretation in skin of color is more difficult given the challenge of detecting erythema, leading to an underestimation of ACD in skin of color.

Contact dermatitis is an altered state of skin reactivity induced by exposure to an external agent. Certainly gender, age, environmental, occupational, and genetic factors are thought to be important in the study of contact dermatitis. The effect of race or ethnicity in this area has been studied less frequently.

Contact dermatitis is divided into two basic types depending on the nature of the underlying etiologic mechanism: irritant and allergic. Contact dermatitis from both irritant and allergic sources comprises 6–10% of all dermatology clinic visits, and allergic contact dermatitis (ACD) is thought to represent about 20% of these cases. ACD therefore is an important dermatologic disease with considerable morbidity and economic impact.

Irritant contact dermatitis (ICD) occurs when a chemical agent induces direct damage to the skin and produces inflammation without a classic "allergic" mechanism. The clinical manifestations can be subtle, such as with a stinging sensation on exposure, or marked, such as with severe chemical burns. The timing varies but is usually within a short period of minutes for a single exposure to days or weeks for multiple exposures. Most irritant reactions seen in the clinic are of moderate severity and are due to cumulative insult with mildly toxic substances such as ordinary soap and water.

ACD occurs when contact with a specific allergen or a closely related chemical substance elicits an immunologic inflammatory response in the allergic individual, usually 24–72 hours after reexposure. A dose-response relationship exists for allergens and for irritants but is more important in the irritant reaction. While, historically, irritant and allergic contact dermatitis were two different entities, irritancy itself is now thought to play an important role in ACD. The presence of more irritants or allergens or the combination of more irritant and allergens potentially influences the allergenicity of a substance.[1,2] Clinically, ACD is inflammation of the skin manifested by varying degrees of erythema, edema, and vesiculation in its acute form, but it also may present as a subacute or chronic eczematous process. Diagnosis of ACD may be suspected based on clinical and historic grounds but can only be diagnosed definitively through use of the patch test procedure. In patch testing, small amounts of the allergens are applied to the skin for a fixed time, and 2–4 days later the skin is examined for the presence of eczematous changes.

The ability of the offending agent to cause contact dermatitis depends on both the nature of the allergen/irritant and the skin's condition. The severity of the symptoms depends on exogenous and endogenous factors. Exogenous factors include the chemical and physical properties of the substance and the frequency of application. Endogenous factors include age, gender, preexisting skin diseases, skin sensitivity, genetics, and probably race and ethnicity.[3]

RACIAL DIFFERENCES IN SKIN PHYSIOLOGY AND PATHOPHYSIOLOGY

Ethnic differences in skin physiology and pathophysiology have been described. The literature supports a racial difference in epidermal melanin content and melanosome distribution in people of color compared with fair-skinned individuals. Other studies have shown differences in hair structure and fibroblast size and structure between black skin and white skin.[4] Probably the two most significant differences in skin physiology that are important to determining the relationship between race and contact dermatitis are barrier function and percutaneous absorption. Studies done on the percutaneous absorption of chemicals into the skin have in many, but not all, cases shown that black skin is generally more impervious than Caucasian skin. Wedig and Maibach observed 30% less absorption of C-dipyrithione in blacks versus Caucasian subjects.[5] Lotte and colleagues also looked at three races and found a slight increase in absorption in Asians and a slight decrease in absorption in blacks compared with the Caucasian population.[6] Additional studies used transepidermal water loss (TEWL) as a measure of barrier function of the skin in terms of the evaporation potential for water. Kompaore and colleagues compared TEWL among Caucasians, blacks, and Asians and found a significantly increased values in blacks and Asians in comparison with Caucasians.[7] Reed and colleagues used TEWL and found that subjects, regardless of race, who had lighter-pigmented skin had a more easily perturbed barrier function and a longer recovery time. Overall, these findings suggest a reduced degree of penetration by a chemical into black skin and an increase in barrier function of those with darker skin; both may help to explain the reduced irritant and allergic response we will discuss later.[8]

CLINICAL PRESENTATION OF ALLERGIC CONTACT DERMATITIS IN SKIN OF COLOR

The most common type of skin allergy is allergic contact dermatitis (ACD), a cell-mediated (type IV) immunologic response driven by T-lymphocytes in response to allergenic small molecules (haptens). Heavy metals, fragrances, preservatives, and topical medications make up the main classes of causative agents. However, the overall incidence of ACD is less than that of irritant contact dermatitis (ICD).

Detecting the occurrence of contact dermatitis in different races and ethnicities presents the first challenge. When suspecting the diagnosis, Fisher has pointed out that the manifestation in blacks may be different from that in whites with ACD, in blacks it being more commonly associated with lichenification and hyperpigmentation versus the vesicular, papular, erythematous response seen in Caucasians. In addition, some of the difficulty in diagnosing ACD in skin of color comes from the perception of erythema, an endpoint in determining contact dermatitis through patch testing.[9] Sherertz and Schwartz have emphasized the fact that patch test interpretation in black skin is more difficult given the challenge of detecting erythema, leading to an underestimation of ACD in skin of color.[10]

SUSCEPTIBILITY TO ALLERGIC CONTACT DERMATITIS IN SKIN OF COLOR

The literature on racial differences in susceptibility to ACD is sparse, largely because few investigators are willing or able to knowingly sensitize test subjects in order to prospectively study the etiology and mechanism of the development of ACD. In the past, several studies have been performed looking at the induction of contact dermatitis among different races. Two such studies have shown a reduced sensitivity for blacks versus Caucasians. Rostenberg and Kanof studied black and Caucasian subjects for the incidence of induced sensitization to dinitrochlorobenzene (DNCB) and paranirosodimethylaniline (PNDA). Each material was tested at a concentration of 1% via open application to a uniform area of skin. One month following the exposure, the subjects were challenged with the chemical to determine if sensitization had occurred. If no sensitization was present, the process was repeated for up to four attempts to induce sensitization.

The two chemicals differed in their ability to sensitize, with DNCB being the less potent sensitizer. With DNCB, the cumulative incidence of sensitization increased gradually, with an increasing number of Caucasian subjects showing positive responses at each treatment number. In contrast, sensitization to PNDA occurred more rapidly, yet similarly to DNCB, the cumulative incidence in Caucasian subjects grew more rapidly, showing that black subjects were more resistant than Caucasians to induced sensitization by these strongly sensitizing chemicals.[11]

Twenty-five years later, these results were corroborated by Kligman. Kligman compared the response of black and Caucasian subjects to several commonly encountered skin allergens. Kligman studied induction of sensitization to *p*-phenylendiamine (PPDA), monobenzyl ether of hydroquinone (MBEH), penicillin A nickel sulfate ($NiSO_4$), penicillin G (Pen G), and neomycin sulfate (NEO) between white people and black people. In this study, the sensitization rates of the weak allergens were statistically higher in white subjects than in black subjects. However, the strongest contact allergen, Pen G, showed little differences in the response between races. From these results, Kligman and colleagues concluded that black skin is less responsive to exogenous insult than white skin, possibly as a result of the difference in the ability of a substance to penetrate through black skin versus white skin.[12]

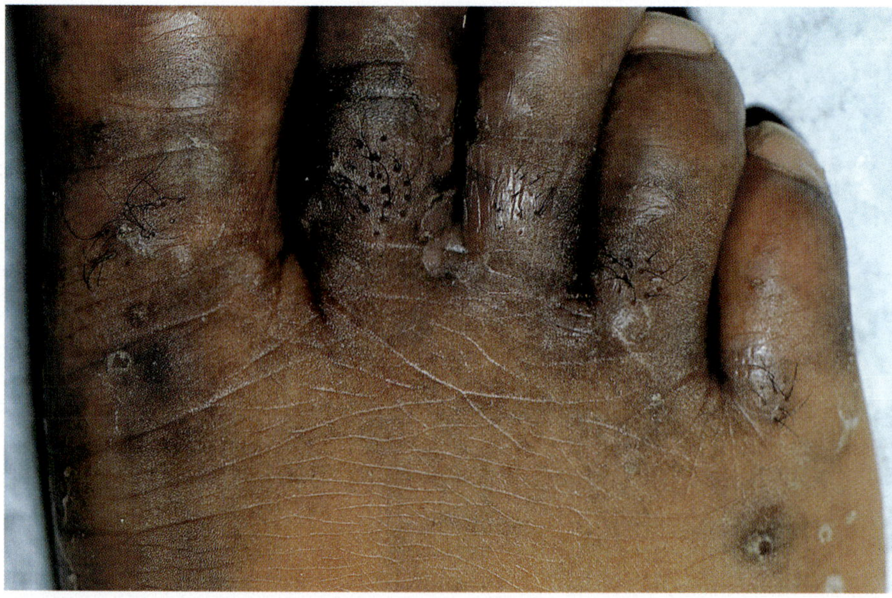

▲ **FIGURE 26-1** Contact dermatitis on the dorsum of the toes and foot of an African-American male with skin type VI.

In contrast, the North American Contact Dermatitis Group[13] reported information on contact dermatitis in approximately 10,000 patients, 10.5% of whom identified themselves as black. These patients had all received patch testing between 1992 and 1998. The percentage of patients with positive patch testing was similar between black and white patients. Additionally, the sites of the dermatitis were similar between races. The hands and face were affected most commonly (Figure 26-1). The most common allergen was nickel, with a comparable response rate to nickel between races. The black population was found to have a higher incidence of contact dermatitis to PPDA, a hair dye allergen, than the Caucasian population (Figure 26-2 A & B). The rates of sensitization in this study were extremely high for the black population, ranging from 7.8–10.6%. Along with the response to nickel sulfate, this was the highest response rate of any allergen tested in the black group. Similar high rates of sensitization and a black predominance were reported in a study on a smaller group of patients by Dickel.[14] Fisher and colleagues had previously reported PPDA to be the most common sensitizer in black patients receiving patch testing.[15]

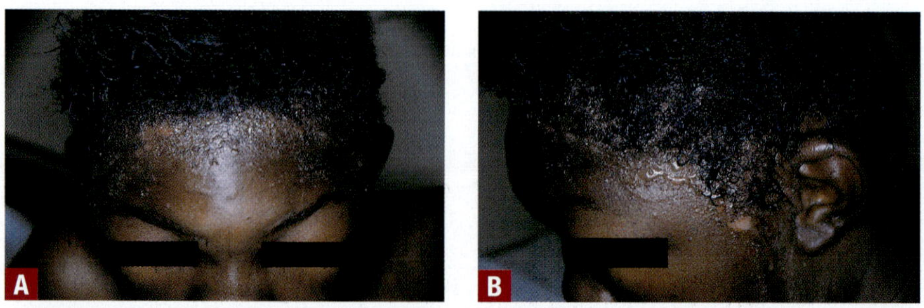

▲ **FIGURE 26-2** Contact dermatitis to *p*-phenylenediamine on the scalp of an African-American female with skin type VI.

While it is possible that biologic and genetic distinctions were contributors to the difference in the incidence of reaction to PPDA, it is more likely that cultural and ethnic differences that lead to different exposure patterns play a larger role. Dickel and colleagues looked at the possibility that racial differences in acetylator genotype and phenotype might explain the higher rates of sensitization to PPDA in the black population.[14] PPDA-sensitive patients theoretically could have differences in their ability to acetylate *N*-acetyltransferase 1 or 2 and that such difference in the acetylation of PPDA could result in a higher or lower allergenicity of PPDA. However, this reasoning alone would not explain differences in the sensitization rates between black and white patients because those two groups have been shown in the past to have similarly high proportions of slow acetylators. Therefore, it is more likely that the differences in PPDA sensitization rates are related to differences in the exposure pattern of the two races. This hair dye component is found in higher concentrations in the darker shades that are used by African-Americans. Therefore, the exposure is not necessarily due to the amount of hair coloring used but rather the concentration of the color used, leading to higher sensitization rates. Another possibility is that the sensitivity shown by black patients represents a cross-sensitization to other chemically related substances that are most often used to treat diseases in African-American patients, such as thiazide diuretics and oral antidiabetic drugs. However, if this were the case, one would expect to find a higher level of sensitization in similarly related allergens, such as benzocaine, which was not the case.[14]

White patients were found to be more sensitive to formaldehyde and formaldehyde-related preservatives, which incidentally are found in cream-based products thought to be used more often in the white population, than to oil-based products thought to be used more often in the black population. Epidemiologic studies like this, however, are by definition retrospective and cannot be controlled for exposure. The assumption made here is that exposure is equivalent among races and that there is no difference in blacks and Caucasians in terms of sensitization to allergens. However, in the real world, to say that exposures are equivalent is an extremely large assumption.

These studies are only able to monitor the elicitation phase, whereas the historical studies such as those by Rostenberg and Kligman were able to examine the actual sensitization process of ACD in naive patients. Those studies show that in experimentally controlled conditions, blacks actually show significantly less sensitivity to induction of sensitization.[11,12]

While the literature comparing the sensitivity to ACD in Caucasians and blacks is limited, the literature on other racial comparisons is even more scarce. Rapaport found that Japanese tend to show a more severe allergic reaction to standard cosmetic ingredients than Caucasians but not a higher incidence.[16] However, the limited data that these studies provide are incomplete because there is no report as to the materials tested. In retrospective studies of patch test subjects in Singapore, a study by Goh found no difference in the incidence of ACD among Chinese, Malays, and Indians within the indigent population.[17,18] Therefore, according to the minimal data available, there is a possible decreased susceptibility among blacks, but no other racial differences in the susceptibility to ACD have been found.

ETHNIC AND CULTURAL PRACTICES AND ALLERGIC CONTACT DERMATITIS

In addition to genetic and biologic differences and exposure rates playing a role in the occurrence of contact dermatitis, racial or ethnic cultural practices are important as well. ACD to PPDA also can found in other ethnic groups owing to their exposure patterns as well. Black henna, used for ceremonial skin painting in the Middle East, North Africa, and the Indian subcontinents, has been found to contain the dye PPDA. Several case reports of ACD after receiving a "henna tattoo" have been published. ACD owing to lawsone, the major allergen in henna is rare, yet the subjects who experienced the reactions almost all had a history of permanent hair dye use in the past, and all had a positive patch test to PPDA.[19–21]

Formaldehyde and related formaldehyde-releasing preservatives have been shown to have a higher rate of sensitization in whites than in blacks. While these chemicals can be found in the industrial setting, they are allergens primarily when found in moisturizers and shampoos. The hypothesis for this finding is that the Caucasian population tends to use more cream-based products, whereas the black population tends to prefer more ointment-based products. Therefore, lower exposure in the black population would lead to lower sensitization rates. However, a decrease in sensitization to chemicals found in similar products has not been demonstrated.[15,22] Conflicting data on several other products, such as quaternuim-15 and neomycin sulfate, signal the fact that additional work is required in this area.

IMPLICATIONS OF POPULATION VARIABILITY IN SKIN TESTING RESPONSE

In order to understand ACD among difference races, clinical testing is very important. However, there is a predominance of volunteers for skin safety testing that are of Caucasian decent. The question then arises, Are clinical laboratories underestimating the ability of skin care and pharmaceutical products to cause contact dermatitis in nonwhite populations? This is therefore an area that warrants additional research.[23,24]

CONCLUSION

ACD in skin of color poses a challenge to clinicians and researchers. Current data on the differences in susceptibility to ACD among races have been inconclusive. Research suggests both an increased and decreased susceptibility of ethnic skin to ACD. Overall, demographic and clinical data support the idea that the prevalence among races is the same. However, reports have shown difference in the types of allergens that sensitize the different racial groups. Given the sparse amount of data, coupled with conflicting studies on contact dermatitis in skin of color, clearly additional investigation is required. Variables that should be the basis of these studies include environmental, cultural, occupational, genetic, individual, and racial differences.

REFERENCES

1. Pedersen LK, Johansen JD, Held E, et al. Augmentation of skin response by exposure to a combination of allergens and irritants: A review. *Contact Dermatitis* 2004;50:265-273.
2. Smith HR, Basketter DA, McFadden JP. Irritant dermatitis, irritancy, and its role in allergic contact dermatitis. *Clin Exp Dermatol* 2002;27:138-146.
3. Krob HA, Fleischer AB, D' Agostino R, et al. Prevalence and relevance of contact dermatitis allergen: A meta-analysis of 15 years of published TRUE test data. *J Am Acad Dermatol* 2004; 51(3):349-353.
4. Taylor SC. Skin of color: Biology, structure, function, and implications for

dermatologic disease. *J Am Acad Dermatol* 2002;46:S41-62.
5. Wedig JH, Maibach HI. Percutaneous penetration of dipyrithione in man: Effect of skin color (race). *J Am Acad Dermatol* 1981;5:433-438.
6 Lotte C, Wester RC, Rougier A, Maibach HI. Racial differences in the in vivo percutaneous absorption of some organic compounds: A comparison between black, Caucasian, and Asian subjects. *Arch Dermatol Res* 1993;284:456-459.
7. Kompaore F, Marty JP, Dupont CH. In vivo evaluation of the stratum cornuem barrier function in blacks, Caucasians, and Asians with two non-invasive methods. *Skin Pharmacol* 1993;6:200-207.
8. Reed JT, Ghadially R, Elias PM. Skin type, but neither race nor gender, influence epidermal permeability barrier function. *Arch Dermatol* 1995;131:1134-1138.
9. Fisher AA. Contact dermatitis in black patients. *Cutis* 1977;20:303-320.
10. Sheretz E, Swartz S. Patch test interpretation of black skin. *Am J Contact Dermatitis* 1993;4:247-248.
11. Rosenberg A, Kanof NM. Studies in eczematous sensitizations: A comparison between the sensitizing capacities of two allergens and between two different strengths of the same allergen and the effect of repeating the sensitizing dose. *J Invest Dermatol* 1941;4:505-516.
12. Kligman AM. The identification of contact allergens by human assay. The maximum test: A procedure for screening and rating contact sensitizers. *J Invest Dermatol* 1966;47:393-409.
13. North American Contact Dermatitis Group. Epidemiology of contact dermatitis in North America: 1972. *Arch Dermatol* 1973;108:537-540.
14. Dickel H, Taylor JS, Evey P, Merk HF. Comparison of patch testing results with a standard series among white and black racial groups. *Am J Contact Dermatitis* 2001; 12:77-82.
15. Fisher AA. New advances in contact dermatitis. *Int J Dermatol* 1977;16:552-568.
16. Rapaport MJ. Patch testing in Japanese subjects. *Contact Dermatitis* 1984;11:9397.
17. Goh CL. Contact sensitivity to topical medicaments. *Int J Dermatol* 1989;28: 25-28.
18. Goh CL. Prevalence of contact allergy by sex, race, and age. *Contact Dermatitis* 1986; 14:237-240.
19. Mohamed M, Nixon R. Severe allergic contact dermatitis induced by paraphenylenediamine in paint-on temporary "tattoos." *Aust J Dermatol* 2000;41: 168-171.
20. Lauchli S, Lautenschlager S. Contact dermatitis after temporary tattoos: An increasing phenomenon. *Swiss Med Wkly* 2001;131:199-202.
21. Le Coz CJL, Lefebvre C, Keller F, Grosshans E. Allergic contact dermatitis caused by skin painting (pseudotattooing) with black henna, a mixture of henna and *p*-phenylenediamine and its derivative. *Arch Dermatol* 2000;136: 1515-1517.
22. DeLeo VA, Taylor SC, Belsito DV, et al. The effect of race and ethnicity on patch test results. *J Am Acad Dermatol* 2002;46: S107-112.
23. Robinson MK, Perkins MA, Basketter DA. Application of a 4-h human patch test method for comparative and investigative assessment of skin irritation. *Contact Dermatitis* 1998;38:194-202.
24. Epstein AM. Health care in America: Still too separate, not yet equal. *N Engl J Med* 2004;351:603-605.

CHAPTER 27

Atopic Dermatitis and Other Eczemas

Nina Desai
Andrew F. Alexis

Key Points

- Atopic dermatitis (AD) is a common inflammatory skin disorder that may affect individuals of any age, race, or ethnicity.
- Genetic, environmental, and cultural factors likely contribute to observed differences in the prevalence of AD in skin of color populations compared with people of European descent.
- Erythema—the clinical hallmark of inflammation in the skin—is more difficult to appreciate in dark-skinned individuals.
- Postinflammatory hyper- and hypopigmentation are of particular concern in skin of color.
- Follicular prominence is a characteristic presentation of AD in patients of African descent and rarely seen in type I–III skin.
- As with other skin types, the mainstay of treatment of AD in skin of color involves recommended bathing practices and judicious use of emollients, topical corticosteroids, and topical immunomodulators.

Atopic dermatitis (AD) is a common inflammatory skin disease that may affect individuals of any age, race, or ethnicity.[1,2] It arises most commonly in childhood or infancy and is characterized by a chronic, relapsing course. While the etiology of AD is incompletely understood, genetic and environmental factors are thought to play important roles in the pathogenesis. The diagnosis of AD is based on a constellation of clinical features, which includes a chronic pruritic eruption that preferentially involves the flexural skin and occurs in conjunction with numerous associated features, such as early age of onset and a personal or family history of atopy (i.e., asthma, hay fever, and AD). Variations in clinical presentation, frequency, cultural perceptions, and response to treatment can be seen among individuals of different racial and ethnic groups.

EPIDEMIOLOGY OF ATOPIC DERMATITIS IN SKIN OF COLOR

Epidemiologic data pertaining to AD in non-Caucasian populations are currently limited. However, several population studies have demonstrated considerable geographic and racial/ethnic variations in the prevalence of AD.[3–5] Based on incompletely understood environmental factors, AD appears to be more common in industrialized nations and urban settings than in developing countries and rural communities.[6] Population surveys in northern Europe, the United States, and Japan have reported prevalence rates of 15.6%, 17.2%, and 21%, respectively, whereas a prevalence of 8.5% was reported in a recent study from southeastern Nigeria.[7–10] However, with increased urbanization and adoption of Western lifestyles, the prevalence of AD appears to be on the rise in developing countries, as it is in more industrialized nations.[10] The International Study of Asthma and Allergies in Childhood (ISAAC) Steering Committee evaluated the frequency of AD among 463,801 children aged 13–14 years from 56 countries.[3] In this 1999 report, a high prevalence of AD was reported in several regions where non-Caucasian individuals predominate, including centers in Africa (Nigeria, Kenya), Asia (Japan, Pakistan), and South America (Paraguay, Chile).

Several epidemiologic studies have shown an increase in the prevalence of AD among blacks and Asian/Pacific Islanders when compared with Caucasians. A recent prospective, 12-month observational study of 182 babies (62 Caucasian, 61 Chinese, and 59 Vietnamese infants) born in Melbourne, Australia, found incidence rates of AD that varied by ethnicity.[5] In this population, AD developed in 21%, 44%, and 17% of the Caucasian, Chinese, and Vietnamese infants, respectively. Because the Caucasian and the Chinese infants were of similar socioeconomical backgrounds, genetic differences likely played a role in the different incidence rates. In contrast, since the Vietnamese infants were of a lower socioeconomic background but of the same racial group as the Chinese infants, environmental factors likely contributed more than genetic factors to this difference in incidence.[5]

AD was found to be more prevalent among Chinese infants born in San Francisco and Honolulu than among the local Caucasian population.[11] Similar findings were shown in London-born black Caribbean children compared with their white counterparts; among London-born black Caribbean children, the prevalence of AD was 16.3% compared with 8.7% in white children.[4] However, a study of Indian and Caucasian preschool children in Leicester, United Kingdom, failed to show any ethnic differences in the prevalence of AD.[12]

The reasons for the observed differences in prevalence may be based at least in part on variations in genetic and environmental factors; however, differences in research methodology between epidemiologic studies must be considered when comparing prevalence rates among populations. Further research into the epidemiology of AD among non-Caucasians is warranted.

GENETICS OF ATOPIC DERMATITIS IN SKIN OF COLOR

Genetic factors are thought to play an important role in conferring susceptibility to AD. Few studies have evaluated racial or ethnic variations in gene expression in AD. However, some studies have yielded variable associations between candidate susceptibility genes and AD in different populations.

An association between atopic eczema/dermatitis syndrome (AEDS) and a variant of the gene encoding chymase (*CMA1*)—a *Bst*XI polymorphism (1903G/A) on the long arm of chromosome 14 (14q11.2)—has been reported previously in a Japanese population.[13] Since mast cell inflammatory mediators, such as tryptase and chymase, are important factors in the pathophysiology of AD and asthma, mast cell chymase has been considered a strong candidate gene for atopy and atopic disease.[13] However, small studies in two Caucasian populations—in Australia and Italy—failed to demonstrate an association between the –1903G/A polymorphism and AEDS. Recent studies have looked at genome-wide linkage analysis in Asian populations with a focus on finding susceptibility genes to AD. Very recent work has also been done looking at the importance of unique filaggrin gene mutations in Asians as Well.[14–16] While these data are limited, they suggest that there may be variable patterns of gene expression among different racial, ethnic, and/or geographic groups.

A recent prospective cohort study by Moore and colleagues evaluated perinatal predictors of AD occurring in the first 6 months of life.[17] In this U.S.-based study of 1005 mothers and their infants, infants born to black or Asian mothers were over two times as likely to be diagnosed with AD as infants born to Caucasian mothers. Among infants born to Hispanic mothers, an increased risk for AD was not found. The increased risk of AD among infants born to black and Asian mothers persisted after control for potential confounding variables, including socioeconomic status and infant feeding patterns. The contribution of genetic versus environmental factors to the observed difference in AD risk in this study is unclear. Further study will be necessary to elucidate the potential role of race and ethnicity in conferring genetic susceptibility to AD.

ENVIRONMENTAL AND CULTURAL FACTORS IN ATOPIC DERMATITIS

Environmental factors likely contribute to observed differences in the prevalence of AD in skin of color populations compared with people of European descent. Some authors have suggested that migration is an increased risk factor for AD. Studies in Hawaii and New Zealand have found higher rates of AD among migrant populations, possibly owing to new or increased allergen exposure after migration or exposure to new environmental triggers associated with urbanization.[18] A study from the New Zealand and Tokelau—a small group of islands in the South Pacific—found a higher prevalence of AD among Tokelauan children who had migrated to New Zealand compared with children who had remained in Tokelau.[19] Variations in infant feeding patterns, antigen exposures, and climactic factors may contribute to observed differences in AD prevalence in different populations. Moreover, cultural differences in diet and household environmental exposures may influence prevalence patterns of AD in different racial/ethnic groups. Cultural practices—including bathing habits, the use of harsh soaps or astringents, or the use of topical home remedies—also may contribute to racial/ethnic variations in disease severity. Further study of the role of environmental and cultural factors in AD is necessary.

CLINICAL PRESENTATION OF ECZEMA IN SKIN OF COLOR

The clinical presentation of AD in skin of color is distinguished by a number of specific features. Most notably, erythema—the clinical hallmark of inflammation in the skin—is more difficult to appreciate in dark-skinned individuals. While this phenomenon is true for all inflammatory diseases of the skin, it is particularly notable in eczematous conditions. In skin of color, acute, subacute, and chronic stages of AD present with various degrees of hyperpigmentation; depending on the skin type, erythema may be subtle or imperceptible (Figure 27-1). For this reason, special attention should be given to recognizing the subtle signs of cutaneous inflammation in dark skin such that the severity of eczema is not underestimated. Second, postinflammatory hyper- and hypopigmentation are of particular concern in skin of color. Typically, AD resolves with pigmentary changes that can last several weeks to many months (Figure 27-2). Often this dyspigmentation can be of equal or greater concern than the dermatitis itself among patients of color. Therefore, early recognition and treatment of AD in skin of color is especially important to minimize or prevent long-term postinflammatory pigment abnormalities. Third, follicular prominence is a characteristic presentation of AD in patients of African descent (Figure 27-3)—rarely seen in type I–III skin. In some patients, multiple 1- to 3-mm follicular papules may be the sole feature of AD. As such, typical morphologic features of eczema, including lichenification, erythema, crusting, and scale, can be absent (Figure 27-4). However, lichenification without follicular prominence is also often seen in dark-skinned patients as it is in Caucasians (Figure 27-5).

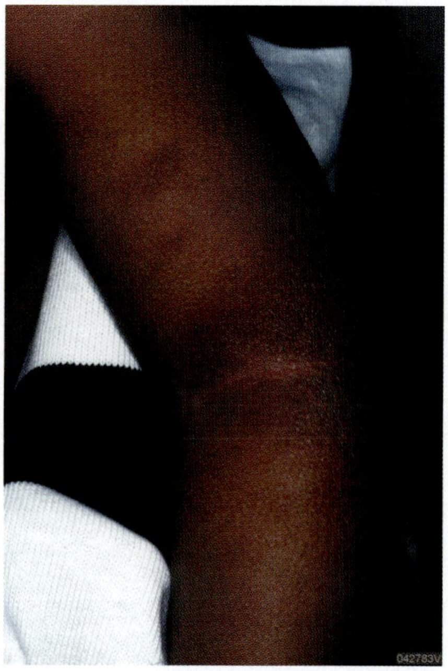

▲ **FIGURE 27-1** Erythema and lichenification in skin of color. Courtesy of DermQuest, *www.dermquest.com*, and Galderma S.A.

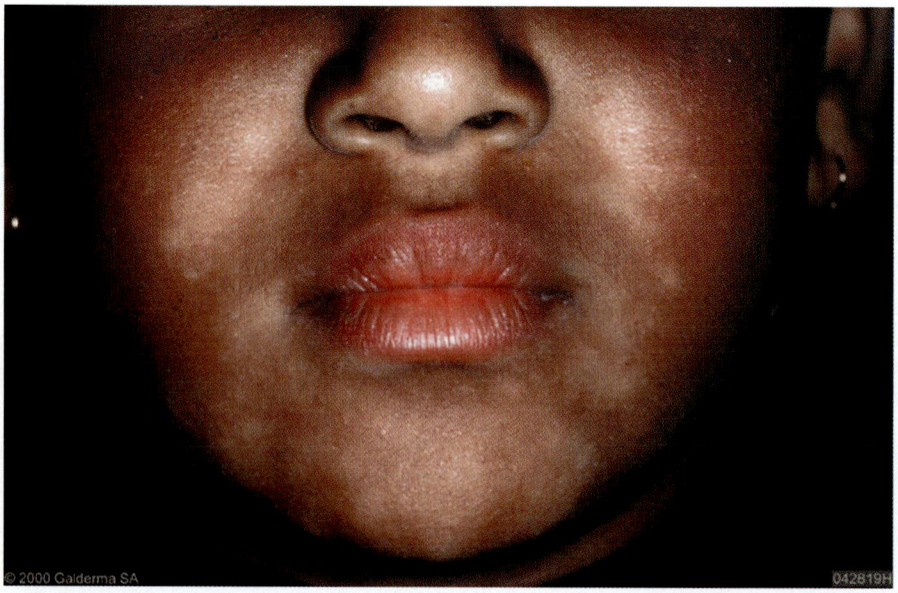

▲ **FIGURE 27-2** Postinflammatory hypopigmentation. Courtesy of DermQuest, *www.dermquest.com*, and Galderma S.A.

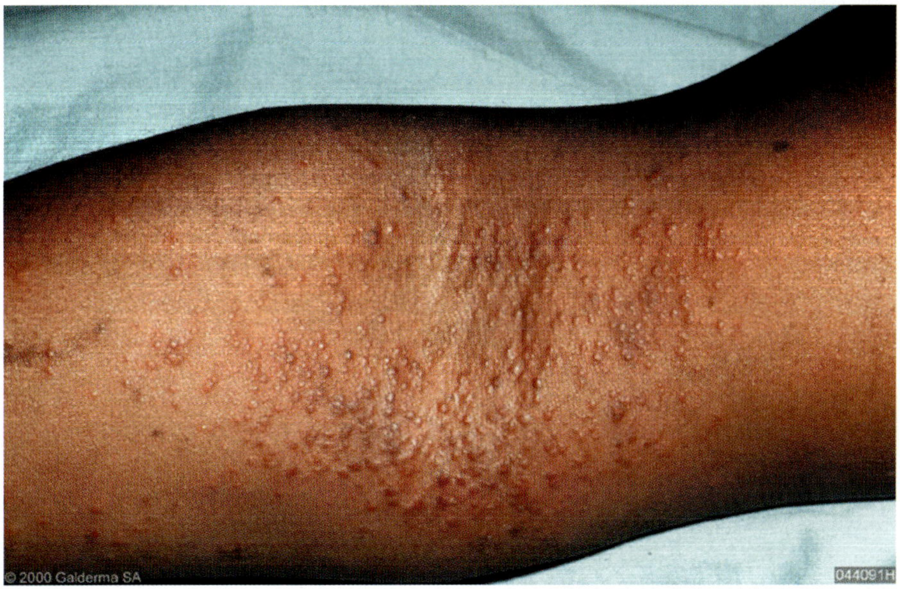

▲ **FIGURE 27-3** Follicular prominence. Courtesy of DermQuest, *www.dermquest.com,* and Galderma S.A.

Racial/ethnic variations in disease severity in AD have been reported. In a longitudinal survey of children with AD in the United Kingdom, blacks were found to be more likely to develop severe AD than their white counterparts.[20] Using the SCORAD (SCORe Atopic Dermatitis) Index, black children were almost six times more likely to develop severe AD than white children, after adjusting for erythema score [odds ratio (OR) = 5.93; 95% confidence interval (CI) 1.9418.12; $P = 0.002$].[20] Of note, without adjusting for erythema scores, no statistically significant difference was found—suggesting that reliance on measuring erythema in darkly pigmented skin can mask disease severity in AD. Further evaluation of potential racial/ethnic differences in AD severity in other populations is warranted.

OTHER ECZEMAS IN SKIN OF COLOR

Other common eczematous conditions such as nummular eczema and asteatotic eczema are also seen frequently in skin of color populations. Differences in epidemiology, clinical presentation, and responses to treatment for these conditions have not been formally studied but appear to be similar across racial/ethnic groups. Nevertheless, cultural variations in the use of emollients, ointments, astringents, and harsh soaps, as well as frequency of bathing, potentially can lead to differences in prevalence and severity of eczematous conditions in different populations.

TREATMENT CONSIDERATIONS IN SKIN OF COLOR

The clinical management of AD in dark-skinned individuals varies only slightly from that in other races. As with other skin types, the mainstay of treatment of AD in skin of color involves recommended bathing practices, judicious use of emollients, and prescribed courses of topical corticosteroids and topical immunomodulators (e.g., tacrolimus and pimecrolimus). Long baths or showers with hot water should be avoided; rather, bathing should be limited to less than 5 minutes with water that is warm or luke warm. The skin should be dabbed dry, leaving some residual moisture, after which a strong emollient is applied promptly.

A child's parents need to be informed that pigmentary changes can persist long after the eczema is treated, and as a result, topical steroids should not be continued in areas where only postinflammatory dyspigmentation remains. Patients and their parents should be reassured that hyper- or hypopigmentation eventually will resolve in most cases. However, in cases of complete depigmentation from severe AD, resolution may not occur. It is important not to cause additional hypopigmentation by the use of potent topical corticosteroids.

Even though treatment among various racial groups is very similar, a study by Janumpally and colleagues found that blacks and Asian/Pacific Islanders were considerably more likely than whites to seek medical care for their AD.[21] In this cross-sectional study using data from the U.S. National Ambulatory Medical Care Survey (NAMCS), blacks and Asian/Pacific Islanders were three and almost seven times more likely to visit a physician for AD, respectively, than whites. These differences were not due to greater overall health care utilization by blacks and Asian/Pacific Islanders because whites had a greater number of per capita visits for all medical and dermatologic conditions during the same time period. Racial/ethnic disparities in patient education, as well as differential

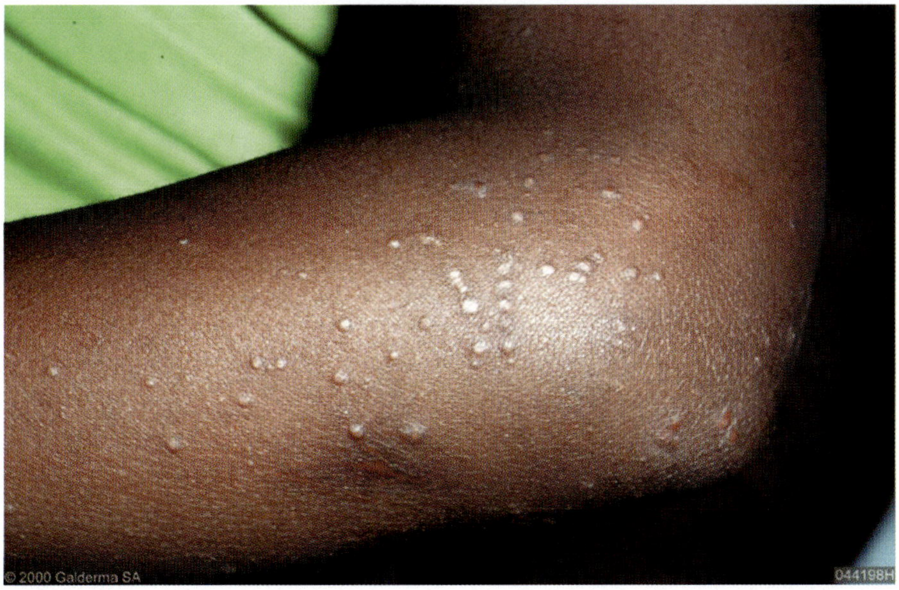

▲ **FIGURE 27-4** Discrete papules without lichenification. Courtesy of DermQuest, *www.dermquest.com,* and Galderma S.A.

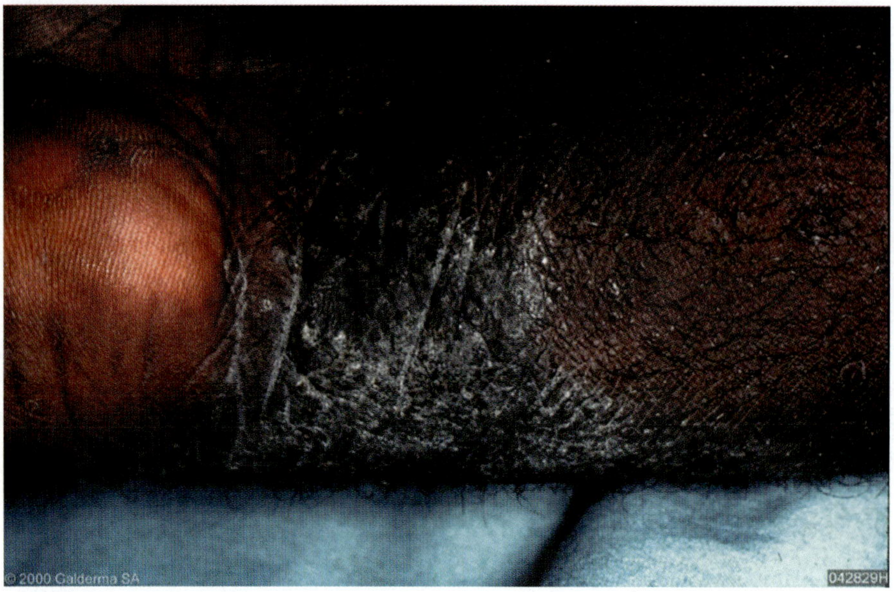

▲ **FIGURE 27-5** Lichenification. Courtesy of DermQuest, *www.dermquest.com*, and Galderma S.A.

cultural responses to AD, may cotribute to the observed differences in health care utilization for AD. It is unclear to what extent (if any) the results of this study reflect racial differences in prevalence and/or severity of AD.

REFERENCES

1. Gawkrodger DJ. Racial influences on skin disease, in Champion RH, Burns DA, Breathnach SM (eds), *Rook/Wilkenson/Ebling Textbook of Dermatology*, Vol 4, 6th ed. Oxford, England, Blackwell Science, 1998, pp 3239-3258.
2. Kefei Kang AMP, Susan T, Nedorost SR, et al. Atopic dermatitis, in Bolognia JJ, Rapini R, et al (eds), *Dermatology*, Vol 1. St Louis, MO, Mosby, 2003, pp 199-214.
3. The International Study of Asthma and Allergies in Childhood (ISAAC) Steering Committee. Worldwide variation in prevalence of symptoms of asthma, allergic rhinoconjunctivitis, and atopic eczema. *Lancet* 1998;351:1225-1232.
4. Williams HC, Pembroke AC, Forsdyke H, et al. London-born black Caribbean children are at increased risk of atopic dermatitis. *J Am Acad Dermatol* 1995;32:212-217.
5. Mar A, Tam M, Jolley D, Marks R. The cumulative incidence of atopic dermatitis in the first 12 months among Chinese, Vietnamese, and Caucasian infants born in Melbourne, Australia. *J Am Acad Dermatol* 1999;40:597-602.
6. Diepgen TL. Atopic dermatitis: The role of environmental and social factors, the European experience. *J Am Acad Dermatol* 2001;45:S44-48.
7. Schultz Larsen F, Diepgen T, Svensson A. The occurrence of atopic dermatitis in north Europe: An international questionnaire study. *J Am Acad Dermatol* 1996;34:760-764.
8. Laughter D, Istvan JA, Tofte SJ, Hanifin JM. The prevalence of atopic dermatitis in Oregon schoolchildren. *J Am Acad Dermatol* 2000;43:649-655.
9. Sugiura H, Umemoto N, Deguchi H, et al. Prevalence of childhood and adolescent atopic dermatitis in a Japanese population: Comparison with the disease frequency examined 20 years ago. *Acta Derm Venereol* 1998;78:293-294.
10. Nnoruka EN. Current epidemiology of atopic dermatitis in southeastern Nigeria. *Int J Dermatol* 2004;43:739-744.
11. Worth R. Atopic dermatitis among Chinese infants in Honolulu and San Francisco. *Hawaii Med J* 1962;22:31-34.
12. Neame RL, Kurinczuk JJ, Graham-Brown RAC. Prevalence of atopic dermatitis in Leicester: A study of methodology and examination of possible ethnic variation. *Br J Dermatol* 1995;132:772-777.
13. Iwanaga T, McEuen A, Walls AF, et al. Polymorphism of the mast cell chymase gene (*CMA1*) promoter region: Lack of association with asthma but association with serum total immunoglobulin E levels in adult atopic dermatitis. *Clin Exp Allergy* 2004;34:1037-1042.
14. Enomoto H, Noguchi E, Iijima S, et al. Single nucleotide polymorphin-based genome-wide linkage analysis in Japanese atopic dermatitis families. *BMC Dermatol* 2007;7:5.
15. Nomura T, Sandilands A, Akiyama M, et al. Unique mutations in the filaggrin gene in Japanese patietns with ichthyosis vulgaris and atopic dermatitis. *J Allergy Clin Immunol* 2007;119(2):434-440.
16. Enomoto H, Hirata K, Otsuka K, et al. Filaggrin null mutations are associated with atopic dermatitis and elevated levels of IgE in the Japanese population: A family and case-control study. *J Hum Genet* 2008;53(7):615-621.
17. Moore MM, Rifas-Shiman SL, Rich-Edwards JW, et al. Perinatal predictors of atopic dermatitis occurring in the first six months of life. *Pediatrics* 2004;113:468-474.
18. Frick O. Predisposing factors in the development of allergy, in Lessof MH, Kemeny DM (eds), *Allergy: An International Textbook*. London, Wiley, 1989, pp 350-352.
19. Waite DA, Tonkin SL, O' Donnell TV. Asthma prevalence in Tokelauan children in two environments. *Clin. Allergy* 1980;10:71-75.
20. Ben-Gashir MA, Hay RJ. Reliance on erythema scores may mask severe atopic dermatitis in black children compared with their white counterparts. *Br J Dermatol* 2002;147:920-925.
21. Janumpally SR, Feldman SR, Gupta AK, Fleischer AB Jr. In the United States, blacks and Asian/Pacific Islanders are more likely than whites to seek medical care for atopic dermatitis. *Arch Dermatol* 2002;138:634-637.

CHAPTER 28

Erythema Chronicum Perstans and Related Disorders

Miguel R. Sanchez
Tameka K. Lane

Key Points

- This disease primarily affects Latin Americans, but it is also seen in blacks and Asians; it is seen rarely in non-Hispanic Caucasians.
- It is also known as dermatitis cenicienta ("ashy dermatosis"), los cenicientos ("the ashen ones"), erythema dyschromicum perstans and erythema chronicum figuratum melanodermicum and pintoid.
- The pathogenesis is elusive and often no etiologic cause can be assigned to the disease.
- Characterized by asymptomatic, progressive, often symmetrically distributed hyperpigmented macules and patches.

Since erythema chronicum perstans was reported initially in 1957 by Osvaldo Ramirez from El Salvador under the name *dermatitis cenicienta* ("ashy dermatosis"), little progress has been made in elucidating its pathogenesis or finding effective treatments.[1] Ramirez called patients with the eruption *los cenicientos* ("the ashen ones"), a term that compares them with Cinderella (*La Cenicienta*), the downtrodden fictional character with the ash-dirtied face.[2] Later, after examining patients in Venezuela, Marion Sulzberger proposed a name change to *erythema dyschromicum perstans,* a more dignified descriptive term and one that calls attention to the erythematous margin of early lesions.[3] The disease also has been referred to in the literature as *erythema chronicum figuratum melanodermicum and pintoid.*[4]

CLINICAL PRESENTATION

Individuals with Fitzpatrick skin types III–VI are predominantly affected. Most diagnosed patients have been Latin Americans, but the disease has been described in Asians, blacks, and rarely, non-Hispanic Caucasians and reported from most regions of the world. There is no clear gender predilection, although several reviews relate a slightly higher incidence in women.[3–5] The disease predominantly affects adults between the second and third decades of life but can occur at any age, including in prepubertal children as young as 2 years of age.[6]

The onset of the disease is insidious, and it usually spreads widely before patients seek medical treatment.[5] The classic clinical presentation is characterized by the rapid eruption of asymptomatic (rarely pruritic), progressive, often symmetrically distributed hyperpigmented macules and patches in shades that range from slate gray to lead-colored to silvery brown in different individuals[7] (Figure 28-1). The lesions may be round, oval, or more commonly polycyclic, and they gradually extend peripherally. They develop over nearly any body part but more commonly arise on the torso and proximal upper extremities, followed by the neck and face, and spread over weeks to months.[8] Oral and genital mucosae, scalp, nails, palms, and soles are excluded. This distinction is useful for differentiating this entity from lichen planus, which frequently involves mucosal surfaces, and secondary syphilis, which commonly affects the palms and soles.[9] The eruption can become considerably widespread and involve a large surface area of the body, leading to considerable cosmetic disfigurement and contributing to profound psychological stress.[6–9]

Early lesions may display a slightly elevated, 1- to 2-mm erythematous margin, indicating that a fleeting inflammatory process leads to the subsequent long-standing pigmentary alteration.[4–9] When present, this finding is particularly helpful in establishing a diagnosis and provides the most characteristic histopathologic changes to confirm the clinical impression, but often the erythema has resolved by the time the patient seeks dermatologic care.[5,7–10]

An incontinentia pigmenti pattern with ashy-colored linear and reticulate patches involving Blaschko's lines on the chest, back, and abdomen has been described.[10] Unilateral eruptions may represent resolving linear lichen planus pigmentosus.[11,12] Cases of ashy dermatosis with concomitant vitiligo or with lichen planopilaris are rare.

A recent series described the findings in 14 children and found an additional 25 children reported in the literature.[6] No trigger factors were identified. In comparison with adults, resolution of pigmentation occurs more frequently, with half of pediatric cases experiencing eventual improvement.[6,13]

PATHOGENESIS

The pathogenesis of the disease remains elusive. Anecdotally reported precipitating factors include exposure to the fungicide chlorothalonil during fumigation of banana plantations, intestinal whipworm infection (for which effective eradication produced lesional remission), orally administered radiographic

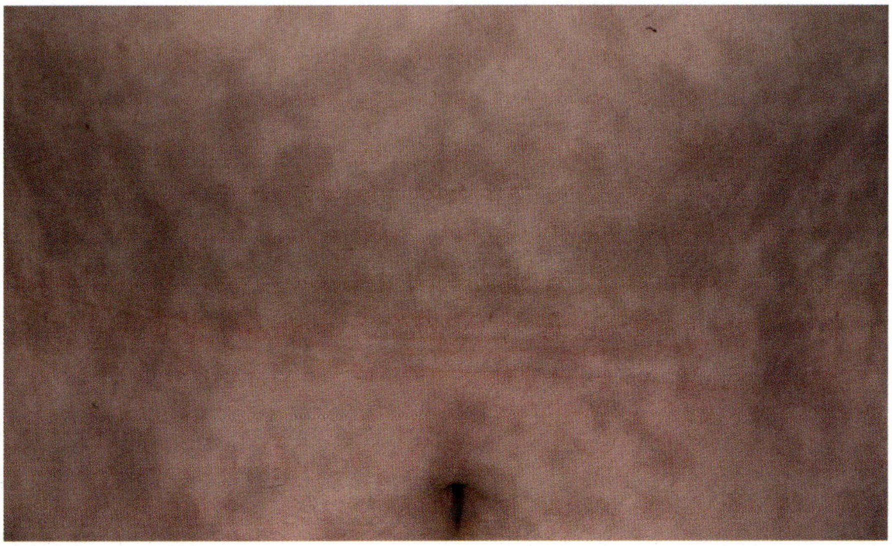

▲ **FIGURE 28-1** Characteristic pigmented patches with a bluish gray hue in a woman with erythema dyschromicum perstans.

contrast media, ingestion of ammonium nitrate, chronic hepatitis C or human immunodeficiency virus (HIV) infection, endocrinopathies, occupational cobalt allergy in plumbers, and intentional ingestion of the fertilizer ammonium nitrite by a truant youth.[3,8] However, in most cases, no apparent cause can be demonstrated, and the etiologic importance of most of these factors is disputable. Some have proposed that erythema dyschromicum perstans is not a specific disease entity but that the lesions constitute a variant of postinflammatory hyperpigmentation and represent the end stage of a nonspecific inflammatory response.[14]

However, immunopathologic investigations of active erythema dyschromicum perstans implicate the role of immune modulation. It has been proposed that an aberrant immune response targeting basal cell layer antigens may initiate the disease process. Miyagawa and colleagues detected increased expression of intercellular adhesion molecule 1 and major histocompatibility complex (MHC) class II molecules (HLA-DR) within the basal cell layer.[15] Ia antigen expression of keratinocytes and pronounced OKT5 and OKT6 staining of Langerhans' cells have been demonstrated. In addition, they identified in strata spinosum and granulosum from erythema dyschromicum perstans lesional skin the presence of thrombospondin receptor CD36, which is ordinarily absent in normal skin but characteristically found in inflammatory cutaneous diseases.[16]

DIAGNOSIS

The diagnosis of erythema dyschromicum perstans relies predominantly on clinical observation and is only supported by nonpathognomonic histopathologic features.[7] The main benefit of a biopsy is usually the exclusion of other diagnoses in consideration rather than confirmation of the diagnosis of ashy dermatosis. Examination of the inflammed, active border reveals mild basal cell layer vacuolar degeneration with occasional scattered colloid bodies, hyperkeratosis, a prominent granular layer, and minimal focal parakeratosis.[5] The superficial dermis may be edematous and shows a mild to moderate, often patchy lichenoid infiltrate of lymphocytes and histiocytes intermingled with melanophages that extends minimally to the middermis, where the pattern is more perivascular.[9] The infiltrate contains both helper/inducer and suppressor/cytotoxic lymphocytes. There is also prominent pigment incontinence in the upper dermis with variable basal cell hypermelanosis. Plasma cells and eosinophils are inconspicuous. In contrast, biopsies from older patches show compact hyperkeratosis and histologic features consistent with postinflammatory dermal hyperpigmentation, including a scant perivascular mononuclear infiltrate with numerous melanin-laden macrophages in the dermis.[7]

The vacuolization of the epidermal basal cells in early lesions suggests that the basal cell layer is a principal target, with the resulting pigment incontinence contributing to the characteristic ashy-gray color. Such a finding has triggered the hypothesis that an aberrant immune response targeting basal cell layer antigens incites the disease process. Inflammation is less severe than that seen in lichen planus but may extend more deeply.[8] Immunofluorescence is similar to that seen in lichen planus, namely, colloid bodies with possible IgM or IgG deposition with complement and fibrin occasionally located at the interface.[8]

DIFFERENTIAL DIAGNOSIS

The differential diagnosis includes a number of eruptions with increased pigmentation. Some of these diseases can be difficult to differentiate clinically and even histopathologically from erythema dyschromicum perstans even by health care providers with experience in pigmentary disorders. A common practice is to clinically diagnose any eruption with an ashy-colored erythema as dyschromicum perstans, but this hue may be produced by a number of factors, including the depth of the melanin in the dermis or deposits of metal salts. While most of these eruptions are merely disfiguring, more serious diseases, such as urticaria pigmentosa and pigmented cutaneous T-cell lymphoma, need to be considered. The presence of Darier's sign in the former and of scaling in the latter helps to exclude ashy dermatosis, but microscopic skin examination is reassuring and valuable in confirming the correct diagnosis.

Hyperpigmentation

Postinflammatory hyperpigmentation is the most common pigmentary problem in persons of color. While seemingly omnipresent in dark tan to brown skin, hyperpigmentation also commonly develops after the active stages of inflammatory or infectious skin diseases or trauma in persons with Fitzpatrick photoskin type III from Hispanic, Native American, Middle Eastern, and Asian backgrounds. Melanogenesis and pigment incontinence are further exacerbated by scratching or rubbing. Notably, the erythema may be unappreciable on visual inspection, so early inflammatory lesions may not be detected by the patient or even the physician.[17]

Although many skin diseases produce demarcated patches and plaques that can heal with increased pigmentation, the ones more frequently misdiagnosed clinically as erythema dyschromicum perstans include pityriasis rosea, nummular eczema, contact dermatitits, lichen planus, drug eruptions, syphilis, and pityriasis lichenoides chronica. Histopathologic examination can help to exclude these diseases if the classic changes of the causative dermatosis are present or if there is absence of dermal melanophages. An important consideration in formulating the treatment plan is that melanogenesis can be sustained for weeks after clinical resolution of inflammation, indicating that there may be value in continuing anti-inflammatory therapy even after signs of inflammation are no longer detectable. Ultraviolet (UV) light worsens and perpetuates hyperpigmentation, so the use of sunblocks or UV-protective clothing is essential. Untreated, pigmentation can persist for many months, especially if there is a dermal component.

Initially described by Degos, idiopathic eruptive macular pigmentation (IEMP) consists of an eruption of discrete, brown, asymptomatic macules on the trunk, neck, and proximal extremities. The disease preferentially affects children and adolescents. The pigmentation is not believed to be preceded by erythema or signs of inflammation.[18] Histopathologically, pigmentation of the basal cell layer and epidermis and prominent dermal melanophages are observed, but there is no lichenoid infiltrate or abnormal number of mast cells.[19] Over months to years, gradual resolution of the pigmentation occurs.[19] Some authors have regarded this disease as a subclinical interface inflammatory process or a variant of pityriasis rosea.[18]

Pityriasis rosea and lichen planus

Pityriasis rosea is a common benign erythematous papulosquamous disease. An initial oval or round, larger, salmon-colored patch with dark red edges (the herald patch) often appears days or weeks prior to involvement of the trunk and proximal extremities. The lesions may appear gray on patients with darker skin shades. However, the eruption usually consists of small, oval patches or barely raised plaques of uniform size with a circumferential collar of fine scale. The lesions are oriented in a "Christmas tree" pattern with their long axes following the lines of cleavage. The incidence is increased in the spring and fall. Typically, the face is spared. Another differentiation is that pruritus is present in 75% of patients, whereas erythema dyschromicum perstans is nearly always asymptomatic. However, in about 20% of patients, the eruption is atypical and more challenging diagnostically. These variants are more common in persons with skin of color. In some of these cases, the lesions may erupt predominantly on the extremities or in the axillae or groin. The lesions may be large (gigantic), urticarial, vesicular, pustular, purpuric, or erythema multiforme–like. The natural history of pityriasis rosea is spontaneous resolution in approximately 6 weeks, in contrast to the persistent hyperpigmentation of ashy dermatosis.

Lichen planus actinicus, also known as *lichen planus tropicus, lichen planus subtropicus,* and *summertime actinic lichenoid dermatitis,* is often considered to be synonymous with lichen planus pigmentosus, but contrary to the former, the later has features that permit its differentiation. This rare condition preferentially affects children and young adults. Most important among these is the predominance of lesions over areas exposed to UV light, a tendency to remit in winter, the presence of erythema in some lesions at the time of diagnosis, and the absence of lesions from intertriginous areas.[20]

Four morphologic patterns have been reported: annular, dyschromic, plaquelike, and pigmented.[20] In the annular form, the lesions are ringlike erythematous papules and plaques that become pigmented. In addition to the histologic changes characteristic of lichen planus, there is significant pigment incontinence (Figure 28-2). The dyschromic type is characterized by small, white, angular papules that coalesce into plaques on the neck and dorsa of the hands. In the classic plaquelike type, the lesions are those of lichen planus, but the distribution is predominantly over sun-exposed areas. Notably, severe pruritus, the Koebner phenomenon, and mucous membrane involvement are not common features of lichen planus actinicus. Lichen planus pigmentosus (LPP) predominates in

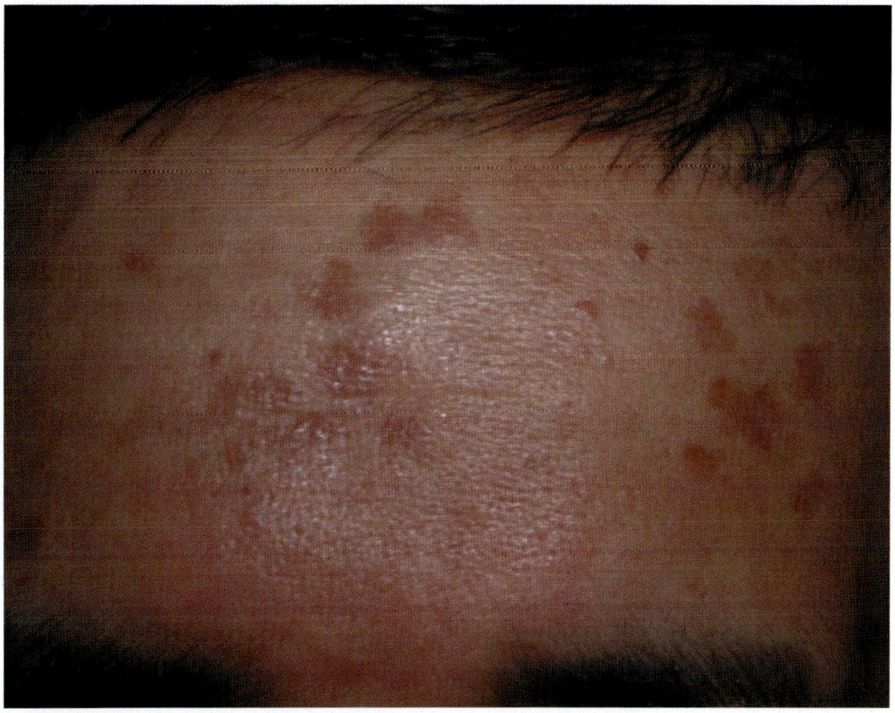

▲ **FIGURE 28-2** Erythematous barely raised papules on the forehead.

Latin American, Middle Eastern, Asian, and other persons with Fitzpatrick phototypes III–V. The eruption consists of oval and round macules and small patches that develop insidiously on sun-exposed body regions, usually the face (especially the preauricular area and temples) and neck and uncommonly the trunk and upper extremities.[21] The lesions can become diffuse. The color is usually brown, but in darker skin shades, the hue may be gray-brown or slate gray. The lesions are pruritic in over half the patients. Reticulate and perifollicular patterns also have been described. In one patient, there was progressive diffuse darkening of the total face. Flexural involvement over the axillae, inframammary folds, and occasionally the groin is present in some patients, and the lesions may be limited to intertriginous areas, prompting the term *lichen planus pigmentosus inversus*[22] (Figure 28-3). Antecedent erythema is reportedly absent. The palms and soles are spared, but lesions may arise on the mucous membranes. Bluish black pigmentation diffusely present bilaterally over the buccal mucosa and lateral borders of the tongue has been described, but it is not certain that these changes do not represent pigmentation that is common in dark-skinned patients. The eruption is symmetric in approximately 90% of patients and is limited to 10% or less of the body surface area in two-thirds of patients, although occasionally the lesions may involve more than 50% of the skin surface.[21]

Linear lichen planus pigmentosus, the combined type of lichen planus pigmentosus and linear lichen planus, is rare. Pigmented macules and patches appear in a zosteriform pattern that seems to follow the lines of Blaschko. The clinical features are similar to those of erythema dyschromicum perstans but can be distinguished, first, by the characteristic distribution and, second, by the older mean age at onset (commonly the fourth to fifth decades for lichen planus

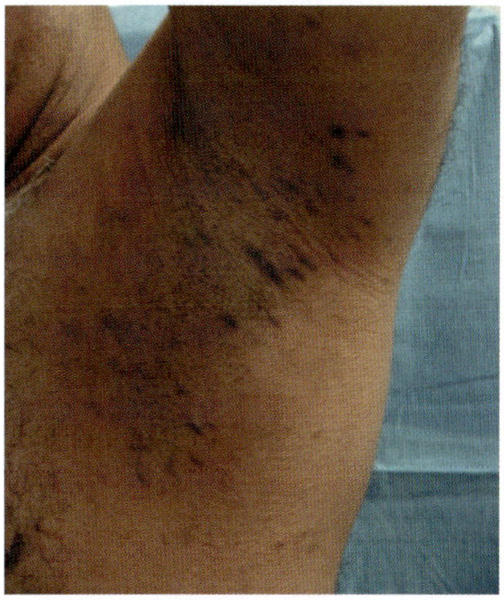

▲ **FIGURE 28-3** Violaceous macules and papules that rapidly became deeply pigmented characteristic of lichen planus pigmentosus.

pigmentosus versus the second to third decades for erythema dyschromicum perstans), and lastly, by the coexistence of classic lichen planus lesion in up to 20% of patients.[21] The course is characterized by exacerbations and remissions that occasionally are accompanied by pruritus. Histopathologic changes consist of a usually perivascular rather than lichenoid mononuclear dermal infiltrate with numerous melanophages in the papillary dermis. Beneath the epidermis, there are densely aggregated eosinophilic bodies surrounded by periodic acid–Schiff (PAS)–positive remnant basement membrane with vacuolar degeneration of the basal layer. The eosinophilic bodies are immunoreactive with keratin, and it has been suggested that they represent denatured epidermal rete ridge damaged by apoptotic changes. Hyperkeratosis and epidermal thinning are present in some cases.

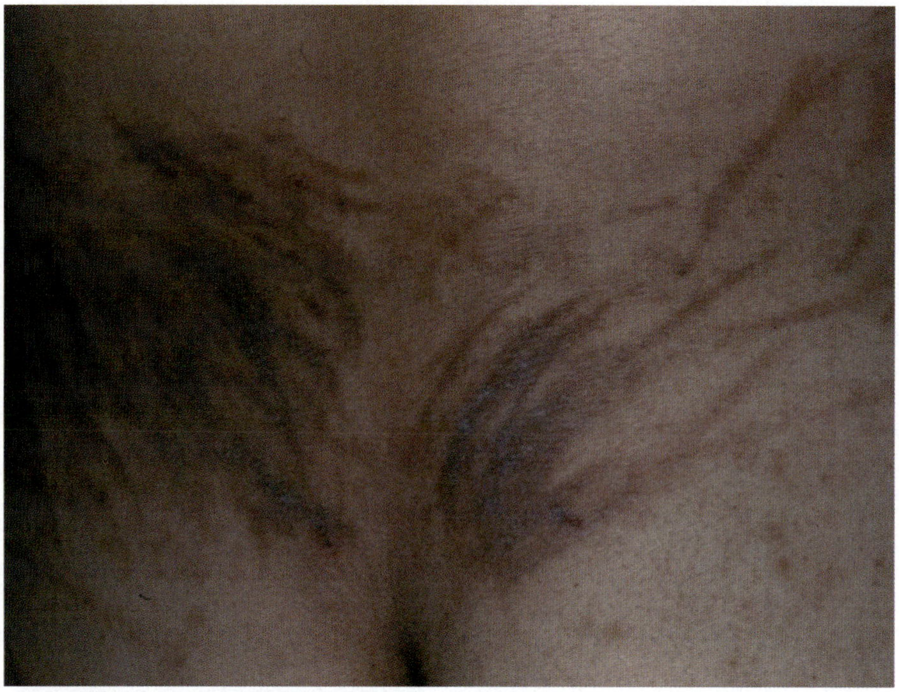

▲ **FIGURE 28-4** Pigmented streaks owing to bleomycin reaction.

Drug-induced pigmentation

Drug-induced pigmentation represents 10–20% of cases of acquired hyperpigmentation.[23] The most common drug eruptions that resemble erythema dyschromicum perstans in darker-skinned persons are fixed drug, erythema multiforme, lichenoid, photosensitive, pityriasis rosea–like, or eczematous reactions. The pathogenesis depends on the agent, and the disorder may result from increased synthesis or incontinence of melanin, tissue deposition of the drug, synthesis of drug-induced pigments, or deposits of iron sometimes after a nonspecific cutaneous inflammation and the lesions are frequently worsened by sun exposure.[23] The most frequently implicated drugs are nonsteroidal anti-inflammatory drugs, antimalarial agents, amiodarone, cytotoxic drugs, heavy metals, psychotropic drugs, and tetracyclines. Minocycline usually causes pigmentation on the face, (especially over areas of prior inflammation, such as acne) or blue-gray pigmentation on the pretibial areas and forearms, or a generalized darkening of the skin that is accentuated on sun-exposed areas. The pigmentation can be diffuse or patchy and may affect nail beds, the sclerae, the conjunctivae, and the oral mucosa. It has been reported that 4% of persons whose cumulative dose exceeds 100 g develop pigmentation.[23] The antimalarial agents chloroquine and hydroxychloroquine can cause a blue-black pigmentation that usually affects the face and anterior aspects of the lower legs. Clofazimine induces a diffuse reddish brown discoloration that accentuates inflammatory lesions. The photosensitive reaction associated with amiodorone can produce a slate-gray pigmentation in some patients. Widespread flagellate pigmented patches can be induced by bleomycin (Figure 28-4). Other therapeutic agents that are notoriously implicated in patients with pigmentary alterations include carbamazepine, chlorpromazine, thioridazine, zidovudine, busulfan, cyclohosphamide, doxorubicin, bismouth, silver, and gold.

The characteristic lesion of a fixed drug eruption is a single or multiple, circular or oval, erythematous, edematous, barely raised, occasionally centrally vesiculating plaque that becomes pigmented on any body region but preferentially on the hands, feet, and trunk (Figure 28-5). There may be stinging, itching, or no symptoms. Plaques commonly develop on the oral and genital mucosae, and mucous membranes may be the only region affected. In the nonpigmented variant, the lesions resolve in 2–3 weeks without residual hyperpigmentation. However, the disease also can present as pigmented

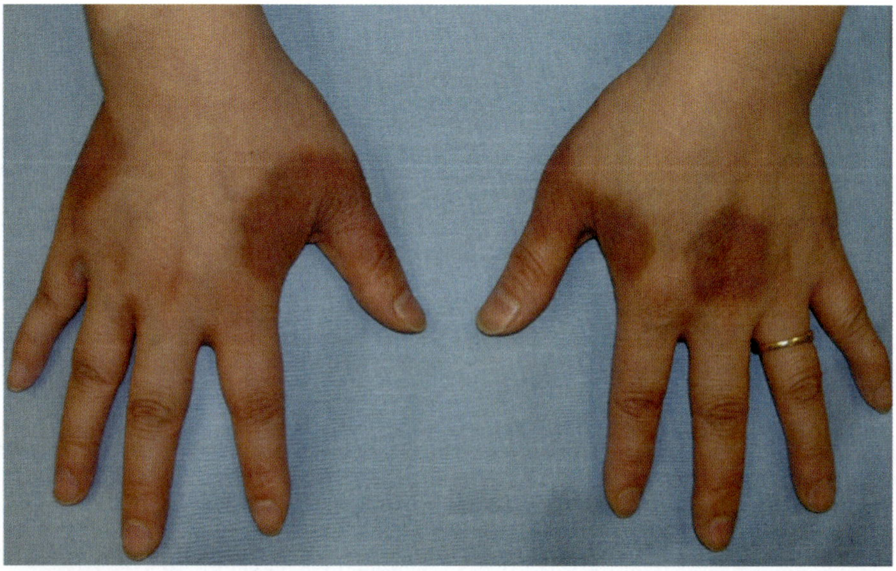

▲ **FIGURE 28-5** Sharply demarcated pigmented patches on the surface of the hands owing to fixed drug eruption.

patches that recur at fixed sites. The pigmentation becomes darker and larger with each recurrence. There is predilection for Blascko's lines, and a linear variant has been reported.[24] Morphologic variants include morbilliform, scarletiniform, multiforme, eczematous, urticarial, and nodular forms. The eruption may be localized, generalized, bullous, or bullous necrotizing. Lesions erupt from 30 minutes to 8 hours after administration of the offending drug but rarely can develop even in the absence of medications. Although this presentation is not characteristic, this reaction should be considered in the evaluation of any patient with discrete, demarcated hyperpigmentation.

Mizukawa and colleagues described a patient who was initially diagnosed as having erythema dyschromicum perstans.[25] However, on immunohistochemical biopsy evaluation, intraepidermal T cells were identified between basal and suprabasal keratinocytes, suggestive of fixed drug eruption. The patient suffered recurrence even after the presumed culpable drug, theophylline, was withheld. The most frequently responsible drugs include the muscle relaxant chlormethanone, antibacterials (especially sulfonamides), nonsteroidal anti-inflammatory agents (particularly piroxicam and mafenamic acid), beta-blockers, carbamazepine, theophylline, and nifedipine.[25] It has been proposed that the drug induces tumor necrosis factor-α–dependent keratinocyte inter-cellular adhesion molecule-1 (ICAM-1) expression in lesional skin, which, in turn, stimulates the activation of T cells that cause selective damage to the epidermis. Recently, it has been suggested that expansion of interleukin 10 (IL-10)–producing CD4+ and CD8+ T cells may be responsible for the spontaneous resolution of the reaction.[26]

Macular Amyloidosis

Macular amyloidosis is a pruritic eruption consisting of dusky-brown or slate-gray macules symmetrically distributed over the upper back and, in some patients, the arms. The characteristic reticulated or rippled pattern of pigmentation was present in less than half the patients in two studies. The deposits contain amyloid-P (a nonfibrillar protein that is identical to serum plasma globulin and inhibits the activity of elastase) and altered keratins. The amyloid is either secreted by disrupted epidermal cells in the basal layer or is the end product of filamentous degeneration of necrotic epidermal cells that have been transformed by macrophages. The deposits are readily demonstrated with stains such as Congo red, periodic acid–Schiff, and crystal violet.

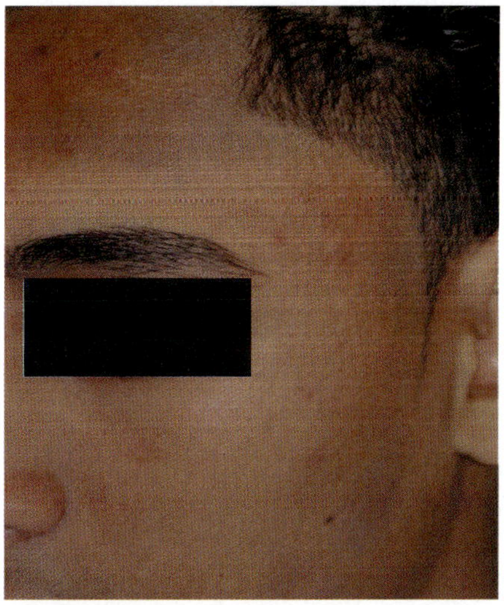

▲ **FIGURE 28-6** Friction melanosis on the face and neck owing to rubbing with an exfoliative scrubber.

Friction Melanosis

The lesions of friction melanosis are single or multiple, irregular, ill-defined, smooth, hyperpigmented patches secondary to repeated frictional trauma with rough materials such as scrub pads, loofahs, nylon towels, brushes, horse hair gloves, and tight clothing or caps (Figure 28-6). It is found in obese people similarly to intertrigo on such areas as the upper thighs where skin rubs skin. It has been reported in some thin devoted Jews from rigid backrests that rub against the lower back during the swaying activity associated with Torah study or *davening* (davener's dermatitis). The pigmentation may be uniform or mottled. Cases may occur owing to rubbing against stretch benches during exercise. These lesions develop more commonly in young adults. The prevalent areas involved are the clavicular zones, acromion, thyroid cartilage, vertebral spines, scapular and suprascapular areas, elbow and epicondyles, ulnar styloid, ulnar aspect of the forearms, forehead, and lateral aspect of the distal thighs.[27]

When amyloid is present histologically, the condition is considered to be a form of macular amyloidosis, but amyloid deposits are not seen histologically in many patients (only 40% in one study).[28] Since in some cases amyloid may be seen in subsequent biopsies, it may appear reasonable to consider this entity as a variant of macular amyloidosis. Furthermore, in one study, amyloid was present in all cases under electron microscopy.[28] However, in contrast to the former, the lesions of frictional melanosis are invariably asymptomatic and persist for longer than the typical 3- to 5-year duration of macular amyloidosis.

Linear Atrophoderma of Moulin

Linear atrophoderma of Moulin presents with discrete, hyperpigmented, well-demarcated patches that may be slightly depressed and follow Blaschko's lines.[29] Early in the course, the atrophic changes may be subtle and not easy to detect clinically. Establishing a diagnosis can be particularly challenging because the only changes present may be irregular hyperpigmentation of the basal epidermis without dermal atrophy, pigment incontinence, inflammation, or alteration of connective tissue.[29] In some reported cases, depending on the stage of evolution, variable findings, such as a perivascular mononuclear infiltrate, sclerosis with thick collagen, decreased elastic fibers, and psoriasiform changes with hyperkeratosis and acanthosis, have been observed.

The contrast between normal and involved skin can be emphasized with an incisional biopsy across the border from lesional to clinically unaffected skin. The lesions first appear during childhood or adolescence and occasionally in early adulthood. Telangiectatic and inflammatory variants have been documented, and some have considered the entity as a linear variant of idiopathic atrophoderma of Pasini and Pierini, with "cliff-drop" edges that distinguish affected and unaffected skin. The differential diagnosis includes pigmented skin conditions that appear in linear distribution or follow Blascko's lines. These include linear lichen planus pigmentosus, linear morphea, Goltz syndrome, linear and whorled nevoid hypermelanosis, a linear epidermal nevus, stage 3 of incontinentia pigmenti, X-linked reticulate pigmentary disorder, and a linear fixed or lichenoid drug eruption.

Confluent and Reticulate Papillomatosis of Gougerot and Carteaud

Confluent and reticulate papillomatosis of Gougerot and Carteaud involves 1- to 5-mm gray-brown, papillated, hyperkeratotic, barely raised papules that form plaques that become confluent into plaques centrally and reticulated at the periphery (Figure 28-7). The first lesions usually appear in the intermammary area, chest, and midback. Subsequent lesions may develop in the neck, axillae,

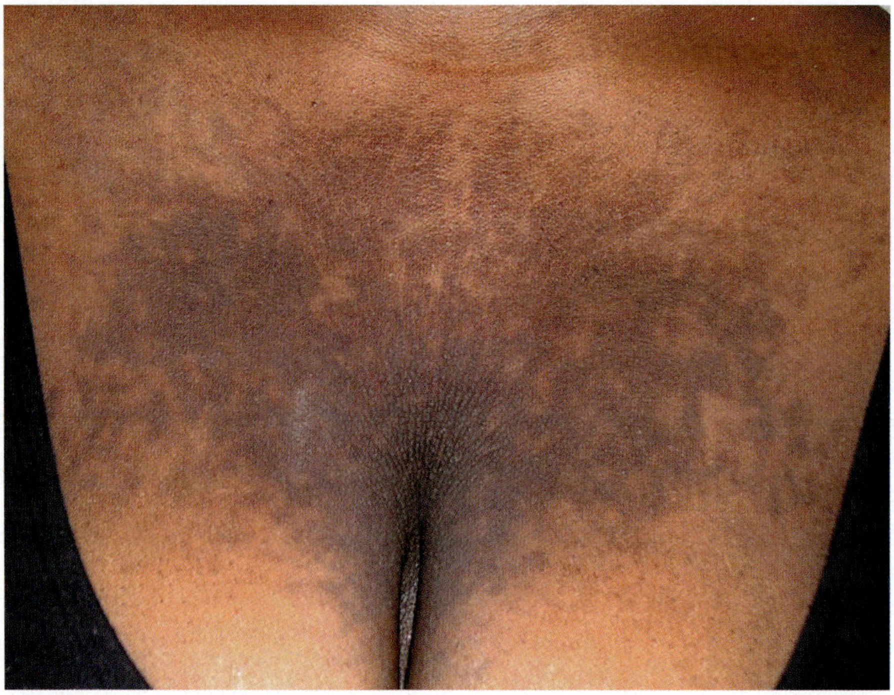

▲ **FIGURE 28-7** Brown papillated papules becoming confluent to form reticulated plaques on chest in confluent and reticulate papillomatosis of Gougerot and Carteaud.

and upper abdomen. The disease is significantly more prevalent in people of darker pigmentation and in young women. Skin biopsies of involved skin show acanthosis, papillomatosis, hyperkeratosis, and an increased number of melanosomes in the stratum corneum. Most cases are sporadic, but familial cases have been described. A role for *Malassezia furfur,* which is frequently cultured from lesions, has been proposed. Some of these patients respond to antifungal therapy, raising speculation that the disease is a variant of pityriasis versicolor on seborrheic areas. However, other patients do not respond to antifungals but to minocycline or azithromycin, and yet others are therapeutically recalcitrant and require tazarotene or systemic retinoids.[30]

Prurigo Pigmentosa

Prurigo pigmentosa is a recurrent inflammatory dermatosis characterized by pruritic, urticarial, erythematous papules and occasionally papulovesices and vesicles arranged in reticular pattern and symmetrically distributed on the back, neck, and chest. The lesions heal within days, resulting in a retiform hyperpigmentation. Most reported cases have been young Japanese women, and the eruption is more common in the spring and summer. One case was caused by an allergy to chrome in a detergent. Skin biopsy of early lesions shows a superficial perivascular infiltrate with neutrophils that invade the epidermis. Spongiosis, ballooning, and necrotic keratinocytes are present.[31] In late lesions, the infiltrate assumes a patchy lichenoid pattern with more eosinophils and lymphocytes than neutrophils. There is epidermal vesiculation and in some cases vacuolar alteration at the dermal-epidermal junction. In the later stage, the epidermis becomes hyperplastic, parakeratotic, and studded with melanin, with melanophages appearing in the dermis.[31] Immunofluorescence is invariably negative. Notably, minocycline or doxycycline is usually effective in resolving symptoms as well as the pigmentation. Dapsone can be used in unresponsive cases.

Acquired Relapsing Blaschko Dermatitis

Acquired relapsing Blaschko dermatitis presents with acquired, hyperpigmented, confluent, unilateral, occasionally scaly papules that become confluent into plaques in a linear arrangement on the trunk and neck and heal spontaneously. Variants with papulovesicles and involvement of the palms and soles have been described. The lesions form a V shape over the spine and an S shape on the lateral and anterior aspects of the trunk because Blasckho's lines assume these configurations over these areas owing to movements of the skin during embryogenesis.[32] The eruption relapses, particularly during times of stress. On histopathologic examination, there is a superficial perivascular infiltrate of lymphocytes and eosinophils.[32] The epidermis is hyperplastic, and spongiosis and mounds of parakeratosis are present. Systemic corticosteroids have been found to be effective.

TREATMENT

Numerous treatments have been proposed for erythema dyschromicum perstans, including antibiotics, clofazimine, oral and topical corticosteroids, keratolytic agents, ascorbic acid, isoniazid, tretinoin, chloroquine, and griseofulvin, but with few exceptions, there are little or no data to support recommendation of these therapies. Clofazimine may be of some modest benefit via its anti-inflammatory and immunomodulatory effects.[33] The drug was found to reduce expression of intercellular adhesion and lymphocyte activation molecules and decreased the mononuclear cell infiltrate. In seeming contradiction, clofazimine exerts both proinflammatory and anti-inflammatory affects. It serves as a hypochlorous acid forager, decreasing neutrophilic inflammation, and modifies monocytes and lymphoid cell function. Specifically, Piquero-Martin and colleagues found that clofazimine improved skin coloration, which correlated with attenuation of venous blood CD4:CD8 ratios.[34] Some have suggested that the drug's induction of a diffuse red-brown coloration helps to mask the pigmented lesions of erythema dyschromicum perstans. The administered dose in a study in which seven of eight patients had good to excellent responses was 100 mg every other day to those weighing under 40 kg and 100 mg daily to those heavier than 40 kg. After 3 months, the dose was reduced to 200 and 400 mg weekly, respectively.[34] Other cases have been treated with doses as high as 300 mg daily, which is associated with greater gastrointestinal intolerance and other adverse effects. Notably, treatment has to be continued for months and usually close to 1 year, and even then there are reports of therapeutic failure, which partly explains the lack of acceptance of the drug as treatment for the disease.

Dapsone also has been investigated in very small series and is reported to hasten resolution of pigmentation.[35] Because of the unavailability of clofazimine in some countries, dapsone has become a more popular treatment. Its effectiveness is possibly mediated through an immunomodulatory effect. Kontochristopoulos and colleagues reported regression of active disease, improvement of pigmentation, and cessation of the disease process with dapsone continued from 2–3 months. An adult dose of 100 mg daily is administered for at least 8–12 weeks.[36]

Hydroquinone is usually ineffective because the melanin deposition is found too deep in the dermis to achieve therapeutic concentrations. Efforts at improving pigmentation with chemical peels and with the Q-switched ruby (694-nm), Q-switched Nd/Yag (1064-nm), and Q-switched alexandrite (755-nm) lasers have been disappointing.

REFERENCES

1. Ramírez CO. *Los Cenicientos: Problema Clínico:* Report of the first Central American Congress of Dermatology, Vols 5-8. San Salvador, CACD, 1957, pp 122-130.
2. Ramirez CO. The ashy dermatosis (erythema dyschromicum perstans): Epidemiological study and report of 139 cases. *Cutis* 1967;3:244-247.
3. Schwartz RA. Erythema dyschromicum perstans: The continuing enigma of Cinderella or ashy dermatosis. *Int J Dermatol* 2004:43;230-232.
4. Osswald SS, Proffer LH, Sartori CR. Erythema dyschromicum perstans: A case report and review. *Cutis* 2001;68:25-28.
5. Pandya AG, Guevara IL. Disorders of hyperpigmentation. *Dermatol Clin* 2000;18: 91-98.
6. Torrelo A, Zaballos P, Colmenero I, et al. Erythema dyschromicum perstans in children: A report of 14 cases. *J Eur Acad Dermatol Venereol* 2005;19:422-426.
7. Sanchez MR. Cutaneous diseases in Latinos. *Dermatol Clin* 2003;21:689-697.
8. Dominguez-Soto L, Hojyo–Tomoka T, Vega Memije E, et al. Pigmentary problems in the tropics. *Dermatol Clin* 1994;12:777-784.
9. Sanchez MR. Dermatologic disease in Hispanics/Latinos, in Halder R (ed), *Dermatology and Dermatological Therapy of Pigmented Skin.* Boca Raton, FL, CRC Press, 2005, pp 357-384.
10. Vega ME, Waxtein L, Arenas R, et al. Ashy dermatosis and lichen planus pigmentosus: A clinicopathologic study of 31 cases. *Int J Dermatol* 1992;31:90-94.
11. Yokozeki H, Ueno M, Komori K, Nishioka K. Multiple linear erythema dyschromicum perstans (ashy dermatosis) in the lines of Blaschko. *Dermatology* 2005;210:356-537.
12. Akagi A, Ohnishi Y, Tajima S, Ishibashi A. Linear hyperpigmentation with extensive epidermal apoptosis: A variant of linear lichen planus pigmentosus? *J Am Acad Dermatol* 2004;50:S78-80.
13. Silverberg NB, Herz J, Wagner A, Paller AS. Erythema dyschromicum perstans in prepubertal children. *Pediatr Dermatol* 2003;20:398-403.
14. Convit J, Piquero-Martin J, Perez RM. Erythema dyschromicum perstans. *Int J Dermatol* 1989;28:168-169.
15. Miyagawa S, Komatsu M, Oluchi T. Erythema dyschromicum perstans: Immunopathologic studies. *J Am Acad Dermatol* 1989;20:882-886.
16. Baranda L, Torres-Alvarez B, Cortes-Franco R, et al. Involvement of cell adhesion and activation molecules in the pathogenesis of erythema dyschromicum perstans (ashy dermatosis): The effect of clofazimine therapy. *Arch Dermatol* 1997;133:325-329.
17. Taylor SC. Enhancing the care and treatment of skin of color: I. The broad scope of pigmentary disorders. *Cutis* 2005;76: 249-255.
18. Sanz de Galdeano C, Léauté-Labrèze C, Bioulac-Sage P, et al. Idiopathic eruptive macular pigmentation: Report of five patients. *Pediatr Dermatol* 1996;13: 274-277.
19. Jang KA, Choi JH, Sung KS, et al. Idiopathic eruptive macular pigmentation: Report of 10 cases. *J Am Acad Dermatol* 2001;44:351-353.
20. Meads SB, Kunishige J, Ramos-Caro FA, Hassanein AM.. Lichen planus actinicus. *Cutis* 2003;72:377-381.
21. Kanwar AJ, Dogra S, Handa S, et al. A study of 124 Indian patients with lichen planus pigmentosus. *Clin Exp Dermatol* 2003;28:481-485.
22. Pock L, Jelinkova L, Drlik L, et al. Lichen planus pigmentosus-inversus. *J Eur Acad Dermatol Venereol* 2001;15:452-454.
23. Dereure O. Drug-induced skin pigmentation: Epidemiology, diagnosis and treatment. *Am J Clin Dermatol* 2001;2:253-262.
24. Megahed M, Reinauer S, Scharffetter-Kochanek K, et al. Acquired relapsing self-healing Blaschko dermatitis. *J Am Acad Dermatol* 1994;31:849-852.
25. Mizukawa Y, Shiohara T. Fixed drug eruption presenting as erythema dyschromicum perstans: A flare without taking any medications. *Dermatology* 1998;197:383-385.
26. Sehgal VN, Srivastava G. Fixed drug eruption (FDE): Changing scenario of incriminating drugs. *Int J Dermatol* 2006:45;897-908.
27. Al-Aboosi M, Abalkhail A, Kasim O, et al. Friction melanosis: A clinical, histologic, and ultrastructural study in Jordanian patients. *Int J Dermatol.* 2004; 43(4):261-264
28. Siragusa M, Ferri R, Cavallari V, Schepis C. Friction melanosis, friction amyloidosis, macular amyloidosis, and towel melanosis: Many names for the same clinical entity. *Eur J Dermatol* 2001;11:545-548.
29. Miteva L, Nikolova K, Obreshkova E. Linear atrophoderma of Moulin. *Int J Dermatol* 2005;44:867-869.
30. Davis MD, Weenig RH, Camilleri MJ. Confluent and reticulate papilloma-tosis (Gougerot-Carteaud syndrome): A minocycline-responsive dermatosis without evidence for yeast in pathogenesis. A study of 39 patients and a proposal of diagnostic criteria. *Br J Dermatol* 2006; 154:287-293.
31. Boer A, Misago N, Wolter M, et al. Prurigo pigmentosa: A distinctive inflammatory disease of the skin. *Am J Dermatopathol* 2003;25:117-129.
32. Megahed M, Reinauer S, Scharffetter-Kochanek K, et al. Acquired relapsing self-healing Blaschko dermatitis. *J Am Acad Dermatol* 1994;31:849-852.
33. Stratigos AJ, Katsambas AD. Optimal management of recalcitrant disorders of hyperpigmentation in dark-skinned patients. *Am J Clin Dermatol* 2004:5:161-168
34. Piquero-Martin J, Perez-Alfonzo R, Abrusci V, et al. Clinical trial with clofazimine for treating erythema dyschromicum perstans: Evaluation of cell-mediated immunity. *Int J Dermatol* 1989;28:198-200.
35. Bahadir S, Cobanoglu U, Cimsit G, et al. Erythema dyschromicum perstans: Response to dapsone therapy. *Int J Dermatol* 2004:43:220-222.
36. Kontochristopoulos G, Stavropoulos P, Pantelos D. Erythema dyschromicum perstans: Response to dapsone therapy. *Int J Dermatol* 1998;37:790-799.

CHAPTER 29

Lichen Amyloidosis

Richard S. Mizuguchi

Key Points

- Amyloidosis is the deposition of amyloid, a group of unrelated proteins, in the extracellular space.
- Amyloidosis is divided into primary systemic and localized cutaneous types.
- Primary cutaneous amyloidosis is subdivided into nodular, macular, and lichen types.
- Ethnic skin, particularly that of Asians, Middle Easterners, and South Americans, seems to be predisposed to developing lichen amyloidosis.
- A review of common dermatologic diagnoses in Asians lists lichen amyloidosis as one of the 12 common skin disorders.
- Treatment is palliative, not curative, and alleviates the symptoms of pruritus.

The term *amyloid* was coined in 1838 by Schneider, a German botanist, to describe cellulose-like substances in plants.[1] *Amyloidosis* refers to the deposition of amyloid, a group of unrelated proteins, in the extracellular space, leading to a pathologic change. Eosinophilic amorphous substances are seen by light microscopy. Amyloid subtypes are composed of 7.5- to 10-nm-wide linear, nonbranching tubular fibrils arranged in meshwork.[2] Each fibril has a β-pleated sheet configuration. The quaternary structure is unknown for all types of amyloid.[3]

The amyloid fibril protein and the mechanism of deposition determine the clinical subtype of amyloidosis. Amyloidosis is divided into primary systemic and localized cutaneous amyloidosis. Localized cutaneous amyloidosis can be further subdivided into nodular, macular, and lichenoid (papular) primary cutaneous amyloidosis and secondary cutaneous amyloidosis. Macular amyloidosis and lichen amyloidosis are thought to be different clinical manifestations of the same disease and can be seen in the same patient. Secondary cutaneous amyloidosis includes sweat gland tumors, dermatofibroma, pilomatrixoma, solar elastosis resulting from psoralen and ultraviolet A (PUVA) therapy, seborrheic keratosis, basal cell carcinoma, Bowen disease, and actinic keratosis.[2]

TABLE 29-1
Common Dermatologic Diagnoses in Asians

20.4	Xerosis
19.3	Pruritus
16.8	Nummular dermatitis
14.2	Dyshidrosis
9.9	Atopic dermatitis
7.1	Melasma
4.5	Photodermatoses
4.2	Psoriasis
3.2	Vitiligo
2.3	Lichen amyloidosis (South Asian)
0.8	Nevus of Ito
2.0	Nevus of Oto

Percentages not available.
Source: Data from Halder R, Nootheti P. Ethnic hair and skin: What is the state of the science. *J Am Acad Dermatol* 2003;48:S143–148.

Freudenthal first introduced the term *lichen amyloidosis* in 1930.[4] Ethnic skin, particularly that of Asians, Middle Easterners, and South Americans, seems to be predisposed to developing lichen amyloidosis.[5–9] A review of common dermatologic diagnoses in Asians lists lichen amyloidosis as one of the 12 common skin disorders (Table 29-1).

PATHOGENESIS

Many factors have been implicated as possible etiologic factors in lichen amyloidosis[10–14] (Table 29-2). The complete characterization of amyloid in lichen amyloidosis remains to be elucidated. In primary localized cutaneous amyloidosis, the amyloid is thought to be derived from keratin peptides of epidermal origin that are formed secondary to necrotic keratinocytes.[20,21] Antikeratin antibodies have been used to confirm the keratin epitopes of primary cutaneous amyloidosis.[22–29]

TABLE 29-2
Possible Etiologic Factors for Lichen Amyloidosis[15–19]

- Prolonged friction (back scratcher use)
- Genetic predisposition
- Epstein-Barr virus
- HIV infection
- Environmental factors

The mechanism of amyloid formation in lichen amyloidosis is unknown and remains controversial. The presence of cytokeratins in primary cutaneous amyloidosis supports Hashimoto's fibrillar body theory of amyloidogenesis. The theory proposes that epidermal basal keratinocytes are transformed to amyloid protein. Cells that undergo apoptosis accumulate tonofilaments and form colloid bodies, which are modified by histiocytes and fibroblasts to form amyloid deposits.[30] This theory is supported by histologic[31] and ultrastructural[32] studies that demonstrate transitional forms between keratinocytes and amyloid. The fibrillar body theory of amyloidosis is further supported by the sequential changes in the antigenic profile from basal keratinocytes to amyloid through cytoid boides.[33] Studies showing amyloid, colloid bodies, and isolated keratin filaments binding amyloid P component and vitronectin further substantiate this theory.

In an alternative theory, Yamagihara suggests that disrupted basal keratinocytes produce and secrete precursor proteins at the epidermal-dermal interface.[34] This theory, known as the *secretion theory,* has been supported by ultrastructural evidence of lamina densa disruption above the amyloid deposits in lichen amyloidosis.[35] Electron microscopic evidence of lamina densa disruption above the amyloid deposits were found in patients with lichen and macular amyloidosis.[21] The deposits contained basement membrane antigens such as types IV and VII collagen, laminin, lamina densa–like substance, and LDA-1 antigen, a basement membrane component.[36]

CLINICAL PRESENTATION

Lichen amyloidosis is characterized by multiple firm, discrete, hyperpigmented and hyperkeratotic, scaly papules that sometimes coalesce to form plaques (Figure 29-1). Pruritus is a prominent feature of lichen amyloidosis. The sites of predilection are the shins or other extensor surfaces of the extremities.[37] Bullous lesions have been described with lichen amyloidosis.[38] However, bullous lesions are seen more frequently in systemic amyloidosis. Generalized lichen amyloidosis occurs very infrequently.[39,40]

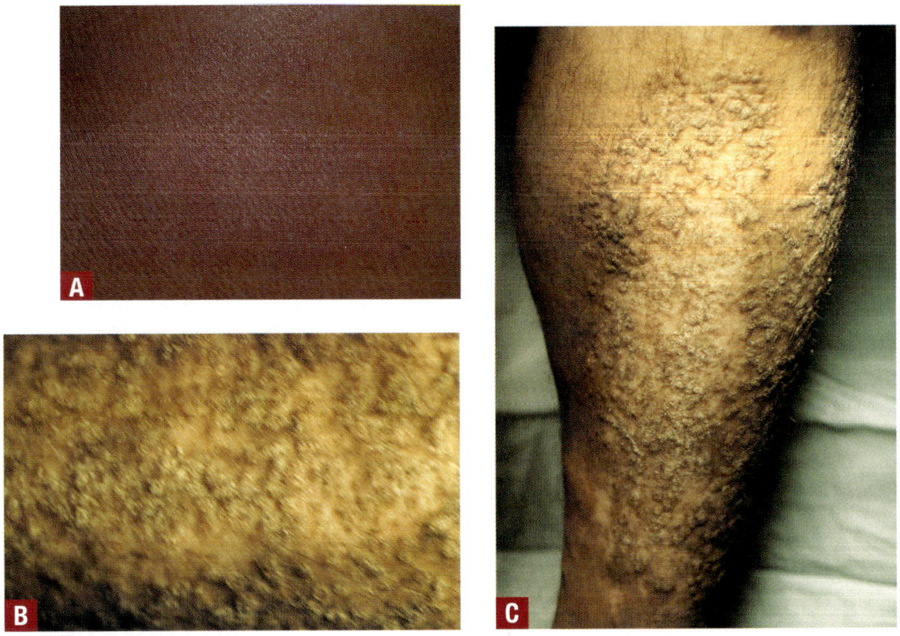

▲ **FIGURE 29-1** Lichen amyloid displaying hyperpigmented and hyperkeratotic, scaly papules coalescing into plaques.

A familial form of primary cutaneous amyloidosis occurs rarely. In all reported cases, inheritance was autosomal dominant. Although most families were of ethnic decent,[41–45] Caucasian families have been reported.[46–50] Therefore, skin phototypes III and IV may not be a predisposing factor in familial macular and lichen amyloidosis.

PATHOLOGY

Amyloid deposits are restricted primarily to the papillary dermis. The deposits may displace the rete ridges. The epidermis above the deposits may show acanthosis or thinning and hyperkeratosis. There are often perivascular lymphohistiocytic infiltrates as well as pigment incontinence (Figure 29-2).

Amyloid can be better visualized using special stains, and Congo red stain is the best. When used with polarized light, amyloid emits a characteristic apple-green birefringence with Congo red stain. Amyloid also may be stained successfully with a variety of other histologic stains[51,52–54] (Table 29-3).

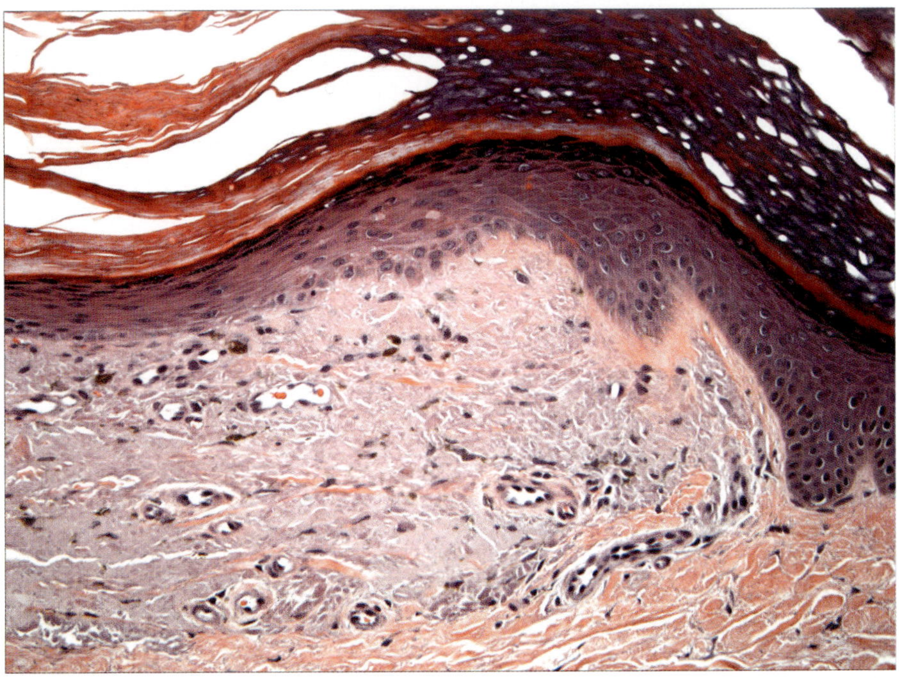

▲ **FIGURE 29-2** Pathology (H&E stain). There is hyperkeratosis with thinning of the epidermis. In the papillary dermis, amyloid deposits are seen. There is a sparse perivascular lymphohistiocytic infiltrate.

TABLE 29-3
Histologic Stains for Amyloid[55–57]

Highman's crystal and methyl violet
Benhold's Congo red stain
O&G stain
Cotton dyes (Pagoda red, RIT, Scarlet No. 5, RIT, Cardinal Red No. 9)
Thiazole dye
Triphenyl-methane dye
PAS method
Sirius red

TREATMENT

Lichen amyloidosis is a chronic skin disorder that does not respond to any one treatment modality. Treatment is palliative, not curative, and alleviates the symptoms of pruritus rather than removing the amyloid deposits (Table 29-4). Possible precipitating and/or aggravating factors such as chronic friction induced by scratching and rubbing should be avoided.[58] In mild cases, topical corticosteroids (with or without occlusion) and intralesional corticosteroids are the first line of treatment.[59] The addition of a keratolytic agent such as urea or salicylic acid may be beneficial. Calcipotriol has been shown to be effective in the treatment of lichen amyloidosis.[53] Tacrolimus also has been reported to have a beneficial effect.[60]

Dimethyl sulfoxide (DMSO) has been known to be effective for the treatment of both lichen and macular amyloidosis, although there are some refractory cases.[52,61–62] Application of 50% or 100% solutions resolves pruritus. Irritant dermatitis and contact dermatitis/urticaria are reported side effects.[53] Phototherapy with UVB and

TABLE 29-4
Treatment of Lichen Amyloidosis[52–54, 58–69]

Remove precipitating and/or aggravating factors
Topical corticosteroids (with or without occlusion cclusion)
Intralesional corticosteroids
Keratolytic agent (urea or salicylic acid)
Calcipotriol
Tacrolimus
Dimethyl sulfoxide (DMSO)
Phototherapy with UVB and photochemotherapy (PUVA)
Systemic retinoids (acitretin)
Cyclosporine
Dermabrasion
Scalpel removal
Q-switched Nd:YAG laser

photochemotherapy (PUVA) should be considered in patients not responding to topical therapy.[54]

As is the case with topical therapy, systemic therapy may be beneficial for some but not all patients. Systemic retinoids, specifically acitretin, have improved the pruritus of lichen amyloidosis and resulted in the flattening of the skin lesions.[63,64] Cyclosporine also has been shown to be effective.

Surgical options include dermabrasion[65] and scalpel removal of amyloid in the epidermis.[66,67] The side effects produced by systemic therapy must be considered when using such therapy.[68] Frequency-doubled Q-switched Nd:YAG laser has been used with some success. It is less invasive than dermabrasion or scapel removal and perhaps should be tried before more invasive treatment modalities.[69] Hyperpigmentation may limit the usefulness of lasers, and a test spot should be done prior to treatment.

Lichen amyloidosis is thought to be purely a cutaneous disease. As such, therapy has been directed at relieving the symptoms of pruritus. Some of the surgical techniques may be directed toward removal of the amyloid from the dermis, although pain and discomfort, as well as hospitalization, may limit the usefulness of these options.

REFERENCES

1. Kyle RA, Gertz MA. Primary systemic amyloidosis: Clinical and laboratory features in 474 cases. *Semin Hematol* 1995; 32:45-59.
2. Breathnach SM. Amyloid and amyloidosis. *J Am Acad Dermatol* 1988;18:1-16.
3. Lambert WC. Cutaneous deposition disorders, in Farmer ER, Hood AF (eds), *Pathology of the Skin*. East Norwalk, CT, Appleton & Lange, 1990, pp 432-450.
4. Wong C-K. History and modern concepts (cutaneous amyloidosis). *Clin Dermatol* 1990;8:1-6.
5. Black MM, Wilkinson DS. Metabolic and nutritional disorders: Amyloid and amyloidosis of the skin, in Rook A, Wilkinson DS, Ebling FJG, et al (eds), *Textbook of Dermatology*, 5th ed. Oxford, England, Blackwell Scientific, 1992, pp 2333-2344.
6. Kibbi AG, Rubeiz NG, Zaynoun ST, Kurban AK. Primary localized cutaneous amyloidosis. *Int J Dermatol* 1992;31: 95-98.
7. Wong CK. Lichen amyloidosis: A relatively common skin disorder in Taiwan. *Arch Dermatol* 1974;110:438-440.
8. Looi LM, Lumpur K. Primary localized cutaneous amyloidosis in Malaysians. *Aust J Dermatol* 1991;32:39-44.
9. Ollague W, Ollague J, Ferretti H. Epidemiology of primary cutaneous amyloidosis in South America. *Clin Dermatol* 1990;8:1-6.
10. Weyers W, Weyers I, Bonczkowitz M, et al. Lichen amyloidosus: A consequence of scratching. *J Am Acad Dermatol* 1997;37: 923-928.
11. Chang YT, Liu HN, Wong CK, et al. Detection of Epstein-Barr virus in primary cutaneous amyloidosis. *Br J Dermatol* 1997;136:823-826.
12. Vaghjimal A, Ahmad H, Soto NE, et al. Lichen amyloidosis in an HIV-infected patient: A case report and review of the literature. *Acta Dermatol Venerol* 1998; 78:399.
13. Buezo GF, Penas PF, Dauden Tello E, et al. Lichen amyloidosis and human immunodeficiency virus infection. *Dermatology* 1995;191:56-58.
14. Goller MM, Cohen PR, Duvic M. Lichen amyloidosis presenting as a papular pruritus syndrome in a human-immunodefieiciency-virus-infected man. *Dermatology* 1997;194: 62-64.
15. Weyers W, Weyers I, Bonczkowitz M, et al. Lichen amyloidosus: A consequence of scratching. *J Am Acad Dermatol* 1997;37: 923-928.
16. Chang YT, Liu HN, Wong CK, et al. Detection of Epstein-Barr virus in primary cutaneous amyloidosis. *Br J Dermatol* 1997;136:823-826.
17. Vaghjimal A, Ahmad H, Soto NE, et al. Lichen amyloidosis in an HIV-infected patient: A case report and review of the literature. *Acta Dermatol Venerol* 1998; 78:399.
18. Buezo GF, Penas PF, Dauden Tello E, et al. Lichen amyloidosis and human immunodeficiency virus infection. *Dermatology* 1995;191:56-58.
19. Goller MM, Cohen PR, Duvic M. Lichen amyloidosis presenting as a papular pruritus syndrome in a human-immunodefieiciency-virus-infected man. *Dermatology* 1997;194: 62-64.
20. Maeda H, Ohata S, Saito Y, et al. Epidermal origin of the amyloid in localized cutaneous amyloidosis. *Br J Dermatol* 1982;106:345-351.
21. Kumakiri M, Hashimoto K. Histogenesis of primary localized cutaneous amyloidosis: Sequential change of epidermal keratinocytes to amyloid via filamentous degeneration. *J Invest Dermatol* 1979;73: 150-162.
22. Huilgol SC, Ramnarin N, Carrington P, et al. Cytokeratins in primary cutaneous amyloidosis. *Australas J Dermatol* 1998; 39:81-85.
23. Yoneda K, Watanabe H, Yanagihara M, Mori S. Immunohistochemical staining properties of amyloids with anti-keratin antiboides using formalin-fixed, paraffin-embeedded sections. *J Cutan Pathol* 1989; 16:133-136.
24. Ortiz-Romero PL, Ballestin-Carcavilla C, Lopez-Estebaranz JL, Iglesias-Diez L. Clinicopathologic and immunohistochemical studies on lichen amyloidosis and macular amyloidosis. *Arch Dermatol* 1994;130:1559-1560.
25. Maeda H, Ohta S, Saito Y, et al. Epidermal origin of the amyloid in localized cutaneous amyloidosis. *Br J Dermatol* 1982;106:345-351.
26. Kobayashi H, Hashimoto K. Amyloidogenesis in organ limited cutaneous amyloidosis: An antitgenic identity between epidermal keratin and skin amyloid. *J Invest Dermatol* 1983;80:66-72.
27. Noren P, Westermark P, Cornwell GG, Murdoch W. Immunofluorescence and histochemical studies of localized cutaneous amyloidosis. *Br J Dermatol* 1983; 108:277-285.
28. Masu S, Hosokawa M, Seiji M. Amloid in localized cutaneous amyloidosis: Immunofluorescence studies with anti-keratin anti-serum especially concerning the difference between systemic and localized cutaneous amyloidosis. *Acta Dermatol Venereol Suppl* 1981;61: 381-384.
29. Kitano Y, Okada N, Kobayashi Y, et al. A monoclonal anti-keratin antibody reactive with amyloid deposit of primary cutaneous amyloidosis. *J Dermatol* 1987; 14:427-729.
30. Hashimoto K. Progress on cutaneous amyloidosis. *J Invest Dermatol* 1984;82:1-3.
31. Black MM, Wilson Jones E. Macular amyloidosis: A study of 21 cases with special reference to the role of the epidermis in its histogenesis. *Br J Dermatol* 1971;84:199-209.
32. Kumakiri M, Hsshimoto K. Histogenesis of primary localized cutaneous amyloidosis: Sequential change of epidermal keratinocytes to amyloid via filamentous degeneration. *J Invest Dermatol* 1973; 73:150-162.
33. Eto H, Hashimoto K, Kobayashi H, et al. Differential staining of cytoid bodies and skin-limited amyloids with monoclonal anti-keratin antibodies. *Am J Pathol* 1984;116:473-481.
34. Yamagihara M, Kitajima Y, Yaoita H, Mori S. Ultrastructural observation of the relationship between amyloid filaments and half desmosomes in macular amyloidosis (abstract). *J Cutan Pathol* 1980; 7:213.
35. Horiguchi Y, Fine JD, Leigh IM, et al. Lamina densa malformation involved in histogenesis of primary localized cutaneous amyloidosis. *J Invest Dermatol* 1992;99:12-18.
36. Horiguchi Y, Fine JD, Leigh IM, et al. Lamina densa malformation involved in histogenesis of primary localized cutaneous amyloidosis. *J Invest Dermatol* 1992; 99:12-18.
37. Wang WJ. Clinical features of cutaneous amyloidoses. *Clin Dermatol* 1991; 8:13-19.
38. Khoo BP, Tay YK. Lichen amyloidosus: A bullous variant. *Ann Acad Med Singapore* 2000;29:105-107.
39. Turse U, Kaya TI, Dusmez D, Ikizoglu G. Case of generalized lichen amyloidosis. *Int J Dermatol* 2003;42:649-651.
40. Yalcin B, Artuz F, Toy GG, et al. Generalized lichen amyloidosis associated with chronic urticaria. *Dermatology* 2003;207:203-204.
41. Ozaki M. Familial lichen amyloidosis. *Int J Dermatol* 1984;23:190-193.
42. Rajagopalan K, Tay CH. Familial lichen amyloidosis: Report of 19 cases in 4 generations of a Chinese family in Malaysia. *Br J Dermatol* 1972;87:123-129.
43. Porto JA, Posse Filho A. Amiloidose cutanea genuina familial. *Bol da Soc Brasil Dermatol Sif* 1960;35:102-103.
44. De Souza AR. Amiloidose cutanea bohlosa familial: Observacao de 4 casos. *Rev Hosp Clin Fac Med Sao Paolo* 1963;18: 413-417.
45. De Pietro WP. Primary familial cutaneous amyloidosis: A study of HLA antigens in

a Puerto Rican family. *Arch Dermatol* 1981;117:639-642.
46. Hartshorne ST. Familial primary cutaneous amyloidosis in a South African family. *Clin Exp Dermatol* 1999;24:438-442.
47. Sagher F, Shanon J. Amyloidosis cutis. *Arch Dermatol* 1963;87:171-175.
48. Vasily DB, Bhaia SG, Uhlin SR. Familial primary cutaneous amyloidosis: Clinical, genetic, and immunofluorescent studies. *Arch Dermtaol* 1978;114:1173-1176.
49. Newton JA, Jagjivan A, Bhogal B, et al. Familial primary cutaneous amyloidosis. *Br J Dermatol* 1985;112:201-208.
50. Bergamo F, Annessi G, Ribuffo M, et al. Familial lichen amyloidosis. *Chron Dermatol* 1997;6:959-961.
51. Highman B. Improved methods for demonstrating amyloid in paraffin sections. *Arch Dermatol* 1946;41:559.
52. Kobayashi T, Yamasaki Y, Watanbe T, Onoda N. Extensive lichen amyloidosis refractory to DMSO. *J Dermatol* 1995; 22:755-758.
53. Ozkaya-Bayazit E, Kavak A, Gungor H, Ozarmagan G Intermittent use of topical dimethyl sulfoxide in macular and papular amyloidosis. *Int J Dermatol* 1998; 37:949-954.
54. Jin AG, Por A, Wee LK, et al. Comparative study of phototherapy (UVB) vs photochemotherapy (PUVA) vs topical steroids in the treatment of primary cutaneous lichen amyloidosis. *Photodermatol Photoimmunol Photomed* 2001;17:42-43.
55. Highman B. Improved methods for demonstrating amyloid in paraffin sections. *Arch Dermatol* 1946;41:559.
56. Prophet EB, Mills B, Arrington JB, et al. *Laboratory Methods in Histotechnology.* Washington, Armed Forces Institute of Pathology, 1992.
57. Yanagihara M, Mehregan AH, Mehregan DR. Staining of amyloid with cotton dyes. *Arch Dermatol* 1984;120: 1184-1185.
58. Hashimoto K, Ito K, Kumakiri M, Headington J. Nylon brush macular amyloidosis. *Arch Dermatol* 1987;123:633-637.
59. Khoo B, Tay Y, Goh C. Calcipotriol ointment vs betamethasone 17-valerate ointment in the treatment of lichen amyloidosis. *Int J Dermatol* 1999;38: 539-541.
60. Castanedo-Cazares JP, Lepe V, Moncada B. Lichen amyloidosis improved by 0.1% topical tacrolimus. *Dermatology* 2002;205: 420-421.
61. Ozkaya-Bayazit E, Kavak A, Gungor H, Ozarmagan G. Intermittent use of topical dimethyl sulfoxide in macular and papular amyloidosis. *Int J Dermatol* 1998; 37:949-954.
62. Pandhi R, Kaur I, Kumar B. Lack of effect of dimethylsulfoxide in cutaneous amyloidosis. *J Dermatol Treat* 2002;13:11-14.
63. Hernandez-Nunez A, Dauden E, Moreno de Vega MJ, et al. Widespread biphasic amyloidosis: Response to acitretin. *Clin Exp Dermatol* 2001;26: 256-259.
64. Reider N, Sepp N, Fritsch P. Remission of lichen amyloidosis after treatment with acitretin. *Dermatology* 1997;194: 309-311.
65. Wong C-K. Treatment (cutaneous amyloidosis). *Clin Dermatol* 1990;8:108-111.
66. Behr FD, Levine N, Bangert J. Lichen amyloidosis associated with atopic dermatitis: Clinical resolution with cyclosporine. *Arch Dermatol* 2001;137:553-555.
67. Teraki Y, Katsuta M, Shiohara T. Lichen amyloidosis associated with Kimura's disease: Successful treatment with cyclosporine. *J Dermatol Treat* 2002;204: 133-135.
68. Harahap M, Marwali RP. The treatment of lichen amyloidosis. *Dermatol Surg* 1998;24:251-254.
69. Liu H-T. Treatment of lichen amyloidosis and disseminated superficial porokeratosis with frequency-doubled Q-switched Nd:YAG laser. *Dermatol Surg* 2000;26:958-962.

CHAPTER 30

Keloids

A. Paul Kelly

Key Points

- Hypertrophic scars and keloidal scars are a major problem for patients with skin of color.
- Keloidal scars are an overgrowth of dense, fibrous tissue that develop as a result of cutaneous injury and invade its surrounding area.
- Hypertrophic scars are also overgrowths of fibrous tissue, but in contrast to keloids, they usually stay within the confines of the precipitating cutaneous injury.
- Keloids differ from hypertrophic scars in osmotic pressure, metabolic activity, and collagen turnover, as reflected in the local concentrations of sodium, magnesium, and calcium, respectively.
- Many theories have been advanced to explain the etiology of keloids, although none have been substantiated.
- Although keloids may be found anywhere on the body, they tend to have a regional predilection, occurring most often on the ears, anterior chest, upper back, and shoulders.
- Although rare, keloids may develop on the eyelids, genitalia, palms and soles, mucous membranes, tongue, and cornea.

SYNONYMS

Cheloide
Keloidal scar
Scarring
Excessive scar tissue
Atypical wound healing

Hypertrophic scars and keloidal scars, which result from complications of cutaneous surgery, trauma, or injury, are an immense problem for patients with skin of color. Hypertrophic scars are an increase in the amount of tissue, usually owing to an increase in the size of cells rather than the number of cells. Keloids are an overgrowth of scar tissue at the site of skin injuries such as surgical incisions, traumatic wounds, vaccination sites, burns, chickenpox, acne, or even minor scratches. They are fairly common in African Americans.

Although keloids are medically benign, they are often psychologically and/or socially devastating for patients. Keloids represent an overgrowth of dense, fibrous tissue that develops as a result of cutaneous injury. Hypertrophic scars usually stay within the confines of the precipitating injury, whereas keloids invade surrounding clinically normal skin. Additional clinical and histologic characteristics distinguish keloidal scars from hypertrophic scars (Table 30-1). However, the medical literature regarding hypertrophic scars and keloidal scars is often confusing because many lesions that are keloidal scars are mislabeled as hypertrophic scars or vice versa. Some patients have both kinds of scars caused by the same traumatic incident. Clinical studies often lump the two disorders together, thus leading to dissemination of incorrect information, which is a practical concern when evaluating therapeutic response.[1]

Keloidal scars and hypertrophic scars are thought to be produced by an overgrowth of fibrous tissue secondary, in most cases, to injury (e.g., lacerations, surgical incisions, ear piercing, vaccinations, herpes zoster, acne lesions, insect bites, and burns) or a deficiency in metalloproteinases. There are, however, a small percentage of patients who develop so-called spontaneous keloids, that is, keloids with no known antecedent trauma or injury. These types of lesions occur most often in patients with a family history of keloids and usually are located in the midchest area. Except for burn patients, most keloids occur in the second or third decade of life, although they can occur anytime from infancy to old age.[2]

Hypertrophic scars usually develop rapidly after cutaneous injury or trauma, whereas keloids develop slowly but continue to enlarge for months to years. In most instances, hypertrophic scars regress with therapy, in contradistinction to keloids, which often recur during therapy or when therapy is discontinued.

HISTORY

Jean Louis Alibert (1768–1837), one of the principal founders of French dermatology, proposed the word *cheloide* (derived from the Greek *chele,* meaning "crab's claw," and *-oid,* meaning "like") in 1806, which he had originally called *cancroide*[3] (Figure 30-1). Alibert later changed the name to *cheloid* to avoid confusion with cancer and its connotation. In the 1825 edition of his text, he wrote a chapter entitled, *"Les cancroides ou keloids,"* using for the first time the word that was adopted by American, English, and German dermatologists.[4] Even though Alibert was the first to describe the clinical characteristics of keloids, Retz, according to Kaposi, had already in the year 1790 described, under the name *darte de graisse,* a cicatrical tumor of the skin, which he thought was of spontaneous origin.[5] Hawkins, in 1835, described lesions that may have been keloids, and Macpherson added to the early literature on keloids.[6,7]

TABLE 30-1
A Comparison of Keloids and Hypertrophic Scars

Characteristics	Keloids	Hypertrophic Scars
Stays in confines of injury	No	Yes
Precipitated by trauma	Not always	Yes
Area of occurrence	Area of little motion	Area of motion
Growth	For extended period	Regresses in time
Symptomatic	Usually	Usually
Response to treatment	Poor	Good
Sodium (osmotic pressure)	Normal	Decreased
Magnesium (metabolic activity)	Increased	Decreased
Calcium (reflects collagen metabolism)	Increased	Decreased
Mucinous ground substance	Abundant	Scanty
Fibroblasts	Few	Numerous
Foreign-body reactions	None	Frequent
Luxol fast blue collagen stain	Reddish	Blue
Mast cells	Increased	Increased
Pathogenesis	Unknown	Unknown
Contain myofibroblasts	No	Yes
Alanine transaminase	Increased	Normal

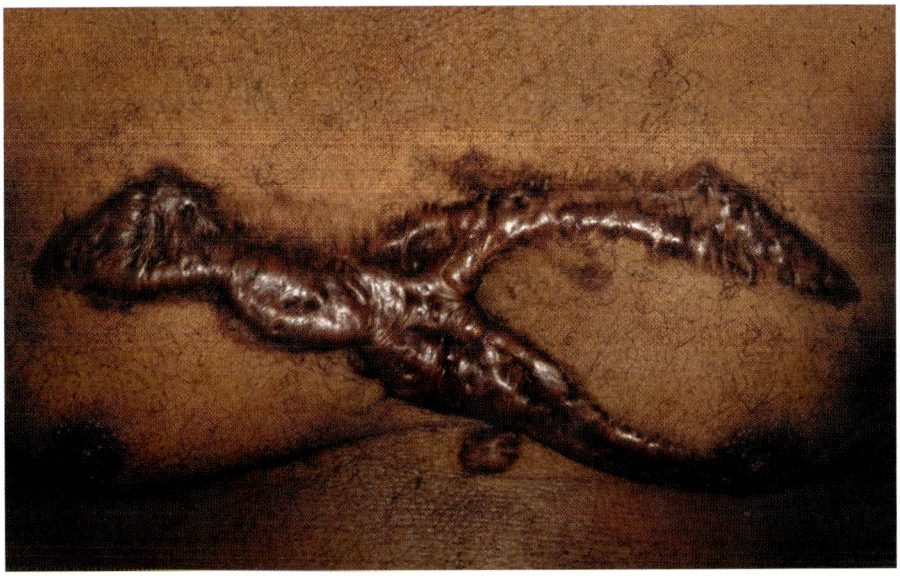

▲ **FIGURE 30-1** A crablike keloid on the midchest of an African American.

The first recorded description of keloid-like scars appears in the Smith papyrus: "[T]he existence of swelling on his breast, large, spreading, and hard, touching them is like touching a ball of wrappings."[8]

Also, the Yorubas recorded their awareness of keloids 10 centuries before Alibert and Retz. Omo-Dare described some of these observations on the character and presentation of keloids. The Yorubas knew, for example, that keloids frequently appear in the same family but that not all members of the family are affected. They knew that there is a time interval between the infliction of trauma that produces a keloid and the appearance of the lesion. Local customs of facial marking and earlobe perforation were usually performed toward the end of the first week of life. However, if there was a delay of the scarification process, according to a Yoruba saying, facial marks made in adolescence and adult life may become keloidal. The Yorubas also knew that once a lesion appeared, it grew and had no effective therapy except when "the Divine Power is suitably appropriated to intervene in bringing about its resolution."[9]

In 1854, Addison introduced the term *true keloid* (arising spontaneously) and labeled Alibert's lesions *false keloids* (those arising at sites of trauma).[10] The lesions he described were probably morphea or scleroderma, and his nomenclature of true keloids and false keloids should be discarded.[11]

Although originally thought to occur only in humans, lesions similar to keloids have been reported in horses, cattle, and dogs and on the feet of vultures and eagles.[12] However, even though these animals may form keloid-like scars, they are not good models for studying wound repair because excessive collagen deposited in animals is reabsorbed when the tissue insult ceases.[13]

EPIDEMIOLOGY

Owing to numerous variables, such as anatomic location, type of trauma, race, age, and gender, the reported incidence of keloids in the general population ranges from a high of 16% of Zairean adults to a low of 0.01% of English Caucasian adults[1] (Table 30-2). Blacks develop keloids more often than whites; however, the reported incidence ratio between the two groups ranges from Brenizer's 2:1 black versus white[14] to Fox's 19:1 ratio.[15] Fox found keloids in 3 of 8382 white patients and 76 of 11,486 black patients.[15] Matas reported the black:white ratio of 9:1[16,17]; Geschichter and Lewis, 6:1[18]; and Cosman and colleagues, 3:1.[12]

TABLE 30-2
Epidemiology

- Incidence varies according to population studied
  - Low of 0.09% in England
  - High of 16% in Zaire
  - Blacks affected 5–16 times more often than whites
  - Asians and Latinos fall in between
- Age of onset averages 22–23
  - Onset after puberty
  - Young skin more taut owing to greater rate of collagen synthesis

In Aruba, however, where more than 3% of the children have keloids, those children of Polynesian ancestry with keloids outnumber the black children who have keloids. Also, in West Malaysia, the lighter-skinned Chinese appear to be slightly more prone to keloid formation than are the darker-skinned Indians and Malays.[19] Arnold and colleagues found that in Hawaii, keloids are five times more common in Japanese and three times more common in Chinese than in Caucasians.[20] It has been reported that Europeans living in the tropics are more likely to develop keloids than those living in more temperate zones, although there has been no subsequent documentation of this observation.[21] The question of why blacks develop keloids and hypertrophic scars more often than whites has had many answers, none of which has been accepted as the sole reason. An interesting theory advanced by Bohrod was based on the principle of long-term social and religious mores for scarification, which, in turn, determined genetic predisposition.[22]

The male:female incidence has been reported to be equal by some investigators, whereas others have reported that the incidence is greater in females.[23] Cosman and colleagues found that the average age of patients at the time of initial treatment was 25.8 years, and the median age at onset was 22.3 years in women and 22.6 years in men.[12] Although it is rare, I have noted the onset of keloids and hypotropic scars in children before their first birthday, as well as in septuagenarians.

ETIOLOGY

Trauma

Many theories have been advanced to explain the etiology of keloids (Table 30-3). In most patients, trauma has been the main, if not the only, precipitating factor. Trauma may be of many different forms, such as simple scratches, abrasions, insect bites, vaccinations, acne papules, chickenpox lesions, surgical procedures, chemical burns, or thermal

TABLE 30-3
Proposed Etiology of Keloids

- Trauma
- Skin tension
- Infection
- Endocrine factors
- Genetic predisposition

burns. Because most people sustain cutaneous trauma, especially on the feet, without developing keloids, and because some keloids arise spontaneously on nontraumatized areas, one may summarize that there is most likely another predisposing variable(s) or factors(s) rather than trauma itself that leads to keloid formation.[24]

Skin Tension

Increased skin tension has been cited as the reason for keloids occurring after surgery.[23,25,26] Cutting across Langer's lines, with a resulting increase in skin tension, also has been suggested. Asboe-Hansen[25] found that with long-standing edema, the mucopolysaccharide content of the skin is maintained at a high level, and this stimulates the deposition of collagen fibers and thus keloid formation.

Increased skin tension also causes the *coiffure keloid,* which forms, in a few cases, on the scalp in response to the tightly braided hair styles found in many parts of Africa and which are increasing in popularity in the United States and worldwide.[27]

Yagi and colleagues introduced the sebum autoimmune mechanism concept of keloid formation. They postulated that after cutaneous trauma, functioning sebaceous glands may secrete sebum intradermally. The sebum then acts as an antigen, initiating an autoimmune granulomatous response that may proceed to keloid formation. These authors cite the virtual absence of keloids on the palms, soles, forehead, and lips, areas that are essentially devoid of sebaceous glands, as further evidence of their theory.[28]

Some investigators[24] have suggested that foreign-body reactions, not the trauma itself, stimulate the formation of keloids or the presence of suture debris or dirt in wounds as probable stimulating factors. Others also have proposed inert material or natural products such as damaged collagen or keratin as causative stimuli.[29]

Infection

Infection, bacterial or viral, has been implicated as a contributing factor in the formation of keloids (Table 30-4). One of the earliest opinions was that the tubercle bacilli caused keloids.[30]

However, in later studies on patients with keloids, not one was found to have clinical evidence of tuberculosis, and the number of positive tuberculin reactions was in the range of that in the normal population.[31] Keloids may appear after chickenpox or herpes zoster infection and after vaccination for smallpox. In the past, there were many inferences[15] that syphilis promoted keloid growth, but of more than a hundred patients with keloids, only one was found to have syphilis.[1]

TABLE 30-4
Infections Associated with Keloids

- Viral infections—higher incidence of keloids after herpes zoster and chickenpox
- Bacterial infections—in the past, tuberculosis and syphilis incriminated; now, no evidence that infections precipitate keloid formation

Endocrine Factors

Keloid formation has been associated with endocrinologic factors, but there is still no definite proof that such factors are of major importance. The thymus, parathyroid, ovary, thyroid, and pituitary, alone or in combination, have been incriminated.[32] Acromegalics have been reported to have a marked susceptibility to keloid formation.[33] Keloids also seem to grow during pregnancy.[34] There seems to be a greater incidence of keloids when there is hyperpigmentation associated with hyperthyroidism, pregnancy, or puberty.[35] It has been postulated that in all the preceding conditions, there is excessive secretion of melanocyte-stimulating hormone (MSH) and increased sensitivity of melanocytes to this MSH, thus explaining why blacks, whose melanocytes may be more reactive to MSH, have a higher incidence of keloids than whites[36] (Table 30-5). The evidence for this supposition is purely circumstantial; keloids are rare on the palms and soles, where the concentration of melanocytes is minimal.

Residues of the thymus gland have been reported in several patients with keloids.[37] Other investigators mention that the thymus may be involved in keloid formation, but to date, there has been no proof of this association.[31]

Hyperthyroidism was mentioned as a possible cause of keloid formation by Justice after he induced keloids in hyperthyroid patients by irritating their skin with "excitant pharmacologic substances," the activity of which was slight.[38] Asboe-Hansen reported that young patients thyroidectomized for Graves disease are apt to form keloids in the surgical wound, and keloids formed after the injection of thyroid extract in thyroidectomized patients.[25] Also, it has been reported that hard fibrous patches, which were probably keloids, regressed in a female patient after unilateral resection of the thyroid gland on that side.[39]

TABLE 30-5
Keloids and Melanocytes

- Not reported in albinos
- Patients with keloids developed vitiligo
  - Keloid regressed in vitiliginous area
- May form with secretion of melanocyte-stimulating hormone (MSH)
  - Face, neck, deltoid area
  - Presternal area, earlobes

Whereas Asboe-Hansen reported that the blood calcium level in most patients with keloids was within normal limits,[25] Pautrier and Zorn found an elevated serum calcium concentration in 9 of 12 patients with keloids, each of whom was noted to have elevated calcium levels in all the keloid tissues.[40] In 1946, Oliver and Barasch reported a parathyroidectomy on a patient with a large keloid and regression of the lesion after surgery.[15] No additional studies have duplicated these findings.

Pituitary secretions have been held responsible for keloid formation, especially since acromegalics have been reported as having an increased susceptibility to the development of keloids. This phenomenon was attributed to the action of growth hormone, which stimulates the formation of new connective tissue, especially collagen fibrils. Keloids seem to be more common in acromegalics, and the keloids seem to grow more rapidly in pregnancy and puberty, times when there is physiologic hyperactivity of the pituitary.[34]

The suggestion of pituitary involvement in keloid formation also has been based on the fact that in states of increased pituitary activity (e.g., pregnancy and puberty), there is an association with increased pigmentation, which, in turn, is based on an increased production of MSH by the pituitary.[34]

Ovarian function also has been associated with keloid formation during puberty, development of growth during pregnancy, and spontaneous resolution after menopause.[41] Geschicter and Lewis's report of increased estrogen content in keloids further supports the ovarian influence,[18] but their findings are somewhat suspect because the results were obtained by assaying an earlobe keloid that had been preserved in formalin for 1–3 years. Solomons found that depression of the ovaries did not alter keloid growth.[42] Also, Vargus, attempting to produce uterine fibroids by administering estrogen to monkeys, was not able to produce cutaneous keloids.[43] The observation that scars and keloids tend to grow during pregnancy supports a pituitary-ovarian influence on keloid formation.[34]

Because keloids seldom occur before puberty, sex hormones may play an important role in their formation. Sex hormone levels have been found to differ between keloids and clinically normal surrounding skin and between keloids and hypertrophic scars. Personen and colleagues found that the diffusion of progesterone from culture medium into tissue is most effective in keloids, with normal skin being the second most effective and hypertrophic scar and the skin surrounding keloids ineffective in taking up progesterone.[44]

Ford and colleagues found that keloids have a high level of androgen binding, whereas estrogen and progesterone receptor binding was essentially undetectable in any of the keloid tissues from males or in keloid tissue from some of the females. They also found that the level of androgen binding in skin adjacent to keloids was elevated, whereas the level in skin adjacent to hypertrophic scars was only 0.1% of that found in keloids.[45]

Mustafa and Abdel-Fattah postulated that estrogen plays a causative role in keloid formation on the basis of a single case of a keloid that enlarged during pregnancy.[34] However, they did not mention that maternal circulating androgens increase during pregnancy, especially in patients carrying a male fetus, nor did they mention the sex of the fetus. Additional evidence favoring the role of androgens is that keloids have a predilection for the chest, upper back, and neck, regions that have an increased rate of dihydrotestosterone metabolism[46] (Figures 30-2 through 30-4).

Krenar's publication suggests that nutritional inadequacy may be the provoking factor in keloid formation.[30] However, malnutrition with protein deficiency seems to decrease fibroplasias.[47,48] Bowesman suggested that adequate nutrition is necessary for keloid formation.[49] Keloid formation is uncommon in acquired immune deficiency syndrome (AIDS) patients.[50]

The relationship between hypertrophic scars and hormonal factors is a subject that needs more research to make definitive determinations.[1]

Genetic Factors

Keloids have a definite familial predisposition, especially in those with multiple lesions.[1,51] Approximately one-third of keloid formers have a first-degree relative with keloids. Also, clinical experience

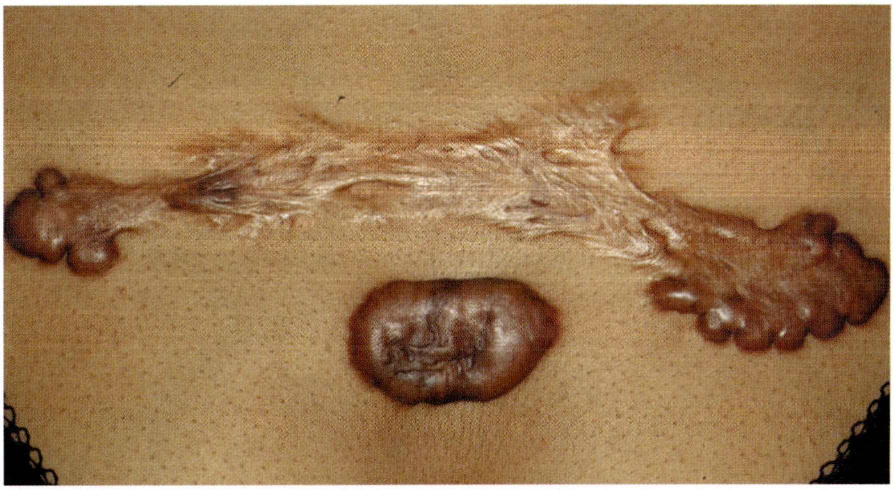

▲ **FIGURE 30-2** Keloid in the midchest area of an African-American woman.

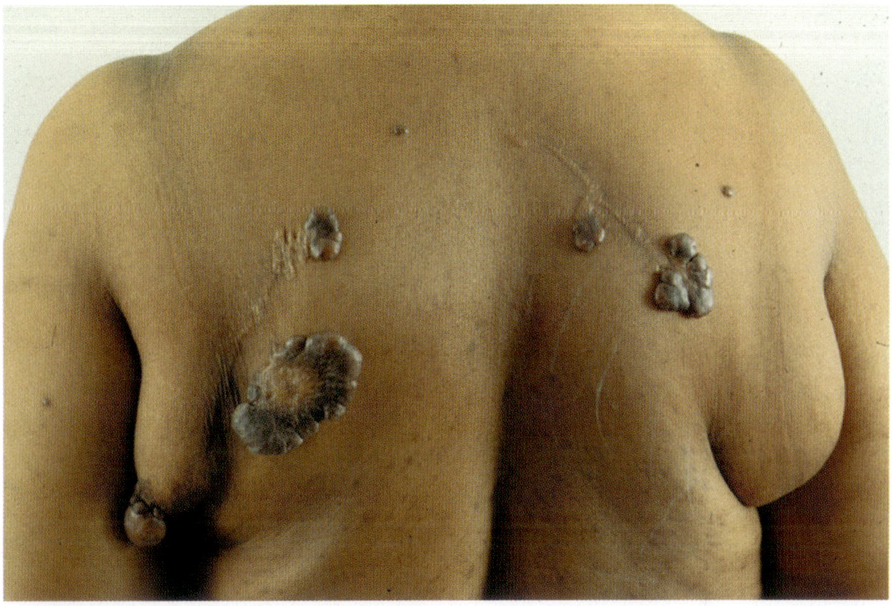

▲ **FIGURE 30-3** Keloids of the upper back of an African-American woman.

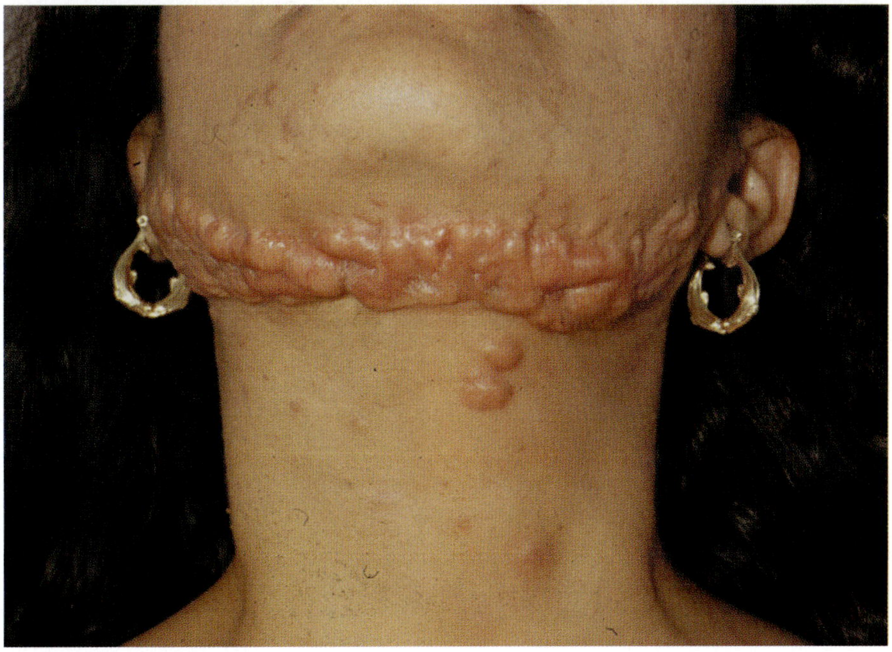

▲ **FIGURE 30-4** Keloid on the anterior neck of a Hispanic woman.

TABLE 30-6
Clinical Findings of Keloidal and Hypertrophic Scars

Keloids	Hypertrophic Scars
• Invade clinically normal skin	• Limited to traumatized area
• May continue to grow for the patient's life, often resistant to therapy	• Usually regress spontaneously in 12–18 months
• Erythematous borders indicate continuing growth	• Usually respond to therapy
• Pruritic, painful, burning	• Rarely grow after 2–3 months
	• Usually asymptomatic

indicates that familial predisposition is more common in blacks. Both autosomal recessive and autosomal dominant patterns of inheritance have been reported.[1] Bloom also mentioned some studies in the German literature that describe congenital keloids, two cases of which were in identical twins.[2] The incidence of keloids in an Italian population was found to be greater in those with HLA-B14 and HLA-BW16 antigens,[52] whereas studies by Cohen and colleagues noted a general HLA-A and HLA-B antigen pattern in patients with keloids.[53]

CLINICAL FINDINGS

Clinical Characteristics

There are several clinical findings that distinguish keloids and hypertrophic scars[1,51–56] (Table 30-6). Although keloids may be found anywhere on the body, they tend to have a regional predilection, occurring most often on the ears (Figures 30-5 through 30-9), anterior chest, anterior neck, upper back, and shoulders. The latter three areas have increased skin tension, and keloids in these locations seem to arise with minimal trauma, are usually flatter with broader bases than keloids elsewhere, and respond less favorably to all modes of therapy. Keloids occur from head to toe and all points in between (Figures 30-10 and 30-11). Keloids on the shoulder and back grow to be larger than keloids elsewhere (Figure 30-12). Abdominal keloids, although rare in men, are common in black women who have had cesarean sections, hysterectomies, or other types of abdominal surgery. Black men who shave develop keloids more often in the beard area than those who do not shave. The flanks seem to be involved more in women than in men[57] (Figure 30-13).

Areas less commonly involved include the face, neck, arms, and lower extremities (Figure 30-14). Midchest lesions are often quite tender (Figures 30-15 through 30-17). Although rare, keloids may develop on the eyelids, genitalia, palms and soles, mucous membranes, tongue, and cornea.[58] Extremity lesions are usual quite taunt[59] (Figures 30-18 through 30-20). Keloids are rare on the oral mucosa.[1] There are two known cases of keloids on the penis, one secondary to circumcision and the other from trauma.[60,61] There are some lesions

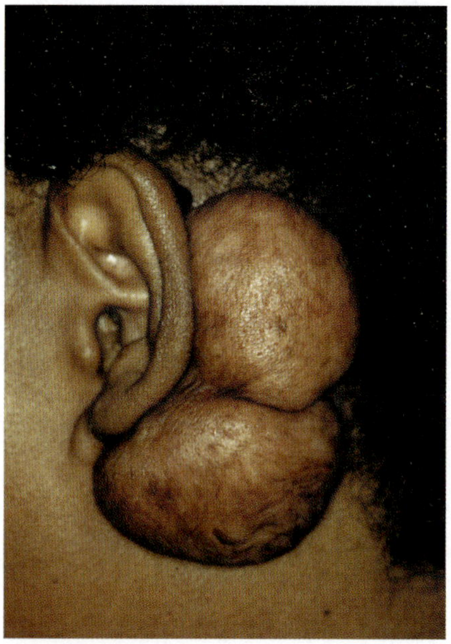

▲ **FIGURE 30-6** Two Large keloids of the left posterior earlobe of an African American woman.

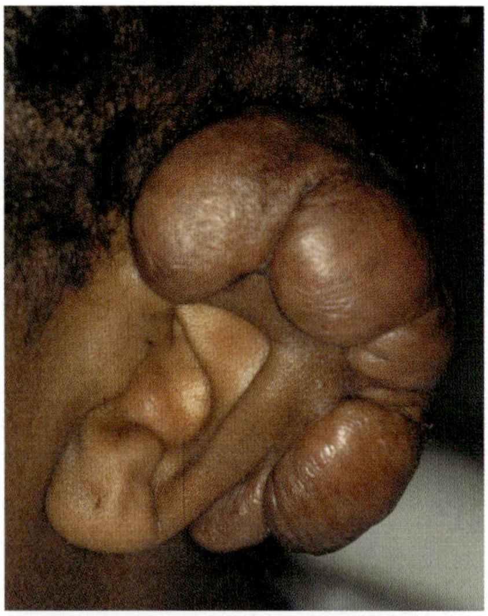

▲ **FIGURE 30-5** Keloids have a regional predilection. They occur most often on the ears but may occur from head to toe and all areas in between.

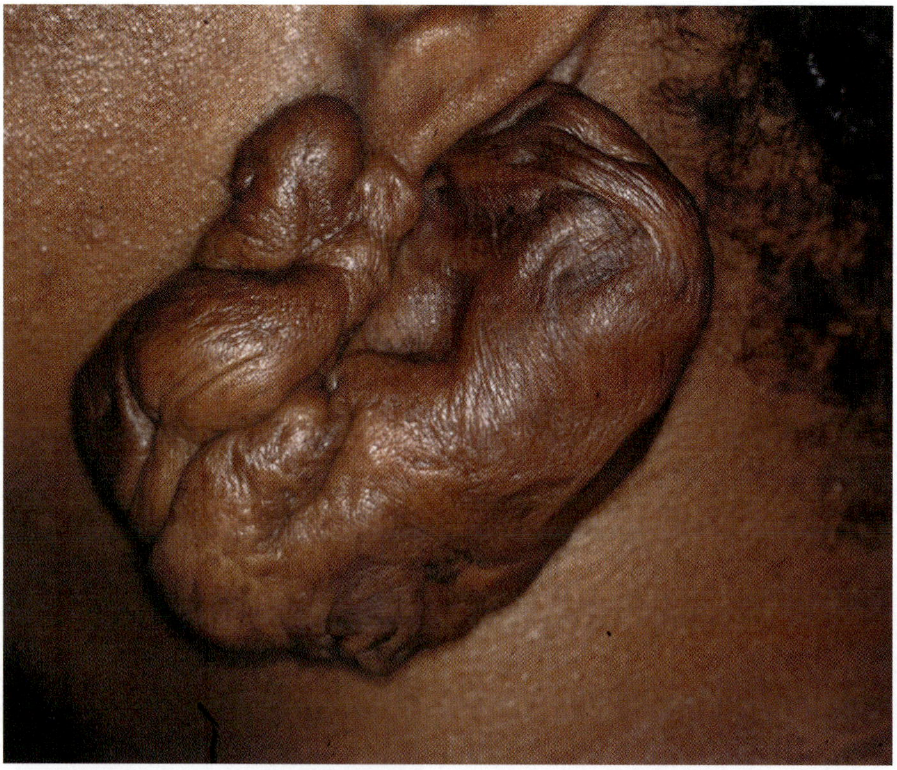

▲ **FIGURE 30-7** Huge keloid wrapped around the left earlobe in a young African American woman.

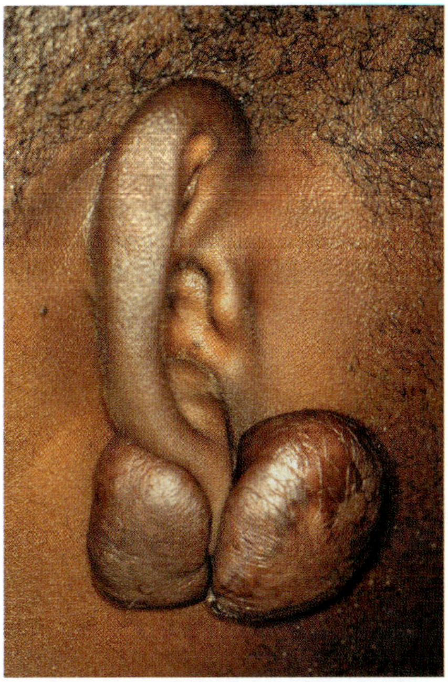

▲ **FIGURE 30-8** Right earlobe with bilateral keloids.

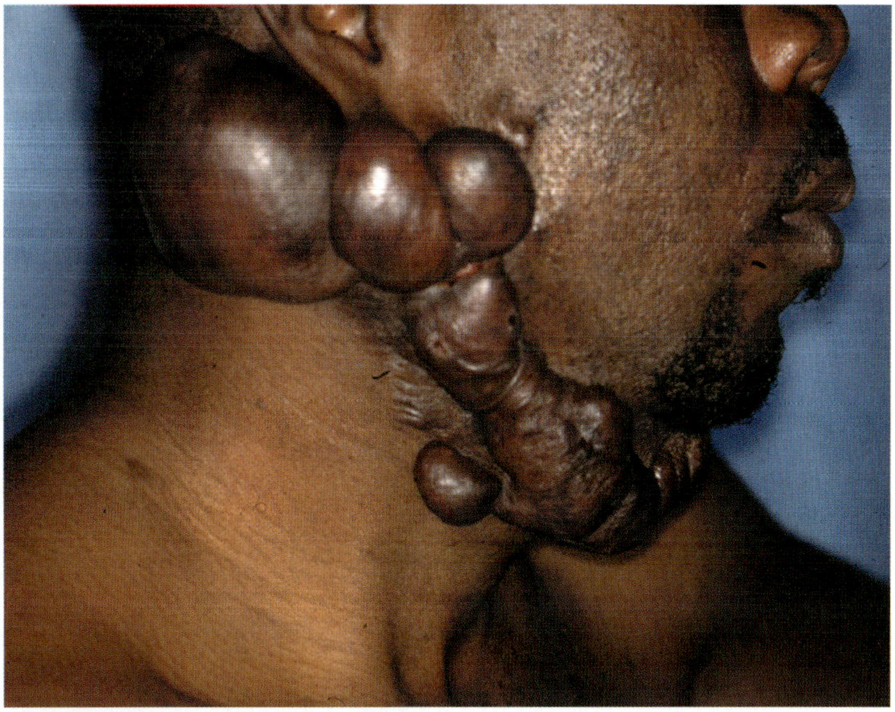

▲ **FIGURE 30-10** Large keloid from head to neck.

that resemble keloids clinically but that are epidermal cysts of the earlobe (Figure 30-21), lipomas of the earlobe (Figure 30-22), and xanthomas[62] (Figure 30-23).

CLINICAL COURSE AND PROGNOSIS

Keloids present as exaggerated growths of scar tissue, extend past the areas of trauma, and once present, tend to continue to enlarge. Sometimes keloids are invaded by sarcoidosis lesions[63,64] (Figure 30-24). In contrast, hypertrophic scars are limited to the traumatized area and regress spontaneously in 12–18 months (Figure 30-25). Both types of lesions are usually asymptomatic, but keloids may be tender, painful, and pruritic or cause a burning sensation. However, cosmetic concern is the main reason patients seek medical intervention. Keloids range in consistency from soft and doughy to rubbery and hard. They project above the level of surrounding skin but rarely extend into the underlying subcutaneous tissue. Even though the overlying epidermis is thinned from pressure, they seldom ulcerate.[57]

Oluwasanmi reported that most keloids occur within a year of the injury or disease that incited their formation, although approximately 20% develop 1–24 years after the first recognizable

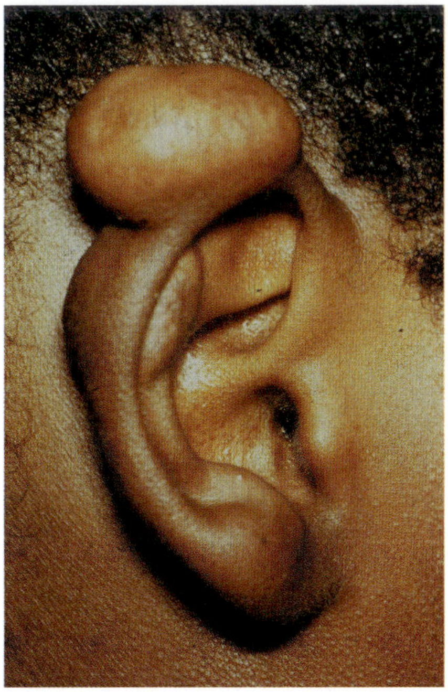

▲ **FIGURE 30-9** A keloid of the superior edge of the right earlobe of an African American woman.

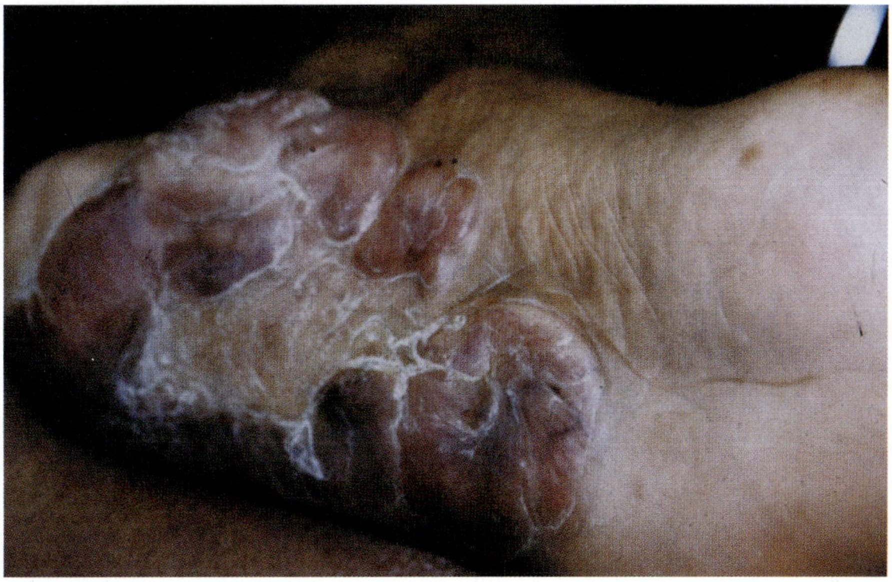

▲ **FIGURE 30-11** Keloid on the sole of the left foot, although it is uncommon for keloids to occur on the feet.

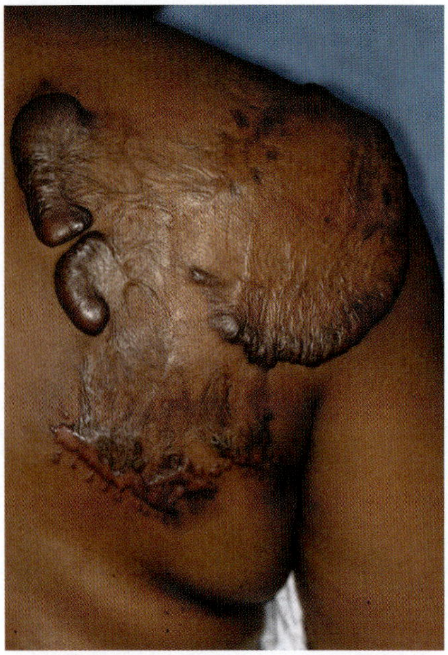

▲ **FIGURE 30-12** Keloids on the shoulder and back often grow to be larger than keloids elsewhere. Also, in this figure, the medial border is violaceous, which means that the keloid is still enlarging.

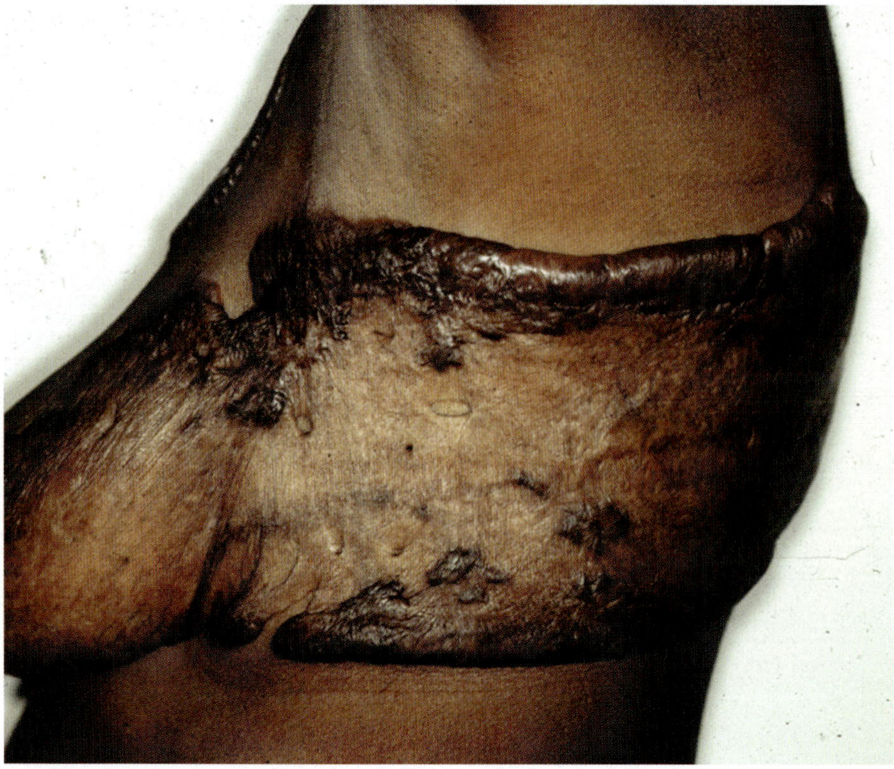

▲ **FIGURE 30-13** Keloid of the left flank and breast of an African-American woman.

injury.[21] The lag period is usually much shorter in lesions that recur after excision.

Initial lesions are often erythematous, become brownish red and then pale in the center as they age, and are often darker at the outer border. They are usually void of hair follicles. Once they are present, the clinical course varies. Most continue to grow for weeks to months and others for years. The growth is usually slow, but keloids sometimes will enlarge rapidly, tripling their size in months. Once they stop growing, keloids are usually asymptomatic and remain stable or involute slightly. Rarely do they regress spontaneously. Spontaneous regression is usually associated with advanced age; it has been reported that one keloid regressed after being present for 40 years.[57]

Keloids may range in size from papules a few millimeters in diameter to football-sized or larger tumors. Those

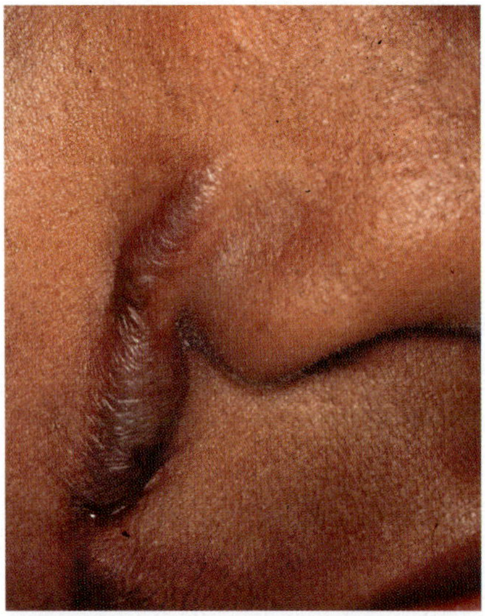

▲ **FIGURE 30-14** Although rare keloids may occur on the face, this figure shows a keloid in the right nasolabial area.

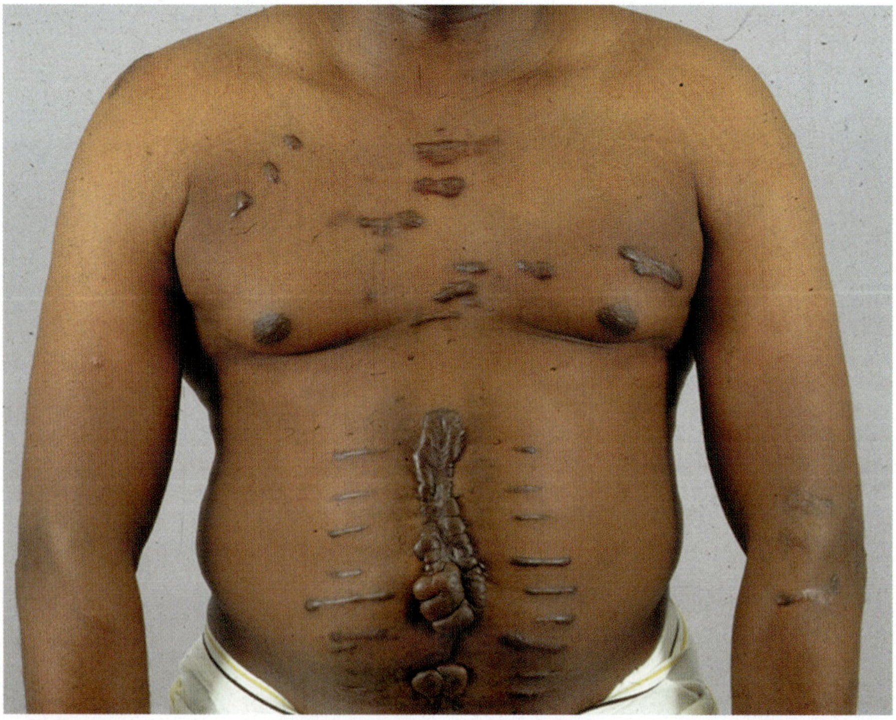

▲ **FIGURE 30-15** Chest and abdominal keloids on an African-American man. The abdominal keloids were secondary to abdominal surgery.

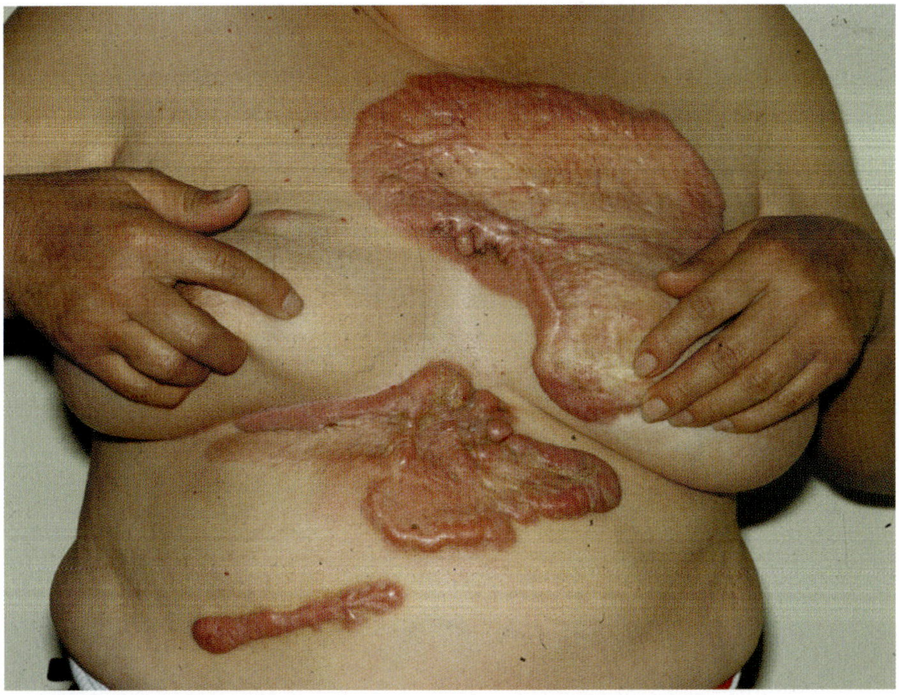

▲ **FIGURE 30-16** Chest, breast, and abdominal keloids on a Hispanic woman.

on the ears, neck, and abdomen tend to be pedunculated, whereas those on the central chest and extremities are usually raised with a flat surface, the base often being wider than the top. Most are round, oval, or oblong with regular margins; however, some have clawlike configurations with irregular borders. Most patients present with one or two keloids, but a few patients, especially those with spontaneous keloids, have multiple lesions, as do those who develop keloids secondary to acne or chickenpox.[59]

Malignant transformation of keloids is rare, and the reported cases are poorly documented. Most patients had had some type of radiation therapy prior to the development of the malignancy.[63] According to Stout, a keloid never develops into malignant hyperplasia, and when a carcinoma does develop within a keloid, it is not a malignant degeneration of the keloid but rather of the overlying epidermis.[64] Thus there appears to be no case reported yet of unequivocally malignant change in an unirradiated keloid. Not only do keloids seem to resist malignancy, but they also seem to be spared in most generalized dermatoses.

PATHOGENESIS

Collagen Synthesis

Electron microscopic studies by Gueft revealed that keloid collagen fibers are thinner and have irregularities of cross-striations, suggesting that keloid collagen is immature.[65] Studies of thermal contraction have demonstrated that, initially, keloid collagen acts like young tissue, which, once formed, proceeds to age the same way as any other newly synthesized collagen.[66]

Harris and Sjoerdsma found that the water content of keloid tissue is uniformly higher than that of clinically normal skin of the same patients, and there is no correlation between the water content and the age of the lesion.[67] Additional findings were that the soluble collagen content and the alpha:beta ratio (single-polypeptide chains:double-peptide chains) are increased in all keloids. The collagen concentration in keloids is normal, but it is lower in recently formed scars. Early hypertrophic scars have the same

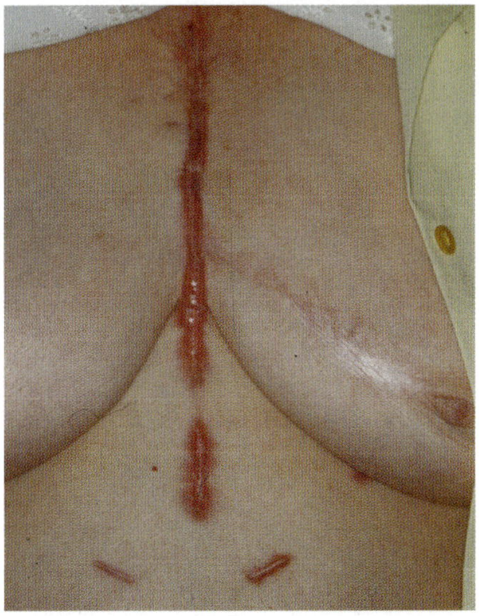

▲ **FIGURE 30-17** Keloids on the midchest of an Asian woman secondary to cardiac surgery.

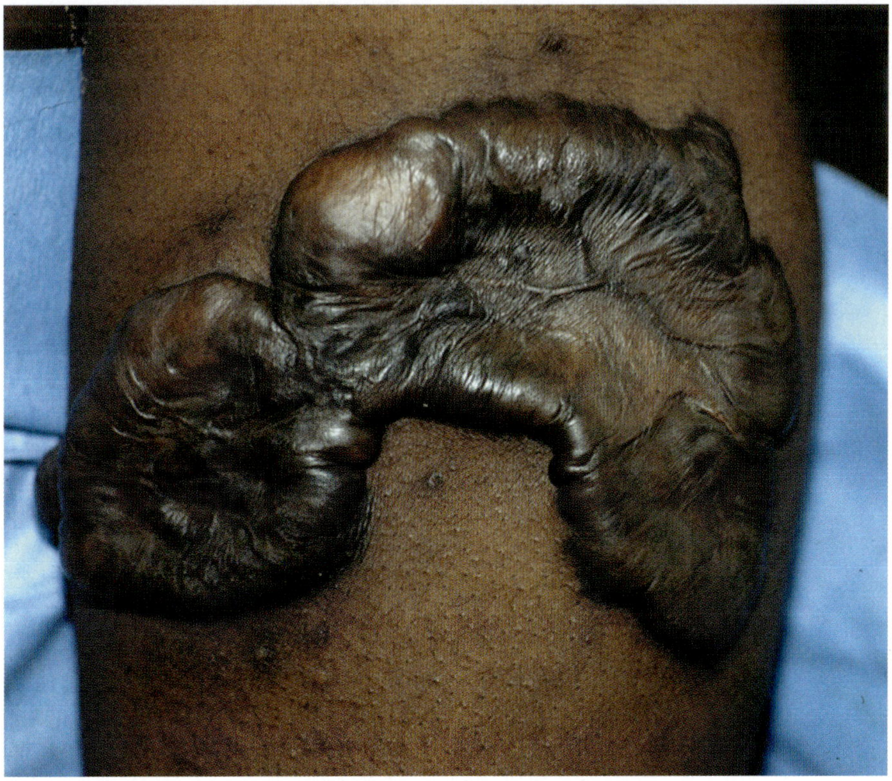

▲ **FIGURE 30-18** Keloid on the medial leg of an African-American man.

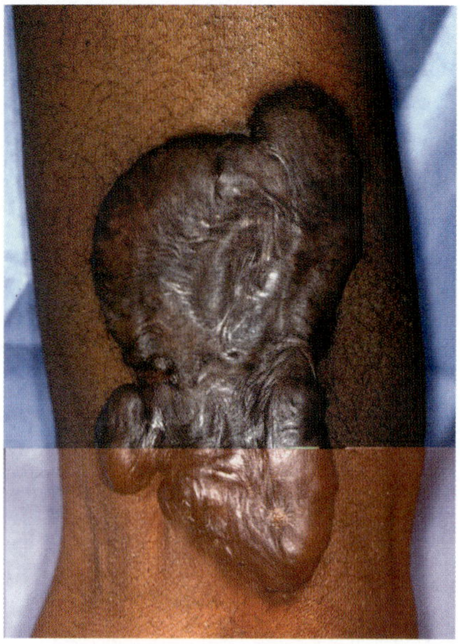

▲ **FIGURE 30-19** Proximal right forearm keloid on an African-American man.

collagen profile as keloids, whereas those more than 87 months old have the same collagen content as normal skin.[68]

Fibronectin

Fibronectin is a glycoprotein synthesized by fibroblasts and an integral factor in fibroblast aggregation. Kischer and Hendrix found that the immunofluorescence reaction of fibronectin is intense in hypertrophic scars and keloids and reflects exactly the conformation of the nodular structure, especially in the upper and middle reticular dermis.[69] There was intense reactivity of fibroconnection in those investigators' hypertrophic scars and keloid cultures, but little or none appeared in the normal skin cultures, suggesting that fibroblasts cultured from keloids and hypertrophic scars may be synthesizing more fibroconnectin than those from normal dermis.[68–70]

Keloid formation seems to be a function of the rate of collagen synthesis or degradation yet does not resemble the conditions involving a change in either collagen synthesis (e.g., active scleroderma, pulmonary fibrosis, liver cirrhosis, and synovial tissue proliferation in inflammatory stages of rheumatoid arthritis) or collagen degradation (e.g., cartilage destruction in rheumatoid arthritis, epidermolysis bullosa dystrophica, and hormonal disturbances such as hyperthyroidism, hyperparathyroidism, and Paget disease of bones). Keloids have an exuberance of dermal proliferation composed mostly of bands of collagen that have increased hyaluronic acid and sulfated glycosaminoglycans.[71]

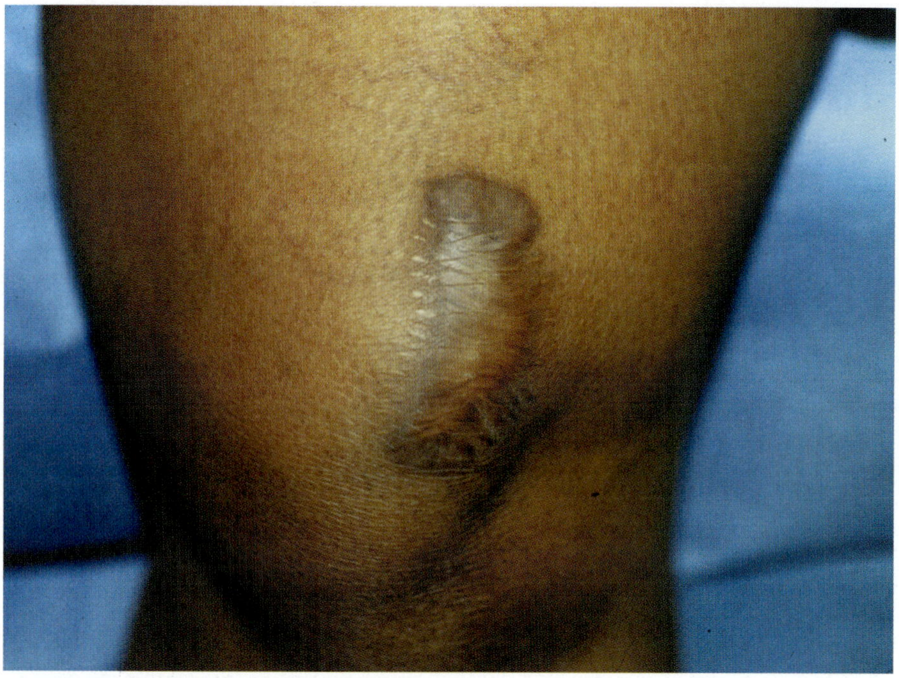

▲ **FIGURE 30-20** Keloid of the left thigh of an African-American man. This keloid has a reddish center that was biopsy-proven sarcoidosis.

There are 25 types of collagen, of which type I and type III are found in the skin. The bulk of skin collagen, as well as that of bone and tendon, is type I, which contains two identical alpha chains designated *alpha 1* and a third chain called *alpha 2*. Type III collagen is composed of three chemical features such as relatively high levels of hydroxyproline and lysine plus some cystine. Type III accounts for more than half the total collagen in

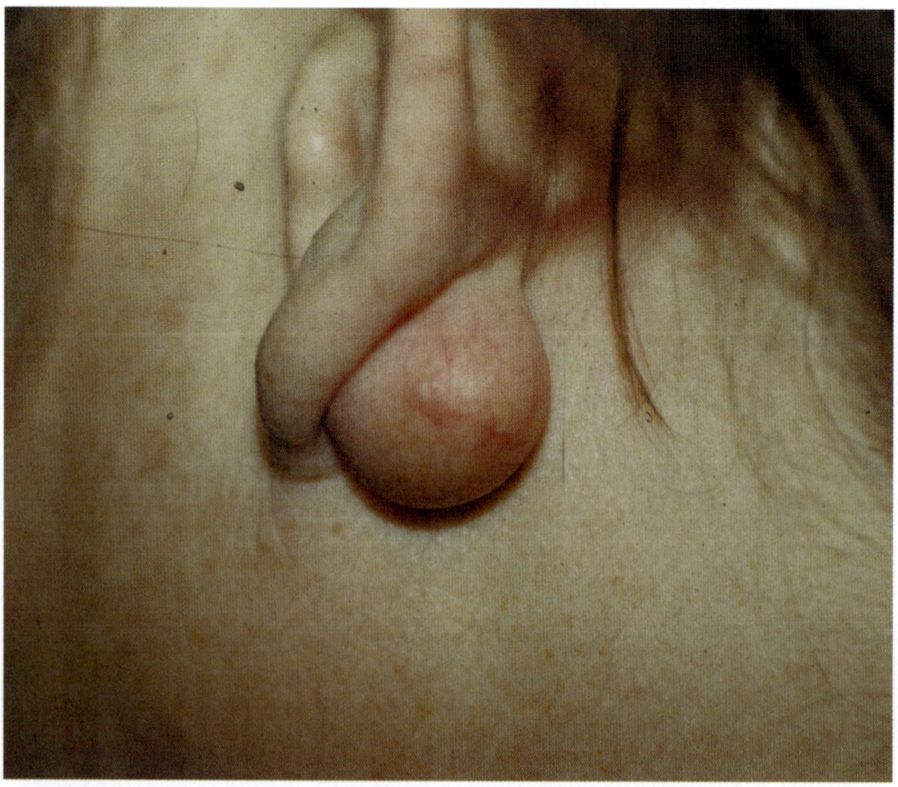

▲ **FIGURE 30-21** An epidermal cyst of the left posterior earlobe in a Hispanic woman.

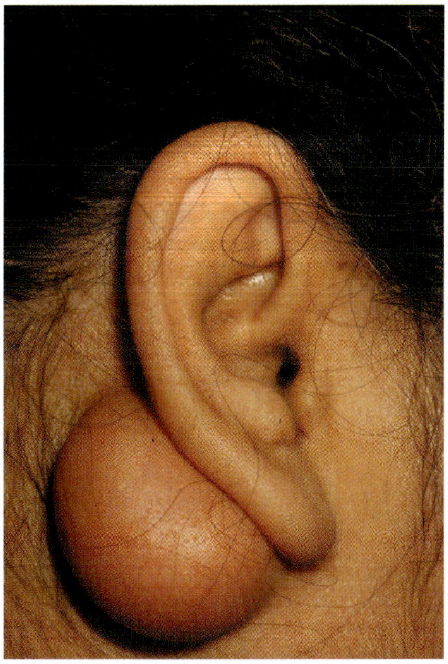

▲ **FIGURE 30-22** A lipoma of the right posterior earlobe in a Hispanic woman.

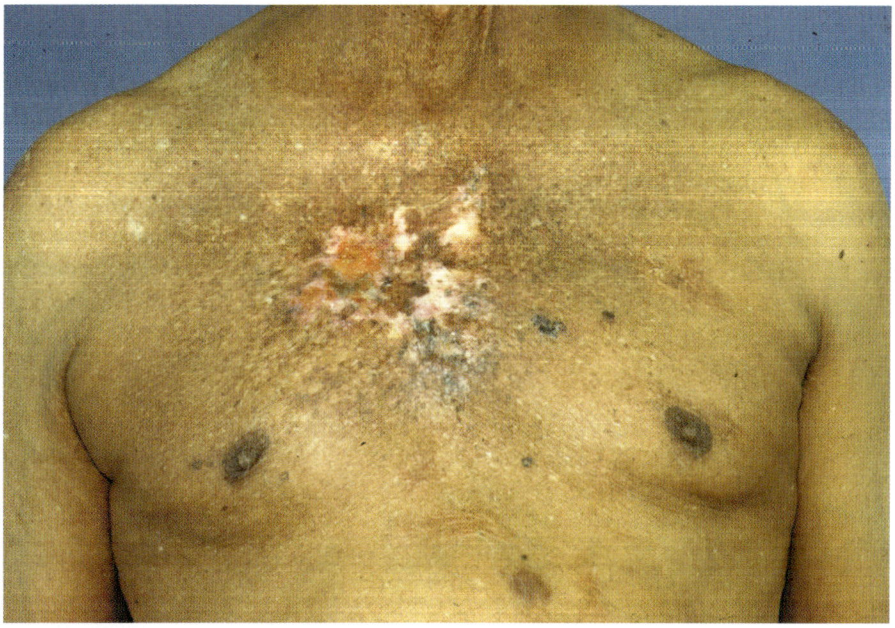

▲ **FIGURE 30-24** An African-American man who developed squamous cell carcinoma in the midchest area secondary to radiation treatment of a large chest keloid.

fetal skin but less than 20% in adult skin.[71,72]

In light of the preceding, one might surmise that keloids have an increase in type I collagen, especially since this type is more resistant to proteolysis than is type III.[73,74] However, studies by Clore and colleagues showed no significant difference in the percentage of type III collagen synthesized by fresh keloid biopsies compared with normal dermis.[75] Likewise, there was no significant difference in the percentage of type III collagen synthesized by keloid fibroblasts compared with normal fibroblasts.[76] These results demonstrate that keloid collagen has the same type distribution as normal dermis and suggests that increased collagen synthesis in keloids is not related to altered collagen types. Also, the increased collagen accumulation in keloids does not appear to result from increased fibroblast proliferation because fibroblasts are sparse on histologic section of older, developing lesions, and keloid DNA content is the same as in normal dermis. McCoy and Cohen have found that sera from keloid patients do not contain a factor that significantly modifies the in vitro growth kinetics or collagen synthesis of keloid-derived or normal dermal fibroblasts.[77]

Studies by McCoy and colleagues demonstrated that altered collagen synthesis by keloid fibroblasts is not related to abnormal cell growth.[78] Keloid

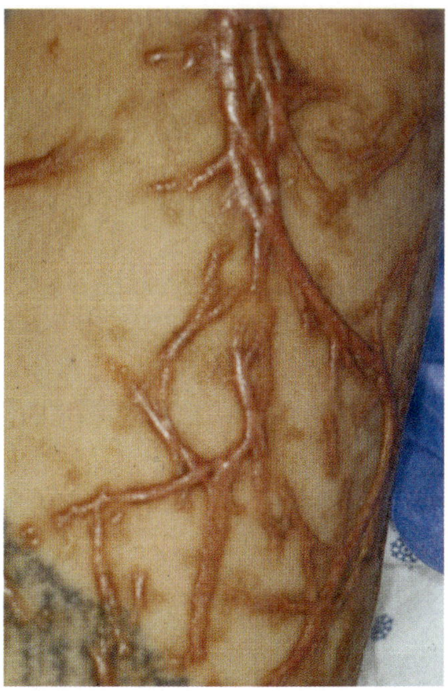

▲ **FIGURE 30-23** Linear xanthomas on the back of a Hispanic man.

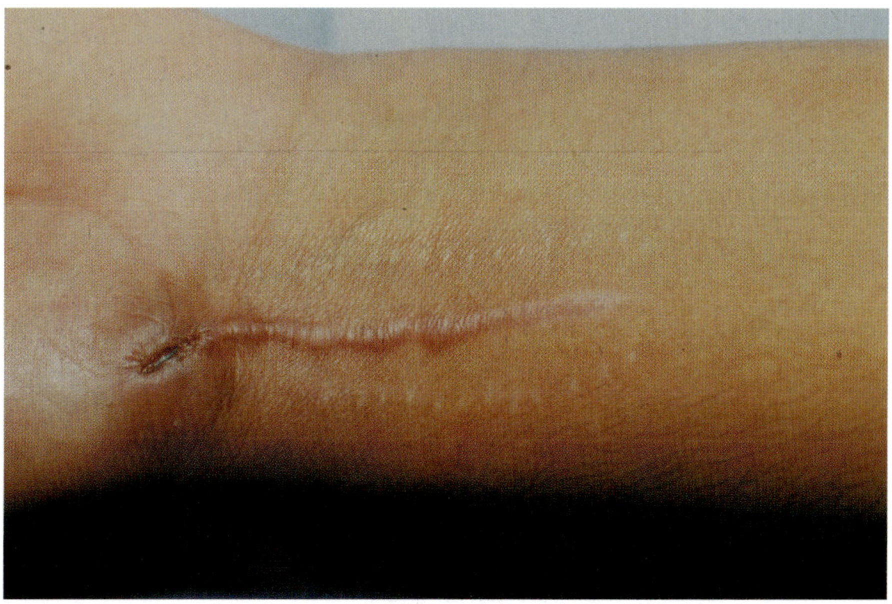

▲ **FIGURE 30-25** Linear hypertrophic scar.

fibroblasts did not exhibit markedly shortened in vitro life spans compared with normal dermal fibroblasts under routine culture conditions. Under sparse growth conditions, however, keloid fibroblasts appeared to lose replicative capacities earlier than normal skin fibroblasts.[79]

An examination of the collagenase produced by explants from normal skin, hypertrophic scars, and keloids cultured in vitro revealed no significant differences in either the amount of the enzyme produced or in the nature of that enzyme. The principal site of collagenase production in keloid specimens appeared to be, as in normal skin, the upper dermal or epidermal layer, with minimal production occurring in the lower fibrous or nodular areas.[80] On the other hand, an examination of the activity of the enzyme collagen synthesis revealed that it is markedly elevated in both keloids and hypertrophic scars in comparison with normal scars and normal skin, suggesting that the rate of collagen biosynthesis is increased in both abnormal scar types in vitro.[80]

Although collagen synthesis is significantly increased in keloids, collagen degradation (i.e., collagenase activity) is also the same or increased compared with that in normal skin and normal scar formation. It would seem as if this increase in collagenase would counterbalance the increase in collagen synthesis; however, Oliver and colleagues found a third factor that influences the collagen production-destruction activity in keloids: tissue α-globulins.[81] Serum α-globulins are known inhibitors of skin collagenase. Patients with keloids have normal serum α-globulins but an increased deposition of the α-globulin α_1 -antitypsin and α_2-macroglobulin in keloid tissue. These investigations postulate that this deposition may, in turn, inhibit the activity of collagenase, causing a decrease in the rate of collagen degradation. In addition, these authors found that women taking oral contraceptives had elevated serum levels of α-globulins, a phenomenon that may explain why pregnant women sometimes experience a growth of existing keloids or hypertrophic scars.[81,82]

Completing the collagenase–α-globulin picture is the phenomenon of intralesional steroids causing keloids to become smaller. After intralesional triamcinolone injections, there is usually a reduction in the size of a keloid as well as a significant reduction of the α_1-antitrypsis deposits.[83] These findings suggest that α-globulins are involved in abnormal scar formation and that the triamcinolone may remove collagenase inhibitors, thereby allowing activation of the collagenase with subsequent breakdown and reabsorption of the excessive collagen.[76]

LABORTORY TESTS

Tissue Cultures

In 1935, Tuma published the first report on tissue culture techniques in the study of keloids.[84] Almost 25 years later, Conway and colleagues found three morphologically distinct cell types in keloid tissue cultures.[85] The most abundant was a small, highly spindle-shaped cell with a high metabolic rate—the *type I fibroblast*. The second type, several times greater in volume with many fine cytoplasmic processes extending from its surface, was called the *type II fibroblast*. The type II fibroblasts migrated more slowly than type I cells and contained a larger number of mitochondria and larger nuclei. The third cell type appeared to be essentially normal fibroblasts.

Conway and colleagues postulated that the type I cell is responsible for the production of the fibrous matrix and the type II cells for absorption of the matrix.[85] This theory is even more plausible in view of the observation that stable and regressing older keloids show a preponderance of cells with abnormally large nuclei (type II fibroblasts) in contrast to recently developed keloids, which usually produce an exuberant growth of type I fibroblasts in tissue culture.

Mucin-like changes have been demonstrated in keloids. However, the condition is not a true endogenous mucinosis and differs histochemically from cutaneous mucinosis. These patients had had previous corticosteroid injections, and the interaction of steroids within the fibrous tissue probably produced these histologic changes.[86] Other histopathologic findings include one case of keloidal calcification and one case of psuedomelanoma.[87,88]

Histopathology

Since keloids and hypertrophic scars have clinical similarities, histopathologic differentiation between them is difficult.[89] Some investigators claim that no clear distinction can be made between the lesions, whereas others have found definite morphologic differences.[90] Blackburn and Cosman reported that keloids have conspicuous bundles of thick, glassy, faintly refractile, pale-staining collagen, a feature absent from hypertrophic scars.[82] In addition, keloid tissue usually has abundant mucinous ground substance, few fibroblasts, and no foreign-body reactions, whereas hypertrophic scars have scanty mucinous ground substance, numerous fibroblasts, and frequent foreign-body reactions.[91]

Another difference between keloids and hypertrophic scars is that Luxol fast blue stains normal collagen blue and keloid collagens reddish. Keloids that develop in skin defects (e.g., burns and cuts) do not have a normal papillary dermis, whereas so-called spontaneous keloids and those that develop from old acne lesions are separated from the epidermis by a fairly normal papillary dermis.[92]

Early forms of fibroblasts persist longer in keloids than in normal scar tissue. In normal wound healing, connective tissue elements regress after the third week, whereas in keloids, fibroblasts proliferate around neovascular formations to form dense masses of collagen. This process can continue for months to years, thus determining the size of the keloids.[93]

Craig and colleagues reported that in keloid tissue, as in normal skin, mast cells are present only in the dermis, never in the epidermis.[94] However, unlike normal skin, where the mast cells are located primarily around adnexal tissue in the superficial dermis, keloid mast cells occur throughout the dermis, interspersed among collagen bundles. Although the concentration of mast cells in keloid dermis is not appreciably different from that in normal skin, the much thicker dermis of a keloid suggests a greater total mast cell number under a given epidermal area.[94]

New elastic tissue formation is often a feature of normal scar tissue formation but not of keloids, which are also deficient in or devoid of lymphatics. Normal lymphatic function is associated with the presence of elastic tissue; lymphatics are not able to function without it.[95]

Keloids have an exuberance of dermal proliferation composed mostly of bands of collagen glycosaminoglycans.[24] Chemical analysis shows the activity of α-naphthyl acid phosphatase to be greater in keloids than in normal skin. The enzymes of the Embden-Meyerhof glycolytic pathway and of other systems relating carbohydrate to amino acid and fatty acid metabolism are more active in keloids and hypertrophic scars than in normal skin. Because of their high water content, collagen fibrils in keloids are bound to hyaluronic acid until they reach maturity.[24] A significant increase in alanine transaminase is found in keloids but not in hypertrophic scars.[96]

Keloids differ from hypertrophic scars in osmotic pressure, metabolic activity, and collagen turnover, as reflected in the local concentrations of sodium, magnesium, and calcium, respectively. Keloids have a higher content of water and soluble collagen than normal skin. They are deficient in lymphatics and associated elastic fibers. These qualities are true of early hypertrophic scars as well, but after 7 months, the two diverge as hypertrophic scars normalize their water and collagen content. Sodium, a measure of osmotic pressure, is normal in keloids and decreased in hypertrophic scars, whereas magnesium, a measure of metabolic activity, is increased in keloids but decreased in hypertrophic scars. Calcium, which reflects collagen metabolism, is increased in keloids and decreased in hypertrophic scars.[97]

DIFFERENTIAL DIAGNOSIS

- Hypertrophic scar
- Lipoma
- Dermatofibrosarcoma protuberans
- Dermatofibroma
- Squamous cell carcinoma
- Fibrotosis

Keloids are usually distinctive enough not to be confused with other cutaneous lesions, although sometimes hypertrophic scars may be difficult to rule out. As mentioned previously, hypertrophic scars remain within the bounds of the initial injury, are not clawlike, and often regress spontaneously.[31] Allergic contact dermatitis secondary to gold earrings may produce keloidal lesions on the earlobes, but histopathologic study of these lesions shows a dense infiltration of lymphoid cells plus the formation of lymphoid follicles rather than dense collagen tissue.[98–101]

TREATMENT

The first rule of keloid therapy is prevention (Table 30-7). Withhold nonessential cosmetic surgery from known keloid formers, close all surgical wounds with minimal tension, make sure that incisions do not cross joint spaces, avoid midchest incisions, and when making incisions, follow the skin creases, if possible. Known keloid formers should apply pressure with a gradient elastic garment or other apparatus for 4–6 months after burns, surgical procedures, or major skin trauma.

TABLE 30-7
Keloid Preventative Measures

- Withhold ear piercing or elective cosmetic surgery from known keloid formers.
- Avoid tattoos.
- Close surgical wounds with normal tension.
- Avoid making cross-joint spaces.
- Avoid midchest incisions.
- Educate patient on postoperative care.

No single therapeutic modality that is best for all keloids (Table 30-8). The type of therapy depends on location, size, and depth of the lesion; age of the patient; and past response to treatment. Treatment can be frustrating for both the patient and the physician. Excision of the lesion is actually the least important part of treatment. More important is the patient's compliance in postoperative therapy.

The lack of uniform treatment guidelines, with no foolproof protocol, is the crux of the problem. In fact, even the optimal time to start treatment is unknown.[57]

Steroid Injections

My treatment of choice for most earlobe keloids and those in locations other than the midchest is corticosteroid injections (Tables 30-9 through 30-11). Steroid injections should be given every 2–3 weeks at least four times prior to surgery. Diagnosis and treatment of keloids are basically the same irrespective of the patient's skin color.

Here are a few therapeutic gems:

1. *Procedures to decrease the pain from injections:* Prior to injection of intralesional steroids, the keloid should be covered with a topical anesthetic such as EMLA, a eutetic mixture of one-half (2%) lidocaine and one-half prilocaine, to help the patient withstand the pain of the injection. This topical anesthesia should be applied an hour before surgery and occluded with a very thin plastic wrap. The lidocaine does not relieve the initial pain of injection but does allow multiple injections with minimal discomfort and prevents most postinjection pain.
2. Another way of making steroid injections less painful is to pretreat the keloid with liquid nitrogen for a 10- to 15-s thaw time. This causes tissue edema, making the injection into the keloid much easier. Freezing for more than a 25-s thaw time often will cause hypopigmentation; triamcinolone injections in strengths of 3 mg/mL or stronger also may cause hypopigmentation of the injected area for 6–12 months. Inform patients of this possibility.
3. *Needle injection procedure:* Since the keloids are often hard, insert the needle deep into the keloid. Slowly remove the needle while injecting the keloid until reaching the dermal-epidermal junction. Here, the steroid goes in easier. Inject with a small 27-gauge needle because larger-bore needles may behave like a punch biopsy.
4. *Intralesional steroid mixture for keloid therapy:* Triamcinolone acetonide should be mixed in equal parts: 10 and 40 mg/mL (Kenalog-10 and Kenalog-40; Squibb). If the keloid is large enough to require multiple injections, a dilution of the Kenalog-10 can be mixed with an equal part of 2% lidocaine.
5. If the response to kenalog injections is minimal to absent after two or three injections, or if the keloids have been injected previously with the same concentration of triamcinolone without improvement, then a higher concentration of steroid is recommended, for example, full-strength triamcinolone acentonide (40 mg/mL).
6. Use a Luer-Lok-type or fixed-needle insulin syringe to prevent the needle from separating from the syringe during injection. To prevent clogging, use nothing larger than a 27-gauge needle for either dosage of triamcinolone. The 40 mg/mL dosage sometimes puddles in the injected sites, forming superficial xanthomatous-like deposits that may have to be removed for optimal cosmetic results.
7. For easy removal of the steroid, use a small curette, or make a nick in

TABLE 30-8
Treatment of Keloids

- No one therapeutic modality is best for all keloids.
- Standard treatment includes intralesional steroids, surgical excision, pressure, radiation, lasers, cryosurgery, and other medical therapies.
- Polytherapy is more successful than monotherapy.
- Excision alone has a 45–100% recurrence rate.

TABLE 30-9
Intralesional Steroid Injections

- Inject triamcinolone acetonide (TAC), 40 mg/mL, with maximum amount of 1–½ mL.
  - Any dose of triamcinolone greater than 3 mg/mL may cause hypopigmentation that may last 6–12 months.
- Use a small-bore (27 or 29 gauge) needle because it does not clog as often as large-bore needles.
- Inject where the skin is wrinkled (pinch the skin for more wrinkling).
  - Epidermal-dermal plane is easier to find.
  - Atrophy also may occur at injection site(s), usually lasting 6–12 months.
  - For preoperative anesthesia and keloid inhibition, inject a mixture of half 40 mg/mL TAC and half 2% xylocaine.
  - Corticosteroids delay wound healing.
  - Wait 2–3 weeks before removing sutures, except for the face, where 10 days are sufficient.
- Following surgical removal with corticosteroid injections is the most common procedure.
  - Wait 2 weeks after suture removal to avoid wound dehiscence.
  - Give corticosteroid to postoperative site every 2–3 weeks.
- Freeze with liquid N_2 for 10–15 seconds for easier injection.
  - Liquid N_2 also provides some anesthesia and edema.
- Inject every 2–3 weeks before surgery.
  - To ease injection pain, apply 2% lidocaine and 2% prilocaine cream thickly under occlusion 1 hour prior to injection.
- Inject inflammatory border surrounding keloid.

the skin and use a strong suction apparatus.

8. Sometimes the base of the keloid is so fibrotic that it is almost impossible to inject. In these cases, insert a large-bore needle into the keloid, and inject the triamcinolone suspension as you slowly withdraw the needle.
9. The steroid solution is under great pressure and often leaks out. To prevent leaking, paint the area around the needle site with a tincture of benzoin, and cover it with a piece of waterproof tape immediately after withdrawing the needle.
10. Inject only the base of the keloid or the lesion itself, not the surrounding tissue; injecting the surrounding areas may cause normal tissue to atrophy and the keloid to sink down to skin level without becoming flat or softer.
11. The initial injection usually produces no visible change in the keloid but often makes it softer and alleviates most symptomlogy.
12. Inform patients that the steroid injections will not narrow the scar, even if it completely flattens.[102–105]

The effect of corticosteroids on collagen synthesis and degradation is not completely understood, but we do know that corticosteroids seem to work better in early keloids. This may be because only the younger fibroblasts can be induced by steroids to produce collagenase.[106] Older cells appeared not to respond to steroids with collagenase production. In addition, cortisol administration in rats causes a rapid disappearance of collagen from the dermis, whereas prednisone, cortisone, and deoxycorticosterone are without effect. This difference indicates that the β-hydroxyl group present in prednisone, cortisol, and triamcinolone is necessary to exert the effect and may explain why triamcinolone injections are helpful in reducing the size of keloids.[103–105]

TABLE 30-10
Multiple Complications with the Use of Systemic Corticosteroid in the Treatment of Keloids

- Severe infections
- Hyperglycemia (not usual)
- Edema
- Osteonecrosis
- Myopathy
- Peptic ulcer disease
- Hypokalemia
- Osteoporosis
- Euphoria
- Psychosis
- Myasthenia gravis
- Growth suppression
- Abrupt discontinuation = adrenal crisis

TABLE 30-11
Intralesional Interferon-alfa-2b

- Inject 1 million units per linear centimeter of postoperative site.
- Repeat 1–3 weeks later.
- Warn patients about flulike symptoms.
  - Premedicate with 500–1000 mg acetaminophen.
  - Take every 6 hours in the evening for pain for 2 days.
  - 18% recurrence with interferon-alfa-2b.
  - 51–100% recurrence with surgery only.

Surgery

If there is no significant regression of the keloid tissue after four injections, or if the keloid no longer responds to further injections, surgery is recommended. The surgical method differs according to the size and location of the lesions:

1. For keloids with narrow bases (<1 cm in diameter), a simple excision followed by undermining of the base and closure with interrupted sutures will suffice. Before closure, the base of the operative site is injected with Kenalog-40 so that the earliest fibroblasts are exposed to steroids. Or surgical anesthesia is provided by one-half 2% lidocaine and one-half triamcinolone, 40 mg/mL, mixed together.
2. For posterior pedunculated earlobe keloids, for which cosmetic appearance is not important, shaving followed by pressure hemostasis is a simple and efficient method of removal.
3. For large, nonpendunculated earlobe keloids and keloids with wide bases on other parts of the body, removal is more complex. First, a half-moon incision approximately one-fifth the size of the lesion is made from one border onto the part of the keloid with the smoothest and flattest-looking surface. The remaining part of the keloid is then excised, and the tip of saved epidermis and superficial dermis is carefully dissected from the underlying white glistening fibrous tissue mass. Triamcinolone, 40 mg/mL, is injected into the base of the surgical site. The overlying skin is then approximated to the undermined borders of the excision with 6-0 nylon interrupted

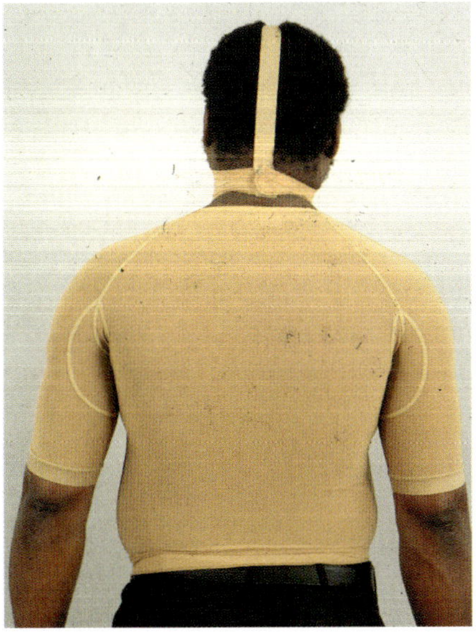

▲ **FIGURE 30-26** A pressure-gradient garment (Jobst) that helps to prevent recurrence of treated keloids.

sutures. The sutures are left in for 10–14 days because earlier removal may cause wound dehiscence. This slow healing is the consequence of the steroid injection. A week after suture removal, the postoperative site is injected with triamcinolone acetonide, 10 mg/mL, every 2 weeks. In most cases, four postoperative injections are sufficient to prevent recurrence.

4. In patients in whom the overlying skin is not smooth enough to be used as a cover for the excised tissue, a tissue expander may be inserted so that the keloid can be excised and closed primarily several months later.[57]

Pressure

Another adjunct for preventing recurrence is the use of a pressure-gradient garment on the postoperative site for at least as 12 hours, preferably 20 hours a day for 4–6 months (Figure 30-26). For earlobe keloids, special pressure earrings or devices may be used. The proposed mechanism of action is outlined in Table 30-12.[107–109]

TABLE 30-12
Keloid Pressure Treatment

- Start pressure garments 1 week after suture removal.
  - Reduces size and thickness of keloids.
  - Reduces intralesional mast cells.
  - Reduces histamine production.
- Combine with a class 1 steroid.

Radiation Therapy

For patients with midchest keloids or a history of keloid recurrence after surgery, radiation therapy is an adjunct modality. A dose of 250 rads is given immediately after surgery, followed by four more treatments at weekly intervals. Other regimens include (1) a single dose of 1000 rads the day after surgery and (2) 300 rads the day after surgery and then thereafter every other day for a total of three treatments.

Fisher and Storck treated more than 300 patients with radiotherapy alone.[110] In a 20-year follow-up, they found that radiotherapy was most effective when used within the first 5 months of keloid formation. Their total dose ranged from 800–2400 rads divided over 2–5 months. They noted better results with postoperative keloids, lacerations, and infections than with scars from burns, scalds, and caustics. More intensive studies by Vanden Brank and Minty produced the following conclusions[111]: Primary irradiation of early keloids that are still cellular, well vascularized, and growing may cause some resolution if more than 1000 rads is given. They found no merit in fractionating the doses. When treating older keloids, primary radiation alone failed to cause resolution, although it did relieve symptoms such as pruritus. Doses of 1000 rads or more may cause atrophy of the irradiated area or radionecrosis, leading to more keloid formation.

Vanden Brank and Minty's studies demonstrated that preoperative radiation was unsatisfactory for reducing keloids, and because of rapid recovery from radiation, there may be superregeneration. Postoperative radiation within 48 hours of surgery was the most effective technique in their series; the optimal dose was between 1000 and 1500 rads. They advocated a margin of 0.5 cm of normal skin. This dose caused atrophy of the subcutaneous tissues, which eventually may lead to squamous cell carcinoma.[111]

Arnold, after protecting the surrounding skin with putty containing bismuth, found that 500 rads every 5 days for four doses starting on the first postoperative day prevents recurrence.[112,113] Shaffer and colleagues evaluated 13 studies of keloids treated with radiation, with a total of 2225 patients having 2592 keloidals scars.[114] They concluded that although all the studies were retrospective and uncontrolled, it appeared that radiation after surgical excision prevented recurrence of keloidal scars in approximately 75% of patients at 1-year follow-up. The most frequently used treatment was supcrficial x-rays of 9 cGy or greater in fractions given within 10 days of surgery.[114]

Young children with keloids either should not be irradiated or, if they are, the metaphyses should be shielded to prevent retardation of bone growth. Even doses of less than 400 rads may cause growth retardation.[24]

Laser Treatment

Abergel and colleagues reported successful treatment of keloids with the Nd:YAG laser.[115] However, I have found that laser therapy (carbon dioxide or Nd:YAG) alone does not prevent keloid recurrence. It must be combined with intralesional steroids during surgery and every 2–3 weeks times four treatments. In addition, pressure therapy should be used as an adjunct to prevent recurrence. A study evaluating the 585-nm pulsed-dye laser for treatment of keloidal scars demonstrated efficacy in reducing subjective symptoms, color, and height in the scars.[116]

Other Treatments

Silicone gel and other dressings (Table 30-13) have been evaluated in 12 studies involving 538 patients with keloidal or hypertrophic scars. Treatment was applied for at least 12 hours. Although most of the studies involved hypertrophic scars, in the one with keloidal scars, 34% of the scars showed flattening after 6 months of continuous gel use.[117]

Ligatures may be used for pedunculated keloids when surgery or corticosteroid injections are either contraindicated or refused by the patient. A 4-0 nonabsorbable suture is tied tightly around the base of the lesion, and a new one is applied every 2–3 weeks. The sutures gradually cut into and strangulate the keloid, eventually causing it to fall off. However, in the southern part of the United States, it was the custom to tie a horse's mane hair around the keloid instead of a suture.[57]

Topical tretinoin applied twice a day may alleviate pruritus and other

TABLE 30-13
Miscellaneous Treatments for Keloids

- Silicone gel sheeting, flurandrenolide (Cordran) tape, or Curad cosmetic pad
  - Start 1 week after suture removal.
- Pentoxifylline (Trental) 400 mg tid
  - Limited success

keloid symptomatology and may cause various degrees of regression. This method seems to be even more effective when combined with a potent topical steroid.[118]

In addition, there have been small studies or case reports using several other modalities. Ultraviolet A1 radiation has been reported to soften and flatten keloids.[119,120] Onwukwe had success with surgical excision combined with methotrexate.[121] Methotrexate induces folic acid deficiency, resulting in poor collagen formation. Methotrexate, 15–20 mg, is given orally in a single dose every 4 days starting a week prior to surgery and is continued for 3–4 months after the postoperative site is healed.

Oral medications such as asiatic acid, penicillamine, colchicine, and β-aminopropionitrile have been combined with surgical excision to prevent recurrence. Numerous other topical, physical, and systemic modalities have been advocated but have been either unsuccessful or proved less effective those mentioned earlier.[57]

Imiquimod is a topical therapeutic agent that behaves as an immune response modulator by inducing interferon-α; interluken-1, interluken-6, and interluken-8; and tumor necrosis factor alpha. In a small 13-patient study by Berman and Kaufman, imiquimod cream was applied to the postoperative site daily for 8 weeks, starting immediately after surgery.[103] Some of these patients experienced marked irritation and had to discontinue the medication for 3–6 days. Imiquimod should not be used on postoperative incision sites, flaps, grafts, large wounds, and wounds under tension for 4–6 weeks because they may splay or dehisce. Also, over half the patients using imiquimod will develop hyperpigmentation of the treated areas.[122]

CONCLUSION

Keloids are benign fibrous growths that result from an abnormal connective tissue response in certain predisposed individuals. Blacks form keloids more often than whites, but the reason for this racial difference is not known. Trauma, foreign-body reactions, infections, and endocrine dysfunction all have been proposed as precipitating factors. Keloids are found most commonly on the earlobes, shoulders, upper back, and midchest. They extend past the area of trauma and, once present, tend to remain stable. Although sometimes pruritic, painful, or tender, they are usually asymptomatic. Keloids often arise during pregnancy and grow more rapidly during pregnancy and are more common after puberty. The Yoruba of West Africa believe that piercing before puberty may prevent keloid formation. Estrogens increase serum α-globulins and are collagenase inhibitors. Histologically, although there have been many therapeutic modalities, most have had limited success. The most commonly used therapeutic approach is a combination of cryotherapy, intralesional steroid injections, surgical excision, and pressure devices.

REFERENCES

1. Datubo-Brown DD. Keloids: A review of the literature. *Br J Plast Surg* 1990;43:70-77.
2. Bloom D. Heredity of keloids: A review of the literature and report of a family with multiple keloids in five generators. *NY State Med J* 1975;56:511-519.
3. Alibert JLM. *Description des Maladies de la Peau Observees a l'Hospital Saint Louis et Exposition des meilleures Methodes suivies pour leur Traitement.* Paris, Barrois Paine et fils, 1806, p 113.
4. Alibert JLM. *Description des Malaides de la Peau Observees a l'Hopital Saint Louis et Exposition des meilleures Methodes suivies pour leur Traitement,* Vol 2. Brussels, Auguste Wahlen, 1825, p 34.
5. Kaposi M. Keloid, in Hebra F, Kaposi M (eds), *Diseases of the Skin Including the Exanthema.* London, New Sydenham Society, 1874, p 272.
6. Hawkins C. Cases of warty tumors of cicatrices. *Med Chir Trans* 1835;19:19.
7. Macpherson J. On tumors of cicatrices. *London Med Gaz* 1844;35:348.
8. Breasted JH. *The Edwin Smith Surgical Papyrus,* Vol 1: *Hieroglyphic Translation and Commentary.* Chicago, University of Chicago Press, 1930, pp 403-406.
9. Omo-Dare P. Yoruban contribution to the literature on keloids. *J Natl Med Assoc* 1973;65:367-406.
10. Addison T. On the keloid of Alibert and on true keloid. *Med Chir Trans* 1854; 37:27.
11. Addison T. On the keloid of Alibert and on true keloid, in Shelley WB, Crissey JT, Stokes JH (eds), *Classics in Clinical Dermatology with Biographical Sketches.* Springfield, IL, Charles C Thomas, 1953, pp 93-94.
12. Cosman B, Crikelair FG, Ju MC. The surgical treatment of keloids. *Plast Reconstr Surg* 1961;27:105-109.
13. Cohen IK, McCoy BJ. Keloid: biology and treatment, in Dineen P, Hildick-Smith G (eds), *The Surgical Wound.* Philadelphia, Lea & Febiger, 1981, pp 123-131.
14. Brenizer AG. Keloid formation in the Negro. *Ann Surg* 1915;61:87.
15. Fox H. Observations on skin diseases in the American Negro. *J Cutan Dis* 1908;26:67.
16. Matas R. The surgical peculiarities of the Negro. *Transact Am Surg Assoc* 1896;14:483.
17. Hazen HH. Personal observations upon skin diseases in the American Negro. *J Cutan Dis* 1914;32:705.
18. Geschicter CF, Lewis D. Tumors of connective tissue. *Am J Cancer* 1938; 25:630.
19. Alhady SM, Sivanantharajah K. Keloids in various races: A review of 175 cases. *Plast Reconstr Surg* 1969;44:564.
20. Arnold HL. Keloids, in Maddon S (ed), *Current Medical Management,* 2nd ed. St Louis, Mo. Mosby, 1975, p 194.
21. Oluwasanmi JO. Keloids in the African. *Clin Plast Surg* 1974;1:179.
22. Bohrod MG. Keloids and sexual selection: A study in the racial distribution of disease. *Arch Dermatol Syphilol* 1937;36:19.
23. Ketchum LD, Cohen IK, Masters FW. Hypertrophic scars and keloids: A collective review. *Plast Reconstr Surg* 1974;53:140.
24. Al-Attar A, Mess S, Thomasen JM, et al. Keloid pathogenesis and treatment. *Plast Reconstr Surg* 2006;117:286-300.
25. Asboe-Hansen G. Hypertrophic scars and keloids: Etiology, pathogenesis, and dermatologic therapy. *Dermatologica* 1960;120:178.
26. Kelly AP. National Medical Association, Section on Dermatology, Lecture, *An Etiological Update on Keloids,* San Antonio, Texas, August 1, 1999.
27. Bayles MA. Coiffure keloids. *Br J Dermatol* 1972;86:415.
28. Yagi KI, Dafalla AA, Osman AA. Does an immune reaction to sebum in wounds cause keloid scars? Beneficial effect of desensidization. *Br J Plast Surg* 1979;32:223-225.
29. Ginarte M, Peteiro C, Toribio J. Keloid formation induced by isotretinoin therapy. *Int J Dermatol* 1999;38:228-229.
30. Krenar J. Keotazce etiologie a kliniky keloidu a hypertrofickych jizer. *Cas Lek Cesk* 1958;97:1619.
31. Garb J, Stone MJ. Keloids: Review of the literature and a report of eighty cases. *Am J Surg* 1942;58:515.
32. Lorber B. Are all diseases infectious? *Ann Intern Med* 1996;125:844-851.
33. O'Connor SM, Taylor CE, Hughes JM. Emerging infectious determinants of chronic diseases. *Emerg Infect Dis* 2006; 12:1051-1057.
34. Moustafa MFH, Abdel-Fattah AMA. Presumptive evidence of the effect of pregnancy estrogens on keloid growth: A case report. *Plast Reconstr Surg* 1975; 56:450-453.
35. Kelly AP, Zheng P, Johnson BL. Mast cells and keloid formation. *J Invest Dermatol* 1996;106:838.
36. Diegelmann RF, Bryant CP, Cohen IK. Tissue (-globulins in keloid formation. *Plast Reconstr Surg* 1977;59:481.
37. Glucksmann A. Local factors in the histogenesis of hypertrophic scars. *Br J Plast Surg* 1951;4:88.
38. Justice J. Beobachtungen und Experiemente zur Atiologie des Keloids. *Arch Dermatol Syphilol (Berl)* 1919; 197:274.
39. Allan JC, Keen P. The management of keloid in the South African Bantu. *S Afr Med J* 1954;28:1034.
40. Pautrier LM, Zorn R. Calcemie teneur en calcium de la peau dans les cheloides et les acnes cheloidinnes. *Bull Soc Franc Dermatol Syphilol* 1931;38:953.

41. Mysliwska J, Trzonkowski P, Bryl E, et al. Lower interleukin-2 and higher serum tumor necrosis factor levels are associated with perimenstrual, recurrent, facial herpes simplex infection in young women. *Eur Cytokine Network* 2000;11:397-406.
42. Solomons B Jr. Keloids and their treatment. *Practitioner* 1952;168:465.
43. Vargus L Jr. Attempt to induce formation of fibroids with estrogens in the castrated female Rhesus monkey. *Bull Johns Hopkins Hosp* 1943;73:23.
44. Personen S, Rintala A, Saivio A, et al. On the [4-^{14}C] progesterone metabolism of keloid and hypertrophic scar. *Scand J Plast Reconstr Surg* 1976;10:173.
45. Ford LC, Kind DF, Lagase LD, et al. Increased androgen binding in keloids: A preliminary communication. *J Dermatol Surg Oncol* 1983;9:545.
46. Cohen IK, Diegelmann RK, Keiser HR. Collagen metabolism in keloid and hypertrophic scar, in Longacre JJ (ed), *The Ultrastructure of Collagen.* Springfield, IL, Charles C Thomas, 1973, pp 199-212.
47. Edgerton MT Jr, Hanrahan EM, Davis WB. Use of vitamin E in the treatment of keloids. *Plast Reconstr Surg* 1951; 8:224.
48. Kobak MW, Benditt EP, Wissler RM, et al. Relationship of protein deficiency to experimental wound healing. *Surg Gynecol Obstet* 1947;85:751.
49. Bowesman C. *Surgery and Clinical Pathology in the Tropics.* Edinburgh, E&S Livingstone, 1960, p 798.
50. Discussions with Wilbert Jordan, M.D., Director, OASIS Clinic, Los Angeles County Department of Health Services, Martin Luther King Jr. Multi-Ambulatory Care Clinics.
51. Marneros AG, Norris JEC, Olsen BR, Reichenberger E. Clinical genetics of familial keloids. *Arch Dermatol* 2001;137: 1429-1434.
52. Laurentaci G, Dioguardi D. HLA antigens in keloids and hypertrophic scars. *Arch Dermatol* 1971;113:1726.
53. Cohen IK, McCoy BJ, Mohanakumar T, et al. Immunoglobulin, complement, and histocompatibility antigen studies in keloid patients. *Plast Reconstr Surg* 1979;63:689.
54. Mowlem R. Hypertrophic scars. *Br J Plast Surg* 1961;4:113.
55. Psillakis JM. Water and electrolyte content of normal skin, scars and keloid. *Plast Reconstr Surg* 1971;47:272.
56. Vanden Brank HA, Minty CC. Radiation in the management of keloids and hypertrophic scars. *Br J Surg* 1960; 47:595.
57. Kelly AP. Keloids. *Dermatol Clin* 1988;6:413-424.
58. Lahav M, Cadet JC, Chirambo M, et al. Corneal keloids: A histopathological study. *Graefes Arch Clin Exp Ophthalmol* 1982;218:256.
59. Koonin AJ. The etiology of keloids: A review of the literature and a new hypothesis. *S Afr Med J* 1964;38:913.
60. Kormoczy BI. Enormous keloid(?) on a penis. *Br J Plast Surg* 1978;31:268.
61. Parsons RW. A case of keloid on the penis. *Plast Reconstr Surg* 1966;37:431.
62. Diegelmann RF, Bryant CP, Cohen IK. Tissue (-globulins in keloid formation. *Plast Reconstr Surg* 1977;59:481.
63. Perez CA, Lockett MA, Young G. Radiation therapy for keloids and plantar warts. *Front Radiat Ther Oncol* 2001 ;35:135-146.
64. Stout AP. Fibrosarcoma, the malignant tumor of fibroblasts. *Cancer* 1966;1:30.
65. Gueft B. Keloids. *Trans Electron Microsc Soc Am* 1965;23:5.
66. Rasmussen DM, Wakin KG, Winkleman RK. Isotonic and isometric thermal contraction of human dermis: III. Scleroderma and cicatrizing lesions. *J Invest Dermatol* 1964;43:349.
67. Harris ED, Sjoersdma A. Collagen profile in various clinical conditions. *Lancet* 1966;1:705.
68. Tuan Tl, DiCesare P, Cheung D, Nimni ME. Keloids and hypertrophic scars, in Nimni ME, Kang AH (eds), *Collagen: Pathobiochemestry.* Boca Raton, FL, CRC Press, 1991, pp 125-136.
69. Kischer CW, Hendrix MJC. Fibronectin (FN) in hypertrophic scars and keloids. *Cell Tissue Res* 1983;231:29.
70. Kischer CW, Wagner HN Jr, Pindur L, et al. Increased fibronectin production by cell lines from hypertrophic scar keloid. *Connect Tissue Res* 1989;26:279-288.
71. Babu M, Diegelmann R, Oliver B. Fibronectim is overproduced by keloid fibroblast during abnormal wound healing. *Mol Cell Biol* 1989;9:1642-1650.
72. Cohen IK, Keiser HR, Sjordsma A. Collagen synthesis in human keloid and hypertrophic scar. *Surg Forum* 1971; 22:488.
73. Tuan TL, Nitcher LS. The molecular basis of keloid and hypertrophic scars formation. *Mol Med Today* 1998; 4:19-24.
74. Bettinger DA, Yager DR, Diegelmann RF, Cohen IK. The effect of TGF-β on keloid fibroblast proliferation and collagen synthesis. *Plast Reconstr Surg* 1996; 98:827-833.
75. Clore JN, Cohen IK, Diegelmann RF. Quantitative assay of types I and III collagen synthesized by keloid biopsies and fibroblasts. *Biochim Biophys Acta* 1979;586:384.
76. Uitto J, Peredja AJ, Abergel RP, et al. Altered steady state ratio of type I/III procollagen mRNAs correlates with selectively increases type I procollagen synthesis in cultured keloid fibroblast. *Proc Natl Acad Sci USA* 1985;82:5935-5943.
77. McCoy BJ, Cohen IK. Effects of various sera on growth kinetics and collagen synthesis by keloid and normal dermal fibroblasts. *Plast Reconstr Surg* 1981;67:505.
78. McCoy BJ, Galdum J, Cohen IK. Effects of density and cellular aging on collagen synthesis and growth kinetics in keloid and normal skin fibroblast. *In Vitro* 1982;18:79.
79. Calderon M, Lawrence WT, Banes AJ. Increased proliferation of keloid fibroblasts wounded in vitro. *J Surg Res* 1996;61:343-347.
80. Garcia-Ulloa AC, Arrieta O. Tubal occlusion infertility due to an excessive inflammatory response in patients with predisposition for keloid formation. *Med Hypoth* 2005;65:908-921.
81. Oliver N, Babu M, Diegelmann R. Fibronectin gene transcription is enhanced in abnormal wound healing. *J Invest Dermatol* 1992;99:579-586.
82. Blackburn WR, Cosman B. Histologic basic of keloid and hypertrophic scar differentiation. *Arch Pathol* 1966;82:65.
83. Schofield JD, Jackson SS. Collagen biosynthesis in normal human skin, normal and hypertrophic scar and keloid. *Eur J Clin Invest* 1975;5:69.
84. Tuma W. Quelques experiences sur la culture des keloids humaines in vitro. *Comp Rendu Assoc Anat* 1935;30:507.
85. Conway H, Gillette RW, Findley A. Observation on the behavior of human keloids in vitro. *Plast Reconstr Surg* 1959; 24:229.
86. Santa Cruz DJ, Ulbright TM. Mucin-like changes in keloids. *Am J Clin Pathol* 1981;75:18.
87. Redmond WJ, Baker SR. Keloidal calcification. *Arch Dermatol* 1983;119:270.
88. Hiss Y, Shafir R. Pseudomelanoma in a keloid. *J Dermatol Surg Oncol* 1978;4:938.
89. Uitto J, Lichentenstein JR. Defects in the biochemistry of collagen in diseases in connective tissue. *J Invest Dermatol* 1976; 66:59.
90. Cohen IK, McCoy BJ, Mohanakumar T, Diegelmann RF. Immunoglobulin, complement, and histocompatibility antigen studies in keloid patients. *Plast Reconstr Surg* 1979;63:689-695.
91. Boyce DE, Ciampolini J, Ruge E, et al. Inflammatory cell subpopulations in keloid scars. *Br J Plast Surg* 2001,54: 511-516.
92. Mehregan AH. *Pinkus' Guide to Dermatohistophathology,* 4th ed. New York, Appleton-Century-Crofts, 1986, p 537.
93. Mancini RE, Quaife JV. Histogenesis of experimentally produced keloids. *J Invest Dermatol* 1962;38:143.
94. Craig SS, DeBloids G, Schwartz LB. Mast cells in human keloid, small intestine and lung by an immunoperoxidase technique using murine monoclonal antibody against tryptase. *Am J Pathol* 1984;124:427.
95. Crockett DJ. Regional keloid susceptibility. *Br J Plast Surg* 1964;17:245.
96. Bhangou KS, Quinlivian JK, Connelly JR. Elastic fibers in scar tissue. *Plast Reconstr Surg* 1976;57:308.
97. King CD, Salzman FA. Keloid scars: Analysis of 89 patients. *Surg Clin North Am* 1970;50:595.
98. Psillakis JM. Water and electrolyte content of normal skin, scars and keloid. *Plast Reconstr Surg* 1971;47:272.
99. Fisher A. Allergic dermal contact dermatitis due to gold earrings. *Cutis* 1987; 39:473-375.
100. Iwatsuki K, Yamada M, Takigawa M, et al. Benign lymphoplasia of the earlobes induced by gold earrings: Immunohistologic study on the cellular infiltrates. *J Am Acad Dermatol* 1987;16:83.
101. Niessen FB, Spauwen PH, Schalkwijk J, Kon M. On the nature of hypertrophic scars and keloids: A review. *Plast Reconstr Surg* 1999;104:1435-1458.
102. Berman B, Flores F. Recurrence rates of excised keloids treated with postoperative triamcinolone acetonide injections or interferon-afla-2b injections. *J Am Acad Dermatol* 1997;137: 755-757.
103. Berman B, Kaufman J. Pilot study of the effect of postoperative imiquimod 5% cream on the recurrence rate of excised keloids. *J Am Acad Dermatol* 2002;47:S209-211.

104. Fitzpatrick RE. Treatment of inflamed hypertrophic scars using intralesional 5-FU. *Dermatol Surg* 1999;25:224-232.
105. Bodokh I, Brun P. The treatment of keloids with intralesional bleomycin. *Ann Dermatol Venereol* 1996;123:791-794.
106. Houck JC, Sharma VK, Carillo A. Control of cutaneous collagenolysis, in Weber G (ed), *Advances in Enzyme Regulation,* Vol 8. New York, Pergamon Press, 1970.
107. Brent B. The role of pressure therapy in the management of earlobe keloids: Preliminary report of a controlled study. *Ann Plast Surg* 1978;1:579.
108. Lawrence WT. Treatment of earlobe keloids with surgery plus adjuvant intralesional verapamil and pressure earrings. *Ann Plast Surg* 1996;37:167-169.
109. Snyder GB. Button compression for keloids of the lobule. *Br J Plast Surg* 1974;27:186.
110. Fisher E, Storck H. X-ray treatment of keloids. *Schweiz Med Wochenschr* 1957; 87:1981.
111. Vanden Brank HA, Minty CC. Radiation in the management of keloids and hypertrophic scars. *Br J Surg* 1960; 47:595.
112. Arnold HL, Graver FH. Keloids: Etiology and management by excision and intensive prophylactic radiation. *Arch Dermatol* 1959;80:772.
113. Borok TL, Bray M, Sinclair I, et al. Role of ionizing irradiation for 393 keloids. *Int J Radiat Oncol Biol Phys* 1998;15:836-870.
114. Shaffer JJ, Taylor SC, Cook-Bolden FA. Keloidal scars: A review with a critical look at therapeutic options. *J Am Acad Dermatol* 2002;46:S63-97.
115. Abergel RP, Dwyer RM, Meeker CA, et al. Laser treatment of keloids: A clinical trial and an in vitro study with Nd:YAG laser. *Lasers Surg Med* 1984;4:291.
116. Alster TS, Williams CM. Treatment of keloid sternotomy scars with 585-nm flashlamp-pumped dye-laser. *Lancet* 1995;345:1198-2000.
117. Mercer NS. Silicone gel in the treatment of keloid scars. *Br J Plas Surg* 1989;12:102-108.
118. Janssen DeLimpens AMP. The local treatment of hypertrophic scars and keloids with retinoic acid. *Br J Dermatol* 1980;103:319.
119. Asawanonda P, Khoo LSW, Fitzpatrick TB, Taylor CR. UV-A1 for keloid. *Arch Dermatol* 1999;135:348-349.
120. Hannuksela-.Svahn A, Grandal OJ, Thorstensen T, Christensen OB. UVA 1 for treatment of keloids (abstract). *Acta Dermatol Venereol* 1999;79:490.
121. Onwukwe MF. Surgery and methotrexate for keloids. *Schoch Lett* 1978;28:4.
122. Berman B, Kaufman J. Pilot study of the effects of postoperative imquimod 5% cream on the recurrence rate of excised keloids. *J Am Acad Dermatol* 2002;47:S209-211.

CHAPTER 31

Bullous Diseases

Mobolaji Opeola
Brittney De Clerk

Key Points

- Pemphigus vulgaris is the most common autoimmune blistering disorder and is caused by antibodies to desmogleins.
- Several variants of pemphigus exist: pemphigus vegetans, endemic pemphigus foliaceus, pemphigus erythematosus, drug-induced pemphigus, IgA pemphigus, and paraneoplastic pemphigus.
- Bullous pemphigoid is seen generally in the elderly and is caused by autoantibodies to two antigens: BPAg1 (230 kDa) and BPAg2 (180 kDa).
- The antigens for bullous pemphigoid are found in the hemidesmosomes of the basal keratinocytes.
- Pemphigoid gestationis is a rare blistering disease occurring during pregnancy that is not well understood.
- Chronic bullous disease of childhood is a rare, acquired autoimmune bullous disease with variable clinical presentation caused by antibodies to BPAg2.
- Treatment of chronic bullous disease of childhood can be complicated by the incidence of glucose-6-phosphate dehydrogenase (G6PD) deficiency within a population.
- The diagnosis and treatment of bullous diseases in patients with skin of color can be influenced by genetic and epidemiologic factors.

Bullous diseases of the skin can be either acquired or autoimmune in nature. The acquired forms result from a defective or missing component of the epidermis or the basement membrane zone. Autoimmune bullous diseases are caused by destruction of native components of the epidermis or basement membrane zone, resulting in breakdown of the integrity of the skin. There are many different kinds of bullous dermatoses. They can be differentiated by their varied clinical, pathologic, immunohistochemical, and serologic features. This chapter explores several of the autoimmune bullous dermatoses that need special consideration in regard to diagnosis and treatment in skin of color.

PEMPHIGUS

Pemphigus is an autoimmune intraepidermal blistering disease with two main variants: pemphigus vulgaris and pemphigus foliaceus. Further subclassification can be made based on clinical, histologic, and etiologic factors, yielding other diagnoses, such as pemphigus vegetans, endemic pemphigus foliaceus, pemphigus erythematosus, drug-induced pemphigus, IgA pemphigus, and paraneoplastic pemphigus. The incidence of each of these variants differs with location and ethnicity, suggesting that environmental and hereditary factors play a role in the pathogenesis of pemphigus. Most studies on pemphigus are done in Europe and North America, but some studies have been performed on skin of color in Asia and South America, and there is a dearth of pemphigus literature from Africa.

Pemphigus Vulgaris (PV)

PV is an intraepidermal autoimmune blistering disease mediated by antibodies directed against components of the keratinocyte cell membrane leading to acantholysis. These tissue-bound antibodies (IgG1 and IgG4) are directed most commonly against desmoglein 3 (130 kDa). In addition to the tissue-bound antibodies, these patients also have circulating antibodies. Disease activity correlates with the circulating antibody titer: The higher the titer, the worse is the disease activity.

Clinically, these patients present classically with generalized flaccid bullae occurring on normal-appearing skin or on an erythematous base (Figure 31-1*A, B*). These bullae demonstrate a positive Nikolsky's sign and rupture to form painful erosions, which can heal into hyperpigmented patches, especially in skin of color. More than 50% of patients have involvement of the mucous membranes, mainly the oral mucosa, but also the eye, esophagus, genitalia, and anus (see Figure 31-1*C, D*). Involvement of the oral mucosa presents as painful erosions on the buccal, gingival, or palatine mucosa.

The mean age of onset of PV is in the fifth decade in North America, Europe, South Africa, and India. However, in Kuwait, the mean age of onset is in the fourth decade.

Diagnosis is made with a skin biopsy (preferably of the edge of a blister) and direct and indirect immunofluorescence studies. Histopathologic analysis of the

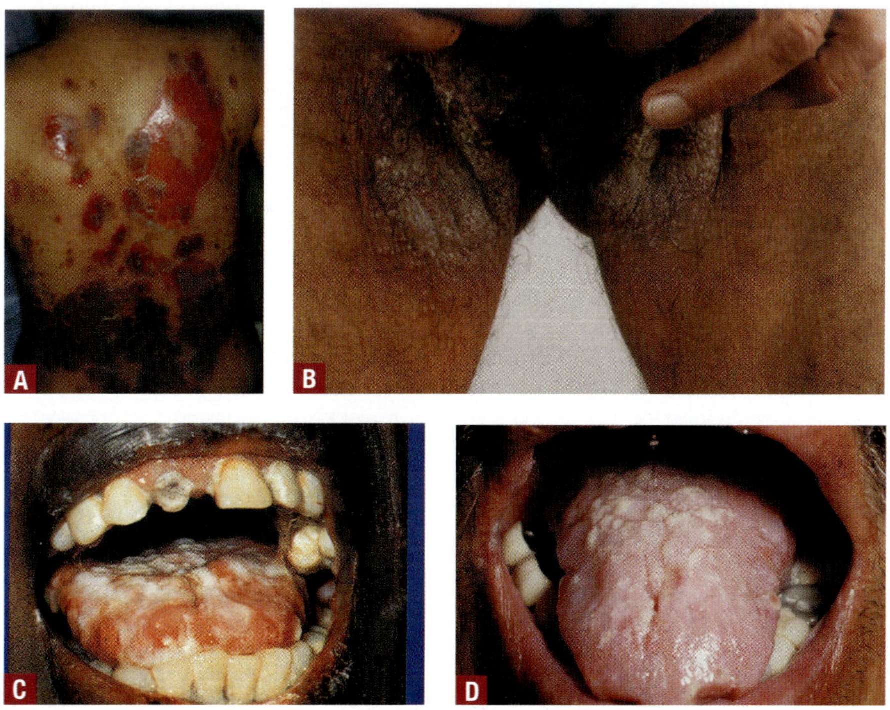

▲ **FIGURE 31-1** *A–D.* Pemphigus vulgaris.

skin will show acantholysis with a suprabasal blister and a mild superficial mixed cellular infiltrate with eosinophils. Direct immunofluorescence (DIF), preferably on perilesional skin, will show a "chicken wire" deposition of intercellular IgG with or without C3 on the surfaces of keratinocytes. The preferred substrate for indirect immunofluorescence (IIF) is monkey esophagus, and it will show circulating antiepidermal IgG antibodies, specifically to desmoglein. The IIF titer is useful for determining the degree of disease activity in PV. The use of an enzyme-linked immunosorbent assay (ELISA) can result in better sensitivity. Although the classic antigen is desmoglein 3, the influence of race on the frequency of anti-desmoglein 1 (antidsg1) in PV has been reported. Most (75–90%) of PV patients from the Indian subcontinent have elevated antidsg1 compared with only 46% of patients of northern European descent and 57% of patients of other races.[1,2] A direct correlation between antidsg3 titers and the severity of oral disease was noted, as well as between antidsg1 titers and the severity of cutaneous disease.[1,3]

Pemphigus Vegetans

This is a vegetating variant of PV presenting in the flexural, intertriginous areas and on the scalp as fungating vegetations or papillomatous lesions.[4] There are two forms: Neumann type (begins and ends as PV) and Hallopeau type (circumscribed lesions with a relatively benign course). Biopsy of a vegetating lesion will show suprabasal acantholysis with pseudoepitheliomatous hyperplasia containing eosinophil microabscesses. The laboratory findings, pathogenesis, and treatment are similar to those of PV.

Pemphigus Foliaceus (PF)

PF is also an autoimmune intraepidermal blistering disease, but the disease activity is in the more superficial portion of the epidermis, resulting in superficial erosions. PF is associated with antibody (IgG1 and IgG4) directed against a keratinocyte cell adhesion molecule called *desmoglein 1* (160 kDa) that is present in the granular layer of the epidermis.

Clinically, these patients present with crusted superficial erosions and transient flaccid bullae that rupture easily in the seborrheic distribution, such as, the face, chest, and back (Figure 31-2). Nikolsky's sign is also positive. Owing to the pathogenesis of PF, there is rarely any mucous membrane involvement because desmoglein 3 (versus desmoglein 1) is expressed more in the mucosal membranes. PF can be induced by intense ultraviolet (UV) light exposure or burn and medications (see "Drug-Induced Pemphigus" below). Therefore, photoprotection may play a role in the management of PF. Summer exacerbations of pemphigus are seen both in India and South Africa.[5]

Some patients in Mali and South Africa presented with pruritus and pustules with hypopyon.[5,6] A rare clinical variant of PF with seborrheic keratosis–like verrucous lesions (mostly in erythrodermic PF) is not uncommon in these countries. Recently, an African-American man was found to have these seborrheic keratosis–like lesions described as multiple, sharply demarcated, hyperpigmented, "stuck on"–appearing verrucous papules and plaques on the back, chest, and neck.[7]

The mean age of onset of PF is in the fourth and fifth decades in North America, Europe, South Africa, Mali, and Kuwait. However, in Tunisia and Brazil, the mean age of onset is in the third decade.

Histologic analysis of a blister edge or verrucous lesion will show acantholysis in the upper epidermis (intragranular layer or subcorneal) and mild mixed dermal infiltrate with eosinophils. DIF will show IgG deposition in the epidermis, mostly in the upper part. IIF using guinea pig esophagus as the preferred substrate will demonstrate the presence of circulating antiepidermal IgG.

Pemphigus herpetiformis is a variant of PF in which the lesions present clinically as clusters of vesicles resembling dermatitis herpetiformis. This clinical variant was seen in 35% of patients in Tunisia presenting with PF.[8]

Fogo Selvagem/Endemic Pemphigus Foliaceus

Endemic PF is described extensively in South America, specifically Brazil. It is an endemic form of PF with both environmental and genetic associations. Clinically, these patients present with flaccid bullae that later evolve into eczematoid, psoriasiform, impetiginous, or seborrheic-like lesions. Incidence is 34 cases per 1 million people in rural Brazil, and it affects children and young adults, with a peak incidence in the second and third decades. Most of these patients live in close proximity to a river. There is a significant association between fogo selvagem and exposure to the *Simulium* (black) fly.[9] In addition to the environmental factors, there is a significant occurrence of endemic PF in family units where multiple, genetically related individuals are affected. A Brazilian study suggests that the pathogenetic antibodies may be IgG4 directed against the EC5 domain of desmoglein 1.[10]

Pemphigus Erythematosus (PE)

PE is a localized form of PF with features of lupus erythematosus. This is also known as *Senear-Usher syndrome.* Erythematous small flaccid vesicles and bullae with crusting on the cheeks (malar region), forehead, sternum, and upper back are seen. Histologically, these patients have epidermal acantholysis with intercellular antibody and antibody deposition along the dermal-epidermal junction (lupus-like). PE patients can have a positive antinuclear antibody (ANA) titer.

Paraneoplastic Pemphigus (PNP)

PNP is an uncommon blistering disorder seen as a paraneoplastic condition in patients with Castleman disease, non-Hodgkin lymphoma, Chronic lymphocytic leukemia (CLL), sarcoma, and thymoma. The cutaneous lesions observed vary from macules to erythema multiforme–like lesions to bullae and erosions. The mucous membrane is also involved in many cases. The range of clinical presentations may be explained by the pathogenesis of this condition. There is a complex immune response with antibody directed against various epidermal and basement membrane proteins, including desmoplakin 1 (250 kDa), envoplakin (190 kDa), bullous pemphigoid antigen 1 (BPAg1; 230 kDa), periplakin (190 kDa), 170-kDa antigen, and desmogleins 1 and 3.[4] A skin biopsy will show epidermal acantholysis, suprabasal clefting, and interface change at the basement membrane. DIF will demonstrate intercellular IgG and C3 in the epidermis, whereas IIF shows circulating antiepidermal IgG on rat bladder or squamous epithelium substrate.

Drug-Induced Pemphigus

PF is the most common form of pemphigus induced by drugs. Various drugs have been implicated, including thiol drugs (e.g., captopril, enalapril, and penicillamine) and nonthiol drugs, [e.g., penicillins, cephalosporins, piroxicam, interleukin 2 (IL-2), nifedipine, and pyrazolone derivatives]. Thiol drugs result in acantholysis of the epidermis without antibody formation, and clinical improvement is likely when the offending drug is

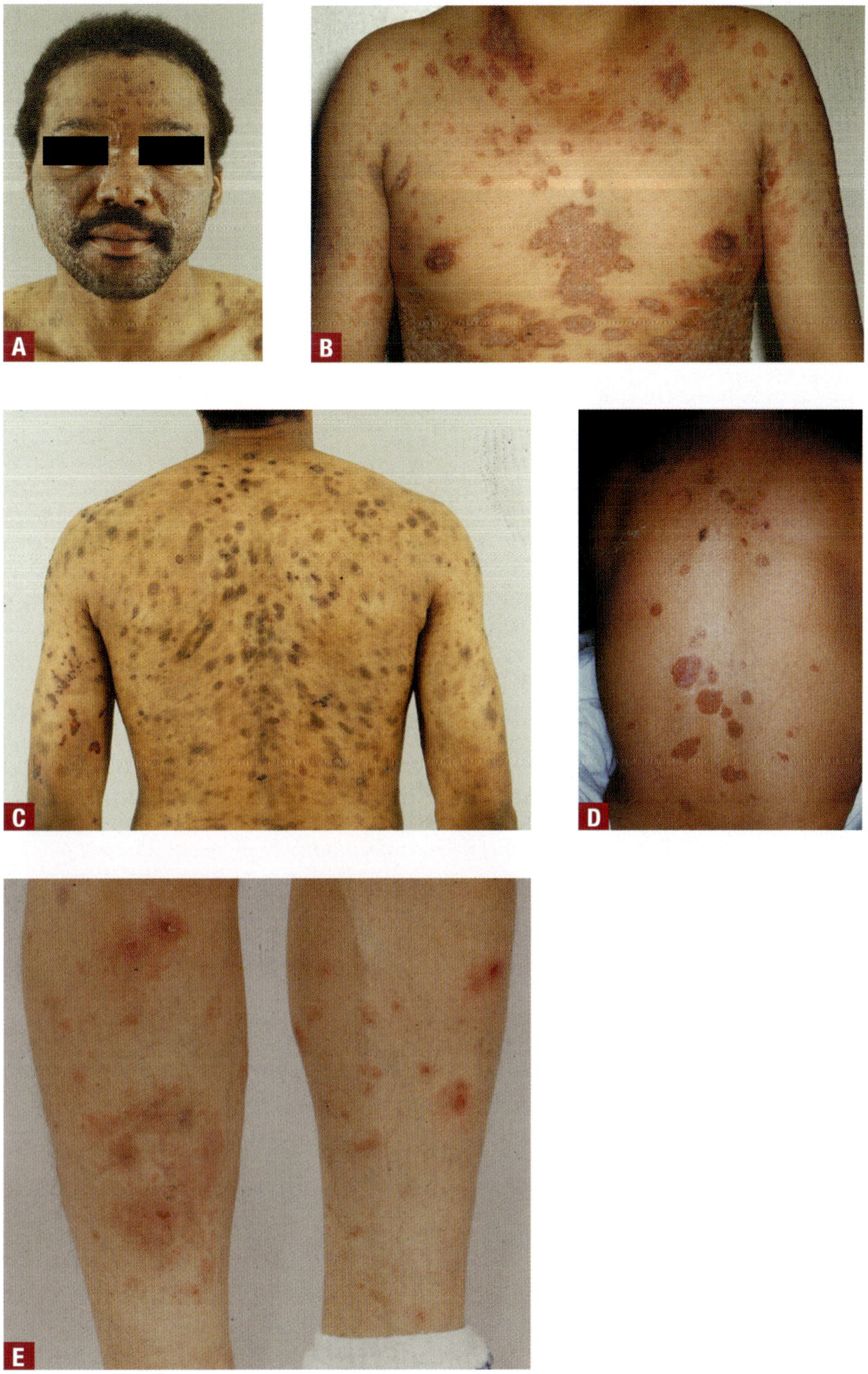

▲ **FIGURE 31-2** *A–E.* Pemphigus foliaceus.

discontinued. Nonthiol, nonsulfur drugs cause induction of antiepidermal antibodies, behaving similar to chronic pemphigus. Idiopathic and drug-induced pemphigus are identical clinically, and diagnosis is made by identification of the causal drug, skin biopsy, and DIF and IIF.

Epidemiology

Epidemiology data on pemphigus are not well documented for most regions, but available data show varying incidence in different regions. PV is reported extensively in Jews and people of Mediterranean descent. The incidence in Europe ranges widely between 0.76 and 9.3 cases per 1 million persons per year. An incidence of about 4.6 cases per 1 million persons per year was reported in Kuwait, 1.6 cases per 1 million persons per year in Saudi Arabia, and 6.7 cases per 1 million persons per year in Tunisia.[11,12]

PV is the more common pemphigus in Europe and North America. In Tunisia, however, PF (44–61%) is more common than PV, and in Mali, most (83%) patients with pemphigus have PF.[6,12,13] In South Africa, PF (76%) is much more frequent than PV in blacks. In South African patients with PV, most (74%) were of Indian origin.[5] Similarly, in Malaysia, Indians of Malaysian origin are more likely to develop PV than any other ethnic groups.[14] Over 90% of pemphigus patients in northern India have PV.[15] This supports the notion that there are hereditary factors contributing to the development of pemphigus.

In Kuwait, evaluation of all bullous diseases showed 47% to be pemphigus, 22% pemphigoid, 19% pemphigoid gestationis, and 7% linear IgA bullous disease.[10] A large percentage (80%) of the pemphigus patients in Kuwait have PV. Similarly, in China, Singapore, and Malaysia, pemphigus is the most prevalent autoimmune bullous disease.[11,16]

The epidemiology of pemphigus in Tunisia is unusual. There is an unusually high rate of 15.5 cases per 1 million persons per year of PF among women aged 25–34 years.[12] Likewise, in Mali, there is a prevalence of PF in women, but most are older than 40 years of age.[6] The high incidence of PF in Tunisian women may be linked to the use of traditional cosmetics containing kohl, henna, and souak.[17]

Genetics

Genetic factors play a role in the development of PV. Several studies have shown linkage of PV with some major histocompatibility complex (MHC) human leukocyte antigen (HLA) class II molecules. In North American and Europe studies, HLA-DR4, -DR6, and -DR14 are associated with PV.[4,8] Various studies in other populations around the world also have documented an association between pemphigus and HLA-DR4, -DR14, -DQB1*0302, and -DQ5 haplotypes.[18–21] Fogo selvagem also has been associated with HLA-DRB1. Although there are differences in the types of pemphigus prevalent in different regions, the genetic predisposition is similar.[22] There is a high incidence of HLA-B8 in South African PF patients.[5]

Prognosis

Unexplained disease flare may be secondary to bacterial or viral superinfection.[23] Morbidity and mortality of PF is usually lower than in PV. This is most likely related to the depth of the blister and presence or absence of extracutaneous manifestations. Mortality in the South African study was reported at 14%, mostly of the PV type.[5] Interestingly, Haouet and colleagues also reported a mortality rate of 14% in Tunisia.[13] Most deaths were related to septicemia and the high doses of steroids used in older treatment regimens. The mortality is more likely due to complications of treatment rather than to the disease itself. Morbidity and mortality are worse in older patients and in patients with extensive disease. In a study of Japanese patients, there was a 5% association rate of internal malignancy with pemphigus, with lung cancer being the most common in pemphigus and gastric cancer in bullous pemphigoid.[24] The ages of onset of malignancy were 64.7 and 69.2 years, respectively.

A special consideration in skin of color is the prevalence of postinflammatory pigment changes, most commonly hyperpigmentation. The more severe or extensive the disease and the longer the duration of disease, the higher are the chances of postinflammatory pigment alterations.

Management

Management of these patients may require a multidiscipline approach, usually with the expertise of a dermatologist, ophthalmologist, and dentist. First line of treatment for pemphigus is oral prednisone (1–1.5 mg/kg per day), which is tapered based on disease activity. Treatment with steroids is usually long term; therefore, side effects need to be monitored. Bisphosphonates, calcium, and vitamin D are useful in these patients to prevent skeletal complications. PF, if limited, can be treated solely with topical steroids. Hydroxychloroquine is also useful in PF. Other steroid-sparing mediations can be used in the management of patients with PV and PF, such as dapsone, tetracyclines with nicotinamide, gold, azathioprine, mycophenolate mofetil, cyclosporine, cyclophosphamide, intravenous immune globulin (IVIG), rituximab, and plasmopheresis.[8,25] In reports from South Africa and India, patients were treated frequently and successfully with dexamethasone-cyclophosphamide pulse treatment. However, owing to the serious side effects of cyclophosphamide, such as hemorrhagic cystitis, transitional cell carcinoma, and gonadal dysfunction, dexamethasone pulse treatment can be used with azathioprine or methotrexate with similar results.[26] Cumulative studies in South Africa reveal that cyclophosphamide may be more effective than azathioprine. With adequate therapy, clinical clearance of cutaneous and mucosal lesions is observed, and there is a significant reduction in the peripheral antiepidermal antibody load.

BULLOUS PEMPHIGOID

Bullous pemphigoid is an autoimmune blistering disease generally seen in the elderly that is characterized by large, tense bullae usually appearing on the trunk and intertriginous and flexor surfaces. Mucosal involvement is rare. The large bullae will rupture, leaving erosions that usually heal spontaneously. Initial skin lesions may consist of only urticarial or eczematous patches and plaques with pruritus that will progress to bullae over time (Figure 31-3). The mean age of onset is between 65 and 75 years, but the disease can occur in children. The frequency varies by geography, but generally it is very rare, with less than 6 cases per 1 million persons per year in all regions reported.[28]

The histology of bullous pemphigoid reveals subepidermal bullae without acantholysis. The inflammatory infiltrate is superficial and rich in eosinophils, although neutrophils occasionally predominate. DIF shows a continuous band of IgG and C3 along the basement membrane zone, best seen in perilesional skin. The antibodies are directed against two antigens present in the hemidesmosomes along the basement membrane: BPAg1 (230 kDa) and BPAg2 (180 kDa). The BPAg1 is completely intracellular, whereas BPAg2 is a transmembrane protein with an extracellular zone. It is now thought that the noncollagenous (NC) 16-Å extracellular portion of BPAg2 serves as the initiating antigen in the disease.[29]

There are numerous options for treatment that vary depending on disease severity. Localized disease can be treated with topical or intralesional corticosteroids. Oral prednisone is used for generalized disease, but side effects of systemic corticosteroids should be weighed, and steroid-sparing agents should be started whenever possible. Tetracycline alone or combined with nicotinamide may be effective. Dapsone may be useful when neutrophils predominate on biopsy. However, use of dapsone is dangerous in populations with a high incidence of glucose-6-phosphate dehydrogenase (G6PD) deficiency. Choices for further immune suppression with steroid-sparing agents include azathioprine, mycophenolate mofetil, cyclosporine, cyclophosphamide, and methotrexate.

When comparing bullous pemphigoid across skin types, one finds that the prevalence varies according to region. Bullous pemphigoid is the most common subepidermal immunobullous disorder in Singapore, accounting for 88% of cases. Epidermolysis bullosa acquisita accounted for 6%, linear IgA dermatosis for 3%, and bullous systemic lupus erythematosis for 3%.[30]

Pemphigoid was seen in 22%, pemphigus gestationis in 19%, linear IgA bullous disease in 7%, lichen planus pemphigoides in 3%, and epidermolysis bullosa acquisita in 2.3%.[11] Bullous pemphigoid proved to have a lower overall prevalence in this study compared with those from Europe and Singapore.[30,33,34] In Kuwait, the estimated incidence of bullous pemphigoid is 2.6 cases per 1 million persons per year.[37]

There are several variants of bullous pemphigoid that have been reported in persons with dark skin. A 24-year-old Ugandan man was found to have a scarring mucocutaneous bullous disease sharing components of both bullous pemphigoid and cicatricial pemphigus. Antibodies to BPAg1, BPAg2, and laminin 5 were found in the patient's serum. He was treated with oral prednisolone and dapsone, leading to healing and some scar formation of the lesions.[38]

One variant of bullous pemphigoid, lichen planus pemphigoides, shows clinical, histologic, and immunologic attributes of both lichen planus and bullous pemphigoid. Three black patients from West Africa near the Senegal River were found to have severe lichenoid erythrodermic bullous pemphigoid that was distinct from classic lichen planus pemphigoides. Their disease was significant in its severity, rapid onset of bullous lesions, and mucosal involvement in two of the three patients. Additionally, they were all found to have the HLA-DR10 haplotype.[39] This case series demonstrates that ethnicity may play a strong role in the incidence, severity, and clinical findings of autoimmune bullous diseases of the skin.

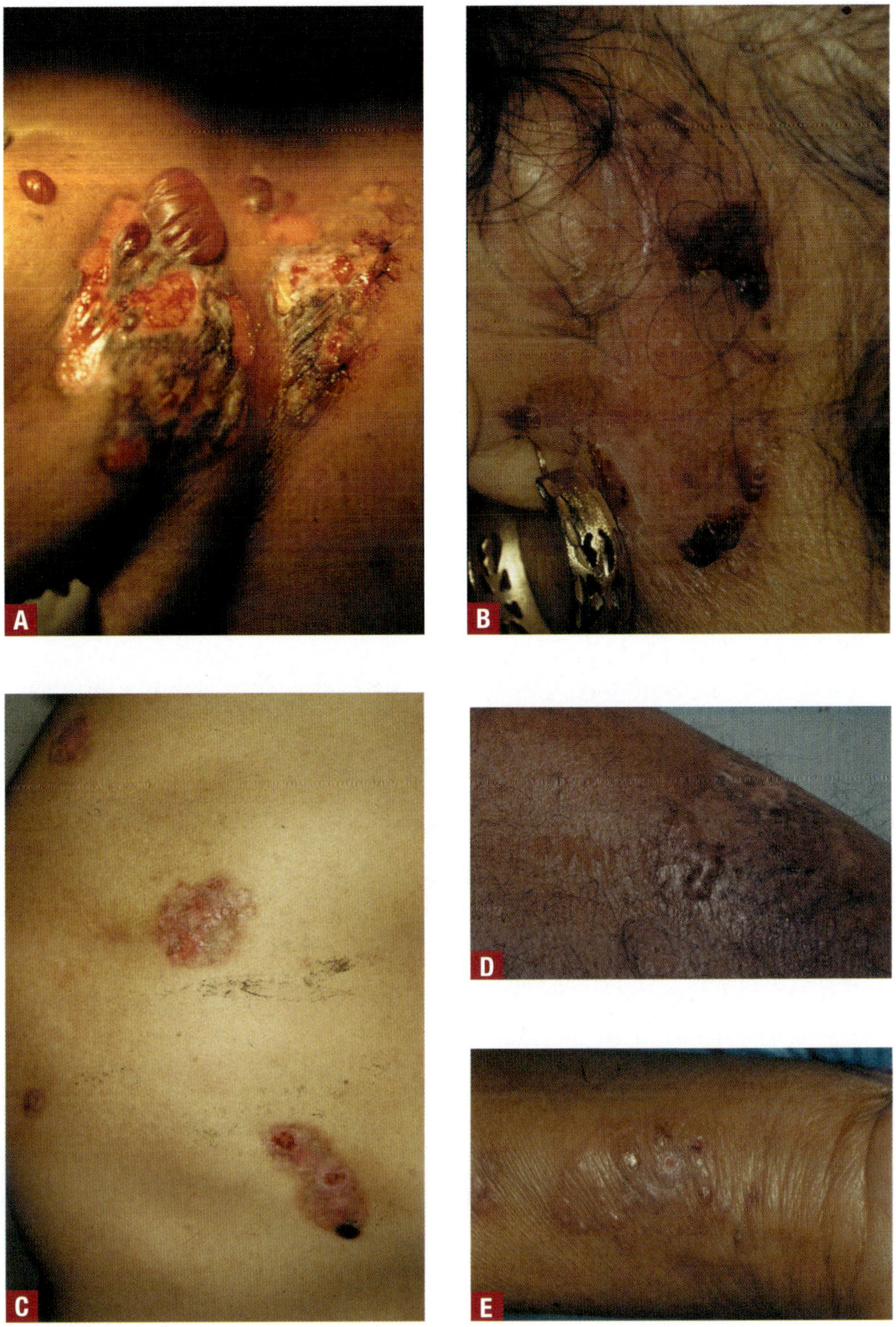

▲ **FIGURE 31-3** *A–E.* Bullous pemphigoid.

Previously, it was thought that bullous pemphigoid was much more rare in the Far East.[13,32] This distribution is similar to that seen in Europe but varies from that in Africa.[33,34] A Ugandan study aimed at defining the incidence of subepidermal blistering diseases (which did not include pemphigus) found that bullous pemphigoid was much more rare in East Africa than in other parts of the world.[35] In contrast, a high frequency of IgA autoantibodies was found in the Ugandan population. Bullous pemphigoid accounted for only 41% of all subepidermal blistering dermatoses in Uganda. The younger patients had a tendency for IgA diseases, whereas the older patients showed for IgG reactivity. A possible explanation for the different frequency of disease is that the Ugandan population is, on average, younger than the East Asian and European populations.

In Kuwait, Nanda and colleagues demonstrated that bullous pemphigoid was more common than IgA dermatoses in patients of Arab ethnicity, proving similar to Singapore. This study, however, also included pemphigus in its analysis and found that pemphigus is the most common autoimmune blistering dermatosis, observed in 47% of patients.

PEMPHIGOID GESTATIONIS

Pemphigoid gestationis (PG), formerly called *herpes gestationis,* is a rare blistering disease occurring during pregnancy, usually beginning in the second or third trimester, and it may recur in the postpartum period. The incidence of this disease varies depending on location or region. PG is described primarily in patients of European descent; therefore, most of the information known about this disease is from this population. There are only a few studies of PG in the nonwhite ethnic population. With literature on PG in ethnic groups being uncommon, literature in American blacks is even less common.

The pathogenesis of this condition is not well understood. It is believed that there are complement-fixing IgG antibodies that bind to BPAg2 (also known as *BP180* or *type XVII collagen*) of the hemidesmosome in the basement membrane.[40,41] Most patients with PG have C3 with or without IgG deposition at the basement membrane and circulating anti–basement membrane IgG antibodies that can detected with the appropriate laboratory tests. This activity at the basement membrane leads to the clinical picture of urticaria and bullae. The antibodies produced in the mother occasionally can cross the placenta, leading to a rare transient blistering or papular disease in the infant.

Clinically, PG presents as very pruritic urticarial papules and plaques that evolve into vesicles and bullae in the pregnant female (Figure 31-4). The lesions tend to occur mostly on the trunk (specifically the abdomen), legs, and arms, with extension to the flexure areas. In addition to the cutaneous lesions, patients can have involvement of the mucous membranes, although this is uncommon.[41,42] A study done in Mexico reported six of eight patients with extensive blistering involving the palms and soles.[45] The disease is usually self-limited, but PG is also known to flare during the postpartum period, with subsequent menstrual periods and pregnancies, and with the use of oral contraceptives.[40,41] Thirteen women with PG were studied by Merchaoul and colleagues in Tunisia, North Africa. Most of the patients (75%) developed exacerbation of cutaneous lesions immediately postpartum. Most of the infants born to these mothers were normal, but there was one case of intrauterine fetal death and another of intrauterine fetal growth retardation (IUGR).[43] Garcia-Gonzalez and colleagues found rare complications in their Mexican study, such as IUGR, oligohydramnios, and eclampsia.[45]

PG has been associated with the presence of HLA-DR3 and -DR4. Shornick and colleagues reported two cases of PG in African-American females, both having the typical historical and clinical features of the disease. HLA typing was done on one of the patients and showed a combination of HLA-DR3 and -DR4, although HLA-DR4 is uncommon in American blacks.[44] The authors suggested that the paucity of HLA-DR4 antigen in African-Americans might explain the infrequent occurrence of PG in this population. All eight patients in the Mexican study by Garcia-Gonzalez and colleagues were shown to have the HLA-DR3/DR4 phenotype.[45] Kuwaiti patients with PG were observed to have a predominance of HLA-DR3 and -DQ2 antigens. No predominance of HLA-DR4 antigen was observed in Kuwait.[46]

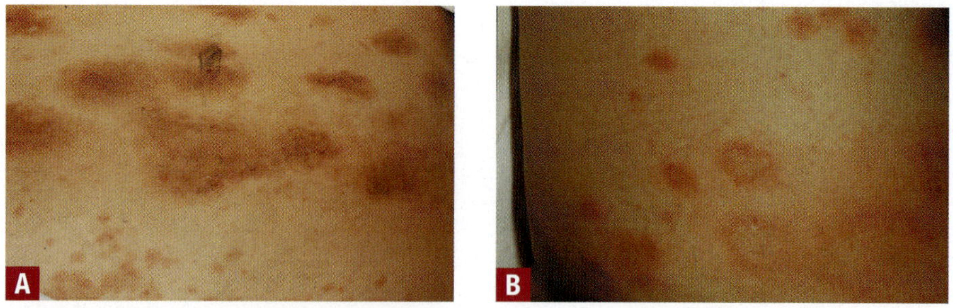

▲ **FIGURE 31-4** *A, B.* Pemphigoid gestationis.

Differential diagnosis for PG includes pemphigus, bullous pemphigoid, and other blistering diseases in pregnancy, such as pruritic urticarial papules and plaques of pregnancy, polymorphic eruption of pregnancy, and impetigo herpetiformis.

A skin biopsy of the urticarial plaques will demonstrate histopathologically a dermal lymphohistiocytic infiltrate with eosinophils, dermal edema, and basal cell necrosis at the dermal papillae.[40] Biopsy of a vesicular lesion will show a subepidermal blister with eosinophils.[41] PG can be diagnosed with a skin biopsy showing the classic histologic feature. DIF performed on skin adjacent to a blister usually shows deposition of C3 (100%) and IgG (25–100%) along the basement membrane. IIF studies shows circulating antibodies in the serum.

Management of these patients is usually undertaken by both an obstetrician and a dermatologist. The treatment of choice for these patients is oral prednisone because other immune-modifying medications may be contraindicated in pregnancy. The dose is adjusted based on disease activity. Addition of pyridoxine, antihistamines, and topical steroids also plays a role in therapy.[4] If disease persists postpartum or flares with menstrual periods or use of oral contraceptives, tetracyclines with nicotinamide, dapsone, plasmapheresis, and steroid-sparing immunosuppressant agents such as azathioprine, methotrexate, cyclophosphamide, and IVIG can be beneficial in some patients.

CHRONIC BULLOUS DISEASE OF CHILDHOOD

Chronic bullous disease of childhood is a rare acquired autoimmune bullous disease with variable clinical presentation. The age of onset is generally between 6 months and 10 years of age. The mean age of onset is during the preschool years.[47] Both cutaneous and mucosal involvement is possible. On physical examination, small vesicles or bullae surround an erythematous to urticarial central base. Lesions typically appear suddenly, usually on the trunk and extremities, with the characteristic "string of pearls" appearance that develops over several weeks. In children, the most common location of the vesicles is on the lower abdomen or genital area. Mucosal lesions may appear on the conjunctivae and in the mouth. The incidence and prevalence of chronic bullous disease of childhood have not been well established.

The disease is best characterized by autoantibodies directed at a 97-kDa component on the extracellular portion of the 180-kDa bullous pemphigoid antigen 2 (BPAg2). Histologically, there is a subepidermal blister with a superficial dermal neutrophilic infiltrate and basal vacuolization. On DIF, linear deposition of IgA and sometimes C3 along the basement membrane will be seen. There is a linear deposition of IgA antibodies along the basement membrane zone principally in the lamina lucida. Dapsone is considered standard therapy for treatment of chronic bullous disease, and it usually results in good control of the disease. Other treatment options for refractory cases are systemic corticosteroids, sulfapyridine, colchicine, and the penicillin family of antibiotics.[48–51] In most cases, spontaneous remission will occur within 2 years of disease onset.

The information pertaining specifically to skin of color on chronic bullous disease of childhood originates primarily from clinical studies performed in Africa and the Middle East. Studies are usually small, and those studies consisting of a mixed population of skin colors are not large enough to draw significant conclusions about differences between the subgroups. A few of the findings were consistent between the studies performed in patients with darker skin compared with those from patients with lighter skin. Physical distribution of lesions remained fairly consistent throughout the studies, with the most severe involvement in the lower trunk and perineum.[52] A slight increased prevalence in females is seen across all skin types.[52] HLA typing revealed an increased incidence in those with HLA-B8, -DR3, and -DQ2 antigens.[48,52,53]

One clinical problem more specific to dark-skinned individuals is G6PD deficiency. The treatment of choice for chronic bullous disease of childhood is dapsone. Sulfapyridine is one of the alternative treatments. Both these medications are contraindicated in persons with G6PD deficiency because of the risk of hemolysis. G6PD deficiency is an X-linked trait that results in increased oxidative stress on erythrocytes with resulting hemolysis.[54] The incidence of G6PD deficiency varies throughout the world, but the highest incidence lies in areas of the world with a high incidence of malaria. It is thought that heterozygotes for the G6PD deficiency mutation have a relative resistance to malaria. The highest prevalence of G6PD deficiency is in Africa, Asia, the Mediterranean, and the Middle East. In African-American males, the prevalence is thought to be 10%. This enzyme deficiency will affect therapy, response to therapy, and most important, side effects to therapy. In patients who are treated with dapsone or sulfapyridine, hemolysis may occur, and patients will need to be treated with alternative therapies. Therefore, most of the research into alternative antimicrobial therapies, including flucloxacillin and oxacillin, has been performed in Africa and the Middle East.[48,51] These semisynthetic, β-lactamase-resistant penicillins have proven to be viable alternatives to the standard therapies with fewer side effects. Additionally, the cost differential may be significant. An analysis of total cost reveals that treatment with a penicillin may be one-quarter to one-fifth that of dapsone or sulfapyridine.[50] This is important from an epidemiologic standpoint, as well as from an economic one. In conclusion, clinical presentation, genotyping, epidemiology, and clinical course are comparable among the spectrum of skin types. However, treatment modalities may differ owing to an increased risk of adverse effects from the commonly used treatments.

REFERENCES

1. Sharma VK. Evaluation of desmoglein enzyme-linked immunosorbent assay (ELISA) in Indian patients with pemphigus vulgaris. *Int J Dermatol* 2006;45:518-522.
2. Harman KE, Gratian MJ, Bhogal BS. A study of desmoglein 1 autoantibodies in pemphigus vulgaris: Racial differences in frequency and the association with a more severe phenotype. *Br J Dermatol* 2000;143: 343-348.
3. Kumar B, Arora S, Kumaran MS. Study of desmoglein 1 and 3 antibody levels in relation to disease severity in Indian patients with pemphigus. *Indian J Dermatol Venereol Leprol* 2006;72:203-206.
4. James WD. Chronic blistering dermatoses, in *Andrew's Diseases of the Skin,* 1oth ed. Philadelphia, Saunders Elsevier, 2006, pp 459-478
5. Aboobaker J, Morar N, Ramdial PK. Pemphigus in South Africa. *Int J Dermatol* 2002;40:115-118.
6. Mahe A, Flageul B, Cisse I. Pemphigus in Mali: A study of 30 cases. *Br J Dermatol* 1996; 134:114-119.
7. Bagheri MM, Alagheband M, Memar OM. Pemphigus foliaceus presenting as eruptive seborrheic keratosis and responding to gold treatment. *J Drugs Dermatol* 2002;1:333-334.
8. Pemphigus Foliaceus, Schwartz MD, 2007, *www.emedicine.com.*
9. Diaz LA. Endemic pemphigus foliaceus (fogo selvagem): II. Current and historic epidemiologic studies. *J Invest Dermatol* 1989;92:4-12.
10. Aoki V. Environmental risk factors in endemic pemphigus foliaceus (fogo selvagem). *J Invest Dermatol Symp Proc* 2004; 9:34-40.
11. Nanda A, Dvorak R, Al-Saeed K. Spectrum of autoimmune bullous diseases in Kuwait. *Int J Dermatol* 2004;43:876-881.
12. Bastuji-Garin S, Souissi R, Blum L. Comparative epidemiology of pemphigus in Tunisia and France: Unusual incidence of pemphigus foliaceus in young Tunisian women. *J Invest Dermatol* 1995;104:302-305.
13. Haouet H, Ben HA, Haouet S. Tunisian pemphigus: Apropos of 70 cases (Experience in the dermatology department of La Rabta Hospital 1974-1992). *Ann Dermatol Venereol* 1996;123:9-11.
14. Adam BA. Bullous diseases in Malaysia: Epidemiology and natural history. *Int J Dermatol* 1992;31:42-45.
15. Kanwar AJ. Pemphigus in North India. *J Cutan Med Surg* 2006; 10:21-25.
16. Adam BA. Bullous diseases: A 7-year survey of experience with 77 patients. *Ann Acad Med Singapore* 1983;12: 19-25.
17. Bastuji-Garin, Turki H, Mokhtar I. Possible correlation of Tunisian pemphigus with traditional cosmetics: A multicenter case-control study. *Am J Epidemiol* 2002;155: 249-256.
18. Brick C. Pemphigus and HLA in Morocco. *Transfus Clin Biol* 2007;14:402-406.
19. Delgado JC, Yunis DE, Bozon MV. MHC class II alleles and haplotypes in patients with pemphigus vulgaris from India. *Tissue Antigens* 1996;48:668-672.
20. Wilson C, Wojnarowska F, Mehra NK. Pemphigus in Oxford, UK, and New Delhi, India: A comparative study of disease characteristics and HLA antigens. *Dermatology* 1994;189:108-110.
21. Glorio R. HLA haplotypes and class II molecular alleles in Argentinian patiensts with pemphigus vulgaris. *J Cutan Med Surg* 2002;6:422-426.
22. Wilson CL, Wojnarowska F, Dean D. IgG subclasses in pemphigus in Indian and UK populations. *Clin Exp Dermatol* 1993; 18:226-230.
23. Zouhair K, el Ouazzani T, Azzouzi S. Herpetic superinfection of pemphigus: 6 cases. *Ann Dermatol Venereol* 1999;126: 699-702.
24. Ogawa H. The incidence of internal malignancies in pemphigus and bullous pemphigoid in Japan. *J Dermatol Sci* 1995; 9:136-141.
25. Tirado-Sanchez A, Leon_Dorantes G. Treatment of pemphigus: An overview in Mexico. *Allegol Immunopathol* 2006;34: 10-16.
26. Rao PN, Lakshmi TS. Pulse therapy and its modifications in pemphigus: A six-year study. *Indian J Dermatol Venereol Leprol* 2003;69: 329-333.
27. Stanley JR. Pemphigus, in Freedberg IM (eds), *Fitzpatrick's Dermatology in General Medicine,* 6th ed. New York, McGraw-Hill, 2003, pp 558-567.
28. Yeh SW, Ahmed B, Sami N. Blistering disorders: Diagnosis and treatment. *Dermatol Ther* 2003;16:214-223.
29. Zillikens D, Rose PA, Balding SD. Tight clustering of extracellular BP180 epitopes recognized by bullous pemphigoid autoantibodies. *J Invest Dermatol* 1997; 109:573-579.
30. Wong SN, Chua SH. Spectrum of subepidermal immunobullous disorders seen at the National Skin Centre, Singapore: A 2-year review. *Br J Dermatol* 2002;147:476-480.
31. Friedman H, Campbell I, Rocha-Alvarez R. Endemic pemphigus foliaceus (fogo selvagem) in native Americans from Brazil. *J Am Acad Dermatol* 1995;32:949-956.
32. Jin P, Shao C, Ye G. Chronic bullous dermatoses in China. *Int J Dermatol* 1993;32: 89-92.
33. Zillikens D, Wever S, Roth A. Incidence of autoimmune subepidermal blistering dermatoses in a region of central Germany. *Arch Dermatol* 1995;131:957-958.
34. Bernard P, Vaillant L, Labeille B. Incidence of autoimmune distribution of subepidermal autoimmune bullous skin disease in three French regions. *Arch Dermatol* 1995; 131:48-52.
35. Mulyowa GK, Jaeger G, Kabakyenga J. Autoimmune subepidermal blistering diseases in Uganda: Correlation of autoantibody class with age of patient. *Int J Dermatol* 2006;45:1047-1052.
36. Capon F, Bharkhada J, Cochrane NR. Evidence of an association between desmoglein 3 haplotypes and pemphigus vulgaris. *Br J Dermatol* 2006; 154:67-71.
37. Nanda A, Al-Saeid K, Al-Sabah H. Clinicoepidemiological features and course of 43 cases of bullous pemphigoid in Kuwait. *Clin Exp Dermatol* 2006;31:339-342.
38. Mulyowa GK, Jaeger G, Sitaru C. Scarring autoimmune bullous disease in a Ugandan patient with autoantibodies to BP180, BO230, and laminin 5. *J Am Acad Dermatol* 2006;54: S43-46.
39. Joly P, Tanasescu S, Wolkenstein P. Lichenoid erythrodermic bullous pemphigoid of the African patient. *J Am Acad Dermatol* 1998;39:691-697.
40. Karz SI. Pemphigoid gestationis (herpes gestationis), in Freedberg IM, et al (eds),

Fitzpatrick's Dermatology in General Medicine, 6th ed. New York, McGraw-Hill, 2003, pp 592-595.
41. Castro LA. Clinical experience in pemphigoid gestationis: Report of 10 cases. *J Am Acad Dermatol* 2006;55:823-838.
42. Mokni M, Fourati M, Karou I. Pemphigoid gestationis: A study of 20 cases. *Ann Dermatol Venereol* 2004;131:953-956.
43. Merchaoui J, Makhlouf T, Sfar R. Obstetrical prognosis of gestational pemphigoid: Study of a series of 13 cases and review of the literature. *J Gynecol Obstet Biol Reprod* 1992;21:963-967.
44. Shornick JK. Herpes gestationis in blacks. *Arch Dermatol* 1984;120:511-513.
45. Garcia-Gonzalez E, Castro-Llamas JBS, Karchmer S. Class II major histocompatibility complex typing across the ethnic barrier in pemphigoid gestationis: A study in Mexicans. *Int J Dermatol* 1999;38:46-51.
46. Nanda A, Al-Saeed K, Dvorak R. Clinicopathological features and HLA tissue typing in pemphigoid gestationis patients in Kuwait. *Clin Exp Dermatol* 2003;28:301-306.
47. Wojnarowska F, Marsden RA, Bhogal B. Chronic bullous disease of childhood, childhood cicatricial pemphigoid, and linear IgA disease of adults. *J Am Acad Dermatol* 1988;19: 792-805.
48. Denguezli M, Ben Nejma B, Nouira R. IgA linear bullous dermatosis in children: A series of 12 Tunisian patients. *Ann Dermatol Venereol* 1994;121:888-892.
49. Banodkar DD, Al-Suwaid AR. Colchicine as a novel therapeutic agent in chronic bullous disease of childhood. *Int J Dermatol* 1997;36: 213-216.
50. Siegfried E, et al. Chronic bullous disease of childhood: Successful treatment with dicloxacillin. *J Am Acad Dermatol* 1998;39: 797-800.
51. Abdulmajeed A, Al-Khawajah M, Al-Sheikh O. Treatment of linear IgA bullous dermatosis of childhood with flucloxacillin. *J Am Acad Dermatol* 2006;54: 652-656.
52. Aboobaker J, Wojnarowska FT, Bhogal B. Chronic bullous dermatosis of childhood: Clinical and immu-nological features seen in African patients. *Clin Exp Dermatol* 1991; 16:160-164.
53. Collier PM, Wojnarowska F, Welsh K. Adult linear IgA disease and chronic bullous disease of childhood: The association with human lymphocyte antigens Cw7, B8, DR3 and tumour necrosis factor influences disease expression. *Br J Dermatol* 1999;141:867-875.
54. Beutler E. G6PD deficiency. *Blood* 1994;84: 3613-3636.

SECTION 4

Hair, Scalp, and Nail Disorders

CHAPTER 32

Acne Keloidalis

A. Paul Kelly

Key Points

- The initial lesions of acne keloidalis (AK) present as a folliculitis and then become keloidal-like papules, many of which coalesce to form one or several plaques.
- AK is problematic for darkly pigmented skin of color patients with coarse, curly hair, usually between puberty and middle age.
- Although the older literature implies that AK only occurs in males, we now know that it can occur in females.
- Therapy can be medical or surgical and/or a combination of both.
- Excision with second-intention healing seems to be the best surgical modality.
- The application of a class I or II topical steroid is the standard medical therapy.

SYNONYMS

- Acne keloidalis nuchae
- Dermatitis papillaris capillitii
- Keloidal folliculitis
- Sycosis nuchae
- Folliculitis keloidis nuchae
- Folliculitis nuchae scleroticans
- Nuchal keloid acne
- Keloid acne
- Folliculitis keloidalis
- Folliculitis barbae traumatica
- Sycosis framboesiformis
- Lichen keloidalis nuchae

Acne keloidalis (AK) refers to the formation of keloidal-like papules and plaques on the occipital scalp and posterior neck almost exclusively in darkly pigmented men with coarse, curly hair who shave.[1] It usually starts after puberty as an acute folliculitis and perifolliculitis that becomes chronic. As the disease progresses, the papules enlarge to form keloidal-like plaques. Also, a scarring alopecia is common in the involved scalp area.

AK was first described by Kaposi in 1869 as *dermatitis papillaris capillitii,* one of the older synonyms for AK.[2] This name was based on the anatomic location of AK; the capillitium is the suboccipital portion of the skin. Three years later, Bazin named the disorder *acne keloidalis,* a designation that still prevails today.[3]

The older literature implies that AK only occurs in males, but we now know that it can occur in females at a ratio of approximately 20:1. Although AK is found predominately in Negroid or darkly pigmented men with coarse, curly hair, the next most common group with AK is Hispanics followed by Asians, while Caucasians develop it least often.[4]

ETIOLOGY AND PATHOGENESIS

The exact cause of AK is unknown or speculative. It is not acne vulgaris, nor is it a true keloid. The AK lesions do not have comedones, as do acne lesions. Acute folliculitis and perifolliculitis usually precede AK. This is followed by chronic folliculitis and then AK. Systemic antibiotics may cure the folliculitis but do not soften or clear the existing keloid-like lesions. AK usually responds to systemic steroid therapy.

George and colleagues found that 15% of their patients had a family history of AK.[5] As in pseudofolliculitis barbae (PFB), shaving short, tightly curled hair, common among darkly pigmented men, and having the new hair growth curve back to penetrate the skin may be the precipitating factor. Other incriminating factors are continuous irritation from shirt collars, chronic low-grade folliculitis, and an autoimmune process.

Goethe and Berger presented histologic evidence that AK is a transepithelial elimination disorder similar to perforating folliculitis,[6] whereas Sperling and colleagues found histologic evidence that AK is a form of scarring alopecia.[7] Their findings also negated an association between PFB and AK.

Burkhart and Burkhart[8] reported that AK represents a variant form of lichen simplex chronicus with fibrotic keloidal scarring rather than acne mechanica, as proposed by Kanable and colleagues.[9] George and colleagues[5] suggested that AK is associated with the male gender seborrheic constitution, early reproduction years, and increased fasting blood testosterone concentrations. Increased mast cell density and dilatation of the dermal capillaries are features that may predispose AK to form on the vascular prominent occipital location.

The use of antiepileptic drugs, causing an increased number of mast cells in the occipital region, and the use of cyclosporine for renal transplant patients both have been cited as causes of AK. Azurdia and colleagues reported on three white men who developed AK lesions on the occipital scalp and nuchal neck after treatment with cyclosporine following organ transplantation.[10] Also, AK-like lesions have been reported on the scalp of an epileptic patient on diphenylhydantoin and carbamazepine. The lesions resolved when the drugs were discontinued.[11]

All these probable AK precipitating factors indicate that the etiology of AK is multifactorial.

PATHOLOGY

Histologically, there are follicular and perifollicular inflammations that change in composition during evolution of the lesions. Initially, the infiltrate is composed of neutrophils and lymphocytes. Fox[12] reported in 1942 that mast cells were predominant in AK. This is significant because mast cells are also increased in keloids and other fibrosing disorders. Mast cells are not increased in darkly pigmented men with coarse, curly hair unless they have fibrotic disease. The folliculitis begins at the upper third of the hair follicle. Sebaceous glands are markedly diminished or absent in all stages of folliculitis. In more advanced lesions, hair follicles are disrupted, and broken hair fragments are surrounded by granulomatous inflammation. Dermal fibrosis and scars are seen as this stage and resemble the collagen fibers in scar tissue rather than those in true keloids.[3]

One follicle can show several stages of inflammation at a given point in time. The lower portion of the follicle, including the matrix, is usually spared until later in the disease process. The shaft that guides the hairs to the surface is lost in the inflammatory process, and these hair fragments proliferate beneath fibrotic tissue and are surrounded by a foreign-body response, producing the tufted hairs seen late in the disease process. Tufted hair folliculitis or polytrichia hairs are characterized by several to 20 or more hairs emerging from a single follicular opening or from large follicular pustules.[6] These hairs have separate follicles in the lower dermis, but the inflammation and scar tissue higher in the dermis seem to cause the amalgamation of hairs into one follicle (Figure 32-1).

Laboratory Studies

Other than histopathology, there are no specific tests for AK. Bacterial cultures should be taken intermittently for any pustular or draining lesions. If pathogens are found, the patient should be treated with the appropriate antibiotics. Herzberg and colleagues[13] found that the follicular lymphocyte infiltrate contained mixed B- and T-cell populations and that the plasma cell immunoglobulins were of a polyclonal nature.

CLINICLAL FINDINGS

AK begins after puberty as firm, dome-shaped papules 2 to 4 mm in diameter on the nape of the neck or the occipital scalp (Figures 32-2 through 32-4). Pustules also may be present in the same areas, but they are usually short-lived because the tops are sometimes scratched off as a result of pruritus of the involved area, or they are traumatized when the hair is combed or brushed. In contradistinction to acne, comedones are not present.

As the disease progresses, more papules may appear, and those already present may enlarge. Some coalesce to form keloid-like plaques, which are usually arranged in a horizontal band-like lesion of the occipital scalp. The plaques are most often only a few centimeters in diameter but sometimes cover most of the occipital scalp (Figure 32-5). Large lesions are usually hairless, and their upper border is often fringed with tufted hairs appearing like doll's hair, as in Figure 32-1. Scarring alopecia and subcutaneous abscesses with draining sinuses also may be present.

The early papular lesions are usually asymptomatic, but the pustular ones are often puritic and may be painful. Also, the larger plaques are usually more painful than the smaller ones. Chronic lesions with abscesses and sinuses may emit an odorous drainage. Even though many lesions are asymptomatic, their appearance is often a cause of tremendous cosmetic concern to the patient.

One explanation provided by Herzberg and colleagues is based on extensive transverse microscopy–histochemistry and electron microscopic analysis. The researchers described the hypothetical sequence of inflammatory events that takes place in AK. The acute inflammation, whether it begins in the sebaceous gland or elsewhere in the region of the deep infundibular or isthmus levels, is a cause or the result of a weakened follicular wall at these levels. This enables the release of hair shafts into the surrounding dermis. The "foreign" hairs incite further acute and chronic granulomatous inflammation. The granulomatous inflammation manifests clinically as a papular lesion. Fibroblasts lay down collagen, and scars form in the region of inflammation. Distortion and occlusion of the follicular lumen by fibrosis leads to hair retention in the inferior follicle and further smoldering granulomatous inflammation and scarring. The scar and granulomatous inflammation manifest clinically as scars and plaques.[13]

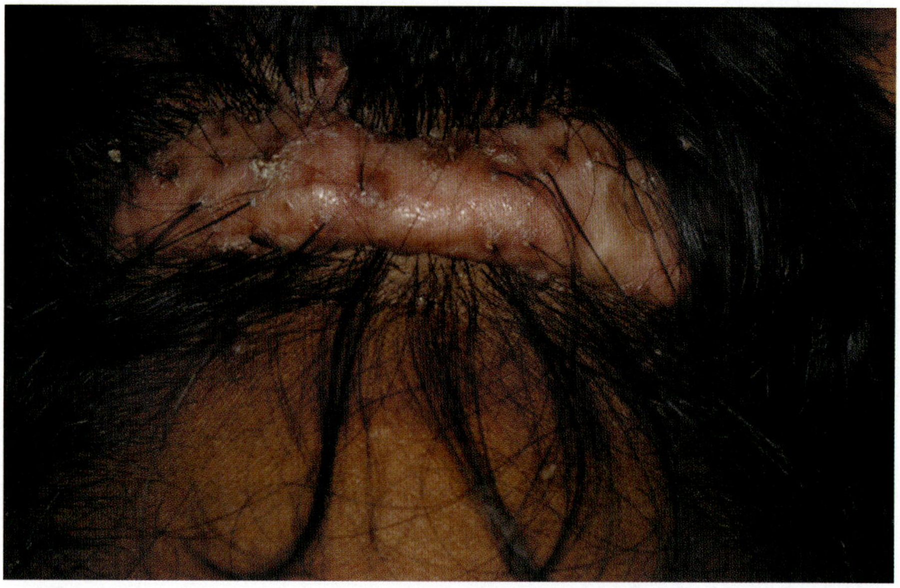

▲ **FIGURE 32-1** A large keloidal hairless plaque with tufted hairs producing doll-like hair on the upper border.

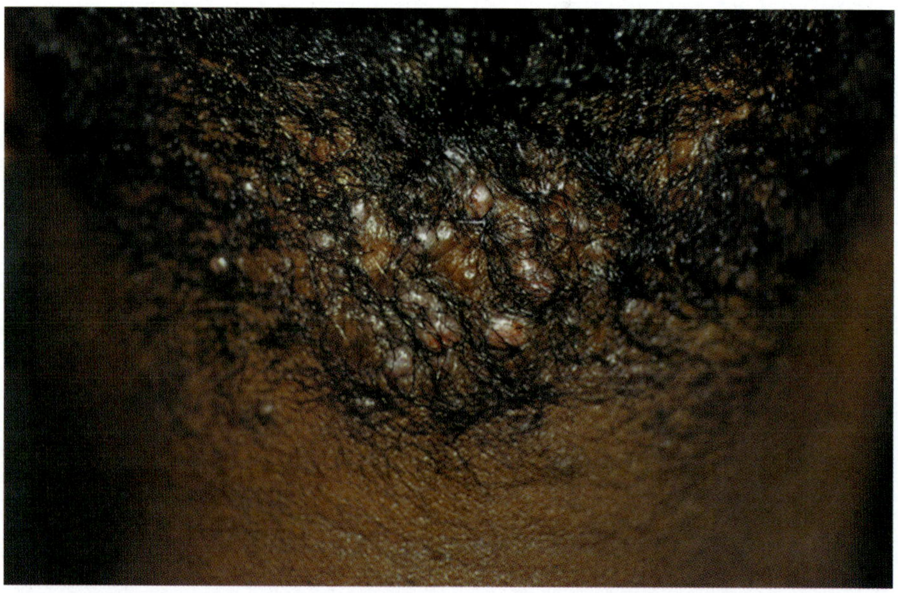

▲ **FIGURE 32-2** All stages of acne keloidalis pustules, dome-shaped papules, and plaques.

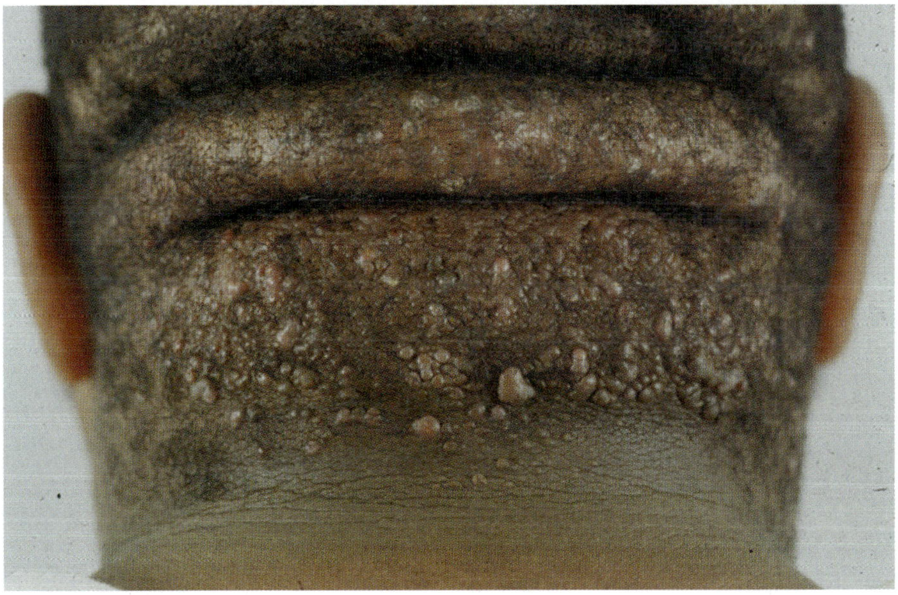

▲ **FIGURE 32-3** Numerous papular lesions on the nucal areas of a darkly pigmented man with coarse, curly hair.

Interestingly, little can be added to Adamson's clinical description of AK written in 1914:

> The eruption occurs on the back of the neck in the form of a raised transverse band at the lower margin of the hairy scalp. The band is usually dusky red in color, smooth and firm to the touch in fact, of keloidal aspect and consistence. It is hairless except at its upper margin, which is abrupt, broken in nodules and fringed with hair tufts, like aigrettes, or the bunches of bristles in a brush. There may be pustules or crusted nodules here and there along the upper border. The lower margin slopes gradually to the normal skin. Usually there are no comedomes or follicular pustules of acne when the patient comes under observation, and there may or may not be a history of acne of the face of youth. Often the patient complains of itching at the site of eruption.[14]

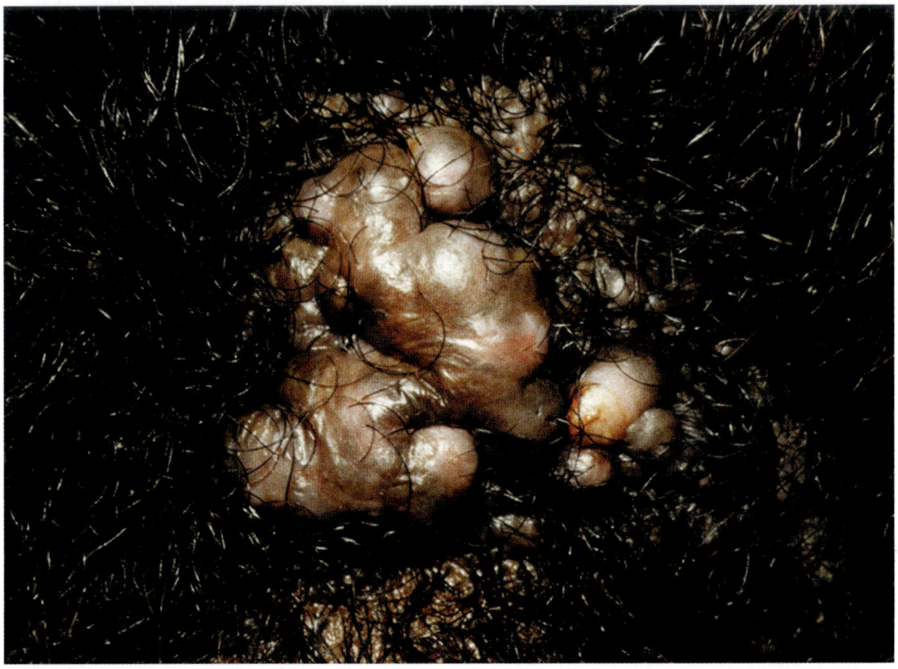

▲ **FIGURE 32-4** Small to large dome-shaped keloid nodules on the posterior occipital area.

DIFFERENTIAL DIAGNOSIS

A diagnosis of AK can be made from the following conditions:

- Keloids-like plaques
- Scarring alopecia
- Acute folliculitis infection
- Perifolliculitis
- Chronic folliculitis and perifolliculitis

Because AK presents a classic picture, in most cases there is no need for a differential diagnosis, but perifolliculitis capitis abscedens et suffodiens, folliculitis, sarcoidosis, and nevus sebaceus of Jadassohn must be ruled out.

COMPLICATIONS

While AK is a medically benign dermatosis, it also can be socially or psychologically debilitating, as for the patient in Figure 32-5. In addition, patients with AK can develop squamous cell carcinoma secondary to radiation therapy.

CLINICAL COURSE AND PROGNOSIS

The course of the disease is usually chronic and often leads to hair follicle destruction and polytrychoid hairs (3–20 hairs coming out of one follicle).[15] The only reported case of familial AK involved a father and all three of his sons, but not his two daughters.[16] It is rare for AK to develop before adolescence or after age 50. Darkly pigmented men with coarse, curly hair seem to have an earlier age of onset of AK, and if the lesions are treated early enough, the prognosis is good for almost complete recovery.

PREVENTION

Patients at risk for developing AK should be made aware that their actions can cause its onset. They should not get their occipital hairline edged with a razor or clippers and avoid tight-fitting shirts, hats, or other clothing that continuously rubs the posterior hairline. However, once the lesions appear, the sooner therapy is initiated, the smaller is the chance of developing large lesions.

TREATMENT

Be aware that certain medications have been associated with the development of AK, especially cyclosporine. Unfortunately, there is no one thera-

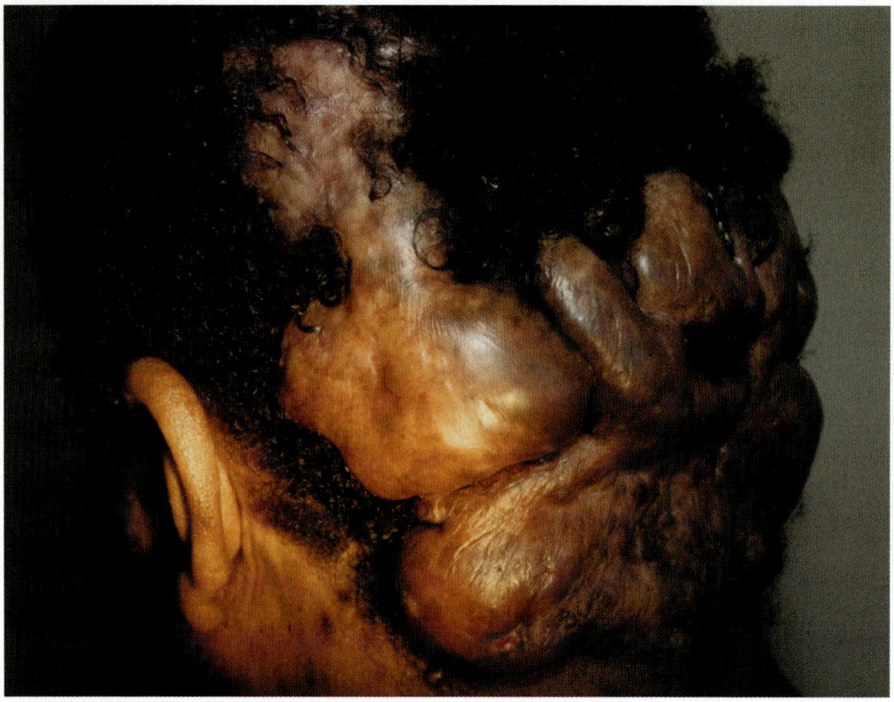

▲ **FIGURE 32-5** A darkly pigmented man with coarse, curly hair with several large keloid-like lesions covering most of the occipital scalp.

peutic modality that cures AK except systemic corticosteroids, which stop the lesional activity and cause a partial or complete regression of any AK lesions. However, when systemic corticosteroids are discontinued, the lesions return in weeks to months, and long-term corticosteroid therapy may lead to many complications, especially adrenal suppression and brittle bones.

Topical Therapy

Topical therapy is sometimes effective in attenuating AK:

- A class I or II corticosteroid gel (e.g., Diprolene or Topicort) or clobetasol foam (Olux) twice a day[17]
- A corticosteroid gel combined with retinoic acid gel applied every night to relieve the symptoms and help flatten existing lesions
- For pustules and other evidence of infection, topical clindamycin (CleocinT) or mupirocin ointment applied on a twice-daily basis until the pustules abate and the inflammation subsides
- Imiquimod (Aldara) applied every day for 5 days, then 2 days off, for 8 weeks

Minor Invasive Therapeutic Techniques

These techniques often attenuate the process but usually are not curative:

- *Injecting corticosteroids into the lesions*
  - Inject a mixture of usually one-half 10 mg/mL triamcinolone acetonide and one-half 40 mg/mL at 3-week intervals using an insulin syringe with a 29-gauge needle.
  - *Note:* Before starting, warn the patient that he or she may develop hypopigmentation in the injection site that may last for 12–18 months.
- *Removing papules*
  - Remove each papule with a hair transplant punch, leaving the postoperative site to close by second-intention healing or close with sutures.
  - *Note:* The punch should extend deep, past the deepest layer of the hair follicle, into the subcutaneous tissue. Superficial removal has a much higher incidence of recurrence.
- *Laser therapy*
  - Laser therapy (carbon dioxide or Nd:YAG) has proven successful in some patients.
  - Preliminary studies show that long-pulse diode laser therapy or long-pulse Nd:YAG lasers may be successful in removing trapped hairs, which then may attenuate the nidus of AK.
- *Cryotherapy*
  - Cryotherapy is helpful for some patients.
  - The AK lesions are frozen for 20+ seconds, allowed to thaw, and then frozen again for 20+ seconds.
  - The morbidity (discomfort and drainage) is greater than with other modalities.
  - When the freeze-thaw time is greater than 25 seconds, the melonocytes are destroyed, and the treated areas often become hypopigmented and may remain so for 12–18 months.

Surgical Removal of Large Lesions

Large linear lesions up to 1 cm in diameter can be excised and closed using a horizontal ellipse with 4-0 sutures. Often the postoperative site may later splay to the diameter of the initial excision, so it is advisable to close the operative site without flexing the posterior neck. When it is necessary to flex the neck to close the excisional defect, the patient will spend a week or more looking upward. Under such tension, the resulting scar splays, often to the size of the amount of area removed and frequently creating an area of alopecia as large as the initial defect. Gloster recommends treating extremely large lesions with multiple-stage excisions.[18]

Procedures for Removal of Larger Lesions

For large lesions that do not respond to medical treatment or minor surgical intervention, the area of AK can be excised to the fascia or to the deep subcutaneous tissue and left to heal secondarily.[19] The technique is as follows:

- For optimal healing, excise a horizontal ellipse of the posterior scalp that includes the posterior hairline and extends to the muscle facia or deep subcutaneous tissue (Figures 32-6 and 32-7).
- Tie off or coagulate all bleeders after excision, and then apply pressure to the postoperative site from 10–15 minutes and check for bleeding again.
- Once the oozing has stopped, apply a topical antibiotic ointment (e.g., mupirocin or Neosporin) twice a day after cleaning the wound with saline or alcohol.
- Instruct the patient to clean the postoperative site twice a day once the dressing is removed.
- *Important:* Do not inject corticosteroids until complete wound healing

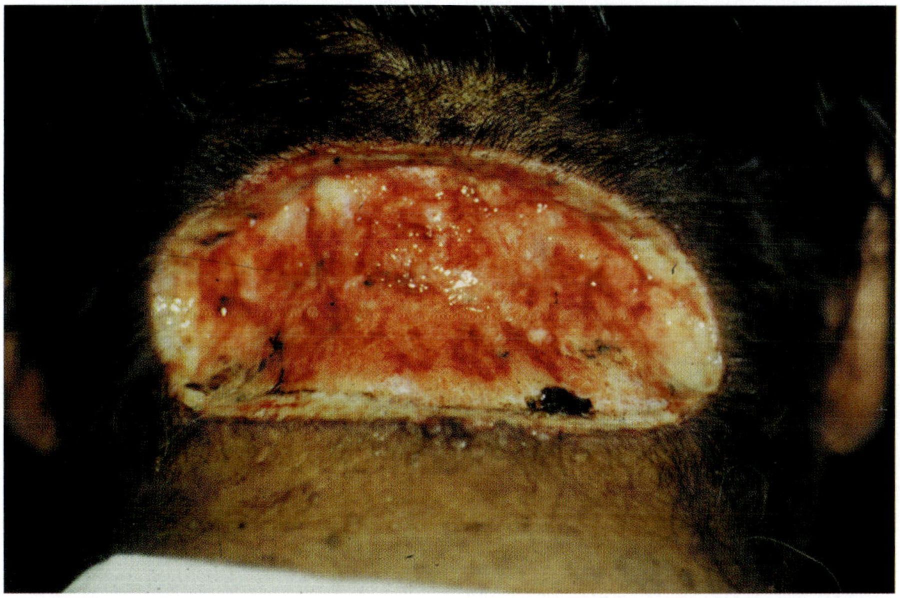

▲ **FIGURE 32-6** A Native American man 5 days after excision and start of second-intention healing. This case shows that people with straight hair also can develop AK.

because it prevents further wound contraction.

- There are poor cosmetic results when a nonhorizontal elliptic excision is used (Figures 32-8 and 32-9) in the following manner: (1) the excision extends above the occipital notch, (2) the lower border of the excision is above the posterior hairline, and (3) intralesional steroids are used prior to the wound becoming healed.

POSTOPERATIVE CONSIDERATIONS

- The postoperative site usually heals in 8–12 weeks.
- Once it is healed, apply retinoic acid–corticosteroid gel preparation every night.

  Note: Excision with grafting is not usually a viable option because it may result in an atrophic non-hair-bearing area.

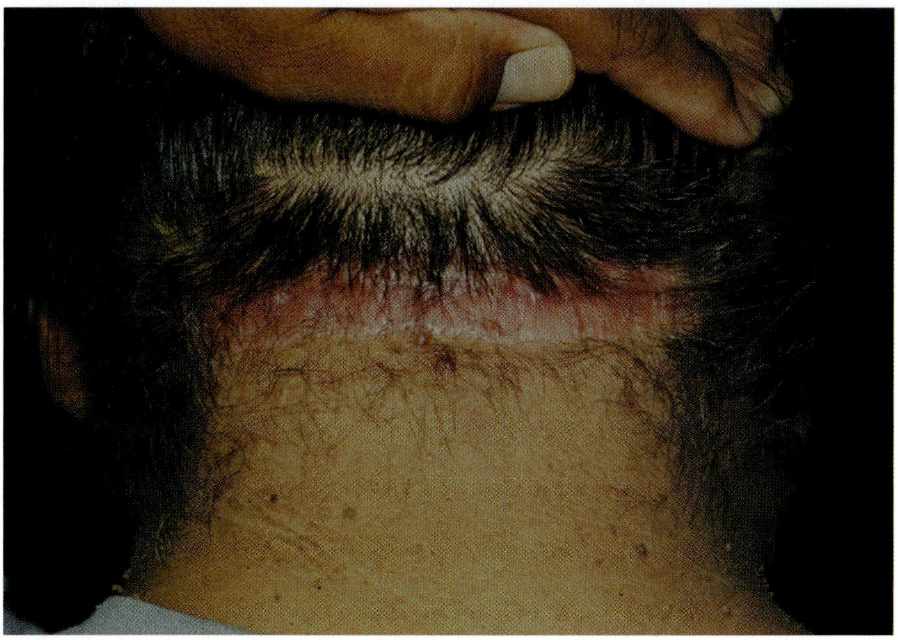

▲ **FIGURE 32-7** One month after second-intention healing of the man in Figure 32-6.

PATIENT PREPARATION FOR THE SURGERY

- Before surgery, tell the patient and his or her caretaker to clean the postoperative site twice a day with alcohol or saline and then to apply an antibiotic ointment.
- Show the patient and caretaker photographs of the stages of healing to help them understand process.
- Explain the level of pain to expect for few days, which acetaminophen is usually sufficient to relieve.
- Tell the patient to immediately start after surgery a 10-day course of a broad-spectrum antibiotic (e.g., erythromycin or cephalosporin) or tetracycline.

CONCLUSION (Table 32-1)

Although the causes of AK are still uncertain, its victims are mainly males. There is help for patients through topical therapy, minor invasive techniques, including some of the recently reported laser therapy and excision. With second intention healing, the postoperative site usually heals completely in 3 months. Second-intention healing gives good to excellent cosmetic results if the lesion is removed with a horizontal elliptic

TABLE 32-1
Overview of Acne Keloidalis

First reported by Kaposi in 1869

Most common synonyms
- Acne keloidalis nuchae
- Folliculitis keloidalis
- Acne keloid

Etiology and pathogenesis
- Found mainly in darkly pigmented men with course, curly hair
- Occurs after puberty or before age 50
- Starts as a chronic folliculitis of the posterior scalp and neck
- Probably related to close shaving & irritation from tight shirt collars or caps

Differential diagnosis
- Folliculitis
- Acne vulgaris
- Keloid
- Nevus sebaceous

Treatment
- Intralesional corticosteroids
- Liquid nitrogen
- Laser therapy
- Excise with secondary-intention closure

Complications
- Once scarring occurs, the skin does not return to normal

logical features of acne keloidalis in a black population. *Int J Dermatol* 1993;32: 714-716.
6. Goethe DK, Berger TG. Acne keloidalis nuchae: A transepithelial elimination disorder. *Int J Dermatol* 1987;26:442-444.
7. Sperling LC, Homoky C, Pratt L, Sau P. Acne keloidalis is a form of primary scarring alopecia. *Arch Dermatol* 2000;136: 479-484.
8. Burkhart CG, Burkhart C. Acne keloidalis is lichen simplex chronicus with fibrotic keloidal scarring. *J Am Acad Dermatol* 1998;39:661.
9. Knable AL, Hanke CW, Gonin R. Prevalence of acne keloidalis nuchae in football players. *J Am Acad Dermatol* 1997; 37:570-574.
10. Azurdia RM, Graham RM, Weismann K, et al. Acne keloidalis in Caucasian patients on cyclosporine following organ transplantation. *Br J Dermatol* 2000;143: 465-467.
11. Malberbe WDF. Dermatome dermaplanning and sycosis nuchae excision. *Clin Plast Surg* 1977;4:289-296.
12. Fox H. Folliculitis keloidalis "a better term than dermatitis papillaris capilliti." *Arch Dermatol Syphilol* 1942;55:112-113.
13. Herzberg AJ, Dinehart SM, Kerns BJ, Pollack SV. Acne keloidalis: Transverse microscopy immunohistochemistry and electron microscopy. *Am J Dermatopathol* 1990;12:109-121.
14. Adamson HG. Dermatitis papillaris capillitti (Kaposi): Acne keloid. *Br J Dermatol* 1914;26:69-83.
15. Luz Ramos M, Munoz Perez MA, Pons A, et al. Acne keloidalis and tufted hair folliculitis. *Dermatology* 1997;194: 71-73.
16. D'Souza P, Iyer VK, Ramam M. Familial acne keloidalis. *Acta Dermatol Venerol* 1998;78:382.
17. Callender VD, Young CM, Haverstock CL, et al. An open label study of clobetasol propionate 0.05% and betamethasone volerate 0.1% foams in the treatment of mild to moderate acen keloidalis. *Cutis* 2005;75:317-321.
18. Gloster HM. The surgical management of extensive cases of acne deloidalis nuchea. *Arch Dermatol* 2000;136:1376-1379.
19. Glenn MJ, Bennett RG, Kelly AP. Acne keloidalis nuchas: Treatment with excision and second-intention healing. *J Am Acad Dermatol* 1995;33:243-246.

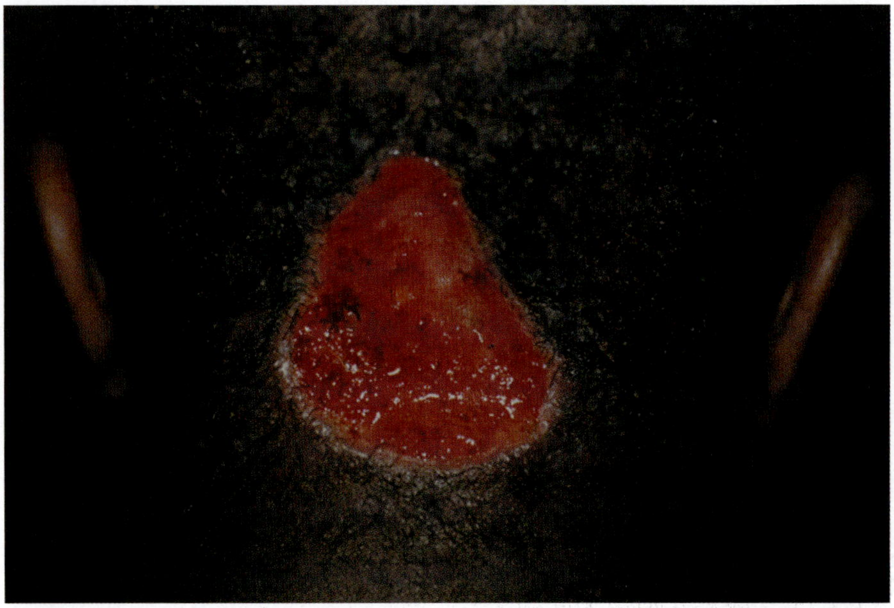

▲ **FIGURE 32-8** After excision of an acne keloidalis lesion that was done in a nonelliptical fashion above the posterior hairline and not below the hair follicles.

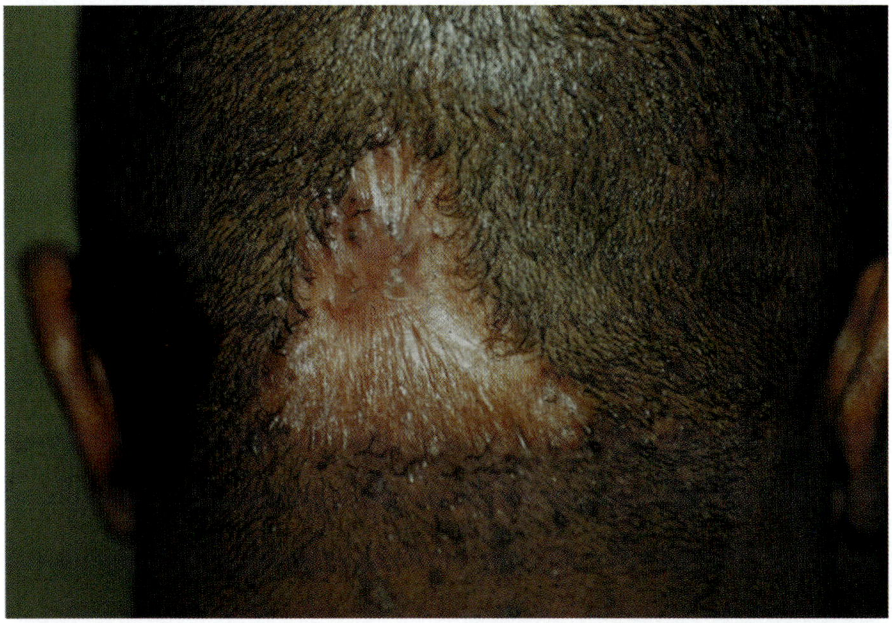

▲ **FIGURE 32-9** Poor healing in the patient in Figure 32-8 owing to direction, depth, and excision above the hairline.

excision that is below the hair follicles, and the posterior hairline is removed in the horizontal elliptic excision.

REFERENCES

1. Kelly AP. Acne keloidalis nuchae. *E-medicine Journal* 2000;2, *www.emedicine.com/derm/topoic558.htm.*
2. Kaposi M. Ueber die sogennante framboesia und mehrere andere arten von papillaren neubildungen der haut. *Arch Dermatol Syphilol* 1869;1:382-423.
3. Cosman B, Wolff M. Acne keloidalis. *Plast Reconstr Surg* 1972;50:25-30.
4. Dinehart SM, Tanner L, Mallory SB, Herzberg AJ. Acne keloidalis in women. *Cutis* 1989;44:250-258.
5. George AO, Akanji AO, Nduka EV, et al. Chemical, biochemical and morpho-

CHAPTER 33

Pseudofolliculitis Barbae

A. Paul Kelly

Key Points

- Pseudofolliculitis barbae (PFB) is a common dermatologic disorder of the hair follicles affecting people with skin of color who shave.
- Darkly pigmented men with coarse, tightly curled hair are especially affected by PFB.
- The primary lesions of PFB are papules and pustules in the beard area that cause cosmetic disfigurement: scarring, postinflammatory hyperpigmentation, secondary infection, and keloid formation.
- Chronic PFB of the shaved areas may produce fine linear depressed scars or so-called grooves.
- The anterior neck, submandibular chin, and lower jaw are the next most common areas for PFB.
- Therapy for PFB with over-the-counter depilatories and/or specific shaving techniques has been used with success, as have topical combination creams.
- Hair-removal lasers and electrolysis can be used for the treatment of PFB, but more study of their effectiveness is needed.

SYNONYMS

- Shave bumps
- Razor bumps
- Barber's bumps
- Barber's itch
- Ingrown hairs
- Folliculitis
- Folliculitis barbae traumatica
- Sycosis barbae
- Pili incarnatii
- Chronic scarring pseudofolliculitis of the Negro beard

Pseudofolliculitis barbae (PFB) is a common inflammatory skin problem of up to 60% of people of color with coarse, tightly curled hair who shave close to the skin[1] (Figure 33-1). It can occur in any race and in either sex. The pubic area (Figure 33-2), scalp, and legs also may develop PFB if they are shaved often.

Strauss and Kligman coined the term *pseudofolliculitis barbae* in 1956.[2] PFB is the bane of existence for affected men, especially those in the military, other law enforcement, or occupations that require workers to be clean shaven.

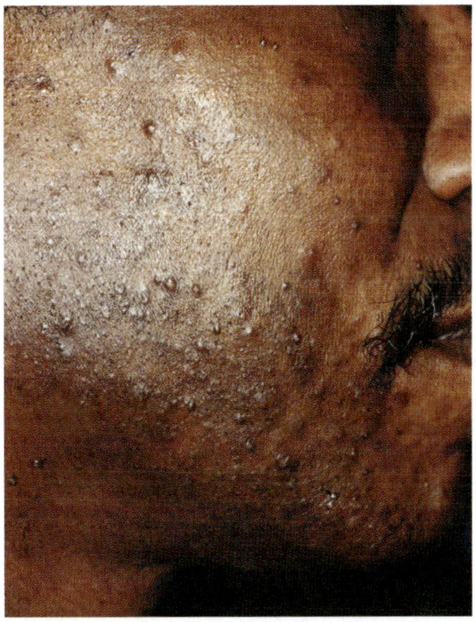

▲ **FIGURE 33-1** Moderate PFB (more than a dozen but less than 100 papules and pustules) of the right cheek and chin of a darkly pigmented man.

EPIDEMIOLOGY AND PATHOGENESIS

The incidence of PFB ranges from approximately 45–85% of the African-American male population. However, PFB can occur in any race and in either sex regardless of whether the person has dark pigmentation or not.

The epidemiology of PFB involves the hair curving as it exits the follicle and penetrating the skin as it grows, causing inflammation (Figure 33-3). Papules with hairs in the center become infected. Complications from chronic PFB may result in hypertrophic scars (Figures 33-4 and 33-5) and keloids (Figures 33-6 and 33-7). On occasion, cutaneous sarcoidosis may develop within the scarred areas.

Tightly curled hair is usually cut at an oblique angle, creating a sharp tip at the distal end that enables the hair to penetrate the skin 1–2 mm from where it exits the follicle. Once the hair penetrates the dermis, an inflammatory reaction ensues. Hair growth usually continues into the dermis, reaching a depth of 2–3 mm. In the dermis it produces an even greater inflammatory reaction, manifested by pustules and papules. The hair reaches the length of 10 mm after a growth period of up to 6 weeks. At this point, a spring action occurs that pulls out the embedded tip. Cutting the hair against the grain and pulling the skin taunt cause transfollicular penetration. When the skin tension is released, the hair retracts below the skin surface. Inflammatory papules develop when the curving hair tips penetrate the hair follicle or the surrounding epidermis.

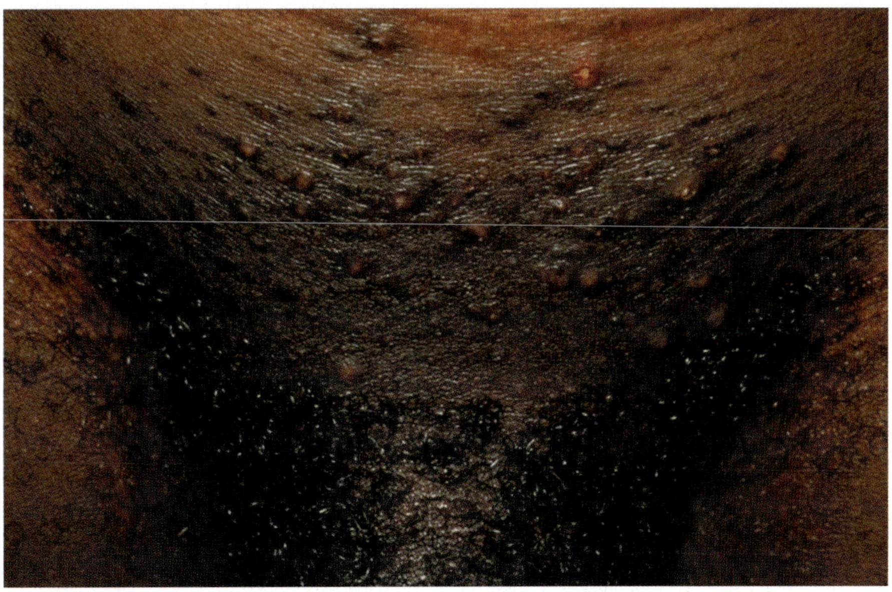

▲ **FIGURE 33-2** A darkly pigmented man with folliculitis secondary to shaving his suprapubic area.

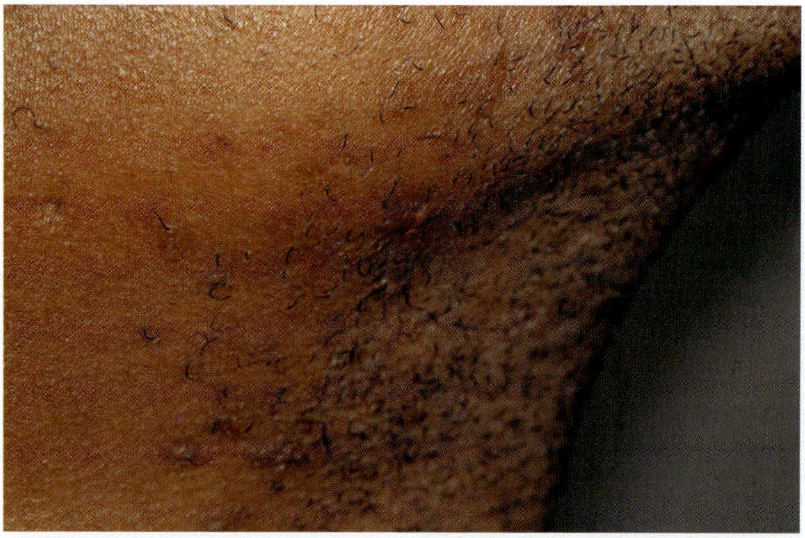

▲ **FIGURE 33-3** A darkly pigmented man with course, tightly curled hair and mild PFB (fewer than a dozen papules) of the right anterior neck and cheek. Note the loop hairs that penetrate the dermis.

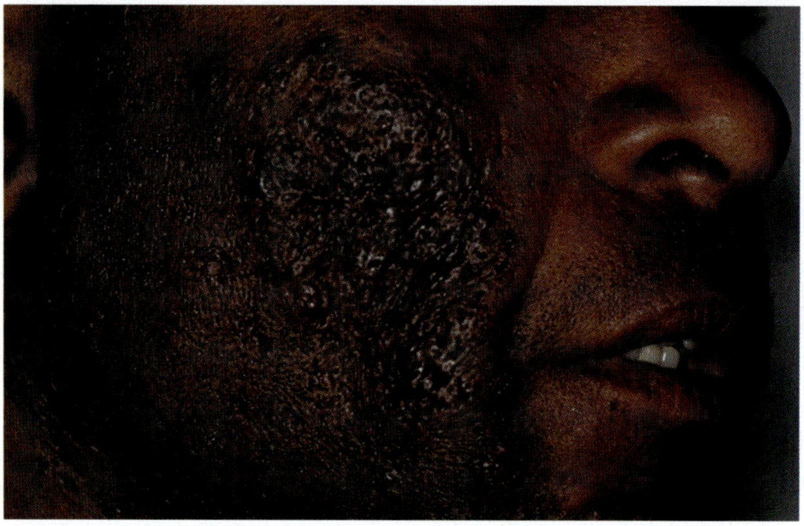

▲ **FIGURE 33-4** PFB of a darkly pigmented man with both moderate PFB in right lateral cheek and scarring on the right medial cheek.

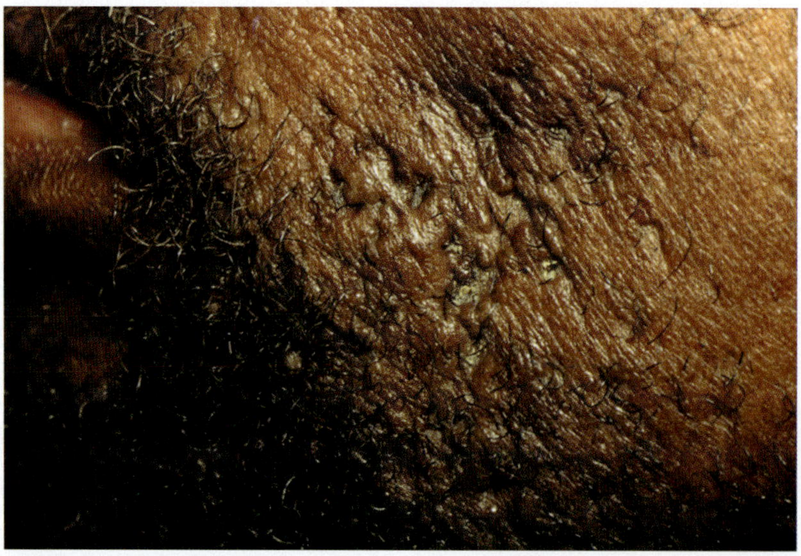

▲ **FIGURE 33-5** A darkly pigmented man with scarring of the left cheek secondary to chronic PFB that he has had for more than 20 years.

CLINICAL FINDINGS

Dermatologists agree that a clinical diagnosis of PFB is not difficult to make.[3] Clinically, PFB lesions are firm, flesh-colored, erythematous or hyperpigmented papules. Pustles and papulopustules are secondary bacterial infections. Chronic PFB may produce grooves (Figure 33-8), preventing the removal of hairs by standard shaving techniques. Chronic lesions may cause postinflammatory hyperpigmentation, although a few have hypopigmentation in the areas of involvement (Figure 33-9). I find that the severity of PFB ranges from mild (less than a dozen papules or pustules) to severe (more than 100 papules or pustules)[4] (Figure 33-10). Perry and colleagues reported that the most common site of involvement for men was the neck and for women the chin[5] (Figures 33-11 and 33-12).

DIFFERENTIAL DIAGNOSIS

- Acne vulgaris
- True folliculitis
- Traumatic folliculitis
- Tinea barbae
- Sarcoidal papules
- Keloids
- Hypotrophic scars

Specifically, in contrast to acne, PFB has no comedones. Also, acne is common on non-hair-bearing, nonshaved areas, unlike PFB. True folliculitis pustules will have a positive bacterial culture, whereas only secondarily-infected PFB lesions will. Traumatic folliculitis, also caused by shaving too closely, presents inflammation of the follicle without evidence of infection and follicular penetration. Lesions of PFB are isolated, whereas those of tinea barbae are confluent and often unilateral. And while sycosis barbae papules may resemble PFB, Halder noted that shaving improves the condition but makes PFB worse.[6] More clinical studies, especially with laser therapy[3] (see Chapter 73), are needed to determine the etiology and best treatment of PFB.

COMPLICATIONS

- Scarring
- Hyperpigmentation
- Hypopigmentation
- Hypotrophic scars
- Keloids
- Sarcoidosis

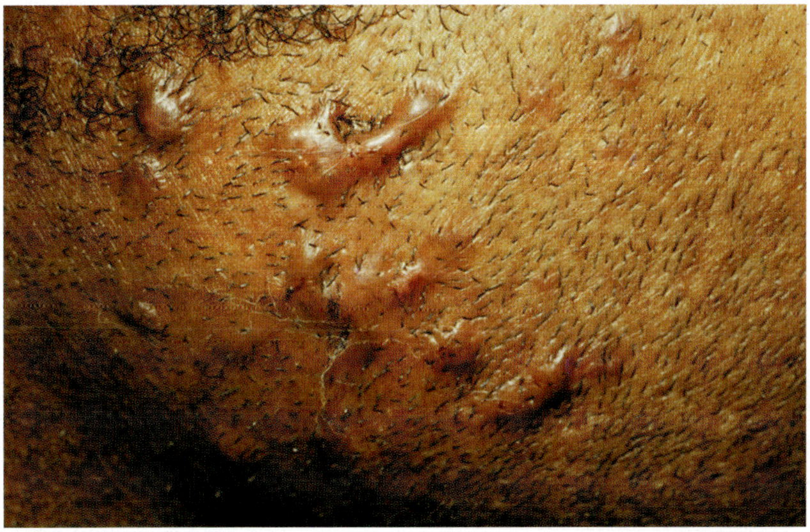

▲ **FIGURE 33-6** Small keloids secondary to PFB in a man with skin of color.

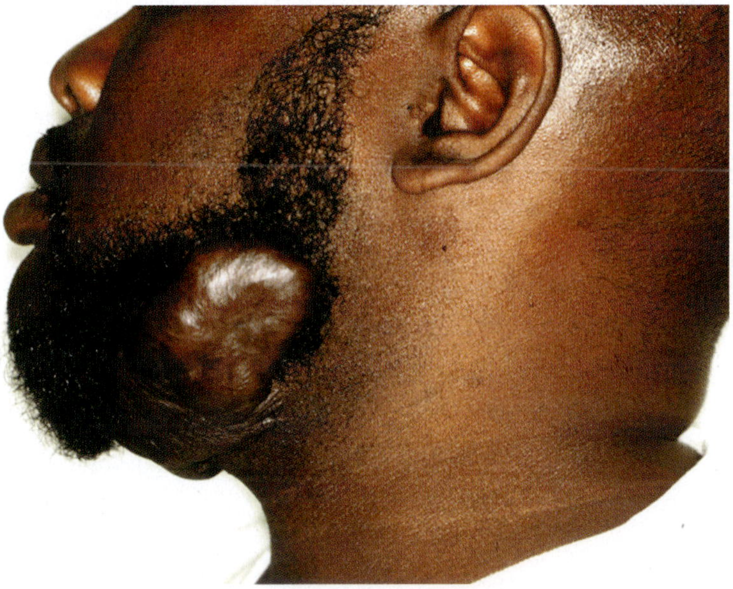

▲ **FIGURE 33-7** A large keloid secondary to PFB on a darkly pigmented man's left cheek and submental area.

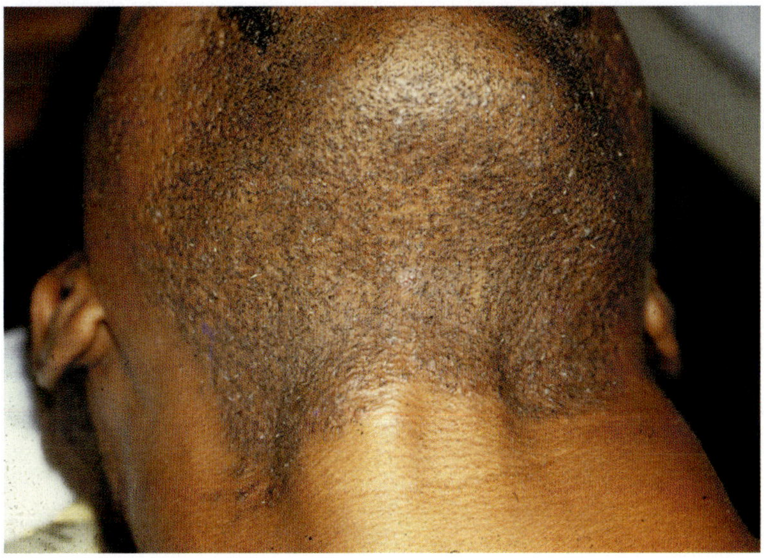

▲ **FIGURE 33-8** Chronic PFB of the anterior neck and chin in a darkly pigmented man. Grooving is present in the submental and anterior neck areas.

CLINICAL COURSE AND PROGNOSIS

There is not a straight trajectory for a prognosis and clinical course for PFB. People of color who have coarse, tightly curled hair and who shave have a greater susceptibility and probability that the disease will worsen. Treatment plans, discussed later, are not failsafe. The prognosis is not good unless the patient either stops shaving or has begun treatment early enough to stop the progression of PFB. The only 100% effective preventive measure is to discontinue shaving, which is not an alternative for many patients.

TREATMENT

Before initiating therapy, counsel patients on the cause of PFB, warning that the only complete cures are cessation of shaving or depilation.[7] However, if they must shave, instruct them not to pull the skin taut and shave only with the grain of the hair. Make sure that the patient understands that the purpose of therapy is to control, not cure, PFB.

Electrolysis is a somewhat tedious, long-term procedure. In darkly pigmented patients with curved hair follicles, the standard electrolysis needle often penetrates the follicle before reaching and destroying the hair bulb. This may set up a nidus for transfollicular penetration. Wax depilation and tweezing also may cause the same postinflammatory hyperpigmentation and mild scarring, especially in darkly pigmented patients.

Epilation is another effective modality.

Laser therapy also has proved effective, though controversial. Kauvar[8] claimed that more than 50% of darkly pigmented patients treated with a diode laser improved. Other researchers[9] have reported a significant decrease in hair growth with long-pulsed diode laser treatment without signs of epidermal damage. Weaver[10] reported that the long-pulse neodymium:yttrium-aluminum-garnet (Nd:YAG) laser with continuous-contact cooling was a safe and effective means of treatment for PFB in both men and women with darker skin. Because the long-pulsed Nd:YAG laser is more painful, the patient may need a topical anesthetic before therapy. The 810-diode laser seems better for lighter skin and the Nd:YAG laser 1064 for the more darkly pigmented. Whatever type of laser is used, dyspigmentation, scarring, crusting, and blistering still may develop.

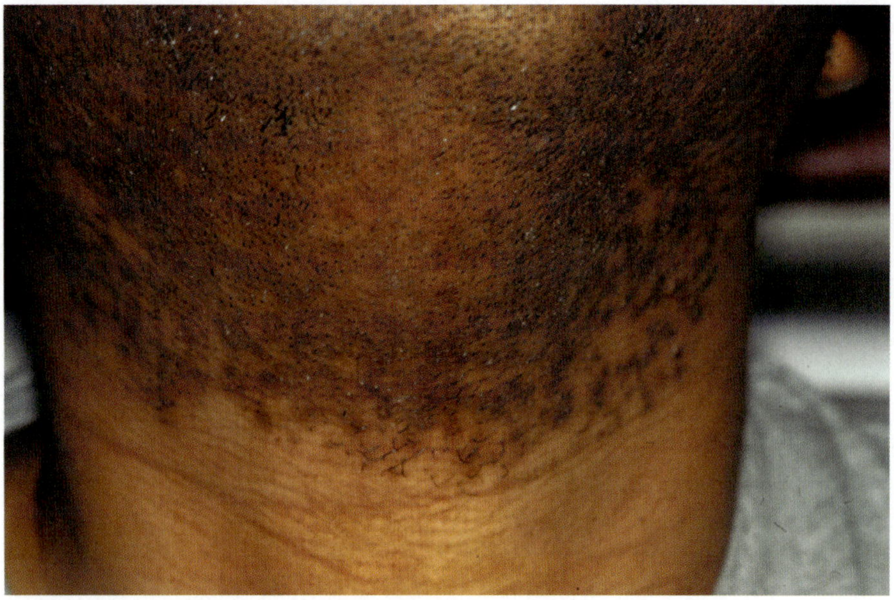

▲ **FIGURE 33-9** Moderate PFB of the anterior neck of a darkly pigmented man. Note the postinflammatory hyperpigmentation.

Surgical depilation is another modality for permanent hair removal, Hage reports.[11] The skin is undermined in all directions and manually everted when making a submandibular incision. The hair bulbs are either electrodesiccated, extracted, or clipped. Unfortunately, the procedure is expensive, and a keloid can develop in patients with such a propensity.

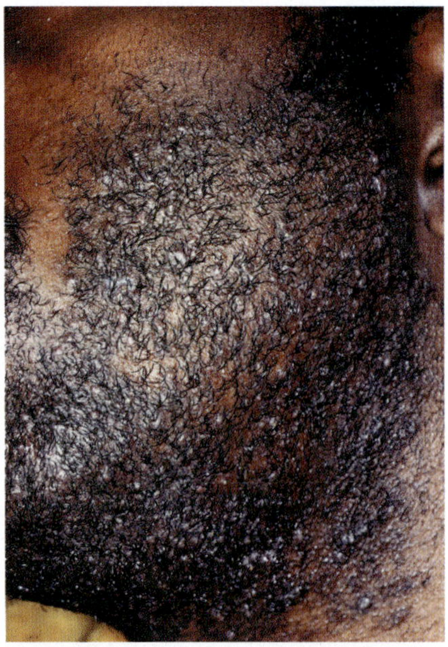

▲ **FIGURE 33-10** Profile of a darkly pigmented man with severe/chronic PFB. Present are numerous papulopustules, grooving, and PIH of the left cheek. Courtesy of Yvonne Knight, M.D., Richmond, VA.

Temporary radiation epilation can relieve the symptoms of PFB and give the skin a chance to improve before applying other therapeutic modalities. Permanent epilation is contraindicated because of the high incidence of skin cancer developing 10–25 years later.

When these procedures are not affordable or impractical, other therapeutic measures are available to attenuate the disease while allowing the patient to shave. Except for mild cases, PFB requires medical intervention during the acute pustular phase, which is often painful and/or pruritic.

I recomment the following therapeutic approach[7]:

1. Advise patients to discontinue shaving for one month for mild cases, 2–3 months for moderate cases, and 3–6 months for severe cases. During this shaving hiatus, the beard can be trimmed with scissors or electric clippers to a minimum length of 1 cm. Inform the patient that the PFB probably will get worse initially after the first week of not shaving, when the shaved hairs are long enough to penetrate the skin, creating more lesions.
2. Use a warm water, saline, or Burrow's solution compress for 10–15 minutes three times a day to soothe the lesions, remove crust, stop drainage secondary to inflammation, and soften the epidermis, allowing easier and earlier release of ingrown hairs.
3. After compressing and releasing the ingrown hairs, apply a topical hydrocortisone cream or lotion (for 3–4 weeks only) to the shaved area.
4. When secondary bacterial infection is present, apply the prescribed systemic antibiotic. In cases that do not improve with these steps, a therapeutic approach of a 5- to 10-day regimen of prednisone, 40–60 mg/day, may be used, provided there are no contraindications. Shaving should not be resumed until all the inflammed lesions have cleared and all the ingrown hairs have been released.

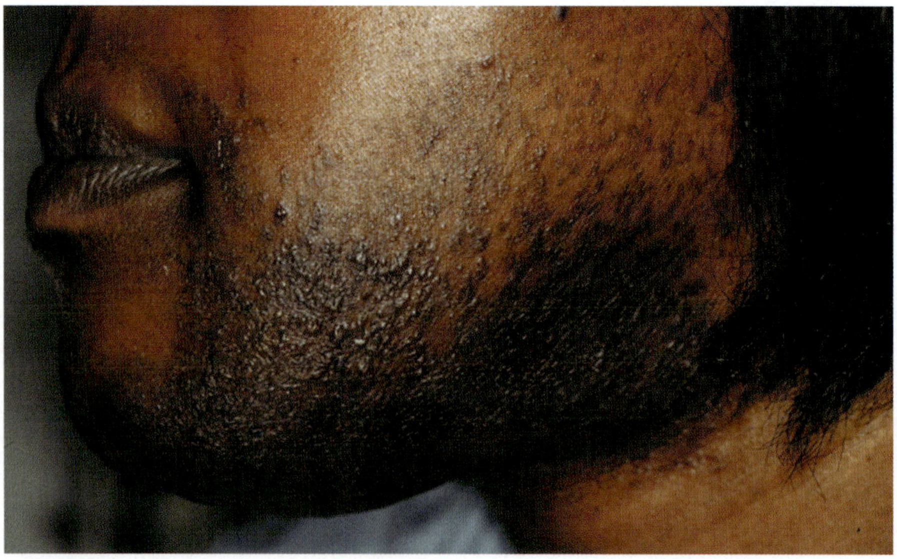

▲ **FIGURE 33-11** Moderate PFB of the left cheek in a darkly pigmented woman with postinflammatory hyperpigmentation.

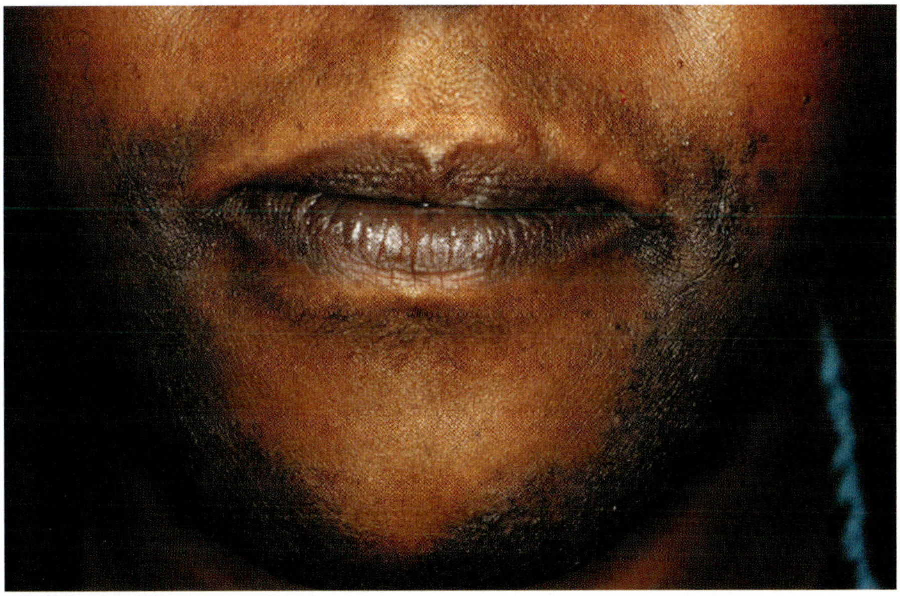

▲ **FIGURE 33-12** The patient from Figure 33-11 showing PFB with postinflammatory hyperpigmentation of the chin and medial cheeks.

For those who must shave, advise the following daily regimen:

1. Ingrown hairs should not be plucked because they may cause irritation or may grow and eventually penetrate the follicular wall.
2. Use electric clippers to remove as much preexisting beard hair as possible without causing irritation.
3. Wash beard area with a wash cloth and then massage with a soft tooth brush or polyester sponge.
4. Rinse the beard area to remove any remaining soap. Apply warm water compresses for approximately 5 minutes.
5. Use any shaving cream, making sure not to let the lather dry. If for any reason it dries, reapply the lather before shaving.
6. Choose a sharp razor that cuts best without irritation. There are shavers on the market made especially for PFB, which interested patients can find by doing a Web search. The PFB (Bump Fighter) razor (American Safety Razor Company, Stanton, VA) with polymer coating of a single-edge blade and foil guard has been reported to cause a significant reduction in the number of PFB lesions.[12] The Norelco Black Pro (Norelco Consumer Products, Stanford, CT) is an electric shaver that seems to help those with mild to moderate PFB.
7. Shave with the grain of the hair, using short strokes while avoiding pulling the skin taut. Twice over one area is usually sufficient.
8. After shaving, rinse the face with warm tap water and then compress with cool water for approximately 5 minutes.
9. Use a magnifying mirror to search for any ingrown hairs. To release them gently, insert a toothpick under the loop or brush the beard area with a soft toothbrush.
10. Apply the most soothing and least irritating aftershave preparation. If burning or itching ensues, a topical hydrocortisone preparation can be used after the aftershave lotion.
11. In those areas where hair growth is haphazard (anterior neck and submandibular area), daily brush of the beard often gives direction to the grain of the hair. Take care to avoid nicks and cuts in order to prevent traumatic folliculitis.

Those who find that shaving worsens their PFB or is too irritating may use chemical depilators. The two basic types are barium sulfide and calcium thioglycolate preparations, both found in powder, lotion, cream, and paste forms. They work by lysing disulfide bonds in the hair. This results in hair with a softer, more brushlike tip, making extrafollicular and transfollicular penetration much more difficult.

Barium sulfide preparations (Magic Shave-Red, Magic Shave-Blue, and Royal Crown Red and Blue) must be mixed with water before being applied as a paste and often leave an odor. Calcium thioglycolate preparations (Magic Shave-Gold, Royal Crown-Supreme, Nair, and Neet) can remain on the skin longer without causing irritation and do not have an offensive odor.

Because embedded hair tips are not affected by depilatories, it usually takes several weeks before clinical improvement is evident. Advise the patient, before using a chemical depilatory, to apply a small amount to the hair-bearing area on the forearm, leave it on for 5–10 minutes, and then wash it off with soap and water. If irritation develops on the test area within 48 hours, the depilatory should not be used on the face or on any area with PFB.

Some of the *adjuncts* to shaving are topical tretinoin, especially early in the onset of the disease. It is thought to work by alleviating hyperkeratosis and toughening the skin.[13] The use of tretinoin does not alter the previously described shaving regimen. Treating the PFB patient with a weekly liquid nitrogen cryospray to cause a light peel is often a helpful. A 10- to 15-second thaw time is usually sufficient. Freezing greater than 25 seconds produces hypopigmentation, which may last 1 year or longer. Glycolic acid and other α-hydroxy acids can be used to reduce hyperkeratosis of the follicular infundibulum and thickening of the stratum corneum.[14] This, in turn, allows the hair to grow our straighter and makes shaving easier. Topical or systemic antibiotics may be necessary to treat secondary infection.

Another product that can function as an adjunct for all the above-mentioned therapeutic regimens is eflornithine hydrochloride cream 13.8% (Vaniqua). It inhibits ornithine decarboxylase, a major enzyme involved in hair cell division, and slows the rate of hair growth. It is applied twice a day and washed off 4 hours after application. Some patients develop an irritant contact dermatitis.

CONCLUSION (Table 33-1)

PFB is essentially a disorder of the beard in darkly pigmented men who shave. It also may develop in other races, in women, and on any hair-bearing area that is closely and frequently shaved. The only permanent cures are beard growth or depilation. All other treatments are aimed at controlling symptoms. An important part of the therapeutic regimen is patient education.

TABLE 33-1
Summary of Pseudofolliculitis Barbae

First reported by Stauss and Kligman in 1956

Most common synonyms
- Shave bumps or razor bumps or folliculitis

Etiology and pathogenesis
- A chronic inflammatory disease that is caused by shaved hairs cut at an oblique angle and growing back into the skin
- Found mainly in darkly pigmented men with course, tightly curled hair
- Pathogenesis: transfollicular and extrafollicular penetration

Clinical findings
- Occurs after puberty but before age 50
- Foreign-body inflammatory reaction surrounding an ingrown hair
- Postinflammatory hyperpigmentation or keloids can result from PFB

Differential diagnosis
- Folliculitis or acne vulgaris
- Sarcoidosis

Prevention and treatment
- Prevention: 100% effective treatment is to discontinue shaving.
- Electric shavers may help because they do not cut as close to the skin as do blades.
- Over-the-counter foil-guard safety razors may be a treatment option.
- Although sometimes difficult for patients to tolerate, chemical depilatories can be used.
- Laser destruction of the hair follicles may cause some scarring.
- Electrolysis may not be effective on curved hair follicles.

Complications
- Once PFB groves, scars, or hyperpigmentation appear, the skin does not return to normal.

REFERENCES

1. Gottlieb JS, Skopit SE, Del Rosso JQ. Pseudofolliculitis barbae. *Journal of AOCD* 2007; *www.aOcd.org/skin/dermatologic_diseases/pseudofolliculitis.htm.*
2. Strauss JS, Kligman AM. Pseudofolliculitis of the beard. *Arch Dermatol Syphilol* 1956;74:533-542.
3. Halder RM, Roberts CI, Noothetic PK, Kelly AP. Dermatological disease in blacks, in Halder RM, (ed), *Dermatology and Dermatological Therapy of Pigmented Skin.* Bora Raton, Florida; Taylor & Francis, 2004, p 336.
4. Kelly AP. Pseudofollicilitis barae and acne keloildalis nuchae. *Dermatol Clin* 2003;21: 645-653.
5. Perry P, Cook-Bolden FE, Rahman Z, et al. Defining pseudofolliculitis barbae in 2001: A review of the literature and current trends. *J Am Acad Dermatol* 2002:46: 3113-3119.
6. Halder RM. Pseudofolliculitis barbae and related disorders. *Dermatol Clin* 1988;6: 407-412.
7. Kelly AP. Pseudofolliculitis barbae, in: Arndt K, LeBoit P, Robinson J, Wintroubt B (eds), *Cutaneous Medicine and Surgery.* Philadelphia, Saunders, 1996, pp 499-503.
8. Kauvar ANB. Treatment of pseudofolliculitis with a pulsed infrared laser. *Arch Dermatol* 2000;136:1343-1346.
9. Jackson BA, Junkins-Hopkins J. Long-pulse diode laser treatment for hair removal in dark skin: Clinicopathologic correlation (abstract). Presented at the *Ethnic Hair and Skin: What Is the State of the Science Conference,* Chicago, September 29-30, 2001.
10. Weaver S, Sagaral E. Treatment of pseudofolliculitis barbae using a long-pulse Nd:YAG laser (abstract). Presented at the *Ethnic Hair and Skin: What Is the State of the Science Conference,* Chicago, September 29-30, 2001.
11. Hage JJ, Bowman FG. Surgical depilation for the treatment of pseudofolliculitis or local hirsutism of the face: Experience in the first 40 patients. *Plast Reconstr Surg* 1991;88:446-451.
12. Alexander AM. Evaluation of a foil-guarded shaver in the management of pseudofolliculitis barbae. *Cutis* 1981;27:534-542.
13. Kligman AM, Mills OH. Pseudofolliculitis of the beard and topically applied tretinoin. *Arch Dermatol* 1973;107:551-552.
14. Perricone NV. Treatment of pseudofolliculitis barbae with topical glycolic acid: A report of two studies. *Cutis* 1993;52: 232-235.

CHAPTER 34

Hair Care Practices

Chemene R. Quinn

Key Points

- African hair is five times more difficult to comb, is more fragile, and has lower stress requirement at breaking than Caucasian or Asian hair.
- It is estimated that 80% of African-American women use chemicals relaxers and/or thermal instruments to straighten their hair. The type and extent of use will vary based on intraracial curl pattern differences.
- Specialized grooming products and procedures are needed to ensure that the African hair maintains its cosmetic value.
- There are no biochemical differences among black, Caucasian, and Asian hair types.
- In black men and women, many of the scalp dermatoses and alopecias are associated with hair care practices.
- Dermatologists should be knowledgeable of the various styling methods and cultural attitudes of patients with textured hair to avoid recommending treatments that may cause further damage or noncompliance.

Hair care in the patient of color can prove to be perplexing to even the most seasoned dermatologist. The variations in hair textures, grooming practices, cultural identity, and even terminology can be overwhelming during a limited office visit.

Human hair is categorized into three groups: Asian, Caucasian, and African. There are no biochemical differences among black, Caucasian, and Asian hair types.[1,2] Many black women and men spend a great deal of time and money grooming their hair, some visiting the hair salon as much as once or twice weekly. Ethnic hair care is a multibillion-dollar industry.[3,4]

This chapter will outline and discuss hair care practices with a focus on the patient of African ancestry. A summation of practical hair care guidelines for clinical reference is provided in Tables 34-1 and 34-2.

TABLE 34-1
Sample Handout for Black Patient Hair Care Recommendations

Practical hair care for patients with African hair

- Cleanse hair every 1–2 weeks. [Chemicals (e.g., chlorine, etc.) should be washed out daily.]
- Use cleansers and conditioners formulated for hair texture (coarse, dry, or damaged hair); avoid choices marketed solely to ethnic or people of color.
- Avoid direct heat more than two times a week.
- Do not apply heat to dirty hair or hair layered with styling products.
- Air dry or wet set your hair rather than blow-drying for styling.
- Get hair trimmed every 8–12 weeks.
- Establish open communication with stylists in your area.
- Use emollients for hair shafts only.
- *Excessive scalp irritation, burns, or hair breakage should be evaluated promptly by a dermatologist knowledgeable in African hair types.*

Additional recommendations based on styling choices

Chemically altered hair

- Schedule a professional touch-up no more than every 6–8 weeks.
- Recommend no-lye chemical relaxers.
- Avoid scalp manipulation prior to chemical service.
- Highlights, cellophanes, and colors should be done by a professional stylist to avoid hair shaft damage.
- Use only a licensed cosmetologists for chemical treatments.
- Promptly seek medical attention for alopecia, burns, or persistent scalp irritation.

Braids, weaves, locks, plaits, and cornrows

- Avoid styles that put tension/traction on the hair.
- Use emollients on the hair shafts only.
- Use "no damage" hair hosiery instead of rubber bands.
- Volume and weigh of extensions should not be excessive.
- Remove and replace braids every 4–6 weeks.

TABLE 34-2
Relaxer Record

Name ______________________________ Tel ____________

Address ____________________ City _____ State ____ Zip Code ________

Description of Hair

FORM	LENGTH	TEXTURE	POROSITY	
☐ wavy	☐ short	☐ coarse	☐ soft	☐ very ☐ less
☐ curly	☐ medium	☐ medium	☐ silky	☐ moderate ☐ least
☐ extracurly	☐ long	☐ fine	☐ wiry	☐ normal ☐ resistant
				☐ lightened

Condition

☐ virgin ☐ retouched ☐ dry ☐ oily ☐ lightened

Tinted with ____

Previously relaxed with (name of relaxer) ______________________

☐ Original sample of hair enclosed

Type of Relaxer or Straightener

☐ whole head ☐ retouch

☐ relaxer ____________strength ☐ straightener __________strength

Results

☐ good ☐ poor ☐ sample of relaxed hair enclosed ☐ not enclosed

Date	Operator	Date	Operator

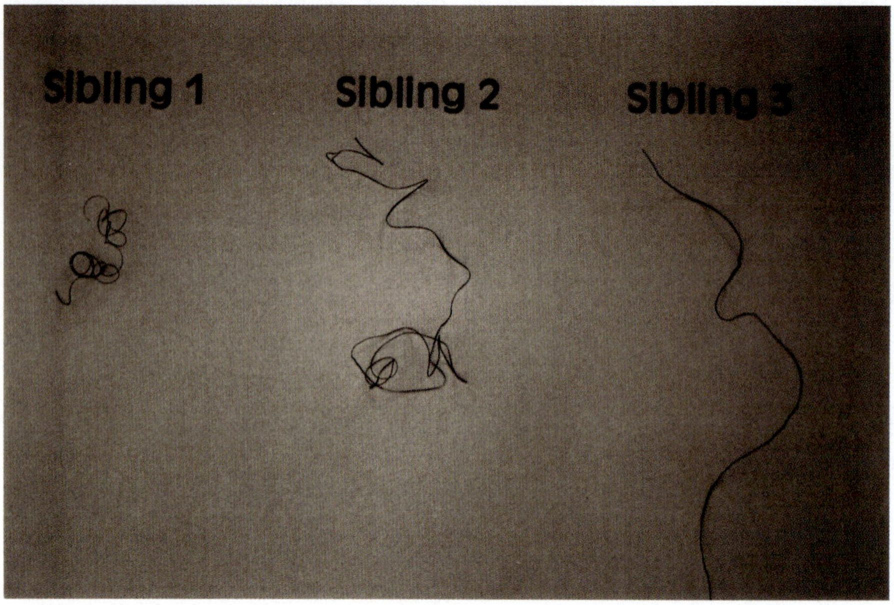

▲ **FIGURE 34-1** Intraracial variability of curl degree in three siblings with unprocessed virgin hair.

TABLE 34-4
Structural Properties of African Hair

- Has a lower radial swelling rate.
  - Percentage on exposure to water
- The composition and structure are the same for the three ethnic types of hair.
- African hair is described as excessively curly.
  - Possessing an elliptical or flattened shape in cross section
  - Spiral curls in its tertiary structure
- Intraethnic variability of ellipicity is increased in African hair.
  - At regions of twists, African hair has a wide variety of shapes.

PHENOTYPE OF AFRICAN HAIR

Since the hair phenotype varies from tightly coiled in sub-Saharan Africa to very straight in northern areas, individuals whose ancestors hailed from the African continent are now a mosaic of other racial and ethnic groups.[5,6] The degree of curl in virgin (untreated) African hair varies tremendously from almost none at all to tightly coiled hair through which a comb cannot be drawn[7] (Figure 34-1). Porter and colleagues have shown that as hair becomes curlier in appearance, it has a lower curve diameter (CD), extends less when strained, and is more susceptible to breakage. These findings suggest that the mechanical fragility of hair increases with higher degrees of curl[8] (Table 34-3).

Because hair texture is not uniform among those of African ancestry, basic hair care practices vary based on the degree of tightness of the curl (CD) or phenotype.

Structural Properties

Studies suggest that African hair has a lower radial swelling rate/percentage on exposure to water, but hair composition and structure do not differ for the three ethnic types of hair.[1,2,9] African hair is described as excessively curly, possessing an elliptical or flattened shape in cross section and spiral curls in its tertiary structure.

Intraethnic variability of the ellipticity is increased in African hair, and at regions of twists, hair of African origin displays a wide variety of shapes[10,11] (Table 34-4). The tensile properties of excessively curly hair indicate that is has a lower strain value at breaking point compared with straight hair.[12] African hair has a tendency to form knots and longitudinal fissures and splits along the hair shaft[13] (Figure 34-2). This complex shaft structure creates the need for specialized grooming products and procedures to ensure that the hair maintains its cosmetic value.[7]

TABLE 34-3
Phenotype of African Hair

- African hair becomes curlier in appearance when
  - It has a lower curve diameter.
  - It extends less when strained.
  - It is more susceptible to breakage.
- Mechanical fragility of African hair increases with higher degrees of curl.

MAINTENANCE TECHNIQUES

Cutting and Trimming of the Hair

African hair grows more slowly and breaks more often than Asian or Caucasian hair.[10] Combing the hair can increase fractures and breaks in natural (virgin) hair as it grows longer. African-American hair tends to develop a high static charge when combed in the dry state, and combed natural hair can remain short for many years without a haircut.[5,7] The constant formation of

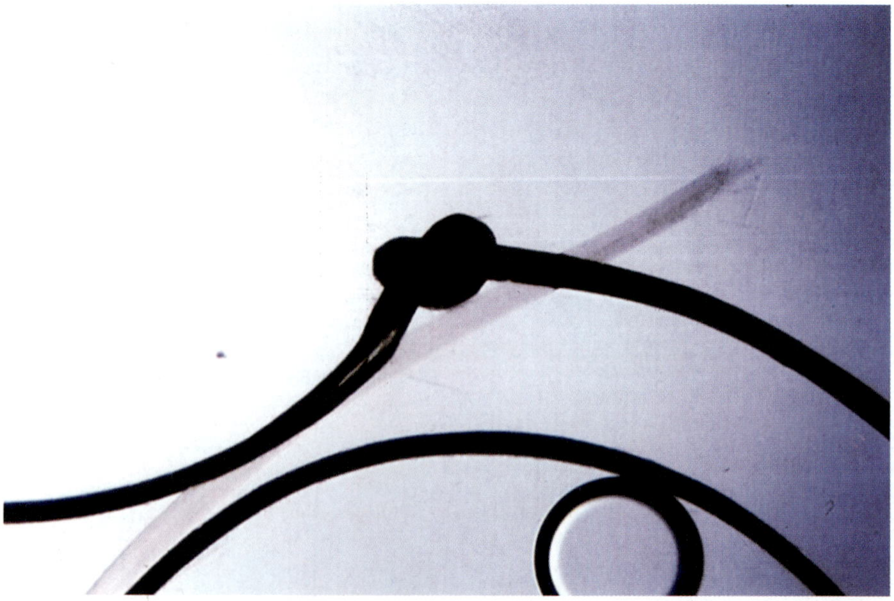

▲ **FIGURE 34-2** A knot forming in a fiber of African hair. Passing a comb through knots will fracture the hair.

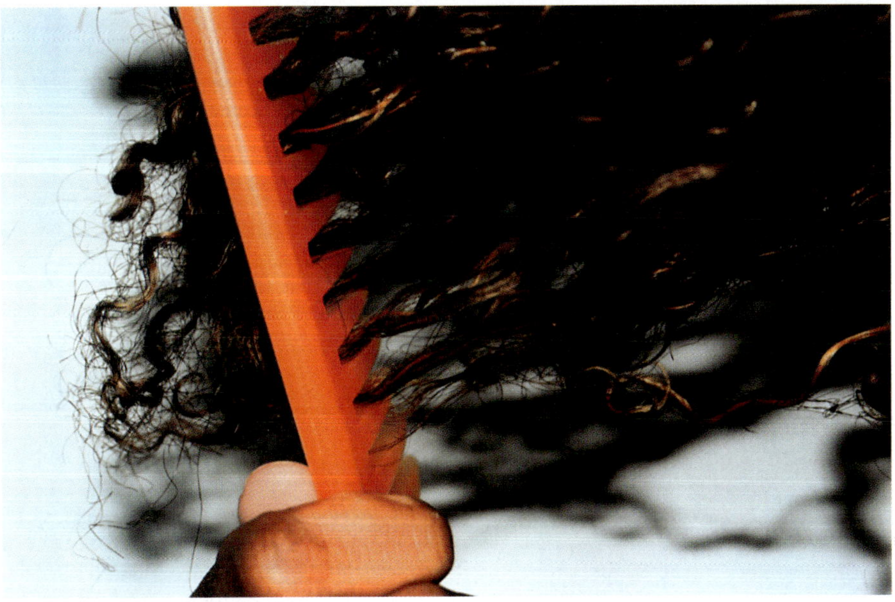

▲ **FIGURE 34-3** Wide-tooth combs or fingers can decrease breakage from combing.

knots will cause hair to break when combed (Figures 34-2 and 34-3). A "steady state" of daily breakage and equivalent new growth can be reached in independence.[5] Black females with tightly coiled hair may be averse to cutting their hair because of the "daily haircut" owing to breakage.

Straightening the hair or allowing it to lock maybe the only way to realize true anagen length potential in textured African hair. Blacks with relaxers, dreadlocks, and twist styles have increased length and decreased breakage. A small study by Whisenant and colleagues found that frequent shampooing and trimming were associated with hair damage in blacks. Yet excessive damage from styling practices may increase the need to cut damaged hair. Further investigation is warranted.[14]

Despite conflicting data, it may be wise to instruct black patients to trim their hair every 8–12 weeks to minimize distal breakage and maximize luster and style maintainance.

Cleansing

Hair cleansing needs differ between straight hair and African hair. African hair has a significantly lower water content than Caucasian or Asian hair and does not become coated with sebum secretion as naturally as straight hair. Tightly coiled hair naturally stands away from the scalp; therefore, excess sebum can increase styling ease.[7,13]

Cleansing agents targeted to this population contain mild amphoteric detergents, detanglers, silicone-based materials, quaternary ammonium compounds, and cationic polymers that will not aggravate the scalp.[12,15]

Conditioning

Heavier conditioning products are required to overcome the higher static charges in African hair.[16] Conditioners function to ease both wet and dry combing; to smooth, seal, and realign damaged areas; to provide protection against thermal and mechanical procedures; and to impart sheen and a silky feel.[12]

Moisturization, Scalp Oils, and Pomades

Many patients will describe this process as "greasing" or "basting" the scalp. The hair is sectioned with a comb in small parts, and a moisturizing agent is applied directly to the exposed scalp and proximal hair shafts. The agent is not washed out. Moisturizing the hair enables combing without the tugging or pulling that can result in breakage. Since the water content in African hair is slightly less than in Caucasian hair, you will find that most black patients use a daily grooming agent.[7,12]

Complications/Treatment/Prevention

SHAMPOOING Black women who shampoo their hair twice weekly or more often have a higher rate of shaft damage; therefore, shampooing can be limited to once every 1–2 weeks.[14] Conditioning shampoos directed toward and marketed to people with damaged or chemically or color-treated hair can decrease breakage in black patients. It has been shown that those containing sphinganine-derived ceramide (i.e., C18-dhCer) bind to and protect virgin and chemically treated African hair from excessive breakage.[17] Excessive exposure to chemicals such as chlorine in pool water should be washed from the hair daily despite the preceding recommendation and a conditioning agent applied to prevent breakage.

Women with hair styled with weaves, relaxers, curly perms, Jheri curls, and braids may opt to shampoo even less frequently so that their hair will not revert back to its natural state. This is not recommended and can promote seborrhea, increase the risk to fungal infection, and create a foul odor.[18] Conditions such as seborrhea, tinea capitis, and psoriasis will necessitate more frequent washing and will be explained in detail in Chapters 22, 36 and 37.

CONDITIONING, MOISTURIZATION, SCALP OILS, AND POMADES Wet hair shafts should be coated with a conditioning agent. To decrease breakage, a wide-tooth comb (see Figure 34-3) or fingertips should be used starting at the ends and advancing proximally to comb the hair.

Overuse of moisturizers can lead to pomade acne involving the forehead (Figure 34-4), scalp oil folliculitis, chronic oil folliculitis, and seborrheic dermatitis. Patients should avoid products that are petrolatum-based. Newer agents containing less occlusive agents are recommended. Moisturizers should be applied to the entire hair shaft, and not to the scalp. Questioning regarding irritation or pruritus and evaluation of the scalp should be performed if a patient feels the need to apply pomades directly to the scalp.

STYLING TECHNIQUES

Thermal Straightening

Blow drying the hair is the process of drying wet hair with repetitive combing in the presence of a hair dryer delivering various degrees of heat. It is used to straighten hair, prepare it for pressing (see below), and to style it. Air drying or wet setting the hair are alternative drying methods that decrease the chance of breakage but despite aggressive use, these styling method may not achieve or maintain the desired styling effect.

Commonly called *pressing* or *hot combing*, thermal straightening is the process that straightens hair using high heat

(~350°F), oils, and metal implements. Flat irons, marcel irons, and curling irons are implements heated by marcel stoves or electrical heat (Figure 34-5) These instruments are used for the styling of virgin or chemically processed hair. Daily use can contribute to excessive dryness, bubble hairs, proximal trichorrhexis nodosa, weathering, trichoptilosis, and chronic breakage.[19]

The straightening effect of thermal styling is temporary and will be reversed with water exposure owing to the temporary rearrangement of hydrogen and disulfide bonds within the hair shaft.[20]

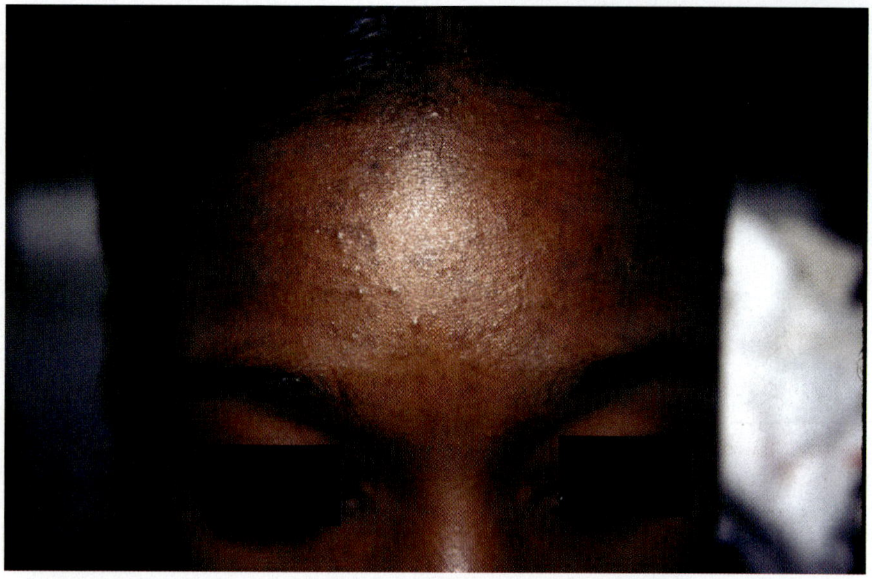

▲ **FIGURE 34-4** Multiple closed comedones of pomade acne on the forehead from hair lubricant use.

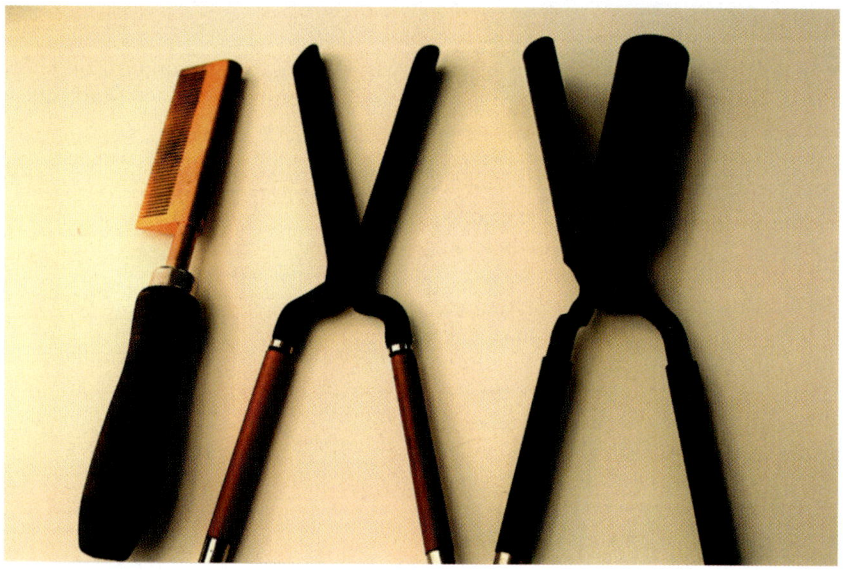

▲ **FIGURE 34-5** Marcel irons. Combs and flat irons straighten hair, and cylindrical devices are used to curl the straightened hair.

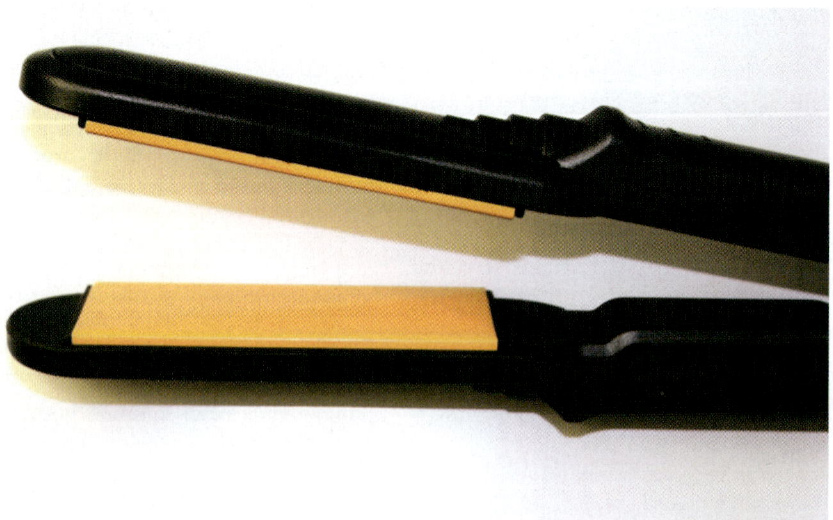

▲ **FIGURE 34-6** Heat-controlled negative-ion ceramic-plated irons with automatic shutdown can be safer and easier to use and give the hair a smoother finish.

COMPLICATIONS/TREATMENT/PREVENTION

Pressing of the hair should not be done more than two times a week. It is not recommended to press hair that has not been properly cleansed and conditioned prior to application of heat. Blacks have a high incidence of repeated daily layering of hair care products and lower frequency of shampooing, which can increase the flammability of hair.[21] Proximal breakage may occur, and a foul odor may emanate from hair when it is not cleansed prior to heat thermal styling. Hairline breakage and thinning can result from excessive use of thermal implements, which in the face of daily perspiration and water exposure, are used to maintain straightness.[20]

It is impractical to counsel every patient to discontinue the use of all thermal devices. Newer ceramic irons that generate negative ions possess adjustable temperature controls, and overheating controlling devices with automatic shutdown are recommended to replace pressing combs (Figure 34-6). These irons, as with other thermal devices, should not be used on damp hair. Communication with hair care professionals in your area can aid your patients in obtaining healthy styles and styling behavior.

Scalp, ear, and neck burns are seen commonly in women who use thermal styling agents and devices (Figure 34-7). The exposure to extreme heat should be avoided by using protective devices, which can be purchased at beauty supply stores (Figure 34-8). Local treatment may be necessary to prevent scarring, keloids, and infections.

Chemical Relaxation or Lanthionization

Mistakenly called "perms," chemical relaxers have been used by male and females of African descent for decades. Seventy percent of African-American females use chemical relaxers.

Chemical relaxers straighten the hair shaft using chemicals that alter the hair's natural texture, and the hair does not revert to virgin state with exposure to water.

Chemical relaxers containing sodium, potassium, or guanidine hydroxides straighten by affecting cysteine disulfide bonds of the hair.[22] Sodium hydroxide (lye-based) relaxers are used mainly in the salon, whereas (no-lye) relaxers are popular for home use. It is widely believed by stylists and patrons that lye-based relaxers have a better straightening effect. Lye-based relaxers have more irritation potential, are cheaper and easier to use, and are preferred by stylists for perceived relaxer performance. Recent laboratory results have indicated greater efficacy for the no-lye (guanidine-based) cream-finished products over lye-based products.[23]

The newly markedly Japanese straightening systems are an extremely harsh relaxing system that requires thermal processing on damp hair. However, I do not recommend them on the African hair type.

Numerous "Comb thru" or S-curl texturizers are marketed to black men and children and those with sensitive scalps. They are less permanent and can be controlled for desired curl relaxation. Non-lye chemicals such as sulfites, lithium hydroxide, and guanidine persist as the active ingredient in these no-lye and no-mix products. The hair shaft is not completely straightened to allow for a looser curl and a more manageable style.[24] Jheri curl or curly perm (Figure 34-9) uses ammonium thioglycolate with a lotion, wrapping the hair on rollers to relax the curl, and then resetting the hair in a curly or wavy pattern. Both styles can be maintained with a glycerin-based lotion moisturizer or spray curl activator that is messy and labor-intensive. A daily leave-in conditioner can be recommended as a more elegant alternative.

The curly shape of the hair is programmed from the bulb and is a "shape memory" material. Reapplication of any of the preceding relaxers to new growth called a "touch-up" is necessary to maintain style as the hair grows and can prevent texture differences that may predispose hair to breakage at areas of transition in texture.[25]

COMPLICATIONS/TREATMENT/PREVENTION

Seventy-three percent of black women complain of breakage, trichoptilosis (the hairs are covered with feather-like projections), and dryness caused by

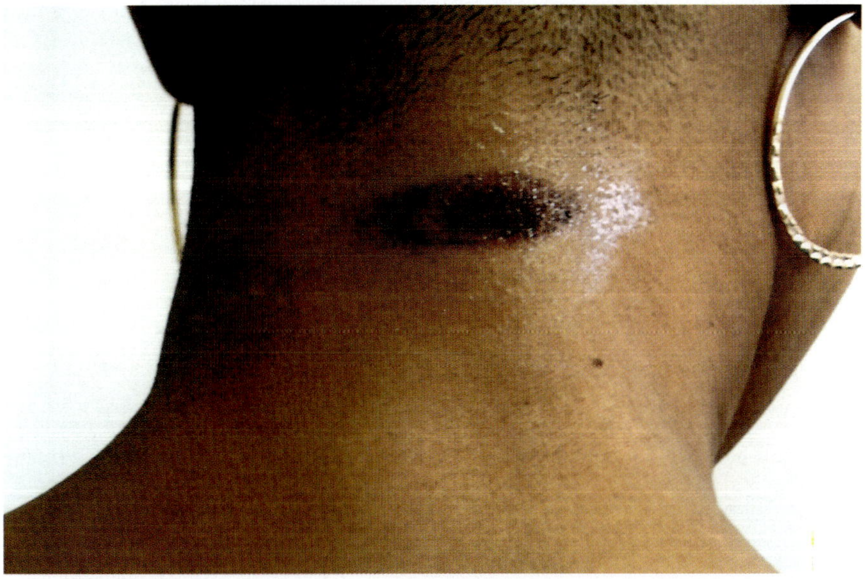

▲ **FIGURE 34-7** Thermal burn after electric curling iron use.

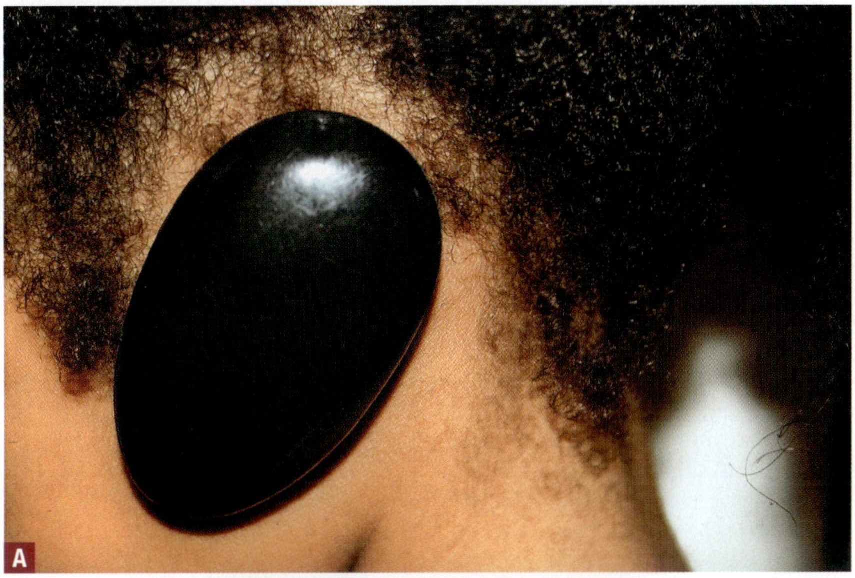

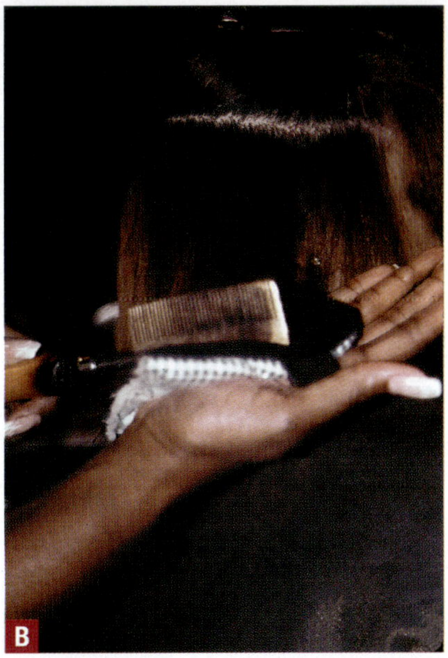

▲ **FIGURE 34-8** Ear protectors (*A*) and handheld devices (*B*) should be used to protect client and stylist from burns during thermal styling.

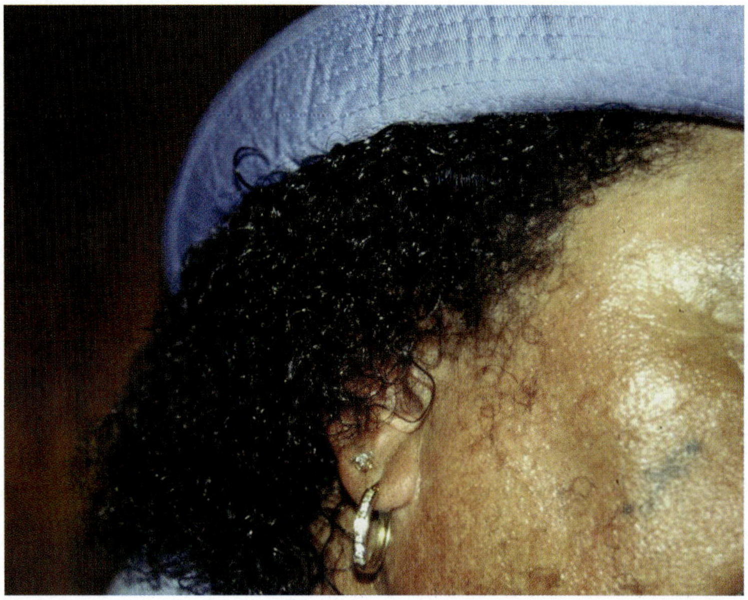

▲ **FIGURE 34-9** A Jheri curl needs a daily curl activator to maintain style, which can be messy and give a greasy appearance.

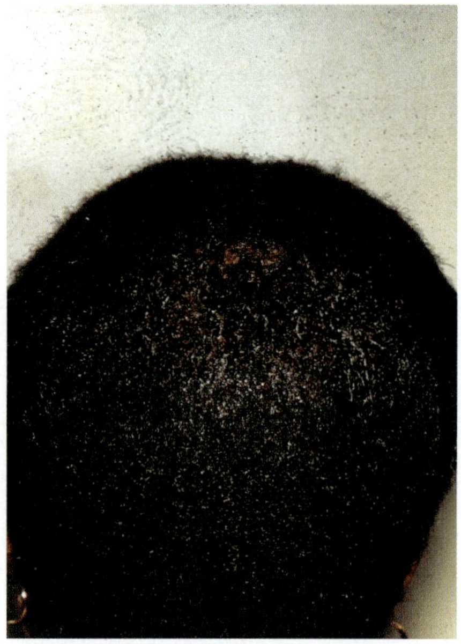

▲ **FIGURE 34-10** Chronic proximal hair breakage in a an adult black woman.

chemical treatments[26–28] (Figure 34-10). Frequency of application of a touch-up should be no more than every 8–12 weeks to minimize breakage and relaxer-induced alopecia and to decrease scalp irritation.[29]

Patients with chemical relaxers should be counseled to avoid scalp irritants or manipulation prior to receiving "touch-ups" (Figure 34-11). Requesting a copy of the patient's salon "relaxer record" can aid in making recommendations when damage to the scalp has occurred (see Table 34-2). It has been suggested that repetitive scalp irritation and burns may play a role in fibrosis and inflammation of the scalp associated with cicatricial and noncicatricial alopecia, although more research is necessary to confirm the association.[30–32] Holloway Barbosa and colleagues revealed, using Sebutape, a noninvasive method to examine molecular events, that although hair is the target of chemical relaxers, sensory irritation of the scalp occurs and may be due to both cytokine-mediated and neurogenic irritation.[33]

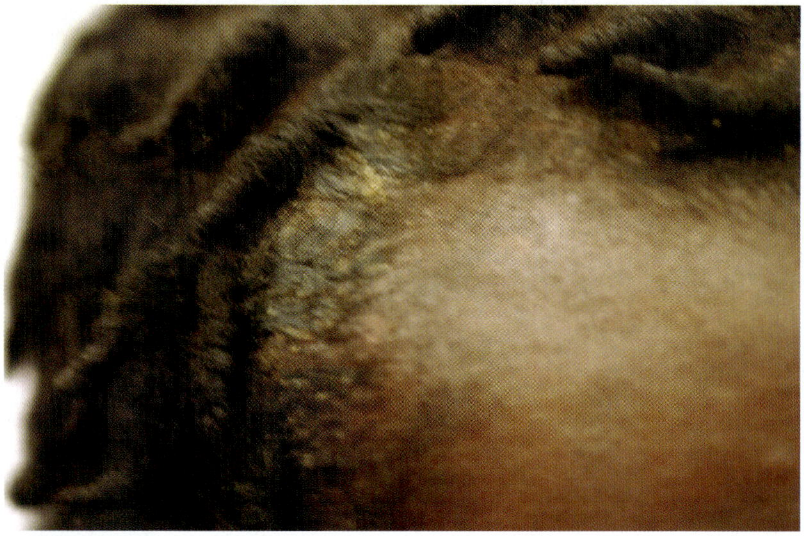

▲ **FIGURE 34-11** Scalp irritation and secondary infection after use of a chemical relaxing agent.

NONPROCESSED OR NATURAL STYLING

Afros

Afros comprise a natural hair style in which the hair is unprocessed and allowed to grow radially from the head (Figure 34-12). Moisturizers and oils are needed to maintain this style. With the Afro style, hair is not combed with a standard comb but rather a "pick" or fingers are used for daily maintenance. The style is most often

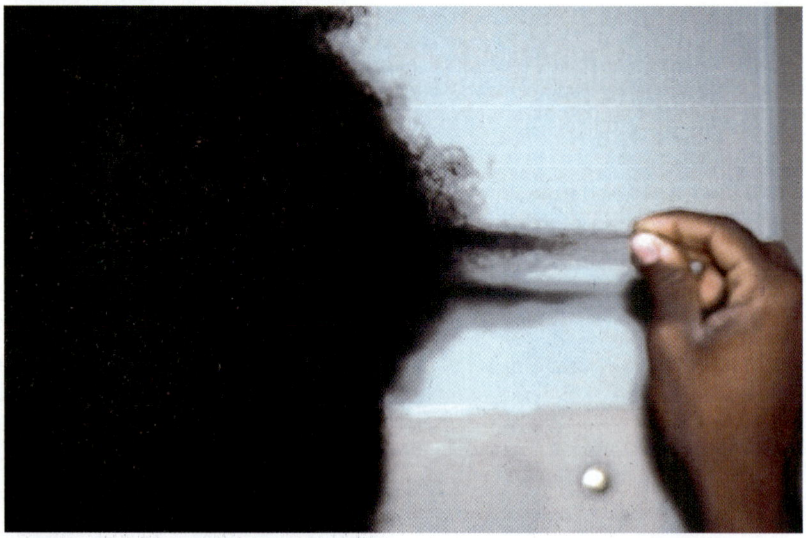

▲ **FIGURE 34-12** Afro style. Extending the curled hairs reveals the actual length.

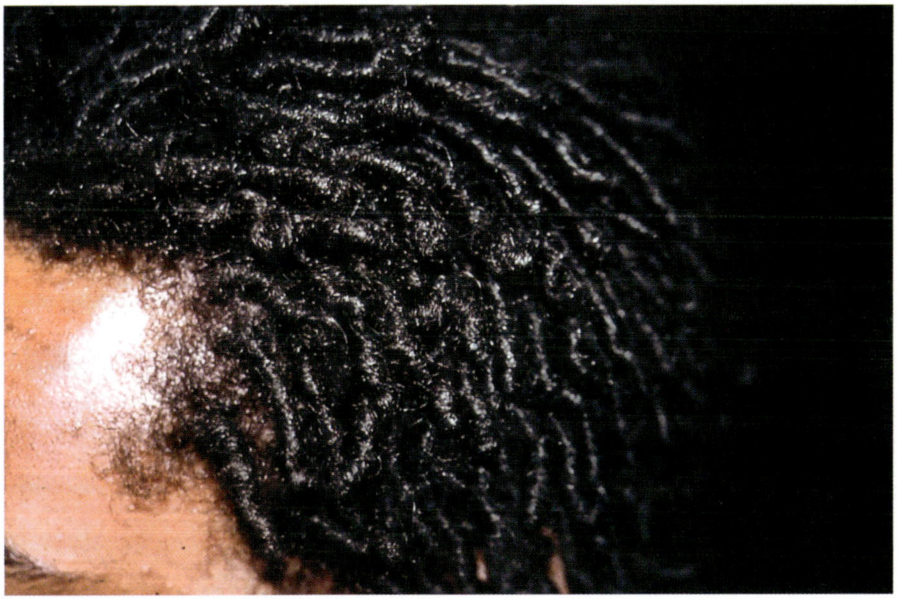

▲ **FIGURE 34-13** Black man with a twist style.

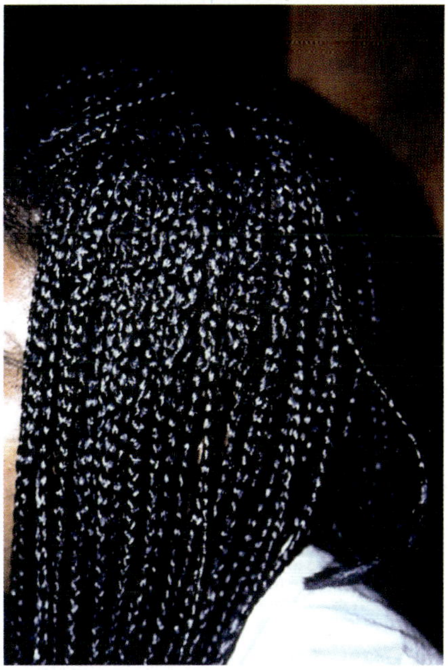

▲ **FIGURE 34-15** Black woman with individual braids.

worn by black men. The frequency of the Afro style in black women may increase as they mature. This may be due to lifestyle changes, retirement, alopecias, hair breakage, or financial constraints.[22] Many middle-age black women who have adopted an Afro express an acceptance and understanding of their hair type that they did not have in their youth, and those no longer in the work force feel less pressure for hair assimilation.

Locks, Twists, and Dreadlocks

Twisting of the hair can help to minimize the bulk of thick hair and redefines the hair shaft's natural curl, making the hair more manageable. Two pieces of hair are twisted around one another to form the twist (Figure 34-13). Locks, which are irreversible, are formed when uncombed hair tangles and mats in to clusters. There are several lock styles, including free form, wrapping, and Sisterlocks.[34]

Miscellaneous Styling

Various molding techniques (e.g., finger waving, freezes, and wraps) are used to obtain hairstyles ranging from a tight hold to a freeze hold (Figure 34-14). These fixatives used are balanced with plasticizers such propylene glycol or glycerin. Styling gel and spritzs used to achieve and maintain these styles, may contain upwards of 64% by weight SD 40 alcohol and should be avoided owing to increased hair shaft dryness and breakage.[13]

Braiding, microbraids, and plaits (a synonym for braiding with southern root derivation) are styled by interlocking three or more pieces of hair to create a three-dimensional section that extends from the head (Figure 34-15). Braiding hair with extensions (the addition of human or synthetic hair) can give an appearance of longer length similar to straight hair. Many women adopt a braid style when implementing an exercise program to avoid styling dilemmas. A cornrow is a stationary braid that lays flat on the scalp. Cornrows and plaits are used commonly under wigs, with weave styles and in children.

Hair weaving can be done for fashion, for therapeutic or prosthetic reasons. Many women believe that a weave style will help them to grow out their hair, cover balding areas or add thickness to their hair, or create style.[34] Sewing, gluing, or braiding is used to hold hair pieces in place (Figure 34-16).

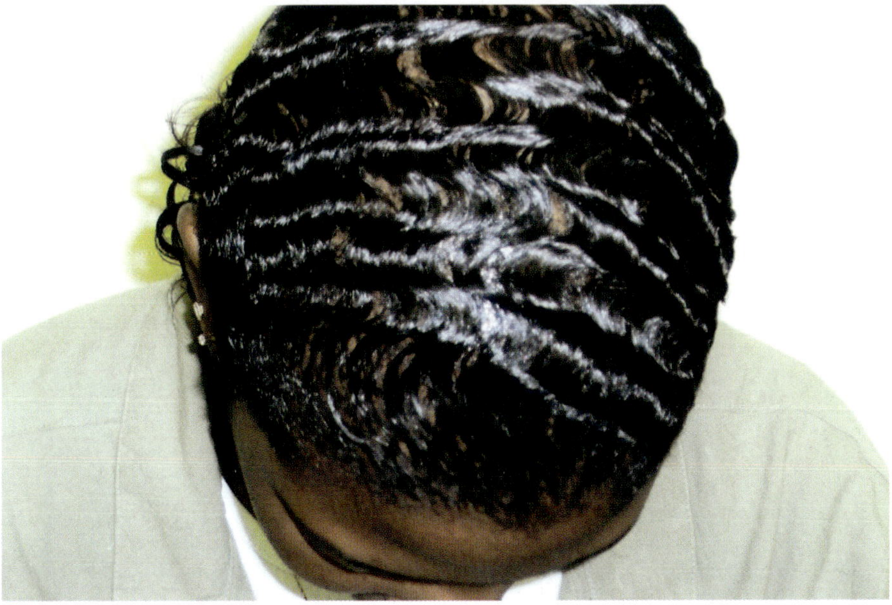

▲ **FIGURE 34-14** Black woman with "freeze" style complaining of alopecia. The molded hairstyle made clinical scalp examination impossible.

COMPLICATIONS/TREATMENT/PREVENTION

Traction folliculitis and resulting traction alopecia are found commonly in black patients with tight hair styles such as twists, locks, weaves, ponytails, braids, extension and hair roller use (Figures 34-17 and 34-18). Loosening of these styles can prevent long-term alopecia.

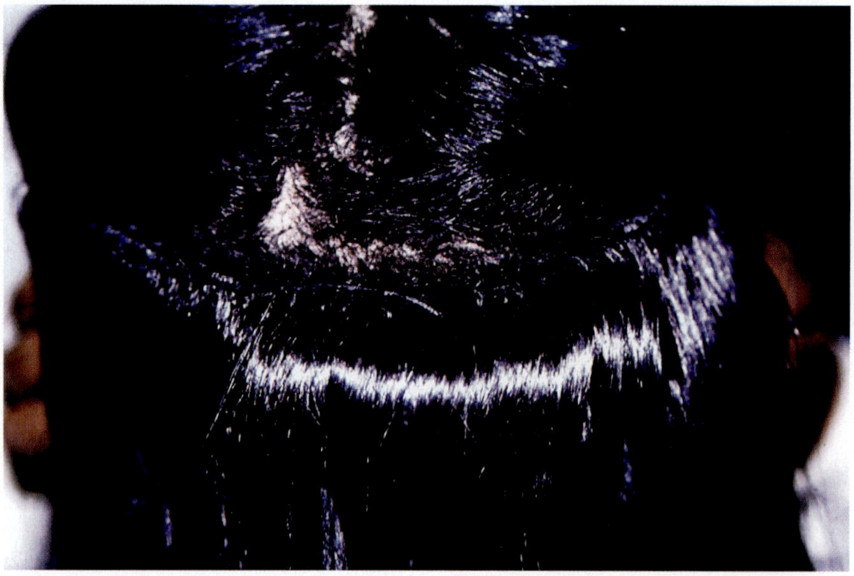

▲ **FIGURE 34-16** Black woman with weave style sewn onto a braided cornrow to add volume and length.

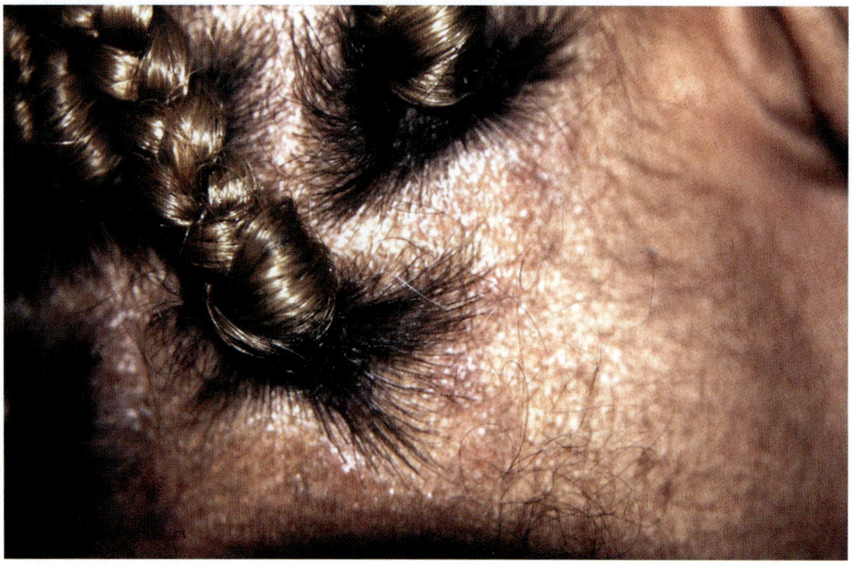

▲ **FIGURE 34-17** *A, B.* Traction folliculitis, erythematous papules and pustules at areas of tension.

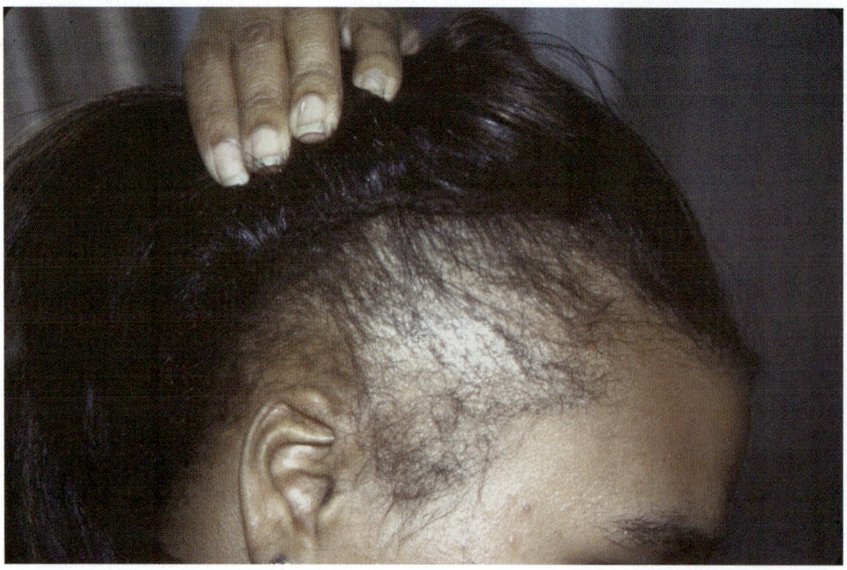

▲ **FIGURE 34-18** Traction alopecia from prolonged weaving of hair.

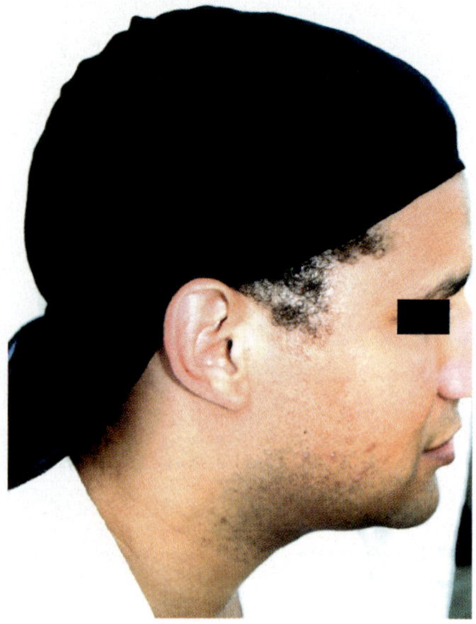

▲ **FIGURE 34-19** Traction "Durag" use by a black man.

Patients should be counseled to avoid hairstyles that are too tight and to loosen their hair overnight as styles permit. Contact or irritant dermatitis to adhesive/glue products (acrylates) and hair extensions can complicate weave styling.

BLACK MEN: SPECIAL CONSIDERATIONS

Originally made as hair protective garments, wave caps or "durags" (Figure 34-19) are worn by black men to physically relax the curl and maintain hair overnight. Durags are also used to maintain neat braid styles in black men and women.

Complications/Treatment/Prevention

Cream and pomade use under "durag" occlusion can cause pomade acne, irritant dermatitis, spread infection, and exacerbate seborrhea. Instruct patients to clean caps and use breathable or mesh fabric to minimize these complications.

Some black men use chemicals to relax, not straighten, the natural curl of their hair. A minority may use chemicals and thermal instruments to achieve straight hair and length. Similar recommendations should be given for hair maintenance as for female patients with such styles.

PEDIATRIC HAIR CARE: SPECIAL CONSIDERATIONS

Braids (plaits) are common in young black girls, and while boys usually wear

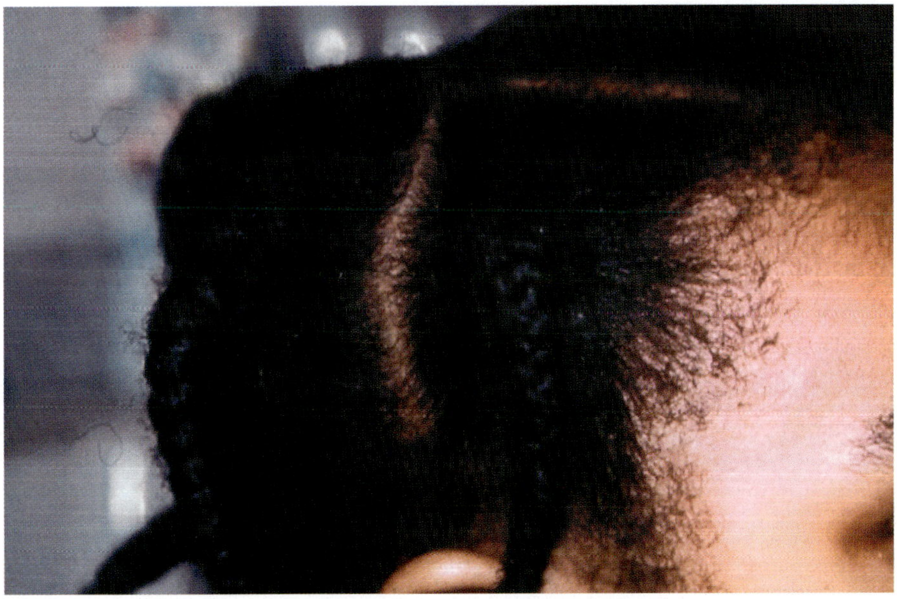

▲ **FIGURE 34-20** A black child with plaits.

Afro styles cropped short, braids and cornrows are increasing in popularity (Figure 34-20). Numerous products are increasingly being marketed for children of African descent that promise straighter and more manageable hair. Chemical relaxers are used quite frequently in the pediatric population and are started as early as 3 years of age in some patients (personal observation).

Complications/Treatment/Prevention

Hair loss in young women is growing at epidemic proportions. Black women from toddler age through adolescence are particularly susceptible to hair breakage. They are at risk for haphazard hair maintenance, experimentation, aversion to hair trimming, and the frequent use of at home chemical and thermal hair products by nonlicensed stylists. Chronic proximal hair breakage is common in children when chemical relaxers are not maintained properly (Figure 34-21). More than 70% of adult black women admit to hot comb use in childhood, and 51% recall suffering from scalp burns as a child.[35]

As mentioned earlier, braids, plaits, and cornrows with sufficient tension can cause traction folliculitis and alopecia (Figure 34-22). Dr. Vera Price recommends that hair be loosened each night and that the part pattern be changed frequently to decrease breakage and thinning. To minimize damage and traction

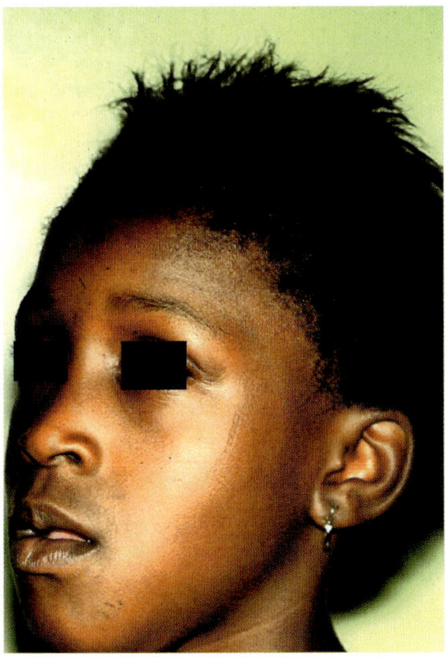

▲ **FIGURE 34-21** Chronic hair breakage from relaxers in a black female child.

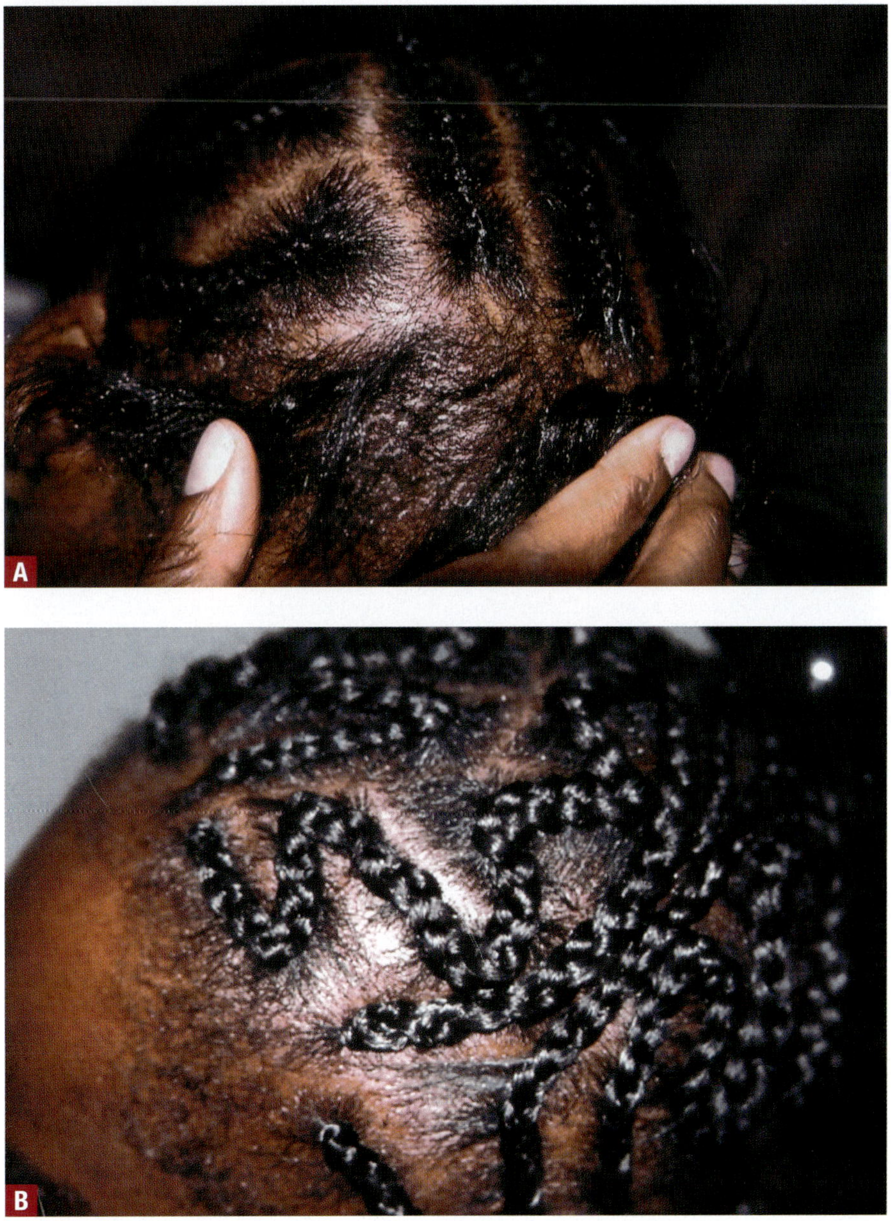

▲ **FIGURE 34-22** *A, B.* Traction alopecia in black children with cornrows.

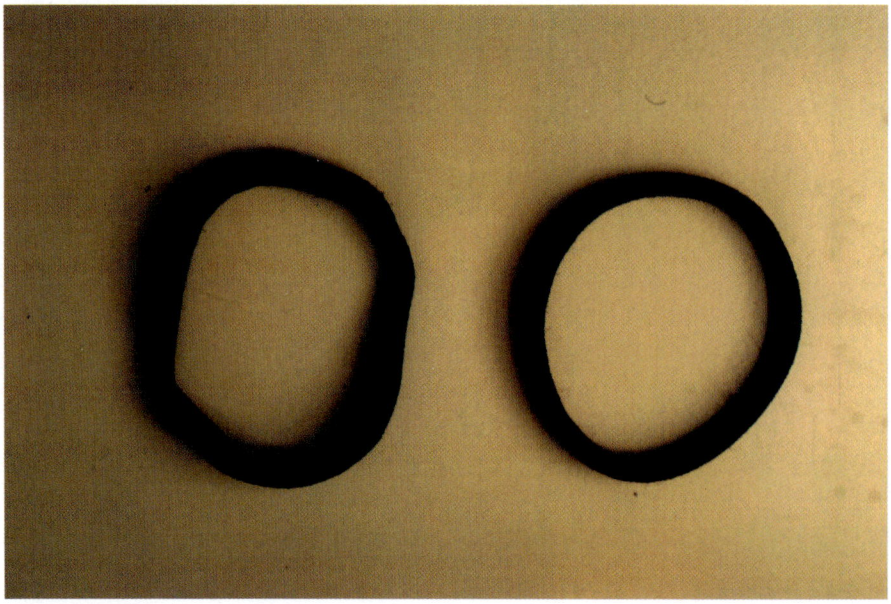

▲ **FIGURE 34-23** Hair bands without metal implements can decrease tension on the scalp and prevent hair shaft breakage.

alopecia, products such as Satin No Damage elastics can be used to gather and hold sectioned hair and ends in place[36] (Figure 34-23). Rubber bands and bands with metal implements should be avoided.

Physicians should discourage the use of chemical styling agents in pediatric patients owing to risks of chemical burns, contact dermatitis, inconsistent hair grooming routines, greater fungal infection susceptibility, and possible cultural identity issues.

REFERENCES

1. Lindelof B, Forslind B, Hedblad M-A, Kaveus U. Human hair form. *Arch Dermatol* 1988:124:1359-1363.
2. Dekio S, Jidoi J. Hair low-sulfur protein composition does not differ electrophorectically among different races. *J Dermatol* 1988;15(5):393-396.
3. Callender VD., McMichael AJ, Cohen GF. Medical and surgical therapies for alopecias in black women. *Dermatol Ther* 2004;17(2):164-76.
4. Grimes PE, Davis LT. Cosmetics in blacks. *Dermatol Clin* 1991;9(1):53-68.
5. Khumalo NP. African hair morphology: Macrostructure to ultrastruture. *Int J Dermatol* 2005;44:10-12S.
6. Taylor SC. As simple as black and white? Colloquium on race/ethnicity/skin color. *J Am Acad Dermatol* 2006;54:1067-1071.
7. Draelos ZD. Understanding African-American hair. *Dermatol Nurse* 1997;9(4): 227-231.
8. Porter CE, Diridollou S, Holloway Barbosa V. The influence of African-American hair's curl pattern on its mechanical properties. *Int J Dermatol* 2005; 44:4-5S.
9. Franbourg A, Hallegot P, Baltnneck E, et al. Current research on ethnic hair. *J Am Acad Dermatol* 2003; 48: 1152-119S.
10. Loussouran G. African hair growth parameters. *Br J Dermatol* 2001;145:294-297.
11. Wickett RR. Presented at *Loreal 1st International Symposium: Ethnic Skin and Hair, Chicago, IL, 2001*.
12. Syed AN. Ethnic hair care products, in Johnson DH (ed), *Hair and Hair Care,* Vol 17. New York, Marcel Dekker, 1997, pp 235-259.
13. Taylor SC. Skin of color: Biology, structure, function, and implications for dermatolgic disease. *J Am Acad Dermatol* 2002;46:41-62S.
14. Whisenant K, Taylor SC. Presented at *Loreal 2nd International Symposium: Ethnic Skin and Hair: New Directions in Research,* Chicago, IL, 2003.
15. Miller JJ, Heymann WR. African-American Hair Care (audiotape).
16. Jachowicz, Wis-Surel, Garcia ML. Relationship between trichoelectric charging and surface modifications of human hair. *J Soc Cosmet Chem* 1985;36;189-212.
17. Bernard BA, Franbourg A, Francois AM, et al. Ceramide binding to African-American hair fibre correlates with resistance to hair breakage. *Int J Cosmet Sci* 2002;24:1-12.
18. Silverberg NB, Weinberg JM, DeLeo VA. Tinea capitis: Focus on African-American women. *J Am Acad Dermatol* 2002;46: 120-124S.
19. Brown VM, Crounse RG, Abele DC. An unusual new breakage of the hair shaft abnormality: "Bubble hair." *J Am Acad Dermatol* 1986;15: 1115-1117.
20. Grimes PE, Davis LT. Cosmetics in blacks. *Dermatol Clin* 1991;9:53-68.
21. Cannel D. Cosmetic/pharmaceutical research: Development, safety, and efficacy of ethnic products. Presented at *Loreal 3rd International Symposium: Ethnic Skin and Hair: Advancing the Scientific Frontier,* Chicago, IL, 2005.
22. McMichael AJ. Hair and scalp disorders in ethnic populations. *Dermatol Clin* 2003;21:629-644.
23. Bryant H, Yang GY, Holloway Barbosa V. Lye vs no-lye relaxers: Comparison of laboratory results an end-user perceptions. Presented at *Loreal 3rd International Symposium: Ethnic Skin and Hair: Advancing the Scientific Frontier*, Chicago, IL, 2005.
24. Proline International, Dallas, Texas, 2006, *www.barberselect.com/products.cfm*.
25. Joyner M. Hair care in the black patient. *J Pediatr Health Care* 1988;2:281-287.
26. Halder RM. Hair and scalp disorders in blacks. *Cutis* 1983;32:378-380.
27. Bulengo-Ransby SM. Chemical and traumatic alopecia from thioglycolate in a black women. *Cutis* 1992;49:99-103.
28. Miller, JJ. Relaxer-induced alopecia. *Am J Contact Dermat* 2001;12:238-239.
29. Thibaut S, Bernard BA. The biology of hair shape. *Int J Dermatol* 2005;44:2-3S.
30. Nicholson AG, Harland CC, Bull RH, et al. Chemically induced cosmetic alopecia. *Br J Dermatol* 1993;128:537-541.
31. Nnoruka NE. Hair loss: Is there a relationship with hair care practices in Nigeria? *Int Soc Dermatol* 2005;44:13-17S.
32. Swee W, Klontz KC, Lambert LA. A nationwide outbreak of alopecia associated with the use of a hair-relaxing formulation. *Arch Dermatol* 2000;136:659-665.
33. Tackey RN, Holloway Barbosa V. Molecular response in the scalp after application of relaxer to the hair. Presented at *Loreal 3rd International Symposium: Ethnic Skin and Hair: Advancing the Scientific Frontier*, Chicago, IL, 2005.
34. Ferrel P. *Let's Talk Black Hair,* Vol 1. Washington, Cornrows & Co, 1996.
35. Cook-Bolden F. Enlist hair stylists in stopping traction alopecia. *Skin & Allergy News*. 2002;33:45.
36. Scunci, a Division of Conair Corporation, Stamford, CT, *www.scunci.com/product_detail.aspx?gid=4&pid=9999999999*.

CHAPTER 35

Alopecia

Chemene R. Quinn

Key Points

- Alopecia is divided into cicatricial and noncicatricial forms.
- Central centrifugal scarring alopecia (CCSA) is responsible for more cases of scarring alopecia than all other forms in African-American women.
- Classification of cicatricial alopecia is confusing and controversial.
- Many disorders have overlapping clinical and histologic features.
- Scalp biopsy and histopathologic evaluation are strongly recommened for diagnosing alopecia in black patients.
- Medical treatment and education on proper hair care practices are imperative in the treatment of alopecia.
- Prompt diagnosis and aggressive treatments are warranted to halt progression of disease and salvage viable hair follicles.

PRIMARY CICATRICIAL ALOPECIAS

Cicatricial alopecia represents a poorly understood group of disorders characterized by a common final pathway of replacement of the hair follicle structure by fibrous tissue.[1] Numerous classification systems have been described. Sperling identified five distinct pathologic forms of scarring alopecia—chronic cutaneous lupus, lichen planopilaris, dissecting cellulitis, acne keloidalis nuchae, and central centrifugal scarring alopecia[2] (Table 35-1). The North American Hair Research Society (NAHRS) classifies the primary cicatricial alopecias by histopathologic findings—lymphocytic, neutrophilic, mixed, and nonspecific.[1] Scalp biopsy remains the "gold standard" for the diagnosis and classification of alopecias. This is especially true in black patients. Numerous classifications with overlapping clinical and histopathologic features impede prompt diagnosis and treatment in this population. Scalp biopsies should be taken from symptomatic hair-bearing areas.[3] The importance of offering patients an immediate scalp biopsy cannot be overemphasized. A detailed discussion on the scalp biopsy technique in black patients is presented at the end of this chapter. Treatment should be based on clinical and histopathology results (Table 35-2). The NAHRS classification system and previous work done by Dr. Sperling have indeed resulted increased interest and volume of scholarly investigation directed toward cicatricial alopecia.

TABLE 35-1
Sperling's Alopecia Classification

- Chronic cutaneous lupus
- Lichen planopilaris
- Dissecting cellulites
- Acne keloidalis nuchae (Folliculitis keloidalis)
- Central centrifugal scaring alopecia

CENTRAL CENTRIFUGAL SCARRING ALOPECIA (CCSA)

Epidemiology, Etiology, and Pathogenesis

CCSA is a poorly understood lymphocytic cicatricial alopecia seen commonly in African-American females and less commonly in black men. CCSA is responsible for more cases of scarring alopecia than all other forms.[4] Formerly called *hot comb alopecia* or *follicular degeneration,* this disorder is not well defined, and the cause is still unknown. It has been proposed that the application of heat, hairstyles that pull too tightly on the scalp, harsh chemical treatments that damage the hair shaft, and family history contribute to the pathogenesis of CCSA.[5]

Clinical Findings

HISTORY Patients complain of hair breakage and paresthesia of the scalp sometimes described as a "pins and needles" sensation, itching, and tenderness. Disease course is as follows: hair breakage and hair thinning followed by hair loss. CCSA is progressive and begins on the crown of the scalp and advances centrifugally to the surrounding areas. Many patients do not seek immediate medical care, and the common presentation is a smooth scalp devoid of hair follicles at the vertex.[6]

PHYSICAL EXAMINATION The early stage of the disease is characterized by central hair breakage, perifollicular hyperkeratosis, erythema, and thinning. Papules and pustules may be present (Figures 35-1 and 35-2). Late disease is characterized by smooth alopecic patches devoid of hair follicles (Figure 35-3).

LABORATORY Histopathology is widely believed to be due to premature desquamation of the inner root sheath (IRS). Horenstein and colleagues found that premature desquamation of the IRS is seen in a variety of cicatricial alopecias and cannot be used alone as a defining feature of CCSA.[7,8] The early stage exhibits a licheniod infiltrate of lymphocytes separated from markedly thinned infundibulum by a prominent zone of alopecia.[9]

Although NAHRS states that laboratory tests are optional, once histopathology confirms a cicatricial alopecia, it is important in black patients to obtain antinuclear antibodies, anti-Ro (SS-A) and anti-La (SS-B) antibodies, hemoglobin, and a white blood cell count to rule out underlying disease states such as lupus erythematosus. Other laboratories studies to consider include platelets, Venereal Disease Research Laboratory test (VDRL), Aspartate aminotransferase (AST), Alanine aminotransferase (ALT), bilirubin, alkaline phosphatase, erythrocyte sedimentation rate, and urinalysis, as indicated. If papules, pustules, or scaling is observed, a KOH, fungal or bacterial culture may reveal an undiagnosed infectious cause.[10]

Differential Diagnosis

- Perifolliculitis capitis abscedens et suffodiens (Dissecting cellulitis)
- Tinea capitis
- Lichen planopilaris
- Chronic cutaneous lupus
- Fibrosing alopecia
- Pseudopelade of Brocq
- End-stage cicatricial alopecia of various inflammatory alopecias
- Sarcoidosis
- Androgenetic alopecia
- Traction alopecia
- Diabetic scalp itch

Prognosis/Clinical Course

Many patients present with end-stage disease, and there is no definitive treatment regimen.

TABLE 35-2

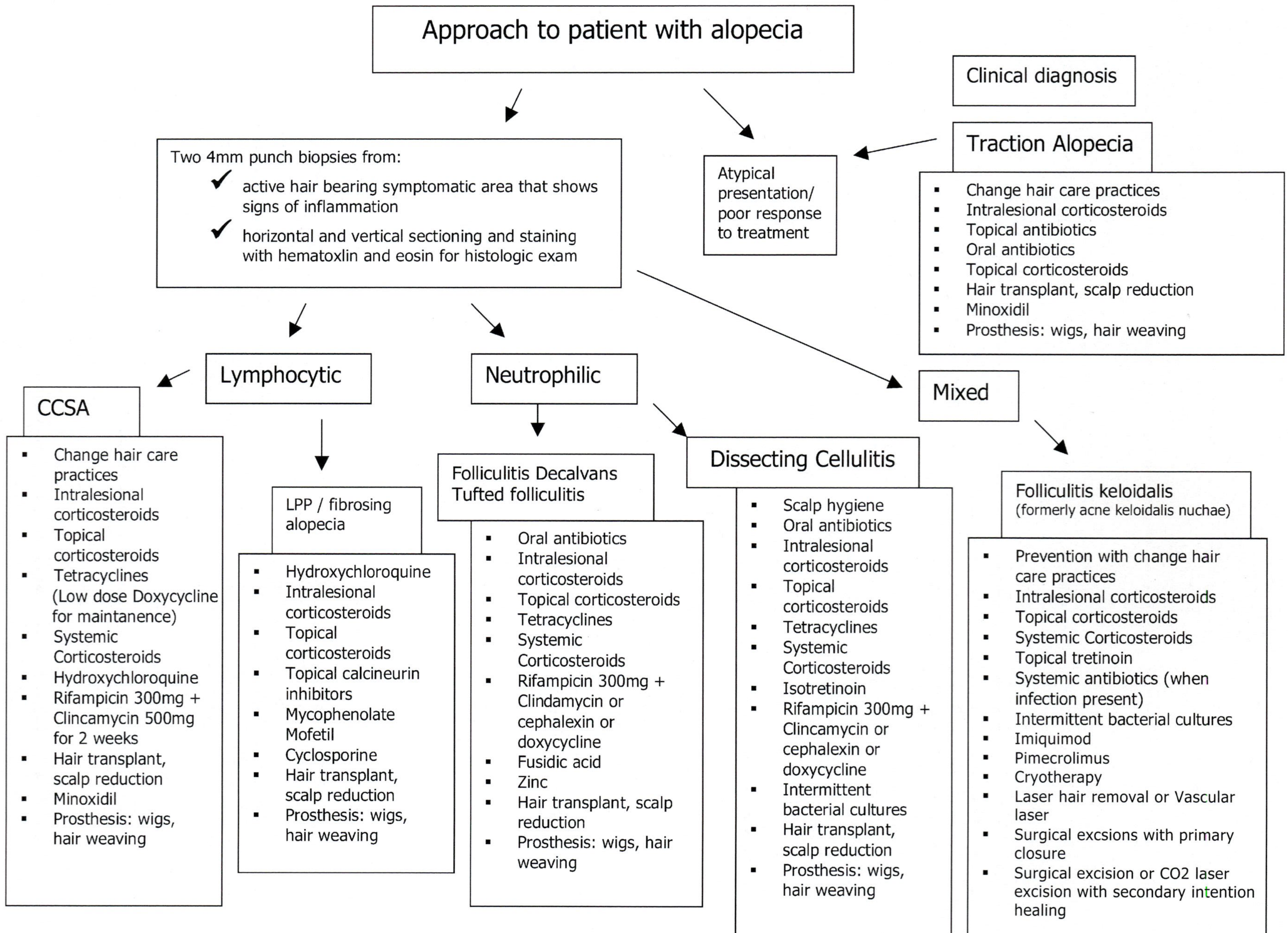

Approach to patient with alopecia
Two 4mm punch biopsies from:
active hair bearing symptomatic area that shows signs of inflammation
horizontal and vertical sectioning and staining with hematoxlin and eosin for histologic exam
Atypical presentation/ poor response to treatment
Clinical diagnosis
Traction Alopecia
Change hair care practices
Intralesional corticosteroids
Topical antibiotics
Oral antibiotics
Topical corticosteroids
Hair transplant, scalp reduction
Minoxidil
Prosthesis: wigs, hair weaving
Lymphocytic
Neutrophilic
Mixed
CCSA
Change hair care practices
Intralesional corticosteroids
Topical corticosteroids
Tetracyclines (Low dose Doxycycline for maintanence)
Systemic Corticosteroids
Hydroxychloroquine
Rifampicin 300mg + Clincamycin 500mg for 2 weeks
Hair transplant, scalp reduction
Minoxidil
Prosthesis: wigs, hair weaving
LPP / fibrosing alopecia
Hydroxychloroquine
Intralesional corticosteroids
Topical corticosteroids
Topical calcineurin inhibitors
Mycophenolate Mofetil
Cyclosporine
Hair transplant, scalp reduction
Prosthesis: wigs, hair weaving
Folliculitis Decalvans
Tufted folliculitis
Oral antibiotics
Intralesional corticosteroids
Topical corticosteroids
Tetracyclines
Systemic Corticosteroids
Rifampicin 300mg + Clindamycin or cephalexin or doxycycline
Fusidic acid
Zinc
Hair transplant, scalp reduction
Prosthesis: wigs, hair weaving
Dissecting Cellulitis
Scalp hygiene
Oral antibiotics
Intralesional corticosteroids
Topical corticosteroids
Tetracyclines
Systemic Corticosteroids
Isotretinoin
Rifampicin 300mg + Clincamycin or cephalexin or doxycycline
Intermittent bacterial cultures
Hair transplant, scalp reduction
Prosthesis: wigs, hair weaving
Folliculitis keloidalis
(formerly acne keloidalis nuchae)
Prevention with change hair care practices
Intralesional corticosteroids
Topical corticosteroids
Systemic Corticosteroids
Topical tretinoin
Systemic antibiotics (when infection present)
Intermittent bacterial cultures
Imiquimod
Pimecrolimus
Cryotherapy
Laser hair removal or Vascular laser
Surgical excsions with primary closure
Surgical excision or CO2 laser excision with secondary intention healing

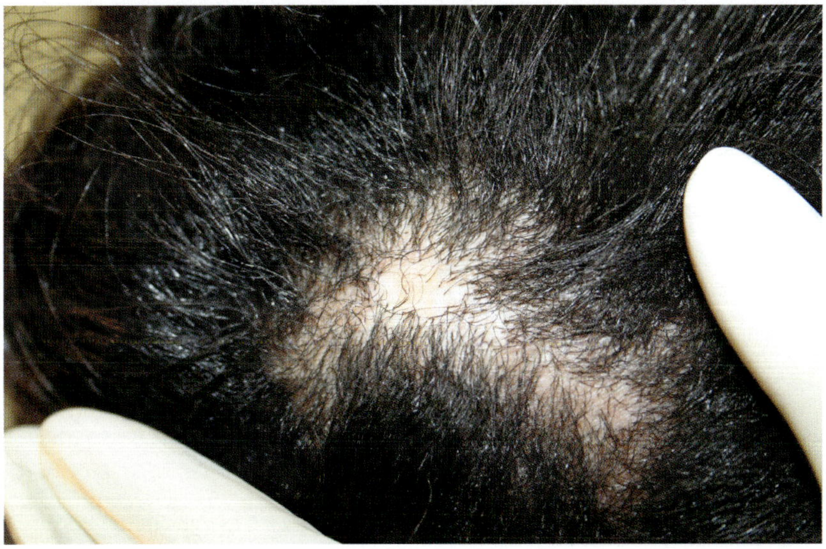

▲ **FIGURE 35-1** Early central centrifugal scarring alopecia.

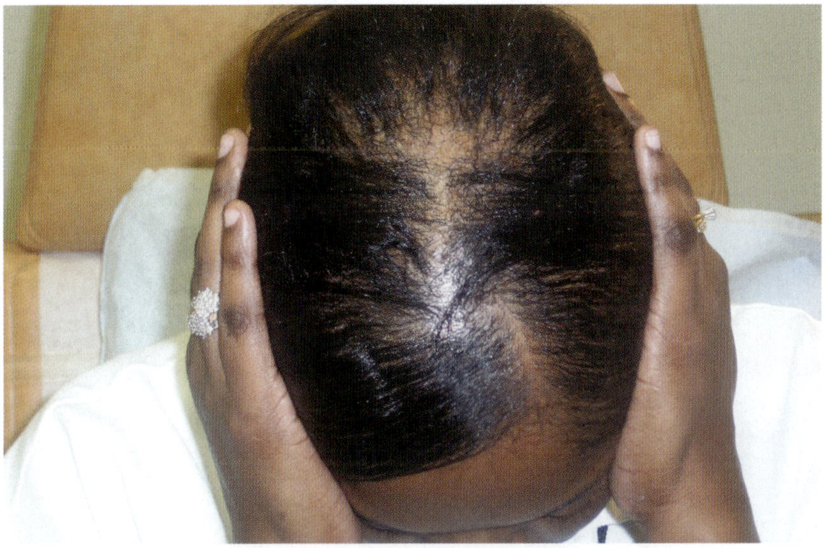

▲ **FIGURE 35-2** Moderate central centrifugal scarring alopecia.

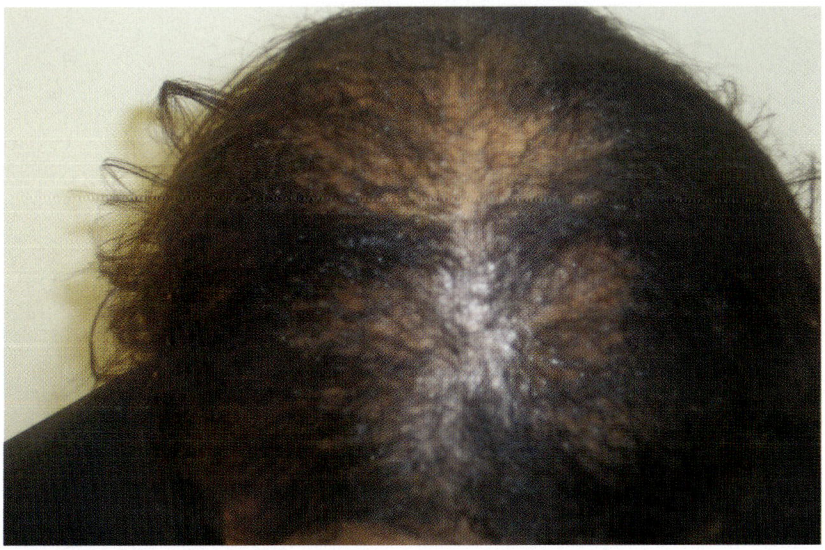

▲ **FIGURE 35-3** Late (end stage) central centrifugal scarring alopecia.

Treatment

Prospective, controlled studies are needed to aid in effective treatment regimens. Treatment recommendations for CCSA have been based on anecdotal reports. Price recommends treatment based on histopatologic classification (i.e., lymphocytic, neutrophilic, mixed).[3]

EARLY DISEASE Aggressive treatment is warranted in the early stage of CCSA to halt progression and salvage viable hair follicles. Intralesional scalp injections of triamcinolone (7.5–10 mg/mL) are helpful if tolerated by the patient (Figure 35-4). Low-dose doxycycline, 20–40 mg, has anti-inflammatory and antibacterial properties and can be useful with combination therapy.

Topical high-potency corticosteroids can be applied for 2 weeks and then tapered to middle-potency agents for maintenance (Dermasmooth/FS Scalp Oil, Hill Dermatceuticals, Sanford, FL, or Luxiq Foam). Foam-based vehicles have shown to be cosmetically acceptable in black patients.[11]

Rifampicin, 300 mg, can be paired with twice-daily cephalexin, 500 mg, for 2 weeks. Mupirocin cream and a high-potency topical steroid can be added for 4 weeks. Minoxidil may be added for maintenance.[12]

Sperling recommends a short tapering course of prednisone, oral tetracycline, and a potent topical corticosteroid for patients with CCSA and pustules.[13] Hydroxychloroquine, 200 mg twice daily, may be helpful in lymphocytic cicatricial alopecias. Patients should have liver function tests and a complete blood count. Retinal examination (baseline and every 3–6 months) should be performed while patients are on therapy.[3] Minoxidil can be helpful as an adjuvant agent to promote hair regrowth and extend the anagen phase in viable hairs.

END STAGE Hair transplants are an excellent option and should be offered to black patients when feasible. Patients should be medically managed and have stable disease for at least 6 months. A test area should be done with a 3- to 4-month wait time to evaluate response. Punch grafting for cicatricial alopecia is used to optimize follicle survival owing to less likely survival in scar tissue.[14] The risk of hypertrophic scars, keloids, and hyperpigmentation should be discussed with patients prior to surgery. The risk of keloids and hypertrophic scar can be reduced by prophylactic use a middle-

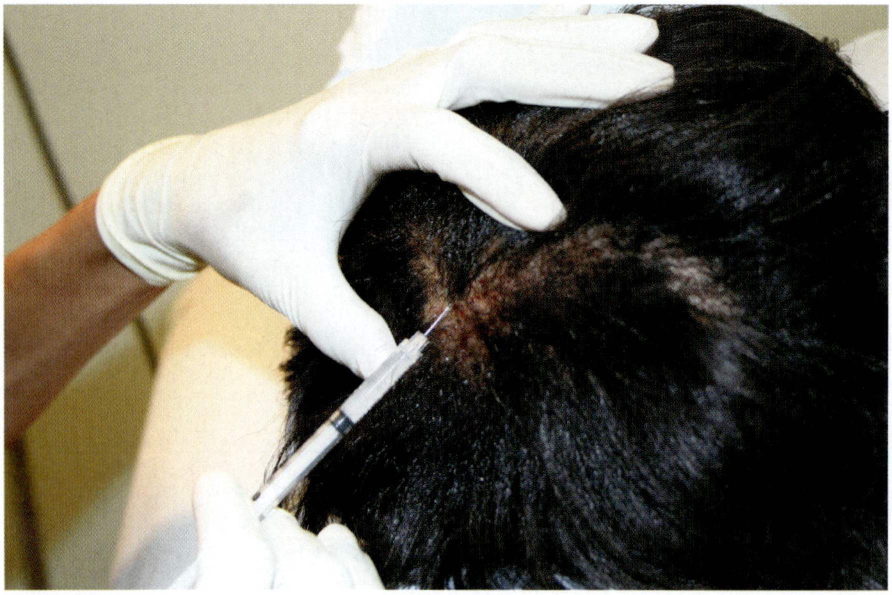

▲ **FIGURE 35-4** Intralesional scalp injection of triamcinolone acetate directly into scalp may halt progression in early disease.

potency corticosteroid immediately postoperatively and a 2-week course of high-potency corticosteroid after suture removal.[14]

Prevention

CCSA may be an end stage of some form of inflammatory disorder; therefore, prompt diagnosis is crucial. Minimize heat, oils, and greases applied directly or close to the scalp. Reduce the frequency of chemical relaxer use to every 6–8 weeks or discontinue entirely.

FOLLICULITIS KELOIDALIS

Synonyms

- Acne keloidalis nuchae
- Acne keloidalis
- Dermatitis papillaris capillitii
- Folliculitis keloidalis nuchae
- Sycosis nuchae
- Acne keloid
- Keloidal folliculitis
- Lichen keloidalis nuchae
- Folliculitis nuchae scleroticans
- Sycosis framboesiformis

Epidemiology, Etiology, and Pathogenesis

Folliculitis keloidalis (FK) was first described by Kaposi as *dermatitis papillaris capillitii,* and later Bazin coined the name *acne keloidalis nuchae.*[19,20] No known cause of FK has been elucidated. FK is an acute folliculitis and perifolliculitis that becomes chronic and progresses into a primary cicatricial alopecia occurring most commonly in black men after puberty.[15] FK represents 0.45–0.7% of dermatoses affecting patients of African origin.[15,16] The female:male ratio is 20:1.[15,17,18] Onset prior to puberty or after age 50 years is extremely rare.[15] There has been one case report of familial acne keloidalis nuchae, and one study found that 15% of FK patients had a family history of FK.[21,22]

Precipitation factors in FK include constant irritation from shirt collars, chronic low-grade folliculitits, seborrhea, hair grooming techniques, and cyclosporine use following organ transplantation.[23,24] Diphenylhydantoin and carbamazepine can produce FK-like lesions that resolve at cessation of therapy (Figures 35-5 and 35-6).

Clinical Findings

HISTORY The typical patient describes lesions that began after a close hair cut or appeared gradually in the occipital scalp and posterior part of the neck. A thorough history should include duration of disease, frequency of flares, past therapeutic treatments and response, hair grooming techniques, use of helmets, and any known allergies.[15]

PHYSICAL EXAMINATION Clinically, examination shows firm, dome-shaped follicular and perifollicular papules on the nape of the neck and occipital scalp (Figures 35-6). With time, the papules may coalesce into keloidal plaques with a bandlike distribution at or below the posterior hairline (Figure 35-7). Alopecia and polytrichia are common. Comedones and acneiform lesions are not present. Acne keloidalis nuchae is a misnomer because there is no acne present, no formation of true keloids, and the condition can involve the entire scalp, leading to permanent alopecia[25,26] (Figure 35-8).

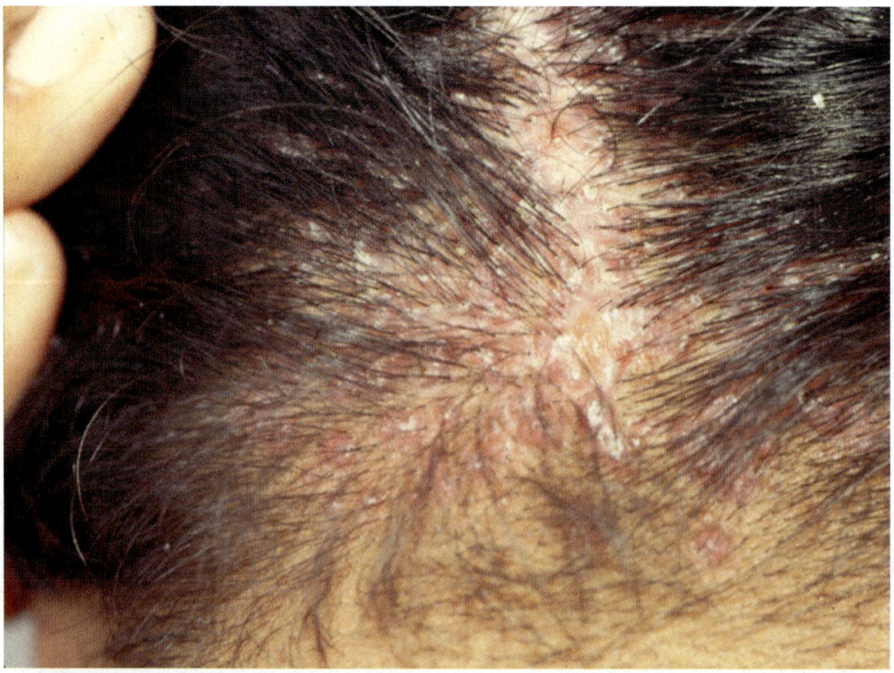

▲ **FIGURE 35-5** Hispanic patient on antiepileptic medication (diphenylhydantoin) showing folliculitis keloidalis.

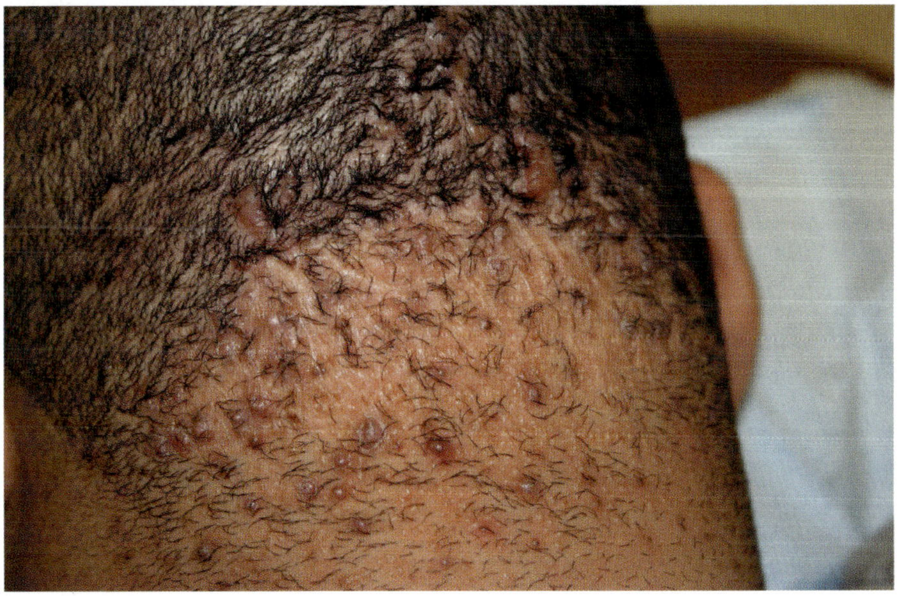

▲ **FIGURE 35-6** Folliculitis keloidalis in a male patient of Caucasian and black descent.

LABORATORY AND OTHER TESTS Bacterial cultures and sensitivities from any pustular or draining lesions should be taken intermittently. If pathogens are present, appropriate antibiotics should be prescribed. KOH with fungal culture and assessment for cervical lymphadenopathy should be performed as clinically indicated and for nonresponsive cases.[27] Histopathologic evaluation is recommended for atypical presentations. Early papular lesions show chronic lymphocytic folliculitis.[4]

Differential Diagnosis

- Perifolliculitis capitis abscedens et suffodiens (dissecting cellulitis)
- Tinea capitis
- Hidradenitis suppurativa
- Acne vulgaris
- Acneiform eruptions
- Folliculitis
- Seborrheic dermatitis
- Regular keloids (when history of trauma exists)
- Folliculitis decalvans-dissecting cellulitis
- Pomade/oil folliculitis
- Pediculosis capitis
- Pseudofolliculitis barbae

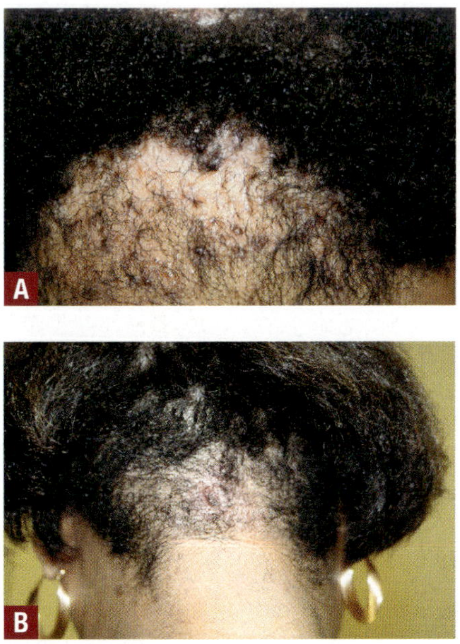

▲ **FIGURE 35-7** *A.* Female patient with bandlike distribution of keloidalis folliculits. *B.* Female patient with folliculitis keloidalis and secondary infection.

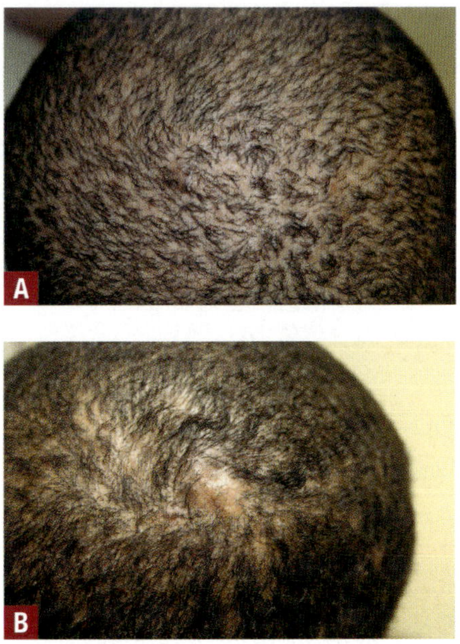

▲ **FIGURE 35-8** *A.* Folliculitis keloidalis involving the entire scalp. *B.* Keloidal scar at vertex scalp with long-term disease.

Complications

- Secondary infection
- Disfiguring keloids
- Extension of disease

Prognosis/Clinical Course

Large lesions can be painful and cosmetically unacceptable. Abscess and sinus formation are possible and may emit a foul odor. Coexistence of other forms of cicatricial alopecia may be observed.

Treatment (Table 35-3)

MEDICAL There is no one therapeutic modality that cures FK. In fact, a combination of treatments seems to be most effective in patients with FK. Systemic corticosteroids will stop the lesional activity and cause a partial or complete regression of any lesions. Long-term side effects and lack of sustained cure limit the efficacy of this treatment approach.

Superpotent corticosteroid gel or foam (Olux Foam, Connetics Corp, Palo Alto, CA) can be applied twice a day for 2 weeks and then tapered to a middle-potency agent (Luxiq Foam, Connetics Corp, Palo Alto, CA) for maintenance.[28] Newer spray formulations may be helpful.

Kelly suggests that retinoic acid (Retin-A, Tazorac), and a class 2 or 3 corticosteroid cream or gel base may be more effective than class 1 or 2 corticosteroids alone.[15] Newer corticosteroids in

TABLE 35-3
Treatment of Keloidalis Folliculitis (FK)/ Acne Keloidalis Nuchae

- No one therapeutic modality will cure FK.
- Superpotent corticosteroid gel or foam.
- Retin-A, Tazorac, and a class II–III corticosteroid.
- If infection suspected, start topical clindamycin foam, gel, or lotion.
- For abscesses and draining sinuses course of prednisone and antibiotics.
- Imiquimod (Aldara).
- Intralesional steroid injections.
- Laser therapy—CO_2, Nd:YAG, or diode.
- Adjunctive laser hair removal.
- Cryotherapy

a foam or spray vehicle may be more cosmetically acceptable than creams.

When pustules or infection is suspected, topical clindamycin (foam, gel, or lotion) should be applied twice daily until the lesions subside. If there is no improvement, a bacterial culture and appropriate systemic antibiotics should be initiated. Large abscesses or draining sinuses may require a short course (7–10 days) of oral prednisone given concomitantly with systemic antibiotics. Imiquimod (Aldara) cream monotherapy for 5 days and then 2 days off for 8 weeks or in combination with pimecrolimus can be effective.[29,30]

Intralesional steroid injections (10–40 mg/mL) administered directly into papules and plaques at 4- to 6-week intervals can be effective.[31] Patients should be warned that the injection sites may become hypopigmented, which may remain for 6–12 months. Injections are easier if the papules are electrodesiccated and curetted first. An application of lidocaine-prilocaine cream or other topical anesthetic mixture under plastic film occlusion 2 hours prior to injection decreases the pain of injections.

Laser therapy (carbon dioxide, Nd:YAG, or diode) has been successful for some patients. Postoperative intralesional triamcinolone injections (10 mg/mL every 2–3 weeks) help to prevent recurrence.[32]

Adjunctive laser hair removal for FK is used to the destroy the tufted hair and minimize scarring. The hair removal laser can reduce growth and inflammation, and hair density will be permanently reduced.[33–35] A combination approach with vascular laser treatment following extensive excision may decrease recurrence.[36]

Cryotherapy also has proven to be successful in some patients. The area is frozen for 20 seconds, allowed to thaw, and then is frozen again a minute later. The morbidity (discomfort and drainage) is greater than with other modalities, and the treated site often becomes hypopigmented and may remain so for 12–18 months. When the thaw time is more than 25 seconds, melanocytes are destroyed, and the treated area often becomes hypopigmented, especially in patients with dark skin.[15]

SURGICAL Excision with primary closure is a surgical treatment modality for the management of extensive cases of FK, and extremely large lesions should be excised in multiple stages.[37] Kelly recommends a horizontal ellipse for excision of larger linear lesions (1 cm or less in diameter) with primary closure. The base of the excision should extend below the hair follicles, and closure of the postoperative site should be done with 4-0 silk sutures[15,30] (Figure 35-9).

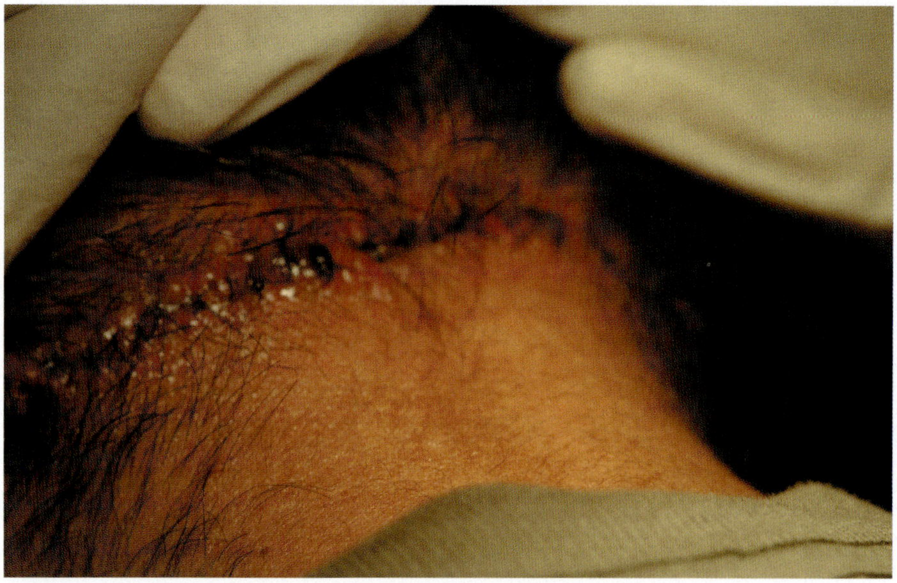

▲ **FIGURE 35-9** Excision with primary closure of folliculitis keloidalis.

Excision with second-intention healing is an excellent option for large lesions that do not respond to medical therapy[38,39] (Figures 35-10 through 35-12). A CO_2 laser in cutting mode has been successful in excising large plaques. Care must be taken to cut below the level of the hair follicles to the deep subcutaneous tissue, and the wound is left to heal by second intention.[40,41] Excision with grafting is not as cosmetically acceptable and is not recommended.[15]

Prevention

The first line of therapy is prevention. Patients should be counseled on preventative measures. Avoidance of close shaving at the hairline, tight-fitting shirts, helmets, or other possible irritation to the scalp is essential to prevent disease progression. As with all cicatricial alopecias, prompt and aggressive treatment should be initiated to prevent loss of viable hair follicles and to lower the chance of developing larger lesions.

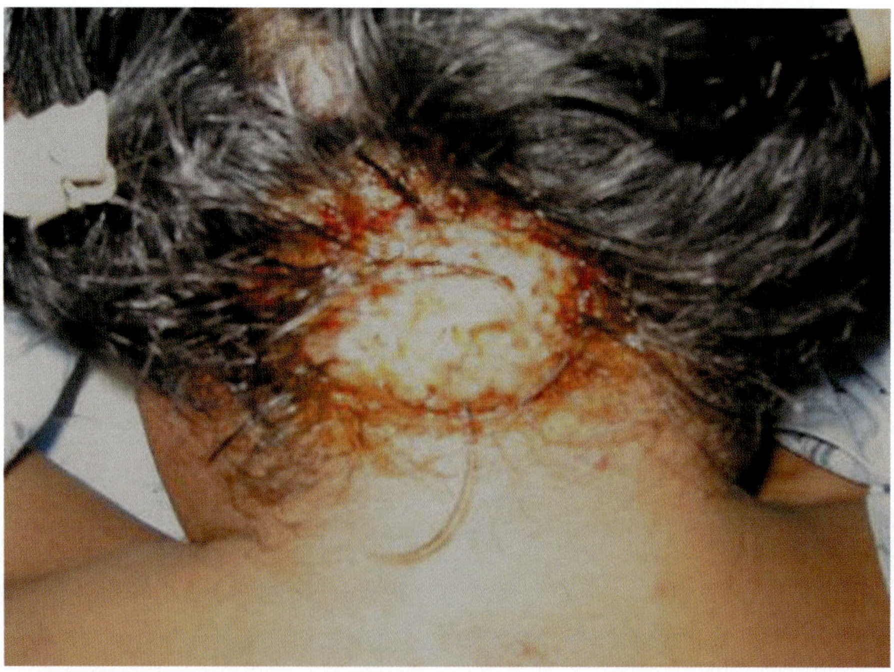

▲ **FIGURE 35-10** Excision and secondary-intention healing (preoperative).

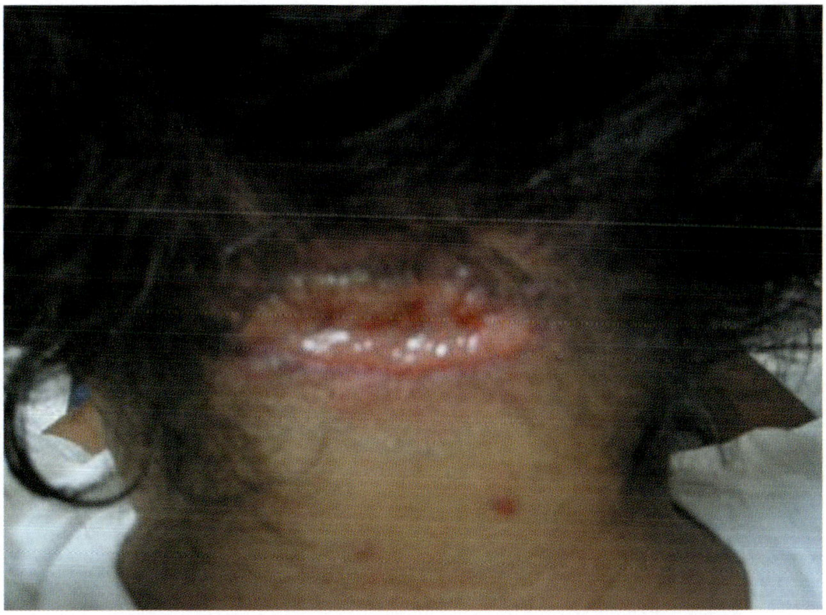

▲ **FIGURE 35-11** Excision and secondary-intention healing (4 weeks postoperatively).

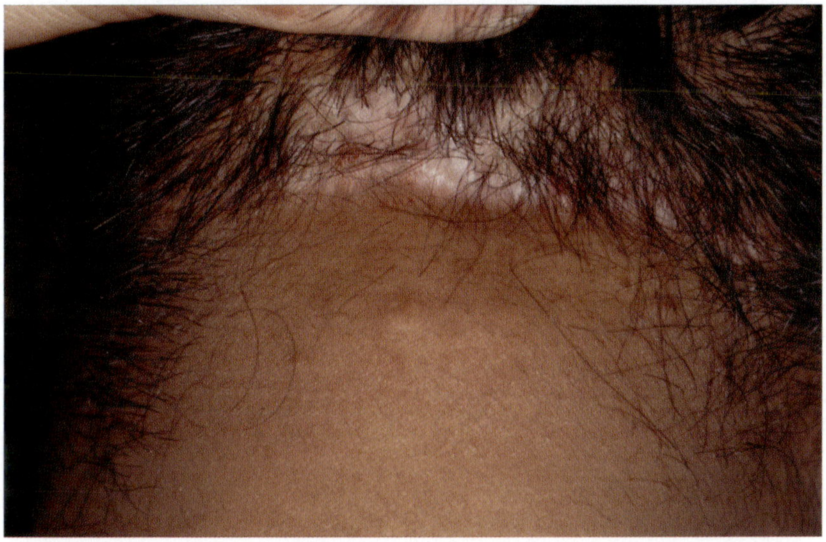

▲ **FIGURE 35-12** Excision and secondary-intention healing (4 months postoperatively).

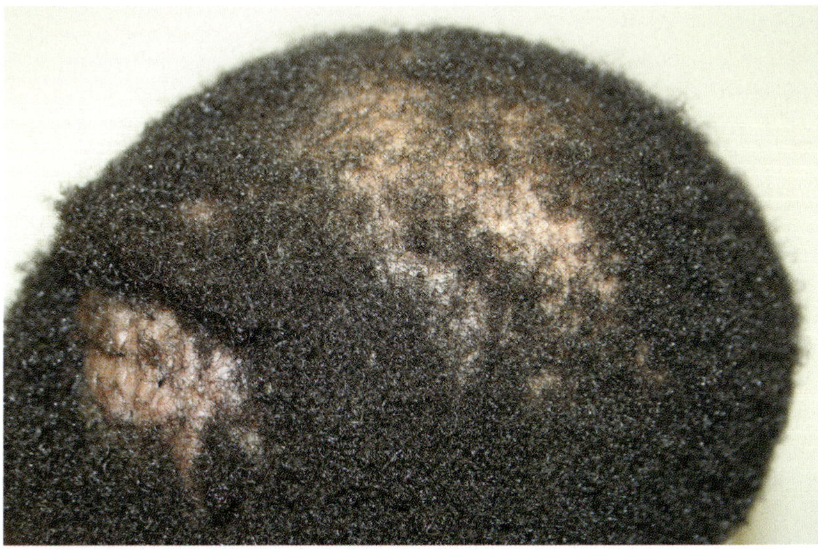

▲ **FIGURE 35-13** Dissecting cellulitis of the scalp.

DISSECTING CELLULITIS OF THE SCALP

Synonyms

- Perifolliculitis capitis abscedens et suffodiens
- Hoffman disease

Epidemiology, Etiology, and Pathogenesis

Most commonly seen in black men in the second to fourth decades, although occasionally seen in females, Hispanics, Caucasians, and Asians, this is a chronic inflammatory disorder of the scalp.[42,43] There is an association with acne conglobata and hidradenitis suppurativa, known collectively as the *follicular occlusion triad*. The common pathogenesis is a destruction of hair follicles and hair follicle retention.

Clinical Findings

HISTORY/PHYSICAL EXAMINATION Dissecting cellulitis is characterized by painful nodules, purulent discharge, burrowing interconnecting abscesses, and cicatricial alopecia. Boggy areas with pustules, nodules, discharging swellings, and patchy hair loss are seen (Figure 35-13). Cerebriform configurations can be a late-term result resembling cutis verticis gyrata.

LABORATORY AND OTHER TESTS Bacterial cultures and sensitivity from any pustular or draining lesions should be taken intermittently. If pathogens are present, appropriate antibiotics should be prescribed. Fungal culture and assessment for cervical lymphadenopathy should be done.

Differential Diagnosis

- Tinea capitis
- Hidradenitis suppurativa
- Folliculitis
- Folliculitis decalvans
- Pomade/oil folliculitis
- Cutis verticis gyrata

Complications

Hair loss can become permanent, and hypertrophic scars and keloids can develop on the scalp. With the chronic inflammation, there is a risk for Marjolins ulcers. Other possible complications include

- Acne conglobata
- Hidradenitis suppurativa
- Tufted folliculitis

Treatment

- Topical corticosteroids
- Intralesional corticosteroids
- Systemic corticosteroids[44]
- Antibiotics
- Dapsone
- Isotretinoin[45,46]
- Oral zinc[43]
- External-beam radiation–induced epilation
- Incision and drainage
- Laser-assisted hair epilation
- CO_2 laser[47]
- Wide surgical excision with split-thickness grafting[48]

Prevention

Scalp hygiene for mild to limited cases and prompt treatment to salvage viable hair follicles constitute prevention strategies.

FOLLICULITIS DECALVANS AND TUFTED FOLLICULITIS

Epidemiology, Etiology, and Pathogenesis

Folliculitis decalvans is a form of recurrent, patchy, painful folliculitis of the scalp causing scarring and hair loss. *Staphylococcus aureus* has been implicated as an etiologic agent.[49] Sperling and colleagues contend that pustules of folliculitis decalvans are a manifestation of either bacterial superinfection or an intense immune response to degenerating follicular components.[50] Prospective, double-blinded studies have not been performed and are needed to quell the debate.

Tufted folliculitis (TF) is an inflammatory scalp disorder characterized by tufting of hair within areas of scarring alopecia and is considered a variant of folliculitis decalvans. TF can be a nonspecific process after a variety of inflammatory scalp conditions. *S. aureus* and nonpathogenic organisms nearly always can be grown from the pustules.[49,51] Tufts of hair with patches of alopecia are commonly associated with other forms of cicatricial alopecia. TF is common in African-American patients with various types of inflammatory alopecias and may be considered an end-stage result.

Clinical Findings

PHYSICAL EXAMINATION Tufted folliculitis is located predominately in the parietal and occipital scalp and presents with an inflamed scalp. Early lesions consist of small areas of perifollicular erythema and pustules. The process extends centrifugally, resulting in patches of cicatrical alopecia. Fully developed lesions consist of tufts of hair with 8–14 hairs emerging from an apparently common dilated follicular opening[52] (Figure 35-14).

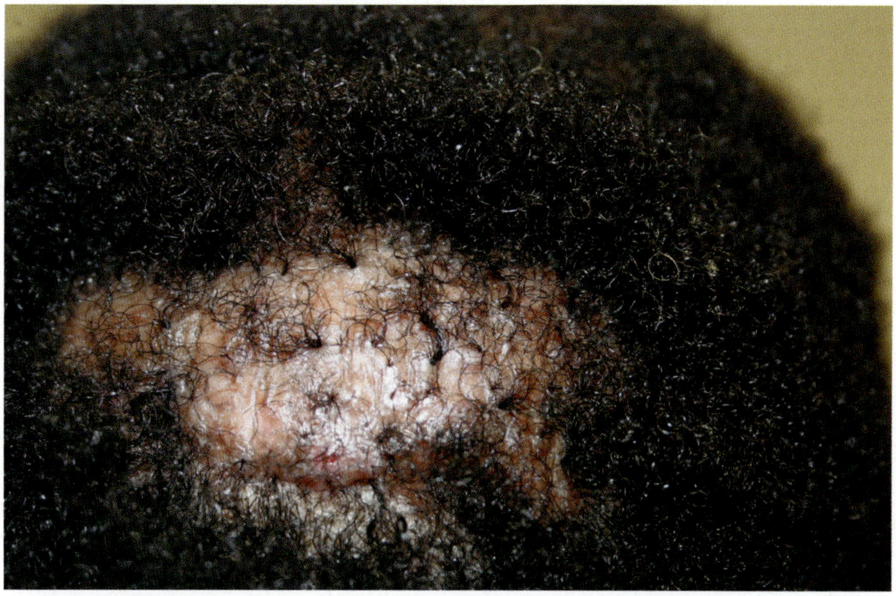

▲ **FIGURE 35-14** Tufted folliculitis. Fully developed lesions have up to 8–14 hairs emerging from an apparently common dilated follicular opening.

LABORATORY AND OTHER TESTS Bacterial cultures and sensitivity should be performed when pustules are present. KOH and fungal cultures should be performed from noninflamed site at baseline if nonresponsive to therapy and prior to use of systemic corticosteroids.

Differential Diagnosis

- Kerion (tinea capitis)
- Dissecting cellulitis
- Folliculitis
- Folliculitis decalvans
- Acne keloidalis nuchae (folliculitis keloidalis)
- Lichen planopilaris (follicular)

Complications

- Secondary infection with abscesses and draining sinuses
- Disfiguring keloids
- Cicatricial alopecia
- Tufted folliculitis

Prognosis/Clinical Course

Treatment, as in most cicatricial alopecias, is difficult. Patients should be counseled that there is no permanent eradication of the disease.

Treatment

Twice-daily oral rifampicin, 300 mg, and twice-daily oral clindamycin, 300 mg, for 10 weeks have been shown to lead to significant improvement and no further extension of lesions.[3] Patients treated with clindamycin should be warned about pseudomembranous colitis. Owing to the rapid emergence of resistance, it is not advisable to use rifampicin alone.[49] Clindamycin may be substituted with oral ciprofloxacin, 750 mg twice daily, or cephalexin, 500 mg four times daily, or doxycycline, 100 mg twice daily, along with rifampicin.[3] Those who are staphylococcus carriers should have their nasal area treated with mupirocin.[3] Fusidic acid and zinc have been reported to be effective in a limited number of patients.[53]

Prevention

Scalp hygiene for mild to limited cases and prompt treatment to salvage viable hair follicles are prevention strategies.

LICHEN PLANOPILARIS AND FIBROSING ALOPECIA

Synonyms

- Follicular lichen planus (LP)
- Lichen planus acuminatus

Epidemiology, Etiology, and Pathogenesis

Lichen planopilaris and its clinical variants have not been noted to be increased in black patients in the literature. It is

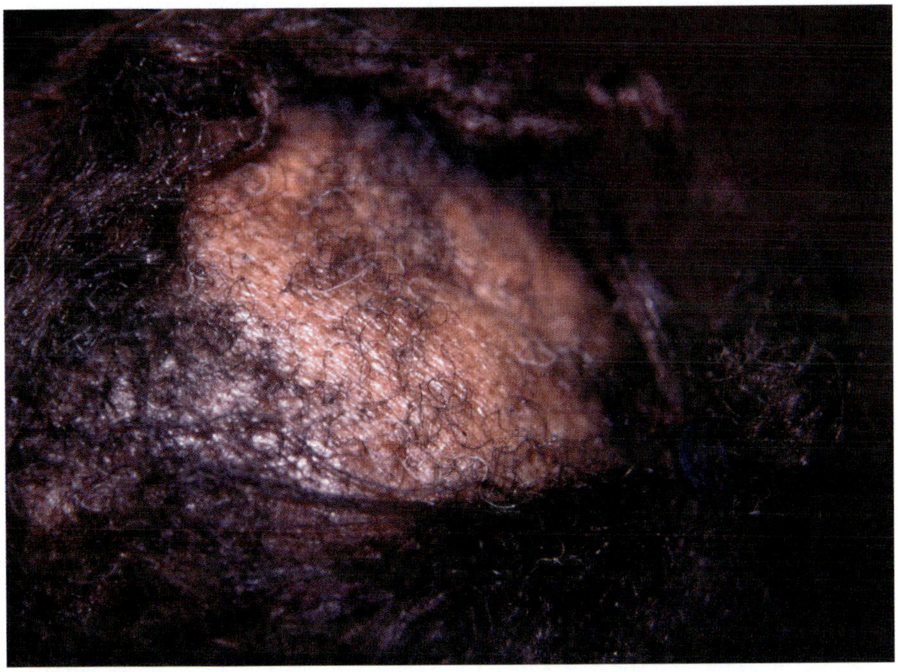

▲ **FIGURE 35-15** Lichen planopilaris. Patient had no systemic findings of lichen planus.

important to mention, owing to the clinical findings, that this disease is closely associated with CCSA and the continued evolution of cicatricial alopecia.

Clinical Findings

PHYSICAL EXAMINATION Cicatricial scalp alopecia, scaling, atrophy, and permanent alopecia with scarring are clinical findings on physical examination (Figure 35-15) Frontal fibrosing alopecia is characterized by a band of frontal/frontoparietal hair alopecia and a marked decrease or complete loss of the eyebrows (Figure 35-16). There is controversy regarding postmenopausal presentation and response to antiandrogens.

LABORATORY AND OTHER TESTS

- Histopathologic examination
- Hepatitis panel

Differential Diagnosis

- Central centrifugal scarring alopecia
- Chronic cutaneous lupus
- Pseudopelade of Brocq
- End-stage cicatricial alopecia of various inflammatory alopecias
- Sarcoidosis
- Androgenetic alopecia
- Traction alopecia
- Diabetic scalp itch

Prognosis/Clinical Course

Many patients develop hair, nail, and/or mucous membrane lesions similar to lichen planopilaris lesions. The lesions may involute spontaneously or go on for years. Mehregan and colleagues reported that the average duration is 18 months.[53a]

Treatment

High-potency topical and intralesional corticosteroids are the mainstay of treatment for primary symptoms and have a positive effect on hair regrowth in the active perimeter of the alopecic patch.[54]

- Tetracycline antibiotics
- Hydroxychloroquine 200 mg twice daily[3]
- Mycophenolate mofetil 0.5 g twice daily and increased to 1 g twice daily for 5 months[3]
- Cyclosporine 3–5 mg/kg per day (usually 300 mg/day)[3,55]
- Finasteride (2.5 mg/day) showed an arrest in the progression of the disease in frontal fibrosing alopecia.[56]
- Thalidomide[57]
- In inactive stage, scalp reduction and hair transplants can be employed.

BIPHASIC ALOPECIAS

With biphasic alopecia, nonscarring hair loss occurs in the early course of the disease, but permanenet hair loss becomes apparent in the later stages.[50]

Traction Alopecia

Traction alopecia (TA) is seen in black men, women, and children (Figure 35-17). TA is a common biphasic alopecia with a temporary noncicatricial phase, but if excessive traction is maintained for extended periods of time, the hair loss may become permanent.[4]

Epidemiology, Etiology, and Pathogenesis

Weaves, braids, chignons, cornrows, rubber band use, and other styles can predispose patients to traction. African-American hair styling techniques can

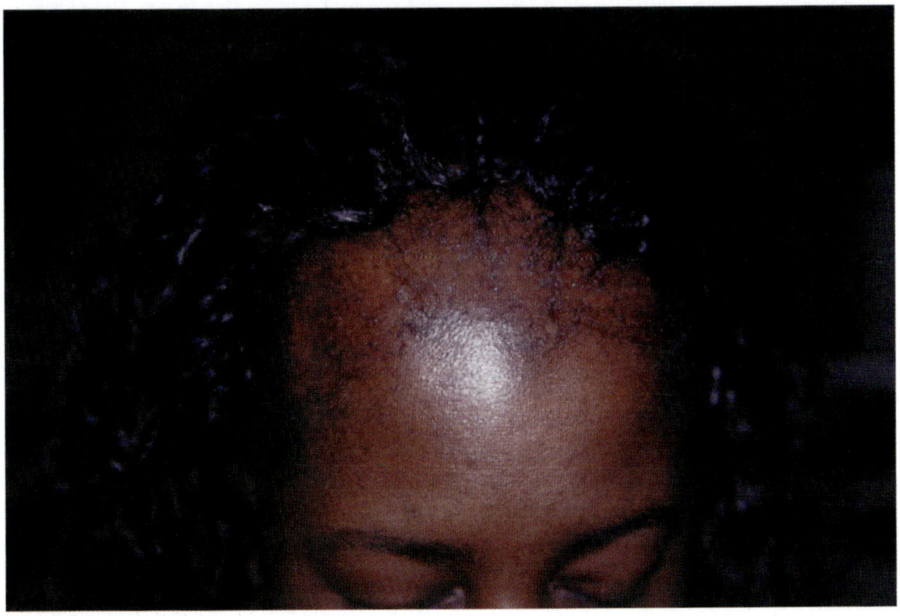

▲ **FIGURE 35-16** Frontal fribosing alopecial is a clinical variant of lichen planopilaris.

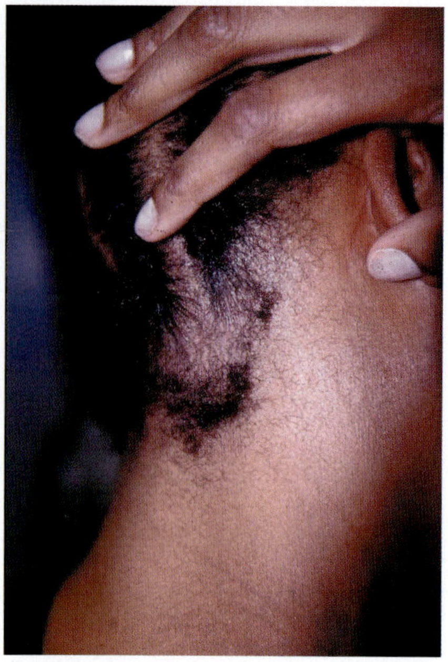

▲ **FIGURE 35-17** Early traction alopecia in a child.

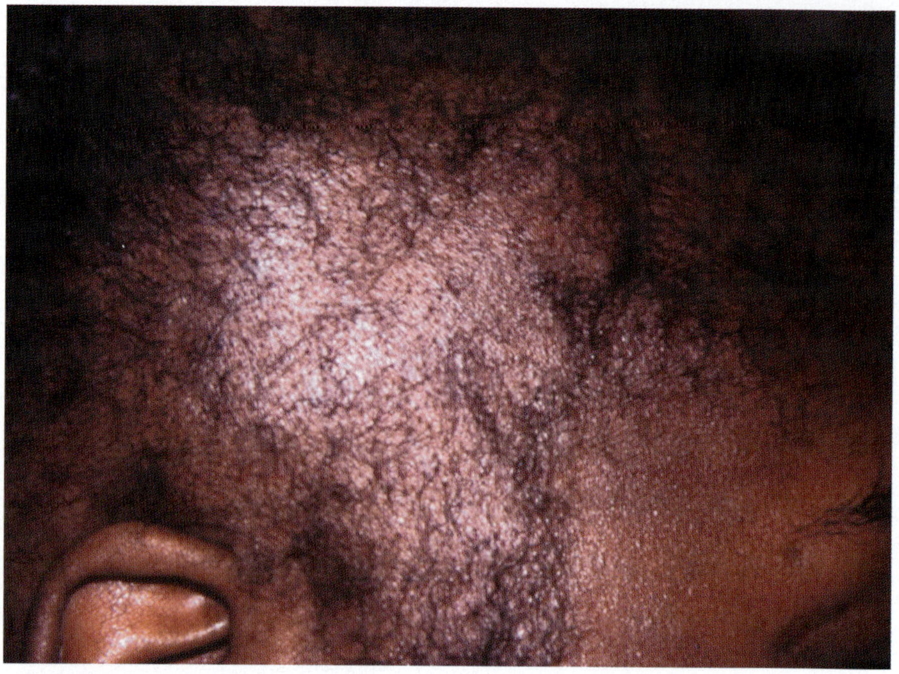

▲ **FIGURE 35-18** Late traction alopecia.

predispose this population to hair shaft damage from traction.[58,59] Early disease presents as a folliculitis and, if the traction is sustained, can progresses to cicatricial alopecia.[60]

Clinical Findings

PHYSICAL EXAMINATION Perifollicular papules and pustules may be present at symmetric areas of traction. The bitemporal area is described most commonly (Figure 35-18). The entire scalp may be involved, and this is dictated by the hair styling technique. Hair casts can be seen with severe cases of traction, and vellus hairs are spared (Figure 35-19).

HISTOPATHOLOGY The acute stage is reversible and resembles a mild form of trichotillomania.[32,61] Fibrosis in the area where terminal follicles were located with a normal number of vellus hairs is considered diagnostic for irreversible (late) TA.[27]

Differential Diagnosis

- Ophiasis (alopecia areata)
- Androgenetic hair loss (female- and male-pattern hair loss)
- CCCA
- Tinea capitis

Treatment

Counsel patients on easing traction and avoiding styles that promote traction. Topical antibiotics (clindamycin lotion) with a topical corticosteroid can be used for early papule lesions.

- Oral antibiotics
- Topical minoxidil
- Intralesional corticosteroids

Follicular unit transplantation, rotation flaps, minigrafting, and micrografting are therapeutic options[60,62] (Figures 35-20 and 35-21).

Prevention

Educating patients on avoiding hair care practices that promote tension can be curative if the process is caught in early stages. Avoid traction and increase the frequency of hair washing to every 1–2 weeks.

Androgenetic Alopecia (Male/female Pattern Hair Loss)

African-American men may display different hair-loss patterns than Caucasion men. It has been observed that black men predominantly exhibit scalp hair loss on the vertex of the scalp. A cicatricial alopecia presentation in black men may be due to the biphasic nature or follicular dropout of pattern hair loss; this also can be an undiagnosed primary cicatricial alopecia.

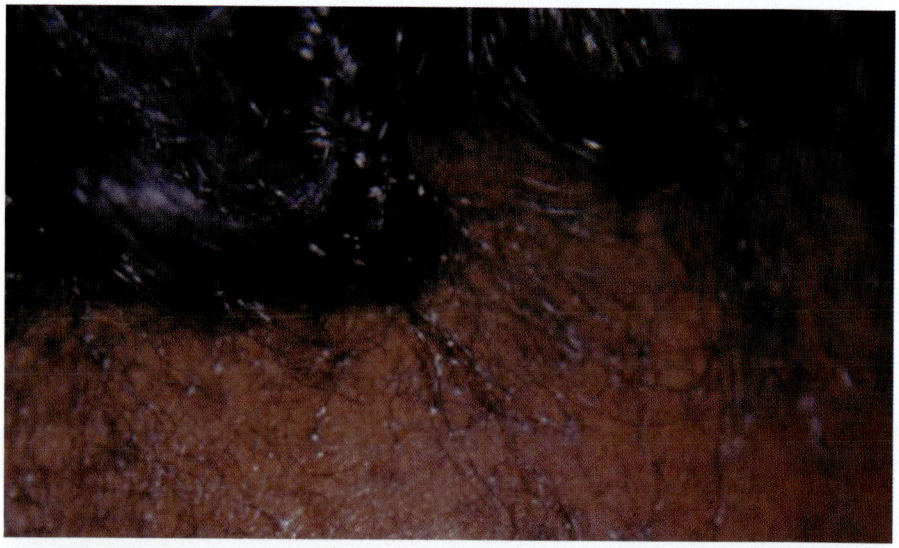

▲ **FIGURE 35-19** Peribulbar casts with extreme traction. Vellus hairs are attached to braid/weave styles, worsening alopecia and contributing to complete hair loss.

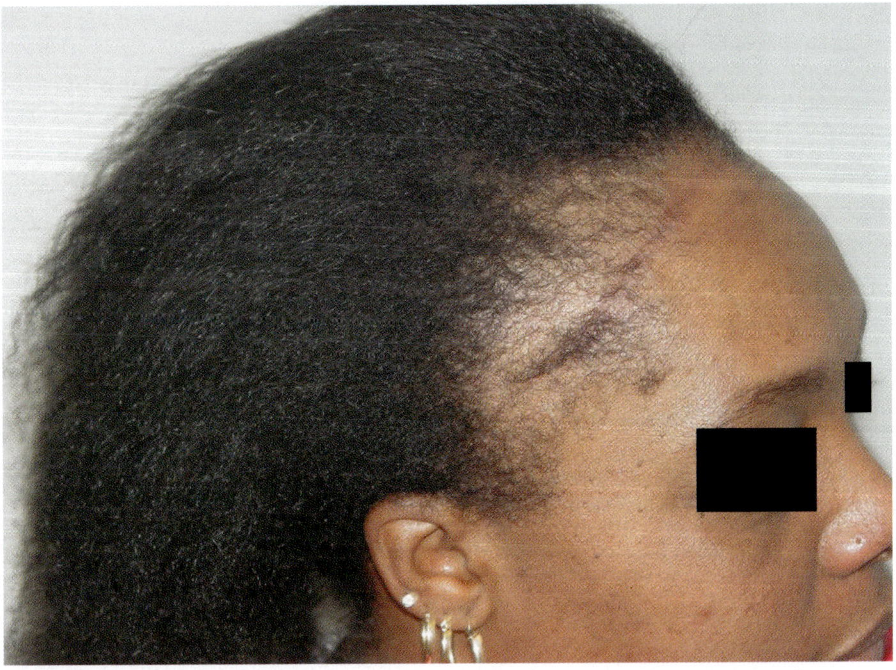

▲ **FIGURE 35-20** Hair transplant for traction alopecia (before). Courtesy of Craig Ziering, MD.

LIPEDEMATOUS ALOPECIA

Epidemiology, Etiology, and Pathogenesis

This is a rare condition of scalp thickening described predominately in black women. The subcutaneous layer is characterized by a boggy scalp with areas of alopecia. High and colleagues speculate that some cases of lipedematous alopecia might represent an unusual late sequela of discoid lupus erythematosus (DLE).[63]

Clinical Findings

PHYSICAL EXAMINATION Lipedematous alopecia begins at the vertex and extends peripherally for 2–10 years before stabilizing.[64] A thick, spongy scalp that results in shortening of hair and variable degrees of diffuse hair loss characterizes the disorder. Paresthesia, itching, and epidermal atrophy can be seen.[65]

LABORATORY FINDINGS Scalp thickness is measured by different techniques, such as introducing a needle, radiographic examination, computed tomography, head ultrasound, and magnetic resonance imaging [increased scalp thickness ranges from 0.9–1.5 cm (normal range 0.5–0.6 cm)].[66,67]

Treatment

Systemic corticosteroids may be effective.[63]

CHRONIC CUTANEOUS LUPUS AND SARCOIDOSIS

Sarcoidosis and lupus erythematosus occur more frequently in black women and are a cause of secondary alopecia (noncicatricial and cicatricial) (Figure 35-22). The incidence of alopecia areata in patients with lupus erythematosus is increased.[68]

Although rare, most reported cases occurred in African-American women. Cutaneous involvement may occur in as many as 25% of cases of systemic sarcoidosis.[69] Scalp sarcoidosis is of variable morphology and may exhibit plaques or nodules of the scalp as well as both cicatricial and noncicatricial alopecia.[69]

Treatment

Treatment for systemic sarcoidosis and lupus is oral glucorticosteroids, and for localized cutaneous disease, topical or intralesional corticosteroids can be very effective. Hydoxychloroquine and other systemic agents such as azathioprine, chlorambucil, methotrexate, and cyclosporine have been used with varying results.

Prevention

Patient with lupus should be counseled regarding photoprotection and sunblock. Tobacco use should be avoided while on hydroxychloroquine therapy.

ADDENDUM

Scalp biopsy is essential for diagnosis in black patients with hair loss. Many dermatologists are reluctant to perform scalp biopsies, and therefore, many alopecias are treated without biopsy-proven pathology.[70]

The NAHRS Workshop is an excellent resource to consult in the initial workup of a patient with suspected cicatricial alopecia. Patients are required to avoid or change hair styles that limit access and should get a full clinical examination of the scalp.

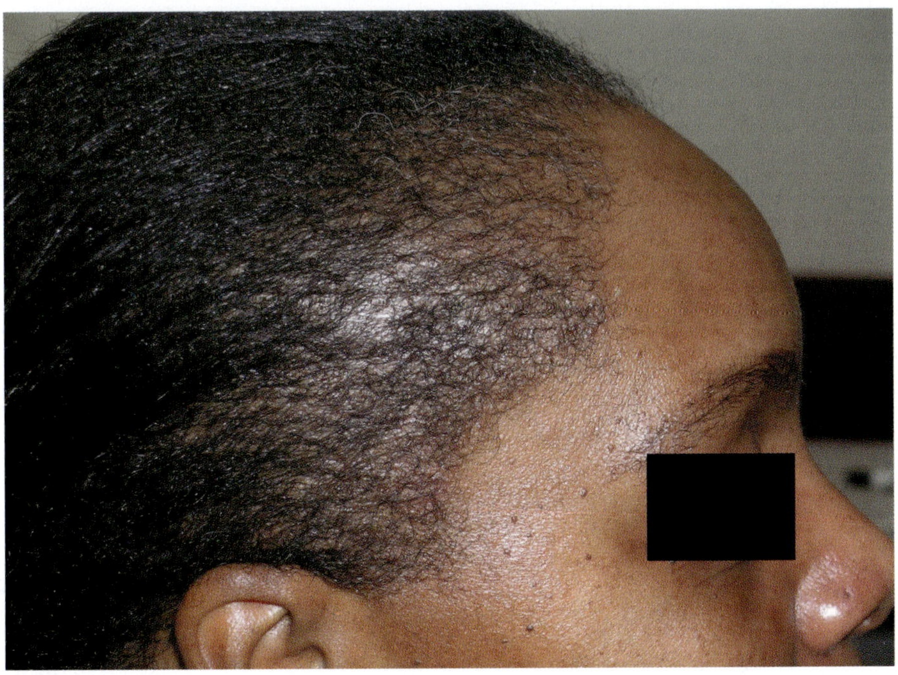

▲ **FIGURE 35-21** Hair transplant for traction alopecia (after). Courtesy of Craig Ziering, MD.

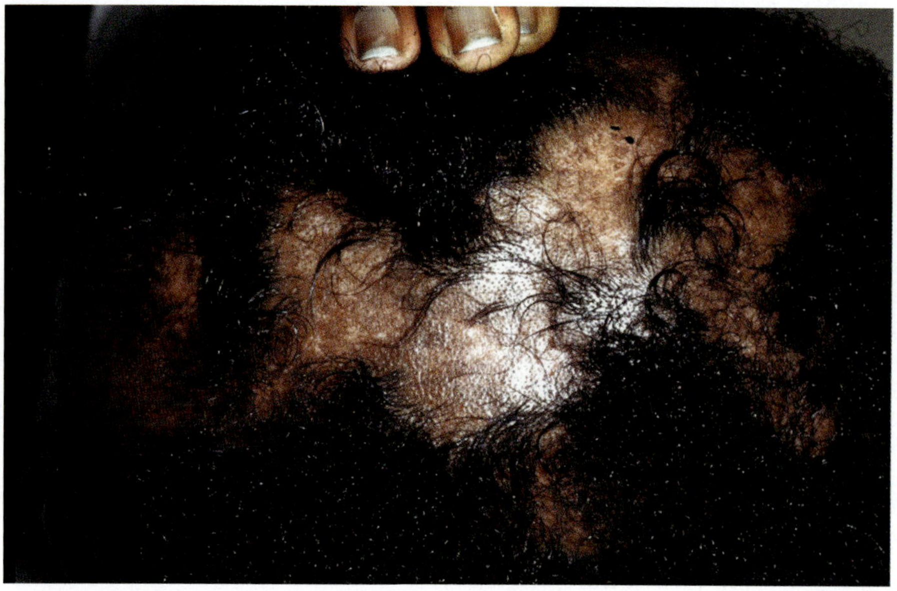

▲ **FIGURE 35-22** Scarring alopecia in a black woman with discoid lupus erythematosus.

Procedure

The areas to be biopsied should be marked with a blue or red China marker. Hairs within the 4-mm field should be clipped (do not shave).[70] Lidocaine 1% with epinephrine 1:1,000,000 is injected with a 30-gauge needle. The area can be prepped with a lidocaine-prilocaine cream (L.M.X.4, Ferndale, Michigan) 20–30 minutes prior to lidocaine administration for needle-averse patients.

To maximize hemostasis in the highly vascular scalp, wait 10–20 minutes to allow for vasoconstrictive effect of the epinephrine.[70] Another approach that may save prep time is to use a circular handle of an instrument to surround the biopsy site and apply firm pressure obtain adequate tamponade of local blood vessels.[71]

The site of the biopsy should be from an active hair-bearing area that shows signs of inflammation (scaling and erythema) and is symptomatic. Avoid hair parts and the frontal portion of the scalp.

Two 4-mm punch biopsies, including subcutaneous fat, cut at the level beneath the hair bulbs should be submitted for horizontal and vertical sectioning and staining with hematoxlin and eosin for histologic examination.[3,70,72] If only a single biopsy specimen is feasible, it may be sectioned either vertically or transversely, and serial step sections should be obtained.[72]

The area is closed with blue-colored monofilament suture. Wound dressings are not necessary and may be problematic.[70] The suture is removed in 5–7 days. Patients must avoid chemical hair treatments and excessive manipulation of the scalp while sutures are in place.

CONCLUSION

The black patient who presents with alopecia can be a vexing clinical problem. Lack of patient education, lack of effective treatments, and cultural barriers are contributing to the dramatic increase in cicatricial alopecia in this population. Proper diagnostic techniques and use of current classification guidelines will aid the physician in determining appropriate treatment plans. Early diagnosis is the key to prevent loss of viable hair follicles, and novel techniques such as video dermoscopy may improve diagnositic capability, extend clinicopathogenetic understating, and improve access to care.[73]

REFERENCES

1. Olsen EA, Bergfeld WF, Cotsarelis G, et al. Summary of North American Hair Research Society (NAHRS)–sponsored Workshop on Cicatricial Alopecia, February 10–11, 2001, Duke University Medical Center, Durham, NC. *J Am Acad Dermatol* 2003;48:103-110.
2. Sperling LC. Scarring alopecia and the dermatopathologist. *J Cutan Pathol* 2001; 28:333-342.
3. Price VH. The medical treatment of cicatricial alopecia. *Semin Cutan Med Surg* 2006;25:56-59.
4. Sperling LC, Cowper SE. The histopathology of primary cicatricial alopecia. *Semin Cutan Med Surg* 2006;25: 41-50.
5. Tackey RN, Holloway Barbosa V. Molecular response in the scalp after application of relaxer to the hair. Presented at *L'Oréal 3rd International Symposium: Ethnic Skin and Hair: Advancing the Scientific Frontier;* Chicago, IL, 2005.
6. Quinn C, Kelly AP. Prevalence of undiagnosed hair and scalp disorders in African-American women presenting to an adult dermatology clinic. Presented at *L'Oréal 2nd International Symposium: Ethnic Skin and Hair: New Directions in Research,* Chicago, IL, 2003.
7. Horenstein MG, Simon J. Investigation of the hair follicle inner root sheath in scarring and nonscarring alopecia. *J Cutan Pathol* 2007; 34(10):762-768.
8. Sperling LC, Cowper SE. The histopathology of primary cicatricial alopecia. *Semin Cutan Med Surg* 2006;25: 41-50.
9. Deyampart NM, Lamb A, Taylor S, et al. Central centrifugal alopecia. *J Am Acad Dermatol* 2004;XX:90S.
10. Martin ES, Elewski BE. Tinea capitis in adult women masquerading as bacterial pyoderma. *J Am Acad Dermatol* 2003;49: 177-179S.
11. George YA, Ravis SM, Gottlieb J, et al. Betamethasone valerate 0.12% in foam vehicle for scalp dermatitis in African-Americans. *Cosmet Dermatol* 2002;15: 23-27.
12. Taylor SC. Practical tips for managing hair disorders in African-Americans females. *Pract Dermatol* 2006;3(7):25-27.
13. Sperling LC. Folliculits decalvans and tufted folliculitis are specific infective diseases that may lead to scarring, but are not a subset of central centrifugal scarring alopecia (letter). *J Am Acad Dermtol* 2001;137:373-374.
14. Callender V. Hair transplant surgery in the treatment of alopecia in women of color. Presented at *L'Oréal 2nd International Symposium: Ethnic Skin and Hair: New Directions in Research,* Chicago, IL, 2003.
15. Kelly AP. Acne keloidalis nuchae. *E-medicine Journal;* available at *www.emedicine.com/derm/topic558.htm;* accessed May 30,2006.
16. Adegbidi H, Atadokpede F, do Ango-Padonou F, Yedomon H. Keloid acne of the neck: Epidemiological studies over 10 years. *Int J Dermatol* 2005;44:49-50S.
17. Ogunbiyi A, George A. Acne keloidalis in females: Case report and review of literature. *J Natl Med Assoc* 2005:97;736-738.
18. Dinehart SM, Tanner L, Mallory SB, et al. Acne keloidalis in women. *Cutis* 1989;44: 250-252.
19. Kaposi M. Ueber die sogennante framboesia und mehrere andere arten von papillaren neubildungen der haut. *Arch Dermatol Syphilol* 1869;1:382-423.
20. Cosman B, Wolff M. Acne keloidalis. *Plast Reconstr Surg* 1972;50:25-30.
21. D'Souza P, Iyer VK, Ramam M. Familial acne keloidalis. *Acta Dermatol Venereol* 1998;78:382.
22. George AO, Akanji AO, Nduka EV, et al. Chemical, biochemical and morphological features of acne keloidalis in a black population. *Int J Dermatol* 1993;32:714-716.
23. Khumalo NP, Jessop S, Ehrlich R. Prevalence of cutaneous adverse effects of hairdressing: A systematic review. *Arch Dermatol* 2006;142:377-383.
24. Azurdia RM, Graham RM, Weismann K, et al. Acne keloidalis in Caucasian patients on cyclosporine following organ transplantation. *Br J Dermatol* 2000;143: 465-467.
25. Grunwald MH, Ben-Dor D, Livni E, Halevy S. Acne keloidalis–like lesions on the scalp associated with antiepileptic drugs. *Int J Dermatol* 1990:29;559-561.

26. Sellheyer K, Bergfeld W. Histopathologic evaluations of alopecias. *Am J Dermatopathol* 2006;28:236-259.
27. Acne keloidalis: A novel presentation for tinea capitis. *Am J Dermatopathol* 2004; 26:140.
28. Callender VD, Young CM, Haverstock CL, et al. An open label study of clobetasol propionate 0.05% and betamethasone valerate 0.12% foams in the treatment of mild to moderate acne keloidalis. *Cutis* 2005;75:317-321.
29. Kelly AP. Pseudofolliculitis barbae and acne keloidalis nuchae. *Dermatol Clin* 2003;21:645-653.
30. Barr J, Friedman A, Baldwin H. Use of imiquimod and pimecrolimus cream in the treatment of acne keloidalis nuchae: P590. *J Am Acad Dermatol* 2005;52:64S.
31. McMichael AJ. Scalp and hair disorders in African-American patients: A primer of disorders and treatments. *Cosmet Dermatol* 2003;16:37-41.
32. Kantor GR, Ratz JL, Wheeland RG. Treatment of acne keloidalis nuchae with carbon dioxide laser. *J Am Acad Dermatol* 1986;14:236-267.
33. McMichael AJ. Hair and scalp disorders in ethnic populations. *Dermatol Clin* 2003;21:629-644.
34. Battle EF Jr, Hobbs LM. Laser-assisted hair removal for darker skin types, in *Dermatologic Therapy: Treatment of Diseases of Ethnic Skin*. Blackwell Publishing, Malden, MA 2004, pp 177-183.
35. Valeriant M, Terracina FS, Messana P. Pseudofolliculitis of the neck and shoulders: A new effective treatment with alexandrite laser. *Plast Reconstr Surg* 2002; 28:333-342.
36. Cook-Bolden F, Swift R, Corbin S. Surgical advances in treating and preventing recurrence of acne keloidalis nuchae. Presented at *L'Oréal 1st International Symposium: Ethnic Skin and Hair*, Chicago, IL, 2001.
37. Gloster HM Jr. The surgical management of extensive cases of acne keloidalis nuchae. *Arch Dermatol* 2000;136:1376-1379.
38. Glenn MJ, Bennett RG, Kelly AP. Acne keloidalis nuchae: Treatment with excision and second-intention healing. *J Am Acad Dermatol* 1995;33:243-246.
39. Califano J, Miller S, Frodel J. Treatment of occipital acne keloidalis by excision followed by secondary intention healing. *Arch Facial Plastic Surg* 1999;4:308-311.
40. Jackson BA. Lasers in ethnic skin: A review. *J Am Acad Dermatol* 2000;48:134138S.
41. Kantor GR, Ratz JL, Wheeland RG. Treatment of acne keloidalis nuchae with carbon dioxide laser. *J Am Acad Dermatol* 1986;14:263-267.
42. Stites PC, Boyd AS. Dissecting cellulitis in a white male: A case report and review of the literature. *Cutis* 2001;67: 37-40.
43. Kobayashi H, Alba S, Tagami H. Successful treatment of dissecting cellulitis and acne conglobata with oral zinc. *Br J Dermatol* 1999;141:37-38.
44. Adrain RM, Arndt KA. Perifolliculitits capitis: Successful control with alternate-day corticosteroids. *Ann Plast Surg* 1980;4: 166-169.
45. Scerri L, Williams HC, Allen BR. Dissecting celullitis of the scalp: Response to isotretinoin. *Br J Dermatol* 1996;134: 1105-1108.
46. Schewach-Millet M, Ziv R, Shapira D. Perifollicultis capitis abscendens et suffodiens treated with isotretinoin (letter). *J Am Acad Dermatol* 1986;15:1291-1292.
47. Glass LF, Berman B, Laub D. Treatment of perifolliculits capitsis abscendens et suffodiens with the carbon dioxide laser. *J Dermatol Surg Oncol* 1989;15:673-676.
48. Bellew SG, Nemerofsky R, Schwartz RA, Granick MS. Successful treatment of recalcitrant dissecting cellulitis of the scalp with complete scalp excision and split-thickness skin graft. *Dermatol Surg* 2003;29:1068-1070.
49. Powell JJ, Dawber RPR, Gatter K. Folliculitis decalvans including tufted folliculitis: Histologic and therapeutic findings. *Br J Dermatol* 1998;140:328-333.
50. Sperling LC, Solomon AR, Whiting DA. A new look at scarring alopecia. *Arch Dermatol* 2000:136;235-242.
51. Powell J. Letter to the editor. *J Am Acad Dermatol* 2006;137:373-374.
52. Annesi G. Tufted folliculitis of the scalp: A distinctive clinico histopathogical variant of folliculitis decalvans. *Br J Dermatol* 1998;138:799-805.
53. Abeck D, Forting HC, Braun-Falco O. Long lasting response to combined therapy with fusidic acid and zinc. *Acta Dermertol Venereol (Stockh)* 1992;72:143-145.
53a. Mehregan DA, Van Hale HM, Muller A. Lichen planopilaris: Clinical and pathologic study of 45 patients. *J Am Acad Dermatol* 1992;27:93-142.
54. Bergfeld WF, Remzi B, Cevasco N. Cicatricial alopecia/lichen planopilaris: The Cleveland Clinic Foundation experience on evaluation, diagnosis, and treatment. *J Am Acad Dermatol* 2004; 50:92.
55. Mirmirani P, Willey A, Price VH. Short course of oral cyclosporine in lichen planopilaris. *J Am Acad Dermatol* 2003;49: 667-671.
56. Tosti A, Piraccini BM, Iorizzo M, Misciali C. Frontal fibrosing alopecia in postmenopausal women. *J Am Acad Dermatol* 2005;52:55-60.
57. George SJ, Hsu S. Lichen planopilaris treated with thalidomide. *J Am Acad Dermatol* 2001;45:965-966.
58. Halder RM. Hair and scalp disorders in blacks. *Cutis* 1983;32:378-380.
59. LoPresti P, Papa CM, Kligman AM. Hot comb alopecia. *Arch Dermatol* 1968:98: 234-238.
60. Callender VD, McMichael AJ, Cohen GF. Medical and surgical therapies for alopecias in black women. *Dermatol Ther* 2004;17:164-176.
61. Sperling LC. *An Atlas of Hair Pathology with Clinical Correlations*. New York, Parthenon, 2003, p 23.
62. Earles RM. Surgical correction of traumatic alopecia in black women. *J Dermatol Surg Oncol* 1986:23;78-82.
63. High WA, Hoang MP. Lipedematous alopecia: An unusual sequela of discoid lupus, or other co-conspirators at work *J Am Acad Dermatol* 2005;53:157-161S.
64. Fair KP, Knoell KA, Patterson JW, et al. Lipedematous alopecia: A clinicopathologic, histologic and ultrastructural study. *J Cutan Pathol* 2000;27:49-53.
65. Mohsin RM, Jackson J. Lipedematous alopecia, a rare form of diffuse hair loss. *J Am Acad Dermatol* 2004;50:90S.
66. Light AE. Histologic study of human scalps exhibiting various degrees of non-specific baldness. *J Invest Dermatol* 1949;13:53.
67. Garn MS, Selby S, Young R. Scalp thickness and fat-loss theory of balding. *Arch Dermatol Syphilol* 1954;70:601.
68. Werth VP, White WL, Sanchez MR, Franks AG. Incidence of alopecia areata in lupus erythematosus. *Arch Dermatol* 1992;128:368-371.
69. Katta R, Nelson B, Chen D, Roenigk H. Sarcoidosis of the scalp: A case series and review of the literature. *J Am Acad Dermatol* 2000;42:690-692.
70. Shapiro J, Madani S. The scalp biopsy: Making it more efficient. *Dermatol Surg* 1999;25:537-538.
71. Whalen JG, Gehris RP, Kress DW, English JC III. Surgical pearl: Instrument tamponade for punch biopsy of the scalp. *J Am Acad Dermatol* 2005;52:347-348.
72. Elston DM, Ferringer T, Dalton S, et al. A comparison of vertical versus transverse sections in the evaluation of alopecia biopsy specimens. *J Am Acad Dermatol* 2005;53:267-272.
73. Ross EK, Vincenzi C, Tosti A. Videodermoscopy in the evaluation of hair and scalp disorders. *J Am Acad Dermatol* 2006;4:58.

CHAPTER 36

Seborrheic Dermatitis

Yvette Andree George

Key Points

- Seborrheic dermatitis is a common concern to patients with skin of color.
- Clinical features of seborrheic dermatitis depend on the age of the individual, the Fitzpatrick skin type, and the presence or absence of concurrent systemic illness.
- Lesions of seborrheic dermatitis in skin of color may be hypopigmented, hyperpigmented, or erythematous in addition to scaly.
- Treatment options are numerous but should be adjusted to the hair grooming practices of the individual with skin of color.

Seborrheic dermatitis is a chronic papulosquamous condition. It is both a superficial and an inflammatory disease that can occur as an isolated condition or in conjunction with other disorders such as blepharitis, acne vulgaris, and ocular rosacea. Several systemic illnesses also have been documented to have an association with seborrheic dermatitis. These systemic illnesses include acquired immune deficiency syndrome (AIDS), zinc deficiency states, and neurologic disorders. Additionally, seborrheic dermatitis is seen frequently in patients who have received psoralen with ultraviolet A (PUVA) therapy.

The etiology of seborrheic dermatitis has remained unclear until recently. Theorized causative factors include *Malassezia globosa* yeast, production of sebum by sebaceous glands, and a genetic susceptibility for an inflammatory response.[31] The presence of the lipophilic *Malassezia* species of yeast had been proposed as a causative agent of seborrheic dermatitis because it has been documented in many cases.[8] However, the *Malassezia* yeast species are also found in normal human skin. Researchers have documented that numbers of *Malassezia* species are also found in individuals without clinical seborrheic dermatitis.[8,31] Supporting the argument of *Malassezia* species as a causative agent is the fact that antifungal medications are efficacious in controlling the condition. Ketoconazole has been demonstrated to reduce the numbers of cutaneous *Malassezia*.[7] Fluconazole (50 mg/day) also has been documented to effectively remove a high percentage of the *Malassezia* species and to produce a clinical improvement in the symptoms of seborrheic dermatitis.[32] Also, recurrence of the clinical findings has been linked to an increase in the numbers of the lipophilic yeast. The increased presence of this yeast and seborrheic dermatitis in AIDS patients has been theorized to relate to a microbial-induced disease in the immunocompromised individuals. Recently, with the use of molecular science and bioinformatics, researchers have identified *M. globosa* as the etiologic agent of seborrheic dermatitis.[31]

Seborrheic dermatitis is easily recognized. However, clinical findings differ based on the Fitzpatrick skin type of the affected individual. Treatment options are numerous but should be adjusted in Fitzpatrick skin types IV–VI based on hair grooming standards. Treatment is usually successful for alleviating symptoms and the clinical manifestations of the disease.

EPIDEMIOLOGY

The occurrence of seborrheic dermatitis in the population is reported at 1–3%.[35] The age range is quite variable and includes infants through adults (Figure 36-1). However, there are two recognized age categories with distinct increases in the rate of occurrence: (Figure 36-2) infancy and the fourth through fifth decades of life. Males are affected more often than females. Seborrheic dermatitis has been reported to occur more often in the African-American population than in the Caucasian population.[1] Another increase in the incidence of seborrheic dermatitis is found in human immunodeficiency virus–positive (HIV1)/AIDS patients, with estimates ranging from 34–83%.[33,48] Higher rates of occurrence also have been found in individuals with diabetes, obesity, malabsorption, Parkinson's disease, and epilepsy (Table 36-1). The role of zinc deficiency in increased rates of seborrheic dermatitis remains controversial.[4,34,47]

ETIOLOGY

The etiology of seborrheic dermatitis has been unclear until recently. Historically, the sebum and lipid levels in individuals with seborrheic dermatitis have gained attention as possible causative factors. Increased lipid content in the skin of some African-Americans compared with Caucasians could account for the higher rates of this skin disease in the African-American community.[7] Similarly, increased sebum has been found in Parkinsonian patients when compared with the levels in other individuals.[6] Another population with increased sebum is newborns. Newborn infants have large and active sebaceous glands, perhaps explaining "cradle cap," which is seen frequently in this population.

TABLE 36-1
Disorders Commonly Associated with Seborrheic Dermatitis[47]

HIV+/AIDS
Diabetes
Obesity
Malabsorption
Parkinson disease
Epilepsy

More recent theories of the cause of seborrheic dermatitis involve immunologic responses of the affected individual. It is suggested that depressed T-cell function leads to increased growth of *Malassezia,* which could account for the high incidence in AIDS patients. It is accepted that seborrheic dermatitis worsens as the AIDS individual's health decreases. Likewise, improvements in the health of these individuals leads to clinical improvements in the appearance of the skin. However, the postulated immunologic link between decreased IgG levels directed against *Malassezia* and seborrheic dermatitis has been questioned.[36,37] Others have reported an increase in natural killer cell activation and increased inflammatory interleukins.[30] This potentially could lead to the inflammation found in seborrheic dermatitis.

Medication-induced seborrheic dermatitis also has been suggested. This is evidenced by the increased incidence of this skin disease in Parkinson patients treated with specific neuroleptic medications.[28,22]

CLINICAL FEATURES

The clinical features of seborrheic dermatitis depend on the age of the individual, the Fitzpatrick skin type, and the presence or absence of concurrent systemic

TABLE 36-2
Clinical Patterns of Seborrheic Dermatitis

Infants: "cradle cap" and "napkin dermatitis"
Adults: hair bearing areas (eyebrows, mustache, eyelid margins)
Skin flexures (nasolabial folds, postauricular fold, axillae and groin)
HIV+/AIDS/Diabetic patients: extensive adult clinical findings, blepharitis, Superinfections

illness (Table 36-2). Manifestations of seborrheic dermatitis in newborn infants include scaling, crusting, and skin that is greasy in appearance. This constellation of clinical findings is referred to as "cradle cap" and is likely related to an overproduction of sebum. Scales are often located throughout the scalp but also can be located on the face, chest, groin, neck, ears, and the eyelids (Figure 36-2). The clinical findings in Fitzpatrick skin types IV–VI can be distinctly different based on reduced visible erythema of involved skin. Instead, the skin may be either hypopigmented or hyperpigmented (Figure 36-1). Severe and generalized seborrheic dermatitis in infancy may represent *Leiner disease,* an exfoliative disorder that occurs in combination with anemia, diarrhea, immunodeficiency, and concomitant bacterial and candidal infections.

Clinical findings of seborrheic dermatitis in the adult population vary by the location of involvement. Common locations include the scalp, face, chest, axillae, submammary area, and groin and gluteal areas. Face and head involvement is most prominent around the eyebrows, perinasal skin, postauricular areas, ears, and eyelids. The face and scalp may be either dry and flaky with white scales or greasy with crusting. The disease may extend from the frontal scalp onto the upper forehead. In Fitzpatrick skin types IV–VI, the skin is often hypopigmented beneath the scale. The perinasal and postauricular skin can appear either hypopigmented, hyperpigmented, or erythematous. Inner ear crusting may be obvious and includes the aural canals. Occasionally, bacterial superinfection occurs. Chest, axillae, groin, and gluteal involvement is usually scaly with hypopigmentation or erythema beneath the scales.

HIV+/AIDS and diabetic patients have clinical findings that are similar to those of other adults with seborrheic dermatitis. However, the skin involvement is often more extensive. Involvement can include blepharitis and occlusion of the meibomian glands, resulting in scaling and burning of the eyelids. Erythema of the eyelids may not be as obvious in ethnic skin. Axillary, extremity, and groin involvement is often diffuse. Bacterial, candidal, and dermatophyte superinfections may be present. Involved skin is more visibly inflamed in those who are immunocompromised. Torso and extremity plaques are moist with extreme erythema that may be visible even in darker ethnic skin.

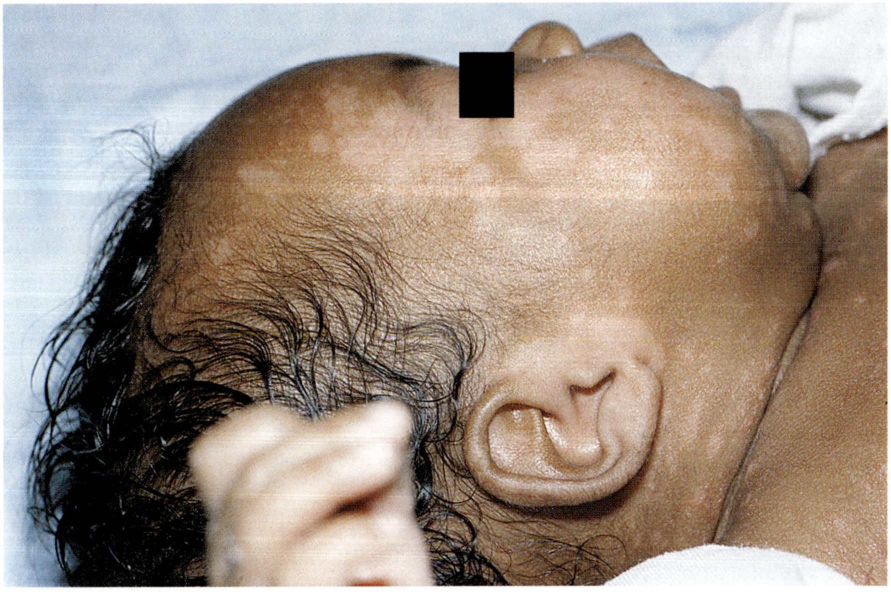

▲ **FIGURE 36-1** Seborrheic dermatitis related hypopigmentation in Fitzpatrick skin type VI.

HISTOPATHOLOGY

The histologic findings of seborrheic dermatitis are consistent with those of other forms of spongiotic dermatitis and include marked spongiosis, acanthosis, and hyperkeratosis. Classic findings also include parakeratosis, neutrophilic infiltrate, and scale crust at the opening of the infundibulum of the hair follicle and psoriasiform hyperplasia of the epidermis. Some degree of elongation of the epidermal ridges is present. The histologic differential diagnosis includes psoriasis. However, the presence of spongiosis in seborrheic dermatitis helps to make this distinction. There are no recognized special stains that are definitive for this diagnosis.

The histologic findings of seborrheic dermatitis in AIDS patients are different from those in immunocompetent

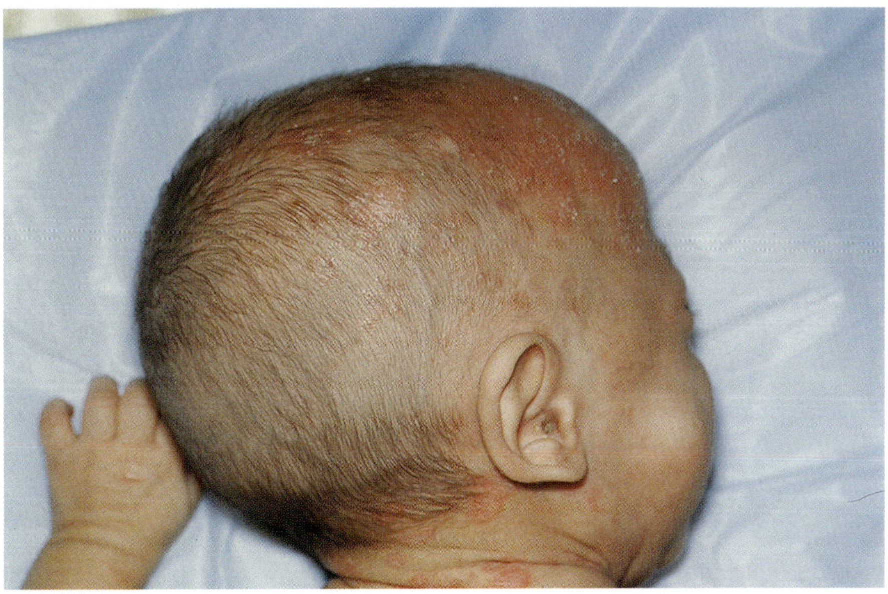

▲ **FIGURE 36-2** Infant displaying extensive "cradle cap".

TABLE 36-3
Histopathologic Differences Between Acquired Immune Deficiency Syndrome–Associated Seborrheic Dermatitis and Classic Seborrheic Dermatitis

Classical seborrheic dermatitis: spongiotic dermatitis, neutrophils at infundibulum of hair follicles
AIDS associated seborrheic dermatitis: necrotic keratinocytes within epidermis, perivascular infiltrates of plasma cells, neutrophils

patients[38] (Table 36-3). In this group of individuals, there are superficial perivascular infiltrates of plasma cells, neutrophils, leukocytoclasia, and keratinocyte necrosis.[38]

ASSOCIATED SYSTEMIC ILLNESSES

The prevalence and severity of seborrheic dermatitis in HIV+/AIDS patients have been well documented.[10,39] The etiology is still undetermined. It has been theorized that there is an increased presence of *Malassezia* and immunologic dysfunction inherent to this systemic illness. However, there are studies that dispute this concept. The prevalence of HIV+/AIDS patients in the ethnic community is significant. It is currently estimated that up to 50% of the HIV+/AIDS males are African-American and approximately 18–20% are Latino.[39,40] Caucasian and other ethnic groups constitute the remainder of cases. In females, the African-American population and Latina population account for a large percentage of cases. Caucasian and other ethnic groups represent the remainder of cases. Therefore, the significance of this skin disease in the ethnic communities should be noted. The high rates of HIV+/AIDS patients and seborrheic dermatitis in African countries also has been documented.

Zinc deficiency can originate from an inherited autosomal recessive trait or be acquired owing to gastrointestinal, renal, or dietary disorders. Acrodermatitis enteropathica is the inherited form of this deficiency that is found in infants. The spectrum of clinical findings includes an erythematous eruption that simulates facial seborrheic dermatitis. However, there is no documented relationship between acquired zinc deficiency and higher rates of seborrheic dermatitis.[34]

Parkinson's disease is a chronic progressive neurologic disorder characterized by tremors, rigidity, bradykinesia, and a disturbance of gait and posture. Many cutaneous clinical findings have been reported, including seborrheic dermatitis and hyperhidrosis. The etiology of these increased rates remains elusive. However, suggested mechanisms include the noted increased sebum excretion rate in Parkinson's patients and a possible induction by the use of chronic neuroleptic medications.[6,28] Many case reports have documented an increased occurrence of seborrheic dermatitis in PUVA-treated patients.[20]

DIFFERENTIAL DIAGNOSIS

The differential diagnosis for seborrheic dermatitis can be separated by the aforementioned distinct age groups that are primarily affected by this skin disease. Skin eruptions in infancy may represent a variety of infection or dermatitis. These include contact dermatitis, atopic dermatitis, tinea capitis, tinea faceii, candidiasis, multiple carboxylase deficiency, biotin-responsive dermatitis, scabies, impetigo, and psoriasis (Table 36-4). Fungal and bacterial cultures, skin biopsy, family history, and laboratory studies can help to distinguish between these various conditions.

The differential diagnosis for adults includes psoriasis, pityriasis rosea, contact dermatitis, systemic lupus erythematosis, atopic dermatitis, candidiasis, rosacea, impetigo, tinea versicolor, and sarcoidosis (Table 36-5). Fungal and bacterial cultures, skin biopsy, and laboratory studies are helpful in determining the etiology of the clinical findings.

TABLE 36-4
Differential Diagnosis of Seborrheic Dermatitis in Children[2]

Contact dermatitis
Atopic dermatitis
Tinea capitis
Tinea faceii
Candidiasis
Multiple carboxylase deficiency
Biotin responsive dermatitis
Scabies
Impetigo
Psoriasis

TABLE 36-5
Differential Diagnosis of Seborrheic Dermatitis in Adults

Psoriasis
Pityriasis rosea
Contact dermatitis
Systemic lupus erythematosis
Atopic dermatitis
Candidiasis
Rosacea
Impetigo
Tinea versicolor
Sarcoidosis

ETHNIC GROOMING PRACTICES

The treatment of scalp seborrheic dermatitis in Fitzpatrick skin types IV–VI requires an understanding of the differences in the structure of the hair, as well as the hair follicle. Equally important is a familiarity with hair styling practices and cultural standards of hair care in the aforementioned groups. Once an understanding of the standard hair care practices is achieved, treatment recommendations can be aligned with those practices, thus enhancing patient compliance.

Textured hair found in many African-Americans is biologically similar to but morphologically different from Caucasian hair. It is oval in shape, flat, and is the most elliptic in cross section.[12] Textured hair grows from a curved hair follicle and appears curly. It has reduced moisture content and therefore is inherently drier than Caucasian hair.[12,49] The tensile strength is lower, and spiraling of the hair makes it more difficult for sebum to be distributed along the length of the hair.[12] These factors lead to increased hair breakage in this population.[49] Therefore, hair washing frequency is usually once weekly or every other week. More frequent washing would lead to a further decrease in moisture content and increased fragility.

Hair styling practices in African-American women are quite varied (Table 36-6). However, approximately 80% are believed to have chemically straightened hair. The chemical relaxers used are sodium (pH 10–14), guanine, and potassium hydroxide. Ammonium thioglycolate (pH 9.4–9.6) also can be used for this purpose. These ingredients break the cysteine disulfide bonds to straighten the hair. These chemical straightening processes may lead to increased hair breakage when compared with non–chemically treated hair.43 Again, daily hair washing should be avoided so as not to exacerbate hair breakage.

Hot combing is a process that allows the straightening of textured hair without the use of chemicals. However, a

TABLE 36-6
Common Hairstyling Practices in African-Americans

Chemical straightening
Weaving synthetic or human hair
Straightening by heat application
Natural locking
Tight braiding

pomade or oil-based hair product is applied to the hair followed by the application of a heated comb that may reach temperatures greater than 150°F. Hot combing may require an hour or more of time to straighten the hair. The straight hairstyle achieved will revert to a curly texture if the hair becomes wet (including with perspiration). Therefore, patients are likely to wash and hot comb once every 2 weeks.

Natural hairstyles are seen primarily in African-American men and a small but increasing number of women. Natural locking of the hair, also termed *dread locks,* is achieved by allowing the natural hair to twist, knot, and matte over time. The hair cannot be combed after this process is complete, which is aided by the application of "dread" wax and keeping the hair dry and tight as the style is developing. Washing the hair is discouraged, although cleaning the scalp with a nonconditioning soap is recommended. Tight braiding of the hair either in cornrows or individual braids (with or without additional synthetic or human hair) is another popular style. Braids may be maintained for extended periods of time without washing or releasing the tension from the hair. Weaving human or synthetic hair into the natural scalp hair may be accomplished by sewing with a thread or bonding to the scalp with glue.

All the aforementioned hairstyles popular in the African-American community have several common features. First, the styles are maintained for extended periods of time ranging from 1 week to 1 month. Loss of the style occurs with hair washing, which necessitates restyling. Finally, hair breakage can occur with the frequent cycle of washing and restyling the hair. Consideration must be given when instructing the patient as to the frequency of hair washing with medicated shampoos, and note should be made of the ability of shampoo to further dry intrinsically dry hair. Medicated solutions and gels also may play a role in reverting a straight hairstyle.

Asian hair has a round hair shaft, is visibly straight, and has the largest diameter with circular geometry as compared with African-American and Caucasian hair.[12] The hair has a higher tensile strength than to Caucasian and African-American hair. It is typically dark in color. Hairstyling methods are used to tighten the hair and create curl. Ammonium and hydrogen peroxide are used to bleach Asian hair and may be combined with agents to perm the hair. Other methods used to obtain curly hair include hot curling irons as well as mousses and gels in combination with heated dryers. All these hairstyles and styling agents may lead to dry hair and increased hair fragility. Therefore, some Asians use coconut oil or milk to condition the hair and reduce fragility.

The hair and styling preferences of Latinos depend on the hair texture. Latinos may have hair that is morphologically similar to textured African-American hair or hair that is identical to straight or curly Caucasian hair. Hair that is similar to textured African-American hair may require all the previously discussed methods to achieve the desired appearance and to maximize manageability. The most commonly used method to achieve this goal is chemical straightening of the hair. The high percentage of individuals with brown/black hair often leads to the use of hydrogen peroxide to bleach the hair or the use of permanent hair dyes. Both these processes, when combined with chemical straightening, can lead to increased fragility. Latino hair that is morphologically similar to Caucasian hair has the same moisture content. Frequent washing is often necessary to reduce the oily appearance.

Native American hair is morphologically similar to Caucasian hair. Therefore, the hair has an intermediate diameter and cross section compared with African-American and Asian hair.[12] The hair has more increased moisture and decreased fragility when compared with African-American hair.[12]

TREATMENT (Table 36-7)

Steroids

Nonfluorinated topical steroids, which address the inflammatory nature of the disorder, are effective in the treatment of scalp, facial, and truncal seborrheic dermatitis. The steroid vehicle is very important when selecting treatment for scalp seborrheic dermatitis in patients who have textured hair. Solutions and gels are often considered to be too drying for textured hair, especially hair that has been chemically straightened. These formulations further dry the innately dry hair of African-Americans, which leads to breakage. Steroid ointments or oils may be preferred with chemically or hot comb straightened hair, braided hair, or natural hair in African-Americans or Afro-Latinos. However, ointments and oils are inappropriate for locked hair because they inhibit the locking process. Steroid foams, lotions, shampoos, and gels are generally useful for natural, non--chemically treated hair of Asians, Native Americans, and Latinos. These vehicles do not give the hair an oily appearance. Steroid foams may be acceptable in chemically straightened ethnic hair for

TABLE 36-7
Treatments for Seborrheic Dermatitis

Medications	Vehicle and/or Name
Topical steroids	Cream, ointment, oil shampoo and foam
Selenium sulfide	Selsun blue, Exsel, Fostex medicated cream, Head and Shoulders
Lithium succinate	
Ketoconazole	Nizoral cream and shampoo
Ciclopiroxolamine	Loprox cream, shampoo, and lotion
Zinc pyrithione shampoo	Head and Shoulders, DHS zinc, Denorex, Pantene Pro V, Zetar, Zincon, and Theraplex Z
Coal tar shampoo	Neutrogena T gel, Duplex T, Denorex extra strength, DHS tar, F/S shampoo, Lonil T, Pentrax, Tegrin, Betatar, Herald tar, Mg 217, Polytar, Reme-T, Tarsum, Theraplex T, Zetar, Tl-seb-T
Salicylic acid	Neutrogena T-sal, Sebulex, DHS-sal, Beta sal, Lonil plus, P & S, Tl-seb, X-seb T plus
Sodium sulfacetamide	Ovace gel, shampoo, and wash
Olive/mineral oil	
Topical immunomodulators	Tacrolimus and pimecrolimus

individuals who do not desire oil based-products.[17] Low- and middle-potency steroid creams and lotions are useful for treatment of facial and body seborrheic dermatitis. High-potency steroid products are discouraged owing to the risk of hypopigmentation and/or atrophy, which may be disfiguring in Fitzpatrick skin types IV–VI.

Antifungal Agents

Ketoconazole is a broad-spectrum antifungal agent that can be used to decrease *Malassezia* species. This broad-spectrum cream also treats *Candida albicans* and most dermatophytes. Ketoconazole is effective in the treatment of facial and truncal seborrheic dermatitis in infants and adults. It is acceptable for Fitzpatrick skin types IV–VI because it does not lead to hypopigmentation. Ketoconazole 2% shampoo is also effective for scalp disease in all skin types. However, the results of shampoo use are often delayed in ethnic patients who shampoo the hair less frequently than other individuals. The use of ketoconazole shampoo also has been noted to worsen the dryness of chemically treated hair. This can lead to increased hair breakage. Shampoo use should be limited to once weekly and combined with moisturizing conditioners.[14] Ciclopiroxolamine is an antifungal 1% cream and shampoo that can treat superficial dermatophyte infections, *Malassezia,* and *Candida.* This medication has anti-inflammatory properties that allow it to be effective against seborrheic dermatitis.[7] The shampoo must not be used too frequently and should be combined with moisturizing conditioners to prevent overdrying and breakage of chemically treated hair. Selenium sulfide has both antifungal and antiseborrheic properties.[47] This product is available as a 1% or 2.5% shampoo. It is effective against *Malassezia.* However, similar to the other shampoos, its frequency of use must be reduced in chemically treated hair.

Other Ingredients

Zinc pyrithione is an active ingredient in some shampoos. This component is noted to be effective against *Malassezia.*[47] It is available as a 1% and 2% shampoo or a 0.25% spray for facial involvement. The recommended use of several times per week is a limiting factor for hair that requires less frequent shampooing. A facial cleansing bar with 2% zinc is effective against facial involvement of this disease.[47] Treatment with coal tar preparations has been considered a mainstay of therapy for seborrheic dermatitis. Shampoos contain 0.4% or 0.5% of the active ingredient. Limiting factors include the odor of the preparation and the reduced frequency of shampoo use in some ethnic groups. Salicylic acid (3%) shampoos are available and beneficial, with the same limitations noted for all antiseborrheic shampoos. Sodium sulfacetamide is available in a 10% face wash and a 10% scalp foam and gel. The lack of alcohol in the scalp foam allows for less drying and breakage when used in chemically treated hair. Olive oil or mineral oil compresses with warm water are helpful for loosening the crusts and scabs on the scalps of infants. This can be combined with a baby shampoo or low-potency steroid for a quicker response. Lithium succinate is a topical ointment that has been used for treatment. This medication interferes with the free fatty acids that are instrumental in the growth of *Malassezia.*[48]

Topical Immunomodulators

Topical tacrolimus and pimecrolimus have been reported to possess antifungal activity.[47] Although not currently approved by the Food and Drug Administration (FDA) for the treatment of seborrheic dermatitis, these agents are being used increasingly for its treatment. As with the topical antifungal preparations, use of these agents avoids the potential side effects associated with topical corticosteroids. A trial of 0.1% tacrolimus ointment in patients with seborrheic dermatitis demonstrated a 70% or greater clearance of the seborrheic dermatitis.[5] A double-blind, vehicle-controlled four-week trial randomized patients with seborrheic dermatitis to pimecrolimus or vehicle. Results revealed that pimecrolimus 1% cream is an effective and well-tolerated treatment for moderate to severe facial seborrheic dermatitis, and efficacy was noted as early as 2 weeks.[44]

An open-label pilot trial of 1% pimecrolimus cream for 16 weeks in the treatment of seborrheic dermatitis in five African-American adults with associated hypopigmentation was performed.[4,5] All subjects in the study noted a marked decrease in the severity of the seborrheic dermatitis, as well as an improvement in the hypopigmentation.

CONCLUSION

Seborrheic dermatitis is a common cutaneous disorder in patients with ethnic skin. In addition to the characteristic flaking and scaling of the face and scalp, postinflammatory changes are common. The structure of the hair, as well as hair and scalp grooming practices, drives the acceptability of treatments for seborrheic dermatitis. Avoidance of shampoo and topical products that dry the hair is important. Preference for medications, such as antifungal agents, that avoid possible side effects such as atrophy and telangiectasias are also preferable in this patient population. Finally, reliance on topical agents in acceptable vehicles to this patient population, such as foam, oils, and/or ointments, is important.

REFERENCES

1. Pierce HE. Treatment of seborrheic dermatitis in the Negro scalp. *J Natl Med Assoc* 1966;58:345-346.
2. Williams MI. Differential diagnosis of seborrheic dermatitis. *Pediatr Rev* 1986;7:204-211.
3. Perniciaro C, Peters MS. Tinea faciale mimicking seborrheic dermatitis in patients with AIDS. *N Engl J Med* 1986;314:315-316.
4. Gupta AK, Bluhm R, Cooper EA, et al. Seborrheic dermatitis. *Dermatol Clin* 2003;21:401-412.
5. Meshkinpour A, Sun J, Weinstein G. An open pilot study using tacrolimus ointment in the treatment of seborrheic dermatitis. *J Am Acad Dermatol* 2003;49:145-147.
6. Mastrolonardo M, Diaferio A, Logroscino G. Seborrheic dermatitis, sebum excretion and Parkinson's disease: A survey of (im)possible links. *Med Hypoth* 2003;60:907-911.
7. Chosidow O, Maurette C, Dupuy P. Randomized, open-labeled, non-inferiority study between ciclopiroxolamine 1% cream and ketoconazole 2% foaming gel in mild to moderate facial seborrheic dermatitis. *Dermatology* 2003;206:233-240.
8. Pechere M, Krischer J, Remondat C, et al. *Malassezia* spp. carriage in patients with seborrheic dermatitis. *J Dermatol* 1999;26:558-561.
9. Basset-Sequin N, Sotto A, Guillot B, et al. Zinc status in HIV-infected patients: Relation to the presence or absence of seborrheic dermatitis. *J Am Acad Dermatol* 1998;38:276-278.
10. Mahe A, Simon F, Coulibaly S, et al. Predictive value of seborrheic dermatitis and other common dermatoses for HIV infection in Bamako, Mali. *J Am Acad Dermatol* 1996;34:1084-1086.
11. Berardesia E, Maibach H. Ethnic skin: Overview of structure and function. *J Am Acad Dermatol* 2003;48:S139-142.
12. Franbourg A, Hallegot P, Baltenneck F, et al. Current research on ethnic hair. *J Am Acad Dermatol* 2003;48:S115-119.
13. Halder RM, Nootheti PK. Ethnic skin disorders overview. *J Am Acad Dermatol* 2003;48:S143-148.
14. McMichael AJ. Scalp and hair disorders in African-American patients: A primer

of disorders and treatment. *Cosmet Dermatol* 2003;16:S337-341.
15. Halder RM. Hair and scalp disorders in blacks. *Cutis* 1983;32:378-380.
16. Joyner M. Hair care in black patients. *J Pediatr Health Care* 1988;2:281-287.
17. George YA, Ravis SM, Gottlieb J, et al. Betamethasone valerate 0.12% in a foam vehicle for scalp seborrheic dermatitis in African-Americans. *Cosmet Dermatol* 2002; 15:23-27.
18. Scott DA. Disorders of the hair and scalp in blacks. *Dermatol Clin* 1988;6: 387-395.
19. Faergemann J. Pityrosporum infections. *J Am Acad Dermatol* 1994;31:S18.
20. Tegner E. Seborrheic dermatitis of the face induced by PUVA treatments. *Acta Derm Venereol (Stockh)* 1983;63:33S.
21. Kenney JA Jr. Dermatoses seen in African-Americans. *Int J Dermatol* 1970;70:110.
22. Binder RL, Jonelis FJ. Seborrheic dermatitis in the neuroleptic induced parkinsonism. *Arch Dermatol* 1983;119: 473-475.
23. Sperling L. Hair density in African-Americans. *Arch Dermatol* 1999;135:656.
24. Smith W, Burns C. Managing the hair and skin of African-American pediatric patients. *J Pediatr Health Care* 1999;13: 72-78.
25. Eisenstat BA, Wormser GP. Seborrheic dermatitis and butterfly rash in AIDS. *N Engl J Med* 1984;311:189.
26. Brownell I, Quan LT, Hsu S. Topical pimecrolimus in the treatment of seborrheic dermatitis. *Dermatol Online J* 2003; 9:13.
27. Martignoni E, Godi L, Pacchetti C, et al. Is seborrhea a sign of autonomic impairment in Parkinson's disease? *J Neural Trasm* 1997;104:1295-1304.
28. Binder RL, Jonelis FJ. Seborrheic dermatitis: A newly reported side effect of neuroleptics. *J Clin Psychiatry* 1984;45: 125-126.
29. Pochi PE, Strauss JS, Mescon H. Sebum production and functional 17-ketosteroid excretion in Parkinsonism. *J Invest Dermatol* 1962;38:45-51.
30. Bergbrant I-M, Johansson S, Robbins D, et al. An immunologic study in patients with seborrheic dermatitis. *Clin Exp Dermatol* 1991;16:331-338.
31. Dawson TL Jr. *Malassezia globosa* and *restricta:* A breakthrough understanding of the etiology and treatment of dandruff and seborrheic dermatitis through whole genome analysis. Presentation at the *21st World Congress of Dermatology*, Buenos Aires, Argentina, 2007, December 15-19, 2007.
32. Zisova LG. Fluconazole and its place in the treatment of seborrheic dermatitis: New therapeutic possibilities. *Folia Med (Plovdir)* 2006;48:39-45.
33. Schwartz RA, Jahusz CA., Janiger CK. Seborrheic dermatitis: An overview. J Am Acad Family Phys 2006;XX:XXX.
34. Abou-Mourad NN, Farah FS, Steel D. Dermatopathic changes in hypozincemia. *Arch Dermayol* 1979;115:956-958.
35. Gupta AK, Bluhm R, Cooper EA, et al. Seborrheic dermatitis. *Dermatol Clin* 2003; 2:40-41.
36. Ashbee HR, Ingham E, Holland KT, Cunliffe NJ. Cell mediated immune response to *Malassezia furfur* serovars A, B, and C in patients with pityriasis versicolor, seborrheic dermatitis and controls. *Exp Dermatol* 1994;3:106-112.
37. Pavry ME, Sharpe GR. Seborrheic dermatitis is not caused by an altered immune response in *Malassezia* yeast. *Br J Dermatol* 1998;139:254-263.
38. Soeprono FF, Schinella RA, Cockerel CT, Comite SL. Seborrheic-like dermatitis of acquired immunodeficiency syndrome. *J Am Acad Dermatol* 1986;14: 242-248.
39. Rosatelli JB, Machado AA, Roselina AM. Dermatoses among Brazilian HIV+ patients: Correlation with the evolutionary phase of AIDS. *Int. J Dermatol* 1997; 36:729-734.
40. Schectman RC, Midgley G, Hay RJ. HIV disease–associated *Malassezia* yeast: A quantitative study of patients presenting with seborrheic dermatitis. *Br J Dermatol* 1995;133:694-698.
41. Laurencin CT, Christensen DM, Taylor ED. HIV/AIDS and the African-American community: A state of emergency. *J Natl Med Assoc* 2008;100:35-45.
42. Santos G, Puga AM, Medina C. HAART, adherence and cultural issues in the US Latino community. *AIDS Read* 2004;14: 526-529.
43. McMichael AJ. Hair breakage in normal and weathered hair: Focus on black patients. *J Invest Dermatol Symp Proc* 2007; 12:6-9.
44. Warshaw EM, Wohlhuter RJ, Liu A, et al. A result of a randomized, double-blinded vehicle controlled efficacy trial of pimecrolimus cream 1% for the treatment of moderate to severe facial seborrheic dermatitis. *J Acad Dermatol* 2007;57:257-264.
45. High WA, Pandya AG. Pilot trial of 1% pimecrolimus cream in the treatment of seborrheic dermatitis in African-American adults with dissociated hypopigmentation. *J Am Acad Dermatol* 2006;54:1083-1088.
46. Nakagawa H, Etol T, Yokata Y, et al. Tacrolimus has antifungal activities against *Malassezia furfur* isoloated from healthy adults and patients with atopic dermatitis. *Clin Drug Invest* 1996;12:245-250.
47. Johnson BA, Nunley JR. Treatment of seborrheic dermatitis. *Am Fam Physician* 2000;6:2703-2710.
48. Cuelenaere C, DeBersaques J, Kint A. The use of lithium succinate in the treatment of seborrheic dermatitis. *Dermatology;* 1992;184:194-197.
49. deSáDias TC, Baby AR, Kaneko TM, Robles Velasco MV. Relaxing/straightening of Afro-ethnic hair: Historical overview. *J Cosmet Dermatol* 2007;6:2-5.
50. Anonymous. Release by NMA. *Newsletter,* February 2007.

CHAPTER 37

Tinea Capitis

Marcy S. Alvarez
Nanette B. Silverberg

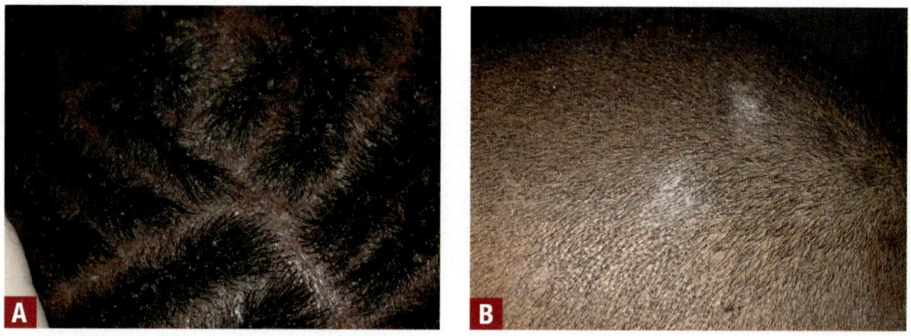

▲ **FIGURE 37-1** Seborrheic-type tinea capitis. ***A.*** In a 4-year-old African-American girl with hyperkeratosis and alopecia marked by widening of the space between the cornrows. ***B.*** Alopecia accompanied by well-circumscribed hyperkeratosis.

Key Points

- Tinea capitis is a common fungal scalp infection affecting school-aged children, usually caused in the United States by *Trichophyton tonsurans*.
- Alopecia and scalp hyperkeratosis in children should raise suspicion of tinea capitis.
- Oral griseofulvin for at least 6 weeks is still the "gold standard" in the treatment of tinea capitis in children; however, reevaluation after therapy is required because there is a growing number of griseofulvin-resistant tinea scalp isolates.
- Family education regarding reduced fungal fomite spread is an integral part of the treatment of tinea capitis.
- Fungal culture and antifungal sensitivities can aid in the treatment of difficult cases.

Tinea capitis (TC) is a dermatophyte infection of the scalp, skin, hair follicles, and hair shafts. Once thought to be rare, TC is now increasingly more common among people of all ages, ranging from neonates to senior citizens. TC is the most common superficial mycotic infection encountered in the pediatric population. Most alarming is its proclivity for children with African and Caribbean hair types. Worldwide, the prevalence of TC continues to increase despite simple methods of diagnosis and effective treatment measures available. This is due in part to the variable clinical presentation, changing epidemiology, and difficulty of elimination of asymptomatic carriers. Recent studies in the United States and Puerto Rico show a point prevalence rate of as high as 13% of school children. These patients are mostly African-American and Hispanic children infected with *Trichophyton tonsurans*.[1] Physicians should maintain a heightened index of suspicion for this potential condition, particularly when treating patients with skin of color. This chapter aims to review the most current information on TC in patients of color, including its diagnosis, treatment, and efforts to control its spread worldwide.

CLINICAL PRESENTATION

TC has five distinctive patterns of clinical disease: noninflammatory (seborrheic) (Figure 37-1), black dot (Figure 37-2), inflammatory (kerion), alopecia areata type, and favus. Recently, a sixth type of TC has emerged, TC caused by *T. beigelii*. In the United States, the prevalence of *T. tonsurans* infection, an endothrix infection of the hair shaft, has been associated with an increase in seborrheic and black dot tinea types. Seborrheic-type TC is the most common type in the United States and appears clinically like seborrheic dermatitis, with scalp erythema, hyperkeratosis, and variable alopecia. Seborrheic dermatitis is not seen in healthy children aged 2–7 years; hence the appearance of seborrhea-like illness in this age group is almost certainly TC. Seborrheic type TC can be mistaken for seborrheic dermatitis or psoriasis, particularly in adults.

In the black dot variant of tinea capitis, hairs are weakened by fungal elements in the hair and are broken midshaft or closer to the scalp, leaving

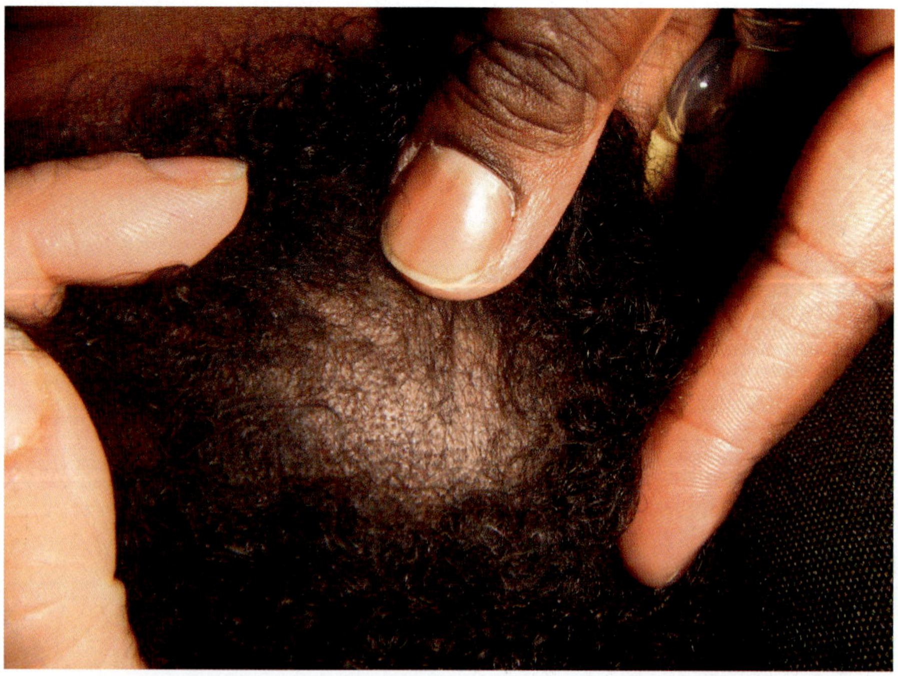

▲ **FIGURE 37-2** Black dot tinea capitis on the scalp of a 1.5-year-old African-American girl.

well-defined patches of studded hair. This so-called black dot tinea also may be known as yellow or red dot tinea as dictated by hair color. The term *black dot* alludes to the epidemiology, that is, infection primarily of African-American and Hispanic children with dark hair. This presentation is common in the suboccipital region of the scalp, and the affected hairs appear gray and feel gritty to the touch. The differential diagnoses for black dot tinea include trichotillomania, traction alopecia, telogen effluvium, and alopecia areata. Lymphadenopathy is uncommon in black dot tinea because it is noninflammatory.

Alopecia areata–type TC presents as smooth alopecia without gritty hairs, hyperkeratosis, or inflammation. While rare, this type should be sought actively in children through culture of all suspected alopecia areata cases. Enlarged occipital nodes should be evaluated on physical examination, but recent studies suggest that they are present in only a third of all pediatric TC patients.[2]

Inflammatory infections (kerion), such as those commonly seen with *Microsporum* species, often reveal scattered perifollicular pustules. Aggressive inflammatory TC appears as a tender, purulent, boggy mass that is often mistaken for cellulitis. Nonscarring and scarring alopecia both can occur. Clinical examination of inflammatory TC usually reveals cervical and/or postauricular lymphadenopathy. Fever, pain, secondary bacterial infection, and abscess formation are further complications that can ensue. These infections tend to resolve over 10 weeks. The immune response can be so intense as to cause scarring alopecia. While in the past *Microsporum* species caused most kerions, currently the species responsible in the United States include *T. tonsurans, T. verrucosum,* and *T. mentagrophytes*. Positive *Trichophyton* skin tests have been elicited in children with kerion production, suggesting a delayed hypersensitivity response to the offending species. The differential diagnosis for inflammatory TC includes impetigo, dissecting folliculitis, and lupus erythematosus.

Favus (tinea favosa) is seen with *T. schoenleinii* and *T. quinckeanum* infections. Favus is a chronic inflammatory form of TC that can lead to cicatricial alopecia, skin atrophy, and scar formation. It is frequently encountered in individuals of African, Mediterranean, and Middle Eastern descent. Scutula, matted clumps of hyphae, and keratin hair debris are the hallmarks of this presentation. Adjacent areas coalesce, leading to a yellow crusty mass that is easily identifiable. Unlike other forms of TC, favus does not remit after puberty. The lesions fluoresce a gray-green color on Wood's lamp examination. Diagnosis is confirmed on microscopy with the presence of the hyphal elements separated by distinctive air tunnels. Infection also can be seen in long hair because hyphal invasion has no affect on hair growth.

White piedra occurs more commonly in subtropical or temperate zones. The white to brown soft nodules found on the hair shaft can be removed easily. Piedra commonly affects the shaft of the hair, whereas TC caused by *Microsporum* and *Trichophyton* species more commonly affect the base. *T. beigelii* infections may appear as white piedra, as seborrheic-type TC, or as some combination of the two. Evidence of any hyperkeratosis or "gray patch" tinea (seborrhea), excoriations secondary to pruritus, alopecia, broken hairs or black dot appearance, cervical lymphadenopathy, pustules, and indurated or boggy plaques should alert the physician to the possibility of TC (Figure 37-3).

Evidence of TC or an id reaction also should prompt a thorough scalp investigation in children because these are often associated with TC cause by *T. tonsurans*.

DEMOGRAPHICS

Age

Historically considered a pediatric disease, TC may be caused by a variety of fungi. Dermatophytes are fungi that derive nutrition from keratin, present only in the skin, hair, and nails. Select fungi show varying preferences for geographic location, age, and race. In the United States, the highest incidence of infection occurs in 3- to 7-year-olds.[3] Worldwide, preadolescent children are affected most commonly as well; however, the age range is highly dependent on region. A recent study in western Africa evaluating symptomatic schoolchildren found an increase in TC cases among 8- to 11-year-olds.[4]

TC also has been described in neonates. An Italian study reported 15 infantile cases of TC caused by *M. canis*.[5] Ismail and colleagues found *T. tonsurans* to be the most common dermatophyte in their London-based infant population with primarily African-Caribbean type hair (91%).[6] In infantile cases, the

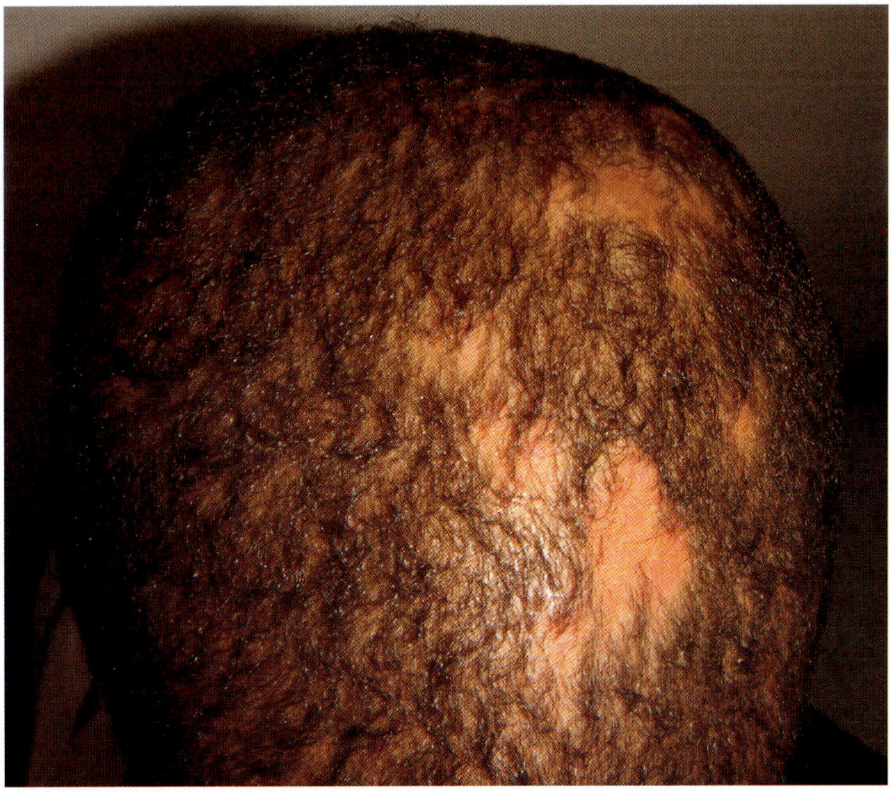

▲ **FIGURE 37-3** Diffuse alopecia and boggy erythematous plaques consistent with a kerion type of tinea capitis. This 4-year-old African-American child also had palpable occipital lymphadenopathy.

primary caregiver should be suspected as the source of infection. African-Caribbean hair type and exposure to an infected individual, rather than socioeconomic status of the patient, are thought to be the primary risk factor for infants.[7]

TC traditionally was thought to be uncommon after puberty, but recent increases in adult and geriatric cases show that this may no longer be the case.[8] The past theory on why adults were less likely to get TC was that pubertal increases in saturated fatty acids in sebum were thought to impart a fungistatic property to the scalp.[9] Investigations into adult infections have been directed predominately at carrier status detection and the relation of affected adult members to index pediatric cases. Some apparently idiopathic adult cases have occurred. One British report discussed two unrelated women who presented with alopecia and hyperkeratosis.[10] Neither patient had direct contact with children or animals, but both frequented the same hairdresser. Fungal cultures grew out *M. canis*. Transmission presumably was due to fomite contamination at the hair salon.

Older studies place the rate of adult infection at less than 3% of all TC cases.[11,12] Recent studies suggest that the rate may be as high as 12.3% in select populations.[8, 13] Typical presentations in adult patients include mild to moderate scaling to well-defined areas of discrete alopecia. Various presentations are possible in adults, particularly in those with immunosuppression or human immunodeficiency virus (HIV) infection.[14] While other superficial cutaneous mycoses are common, few reports of HIV associated TC exist. Di Silverio and colleagues postulate that the overgrowth of *Pityrosporum* species on the scalp of HIV patients may have a protective role.[15,16]

Gender

Incidence and type of TC may vary by sex. In Spain over the past 20 years, *M. audouinii* has a ratio as high as 5:1 of male to female cases.[3] For children in the United States, *Trichophyton* infections do not appear to have a gender preference.

Sexual predilection is most evident in adult populations, particularly with *Trichophyton* infections. Women account for 66–94% of adult TC cases seen worldwide.[8] Most of the reported cases in adults have involved women with African-Caribbean hair types; however, Asian women also have been affected. In a 20-year survey by Bronson and colleagues, women were observed to be infected six times more frequently than men.[17] A French study found 75% of their population to consist of women.[13] Hormonal regulation, alterations of the endocrine system, and immune deficiency are thought to play a role. Postmenopausal women are noted to have a higher rate of infection with *Trichophyton* species. Kalaman and colleagues suggest the decreased production of triglyceride-rich sebum may be a predisposing factor in postmenopausal TC.[18] The lipase activity of *Pityrosporum ovale* is thought to have a protective role in combating scalp dermatophyte infections.[19,20] Some postulate that closer contact and increased exposure to infected children may explain the gender difference. Female caretakers of infected children have been demonstrated to have higher rates of tinea corporis in addition to higher rates of asymptomatic TC infections.[8,13,21] While children may infect their parents and grandparents, grandparents and parents also may infect their kids. Thus pediatric cases that are difficult to eradicate require full family evaluation and cultures. Furthermore, clinicians need to maintain a higher level of suspicion when seeing adult females, particularly African-American women, with seborrhea or scalp psoriasis.

Racial Distribution

The predominance of literature about TC in people of African-American origin is striking. More than 90% of reported TC cases in the United States occur in African-American populations, and there has been a rate of growth of TC cases in the African-American community roughly 10 times greater than in the Caucasian population. This racial penchant is most apparent in lower socioeconomic communities, where there is overcrowding, and children are often living in households with index cases. Although hairstyling practices such as pomades, braiding, and hair covering have been thought to affect disease incidence, a recent multicenter study by Sharma and colleagues demonstrated no positive association between these practices and acquisition of TC.[2]

Latinos are also frequently affected by scalp dermatophytoses. In a New York study evaluating a predominantly Puerto Rican population, *T. tonsurans* and *T. rubrum* were the most frequent isolates.[22] Zoophilic infections with *M. canis* continue to dominate in South American countries such as Peru and Argentina.[23–27] Pediatric studies in Brazil are more variable, showing an increase and predominance of *M. canis* in the south and southeast and *T. tonsurans* in the north and northeast.[25]

EPIDEMIOLOGY

Tinea infections are caused by keratinophilic fungi which inhabit the stratum corneum, follicular orifice, and hairs down to the area of initial keratinization (Adamson's fringe). They rarely invade into the deeper epidermal layers. Systemic infection is seen only in cases of severe immunodeficiency and HIV infection and generally only with *Trichosporum* species, that is, nondermatophytes. Scalp or hair trauma is thought to contribute to acquisition of the disease. Colonization alone is not sufficient to cause infection. Carrier states, defined as colonization with little to no symptomatology, may play a large role in the spread of the disease.

Dermatophytoses are classified according to the area they affect clinically. Infections of the scalp, face and neck, and body and feet are termed *tinea capitis, faciei or barbae (in men), corporis,* and *pedis,* respectively. Although there are over 40 species of dermatophyes, only a dozen are implicated in clinical disease of the scalp. *Trichophyton* and *Microsporum* species account for most cases of TC, the former being far more common in current clinical practice in the United States.

Based on host preference, dermatophytes are further classified as anthropophilic (human), zoophilic (animal), and geophilic (soil). Anthropophilic infections are mainly noninflammatory in nature, whereas zoophilic infections are known to produce marked inflammation. Geophilic fungi such as *M. gypseum* and *M. fulvum* have a worldwide distribution but rarely cause TC.

In rural areas or households with animals such as cats, dogs, or cattle, the zoophilic fungi should be considered. Inquiries about the presence of animals should be made in all suspected tinea cases. *M. canis* is transmitted by dogs and cats, especially kittens, and *T. verrucosum* by cattle. Cats have been shown to be important sources of contagion in Greek, Spanish, and Italian studies.[28–31] *M. canis* is virtually unheard of in Finland, where the country is too cold to support an outdoor cat population.[32]

Dermatophytoses of the scalp are also divided based on hair invasion patterns.

Three types of hair invasion are noted: endothrix, ectothrix, and favus. In endothrix invasions, the hyphae infect the scalp and move down the hair shaft, finally penetrating in the shaft. While the cuticle surface remains intact, the hyphae convert into the infectious arthroconidia or spores. Many *Trichophyton* species produce endothrix infections, namely, *T. tonsurans*, *T. violaceum*, *T. soudanense*, *T. gourvilii*, and *T. yaoundei*.

Ectothrix infections, usually caused by *Microsporum* species, invade the hair shaft in much the same way as endothrix infections. However, these hyphae then penetrate back through the cuticle to develop into the infectious spores both within and outside the hair shaft. Spore sizes range from small (2–3 μm) to large (up to 10 μm). Unlike the hidden spores of endothrix infections, many ectothrix infections will fluoresce under Wood's light. Other species known to cause this type of invasion include *T. verrucosum* and *T. mentagrophytes*.

T. schoenleinii produces a specific type of chronic endothrix invasion known as *favus*. No spores are formed. Instead, the hyphae grow within the hair shaft to create characteristic air spaces. A characteristic honeycomb appearance can be seen on microscopy.

Epidemiologic Shifts and Worldwide Trends in TC

In the United States, two distinct epidemics of TC occurred over the last half century. In the 1940s and 1950s, *M. audouinii* was the most commonly observed pathogen. Mostly affecting white boys, this agent could be identified with the use of a Wood's lamp. In the 1950s, *T. tonsurans* came into the United States with immigrants from Puerto Rico, the Caribbean, South America, Mexico, and other Central American nations.[33–35] Soon, *T. tonsurans* replaced *M. audouinii* as the most common cause of TC. Current surveys show the percentage of TC cases caused by *T. tonsurans* to be upwards of 94% across the United States, Puerto Rico, and Trinidad.[36–38]

Canada and western Europe have recently exhibited parallel epidemiologic increases in the incidence of anthropophilic species. In Canada, Gupta and colleagues observed a major increase in the incidence of *T. tonsurans* over an 11-year period.[39] Once accounting for only 9% of fungal scalp infections, the number of confirmed *T. tonsurans* cases rose to 76%. Over 90% of the observed TC cases in the United Kingdom are now attributed to *T. tonsurans*.[39–42] A survey in Spain from 14 different regions showed *T. tonsurans*, followed by *T. violaceum*, to be the most frequent pathogens.[43] The precipitous rise is believed to be related to increases in travel and immigration from endemic areas. In Spain, most cases have been traced to people of North African origin.

In parts of South America, Latin America, Mexico, and Europe, *M. canis* infections still predominate.[38] Northeastern Spain experienced a drastic increase in *M. canis* infections over the 20-year period of 1977–1997 from 25–90%.[31] *M. canis* accounts for more than 54% of TC infections in eastern Europe, whereas *T. tonsurans* is isolated in less than 5% of eastern European cases.[44] Worldwide trends indicate a slight predilection of *M. canis* for male children,[31,45–47] although predominance in female populations has been seen in some studies, primarily where older patients are involved.[48–51]

In Africa, *T. violaceum* is the main dermatophyte seen in countries such as Rwanda, Ethiopia, Libya, and Jordan.[38,49,51–56] The extent of infection is epidemic in some parts of Africa. The recently observed change in etiology of African infections from *T. schoenleinii* to *T. violaceum* has been attributed to increased immigration from the Mediterranean.[55] Recent upswings of *T. violaceum* infection in New Zealand, Spain, and Italy have been traced to African immigrants.[43,57–59]

T. soudanense is endemic on the western coast of Africa.[60] In a 1-year cross-sectional study by Menan and colleagues, 1913 African school children were examined. Of these, 227 children with scalp symptoms suggestive of TC were examined, 95% of whom were mycologic-positive. More than 63% grew *T. soudanense*, and 31% were positive for *M. langeronii*. Boys in the age range of 8–11 years of age were affected most commonly. Because asymptomatic children were not cultured, the prevalence rate of 11.3% for this region may be grossly underestimated because carrier states went unaccounted.

Sporadic cases of *T. soudanense* have been reported in other parts of Europe and the United States. Markey and colleagues reported two cases of *T. soudanense* TC in adopted Liberian sisters.[61] The appearance of *T. soudanense* outside endemic Africa is not surprising because most cases can be traced to exposure to people of African origin or present in recent immigrants.[61,62]

M. langeronii is the most common causative species of TC in the Central Africa Republic.[63] It is identified in 98% of culture-positive cases, and boys are affected more commonly. In Nigeria, *M. audouinii* still persists and has been linked to a recent report of an outbreak of children with TC.[64]

T. rubrum, while a common cause of tinea elsewhere on the body, rarely infects the scalp. Recent reports have been associated with adult cases of TC. Schwinn and colleagues reported the relative frequency among adult *T. rubrum* TC to be as high as 10% compared with less than 1% of childhood cases.[65] Although the absolute case numbers are low, given the ever-increasing incidence of onychomycosis caused by *T. rubrum*, incidence may rise in the future.

T. beigelii has been found to be a source of tinea pedis and onychomycosis in Mexican children who wear loose sandals that allow exposure to soil. Recently, three cases of *T. beigelii* hair infections in Mexican children presented in our New York clinic. Two children presented with hair concretions that appeared to the referring clinician as lice, and the third child had classic TC. The infections responded to topical ketoconazole shampoo and oral itraconazole therapy.

Contagion

Understanding the transmission of TC is an important step in the eradication process. Transmission may occur via human-to-human spread with actively infected persons or carriers, fomites, animal vectors, or soil. Anthropophilic species prove to be the most difficult to control owing to their varied clinical presentation and highly infectious nature. These species are able to remain viable for long periods as fomites on hairbrushes, linens, playmats, and clothing. Many reports have implicated household items such as dolls, combs and brushes, clothing, bedding, towels, and toys as causative agents of spread.[66,67] Although it seems virtually impossible, MacKenzie and colleagues have even demonstrated airborne transmission.

Examination into the possible correlation of hairstyling practices was a focus of a 2-year cohort study from southeast London.[41] Although the pediatric population was not predominantly of pigmented skin, 91% of TC cases were seen in children with African-Caribbean hair types, with a male predominance of 68%. The most common isolate was *T. tonsurans*. Since short hairstyles for men were in vogue at the time of the study, the use of clippers was more popular than plaiting or the use of traditional scissors. Viable fungal elements were isolated from some of the clippers and razors commonly used on the boys to produce their desired hairstyles. In a report by Takwale and colleagues, the acquisition of *M. canis* TC in two elderly women was presumably from the hairdresser because both visited the same salon within a short period of time.[68]

An Indian study evaluated the use of oils in both men and women because the incidence of TC in this region of the world is rare.[69] Customary use of mustard, coconut, and amla oils imparts a fungistatic property to the hair derived from the percentage of unsaturated and saturated fatty acids contained in the individual oil. Amla oil was found to be the most protective against *M. canis, M. gypseum,* and *T. rubrum*. Mustard oil proved to be the least effective.

Sharma and colleagues evaluated the hair-grooming practices in a 90% African-American population with clinical evidence of TC against age-, sex-, and race-matched controls.[2] This study did not find an association between the sharing of combs and brushes, the use of oils and gels, or the frequency of shampooing, as suggested by other studies. Use of conditioners showed some statistical significance in preventing TC acquisition in the univariable model but not in the multivariable model, suggesting the need for further testing to determine if their use is of importance. A studies by Ghannoum and colleagues also failed to show a correlation between hair braiding practices or the use of oils and creams rinses in their TC population.[1]

Carriers and Fomites

Asymptomatic carriers in the home and at school may aggravate epidemic spread of TC. In the past, the incidence of scalp carriage was grossly underestimated. New studies are looking into its prevalence, its role in spread of the infection, and progression toward clinical symptomatology. In 1954, Mullins reported a family with three generations of *T. tonsurans*–positive TC, raising the suspicion of the home as a major factor in disease transmission.[70] Subsequent studies confirmed the presence of asymptomatic carriers in close association with index cases. Depending on the species, index cases were 34–45% more likely to have infected relatives compared with controls.[71,72] Studies show siblings of infected school-aged children were 9.4 times more likely to be infected.[73]

Classmates and playmates at school are suspected to play a role in the transmission of scalp dermatoses. It is believed that carriers within the classroom may be more important in the spread of infection than index cases. These carriers have been demonstrated to remain culture-positive and symptom-free for as long as 8 months.[74–76] Whether this indicates a chronic carrier state or successive, transient reinfections, the potential to shed infectious spores over long periods of time may pose a larger threat than once believed.

A study of African-American elementary school children in Philadelphia revealed a 14% prevalence rate of asymptomatic carriage of *T. tonsurans*.[77] After treatment of index cases, three classrooms continued to have an increase in the number of carriers. Clusters of friends and siblings of index cases also showed a higher chance of infection.[75,78] These findings are in sharp contrast to an earlier London-based study by Midgely and colleagues in which the carrier state was 12–30% in classrooms but decreased or eventually disappeared after eradication of index cases.[78] This finding was not reproduced in studies by Williams and colleagues and Ali-Shtayeh and colleagues, suggesting that other sources of infection may be important, such as home exposures.[77,79]

In the United States, asymptomatic carrier rates for *T. tonsurans* infections among African-American school children is estimated to be around 8–15%.[73,75,77,78] *T. tonsurans* is often isolated in carrier states, even when it is not the predominant pathogen in the region. In a Spanish study examining 10,000 school children, although *M. canis* was the most common isolate in symptomatic cases, *T. tonsurans* was detected more frequently in scalp carriers.[80] This likely relates to the less inflammatory nature of *Trichophyton* infections.

In poor families, the lack of medical attention coupled with the recycling of clothing, toys, and other personal items increases the chance of fomite spread. Inner-city practices of purchasing used toys have been associated with TC transmission.

SPECIAL CLINICAL SITUATIONS

In immunosuppressed and HIV-infected patients, the clinical presentation is highly varied. Reports show that some presentations may resemble bacterial folliculitis, folliculitis decalvans, dissecting cellulitis, and the scarring related to lupus erythematosus.[81–83] Cases also have ranged in clinical appearance from unusual species such as *T. rubrum,* to pyoderma-like pictures, to suppurative inflammatory granulomas.[16,84]

DIAGNOSIS AND TREATMENT

Laboratory Evaluation and Testing

Diagnosis of TC based on clinical examination alone is usually possible but sometimes can be difficult. It is therefore desirable to have an effective tool for relatively rapid confirmation of diagnosis. A delay in diagnosis can lead to unnecessary procedures, inefficient treatment attempts, or spread of the condition. Wood's lamp, while still useful, has limited utility in today's age in detecting the dermatophyte infections most common in the United States. Direct light microscopy of hair or keratinocyte scrapings of the scalp examined under adjunctive stains is a simple in-office procedure that can confirm the diagnosis. In-office or laboratory fungal cultures may be used in conjunction to help isolate and confirm the causative agent but can take 3–4 weeks to grow and identify the causative species. Biopsy is rarely needed and should be reserved for cases of treatment failure or when proper attempts at direct microscopy and culture fail to reveal the diagnosis.

Wood's Lamp

The Wood's lamp is a safe, easy-to-use means of detection for some dermatophyte infections. The light emits a long-wave ultraviolet radiation (maximum of 365 nm). When *Microsporum* ectothrix infections prevailed in the United States, examination under the Wood's lamp could easily detect infected hairs. With the rise of nonfluorescing endothrix infections with *Trichophyton* species, physicians can no longer solely rely on this screening method. Species known to fluoresce include *M. audouinii, M. ferrugineum,* and *T. schoenleinii*. The infected hairs in favus fluoresce yellow, whereas most *Microsporum* species emit a bright green color.

Microscopy and Culture

There are many ways to obtain an adequate specimen for culture, but particular emphasis should be placed on child-friendly techniques. In the past, plucking clinically affected hairs or scraping the scalp with a blade was performed to obtain a sample. This can be difficult, uncomfortable, and unwelcome in a wary pediatric patient. Tweezing or plucking the hairs can yield poor results because infected hair can break mid-shaft. This is particularly problematic in endothrix infections. Other efforts to obtain suitable specimens include the use of toothbrushes, moist cotton swabs, hairbrushes, moistened gauze, and adhesive tape, all of which will attract hyperkeratotic flakes and broken endothrix-infected hairs.

Friedlander and colleagues compared the use of the cotton swab technique with that of the toothbrush method.[85] Children with untreated TC had cultures obtained from two areas of affected scalp. One group of specimens was obtained by rubbing a sterile toothbrush over the affected areas. The second group of specimens was collected with a moistened cotton-tipped applicator. The specimens were subsequently inoculated on Mycosel medium and incubated either in the office or in the laboratory and were observed for 3 weeks. The authors concluded that use of the cotton swab technique to obtain samples was efficient, effective, and viewed as "friendly" by children. The toothbrush technique has been demonstrated to have a very good yield in other pediatric studies.[75]

Identification of the pathogen with the use of direct microscopy can be performed easily in the office. Hairs obtained from the scalp are mixed with 10–20% potassium hydroxide (KOH), heated, and examined under a microscope. KOH reduces the adhesion of corneocytes, thinning and flattening the stratum corneum, so hyphae are more easily visible. Direct observation of endothrix or ectothrix invasion of the hair also can be seen. Other commercially available stains used in fungal microscopy include Swartz-Lamkin, which stains fungal elements blue, and Calcaflour white solution (Fungi-Fluor, Polysciences, Inc., Warrington, PA), a stain that binds nonspecifically to cellulose and chitin found in fungal cell walls. Under fluorescent microscopy, a blue-white or apple green color can be seen depending on the filter used. The sensitivity and specificity of this fluorescent brightener were 76% and 58%, respectively, according to studies done by Honig and colleagues.[86]

When precise identification of the pathogen is desired, isolation in culture should be performed. There are many commercially available culture media, including Mycosel, Mycobiotic (Sabouraud's agar with cyclohexamide and chloramphenicol), Dermatophyte Identification Medium (DIM), and Dermatophyte Test Medium (DTM).[87,88] Equipped with a color indicator, the latter test medium turns red in the presence of both dermatophytes and some nondermatophytes. Growth on culture medium may take weeks. McLean and colleagues found that culture alone would have missed 33.2% of actual TC cases, whereas solely performing direct mount would have missed only 10.4% of cases.[89] While increased experience in microscopy and culture isolation yields higher positive results, the utility of in-office dry mount cannot be overemphasized.

Treatment

The goal of TC therapy is to achieve a complete cure. Ideal therapies are rapidly effective, easily tolerated, and cost the patient little. Unlike most superficial dermatophytoses, TC does not respond to topical therapy alone; systemic therapy is needed to penetrate into the hair shaft and eradicate the infectious spores. Topical therapy is used adjunctively in index cases, as well as in other household members. Topical shampoos and antifungal solutions have been shown to lower the number of shedding arthroconidia and may be initiated safely to reduce contagion.

Therapy of TC requires clinical and mycologic cures. If both are achieved, recurrences are unlikely. Careful cleaning of brushes, combs, and bedding should help to prevent reacquisition of disease from one's own fomites. Recurrences may or may not respond to therapy as well as the first infectious episode. Furthermore, patients who aren't fully cured remain potentially infectious.

Oral Therapies

GRISEOFULVIN Currently, griseofulvin is the mainstay of therapy. First used in 1958, it has remained the "gold standard" of treatment to which all others therapies for TC are compared.[90] Griseofulvin has a good safety profile and is well tolerated. Griseofulvin is derived from a *Penicillium* species, but no known cross-allergy with penicillin or the cephalosporins has been observed. Griseofulvin is a fungistatic drug that inhibits cell wall synthesis and interferes with spindle microtubule function and DNA production. It is absorbed moderately from the gut, and its uptake is enhanced with fatty food intake. Griseofulvin has a low affinity for keratin and thus requires continuous administration.[91,92]

The most commonly observed adverse events known to occur with griseofulvin are headache and gastrointestinal upset. These side effects occur even less commonly in pediatric populations. More severe, but rare, reactions that have been documented include hepatotoxicity, neutropenia, leukopenia, photosensitivity, drug rashes, urticaria, proteinuria, erythema multiforme, and a serum sickness–like reaction.[93] Id reactions, hypersensitivity responses to the dermatophyte, are often noted shortly after initiation of griseofulvin but do not necessitate discontinuation of therapy. The need for baseline or periodic laboratory monitoring is controversial, but most authors agree that short courses lasting less than 3 months do not require monitoring in healthy children.[94] Rated pregnancy category C, griseofulvin should not be taken by pregnant women.

According to the *Physician's Desk Reference,* griseofulvin is dosed at 5–11 mg/kg per day.[95] However, problematic absorption of the micronized liquid and relative resistances of today's fungi to the drug have necessitated dosing at 20–25 mg/kg per day of the liquid and approximately half that dose if using ultramicronized tablets. Therapy should be continued until clinical and mycologic cure are achieved. This usually takes 6–8 weeks. However, therapy in severe cases may continue upwards of 3 months. When therapy is this prolonged or rapid relapse is noted, alternative drugs may be chosen.

With increasing incidence of disease and documented cases of resistance, a search for alternative medications is underway. Whereas griseofulvin remains the "gold standard" of treatment, alternative systemic antifungals are being investigated both in the United States and abroad. These promising antifungals, including itraconazole, fluconazole, and terbinafine, aim to shorten the length of therapy, improve clinical efficacy and tolerability, and decrease the potential for adverse side effects.

ITRACONAZOLE Itraconazole, a triazole antifungal, is extremely lipophilic and keratinophilic, concentrating in hair, nails, and skin 3- to 10-fold more than in plasma.[96,97] Effective antimycotic concentrations have been measured in the skin for up to 4 weeks after termination of the medication, lending itself to short courses of therapy or pulsed therapy. Dosage is usually 3–5 mg/kg per day for 4–6 weeks taken with meals. Other dosing schedules such as pulses every 2–3 weeks or 100-mg capsules each day irrespective of weight have been shown to be effective in TC therapy for some children. Itraconazole is available in capsule and liquid forms. The liquid form is intended for HIV-infected patients; it is known to cause severe diarrhea in long-term pediatric use owing to cyclodextrin. Cyclodextrin also has been associated with pancreatic carcinomas in laboratory animals. Difficulty in having a child take a capsule is universal regardless of medication; however, capsules may be opened into orange juice for easier ingestion. Owing to the short course of therapy, routine complete blood counts and hepatic enzyme monitoring are not necessary unless long-term usage is required (i.e., exceeding 3 months).

FLUCONAZOLE Fluconazole has been approved for therapy of pediatric fungal infections, including oral candidiasis, and thus has an exceptional safety profile. Fluconazole has been shown to be efficacious in the treatment of TC in doses of 6 mg/kg per day for up to 6 weeks.[96,97] In two studies, once-weekly dosing of 8 mg/kg for up to 12 weeks was shown to produce a complete cure in patients with *Trichophyton* infections. *Microsporum* species also showed high cure rates with a similar dosing regimen, but longer treatment durations may be necessary.

Recent clinical reports have found fluconazole to be safe in children. The most commonly reported side effects included mild to moderate gastrointestinal upset. Although rare, liver function abnormalities have been found. The drug is available in both capsule and suspension forms. It is highly water soluble and well absorbed. Its bioavailability is not affected by food intake.

TERBINAFINE The recommended dosage for terbinafine is 3–6 mg/kg per day up to 8 weeks. *Trichophyton* species are known to respond in 2–4 weeks, whereas *M. canis* infections may require longer therapy to achieve mycologic and clinical cures.[96,97] Only a tablet form is available, and the tablets are not crushed easily. Its pharmacokinetics is not altered with the administration of food. It is recommended to monitor liver enzymes and complete blood count if treatment is warranted for longer than 3 months.

Efficacy (Table 37-1)

Where cost is concerned, griseofulvin and terbinafine are the least expensive forms of therapy in tablet form. Only griseofulvin, itraconazole, and fluconazole are available in pediatric liquid formulations, which are ideal in pediatric medicine. The liquid form of griseofulvin, while costly, may result in increased compliance in smaller children, whereas the tablet has superior gut absorption. In addition to the inability of the azole antifungals to show greater efficacy than the "gold standard," the price of itraconazole and fluconazole remain relatively higher. Fluconazole liquid is the

TABLE 37-1
An Overview of Oral Antifungals Used for Pediatric Tinea Capitis

Drug	Formulations Available	Efficacy/Facts	Recommended Dose	Side Effects	Labs
Griseofulvin	Micronized and ultramicronized tablets Micronized oral suspension	Take with fatty food Bitter tasting Hepatic metabolism	5–11 mg/kg/d in the PDR 10–25 mg/kg/d for 8–10 weeks in clinical practice	Headache GI disturbances Rash Malaise Photosensitivity*	No labs in healthy children CBC, LFT after 3 months of use
Fluconazole	Tablet Capsule Oral suspension	Approved for pediatric candidiasis Kids > 6 months Absorbs without food Pleasant taste Hepatic metabolism	6 mg/kg/d for 3–6 weeks	Diarrhea Headache Rash P450 drug interactions†	No labs in healthy children CBC, LFT after 3 months of use
Itraconazole	Capsule Oral solution (with cyclodextrin stabilizer)	Hepatic metabolism	3–5 mg/kg/d for 4–6 weeks or 100 mg/d or pulsed dose every 2–3 weeks	Diarrhea Headache Rash Alopecia P450 drug interactions†	No labs in healthy children CBC, LFT after 3 months of use
Terbinafine	Tablets	Hepatic metabolism	3–6 mg/kg/d for 4–8 weeks	Diarrhea Headache Rash Dysgeusia P450 drug interactions†	No labs in healthy children CBC, LFT after 3 months of use

*Contraindicated in systemic lupus erythematosus, hepatic porphyrias, hepatitis, and severe liver disease.
†Contraindicated in liver disease and hepatitis.

most easily tolerated in pediatric populations owing to its pleasant taste.

While these newer antifungals have an excellent safety profile, their appeal lies in the shorter duration of therapy and potential for decreased side effects. Further studies are necessary to determine optimal dosage, efficacy, and safety in children, infants, and immunosuppressed patients.

In conjunction with systemic therapy, shampoos and other antimycotic agents have been used to help augment the response. Concerns about compliance, systemic side effects, and absorption variability in these oral medications have led to further investigation into suitable adjunctive therapies to reduce the course of disease.

Shampoos

Antifungals shampoos have been shown to be beneficial as both adjuvant therapy, for sole use in household members who may act as carriers, and to prevent acquisition by friends and family members. Regardless of the dermatophyte, it is postulated that regular use decreases the spore load and shedding of infectious arthroconidia. Thus 1% econazole nitrate, 4% povidine-iodine shampoo and even basic conditioners have been shown to have some beneficial effects.[2,76] Selenium sulfide 2.5% and ketoconazole 2% have been shown to be highly effective when used three times a week.[76,98] When used in conjunction with griseofulvin, topical selenium sulfide produced mycologic cures at 2 weeks of therapy. It is recommended that patients leave the shampoo on for 5 minutes before rinsing. Greer evaluated the daily use of ketoconazole 2% shampoo in 15 black children with *T. tonsurans* TC.[99] A total of 33% achieved complete cure with the use of ketoconazole 2% shampoo alone and remained culture-negative at a 12-month follow-up. By 2 weeks, all spore load counts decreased by 50%. Furthermore, cure rates with the addition of griseofulvin after an 8-week shampooing period were achieved faster than with griseofulvin alone. Zinc pyrithione shampoo has the ability to normalize the ultrastructure of the stratum corneum and may play a role in the treatment of hyperkeratotic or seborrheic presentations of TC.[100]

Other Therapies

Some clinicians use corticosteroids to try to reduce scarring alopecia when extensive scalp inflammation is observed. The benefits of oral or intralesional corticosteroids in the treatment of inflammatory TC are limited. In a study by Ginsburg and colleagues, griseofulvin with intralesional corticosteroid was compared with griseofulvin alone.[101] The study looked at a predominantly female black pediatric population with *T. tonsurans*–positive kerion infections. The parameters evaluated included time to negative culture, time of onset of new hair growth, complete regrowth of hair, and time to scalp clearing. No significant benefit from corticosteroid was observed.

The need to quarantine infected children or those undergoing treatment is under debate. The extended course of the disease, even when therapy has been instituted, precludes children from being kept out of school until TC cure is effected. Further information is needed about the transmission of TC. While index cases are more apparent, carriers in the home and at school are suspected to have as much or a greater role in the spread in the disease. Even when laws are in place to remove TC-positive children from school, they are often not applied. Ectothrix species, while considered more contagious, may deserve greater consideration with regard to isolation measures. Viguie-Vallanet and colleagues noted the rapid spread of *M. langeronii* in kindergarten children in a Paris suburb.[102] In one center, the source was believed to be an African child from an endemic area; the other focus involved a child born in France of African descendants. The authors treated both symptomatic and carrier children. They reported control of the epidemic with no relapse at 1-year follow-up.

CONCLUSION

Tinea capitis continues to be a formidable disease despite recent advances in medical treatment and ease of diagnosis. The rising incidence of the carrier status in cohabitants and school peers presents another challenge in the control of the disease. Given its ubiquity and ability to produce a diverse array of clinical signs and symptoms, physicians need to have increased clinical suspicion when presented with scalp or relevant skin complaints. Suggestions to add TCs to the public health agenda are worth consideration because the potential for permanent scarring, hair loss, and risk of spread is great.[103] Further studies are needed to evaluate which measures can reduce the proclivity of this disease for African and Hispanic populations. Efforts to improve cleanliness of schools and barbershops and to reduce infectivity in living conditions in endemic areas may decrease the incidence. In areas where zoophilic species dominate, control of animal vectors is of high importance. Carrier and fomite spread should be carefully evaluated in each index case's environment. In pediatric patients, the goal of treatment is to find a medication with short duration, minimal side effects, pleasant taste, and ease of availability. Patients and parents need to be counseled that clinical clearance of disease is not equivalent to cure unless mycologic clearance is complete. Trends in fungal species and shifts in age groups of TC cases should be carefully monitored. Clinicians should maintain a high degree of suspicion in patients from infancy to senescence.

REFERENCES

1. Ghannoum M, Isham N, Hajjeh R, et al. Tinea capitis in Cleveland: Survey of elementary school students. *J Am Acad Dermatol* 2003;48:189-193.
2. Sharma V, Silverberg NB, Howard R, et al. Do hair care practices affect the acquisition of tinea capitis? A case-control study. *Arch Pediatr Adolesc Med* 2001;155:818-821.
3. Elewski BE. Tinea capitis: A current perspective. *J Am Acad Dermatol* 2000;42:1-20.
4. Menan EI, Zongo-Bonou O, Rouet F, et al. Tinea capitis in schoolchildren from Ivory Coast (western Africa): A 1998-1999 cross-sectional study. *Int J Dermatol* 2002;41:204-207.
5. Romano C, Gianni C, Papini M. Tinea capitis in infants less than 1 year of age. *Pediatr Dermatol* 2001;6:465-468.
6. Ismail F, Fuller C, Moore M. Infants with tinea capitis: Experience from the GKT Medical School Mycology Department. *Pediatr Dermatol* 2003;20:283-284.
7. Raimer SS, Beightler EL, Hebert AA, et al. Tinea faciei in infants caused by *Trichophyton tonsurans*. *Pediatr Dermatol* 1986;3:452-454.
8. Silverberg NB, Weinberg JM, DeLeo VA. Tinea capitis: Focus on African-American women. *J Am Acad Dermatol* 2001;46: S1204.
9. Rothman S, Smiljanic A, Shapiro AL, et al. The spontaneous cure of tinea capitis at puberty. *J Invest Dermatol* 1947;8:81-98.
10. Takwale A, Agarwal S, Holmes SC, et al. Tinea capitis in two elderly women: Transmission at the hairdresser. *Br J Dermatol* 2001;144:898-900.
11. Pursley TV, Raimer SS. Tinea capitis in the elderly. *Int J Dermatol* 1986;19:220.
12. Terragni L, Lasagni A, Oriani A. Tinea capitis in adults. *Mycoses* 1989;32:482-486.
13. Cremer G, Bournerias I, Vandemeuleubroucke E, et al. Tinea capitis in adults: Misdiagnosis or reappearance? *Dermatology* 1997;194:8-11.

14. Lateur N, Andre J, De Maubeuge J, et al. Tinea capitis in two black african adults with HIV infection. *Br J Dermatol* 1999; 140:722-724.
15. Di Silverio A, Brazzelli V, Brandozzi G, et al. Prevalence of dermatophytes and yeasts (*Candida* spp., *Malassezia furfur*) in HIV patients: A study of former drug addicts. *Mycopathologia* 1991;114:103-107.
16. Bargman H. *Trichophyton rubrum* tinea capitis in an 85-year-old woman. *J Cutan Med Surg* 2000;4:153-154.
17. Bronson DM, Desai DR, Barsky S, et al. An epidemic of infection with *Trichophyton tonsurans* revealed in a 20-year survey of fungal infections in Chicago. *J Am Acad Dermatol* 1983;8:322-330.
18. Kamalan A, Thambiah AS. Histological study in tinea capitis. *Mykosen* 1981;24: 431-441.
19. Plewing G. *Pityrosporum* in normal sebaceous follicles, comedones, acneifrom eruptions and dandruff. *Mykosen* 1978; S1:155-163.
20. Weary PE. *Pityrosporum ovale:* Observations on some aspects of host-parasite interrelationship. *Arch Dermatol* 1968;98:408-422.
21. Leeming JG, Elliott TS. The emergence of *Trichophyton tonsurans* tinea capitis in Birmingham, U.K. *Br J Dermatol* 1995; 133:929-931.
22. McLean T, Levy H, Lue YA. Ecology of dermatophyte infections in South Bronx, New York, 1969 to 1981. *J Am Acad Dermatol* 1987;16:336-340.
23. Fernandes NC, Akiti T, Barreiros MG. Dermatophytoses in children: Study of 137 cases. *Rev Inst Med Trop Sao Paulo* 2001;43:83-85.
24. Dias T, Fernandes Ode F, Soares AJ, et al. Tinea capitis in children from Goiania, Brazil. *Rev Soc Bras Med Trop* 2003;36: 653-655.
25. Brilhante RS, Paixao GC, Salvino LK, et al. Epidemiology and ecology of dermatophytoses in the city of Fortaleza: *Trichophyton tonsurans* as important emerging pathogen of tinea capitis. *Rev Soc Bras Med Trop* 2000;33:417-425.
26. Davel G, Perrotta D, Canteros C, et al. Multicenter study of superficial mycoses in Argentina. EMMS Group. *Rev Argent Microbiol* 1999;31:173-181.
27. Vidotto V, Garcia R, Ponce LM, et al. Dermatophytoses in Cusco (Peru). *Mycoses* 1991;34:183-186.
28. Maraki S, Tselentis Y. Survey on the epidemiology of *Microsporum canis* infections in Crete, Greece over a 5-year period. *Int J Dermatol* 2000;39:21-24.
29. Koussidou-Eremondi T, Devliotou-Panagiotidou D, Mourellou-Tsatsou O, et al. Tinea capitis in children in northern Greece during the period 1981-1995. *Mycoses* 1999;42:319-322.
30. Romano C. Tinea capitis in Siena, Italy: An 18-year survey. *Mycoses* 1999;42: 559-562.
31. Rubio-Calvo C, Gil-Tomas J, Rezusta-Lopez A, et al. The aetiological agents of tinea capitis in Zaragoza (Spain). *Mycoses* 2001;44:55-58.
32. Lehenkari E, Silvennoinen-Kassinen S. Dermatophytes in northern Finland in 1982-1990. *Mycoses* 1995;38:411-414.
33. Rudolph AH. The clinical recognition of tinea capitis from *Trichophyton tonsurans*. *JAMA* 1979;242:1770.
34. Georg GH. *Trichophyton tonsurans* ringworm: A new public health problem. *Public Health Rep* 1952;67:53-56.
35. Provost E. Nonfluorescent tinea capitis in Charleston, SC. *JAMA* 1979;242: 1765-1767.
36. Foster KW, Ghannoum MA, Elewski BE. Epidemiologic surveillance of cutaneous fungal infection in the United States from 1999 to 2002. *J Am Acad Dermatol* 2004;50:748-752.
37. Moore MK, Suite M. Tinea capitis in Trinidad. *J Trop Med Hyg* 1993;96: 346-348.
38. Ghannoum MA, Elewski, B. Etiology of tinea capitis in the United States and Puerto Rico, Latin America and Mexico, and India. *J Am Acad Dermatol* 2004; 50:100.
39. Gupta AK, Summerbell RC. Increased incidence of *Trichophyton tonsurans* tinea capitis in Ontario, Canada between 1985 and 1996. *Med Mycol* 1998;36: 55-60.
40. Child FJ, Fuller LC, Higgins EM, et al. A study of the spectrum of skin disease occurring in a black population in southeast London. *Br J Dermatol* 1999; 141:512-517.
41. Fuller LC, Child FC, Midgley G, et al. Scalp ringworm in southeast London and an analysis of a cohort of patients from a paediatric dermatology department. *Br J Dermatol* 2003;148:985-988.
42. Fuller LC, Child FC, Higgins EM. Tinea capitis in southeast London: An outbreak of *Trichophyton tonsurans* infection. *Br J Dermatol* 1997;136:139.
43. Monzon de la Torre A, Cuenca-Estrella M, Rodriguez-Tudela JL. Epidemiological survey of dermatophytosis in Spain (April–June 2001) *Enferm Infect Microbiol Clin* 2003;21:477-483.
44. Tietz HJ, Czaika V, Ulbricht HM, et al. Tinea capitis in Germany: A survey in 1998. *Mycoses* 1999;42:73-76, 1999.
45. Pereiro Miguens M, Pereiro M, Pereiro M Jr. Review of dermatophytoses in Galicia from 1951 to 1987, and comparison with other areas of Spain. *Mycopathologia* 1991;113:65-78.
46. Khorsravi Khosravi AR, Aghamirian MR, Mahmoudi M. Dermatophytoses in Iran. *Mycoses* 1994;37:43-48.
47. Ravits MS, Himmelstein R. Tinea capitis in the New York City area. *Arch Dermatol* 1983;119:532-533.
48. Shtayeh MS, Arda HM. Incidence of dermatophytosis in Jordan with special reference to tinea capitis. *Mycopathologia* 1985;92:59-62.
49. Shtayeh MS, Arda HM. A study of tinea capitis in Jordan (West Bank). *J Trop Med Hyg* 1986;89:137-141.
50. Shockman J, Urbach F. Tinea capitis in Philadelphia. *Int J Dermatol* 1983;22: 521-524.
51. MacDonald E, Smith EB. The geography of dermatophytes. *Dermatol Clin* 1995;2:85-89.
52. Bugingo G. Causal agents of tinea of the scalp in the region of Butare (Rwanda). *Ann Soc Belg Med Trop* 1993;73:67-69.
53. Jahangir M, Hussain I, Khurshid K, et al. A clinico-etiologic correlation in tinea capitis. *Int J Dermatol* 1999;38: 275-278.
54. Korstanje MJ, Staats CG. Tinea capitis in northwestern Europe 1963-1993: Etiologic agents and their changing prevalence. *Int J Dermatol* 1994;33: 548-549.
55. Singal A, Rawat S, Bhattacharya SN, et al. Clinico-myocological profile of tinea capitis in North India and response to griseofulvin. *J Dermatol* 200128:22-26.
56. Kumar AG, Lakshmi N. Tinea capitis in Tirupati. *Indian J Pathol Microbiol* 1990; 33:360-363.
57. Lamb SR, Rademaker M. Tinea due to *Trichophyton violaceum* and *Trichophyton soudanense* in Hamilton, New Zealand. *Australas J Dermatol* 2001;42:260-263.
58. Romano C, Massai L, Difonzo EM. Dermatophytosis due to *Trichophyton violaceum* in Tuscany from 1985 to 1997. *Mycoses* 2000;43:169-172.
59. Ellabib MS, Agaj M, Khalifa Z, et al. *Trichophyton violaceum* is the dominant cause of tinea capitis in children in Tripoli, Libya: Results of a two year survey. *Mycopathologia* 2002;153:145-147.
60. Menan EI, Zongo-Bonou O, Rouet F, et al. Tinea capitis in schoolchildren from Ivory Coast (western Africa): A 1998-1999 cross-sectional study. *Int J Dermatol* 2002;41:204-207.
61. Markey RJ, Staat MA, Gerrety MJ, et al. Tinea capitis due to *Trichophyton soudanense* in Cincinnati, Ohio, in internationally adopted children from Liberia. *Pediatr Dermatol* 2003;20:408-410.
62. Rubben A, Krause H. Tinea superficialis capitis due to *Trichophyton soudanense* in African immigrants. *Mycoses* 1996;39: 397-398.
63. Testa J, Kaimba C, Georges A, et al. Epidemiology of tinea capitis in Bangui (Central African Republic). *Bull Soc Pathol Exot* 1992;85:395-396.
64. Haedersdal M, Stenderup J, Moller B, et al. An outbreak of tinea capitis in a child care centre. *Dan Med Bull* 2003; 50:83-84.
65. Schwinn A, Ebert J, Brocker EB. Frequency of *Trichophyton rubrum* in tinea capitis. *Mycoses* 1995;38:1-7.
66. Hebert AA, Head ES, MacDonald EM. Tinea capitis caused by *Trichophyton tonsurans*. *Pediatr Dermatol* 1985;2:219-223.
67. MacKenzie DWR, Burrows D, Walby AL. *Trichophyton sulphureum* in a residential school. *Br Med J* 1960;2:1055-1058.
68. Takwale A, Agarwal S, Holmes SC, et al. Tinea capitis in two elderly women: Transmission at the hairdresser. *Br J Dermatol* 2001;144:898-900.
69. Garg AP, Muller J. Inhibition of growth of dermatophytes by Indian hair oils. *Mycoses* 1992;35:363-369.
70. Mullins JF. *Trichophyton tonsurans* infection in tinea capitis survey. *AMA Arch Dermatol Syphilol* 1954;69:438-440.
71. Reid BJ, Shimkin MB, Blank F. Study of tinea capitis in Philadelphia using case and control groups. *Public Health Rep* 1968;83:497-502.
72. Babel DE, Baughman SA. Evaluation of the adult carrier state in juvenile tinea capitis caused by *Trichophyton tonsurans*. *J Am Acad Dermatol* 1989;21:1209-1212.
73. Vargo K, Cohen BA. Prevalence of undetected tinea capitis in household members of children with disease. *Pediatrics* 1993;92:155-157.
74. Ive FA. The carrier stage of tinea capitis in Nigeria. *Br J Dermatol* 1966;78: 219-221.
75. Sharma V, Hall JC, Knapp JF, et al. Scalp colonization by *Trichophyton tonsurans* in an urban pediatric clinic: Asymptomatic

carrier state. *Arch Dermatol* 1988;124: 1511-1513.
76. Neil G, Hanslo D, Buccimazza S, et al. Control of the carrier state of scalp dermatophytes. *Pediatr Infect Dis J* 1990;9:57-58.
77. Williams JV, Honig PJ, McGinley KJ, et al. Semiquantitative study of tinea capitis and the asymptomatic carrier state in inner-city school children. *Pediatrics* 1995;96:265-267.
78. Midgely G, Clayton YM. Distribution of dermatophytes and *Candida* spores in the environment. *Br J Dermatol* 1972; 86:69-77.
79. Ali-Shtayeh MS, Salameh AA, Abu-Ghdeib SI, et al. Prevalence of tinea capitis as well as of asymptomatic carriers in school children in Nablus area (Palestine). *Mycoses* 2002;451:88-94.
80. Cuetara MS, Del Palacio A, Pereiro M, et al. Prevalence of undetected tinea capitis in a prospective school survey in Madrid: Emergence of new causative fungi. *Br J Dermatol* 1998;138:658-660.
81. Pipkin JL. Tinea capitis in the adult and adolescent. *Arch Dermatol Syphilol* 1952; 66:9-40.
82. Sperling LC. Inflammatory tinea capitis (kerion) mimicking dissecting cellulitis: Occurrence in two adolescents. *Int J Dermatol* 1991;30:190-192.
83. Lateur N, Andre J, De Maubeuge J, et al. Tinea capitis in two black african adults with HIV infection. *Br J Dermatol* 1999; 140:722-724.
84. Martin ES, Elewski BE. Tinea capitis in adult women masquerading as bacterial pyoderma. *J Am Acad Dermatol* 2003;49: S177-179.
85. Friedlander SF, Pickering B, Cunningham BB, et al. Use of the cotton swab method in diagnosing tinea capitis. *Pediatrics* 1999;104:276-279.
86. Honig PJ, Sullivan K, McGowan KL. The rapid diagnosis of tinea capitis using calcofluor white. *Pediatr Emerg Care* 1996;12:333-335.
87. Allen AM, Taplin D, Lowy JA, et al. Skin infections in Vietnam. *Milit Med* 1972;137:295-301.
88. Gromadzki S, Ramani R, Chaturvedi V. Evaluation of new medium for identification of dermatophytes and primary dimorphic pathogens. *J Clin Microbiol* 2003;41:467-468.
89. McLean T, Levy H, Lue YA. Ecology of dermatophyte infections in South Bronx, New York, 1969 to 1981. *J Am Acad Dermatol* 1987;16:336-340.
90. Williams DI, Marten RH, Sarkany I. Oral treatment of ringworm with griseofulvin. *Lancet* 1958;2:1212-1213.
91. Epstein WL, Shah VP, Riegelman S. Griseofulvin levels in stratum corneum. *Arch Dermatol* 1960;81:662-666.
92. Sobue S, Sekiguchi K, Nabeshima T. Intracutaneous distributions of fluconazole, itraconazole, and griseofulvin in Guinea pigs and binding to human stratum corneum. *Antimicrob Agents Chemother* 2004;48:216-223.
93. Colton RL, Amir J, Mimouni M, et al. Serum sickness-like reaction associated with griseofulvin. *Ann Pharmacother* 2004;38:609-611.
94. Sheretz E. Are laboratory studies necessary for griseofulvin therapy? *J Am Acad Dermatol* 1990;22:1103.
95. Fleming H, Murray L (eds). *Physicians' Desk Reference,* 58th ed. Montvale, NJ, Thomson, 2004.
96. Chan YC, Friedlander SF. New treatments for tinea capitis. *Curr Opin Infect Dis* 2004;17:97-103.
97. Gupta AK, Adam P, Dlova N, et al. Therapeutic options for the treatment of tinea capitis caused by *Trichophyton* species: griseofulvin versus the new oral antifungal agents, terbinafine, itraconazole, and fluconazole. *Pediatr Dermatol* 2001;18:433-438.
98. Allen HB, Honig PJ, Leyden JJ, McGinley KJ. Selenium sulfide: Adjunctive therapy for tinea capitis. *Pediatrics* 1982;69: 81-83.
99. Greer, DL. Successful treatment of tinea capitis with 2% ketoconazole shampoo. *Int J Dermatol* 2000;39:302-304.
100. Warner RR, Schwartz JR, Boissy Y, Dawson TL Jr. Dandruff has an altered stratum corneum ultrastructure that is improved with zinc pyrithione shampoo. *J Am Acad Dermatol* 2001;45: 897-903.
101. Ginsburg CM, Gan VN, Petruska M. Randomized controlled trial of intralesional corticosteroid and griseofulvin vs griseofulvin alone for treatment of kerion. *Pediatr Infect Dis J* 1987;6: 1084-1087.
102. Viguie-Vallanet C, Savaglio N, Piat C, Tourte-Schaefer C. Epidemiology of *Microsporum langeronii* tinea capitis in the Paris suburban area: Results of two school and familial surveys. *Ann Dermatol Venereol (Stockh)* 1997;124: 696-699.
103. Lamagni T, Evans B, Campbell C. Tinea capitis should be on the public health agenda. *Br Med J* 2000;321:451.

CHAPTER 38

Nail Disorders

Nathaniel J. Jellinek
C. Ralph Daniel, III

Key Points

- Longitudinal melanonychia (LM) is common in darker skin types, usually as a result of melanocyte activation.
- Atypical LM may indicate nail apparatus melanoma (NAM).
- Evaluation of LM for NAM includes a detailed history and physical examination, examination of all 20 nails, use of dermoscopy, and often a nail matrix biopsy.
- NAM has a worse prognosis than its cutaneous counterpart in large part owing to delayed diagnosis.
- Lichen planus may cause irreversible scarring nail disease. Prompt treatment is imperative.
- Lichen planus commonly causes LM in persons of color.
- Psoriasis of the nail unit is difficult to treat primarily because of difficult medication bioavailability.
- Psoriasis and lichen planus both may exist as a primary nail disease without cutaneous disease.
- Onychomycosis is the most common nail disorder.

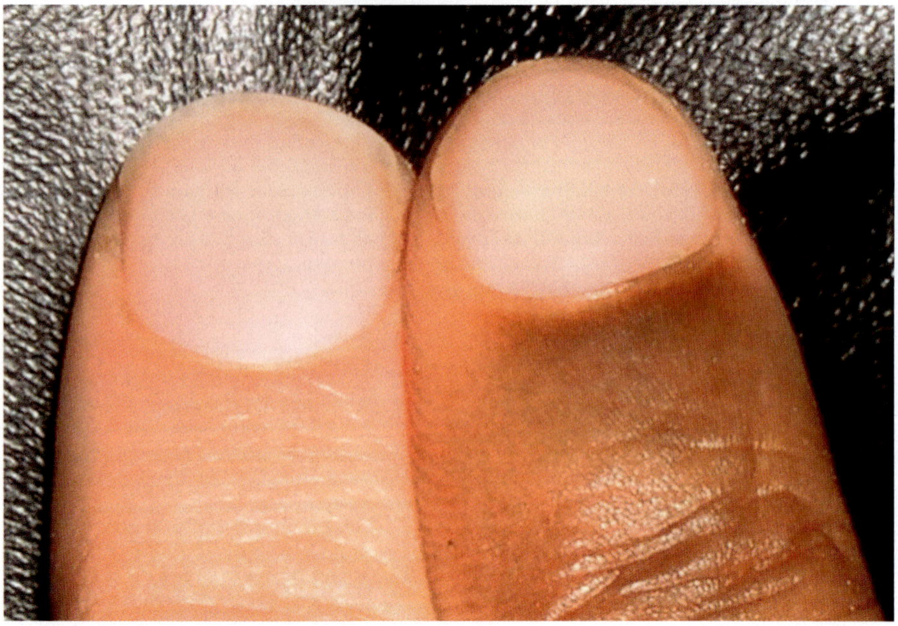

▲ **FIGURE 38-1** Skin phototype II (*left*) and V (*right*) index fingernails. The nail bed color is identical despite the different finger skin colors.

Examination of the nails is an important part of every dermatologic examination in every skin phototype. In skin of color, there is very little in the way of unique nail disease. Nail unit melanocytes may or may not be quiescent, and the clinical appearance of nails of different skin phototypes is closer than perhaps on any other cutaneous structure (Figure 38-1). In darker skin types, these melanocytes are more predisposed to activation and production of melanin pigment, which commonly presents as longitudinal melanonychia (Figure 38-2). This chapter highlights the examination of nails in skin of color, featuring longitudinal melanonychia (LM) and nail apparatus melanoma (NAM), as well as inflammatory and infectious nail diseases (e.g., psoriasis, lichen planus, and onychomycosis).

LONGITUDINAL MELANONYCHIA AND NAIL APPARATUS MELANOMA

Melanonychia simply refers to brown or black nail pigmentation, not necessarily a brown or black nail caused by melanin pigment[1] (Figures 38-3 and 38-4). Longitudinal melanonychia (LM) is a characteristic presentation that may be seen in all races, the prevalence of which varies based on ethnicity and skin phototype. LM is significant because it may be the first presenting sign of nail apparatus melanoma (NAM.) The differential diagnosis for LM is broad[1] (Table 38-1) and includes exogenous pigmentation, bacterial pigment, mycotic pigment (Figure 38-5), melanin, and blood (Figure 38-6). This latter fact becomes important in evaluating LM because one of the most common causes across all skin phototypes is trauma-related hemorrhage. And this is further complicated

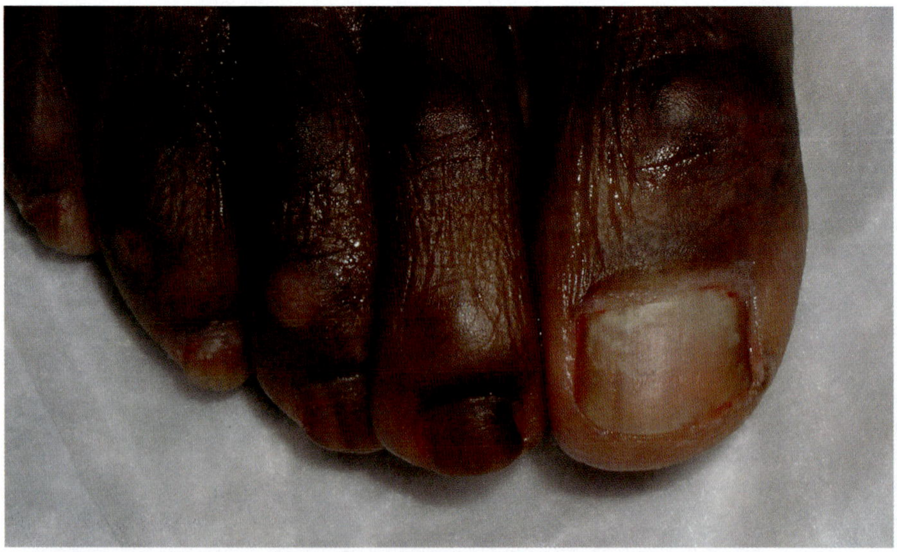

▲ **FIGURE 38-2** Multiple pigmented bands on all five toes in a patient with skin phototype V. Also present is superficial white onychomycosis on the great toenail.

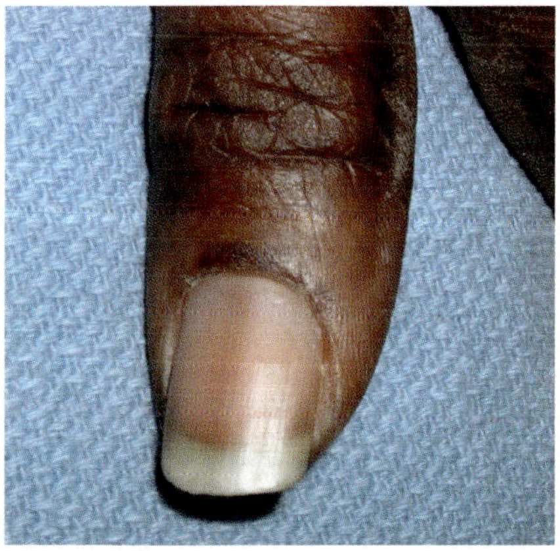

▲ **FIGURE 38-3** Faint, single longitudinal pigmented band on a thumbnail.

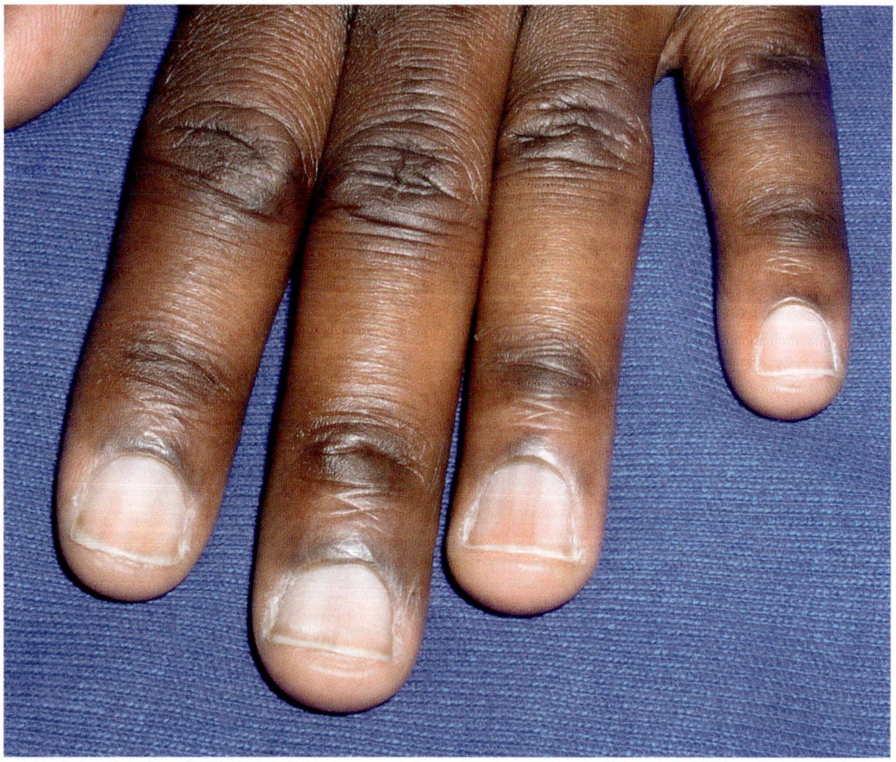

▲ **FIGURE 38-4** Multiple pigmented bands on all four fingernails.

because the presence of blood does not rule out the diagnosis of melanoma and indeed may represent tumor-associated hemorrhage. The approach to LM therefore must be thorough and include an understanding of the broad differential diagnosis as well as a methodical diagnostic plan.

LM is common in darkly pigmented individuals and less common in Caucasians. The spectrum of LM prevalence parallels that of skin color; it is found at some point in time in 10–20% of Japanese people,[2] in 77% of African-Americans older than 20 years of age, and nearly 100% of them by 50 years of age.[3,4] LM is more common on frequently used digits, particularly the thumb and index finger, as well as the hallux. As with cutaneous pigmentation, LM may be congenital or acquired, stable or evolving, uniform and regular or irregular, homogeneous or heterogeneous, and may be associated with a variety of signs (discussed below). Probably the most common cause of LM in people of color is physical stimuli directly to the proximal nail apparatus, in essence triggering melanocytic activation. Robert Baran has termed this *frictional melanonychia*,[5] which may be compared with postinflammatory hyperpigmentation or postrubbing skin pigmentation. Diffuse melanonychia, as opposed to LM, is never considered normal, may be congenital,[3] may be triggered by drugs, may represent underlying nevi or melanoma, or may follow a systemic disease and has been described in Addison disease, with elevated

TABLE 38-1
Differential Diagnosis of Longitudinal Melanonychia

Melanocyte activation
Lentigo
Nevus
Melanoma
Hemorrhage
Mycotic pigment
Bacterial pigment
Exogenous causes

Source: Data from Haneke E, Baran R. Longitudinal melanonychia. *Dermatol Surg* 2001;27:580-584.

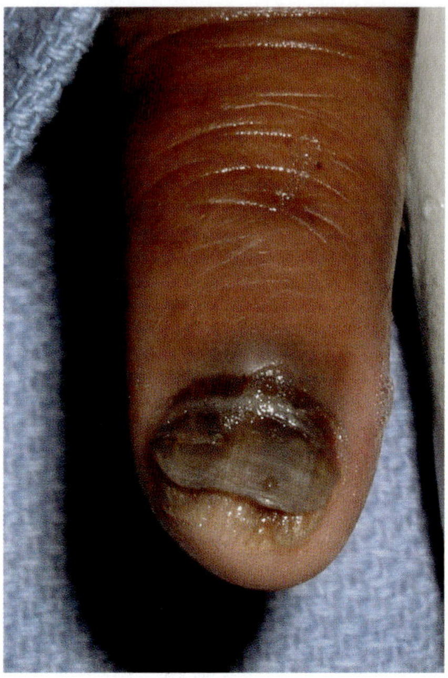

▲ **FIGURE 38-5** Near-complete melanonychia caused by tinea unguium (*T. rubrum*).

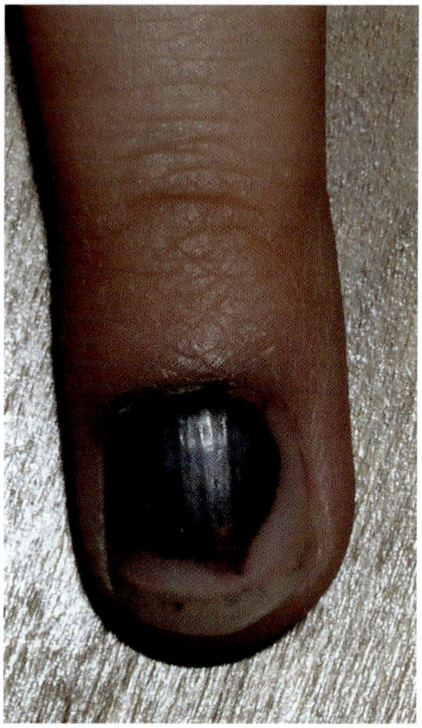

▲ **FIGURE 38-6** Melanonychia from trauma-associated hemorrhage in a child with skin phototype IV.

TABLE 38-2
Nail Pigmentation

A study of "normal pigmentation" of the nails of 296 consecutive people of African ancestry revealed the following data[4]:

- Pigmentation usually occurs in the form of LM and is a normal, common finding in most cases.
- Increasing age is associated with a higher prevalence LM, with increasing numbers of nails involved.
- There is no difference in the nail pigmentation between male and female gender.
- On each nail there may be one or several bands, varying from thin to several millimeters wide.
- The bands vary in depth of color. The bands tends to be darker in persons with darker skin types.
- LM in these individuals may be present in any portion of the nail but most commonly occupies the central area or lateral margins.
- The pigment particles are found scattered throughout the onychocytes but are concentrated in the deeper layers (corresponding to the distal matrix).

melanocyte-stimulating hormone levels, and with psoralen with ultraviolet A (PUVA) treatment[6] (Table 38-2).

Prevalence rates and digit specificity of LM parallel those of nail apparatus melanoma (NAM) (Figure 38-7). Both occur most commonly on the thumb, hallux, and index finger. The nail unit is a relatively rare location for primary melanomas in Caucasians, accounting for only 1–3% of all melanomas,[7,8] although it accounts for between 20% and 25% of all acral melanomas.[9] In dark-skinned Puerto Rican, Japanese, Hawaiian, and Native American populations, it accounts for a substantially higher percentage ranging from 8–33%[10–13]; in people of Japanese and Chinese ancestry, the percentage range is 17–23%, and in African-Americans, up to 25%.[14] In all populations, it carries a poorer prognosis than cutaneous melanoma, with the 5-year survival rate ranging from 16–87%.[15] In part, this is due to delayed diagnosis. In addition, there are some who contend that melanomas of the nail unit are more aggressive malignancies—that they metastasize earlier than cutaneous melanoma, with worse survival rates, stage-for-stage, thickness-for-thickness, than cutaneous melanomas.[16,17] For all races, then, and particularly patients of darker skin types, in whom LM is more common, examination and evaluation for LM, with the suspicion of NAM, are crucial.

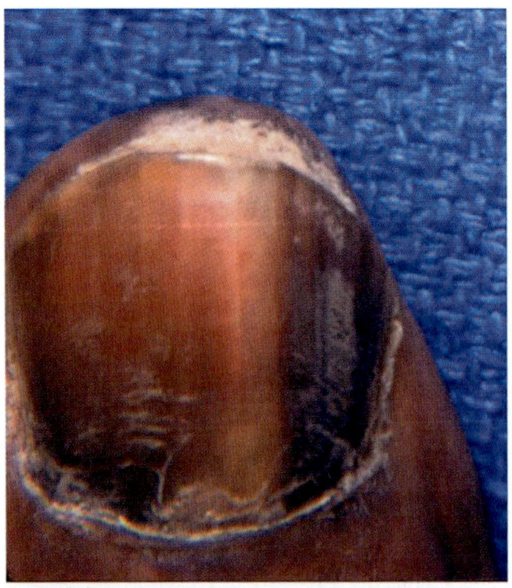

▲ **FIGURE 38-7** Nail apparatus melanoma featuring irregular brown and black longitudinal pigmented bands, a ragged cuticle, and early Hutchinson's sign. Courtesy of Richard Scher, M.D.

The workup starts with a detailed history. Important aspects include the onset, timing, and evolution of the pigmentation. Evolving pigmentation is more suspect than stable melanonychia. A history of trauma may explain hemorrhage; however, trauma has been linked (at least anecdotally) with NAM.[18–20] A family history of LM, associated labial or genital pigmentation, or even a past medical history of related disease (e.g., multiple gastrointestinal hamartomatous polyps) raises the possibility of Laugier-Huntziger syndrome or Peutz-Jeghers syndrome. Family history of multiple atypical nevi or familial melanoma and a personal history of melanoma are all risk factors.[20] Detailed history of medications that may trigger LM, such as minocycline, antimalarial agents, or one of several chemotherapy agents, also may be important.[21] And a careful review for any exogenous source of pigment (e.g., henna or silver nitrate) should be elicited.[1]

Examination of the nails should be equally detailed. All 20 nails need to be evaluated, without polish and with good lighting. Careful full-body examination for multiple atypical nevi is important to elicit a risk factor for melanoma. A single involved nail, particularly of the thumb, hallux, or index finger, is more suspicious. Multiple nails involved at once are more reassuring, although there are few reports of simultaneous melanoma on more than one digit.[22] Evaluation for Hutchinson's sign includes an examination of the proximal and lateral nail folds and eponychium. While a true Hutchinson's sign usually represents radial-growth-phase melanoma, distinguishing true from pseudo-Hutchinson's sign generally requires a biopsy.[23]

Dermoscopy of LM is helpful. This technique was elegantly reported by Ronger and colleagues under oil immersion in 148 consecutive cases of longitudinal melanonychia.[24] Melanomas were significantly associated with a brown background color and the presence of irregular longitudinal lines (in their color, spacing, thickness, and parallelism) a micro-Hutchinson sign, and in one case, blood spots. These dermoscopic patterns helped to differentiate melanomas from nail matrix nevi, lentigines, drug-induced pigmentation, and ethnic-type pigmentation. Others have described dermoscopic Hutchinson's sign on the hyponychium, with excellent sensitivity for melanoma, although the specificity was less accurate.[25] In contrast to the skin, blood under the nail may show pseudopod formation, appearing like budding globules off of a darker red-black macule.[26] Johr and Izakovic published a case series using dermoscopy for the evaluation of pigmentation of the nail unit.[27] They found that color asymmetry (including black dots), irregular diffuse dark pigmentation, and (micro-) Hutchinson's sign were important dermoscopic signs for melanoma. Others have suggested using water-soluble gels as the dermoscopic medium for nail examination in place of immersion or mineral oil.[28] We have found that end-on dermoscopy (Figure 38-8) may provide valuable information as to the origin of the pigmentation. Distal matrix pigmentation, which accounts for approximately 90% of cases of LM, projects onto the undersurface of the free edge of the nail plate, whereas proximal matrix pigmentation projects onto the superficial surface of the nail plate. This finding has important prognostic information because proximal matrix biopsies are more likely to leave a permanent dystrophy than distal matrix biopsies.

Biopsy of the nail unit for melanoma must include the matrix because only a small minority of NAMs arise from melanocytes in the nail bed, nail folds,

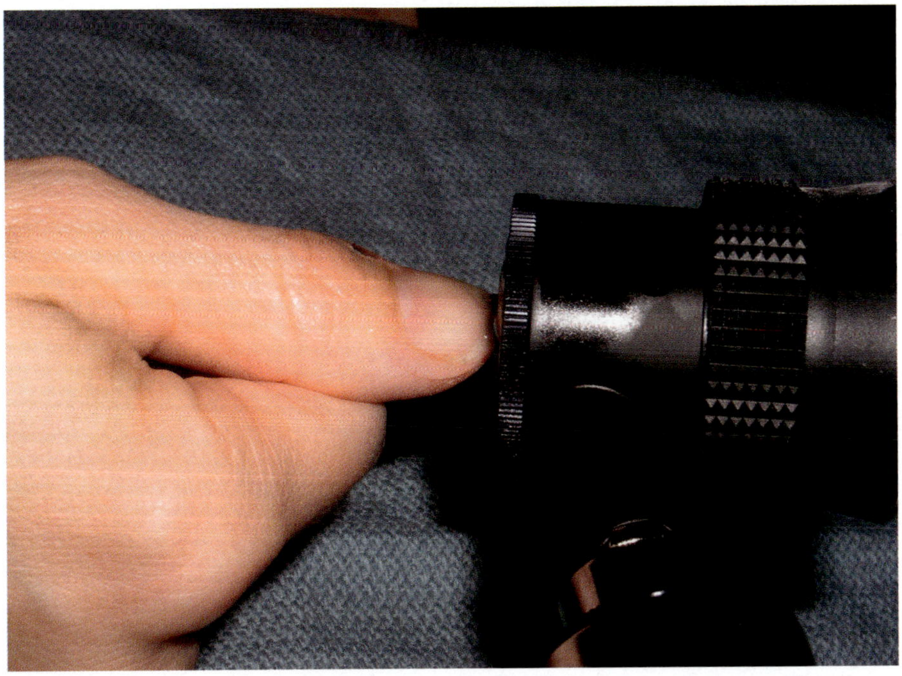

▲ **FIGURE 38-8** End-on dermoscopy allows localization of nail pigment—to the superficial plate (proximal matrix origin) or undersurface of the plate (distal matrix origin).

or hyponychium.[29] Table 38-3 shows a proposed algorithm for biopsy of LM.

Pathology of LM may be quite illustrative. In cases of onychomycosis (see Figure 38-3), histology may show multiple fungal elements, including septate hyphae in dermatophyte infection, pseudohyphae and budding spores in yeast infection, and a number of elements with the range of nondermatophyte mold infections. Hemorrhage may be observed, although typical iron staining (such as Prussian blue) is negative in the nail plate. (The hemoglobin is not metabolized in the nail plate and hence not appreciated with this stain.) Instead, benzadine (for hemoglobin) is the preferred test for nail plate hemorrhage.[30]

In cases of LM of matrix melanocyte origin, there are several possible diagnoses. LM originating from the matrix without melanocytic hyperplasia traditionally has been called *melanocytic activation*. More recently, the term *melanotic macule of the nail* has been proposed for this entity.[31] Melanocytic hyperplasia may represent a lentigo (as in Laugier-Hutziger syndrome), a nevus (most of which are of the junctional variety), melanoma in situ, or melanoma. Distinguishing lentigo from nevus may be difficult because nesting in matrix nevi may be inconspicuous; therefore, some prefer to label all benign matrix hyperplasia as nevus, eschewing the diagnosis of lentigo.[31] As the most sinister diagnosis, and often the most challenging to diagnose, NAM deserves further mention. A detailed discussion of NAM histology follows.

Melanomas and melanomas in situ are characterized by poorly circumscribed proliferations of atypical melanocytes with varying degrees of upward growth. Single melanocytes predominate over nests. Nuclear enlargement with a coarse chromatin pattern is common. Mitoses vary but may not be prominent.[32] Nodular melanomas by definition lack a radial growth phase and grow vertically early in the disease. Unusually, the melanomas may be associated with formation of cartilage and partly mineralized osteoid-like material.[33] This osteocartilaginous differentiation may delay or mask diagnosis, particularly if radiologic studies are performed before or in place of tissue diagnosis.

Immunohistochemistry may be helpful in ambiguous cases. S-100, HMB-45, Mart-1, and Melan-A are all accurate markers for cells of melanocytic origin. The distribution of melanocytes in vertical sections of the matrix has shown and reinforced (through regular and immunohistochemical studies) that the melanocytes are located in a suprabasal (rather than basal) position,[34] which again may be misrepresented as pagetoid upward growth and malignancy when it is simply the normal histologic

TABLE 38-3
Algorithm for Longitudinal Melanonychia

Longitudinal melanonychia
↓
Dermoscopy and end-on dermoscopy of free margin
↓
Dorsal plate pigment (proximal matrix) ←——→ Ventral plate pigment (distal matrix)

Dorsal plate pigment (proximal matrix)
↓
>3 mm wide ← → <3 mm wide
- >3 mm wide → Matrix shave biopsy, multiple 3 mm punch biopsies, longitudinal biopsy with flap reconstruction, or en bloc excision
- <3 mm wide → 3 mm punch biopsy, matrix shave, or longitudinal excision

Ventral plate pigment (distal matrix)
↓
>3 mm wide ← → <3 mm wide
- >3 mm wide → Matrix shave, tangential excision, longitudinal biopsy with flap reconstruction, or en bloc excision
- <3 mm wide → 3-3.5 mm punch biopsy or longitudinal biopsy

pattern. In this sense, then, immunohistochemistry may be good at identifying the cells in question, but more traditional criteria, such including cellular morphology, necrosis, and mitotic activity, can be more crucial to diagnosing melanoma.

Once the biopsy has been performed and a diagnosis made, certainly melanoma and melanoma in situ deserve further workup and prognostic evaluation. A more in-depth discussion of NAM, its treatment, and prognosis follows below. Most of the published data regarding NAM is based on a racially mixed population, that is, not simply patients with skin of color. Where exceptions to this exist, they are noted below.

NAM generally a disease of older individuals, with the mean age of diagnosis in the 60s. It is rare in children, with only six cases reported in the literature over the last 35 years.[35,36] Men and women have nearly equal incidence.[37] As noted earlier, nearly 70% of these tumors are found on the thumb or hallux,[8] perhaps because these digits represent a large proportion of the total amount of nail matrix tissue, perhaps because of trauma, or perhaps because of other, as of yet unexplained causes.[38,39] It is unlikely that ultraviolet exposure is extensively involved in the etiology. The nail plate allows a small amount of ultraviolet A (UVA) penetration and blocks almost all UVB rays,[40] so the nail bed receives very little of the damaging UV exposure.

NAMs are diagnosed later than their cutaneous counterparts, with mean delays ranging from an average of 9–23 months.[41–44] They tend to be asymptomatic. The anatomy is a hindrance in early diagnosis for several reasons. The nail plate may alter light reflectance of the pigment (the Tyndall effect). Many patients assume that the changes are caused by trauma or are simply subungual hemorrhage, a theory occasionally supported by their physicians.[45] From 15–65% have been reported to be amelanotic,[12] although we contend that this number is closer to 30%.

Two-thirds of NAMs present as nail unit pigmentation, including LM. Alternatively, they may present as a subungual tumor, nail plate changes, or inflammatory disease of the nail unit. Bleeding is a late presentation. The widely prevalent condition of onychomycosis may mask changes of underlying melanoma, making them more difficult to observe. Similarly, there may be secondary fungal infection of a dystrophic nail, so fungal tests (e.g., KOH, culture, or nail clipping for periodic acid–Schiff staining) could be misleading. Hence the differential diagnosis for such a presentation is broad, with widely variable and occasionally subtle appearances (see Table 38-1). Consequently, in any lesion that presents suspiciously or in any potentially malignant condition that persists despite treatment, biopsy is warranted. And given the severity of the diagnosis, some advise biopsy of all acquired LMs in adults to rule out NAM,[1] although this may not be practical.

As a result of the difficulties in diagnosis, NAMs are significantly thicker than cutaneous melanomas at the time of diagnosis. The average Breslow depth ranges from 3.5–4.7 mm,[8,15] and 80% are deeper than 1.5 mm.[41] From 60–70% are invasive to Clark level IV or V, and one-quarter of patients at presentation have lymph node or distant metastases.[41,46] This is in stark contrast to cutaneous melanoma, in which only approximately 2% of patients present with distant metastases. There is a proportionally dismal prognosis: In one study of 54 patients with 5-year follow-up, 26 died of disseminated metastatic disease.[41] In most other series, all of which have been limited by the rarity of disease, the 5-year survival rates have been poor, ranging from 20–60%.[47] Correspondingly, late changes and poor prognostic factors are disproportionately present at the time of diagnosis. One report of 46 patients showed 28% of tumors with ulceration, 11% with bony invasion, and 50% with nail destruction.[46] With more encouraging statistics, a more recent study of NAM in Japanese patients compared survival rates in the time periods 1969–1982 and 1983–1993.[48] The 5-year survival rates increased from 53–87%, respectively. The authors credited this dramatic progress to greater public awareness (and discovery of thinner melanomas) and to the introduction of improved chemotherapy.

All melanoma subtypes have been reported to present as NAM, although acral lentiginous type has been most frequent, followed by superficial spreading type. Histopathologically, the tumor most often originates in the nail matrix, although every nail subunit (except the plate) contains melanocytes and hence may present with melanoma. The histopathologic normal variants can make accurate and confident diagnosis difficult for those unfamiliar with nail apparatus histology. The distribution and number of melanocytes in the nail matrix differ from those in other epithelium. Specifically, they may be found irregularly distributed basally or suprabasally, sometimes clustered in small groups of three to four cells.[34] Normal melanocytic nevi in children even may show potentially misleading features.[49] They may have large melanocytes with abundant cytoplasm and a dark, variably sized and shaped nucleus, occasionally showing spindle-shaped melanocytes or transepidermal migration of isolated melanocytes or even nests of melanocytes. Some nuclear atypia is considered by some in benign nevi as well. The upward growth in nevi may be incorrectly interpreted as pagetoid scatter, leading to the misdiagnosis of melanoma in situ.[38]

Melanoma is viewed by many as a systemic disease, with increased likelihood of widespread pathology related to tumor depth, ulceration, and perhaps tumor subtype or location. Local tumor removal with clear margins is advocated by all, but primary extirpation with wider rather than narrower margins has lost favor in the face of absent survival benefit.[19] Accurate local excision, then, is appealing, with staging for lymph node and distant metastasis a mandatory preoperative task.

Once the diagnosis of NAM is made, the patient must be staged. Quantifying the extent of melanoma is essential for determining the appropriate treatment and for assessing prognosis. There are no current data to suggest a different approach to staging patients with NAM versus cutaneous melanoma. Historically, there have been fewer in situ tumors, and the average depth has been deeper. Still, today, lymph node involvement and distant metastasis are more likely to be present, although most evidence suggests that this perception is strictly related to tumor depth rather than to more sinister inherent tumor behavior. The most recent TNM staging system published by the American Joint Committee on Cancer (AJCC)[50] reinforces that tumor depth (Breslow thickness) is the most important prognostic indicator in primary melanoma, with stratification cutoffs at less than 1, 1–2, 2–4, and greater than 4 mm. Microscopic ulceration is the next most significant adverse prognostic indicator. The number of lymph nodes involved supersedes size of lymph nodes as a negative factor. Indeed, the AJCC staging system incorporates micrometastases to the lymph node in its newest classification. Since this information may be gathered only through lymph node biopsy, current practice includes the use of sentinel lymph node biopsy as a staging technique, although its import at this point is theoretical; there is as yet no conclusive data that sentinel lymph node biopsy improves overall survival.[51] Palpable lymphadenopathy in the presence of NAM, as in cutaneous melanoma, dictates either sentinel lymph node biopsy or complete lymph node dissection. Currently, there is a range of therapeutic strategies, although most suggest sentinel lymph node biopsy for patients with tumors at least 1 mm in thickness or Clark level IV.[52,53] Future data should clarify patient selection and more specific indications for and benefits of sentinel lymph node biopsy.

Therapy for NAM is primarily surgical. Over the past 20 years, there has been a movement toward smaller surgical margins,[19] and this has been extended to include tumors of the nail unit. Historically, digital (including nail unit) melanomas were treated with digital amputation. Ten years ago, amputation at various levels was proposed in an effort to decrease disability without affecting survival.[46] More recently, there have been publications advocating more distal levels of amputation or simply excision with 1- to 2-cm margins, sparing amputation.[54] NAM in situ is treated adequately with total excision of all nail tissues without amputation.[55] For invasive tumors, some have proposed digit-sparing "functional" surgery.[54] And in the last several years, proponents of Mohs surgery have provided evidence of its usefulness in the therapy of NAM and NAM in situ.[45,56]

Digital amputation for NAM has been performed anywhere from the level of the metacarpal/metatarsal bones to the distal phalanx. A recent study evaluated the survival rates between two groups of patients, those with an amputation in or proximal to the distal interphalangeal joint and those with less radical "functional" surgery.[54] A retrospective comparative analysis of these two treatment groups of 31 patients showed no survival difference between them at a median follow-up of 54 months.

Most data do not support radiologic or lymph node staging for in situ melanomas or nonulcerated melanomas of less than 1 mm depth, particularly if the Clark level is I–III. These recommendations may change with further data. For all other tumors, sentinel lymph node biopsy and preoperative radiologic screening for distant metastasis generally are recommended. For all patients, regardless of their Breslow thickness or tumor specifications, a review of systems; complete examination of the entire skin, nails, and mucosa; physical examination for lymphadenopathy and hepatosplenomegaly; and careful follow-up are recommended.

Other treatments for NAM include isolated regional perfusion of chemotherapy. While imiquimod, radiotherapy, melanoma vaccines, and even single thermal neutron capture have been advocated for melanomas elsewhere, there are no specific data for their use in the nail unit. Currently, with the exception of regional perfusion chemotherapy, there are no data for use of these therapies outside the indications for treatment of melanomas in other anatomic areas. Isolated regional perfusion of melphalan and other chemotherapeutics has been reported for adjuvant therapy (with ampution) for invasive NAM.[44] Initial studies showed positive results, boasting increases in survival of 15–35%.[43,44] Subsequent data have called into questioned this survival benefit, with two more recent studies showing no improvement in survival between patients treated with amputation and others treated with amputation plus isolated regional perfusion with chemotherapy and mild hyperthermia.[57] Some argue that this treatment decreases the rate of regional recurrence.[43] In a small case series, systemic treatment with dacarbazine, vincristine, and nitrosourea has been credited with improving prognosis.[48]

Overall, prognosis in cases of NAM is poor, although there are trends to show that this is improving, namely, from earlier diagnosis and more in situ and superficial tumors. Surgical extirpation remains a challenge. Whichever technique the surgeon uses, from Mohs surgery to digital amputation, the goal is the same—tumor-free margins. Evaluation for metastasis must be approached on a patient-to-patient basis, with guidelines that are continuously evolving. Chemotherapy remains an adjuvant therapy or palliative therapy. Careful follow-up for local recurrence, second primary tumors, and lymph node and distant metastasis is required and lifelong.

LICHEN PLANUS

Lichen planus (LP) is a common inflammatory skin disease that affects approximately 1% of the U.S. population.[58] Ten percent of patients with LP demonstrate nail disease, whereas a small proportion of them have nail disease in isolation.[59] LP may involve any or all subunits of the nail, including the matrix, bed, and nail folds, and may display protean signs. In bullous LP of the nail unit, it classically presents with nail pain. It also represents a potential onychologic emergency, with rapid nail unit scarring and development of dorsal pterygium. In skin of color, LP varies in ways that are consistent with other cutaneous and nail diseases: The cutaneous erythema tends to be more violaceous and, for those unaccustomed to its examination, may appear subtle. Because the nail bed contains normally quiescent melanocytes and closely resembles the nail bed in other races, the changes are remarkably similar. Of note, hyper- and hypopigmentation of the nail folds are characteristic in darker skin phototypes. And as a follow-up to the preceding section, longitudinal melanonychia owing to melanocytic activation may be triggered by LP (Figure 38-9).

An understanding of the possible presentations, as with psoriasis of the nail unit, is aided by comprehension of the different roles of nail subunits[59] (Table 38-4). The nail matrix, responsible for nail plate production, is capable of producing a wide spectrum of plate abnormalities, with proximal matrix (responsible for the superficial plate) producing pitting, ridging, grooving, and trachyonychia, and distal matrix (responsible for the undersurface of the plate) producing leukonychia and erythronychia.

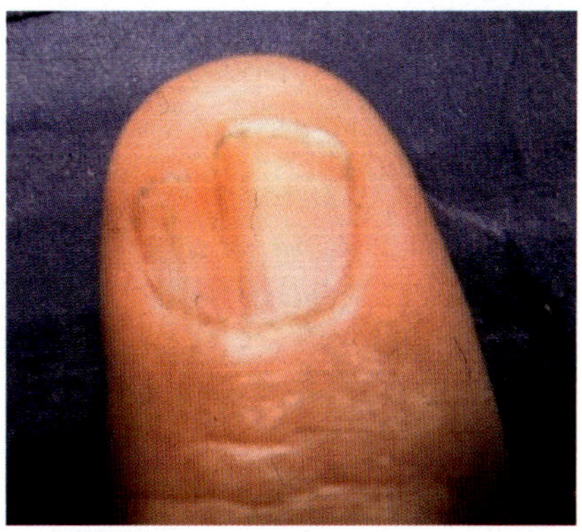

▲ **FIGURE 38-9** Lichen planus demonstrating longitudinal ridging, nail plate thinning, proximal nail bed erythema, and longitudinal melanonychia.

TABLE 38-4
Presentation of Nail Lichen Planus

Ridging	Subungual hyperkeratosis	Wickam's striae
Onychorrhexis	Hyperpigmentation	Hyperpigmentation
Pitting	Hypopigmentation	Hypopigmentation
Koilonychia		
Longitudinal erythronychia		
Leukonychia		
Onychauxis		
Nail plate thinning		
Trachyonychia		
Scarring		
Anonychia		
Pterygium		

TABLE 38-5
Treatment of Nail Lichen Planus

First line
- Irritant-avoidance regimen
- Intralesional corticosteroids
  - 2.5-5 mg/mL triamcinolone, injected into the matrix, with treatments monthly until clear, then tapered gradually

Second line
- Systemic corticosteroids
  - 0.75–1.0 mg/kd/d prednisone continued for several weeks until clinical improvement is evident, then tapered gradually

Third line
- Topical corticosteroids (potent, under occlusion)
- Systemic retinoids
- Systemic griseofulvin
- Topical PUVA

Extensive involvement of both may produce scarring, with resulting dorsal pterygium and/or anonychia (Figures 38-10 and 38-11). Nail bed disease may produce onycholysis, with nail bed hyperkeratosis presenting occasionally as a yellow discoloration.

Treatment of nail unit LP is no different in patients with skin of color. While mild disease such as superficial pitting may not require therapy, more severe, particularly scarring disease requires prompt intervention with corticosteroids, either intralesionally (preferred by us) or systemically.[60] It is important to emphasize that trauma may worsen the disease (Koebner phenomenon) and that gentle nail care is important in any treatment; we recommend an irritant-avoidance regimen to all patients with nail unit LP.[61] Table 38-5 shows treatments for moderate to severe LP divided into first-, second-, and third-line therapies.

PSORIASIS

Psoriasis has many similarities with LP in relation to the nail unit. It is common, affecting approximately 1–2% of the U.S. population (more common with a first-degree family history of disease), with anywhere between 10–50% demonstrating nail disease.[62] As with LP, nail disease in psoriasis may present in isolation of cutaneous disease, with involvement of the different anatomic subunits responsible for the widely variable clinical manifestations. Unlike LP, however, psoriasis does not cause dorsal pterygium and in only rare cases of pustular disease causes scarring and anonychia. Psoriasis vulgaris is just one variant with possible nail disease. Several other diseases present with psoriasiform (and occasionally overlapping or identical) nail findings (Table 38-6). Specifically, several diseases are characterized by pustular changes of the distal phalanx and nail unit, including acrodermatitis continua of Hallopeau.

Table 38-7 reviews the clinical manifestations of nail psoriasis divided by subunit involvement. Matrix involvement is responsible for the primary plate

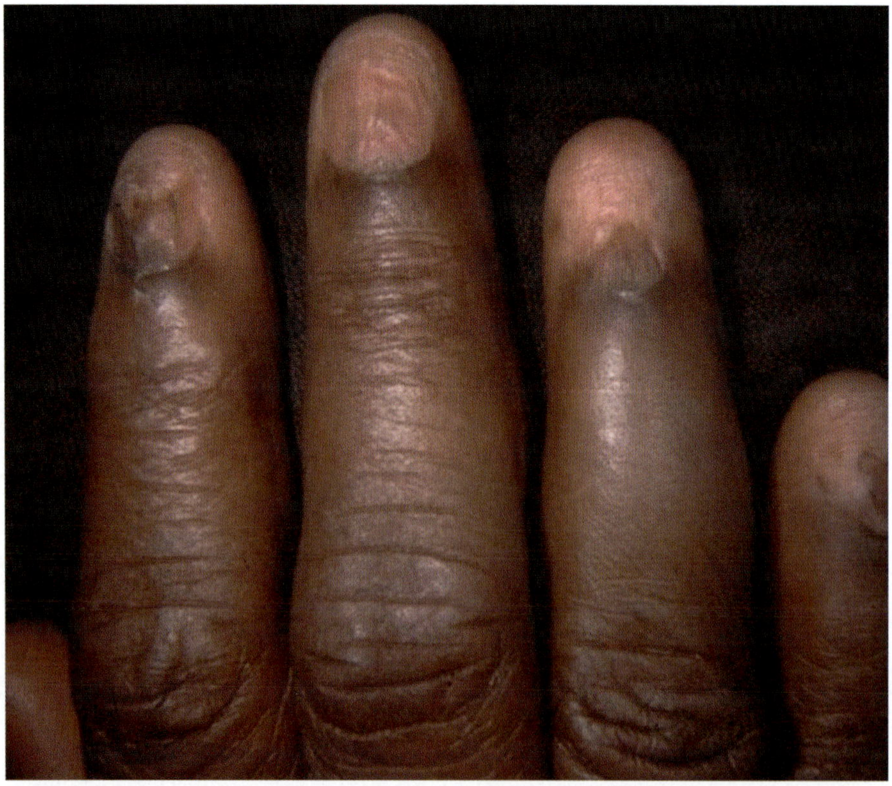

▲ **FIGURE 38-10** Lichen planus demonstrating multiple changes in the same patient: dorsal pterygium, nail plate thinning and ridging, as well as melanonychia (second fingernail).

TABLE 38-6
Psoriasiform Nail Diseases

Psoriasis vulgaris
Nail psoriasis
Pustular psoriasis
Acrodermatitis continua of Hallopeau
Reiter's syndrome
Paraneoplastic acrokeratosis (Bazex syndrome)
Pityriasis rubra pilaris

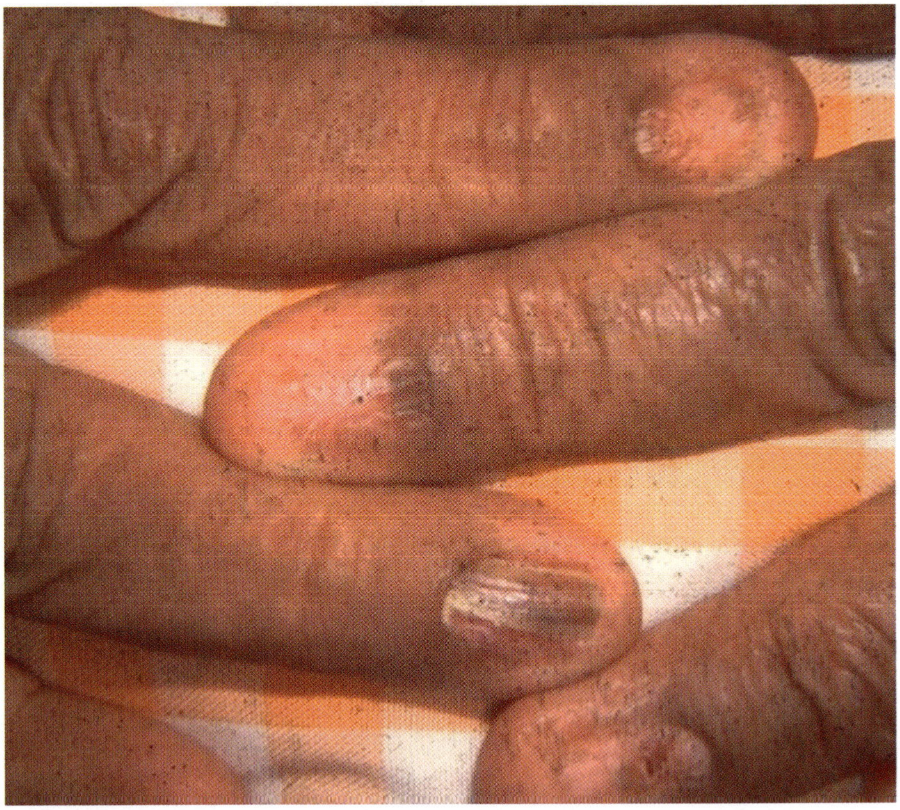

▲ **FIGURE 38-11** Lichen planus demonstrating multiple changes in the same patient: dorsal pterygium, anonychia, longitudinal ridging, as well as melanonychia (second nail from bottom).

abnormalities, including the classic pitting (from proximal matrix involvement), with nail bed involvement responsible for "oil spots," onycholysis, and hyperkeratosis (Figures 38-12 and 38-13). Of note, 80–90% of patients with psoriatic arthritis have nail disease at some time; hence careful evaluation of the joints, particularly the nearby interphalangeal and metacarpophalangeal joints, is appropriate when evaluating patients with psoriasis and nail disease.

Treatment of nail unit psoriasis is no different in patients with skin of color. While mild disease such as superficial pitting may not require therapy, more severe disease may require more aggressive therapy. Nail matrix disease tends to be more responsive to all forms of therapy than nail bed disease. The problem with topical medications, as with other nail conditions such as onychomycosis, is medication bioavailability. Hence intralesional corticosteroids tend to provide more benefit, without systemic side effects. Table 38-8 displays psoriasis treatments, divided into first-, second-, and third-line therapies. As with LP, it is important to emphasize that trauma may worsen the disease (Koebner phenomenon) and that gentle nail care is important in any treatment; we recommend an irritant-avoidance regimen[61] to all patients with nail psoriasis.

TABLE 38-7
Presentation of Nail Psoriasis

Nail Matrix Disease	Nail Bed Disease	Hyponychium Disease	Nail Fold Disease
Pitting	Onycholysis Subungual	Onycholysis Subungual	Cutaneous psoriasis
Ridging	hyperkeratosis	hyperkeratosis	Pustules
Onychorrhexis	Oil spots		
Trachyonychia	Erythema		
Nail plate crumbling	Splinter		Inflammation from
Spotted lunula	hemorrhages		underlying psoriatic
Red lunula			arthritis
Leukonychia			
Beau's lines			
Onychomadesis			

TABLE 38-8
Treatment of Nail Psoriasis

First line
- Irritant-avoidance regimen
- Topical corticosteroids
- Intralesional corticosteroids
  - 2.5–5 mg/mL triamcinolone, injected into the matrix, with treatments monthly until clear, then tapered gradually

Second line
- Topical cyclosporine
- Topical tazarotene
- Topical 5-fluorouracil
- Systemic retinoids
- Phototherapy

Third line
- Topical keratolytics
- Systemic methotrexate
- Systemic cyclosporine
- Biologic (injectable) agents
- Radiation therapy

ONYCHOMYCOSIS

Onychomycosis is the most common nail disorder that presents to the dermatologist's office, accounting for almost 50% of nail visits. Onychomycosis caused by dermatophyte fungi is called *tinea unguium*. The incidence of onychomycosis increases with age. This is perhaps due to repeated nail trauma and exposure over time. Zaias has shown that the tendency to get distal subungual onychomycosis may be inherited in an autosomal dominant fashion with incomplete penetrance.[63,64] When children have the disorder, there is usually a parent with the same.

The foot appears to be a reservoir for fungus.[65] Zaias has written[66] and taught that almost all individuals with onychomycosis have preceding tinea pedis. The pedal disease, however, may not present as obvious infection coexisting

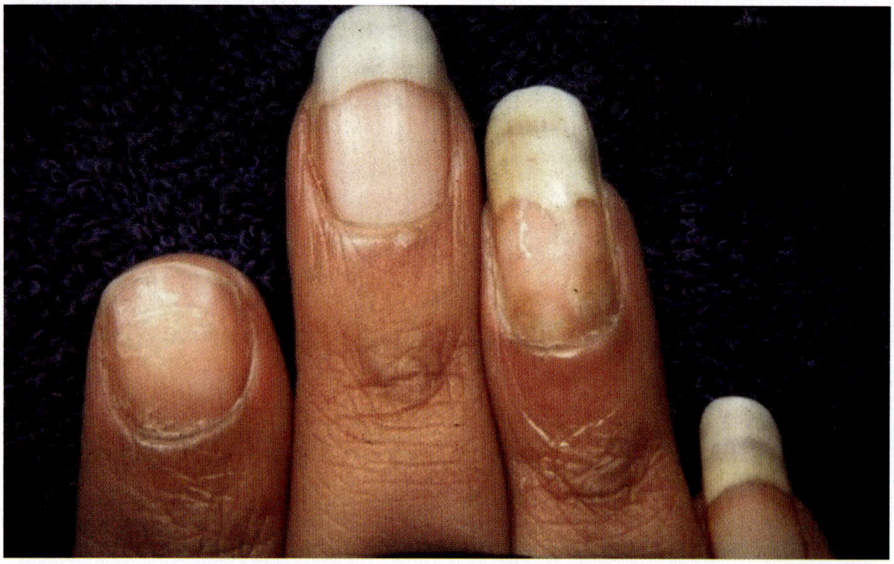

▲ **FIGURE 38-12** Psoriasis demonstrating oil spots and distal onycholysis.

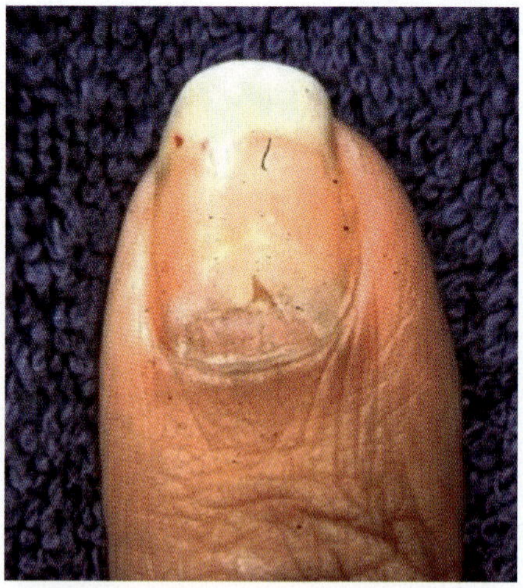

▲ **FIGURE 38-13** Psoriasis demonstrating onychomadesis.

with the nail disease. However, if one looks very closely, a "corneal collarette remnant of a minute vesicle, which may be asymptomatic but KOH positive" will be found on the foot of those with tinea unguium.[66] It is therefore helpful when evaluating for the presence tinea unguium to ask the patient if he or she knows of a past history (preceding nail involvement) of "athlete's foot" and for the doctor to examine patients under magnification that appear to have no coexisting tinea pedis.

The pathogenic sequence of events involves repeated micro- or macrotrauma (from tight shoes, high heels, stubbing the toe, exercise, etc.) that breaks the seal between the nail plate and the hyponychium or other periungual structure, allowing the fungus to enter the nail apparatus from the foot. Once the fungus has established a primary infection as tinea pedis (±tinea unguium), it may then infect other areas of the body.

> There is no need to look for an exogenous source of infection from direct or indirect contact with other persons. The nearest and most abundant source is within the foot itself. It cannot be denied that organisms may be recovered from the socks and shoes, but these represent merely an overflow of infectious elements from the foot itself.[67]

Trychophyton rubrum is the most common etiologic agent, with *T. mentagrophytes* second most common. Nondermatophyte pathogens are uncommon as the primary cause, although the prevalence varies by geography. *Candida,* too, is an unlikely primary pathogen in an immunocompetent host.

Potassium hydroxide (KOH) examination and fungal cultures are used commonly for diagnosis and still comprise the diagnostic "gold standard."[68] A recent study of 341 patients examined longitudinally looked at repeated KOH and culture results in onychomycosis patients who declined treatment to study the accuracy of data obtained in the initial direct microscopic and culture studies used for and strongly relied on in routine diagnosis.[69] Including dermatophyte and nondermatophyte molds (NDMs), this study demonstrated that KOH and culture were 83.9% sensitive for indicating true fungal etiology based on the initial specimens. Recent evidence also suggests that nail plate clipping, histologic processing, and staining with periodic acid–Schiff (PAS) stain may be more sensitive (92%), with a superior negative predictive value (77%), than traditional KOH and culture technique when diagnosing onychomycosis.[70] Based on data currently available, both PAS and KOH plus culture are accepted diagnostic techniques, with comparable accuracy.

There are several clinical patterns that are encountered frequently (Table 38-9). Distal and lateral subungual onychomycosis (DLSO) is encountered most commonly. Superficial white onychomycosis (SWO; see Figure 38-2), unlike DLSO and proximal subungual onychomycosis (PSO), which are caused most commonly by *T. rubrum,* is classically caused by *T. mentagrophytes.*

Possibly confounding the situation in individuals with skin of color who have a predisposition to LM, onychomycosis also may present as melanonychia[1] (see Figure 38-5). Unlike NAM, this pigmentation tends to be wider distally and narrower proximally, occasionally with pointed extensions proximally.[1] Multiple fungi have been reported to cause LM, including *T. rubrum,*[71] *Fusarium solani,*[72] *Candida,*[73] *Exophiala dermatitidis,*[74] and *Wangiella dermatitidis,*[75] as well as black molds such as *Scytalidium dimidiatum, Aspergillus niger,* and *Alternaria alternata.*[1]

Treatment of onychomycosis can be trying. Systemic treatments such as terbinafine and itraconazole offer the highest likelihood of a cure but carry higher risks of adverse effects than the less effective topical treament. However, even the best long-term results are imperfect, and relapse rates are frustratingly high. In the United States, both systemic terbinafine and itraconazole are approved by the Food and Drug Administration (FDA) for treatment of onychomycosis. Pooled meta-analysis data suggest that at 1 year, terbinafine is more effective than itraconazole.[76] Other meta-analyses support this finding.[77] Longer-term data have shown that at 18 and 54 months, terbinafine

TABLE 38-9
Types of Onychomycoses

Distal and lateral subungual onychomycosis
Total dystrophic onychomycosis
Superficial white onychomycosis
Proximal subungual onychomycosis

provides a mycologic cure in 53% and 42% of patients, respectively, versus mycologic cure rates after itraconazole treatment in 38% and 18% of patients, respectively.[78] In these same data, itraconazole-treated patients relapsed twice as often as terbinafine-treated patients. Systemic treatment with fluconazole and griseofulvin usually has yielded disappointing results.

Topical treatments uniformly offer low cure rates. This is likely because onychomycosis is primarily a nail bed (rather than nail plate) disease, and topical treatments lack adequate bioavailability. Single- or few-digit onychomycosis can be treated with physical or chemical plate avulsion followed by topical therapy to increase the likelihood of cure. In all cases, thinning, debridement, or removal of the obstacle nail plate increases medication bioavailability.

REFERENCES

1. Haneke E, Baran R. Longitudinal melanonychia. *Dermatol Surg* 2001;27: 580–584.
2. Kopf AW, Waldo E. Melanonychia striata. *Australas J Dermatol* 1980; 21:59-70.
3. Leyden JJ, Spott DA, Goldschmidt H. Diffuse and banded melanin pigmentation in nails. *Arch Dermatol* 1972;105:548-550.
4. Monash S: Normal pigmentation in the nails of the Negro. *Arch Dermatol* 1932; 25:876-881.
5. Baran R. Personal communication, in Scher RK, Daniel CR III (eds), *Nails: Diagnosis, Therapy, Surgery*, 3rd ed. Philadelphia, Elsevier Saunders, 2005.
6. Zaias N. *Pigmentation: The Nail in Health and Disease*, 2nd ed. Norwalk, CT, Appleton and Lange, 1990, pp 175-182.
7. Banfield CC, Redburn JC, Dawber RP. The incidence and prognosis of nail apparatus melanoma: A retrospective study of 105 patients in four English regions. *Br J Dermatol* 1998;139:276-279.
8. Park KG, Blessing K, Kernohan NM. Surgical aspects of subungual malignant melanomas. The Scottish Melanoma Group. *Ann Surg* 1992;216:692-695.
9. Muchmore JH, Krementz ET, Carter RD, et al. Isolated regional perfusion for treatment of limb melanoma in the American black. *Am Surg* 1989;55:232-237.
10. Takematsu H, Obata M, Tomita Y, et al. Subungual melanoma: A clinicopathologic study of 16 Japanese cases. *Cancer* 1985;55:2725-2731.
11. Hinds MW. Anatomic distribution of malignant melanoma of the skin among non-Caucasians in Hawaii. *Br J Cancer* 1979;40:497-499.
12. Pantoja E, Llobet RE, Roswit B. Melanomas of the lower extremity among native Puerto Ricans. *Cancer* 1976;38:1420-1423.
13. Black WC, Wiggins C. Melanoma among southwestern American Indians. *Cancer* 1985;55:2899-2902.
14. Thai KE, Young R, Sinclair RD. Nail apparatus melanoma. *Australas J Dermatol* 2001;42:71-81.
15. Levit EK, Kagen MH, Scher RK, et al. The ABC rule for clinical detection of subungual melanoma. *J Am Acad Dermatol* 2000; 42:269-274.
16. Quinn MJ, Thompson JE, Crotty K, et al. Subungual melanoma of the hand. *J Hand Surg (Am)* 1996;21:506-511.
17. Glat PM, Spector JA, Roses DF, et al. The management of pigmented lesions of the nail bed. *Ann Plast Surg* 1996;37:125-134.
18. Mohrle M, Hafner HM. Is subungual melanoma related to trauma? *Dermatology* 2002;204:259-261.
19. O'Toole EA, Stephens R, Young MM, et al. Subungual melanoma: A relation to direct injury? *J Am Acad Dermatol* 1995; 33:525-528.
20. Kechijian P. Subungual melanoma in situ presenting as longitudinal melanonychia in a patient with familial dysplastic nevi. *J Am Acad Dermatol* 1991;24:283.
21. Lateur N, Andre J. Melanonychia: diagnosis and treatment. *Dermatol Ther* 2002; 15:131-141.
22. Leppard B, Sanderson KV, Behan F. Subungual malignant melanoma: Difficulty in diagnosis. *Br Med J* 1974;1: 310-312.
23. Baran R, Kechijian P. Hutchinson's sign: A reappraisal. *J Am Acad Dermatol* 1996; 34:87-90.
24. Ronger S, Touzet S, Ligeron C, et al. Dermoscopic examination of nail pigmentation. *Arch Dermatol* 2002;138:1327-1333.
25. Kawabata Y, Ohara K, Hino H, Tamaki K. Two kinds of Hutchinson's sign, benign and malignant. *J Am Acad Dermatol* 2001; 44:305-307.
26. Haas N, Henz BM. Pitfall in pigmentation: Pseudopods in the nail plate. *Dermatol Surg* 2002;28:966-967.
27. Johr RH, Izakovic J. Dermatoscopy/ELM for the evaluation of nail-apparatus pigmentation. *Dermatol Surg* 2001;27: 315-322.
28. Gewirtzman AJ, Saurat JH, Braun RP. An evaluation of dermoscopy fluids and application techniques. *Br J Dermatol* 2003;149:59-63.
29. Jellinek NJ. Nail matrix biopsy of longitudinal melanonychia: diagnostic algorithm including the matrix shave biopsy. *J Am Acad Dermatol* 2007;56(5):803-810.
30. Hafner J, Haenseler E, Ossent P, et al. Benzidine stain for the histochemical detection of hemoglobin in splinter hemorrhage (subungual hematoma) and black heel. *Am J Dermatopathol* 1995;17:362-367.
31. Husain S, Scher RK, Silvers DN, Ackerman AB. Melanotic macule of nail unit and its clinicopathologic spectrum. *J Am Acad Dermatol* 2006;54:664-667.
32. High WA, Quirey RA, Guillen DR, et al. Presentation, histopathologic findings, and clinical outcomes in 7 cases of melanoma in situ of the nail unit. *Arch Dermatol* 2004;140:1102-1106.
33. Giele H, Hollowood K, Gibbons CL, et al. Subungual melanoma with osteocartilaginous differentiation. *Skeletal Radiol* 2003;32:724-727.
34. Perrin C, Michiels JF, Pisani A, Ortonne JP. Anatomic distribution of melanocytes in normal nail unit: An immunohistochemical investigation. *Am J Dermatopathol* 1997;19:462-467.
35. Buka R, Friedman KA, Phelps RG, et al. Childhood longitudinal melanonychia: Case reports and review of the literature. *Mt Sinai J Med* 2001;68:331-335.
36. Antonovich DD, Grin C, Grant-Kels JM. Childhood subungual melanoma in situ in diffuse nail melanosis beginning as expanding longitudinal melanonychia. *Pediatr Dermatol* 2005;22:210-212.
37. Rigby HS, Briggs JC. Subungual mela noma: A clinicopathological study of 24 cases. *Br J Plast Surg* 1992;45:275-278.
38. Banfield CC, Dawber RP. Nail melanoma: A review of the literature with recommendations to improve patient management. *Br J Dermatol* 1999;141:628-632.
39. Krull EA. Malignant melanoma, in Krull EA, Baran R, Haneke E (eds), *Nail Surgery: A Text and Atlas.* Philadelphia, Lippincott Williams & Wilkins, 2001, pp 305-315.
40. Parker SG, Diffey BL. The transmission of optical radiation through human nails. *Br J Dermatol* 1983;108:11-16.
41. Blessing K, Kernohan NM, Park KG. Subungual malignant melanoma: Clinicopathological features of 100 cases. *Histopathology* 1991;19:425-429.
42. Shukla VK, Hughes LE. Differential diagnosis of subungual melanoma from a surgical point of view. *Br J Surg* 1989;76: 1156-1160.
43. Vrouenraets BC, Kroon BB, Klaase JM, et al. Regional isolated perfusion with melphalan for patients with subungual melanoma. *Eur J Surg Oncol* 1993;19:37-42.
44. Baas PC, Hoekstra HJ, Schraffordt Koops H, et al. Isolated regional perfusion in the treatment of subungual melanoma. *Arch Surg* 1989;124:373-376.
45. Brodland DG. The treatment of nail apparatus melanoma with Mohs micrographic surgery. *Dermatol Surg* 2001;27: 269-273.
46. Heaton KM, el-Naggar A, Ensign LG, et al. Surgical management and prognostic factors in patients with subungual melanoma. *Ann Surg* 1994;219:197-204.
47. Spencer JM. Malignant tumors of the nail unit. *Dermatol Ther* 2002;15:126-130.
48. Kato T, Suetake T, Sugiyama Y, et al. Epidemiology and prognosis of subungual melanoma in 34 Japanese patients. *Br J Dermatol* 1996;134:383-387.
49. Goettmann-Bonvallot S, Andre J, Belaich S. Longitudinal melanonychia in children: A clinical and histopathologic study of 40 cases. *J Am Acad Dermatol* 1999;41:17-22.
50. Balch CM, Buzaid AC, Soong SJ, et al. Final version of the American Joint Committee on Cancer staging system for cutaneous melanoma. *J Clin Oncol* 2001; 19:3635-3648.
51. Johnson TM, Sondak VK, Bichakjian CK, Sabel MS. The role of sentinel lymph node biopsy for melanoma: Evidence assessment. *J Am Acad Dermatol* 2006; 54: 19-27.
52. McMasters KM, Reintgen DS, Ross MI, et al. Sentinel lymph node biopsy for melanoma: Controversy despite widespread agreement. *J Clin Oncol* 2001;19: 2851-2855.
53. Perrott R, Glass L, Reintgen D, Fenske N. Reassessing the role of lymphatic mapping and sentinel lymphadenectomy in the management of cutaneous malignant melanoma *J Am Acad Dermatol* 2003;49: 567-588.

54. Moehrle M, Metzger S, Schippert W, et al. "Functional" surgery in subungual melanoma. *Dermatol Surg* 2003;29:366-374.
55. Abimelec P, Dumontier C. Basic and advanced nail surgery: 2. Indications and complications, in Scher RK, Daniel CR (eds), *Nails: Diagnosis, Therapy, Surgery,* 3rd ed. Philadelphia, Elsevier Saunders, 2005 pp 291-308.
56. Banfield CC, Dawber RP, Walker NP, et al. Mohs micrographic surgery for the treatment of in situ nail apparatus melanoma: A case report. *J Am Acad Dermatol* 1999; 40:98-99.
57. Lingam MK, McKay AJ, Mackie RM, Aitchison T. Single-centre prospective study of isolated limb perfusion with melphalan in the treatment of subungual malignant melanoma. *Br J Surg* 1995;82: 1343-1345.
58. Shiohara T, Kano Y. Lichen planus and lichenoid dermatoses, in Bolognia J, Jorizzo J, Rapini R (eds), *Dermatology,* Vol 1. St Louis, MO, Mosby, 2003, pp 175-198.
59. Tosti A, Peluso AM, Fanti PA, Piraccini BM. Nail lichen planus: Clinical and pathologic study of twenty-four patients. *J Am Acad Dermatol* 1993;28:724-730.
60. de Berker D, Baran R, Dawber RPR. The nail in dermatological diseases, in Baran R, Dawber RPR, de Berker D, et al (eds), *Baran and Dawber's Diseases of the Nails and Their Management,* 3rd ed. Oxfoed, England, Blackwell Science, 2001, pp 197-204.
61. Daniel CRIII. Simple onycholysis, in Scher RK, Daniel CR III (eds), *Nails: Diagnosis, Therapy, Surgery,* 3rd ed. Philadelphia, Elsevier Saunders, 2005, pp 97-98.
62. Tosti A, Piraccini BM. Dermatological diseases, in Scher RK, Daniel CR III (eds), *Nails: Diagnosis, Therapy, Surgery,* 3rd ed. Philadelphia, Elsevier Saunders, 2005, pp 105-121.
63. Zaias N, Tosti A, Rebell G, et al. Autosomal dominant pattern of distal subungual onychomycosis caused by *Trichophyton rubrum. J Am Acad Dermatol* 1996;34:302-304.
64. Faergemann J, Correia O, Nowicki R, Ro BI. Genetic predisposition: Understanding underlying mechanisms of onychomycosis. *J Eur Acad Dermatol Venereol* 2005;19: 17-19.
65. Daniel CR III, Jellinek NJ. The pedal fungus reservoir (editorial). *Arch Dermatol* Arch Dermatol. 2006;142:1344-1346.
66. Zaias N, Rebell G. Chronic dermatophytosis caused by *Trichophyton rubrum. J Am Acad Dermatol* 1996;35:S17-20.
67. Strauss JS, Kligman AM. An experimental study of tinea pedis and onychomycosis of the foot. *AMA Arch Dermatol* 1957;76:70-79.
68. Daniel CR III, Elewski BE. The diagnosis of nail fungus infection revisited. *Arch Dermatol* 2000;136:1162-1164.
69. Summerbell RC, Cooper E, Bunn U, et al. Onychomycosis: A critical study of techniques and criteria for confirming the etiologic significance of nondermatophytes. *Med Mycol* 2005;43:39-59.
70. Weinberg JM, Koestenblatt EK, Tutrone WD, et al. Comparison of diagnostic methods in the evaluation of onychomycosis. *J Am Acad Dermatol* 2003;49:193-197.
71. Perrin C, Baran R. Longitudinal melanonychia caused by *Trichophyton rubrum:* Histochemical and ultrastructural study of two cases. *J Am Acad Dermatol* 1994;31: 311-316.
72. Lee HJ, Koh BK, Moon JS, et al. A case of melanonychia caused by *Fusarium solani. Br J Dermatol* 2002;147:607-608.
73. Gautret P, Rodier MH, Kauffmann-Lacroix C, Jacquemin JL. Case report and review: Onychomycosis due to *Candida parapsilosis. Mycoses* 2000;43:433-435.
74. Hata Y, Naka W, Nishikawa T. A case of melanonychia caused by *Exophiala dermatitidis. Nippon Ishinkin Gakkai Zasshi* 1999;40:231-234.
75. Matsumoto T, Matsuda T, Padhye AA, et al. Fungal melanonychia: Ungual phaeohyphomycosis caused by *Wangiella dermatitidis. Clin Exp Dermatol* 1992;17: 83-86.
76. Crawford F, Young P, Godfrey C, et al. Oral treatments for toenail onychomycosis: A systematic review. *Arch Dermatol* 2002;138:811-816.
77. Haugh M, Helou S, Boissel JP, Cribier BJ. Terbinafine in fungal infections of the nails: A meta-analysis of randomized clinical trials. *Br J Dermatol* 2002;147:118-121.
78. Sigurgeirsson B, Olafsson JH, Steinsson JB, et al. Long-term effectiveness of treatment with terbinafine vs itraconazole in onychomycosis: A 5-year blinded, prospective follow-up study. *Arch Dermatol* 2002;138: 353-357.

SECTION 5

Sebaceous and Sweat Gland Disorders

CHAPTER 39

Acne

Susan C. Taylor
Pamela Summers

Key Points

- Acne vulgaris is a disorder that is seemingly common in skin of color populations, including those of African, Asian, and Latin descent.
- Although few studies examine possible differences in the pathogenesis of acne vulgaris in racial and ethnic groups, it is likely that the pathogenesis is similar in all groups.
- Individuals with darker skin tones and acne frequently present with a chief complaint of hyperpigmentation, which is often referred to as *dark marks, blemishes, scars, spots, discolorations, blotches, descoloracions*, or *Mecheta.*
- Hyperpigmented macules may be the predominant lesion found in the skin of color patient with acne.
- Whereas comedonal acne occurs commonly in some skin of color individuals, nodulocystic acne is felt to occur less frequently in this population.
- By and large, treatment regimens for acne vulgaris in skin of color patients are similar to those for white patients, but it is important to avoid topical medications that lead to dryness or irritation and subsequent postinflammatory hyperpigmentation.
- Various maneuvers to improve tolerability to potentially drying topical agents can be instituted for the skin of color patient.
- Oral agents, including antibiotics and retinoids, are effective for skin of color patients with acne.

The diagnosis and treatment of acne vulgaris are a frequent reason for visits by patients to the dermatologist's office. This disease affects 40–50 million people in the United States, and it is commonly seen from the preteen years through age 50.[1,2] Acne often has a negative psychological impact on patients, affecting their self-esteem and self-confidence.[3,4] Furthermore, it may lead to permanent scarring. Since individuals with skin of color represent a greater proportion of the U.S. population, dermatologists will be faced with increasing numbers of individuals with this disease. Acne vulgaris patients with skin of color present with differences in the chief complaint, clinical presentation, precipitating and exacerbating factors, long-term sequelae, treatment, and subsequent adverse events (Table 39-1). This chapter provides a comprehensive review and discussion of these differences.

TABLE 39-1
Differences in Acne Vulgaris in Skin of Color Populations versus White Populations

- Chief complaint (hyperpigmentation)
- Clinical presentation
  - Infrequent cystic acne
- Precipitating and exacerbating factors
  - Pomade acne
- Long-term sequelae
  - Scar formation, including keloidal and ice pick
- Treatment protocols
  - Concomitant treatment of hyperpigmentation
  - Avoidance of irritation
- Adverse events from treatment
  - Hyperpigmentation

EPIDEMIOLOGY

Acne vulgaris is a disorder that is seemingly common in skin of color populations, including those of African, Asian, and Latin descent[5] (Table 39-2). Although exact information on the epidemiology of acne in skin of color patients is limited, health care utilization data provide an indication of the frequency with which patients seek health care for this inflammatory disorder. For the African-American population, clinic and private practice visits for acne have been chronicled since the beginning of twentieth century. In 1908, Fox reported that 4.6% of black patients and 7.4% of white patients presented for treatment of acne.[6] By 1914, the numbers had increased, and Hazen found that 8.4% of black patients as compared with 9.0% of white patients presented with acne vulgaris.[7] In the later part of the twentieth century, surveys from 1965 and 1983 showed that 9.0% and 27.7% of black patients, respectively, presented with acne as compared with 18.0% and 29.5% of white patients.[8,9] At the conclusion of the twentieth century, acne vulgaris was the most common diagnosis in blacks seeking health care, accounting for 15.7% of the diagnoses, as reported by the National Ambulatory Care Survey (NAMCS) for 1993–2002.[5] In a survey of the black pediatric population in Miami, Florida, 49.3% of black children versus 50.7% of white children presented with acne vulgaris, making it the fourth most common dermatologic diagnosis in childeren.[10] Similar statistics have been identified for European black populations, with a 1996 survey from London, England, reporting acne as the primary cutaneous disease in 13.7% of patients.[11] In the black African-Caribbean population, the diagnosis of acne vulgaris was 29.21% in a practice survey from Kingston, Jamaica.[12] In Guadeloupe, 19.5% of African-Caribbean patients presented with acne vulgaris as compared with between 7.1% and 10.4% of Caucasians on the island.[13]

TABLE 39-2
National Ambulatory Care Survey Data (1993–2002) for Diagnosis of Acne

RACE/ETHNICITY	PERCENTAGE
Whites	11.8%
Blacks	15.7%
Asians	15.1%
Latinos	14.2%

Acne vulgaris is purportedly less common in the Asian population than in the white population.[14] However, it was the leading dermatologic diagnosis for Asians in the United States, occurring in 15.1% of these patients, as reported by the NAMCS for 1993–2002.[5] Similarly, in Asia, the National Skin Center in Singapore (NSCS) indicated that acne was the second most common diagnosis among their patients, occurring in 10.9% of Asians.[15] The same survey found that 3.1% of the pediatric Asian population presented with acne, making it the eighth most common cutaneous diagnosis in this group.

A survey of Latino patient visits in the United States demonstrated acne vulgaris to be the most common diagnosis in this population.[16] According to NAMCS, acne represented 14.2% of primary diagnosis in Latinos.[5] In a Middle East pediatric population from Kuwait, acne was a common diagnosis, with 10.5% of patients presenting for dermatologic care.[17]

As survey data indicate, acne vulgaris is a cutaneous disorder for which patients of color frequently seek dermatologic care. Therefore, it is important that health care providers fully understand this disease entity when serving the skin of color population.

PATHOGENESIS

Although few studies examine possible differences in the pathogenesis of acne vulgaris in racial and ethnic groups, it is likely that the pathogenesis is similar in all groups. Acne is a disease of the pilosebaceous follicle, with abnormal follicular keratinocyte desquamation resulting in the development of a follicular plug.[18] Androgen-stimulated increased sebum production and proliferation of the microorganism *Propionibacterium acnes* occur within the follicular plug.[18,19] An inflammatory response ensues.[18]

There are no data that support differences in either the desquamation of the pilosebaceous epithelium or in the proliferation of *P. acnes* between racial or ethnic groups. There are inconclusive data suggesting a difference in sebaceous gland size or activity. Nicolaides concluded that the production of sebum was greater in blacks, but his methodology was deemed flawed.[20] Kligman measured the surface sebum levels in five black and five white subjects during a 4-hour time period and concluded that blacks had greater surface sebum levels than whites.[21] Forehead biopsies from two of the black subjects with moderate or high levels of surface sebum showed they had appreciably larger sebaceous glands when compared with the biopsies from two white subjects who generated low amounts of sebum. However, other studies did not support this conclusion.[4] It is difficult to conclude that individuals of skin of color produce greater amounts of sebum than whites given the small number of studies with small patient populations. Additionally, most studies do not include races other than blacks and whites.

CLINICAL PRESENTATION

The clinical presentation of acne vulgaris in skin of color patients often varies compared with white patients. Individuals with darker skin tones and acne frequently present with a chief complaint of hyperpigmentation, which they refer to as *dark marks, blemishes, scars, spots, discolorations, blotches, descoloracions,* or *Mecheta* (Table 39-3). Hyperpigmented macules may be the predominant lesion found in the skin of color patient with acne (Figure 39-1). Of the 313 patients studied at the Skin of Color Center in New York, hyperpigmented macules were seen in 65.3% of black patients, 52.7% of Hispanic patients, and 47.4% of Asian patients, including Indians and Pakistanis[4] (Table 39-4). In this situation, patients are seeking treatment for the hyperpigmentation and view the active acne lesions as secondary or even unimportant. It is often a challenge for the dermatologist to persuade patients of the necessity of concurrent treatment of both the acne and the hyperpigmentation. It is important that any treatment regimen in this situation include a lightening agent as well as agents for the treatment of acne.

TABLE 39-3
Terms Frequently Used for the Chief Complaint of Acne

Dark marks
Blemishes
Discolorations
Scars
Spots
Descoloracions
Blotches
Mecheta

TABLE 39-4
Presence of Hyperpigmented Macules, Skin of Color Center Study

Acne Hyperpigmented Macules	Percentage
Blacks	65.3%,
Hispanics	52.7%
Asians	47.4%

All the characteristic lesions of acne vulgaris may be seen in individuals with skin of color, including open and closed comedones, papules, pustules, nodules, and cysts (Figure 39-2). In the skin of color population of African descent, hair care practices and product selection may have an impact on the clinical presentation of acne vulgaris. Comedonal acne involving the forehead and temples owing to hair pomade, also termed *hair oil, grease, food, moisturizer,* and *styling agents,* is not uncommon in this population[3,4,22] (Table 39-5). Hair pomades are products containing various types of oils, including olive, vegetable, mineral, castor, mink, tea tree, coconut, and other nut oils, that are applied to textured hair to improve manageability and styling. Clinically, pomade acne is characterized by multiple closed comedones and occasionally papulopustules in areas such as the forehead and temples, where the pomade seeps from the scalp. In a study conducted at the Skin of Color Center in New York, 46.2% of patients reported use of pomade or oil-based hair care products.[4]

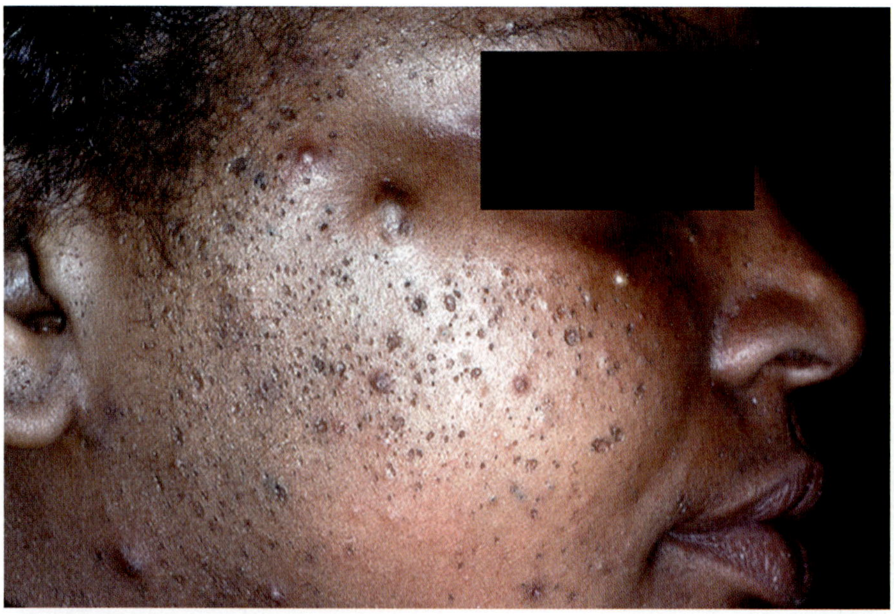

▲ **FIGURE 39-1** Papules, ice pick scars, pustules, open comedones, and postinflammatory hyperpigmentation.

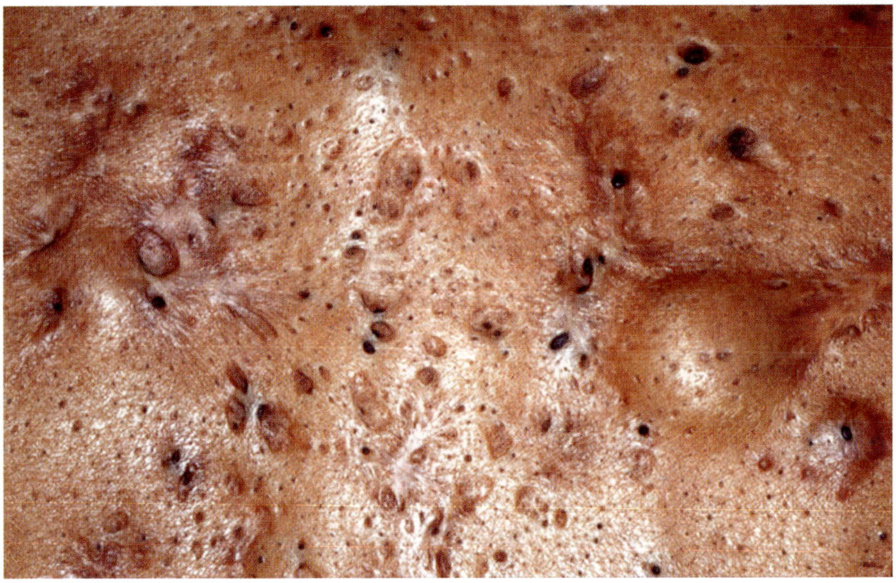

▲ **FIGURE 39-2** Acne, upper back. Papules, nodules, cysts, open and closed comedones, and hypertrophic scars.

Whereas comedonal acne occurs commonly in some skin of color individuals, nodulocystic acne is felt to occur less frequently in this population. Wilkins examined the type of acne lesion present in 4000 incarcerated men and found that blacks had less nodulocystic acne (0.5%) than whites (5%).[23] The occurrence of nodulocystic acne in Latinos was comparable with that of whites.[4] Taylor and colleagues reported at least one cystic lesions in 18% of blacks, 25.5% of Hispanics, and 10.5% of Asians in a study of 313 individuals of color.[4]

Another type of acne seen in black skin is acne conglobata.[24] This form of acne is seen commonly in men and typically is found on the face, neck, chest, and back. Patient presents with comedones, cysts, nodules, and abscesses with draining sinus tracts that may heal with scarring. When acne conglobata, hidradenitis suppurative, and dissecting cellulitis are observed together, it is termed the *follicular occlusion triad*. This triad is not uncommon in the black population.[24]

A sequelae of acne in people of color is the spectrum of scarring, including atrophic, ice pick, and keloidal scarring.[3,4] However, scarring is reportedly less prevalent in blacks than in other racial groups, and this is felt to be related to the lower prevalence of nodulocystic acne in blacks.[4] One study reported scarring in 5.9% of black, 21.8% of Hispanic, and 10.5% of Asian/other patients.[4] When present, ice pick scarring is a sequelae of facial acne; atrophic scarring, chest, back and jawline acne; and keloidal scarring, chest, back, and jawline acne. Given the long-lasting and devastating impact that keloidal scarring can have on patients, the risk of this type of scarring should motivate dermatologists to treat inflammatory acne early and aggressively in this patient population.

HISTOLOGY

When viewed histologically, blacks have been found to have greater inflammation than whites within acne lesions despite appearing noninflammatory clinically.[25] Halder and colleagues demonstrated that comedonal lesions exhibited striking inflammation with polymorphonuclear leukocyte infiltrates. Papular and pustular lesions included multinucleated giant cells that were dispersed beyond the actual papule or pustule. The authors suggested that the inflammatory nature of these lesions is what leads individuals with darkly pigmented skin to develop postinflammatory hyperpigmentation on resolution of the acne.[25]

TREATMENT

By and large, treatment regimens for acne vulgaris in skin of color patients are similar to those for white patients. The goal of acne therapy is to reduce follicular hyperkeratosis, bacteria, sebum production, inflammation, and postinflammatory hyperpigmentation.[3,4] Achieving these goals necessitate an evaluation of the patient's skin type and potential for sensitivity, current skin regimen (including cleansing, toning, and moisturizing products), previous treatments, results, and sequelae.[3] Taylor and colleagues have classified skin of color into three categories to assist in the selection of topical therapeutic agents:

1. Dry/sensitive skin and/or skin with a significant propensity to irritant reactions
2. Normal skin and/or skin with minimal propensity to irritant reactions
3. Oily skin and/or no propensity to irritant reactions[4]

Selection of appropriate agents may be enhanced by taking skin type into consideration (Table 39-6). For example, patients with dry skin are more likely to experience irritation secondary to

TABLE 39-5
Hair Pomades

African Pride African Miracle Castor & Mink Oil
All Ways Natural Castor Oil Conditioning Hair Dress Formula for Maximun Shine and Body
Black n Sassy Tea Tree Oil Triple Gro for Growth Condition & Healthy Hair
DAX Pomade with Lanolin Compounded with Vegetable Oils, Bergamot, Olive Oil and Castor Oil
Doo Gro Mega Thick Growth Oil
Gabels Lemon Pomade
Johnson Products Ultra Sheen Hair Food
Murray's Superior Hair Dressing Pomade
Vigorol Indian Hemp Hair & Scalp Conditioning Treatment
Soft Sheen Carson Sporting Wave Maximum Hold Pomade
L'Oreal Natures Therapy Mega Moisture Slick Moisturizing Pomade
D:FI D:tails Pomade for Hold & Shine
Sebastian Collection Grease Pomade for Flexible Hold
KMS Hair Play Defining Pomade Medium, Flexible Control, High Shine

TABLE 39-6
Compatibility of Topical Agents for Skin of Color

	Oily and/or No Propensity to Irritation	Normal and/or Little Propensity to Irritation	Dry/Sensitive and/or Great Propensity to Irritation
Retinoid/retinoid analogue	Adapalene solution 0.1%, pledgets 0.1%, or gel 0.1%, 0.3% Tazarotene gel 0.05% or 0.1% Tretinoin gel 0.025% or 0.01%	Adapalene gel 0.1% or cream 0.1% Tazarotene cream 0.1% Tretinoin cream 0.025% or microsphere 0.1%	Adapalene cream 0.1% or gel 0.1% Tazarotene cream 0.05% Tretinoin cream 0.025% or microsphere 0.04%
Antibiotics	Clindamycin solution or pledgets Erythromycin solution, pledgets, or gel Erythromycin–benzoyl peroxide Clindamycin–benzoyl peroxide	Clindamycin gel Erythromycin gel	Clindamycin lotion Sulfacetamide lotion
Other	Azeleic acid Benzoyl peroxide 6–10% Salicylic acid 3%	Azeleic acid Benzoyl peroxide 3–6% Salicylic acid 3%	Benzoyl peroxide 2.5–3%

Source: Adapted with permission from Taylor SC, Cook-Bolden F, Rahman Z, Strachan D. Acne vulgaris in skin of color. *J Am Acad Dermatol* 2002;46:S98–106.

topical medications, especially during the winter months or in areas of low humidity. Hence cream formulations are appropriate for this type of patient during the winter months, but a regimen may include a gel formulation during the hot and humid summer months.[4]

It is important to query the skin of color patient regarding over-the-counter skin care product use. Toners and astringents containing witch hazel, alcohol, and other ingredients that are potentially drying may decrease the tolerability of topical medications. Moisturizing products containing oils, cocoa butter, shea butter, and petrolatum commonly used in this population may exacerbate acne.

Treatment of acne vulgaris in skin of color populations includes over-the-counter (OTC) and prescription treatments that are designed to target the pathophysiologic mechanisms of acne. OTC agents are often mildly comedolytic and antimicrobial. Prescription therapy includes topical and systemic retinoids, topical and systemic antibiotics, and anti-inflammatory and hormonal agents.[4,26] Although all agents may be used in skin of color patients, these patients may be particularly susceptible to certain adverse events. Hence avoidance of contact irritant dermatitis owing to its potential for causing further hyperpigmentation is very important. Additionally, consideration must be given to concomitant treatment of hyperpigmented macules.

Topical Therapy

Topical therapeutic agents commonly prescribed for the treatment of acne vulgaris include benzoyl peroxide, azelaic acid, erythromycin, clindamycin, combination benzoyl peroxide–erythromycin, benzoyl peroxide–clindamycin, and retinoids (see Table 39-6). In the selection of topical agents for the treatment of acne, efficacy and tolerability of the agent are primary considerations. Secondary considerations include ability to treat or minimize hyperpigmented macules and maximizing penetration of other therapeutic agents.

Benzoyl peroxide preparations are available in various formulations, vehicles, and concentrations. These agents reduce the population of *P. acnes,* and there are no associated reports of resistance.[27] Formulations include cleansers, solutions, creams, pledgets, and gels with or without microspheres or ingredients such as urea which may improve tolerability. Benzoyl peroxide preparations vary in concentration of the active ingredient from 2.5–10%, with higher concentrations having the potential for excessive drying and irritation. Higher concentrations are most appropriate for oilier skin. Although benzoyl peroxide preparations may bleach clothing, they have no bleaching or lightening effect on hyperpigmented macules.

Benzoyl peroxide 5% may be combined with an antibiotic such as erythromycin 3% or clindamycin 1%. These combinations have been shown to be more effective in decreasing inflammatory and noninflammatory acne lesions than either agent alone.[28,29] As with benzoyl peroxide alone, combination products may produce excessive dryness and irritation of skin of color.

Azelaic acid is a dicarboxylic acid that has been shown to have mild anti-inflammatory and comedolytic effects, as well as activity as a tyrosinase inhibitor.[30] Efficacy in the treatment of inflammatory and noninflammatory acne, as well as in the treatment of hyperpigmentation, has been demonstrated.[31,32] Therefore, it is an agent that may address both the components of active acne and hyperpigmentation in the skin of color patient. Dryness and irritation are potential adverse events with this agent. Finally, clinical experience reveals that the efficacy of azelaic acid is mild to at most moderate in the treatment of both acne and hyperpigmentation compared with other agents.

Retinoids are a preferred treatment for acne vulgaris in the skin of color population. The mechanisms of action of retinoids include inhibition of TLR-2 receptors, thus reducing inflammation; reduction of the formation of hyperproliferative keratins, thus reducing microcomedone formation; and inhibition of AP-1 pathway, thus reducing inflammation and possibly scarring. Each of the three retinoids available in the United States—adapalene, tazarotene, and tretinoin—has been demonstrated to be effective in the treatment of both inflammatory and noninflammatory acne. Likewise, efficacy in the treatment of hyperpigmentation has been demonstrated with several of the retinoids, including 0.1% and 0.025% tretinoin cream, 0.1% adapalene gel, and 0.1% tazarotene cream.[33–39] These properties make the retinoids well suited for the concomitant treatment of both acne and hyperpigmentation in the skin of color population.

Retinoid dermatitis, characterized by dryness, peeling, and erythema of the skin, has been well described with the use of any retinoid or retinoid analogue. Both the concentration of the retinoid and its vehicle may have an impact on the dermatitis. Two of the retinoids—tazarotene and tretinoin—are formulated in at least two different concentrations (0.05% and 0.1% for tazarotene and 0.04%, 0.025%, 0.01%, and 0.025% for tretinoin), with the lower concentration(s) having less potential for irritation. All three retinoids have cream formulations that are generally less drying than their gel formulations. However, each of the retinoids still has the potential of causing irritation, dryness, and peeling of the skin, which may precipitate further hyperpigmentation.

There are various maneuvers that can improve tolerability to potentially drying topical agents including retinoids (Table 39-7) These include initiating treatment with the lower concentration of the agent, as well as with an every-other-day dosing schedule with a gradual increase to daily application.[3,4] Cream and lotion formulations of the topical medication are preferable for initiation of therapy. The use of moisturizing agents before and/or after application of the topical agent may improve tolerability but dilute the concentration of the active ingredient. The application of a small amount of the agent on the order of a "pea size" amount that is spread uniformly over a completely dry face is also recommended to improve tolerability. Avoidance of astringents, toners, and harsh soaps and cleansers is important, substituting nondrying and gentle cleansers.[4]

Instituting therapy for hyperpigmentation along with acne treatment is not contraindicated in the skin of color patient. In addition to azelaic acid and the retinoids, which have been discussed, hydroquinone preparations containing 3% and 10% concentrations may be used in addition to a 2% OTC preparation.[4] Irritation is a possible side effect of higher concentrations of hydroquinone.

TABLE 39-7
Maneuvers to Improve Tolerability of Topical Therapeutic Agents

- Initiate treatment with the lowest concentration of the medication.
- Limit application initially to every other day.
- Begin treatment with a cream or lotion formulation.
- Apply a small amount of the medication on the order of a "pea sized" amount.
- Spread uniformly over a completely dry face.
- Avoid astringents, toners, harsh soaps, and cleansers.
- Use nondrying, gentle cleansers no more than twice daily.
- Use moisturizers before and/or after application of the topical agent.

Adjunctive therapies, such as chemical peels and microdermabrasion, are useful in the acne patient with hyperpigmentation. Glycolic acid in concentrations of 35–70% and salicylic acid in concentrations of 20–30% are used commonly. Grimes demonstrated improvement of acne in 67% of patients and in postinflammatory hyperpigmenation in 80% of patients treated with a series of five salicylic acid peels at 2-week intervals.[40]

Additionally, sun protection factor 15 or higher sunscreen has been suggested to be important in the daily regimen of skin of color patients.[4] Daily use of sunscreen can aid in the treatment of postinflammatory hyperpigmenation because it takes a longer period of time for this condition to resolve if the patient is continually exposed to ultraviolet radiation.

Oral Antibiotics

The selection of oral antibiotics for the skin of color population does not vary greatly from that for the white population.[4] Antibiotics are used for their anti-inflammatory as well as bactericidal and static properties. Selection includes the tetracycline family of medications, including tetracycline, doxycycline, and minocycline. Generally, adverse effects of oral antibiotics do not vary among ethnic backgrounds.[4] In addition to the well-recognized adverse events of gastrointestinal distress, rash, urticaria, and candidal vaginitis, hyperpigmentation and a lupus-like syndrome have been reported with the minocycline class of antibiotics. The later two adverse effects may be of particular concern for the skin of color population, in whom lupus and hyperpigmentation are already common problems. Other oral antibiotics prescribed for the treatment of acne vulgaris include erythromycin, cefadroxil and trimethoprim-sulfamethoxyzole.[26] Antibiotic resistance by *P. acnes* is an emerging problem, with oral erythromycin displaying the most resistance, which is succeeded by clindamycin, tetracycline, and doxycycline.[29]

Isotretinoin

Isotretinoin is an effective agent in the treatment of acne vulgaris because it targets all the pathophysiologic mechanisms of acne: sebum production, follicular hyperkeratinization, *P. acnes,* and inflammation. It is often reserved as the last treatment option for acne because of its potential adverse effects.[26,37]

Isotretinoin can be used safely in individuals with skin of color.[41] Between 1990 and 1997, 17% of acne visits resulted in treatment with isotretinoin.[42] According to IMS National Diagnosis and Therapeutic Index data, African-Americans are seemingly prescribed isotretinoin less often that would be expected.[43] In 1999, only 2.4% of African-Americans received treatment with isotretinoin, although 7.7% of African-Americans presented to physicians with a diagnosis of acne vulgaris. In contrast, Hispanic and Asian isotretinoin prescriptions more closely reflected their office visits for acne vulgaris (4.9% prescriptions per 4.7% of Hispanic office visits, 4.4% presecriptions per 4.0% of Asian office visits).[43] A study by Fleischer and colleagues supports this finding, and the authors found that blacks (3.9%) are less likely to be subscribed isotretinoin for acne treatment than whites (93%).[42] Fleisher postulated that the higher cost of the medication, lack of confidence in the health care system, opposing view of the risk:benefit ratio of treatment, or an overall decreased amount of visits to the dermatologist's office may account for the difference.

Hormonal Therapy

Hormonal therapy is used in women to combat the androgenetic stimulation of the sebaceous glands. Agents used include oral contraceptives and androgen-receptor blockers (e.g., spironolactone, flutamide, and cyproterone acetate).[3,19]

CONCLUSION

Acne vulgaris patients with skin of color present with differences in the chief complaint, clinical presentation, precipitating and exacerbating factors, long-term sequelae, therapeutic needs, and adverse events. Despite these differences, acne vulgaris can be treated effectively in skin of color patients.

REFERENCES

1. White GM. Recent findings in the epidemiologic evidence, classification, and subtypes of acne vulgaris. *J Am Acad Dermatol* 1998;39:S34-37.
2. Lookingbill DP. *Principles of Dermatology,* 3rd ed. Philadelphia, Saunders, 2000.
3. Callender VD. Acne in ethnic skin: Special considerations for therapy. *Dermatol Ther* 2004;17:184-195.
4. Taylor SC, Cook-Bolden F, Rahman Z, Strachan D. Acne vulgaris in skin of

color. *J Am Acad Dermatol* 2002;46: S98-106.
5. U.S. Census Bureau. National Center for Health Statistics. National Ambulatory Medical Care Survey (NAMCS). Generated using Data Ferret, August 2002; http://dataferrett.census.gov/.
6. Fox H. Observations on skin diseases in the Negro. *J Cutan Dis* 1908;26:67-79.
7. Hazen H. Personal observations upon skin diseases in the American Negro. *J Cutan Dis* 1914;23:704-706.
8. Kenney JA. Management of dermatoses peculiar to Negroes. *Arch Dermatol* 1965; 91:126-129.
9. Halder RM, Grimes PE, McLaurin CI, et al. Incidence of common dermatoses in a predominantly black dermatologic practice. *Cutis* 1983;32:388, 390.
10. Schachner L, Ling NS, Press S. A statistical analysis of a pediatric dermatology clinic. *Pediatr Dermatol* 1983;1:157-164.
11. Child FJ, Fuller LC, Higgins EM, et al. A study of the spectrum of skin disease occurring in a black population in southeast London. *Br J Dermatol* 1999;141:512-517.
12. Dunwell P, Rose A. Study of the skin disease spectrum occurring in an Afro-Caribbean population. *Int J Dermatol* 2003; 42:287-289.
13. Mahe A, Mancel E. Dermatological practice in Guadeloupe (French West Indies). *Clin Exp Dermatol* 1999;24:358-360.
14. Lee CS, Lim HW. Cutaneous diseases in Asians. *Dermatol Clin* 2003;21:669-677.
15. Chura-ty G, Goh CL, Koh SL. Pattern of skin diseases at the National Skin Center (Singapore) from 1989-1990. *Int J Dermatol* 1992;31:555-559.
16. Sanchez MR. Cutaneous diseases in Latinos. *Dermatol Clin* 2003;21:689-697.
17. Nanda A, al-Hasawi F, Alsaleh QA. A prospective survey of pediatric dermatology clinic patients in Kuwait: An analysis of 10,000 cases. *Pedriatr Dermatol* 1999; 16:6-11.
18. Freedberg IM, Eisen AZ, Wolffet K, et al (eds). *Fitzpatrick's Dermatology in General Medicine.* New York, McGraw-Hill, 2003.
19. Haider A, Shaw JC. Treatment of acne vulgaris. *JAMA* 2004;292:726-735.
20. Nicolaides N, Rothman S. Studies on the chemical composition of human hair fat: II. The overall composition with regard to age, sex and race. *J Invest Dermatol* 1953;21:9-14.
21. Kligman AM, Shelley WB. An investigation of the biology of the human sebaceous gland. *J Invest Dermatol* 1958;30: 99-125.
22. Plewig G, Fulton JE, Kligman AM. Pomade acne. *Arch Dermatol* 1970;101: 580-584.
23. Wilkins JW Jr, Voorhees JJ. Prevalence of nodulocystic acne in white and Negro males. *Arch Dermatol* 1970;102:631-634.
24. Halder RM, Brooks HL, Callender VD. Acne in ethnic skin. *Dermatol Clin* 2003;21:609-615.
25. Halder RM, Holmes YC, Bridgeman-Shah S, Kligman AM. A clinicopathological study of acne vulgaris in black females. Abstracts for the 1996 Annual Meeting Society for Investigative Dermatology. *J Invest Dermatol* 1996; 106:888.
26. Lebwohl MG, Heymann WR, Berth-Jones J, Coulson I. *Treatment of Skin Disease: Comprehensive Therapeutic Strategies.* St Louis, MO, Mosby, 2002 pp 6-13.
27. Gollnick H, Cunliffe W, Berson D, et al. Management of acne: A report from a global alliance to improve outcomes in acne. *J Am Acad Dermatol* 2006;49:S1-67.
28. Leyden JJ. Topical treatment for the inflamed lesion in acne, rosacea, and pseudofolliculitis barbae. *Cutis* 2004;73:4-5.
29. Leyden JJ. Antibiotic resistance in the topical treatment of acne vulgaris. *Cutis* 2004;73:6-10.
30. Gollnick HP. Azelaic acid 15% gel in the treatment of acne vulgaris: Combined results of two double-blind clinical comparative studies. *J Dtsch Dermatol Ges* 2004;2:841-847.
31. Fitton A, Goa KL. Azelaic acid: A review of its pharmacological properties and therapeutic efficacy in acne and hyperpigmentary skin disorders. *Drugs* 1991; 41:780-798.
32. Balina LM, Graupe K. The treatment of melasma: 20% azelaic acid versus 4% hydroquinone cream. *Int J Dermatol* 1991; 30:893-895.
33. Bulengo-Ransby SM, Griffiths CE, Kimbrough-Green CK, et al. Topical tretinoin (retinoic acid) therapy for hyperpigmented lesions caused by inflammation of the skin in black patients. *N Engl J Med* 1993;328:1438-1443.
34. Halder RM. The role of retinoids in the management of cutaneous conditions in blacks. *J Am Acad Dermatol* 1998;39: S98-103.
35. Jacyk WK. Adapalene in the treatment of African patients. *J Eur Acad Dermatol Venereol* 2001;15:S37-42.
36. Czernielewski J, Poncet M, Mizzi F. Efficacy and cutaneous safety of adapalene in black patients versus white patients with acne vulgaris. *Cutis* 2002;70: 243-248.
37. Tu P, Li GQ, Zhu XJ, et al. A comparison of adapalene gel 0.1% vs tretinoin gel 0.025% in the treatment of acne vulgaris in China. *J Eur Acad Dermatol Venereol* 2001;15:S31-36.
38. Zhu XJ, Tu P, Zhen J, Duan YQ. Adapalene gel 0.1%: Effective and well tolerated in the topical treatment of acne vulgaris in Chinese patients. *Cutis* 2001;68: S55-59.
39. Grimes P, Callender V. Tazarotene cream for postinflammatory hyperpigmentation and acne vulgaris in darker skin: A double-blind, randomized, vehicle-controlled study. *Cutis* 2006;77:45-50.
40. Grimes PE. The safety and efficacy of salicylic acid chemical peels in darker racial-ethnic groups. *Dermatol Surg* 1999;25: 18-22.
41. Kelly AP, Sampson DD. Recalcitrant nodulocystic acne in black Americans: Treatment with isotretinoin. *J Natl Med Assoc* 1987;79:1266-1270.
42. Fleischer AB Jr, Simpson JK, McMichael A, Feldman SR. Are there racial and sex differences in the use of oral isotretinoin for acne management in the United States? *J Am Acad Dermatol* 2003;49:662-666.
43. *IMS National Diagnosis and Therapeutic Index, 1999.*

CHAPTER 40

Hidradenitis Suppurativa

Shari Hicks-Graham

Key Points

- Hidradenitis suppurativa is a chronic inflammatory disorder affecting the apocrine skin.
- The pathogenesis is multifactorial and includes hyperkeratosis of the follicular infundibulum with subsequent rupture of the hair follicles and abscess formation.
- Painful, fluctuant nodules with scarring in the axillary and inframammary regions, groin, and buttocks are typically seen.
- Treatment is quite challenging and includes topical astringents, oral antibiotics, hormonal therapies, retinoids, biologic agents, and surgical excision.

Hidradenitis suppurativa (HS) is a chronic inflammatory disorder affecting apocrine sweat gland–bearing skin. It is also known as *Verneuil's disease* or *acne inversa.* Painful subcutaneous nodules and sinus tracts in the axillae, mammary areas, and perineum are characteristic of this disease. These lesions often drain serosanguineous fluid, become fluctuant, and subsequently develop disfiguring plaquelike or keloidal scars. HS is a member of the follicular occlusion triad that also includes acne conglobata and dissecting cellulitis of the scalp. If a pilonidal sinus is also present, the constellation of findings is termed the *follicular occlusion tetrad.* Diagnosis is based on clinical presentation. Treatment is determined by extent of disease and ranges from conservative measures for immediate relief of pain, systemic antibiotics, other medical therapies, and lastly, wide surgical excision. This condition is challenging to both physician and patient alike because of the typical waxing and waning course and therapeutic resistance. Lastly, the associated pain, odorous discharge, and physical disfigurement often lead to social isolation and a high degree of morbidity. Thus novel treatment approaches are both exciting and extremely necessary. African-Americans have a higher incidence than Caucasians and Hispanics.

HISTORY

Velpeau provided the first description of HS in 1839 when he reported a patient with an inflammatory disorder of the skin affecting the axillary, mammary, and perianal regions.[1] Later, a French surgeon noted that the disorder represented an infection of the sweat glands.[2] The association of hidradenitis specifically with the apocrine glands was made by Schiefferdecker in 1922.[3] The histology of hidradenitis detailed in 1932 indicated that obstruction of the apocrine glands is the initiating feature of the disease.[4]

EPIDEMIOLOGY

The incidence of HS is difficult to determine because of its high rate of misdiagnosis. Studies have reported incidences from 1 per 1000 dermatology patients to 1 per 300 adults.[5,6] One study from Denmark noted the 1-year point prevalence to be as high as 4.1%, with women being affected three times more often than men.[7] In most cases, HS starts at or soon after puberty. The peak onset is between the ages of 15 and 30, coinciding with the postpubertal increase in androgen levels.[8] It is extremely rare for the condition to be present in individuals over the age of 40 or in prepubertal children. A familial autosomal dominant form of HS has been reported with variable gene penetrance.[9]

There is some evidence that the disease may be more common in African-Americans than in Caucasians.[10] It is possible that this relates to anatomic differences in the apocrine gland structure of African descendants, but more research is needed to substantiate this evidence.

PATHOGENESIS

The pathogenesis of HS remained relatively unclear until more detailed studies were performed in the 1990s. Investigators examined the resected axillary lesions of hidradenitis patients and found that the most common histologic feature were sinuses or cystic structures lined by stratified squamous epithelium in the dermis.[11] Inflammation was seen in the apocrine glands in only a third of patients. The authors concluded that plugging and subsequent rupture of the hair follicles were the initiating events in hidradenitis. Two subsequent studies[12,13] supported their findings, and the fundamental initiating factor in HS was established: hyperkeratosis of the infundibulum, giving rise to comedo-like impactions.[14] The subsequent rupture of the plugged hair follicle causes keratin, bacteria, sebaceous material, and hair to spill into the connective tissue, causing abscess formation. This inflammatory reaction ensues along with secondary occlusion of the apocrine gland, ductal dilatation, and gland stasis. Skin flora multiply within the environment supported by nutrient-rich apocrine sweat.[15] This superinfection contributes to cellulitis, tissue destruction, and pain.[16] This cascade of events differs from the early belief that hidradenitis is primarily a disease of the apocrine glands. Instead, it represents an infundibulofolliculitis.[17] No confirmatory test for HS has been established.

Despite this improved pathogenetic understanding, the stimulus for the initial infundibular plugging remains elusive.[8] Disorderly follicular keratinization resulting from androgen excess is thought to be related to HS. Apocrine sweat containing dihydroepiandrosterone sulfate is also known to stimulate sebaceous activity, possibly contributing to follicular blockage. Obesity and tight clothing have been associated and are known to exacerbate the disease, likely owing to the shearing forces of skin-on-skin contact in affected areas.

One study examined glucose tolerance, lymphocyte populations, and human leukocyte antigen (HLA) types in 27 patients with untreated hidradenitis suppurativa.[18] Twenty-two percent of patients had an increased incidence of impaired glucose tolerance. Seven patients with moderate or severe clinical disease had a marked reduction in T-lymphocytes, and these patients had an increased frequency of HLA-A1 and HLA-B8. This association suggests that these factors may predispose the patient to more severe disease, but further research is needed.

The role of microbiologic flora in the pathogenesis of HS is very controversial. It is difficult to meaningfully characterize the flora and the value of the bacterial culture in HS. First, resident skin bacteria may contaminate the culture results.[19] One study evaluating the culture results of samples obtained by carbon dioxide laser surgery indicated that coagulase-negative staphylococci and *Staphylococcus aureus* were the species found most frequently.[19] However, another study found negative cultures in half the patients treated for perianal and perineal disease.[10] In the positive cultures, a number of species including *S. epidermidis, Escherichia coli, Klebsiella, Proteus*, alpha streptococci, anaerobes, and diptheroids were isolated. Others have reported *Streptococcus milleri* to be a pathogenetic organism in perineal hidradenitis, correlating with severity of disease.[16] *Chlamydia trachomatis* and *Bilophila wadswothia* also have been implicated.[20,21] Despite this, response to antibiotic therapy is usually suboptimal in HS, supporting the concept that the inflammation associated with the disease relates more to a structural problem with the hair follicle than to a bacterial infection itself.

Three early studies examined apocrine gland structure and function by race. One unblinded study published by Schiefferdecker in 1922 with 16 subjects (3 black, 1 Chinese, and 12 white Germans) concluded that the black race had increased numbers and larger apocrine glands than either the Chinese or the white race.[22] A second study reviewed over 1100 histologic sections of both white and black subjects from four apocrine-bearing areas of the body (excluding the axilla). Apocrine glands reportedly occurred three times more in the black subjects than in the white subjects.[23] One other study, published in 1960, examined apocrine gland size and function in 30 black and white subjects.[24] The black subjects were determined to have larger and more productive apocrine glands than the white subjects. Nevertheless, this finding was subjectively based on the assessment of apocrine sweat production being "more turbid with a unique odor" compared with white subjects. Although these studies offer possible explanations for the reported higher incidence of HS in individuals of African descent, controlled, blinded investigations about the pathophysiology of HS are still necessary.

CLINICAL FEATURES

Initial findings on physical examination include subcutaneous nodules and sterile abscesses located on any of the anatomic regions bearing apocrine glands. Specifically, the areas most frequently affected include the axillae and inguinal-perineal regions, buttocks, and mammary and inframammary regions (Figures 40-1 and 40-2). The periumbilical region, scalp, face, external auditory meatus, neck, shoulders, and thighs also may be involved.[8] The abscesses may spontaneously drain volumes of malodorous serosanguineous and purulent discharge

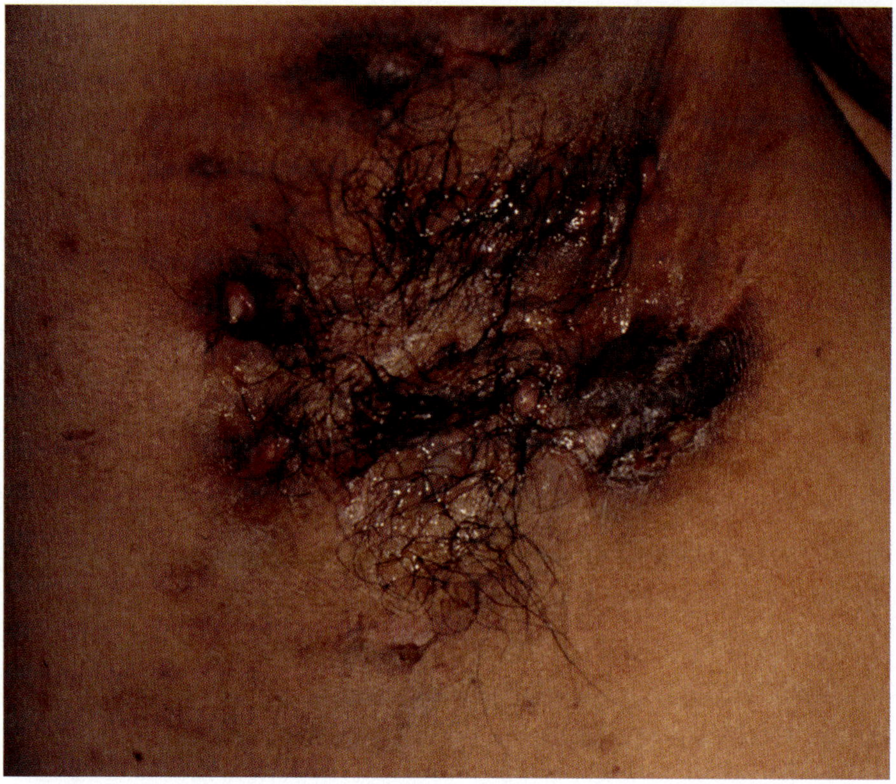

▲ **FIGURE 40-1** Axillae affected by HS. Nodules, keloidal-like scarring, plaques, and draining sinuses.

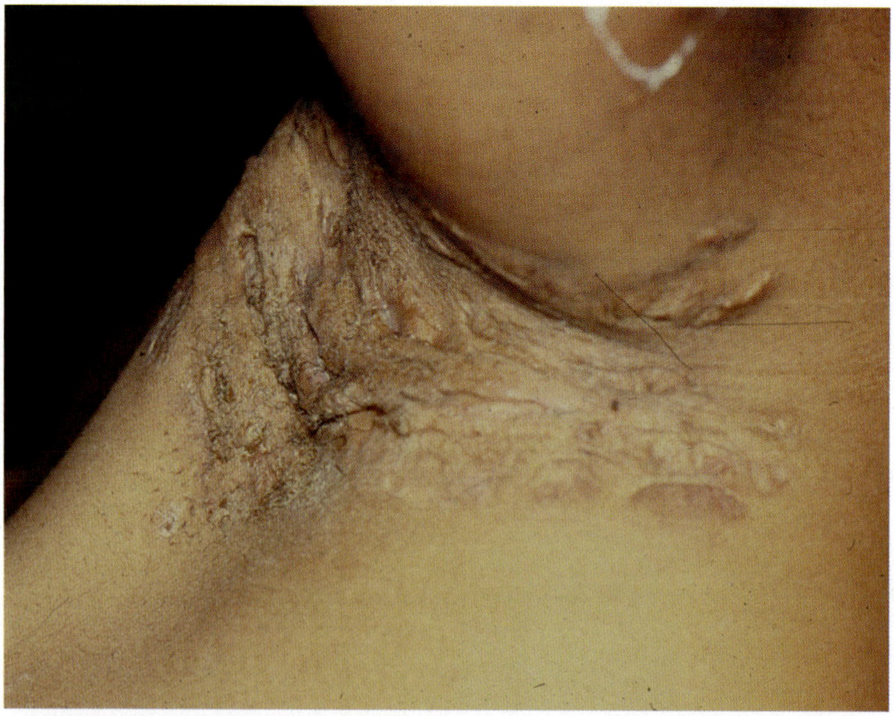

▲ **FIGURE 40-2** Perineal region affected by HS. Indurated hyperpigmented plaques with hemorrhagic draining nodules and sinuses.

(Figure 40-4). These wounds may heal but typically do not and may recur over time. Characteristically, sinus tracts, cavities, and fistulas develop within hard, fibrotic plaques. Dyschromia of overlying skin is frequently associated.

Pain and tenderness associated with the lesions of HS may substantially limit mobility.[25] Simple activities of daily living are compromised as a result of the damage caused by the inflammation and scarring. The embarrassment caused by the foul odor and appearance of the lesions may be extremely troublesome. The burden of this disease may be tremendous because it often limits social interaction and the ability to perform work reliably. This routinely contributes to poor self-esteem and financial difficulties.

The extent of involvement is extremely variable. Disease may be mild in limited areas or involve multiple sites extensively. Remission and relapse are quite common. One British study published in 2000 investigated the natural history of HS by surveying 156 individuals diagnosed with the disease at three different hospitals.[26] The average patient age and age at disease onset were 40.1 and 21.8 years, respectively. Average disease duration was 18.8 years. There was evidence that in women the condition eased or subsided after menopause. Menstruation aggravated the disease in 44% of women. Thirty-eight percent of patients reported a positive family history of the disorder. The average duration of painful boils was approximately 7 days. Over half the patients acknowledged the presence of permanently painful boils that failed to subside and developed an average of two boils per month. Aggravating factors included sweating, heat, stress, fatigue, tight clothing, or friction. Factors that could improve the condition consisted largely of medical treatments and lifestyle measures such as swimming or baths. Almost a quarter of the patients failed to find anything at all to help their condition despite the typically long duration of disease.

Several complications of HS, including hypoproteinemia and iron-deficiency anemia, are possible owing to the chronicity of the inflammation and drainage.[27] In addition, intestinal keratitis, osteomyelitis, fistulas to pelvic organs, amyloidosis, and even death have been reported.[28,29]

The association of squamous cell carcinoma with HS has been documented. One study reported an incidence of 3.2% in 125 cases of hidradenitis.[30] Another investigation reviewing 2119 patients with HS over a time period of 33 years estimated that the relative risk of developing nonmelanoma skin cancer (defined as squamous cell carcinoma) was increased among patients with HS.[31] One report found that the average age at diagnosis of squamous cell carcinoma arising within HS was 47 years, with a male predominance.[32] The perineal, gluteal, and perianal regions were affected most frequently.

Several other disorders also have been associated with HS. The follicular occlusion triad, for example, includes dissecting cellulitis of the scalp, acne conglobata, and hidradenitis suppurativa (Figure 40-3).[33] Pilonidal sinus also has been added, forming the follicular occlusion tetrad. Many reports of simultaneous Crohn's disease and HS have been published, and some authors suggest that the two may be related.[34,35]

DIFFERENTIAL DIAGNOSIS

Early diagnosis of HS may be difficult because of its resemblance to other conditions.[8] Acne, epidermoid cysts, dermoid cysts, cellulitis, erysipelas, furuncles, and carbuncles. All may resemble HS and should be included in the differential diagnosis. Dermatoses that produce sinuses and fistulas, such as lymphogranuloma venereum, granuloma inguinale, actinomycosis, cutaneous tuberculosis, cat scratch disease, tularemia, chronic pyoderma gangrenosum, and Crohn disease, should be considered. The physical examination and history are usually sufficient for differentiating these conditions, but culture results, possible skin biopsy, and colonoscopy may be necessary.

HISTOLOGY

The pathologic findings in HS are quite heterogeneous. One prospective study detailing the histologic findings of 60 biopsy specimens with hidradenitis indicated that apocrine glands were involved in only a minority of cases.[36] The disease appears to be predominantly follicular, with apocrine primary involvement present in a minority of patients. Secondary involvement of apocrine glands and eccrine glands was found in 12% and 25% of all specimens, respectively. Specimens demonstrate poral occlusion with and without folliculitis, sinus tracts, epithelial cysts, abscesses, apocrinitis, diffuse dermal inflammation, pyogenic granuloma, and scarring.

TREATMENT

A number of treatment options, both medical and surgical, are available for hidradenitis suppurativa (Table 40-1). The particular treatment regimen must be based on disease severity and should be discussed thoroughly so that expectations are clearly understood between both physician and patient. Patient education regarding the natural history of this chronic relapsing and remitting disorder must be provided in order for compliance to be optimized.

Initially, mild disease may be treated with conservative measures such as Sitz baths, whirlpool therapy, topical cleansers, and aluminum acetate soaks. Loose clothing is advised for all patients, and weight loss should be suggested for obese patients. Antibiotics may be employed as an adjunctive measure, but they do not have the sole capability to control the disease.[37] Topical clindamycin is the only antibiotic shown to be beneficial for HS in a prospective, randomized, controlled trial.[38] Systemic tetracycline was shown to be equally as effective in a study published in 1998.[39] Oral doxycycline and minocycline also may be of benefit, although the efficacy

TABLE 40-1
Treatment Options

Explain disease and treatment options to patient and emphasize prevention

Mild disease:
- Sitz baths
- Whirpool Rx
- Gentle cleansers
- Aluminum acetate soaks
- Loose clothing
- Weight loss (obese patients)
- Topical antibiotics (clindamycin)

Moderate disease:
- Oral doxycyline or minocycline
- Broad-spectrum antibiotics based on culture results
- Hormonal Rx (cyproterone acetate)
- Leuprolide
- Cryotherapy

Severe disease:
- Systemic retinoids (isotretinoin)
- Systemic corticosteroids (prednisone)
- Cyclosporine
- Biologics (infliximab)
- Surgery (I&D)
- Surgery (excision of apocrine gland area)
- Split-thickness skin grafts
- Second-intention healing
- Carbon dioxide laser

has never been proven in a clinical trial. For more severe disease located in the perineum, broad-spectrum antibiotics may be necessary initially but should be tailored as much as possible to culture results.

Hormonal therapy also may be helpful through an unknown mechanism. In particular, cyproterone acetate, an antiandrogen, has been associated with disease improvement in European trials.[40,41] Leuprolide, a synthetic gonadotropin-releasing hormone, has been demonstrated to improve HS in some patients.[42] Glucocorticoids are temporarily helpful in reducing the inflammation associated with some of the lesions but are associated with suppression of the hypothalamic-pituitary axis among other unwanted side effects. Prednisone at a dose of 60–80 mg/day usually causes dramatic improvement, but the disease usually flares when the prednisone is discontinued.

Retinoids have been employed for treatment of hidradenitis with variable success. Isotretinoin, well known for its ability to substantially improve nodulocystic acne, has been very inconsistent as a therapy for HS. Several studies report mixed results regarding the efficacy of isotretinoin as a treatment for HS.[43–47] One retrospective study of the long-term results using low-dose (0.5–0.67 mg/kg per day) isotretinoin in the treatment of 68 patients with HS demonstrated that 23.5% of patients experienced clearance of their disease, and 16.2% of patients maintained their improvement through the follow-up period (mean duration 57 months).[48] The authors concluded that monotherapy with isotretinoin usually has a limited therapeutic effect for patients with HS. There is no established dosing guideline for use in HS, and the side effects of lipid and hepatic dysfunction and teratogenicity must be considered. The successful treatment of HS and nodulocystic acne with acitretin for maintainance after improvement with two courses of isotretinoin also has been reported.[49]

Cyclosporine also may be considered for its anti-inflammatory properties. It is best reserved for short-term therapy of sudden, severe flares of disease because of its severe side-effect profile, including renal dysfunction, hypertension, and hematologic abnormalities.[50] This potent immunosuppressant was reported to be beneficial in a patient suffering from both hidradenitis suppurativa and pyoderma gangrenosum[51]; however, caution is required in the presence of infection.

Biologic therapies are emerging as a targeted immune-modulating approach for the treatment of many dermatologic diseases, including HS. Several reports have been published regarding the successful use of monoclonal antibody against tumor necrosis factor in the treatment of Crohn's disease associated with HS[52–55]; however, the optimal dosing schedule and duration of therapy have not been determined. In addition, finasteride (5 mg/day for 12–16 weeks) was found to be successful in a few patients.[56] A somewhat newer therapy involves treating the patient with the biologic infliximab, 5–10 mg/kg at weeks 0, 2, and 6, followed by maintenance dose every 4 weeks.

Short-contact photodynamic therapy using topical 20% 5-aminolevulinic acid has been reported as a possible treatment for HS.[57] Additionally, physically destructive modalities such as cryotherapy have been used to treat a limited number of persistent painful nodules of HS.[58] Pain, prolonged healing time, and risk of infection are potential drawbacks of this type of procedure.

Surgery is a viable alternative for the treatment of severe HS affecting a patient capable of undergoing the physical demands of surgery and the subsequent wound care. Incision and drainage may be used to manage acute symptoms but are associated with a very high incidence of recurrence.[8] The unroofing of sinus tracts also may be performed to manage acute disease. General anesthesia is required while the sinus tracts are unroofed and curetted, with the epithelialized floor remaining intact. Aggressive postoperative wound care is essential. Unfortunately, recurrence rates are high with both the aforementioned surgical options; thus they are best regarded as a bridge to more definitive therapy. In my experience, surgical excision of the apocrine gland–bearing areas, especially the axillae, in early HS seems to prevent the development of severe disease.

Local excisions are performed as a means to control local infection without the associated morbidity of an extensive wide excision. One study reported that an overall complete cure rate of 14.7% was achieved with localized

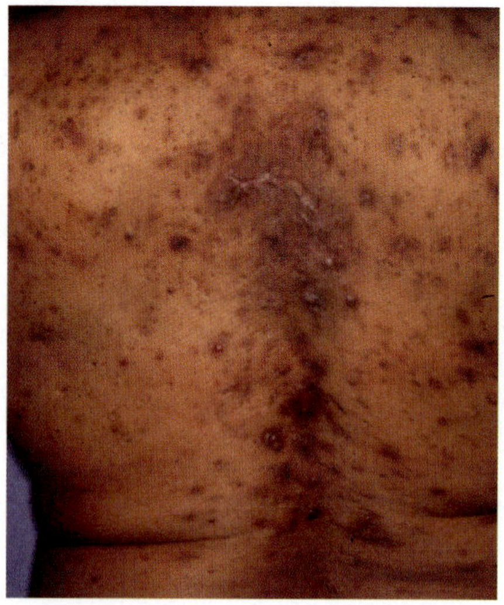

▲ **FIGURE 40-3** Back with nodules and sinus tracts typical of HS.

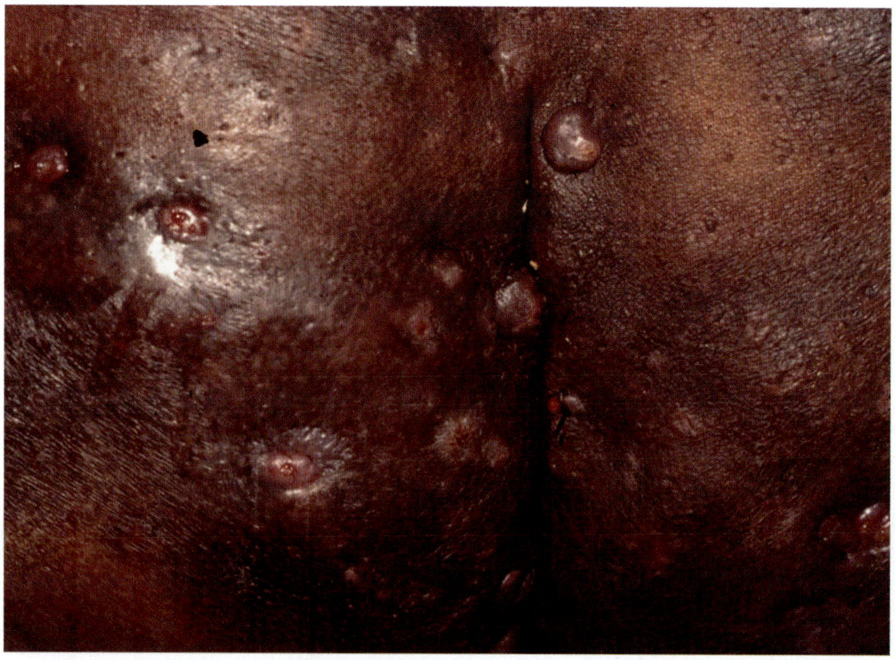

▲ **FIGURE 40-4** Buttocks with fluctuant nodules and indurated plaques.

surgical excision.[59] Seven percent experienced cure in the region treated but with subsequent recurrence in another region. Although high rates of recurrance are associated with this procedure, patient satisfaction is high, with 68% of patients reporting it to be superior to other treatments experienced.

Wide excision of all involved apocrine gland–bearing skin is the most successful treatment of hidradenitis, offering definitive therapy that may be accomplished safely.[8] Regional or general anesthesia is required, and the entire affected area should be resected to normal-appearing deep fascia or at least 5 mm of subcutaneous fat to ensure that all apocrine glands have been removed.[15] The wound may be closed primarily, covered with split-thickness skin grafts, or flaps. Alternatively, the operative defect may heal via secondary intention, generally within 3–8 weeks. Meticulous wound care is mandatory to ensure proper healing of the site, yet typical anatomic areas of involvement such as the perineum make this task challenging.

Carbon dioxide laser surgery also has been studied as a treatment for HS and was found to be fast and efficient.[60,61] Mean healing time was 4 weeks. In the majority of subjects, a step-wise horizontal vaporization technique was used to remove diseased tissue. In the second study, 22 of 24 patients were cured.[60] Although the procedure was associated with successful cure of the treated sites, de novo recurrences in sites beyond the surgical margins occurred.

The Hidradenitis Suppurativa Foundation, Inc. (HSF), is a nonprofit public benefit corporation dedicated to improving the quality of life and quality of care for individuals and families affected by hidradenitis suppurativa and may be a source of great help to patients in need with this disease.

REFERENCES

1. Velpeau A. Aissele, Dictionnaire de Medicine, on Repertoire General des Sciences Medicales sons le Rapport Theorique et Pratique Behcet Jeune Z (ed) 2:91, 1839.
2. Verneuil A. Etudes sur les tumeurs de la peau de quelque maladies des glandes sudoripares. *Arch Gen Med* 1954;94: 693-705.
3. Schiefferdecker B. *Die Hautdrusen des Menschen, und der Saugetiere, ihre Histologische und rassenanatomische Bedeutung Sowie die Muscularis Sexualis.* Stuttgart, E Schweizerbart, 1922.
4. Brunsting HA. Hidradenitis suppurativa: Abscess of the apocrine sweat glands. *Arch Dermatol Syphilol* 1939;39: 108-120.
5. Lookingbill DP. Yield from a complete skin examination. *J Am Acad Dermatol* 1988;18:31-37.
6. Fitzimmons JS, Guilbert PR, Fitzimmons EM. Evidence of genetic factors in hidradenitis suppurativa. *Br J Dermatol* 1985;113:1-8.
7. Jemec GB, Heidenheim M, Nielsen NH. The prevalence of hidradenitis suppurativa and its potential precursor lesions. *J Am Acad Dermatol* 1996;35:191-194.
8. Singer M, Cintron JR. Hidradenitis suppurativa. *Semin Colon Rectal Surg* 2003; 14:186-195.
9. von der Werth JM, Williams HC, Raeburn JA. The clinical genetics of hidradenitis suppurativa revisited. *Br J Dermatol* 2000;142:947-953.
10. Thornton JP, Abcarian H. Surgical treatment of perianal and perineal hidradenitis suppurativa. *Dis Colon Rectum* 1978; 21:573-577.
11. Yu CCW, Cook MG. Hidradenitis suppurativa: A disease of follicular epithelium, rather than apocrine glands. *Br J Dermatol* 1990;122:763-769.
12. Attanoos RL, Appleton MA, Douglas-Jones AG. The pathogenesis of hidradenitis suppurativa: a closer look at apocrine and apoeccrine glands. *Br J Dermatol* 1995; 133:254-258.
13. Jemec GBE, Hansen U. Histology of hidradenitis suppurativa. *J Am Acad Dermatol* 1996;34:994-999.
14. Jansen T, Plewig G. Acne inversa. *Int J Dermatol* 1998;37:96-100.
15. Parks RW, Parks TG. Pathogenesis, clinical features and management of hidradenitis suppurativa. *Ann R Coll Surg Engl* 1997;79: 83-89.
16. Highet AS, Warren RE, Weekes AJ. Bacteriology and antibiotic treatment of perineal suppurative hidradenitis. *Arch Dermatol* 1988;124:1047-1051.
17. Boer J, Weltevreden EF. Hidradenitis suppurativa or acne inversa: A clinicopathological study of early lesions. *Br J Dermatol* 1996;135:721-725.
18. O'Loughlin S, Woods R, Kirke PN, et al. Hidradenitis suppurativa: Glucose tolerance, clinical, microbiologic, and immunologic features and HLA frequencies in 27 patients. *Arch Dermatol* 1988;124:1043-1046.
19. Lapins J, Jarstrand C, Emtestam L. Coagulase-negative staphylococci are the most common bacteria found in cultures from the deep portions of hidradenitis suppurativa lesions, as obtained by carbon dioxide laser surgery. *Br J Dermatol* 1999; 140:90-95.
20. Bendehan J, Paran H, Kolman S, et al. The possible role of *Chlamydia trachomatis* in perineal suppurativa hidradenitis. *Eur J Surg* 1992; 158:213-215.
21. Baron EJ, Curren M, Henderson G, et al. *Bilophila wadsworthia* isolates from clinical specimens. *J Clin Microbiol* 1992; 20: 1882-1884.
22. Schiefferdecker P. The skin glands of humans and mammals, their biology and race: Anatomical meaning (translated from German). Dsaael be (vollkomin.Mitt.) *Zoologica* 1922;72:1-154.
23. Homma H. On apocrine sweat glands in white and negro men and women. *Bull Johns Hopkins Hosp* 1926;38:365-371.
24. Hurley HJ, Shelley WB. The physiology and pharmacology of the apocrine sweat gland, in Hurley HJ, Shelley WB (eds), *The Human Apocrine Sweat Gland in Health and Disease.* Springfield, IL, Charles C Thomas, 1960, pp 22-77.
25. von der Werth JM, Jemec GB. Morbidity in patients with hidradenitis suppurativa. *Br J Dermatol* 2001; 144: 809-813.
26. von der Werth JM, Williams HC. The natural history of hidradenitis suppurativa. *J Eur Acad Dermatol Venereol* 2000;14: 389-392.
27. Ramasastry SS, Conklin WT, Granick MS. Surgical management of massive perianal hidradenitis suppurativa. *Ann Plast Surg* 1985;15:218-223.
28. Banerjee AK. Surgical treatment of hidradenitis suppurativa. *Br J Surg* 1992; 79:863-866.
29. Moschella SA. Hidradenitis suppurativa: Complications resulting in death. *JAMA* 1966;198:201-204.
30. Jackman RJ. Hidradenitis suppurativa: Diagnosis and management of perianal manifestations. *Proc R Soc Med* 1959;52: 110-112.
31. Lapins J, Ye W, Nyren O, Emtestam L. Incidence of cancer among patients with hidradenitis suppurativa.*Arch Dermatol* 2001;137:730-734.
32. Perez-Diaz D, Calvo-Serrano M, Martinez-Hijosa E. Squamous cell carcinoma complicating perianal hidradenitis suppurativa. *Int J Colorectal Dis* 1995;10: 225-228.
33. Self SJ, Montes LFL. Follicular occlusion triad. *South Med J* 1979;63:156-160.
34. Burrows NP, Jones RR. Crohn's disease in association with hidradenitis suppurativa. *Br J Dermatol* 1992;126:523.
35. Gower-Rousseau C, Maunoury V, Colombel JF, et al. Hidradenitis suppurativa and Crohn's disease in two families: A significant association? *Am J Gastroenterol* 1992; 87:928.
36. Jemec GB, Hansen U. Histology of hidradenitis suppurativa. *J Am Acad Dermatol* 1996;34:994-999.
37. Harrison BH, Kumar S, Read GF, et al. Recurrence after surgical treatment of hidradenitis suppurativa. *Br Med J Clin Res* 1987;294:487-489.
38. Clemmensen OJ. Topical treatment of hidradenitis suppurativa with clindamycin. *Int J Dermatol* 1983;22:325.
39. Jemec GBE, Wendelboe P. Topical clindamycin versus systemic tetracycline in the treatment of hidradenitis suppurativa. *J Am Acad Dermatol* 1998; 39:971-974.
40. Sawers RS, Randall VA, Ebling FJ. Control of hidradenitis suppurativa in women using combined antiandrogen (cyproterone acetate) and oestrogen therapy. *Br J Dermatol* 1986; 115:269-274.
41. Mortimer PS, Dawber RP, Gales MA, et al. A double-blind controlled cross-over trial of cyproterone acetate in females with hidradenitis suppurativa. *Br J Dermatol* 1986;115:263-268.
42. Camisa C, Sexton C, Friedman C. Treatment of hidradenitis suppurativa with combination hypothalamic-pituitary-ovarian and adrenal suppression: A case report. *J Reprod Med* 1989; 24:543-546.
43. Jones DH, Cunliffe WJ, King K. Hidradenitis suppurativa: Lack of success with 13-*cis*-retinoic acid (letter). *Br J Dermatol* 1982;107:252.
44. Dicken CH, Powell ST, Spear KL. Evaluation of isotretinoin treatment of

hidradenitis suppurativa. *J Am Acad Dermatol* 1984;11:500-502.
45. Norris JFB, Cunliffe WJ. Failure of treatment of familial widespread hidradenitis suppurativa with isotretinoin. *Clin Exp Dermatol* 1986;11:579-583.
46. Boer J. Isotretinoin-induced remission of hidradenitis suppurativa, in Orfanos CE, Stadler R, Gollnick H (eds), *Dermatology in Five Continents.* World Congress of Dermatology. Berlin, Springer Verlag, 1988, pp 1152-1153.
47. Brown CF, Gallup DG, Brown VM. Hidradenitis suppurativa of the anogenital region: Response to isotretinoin. *Am J Obstet Gynecol* 1988;158:12-15.
48. Boer J, van Gemert MJP. Long-term results of isotretinoin in the treatment of 68 patients with hidradenitis suppurativa. *J Am Acad Dermatol* 1999; 40: 73-76.
49. Scheman AJ. Nodulocystic acne and hidradenitis suppurativa treated with acitretin: A case report. *Cutis* 2002;69: 287-288.
50. Lebwohl M, Ellis C, Gottlieb A, et al. Cyclosporine consensus conference: With emphasis on the treatment of psoriasis. *J Am Acad Dermatol* 1998; 39:464-475.
51. Buckley DA, Rogers S. Cyclosporin-responsive hidradenitis suppurativa. *J R Soc Med* 1995;88:289-290.
52. Roussomoustakaki M, Dimoulios P, Kritikos HD, et al. Hidradenitis suppurativa associated with Crohn's disease and spondyloarthropathy: Response to anti-TNF therapy. *J Gastroenterol* 2003; 38:1000-1004.
53. Lebwohl, B, Sapadin AN. Infliximab for the treatment of hidradenitis suppurativa. *J Am Acad Dermatol* 2003; 49:S275-276.
54. Adams DR, Gordon KB, Devenyi AF, et al. Severe hidradenitis suppurativa treated with infliximab infusion. *Arch Dermatol* 2003;139:1540-1542.
55. Sullivan TP, Welsh E, Kerdel FA, et al. Infliximab for hidradenitis suppurativa. *Br J Dermatol* 2003;149:1046-1049.
56. Farrell AM, Randall VA, Vafaee T, et al. Finasteride as a therapy for hidradenitis suppurativa. *Br J Dermatol* 1999; 141: 1138-1139.
57. Gold M, Bridges TM, Bradshaw VL, et al. ALA-PDT and blue light therapy for hidradenitis suppurativa. *J Drugs Dermatol* 2004;3:S32-35.
58. Bong JL, Shalders K, Saihan E. Treatment of persistent painful nodules of hidradenitis suppurativa with cryotherapy. *Clin Exp Dermatol* 2003; 28:241-244.
59. Jemec GB. Effect of localized surgical excisions in hidradenitis suppurativa. *J Am Acad Dermatol* 1988;18:1103-1107.
60. Lapins J, Sartorius K, Emtestam L. Scanner-assisted carbon dioxide laser surgery: A retrospective follow-up study of patients with hidradenitis suppurativa. *J Am Acad Dermatol* 2002; 47:280-285.
61. Lapins J, Marcusson JA, Emtestam L. Surgical treatment of chronic hidradenitis suppurativa: CO_2 laser stripping-secondary intention technique. *Br J Dermatol* 1994;131:551-556.

SECTION 6

Skin Cancer

CHAPTER 41

Melanoma in Skin of Color

Seaver L. Soon
Carl V. Washington, Jr.

Key Points

- By 2050, African-Americans, Hispanics, and Asians will constitute almost half the U.S. population.
- Melanoma impact varies considerably along the lines of race, class, and ethnicity.
- There is an inverse relationship between melanoma and skin color.
- Melanoma distribution in blacks and Asians is directed to sites of the palms, soles, and nail beds.
- Acral tumors constitute 30–70% of melanomas in blacks, Asians, and Hispanics whereas only 1–9% of whites have acral melanomas.
- There were 55,000 invasive cases in 2004 with 8000 deaths.
- Subungual melanoma exhibits a preponderance in dark-skinned individuals.

Melanoma represents a significant disease burden in the United States, with an estimated 55,000 invasive cases occurring in 2004, resulting in approximately 8000 deaths.[1] This impact varies considerably along the lines of race, class, and ethnicity, as expressed in the broader social context, and as such, the relationship between these variables and melanoma outcome in minority populations is of clinical and social importance.

Since melanoma is predominantly a cancer of white populations, it is perhaps expected that most clinical research and public awareness campaigns promulgate the melanoma experience in Caucasians. This body of knowledge includes such risk factors as red hair, inability to tan, propensity to freckle and to sunburn, and such prototypical clinical presentations as the irregular, changing pigmented lesion on the trunks of men and lower legs of women.

While important for public health, these data may not be specifically relevant to the melanoma experience in persons of color and, furthermore, may inadvertently suggest that melanoma is not a health threat to these populations. U.S. Census data regarding increasing racial heterogeneity underscore the need for research focusing on the clinical and epidemiologic features of melanoma in ethnic populations.

By 2050, Hispanic, African, and Asian Americans, respectively, will comprise 24%, 15%, and 8% of the U.S. population, whereas Caucasians will comprise approximately 50%.[2] Considering the time period 2000–2050, these figures represent a population percentage increase of 188% for Hispanics, 71% for African-Americans, 213% for Asian Americans, and only 7% for Caucasians.[2] Internationally, 20% of the world's melanoma occurs in black and Asian populations.[3] In coming years, knowledge of the clinical expression of melanoma in persons of color will become increasingly relevant for dermatologists and others interested in the health status of minorities.

This chapter considers the epidemiology, clinical features, treatment, and prognosis of acral melanoma in ethnic populations. The findings suggest that the expression of melanoma in minority populations is distinct from that in Caucasians and is typified by lower incidence rates, a characteristic anatomic distribution, advanced stage at presentation, and poorer overall prognosis.

An inverse relationship exists between melanoma incidence and degree of skin pigmentation. Incidence is highest among whites, intermediate among Hispanics, and lowest among Asians and blacks.[4–9]

According to U.S. National Cancer Institute's Surveillance, Epidemiology, and End Results (SEER) data, U.S. melanoma incidence (1997–2001) was 20.3 per 100,000 in Caucasians, 4.3 per 100,000 in Hispanics, 1.9 per 100,000 in Native Americans, 1.4 per 100,000 in Asian Americans, and 1.0 per 100,000 in African-Americans.[1] SEER data (1992–2001) further depict rapidly increasing incidence rates among lightly pigmented racial groups (whites: 16.3 per 100,000 in 1992 versus 21.2 per 100,000 in 2001; Hispanics: 3.3 per 100,000 in 1992 versus 4.3 per 100,000 in 2001), whereas incidence rates in darkly pigmented racial groups are comparatively stable (Asians: 1.0 per 100,000 in 1992 versus 1.4 per 100,000 in 2001; blacks: 0.6 per 100,000 in 1992 versus 0.7 per 100,000 in 2001).[1]

The lower incidence observed in Hispanics, Asians, and blacks most likely results from the protective effect of darker skin pigmentation. The U.S. age-adjusted mortality rate (1997–2001) was 3.0 per 100 000 in whites, 0.8 per 100,000 in Hispanics, 0.5 per 100,000 in Native Americans and blacks, and 0.4 per 100,000 in Asians.[1] Melanoma incidence and mortality thus vary significantly across different ethnic populations.

The preferred anatomic site and histologic subtype of melanoma similarly differs along the lines of ethnicity. Among elderly Caucasians, melanoma predominates on the frequently sun-exposed head and neck with a high proportion of lentigo maligna subtype, whereas in young Caucasians, melanoma shows a predilection for the relatively sun-protected trunk in men and trunk and legs in women, with a greater representation of the superficial spreading melanoma subtype.[10]

Melanoma distribution in Asians and blacks, by contrast, is weighted toward the sun-protected sites of the palms, soles, and nail bed.[11] An analysis of the California Cancer Registry (n = 18,855) reported that melanoma occurred on the lower extremity in only 9% of whites compared with 50% of blacks, 36% of Asians, and 20% of Hispanics.[7] It is of interest, however, that tumor distribution among Hispanics varies according to the degree of skin pigmentation. Lightly pigmented Hispanics exhibit an anatomic distribution identical to that of whites, whereas darkly pigmented Hispanics exhibit a tumor distribution reminiscent of blacks.[8]

Numerous studies report that the most common histologic subtype on the hands and feet is acral lentiginous melanoma.[7,12–20] Although often deemed interchangeable, the terms *acral lentiginous melanoma* and *acral melanoma* are not synonymous. Acral lentiginous melanoma is a histologic designation, whereas acral melanoma is an anatomic designation. Acral melanoma thus encompasses both acral lentiginous melanoma and other histologic subtypes of melanoma (e.g., superficial spreading and nodular melanoma) that may arise in acral locations.

EPIDEMIOLOGY

Acral Melanoma

Acral tumors constitute 30–70% of melanomas in black, Asian, and Hispanic populations and only 1–9% in Caucasians.[6,8,12,17,19,21–30] Large case series report that the mean age of presentation of acral melanoma is during the sixth decade of life compared with the fifth decade for nonacral lesions.[27] The peak incidence of acral melanoma varies across different racial groups, with earlier incidence observed in more lightly pigmented groups. Reported peak incidence is in the fourth to the sixth decades for Hispanics[29,31,32]; in the sixth decade for Chinese,[33–35] Japanese,[26,36] and South Africans of mixed ancestry[37]; and in the seventh decade for Indians[38] and for American,[12,24,25,30,38–40] Carribean,[41] and South African[18] blacks.

It is of interest that the absolute incidence of acral melanoma is almost identical between African and Caucasian Americans (1.7 per 100,000 and 2.0 per 100,000, respectively). The observed racial difference in acral melanoma prevalence results from the proportionally decreased occurrence of nonacral lesions in ethnic populations.[42] The incidence of acral melanoma has further remained static over the past half-century, which contrasts sharply with the escalating rates of nonacral melanoma.[11,23,41,43]

This peculiar epidemiologic pattern, in conjunction with its development on the infrequently sun-exposed sites of the palms and soles, historically has suggested an etiologic role other than solar radiation in acral melanoma.[5] Recent population-based studies in the United States, however, suggest a positive association between ultraviolet (UV) index and increasing incidence and mortality among black men ($p < 0.05$), with a nonsignificant association observed among black women and Hispanics of both sexes.[6,11]

Although preliminary, these results suggest that solar radiation may play a greater than expected role in the development of melanoma in darkly pigmented populations. Additional etiologic theories in acral melanoma include the effect of long-term chronic trauma on benign acral nevi (given the preponderance of acral melanoma on the pressure-bearing heel and ball of the foot),[44] malignant transformation of unstable foci of acral melanocytes,[45] and the relative paucity of free-radical scavenging melanin on the palms and soles in persons of color.[3] None of these explanations appears satisfactory, however, and the pathogenetic sequence of acral melanoma should be considered unknown.

Subungual Melanoma

Like acral melanoma, subungual melanoma exhibits a preponderance in dark-skinned individuals. Subungual melanoma represents 15–20% of melanoma in African-Americans,[46,47] 10–31% in Asians,[46,48–51] and 33% in Native Americans.[52] The peak incidence in subungual melanoma occurs in the fifth to seventh decades.[53] By contrast, results from the Sydney Melanoma Unit database (1950–1994) suggest that subungual melanoma accounts for 0.31% of melanoma in predominantly Caucasian populations (38 per 11,500 melanoma cases; all cases occurred in whites).[54]

CLINICAL FEATURES AND DIAGNOSIS

Acral Melanoma

Acral melanoma in ethnic populations presents commonly as an asymmetric, enlarging, dark brown or black macule/patch with irregular, notched borders, variegated colors, and a diameter greater than 6 mm[55] (Figure 41-1). Although this description echoes the experience in Caucasians, reports in Hispanics highlight the appearance of flecked gray-white areas in many tumors,[32] whereas those in blacks underscore the presence of papillomatous, verrucous, or hyperkeratotic plaques[12] (Figures 41-2 and 41-3). In case series reflecting the acral melanoma experience in Chinese,[33,35] Japanese,[26] Hispanic,[32] and American[12,20] and African blacks,[18,39] a significant proportion of tumors present with an unusually large surface area (generally > 3 cm in diameter) and with signs of advanced local disease, including pain, crusting, bleeding, and nonhealing ulceration.

In terms of site distribution, case series in ethnic populations report predominance of plantar over palmar melanoma (approximate ratio 17:1) and of palmoplantar lesions over subungual lesions (approximate ratio 4:1).[26,27,29,32,33,35,56] Among volar lesions, the most common sites on the sole appear to be the heel and the ball of the foot, whereas no site predilection is obvious on the palm.[18,26,32,39,56] Melanoma of mucocutaneous surfaces is also proportionally more common in pigmented rather than white populations (in which prevalence is less than 10%). In one series involving U.S. blacks ($n = 80$), 44% of female subjects developed mucosal melanoma—including lip, palate, nasal, ocular, vulvar, vaginal, cervical, and anorectal surfaces—compared with only 10% of male subjects.[25]

Oral, nasal, and ocular melanoma exhibited a favorable prognosis relative to cutaneous melanoma, whereas vulvovaginal and anorectal melanoma

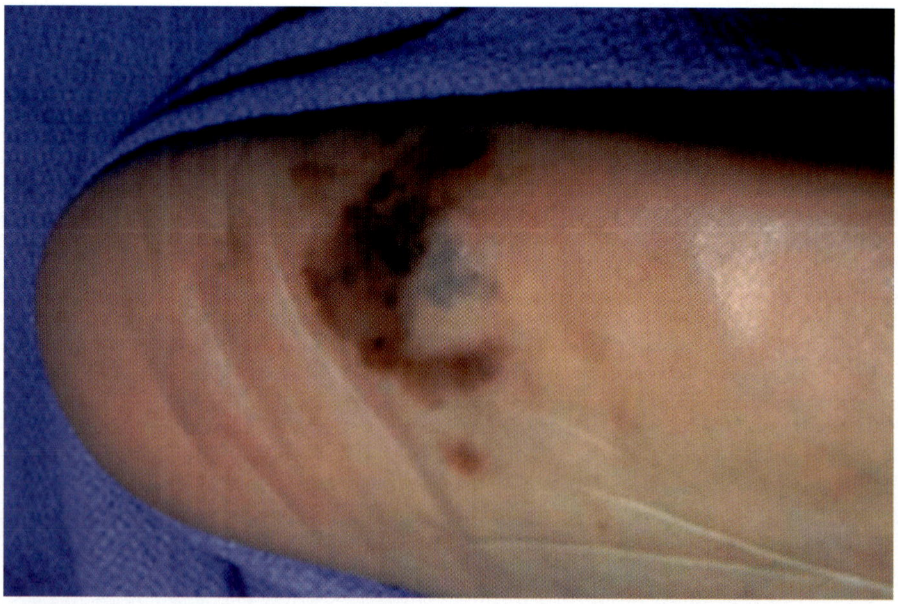

▲ **FIGURE 41-1** Acral melanoma. Ill-defined, asymmetric patch with irregular pigmentation on the heel of the foot.

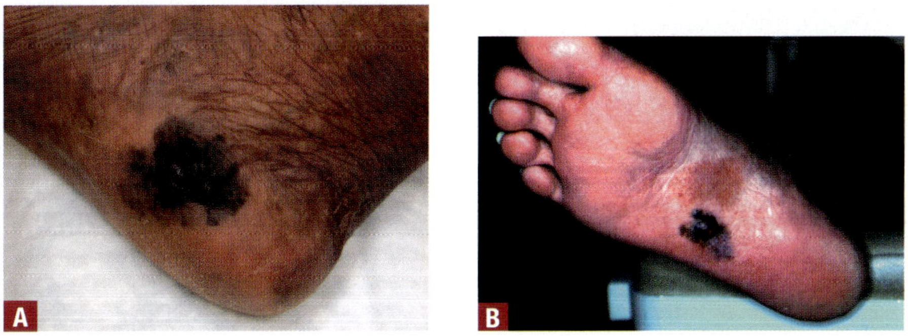

▲ **FIGURE 41-2** ***A.*** Advanced acral melanoma. Irregular patch with central verrucous nodule on the heel of a foot. ***B.*** Advanced acral melanoma. Long-standing patch with central nodule indicating vertical growth phase.

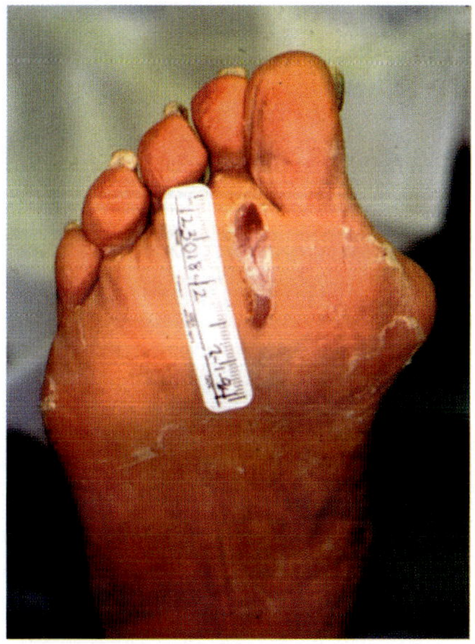

▲ **FIGURE 41-4** Acral lentiginous melanoma presenting as a callous. Note pigmentation of the skin along the lateral edge of the hyperkeratotic plaque.

showed the worst prognosis. In addition to acral melanoma, women of African, and perhaps of other non-European, ancestry may be at increased risk of developing mucosal melanoma.[25]

One challenge in the dermatology of skin of color is the differentiation between benign pigmentation or melanocytic neoplasms and their malignant counterparts. Hyperpigmented macules of the palmoplantar creases, for example, occur in 60% of African-American adults and may measure from 2 mm to several centimeters in diameter.[55] Acral nevi are also more common in darker-pigmented races. One series (n = 251) examining African-Americans reported an average of eight nevi per patient, with only 2% of their population showing no nevi whatsoever. In this series, darkly pigmented blacks possessed fewer nevi and exhibited clustering of their nevi and increased mottled pigmentation on the palmoplantar surface.[56]

By contrast, lightly pigmented blacks possessed more numerous nevi with a greater proportion scattered over the body and relatively fewer on the palms and soles.[57] A Japanese series (n = 23,165) reported a 3% prevalence of plantar nevi with a scattered distribution on the sole.[19]

Hyperpigmented macules of the palmoplantar creases, nevi, and mottled hyperpigmentation should not exhibit the classic morphologic features of acral melanoma. A diameter of 7 mm or more has been proposed as a screening threshold for plantar melanoma in Asians, although smaller, biopsy-proven acral melanomas have been reported.[22,58] Additional considerations in the differential diagnosis of acral melanoma include angioma, hematoma, pyogenic granuloma, ulcer, and digital ischemia.

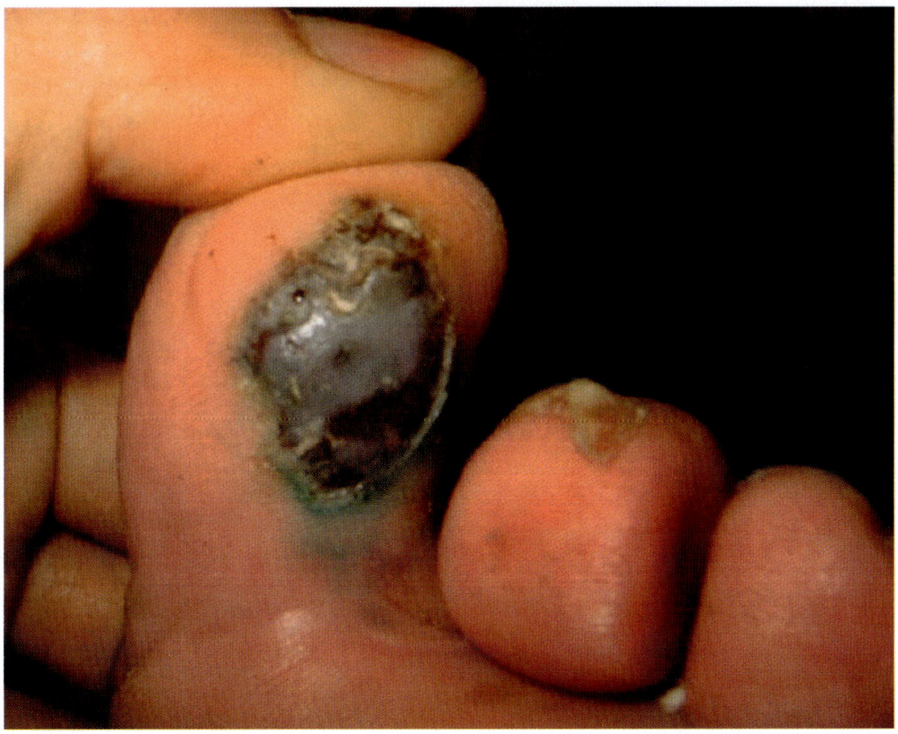

▲ **FIGURE 41-3** Advanced acral melanoma. Advanced tumor demonstrating ulceration, crusting, and bleeding

One series of acral melanoma (n = 18) reported that 39% assumed the morphology of benign hyperkeratotic dermatoses, including large verruca, calluses, and dermatophyte infections[59] (Figure 41-4). This hyperkeratotic acral melanoma variant may be associated with diagnostic delay and significantly poorer prognosis.[13,59,60] Lesions suspicious for melanoma require excisional biopsy or carefully planned incisional biopsy. Shave biopsies should be avoided because the thick stratum corneum of the palms and soles may result in failure to sample deeper, diagnostic pathology.

Subungual Melanoma

Subungual melanoma refers to melanoma of the nail bed and nail matrix. It presents clinically as a solitary brown or black longitudinal pigmented band of the nail (melanonychia striata) with irregular borders and variegated colors that increases in width to eventually involve the entirety of the nail bed[55] (Figure 41-5). *Hutchinson's sign* refers to pigment extension to the periungual skin and, when present, may increase the index of

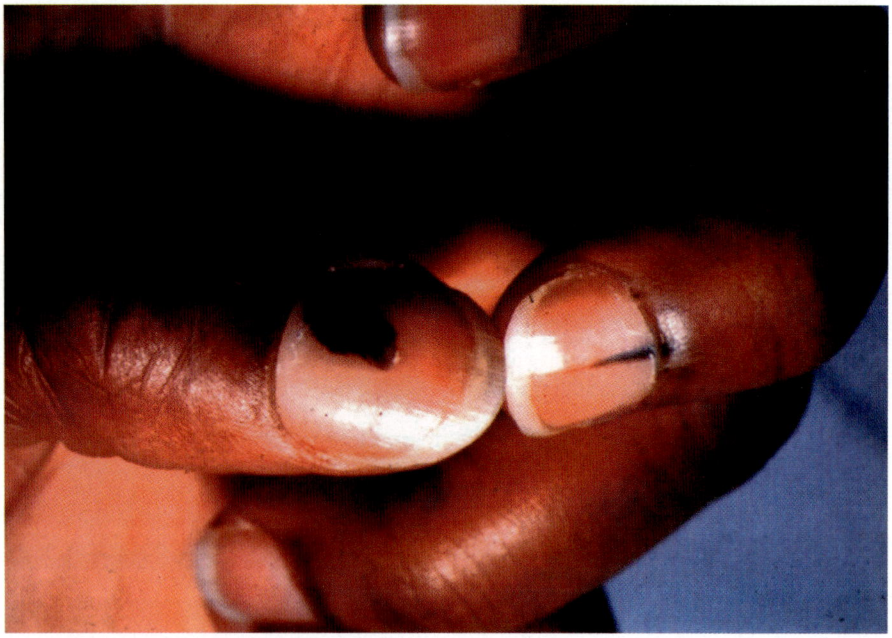

▲ **FIGURE 41-5** Early subungual melanoma. Early melanonychia striata of the third digit. Note coincidental subungual hematoma of the thumb.

suspicion for melanoma (Figure 41-6). Tumor progression to the vertical growth phase results in dystrophy, elevation, and eventually fracture of the nail plate, revealing a friable, ulcerated, and bleeding mass.[26,33,35,47,54] Among both white and ethnic populations, several studies indicate the predominance of hand over foot lesions and of the thumbnail and great toenail over the nails of other digits.[26,27,33,50,54] As in acral melanoma, the most common histologic pattern is acral lentiginous melanoma.[47,50,54,61]

Since misdiagnosis of early subungual melanoma is common, a Japanese study investigated the clinical features of early subungual melanoma (Clark's level I and early Clark's level II) to aid in early detection.[50] Melanonychia striata was the first sign of disease in all patients. Longitudinal pigment streaks, however, are present in approximately 11% of the general population in Japan[62] and in up to 100% of African-Americans aged over 50 years.[53] The following traits may help to differentiate benign pigmented bands from those suspicious for subungual melanoma in ethnic populations: (1) onset after midadulthood, (2) diameter greater than 6 mm, (3) variegated brown or homogeneously black coloration, and (4) Hutchinson's sign.[50] Rapid change also may be added to this list. It is of interest that although Hutchinson's sign is traditionally considered a marker of late disease, it was present in all five patients with *in situ* subungual melanoma in this series.[50]

Considerations in the differential diagnosis of melanonychia striata include lentigo and melanocytic nevus of the nail matrix or nail bed. Pigment bands of this origin, however, are rarely more than 4 mm in diameter (dysplastic or congenital nevi may attain or exceed this size). Systemic causes of nail pigmentation include Addison disease, Peutz-Jeghers syndrome, and ingestion of 5-fluorouracil, phenothiazines, silver, or arsenic.[50] Additional considerations include pyogenic granuloma, radiodermatitis, onychotillomania, squamous cell carcinoma, epithelioma cuniculatum, porocarcinoma, metastatic bronchogenic carcinoma, traumatic hematoma, and onychomycosis.[53] The most common misdiagnoses for subungual melanoma are hematoma and onychomycosis. Fortunately, a hematoma will migrate away from the proximal nail fold over a 4-week observation period, and in the case that this movement does not occur, a biopsy may be warranted.[63] In the same way, a 3- to 4-month course of antifungal therapy should yield a reassuring clear plane of nail at the proximal nail fold, and failure to respond to adequate antifungal treatment may warrant reconsideration of the diagnosis.[13]

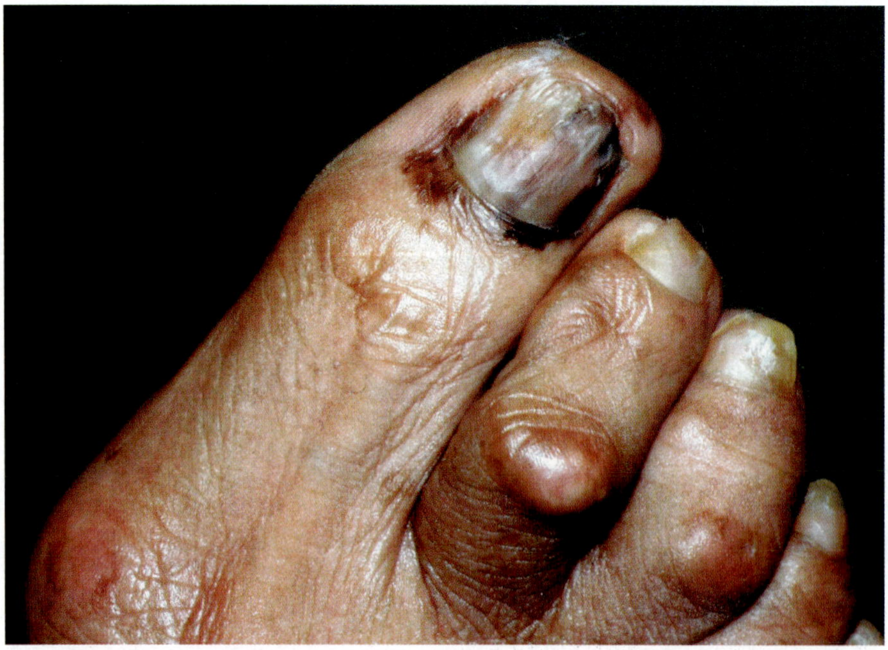

▲ **FIGURE 41-6** Subungual melanoma with Hutchinson's sign. Subungual melanoma demonstrating pigment extension onto proximal and lateral nail folds, as well as the hyponychium.

TREATMENT

Acral and Subungual Melanoma

No randomized studies examining the outcome of acral melanoma in ethnic populations exist. Reported standard treatment for acral melanoma includes wide excision, with or without sentinel lymph node dissection (SLND) and adjuvant therapy. Excision on the plantar surface requires the construction of a durable and functional weight-bearing surface that simulates the normal anatomic structures that withstand pressure and shearing forces while simultaneously allowing for satisfactory local disease control.[18] Where possible, preservation of a portion of the heel or ball of the foot to bear pressure while walking and the fascia of the deep tendons as a base for skin grafting is recommended.[64]

Most studies report excision with 3-cm margins down to the heel fat pad, small muscles, or plantar fascia of the sole, followed by defect closure using split-thickness skin graft.[17,39,63,65] Orthotic footwear should be recommended routinely to decrease sheer force and pressure on the graft site. Hyperkeratoses may develop at the interface between graft and normal skin but respond well to mechanical debridement.[17]

In broad tumors, a 2-cm margin may be used to preserve a functional plantar weight-bearing surface, whereas primary amputation may be indicated in locally advanced disease with bony infiltration.[17] Sentinel lymph node biopsy may be offered to patients with tumor thicknesses greater than 1 mm for staging purposes and to inform the decision to embark on adjuvant therapy.

Reported adjuvant treatments in U.S. blacks with acral melanoma include isolated limb perfusion with melphalan chemotherapy[66] and melanoma immunotherapy. Reported indications for regional limb perfusion include thicker primary acral melanoma (Breslow thickness > 2 mm) and recurrent melanoma without visceral mestastases.[12,17,39]

One series involving black patients with stage I acral melanoma ($n = 15$) reported a survival benefit of excision and regional limb perfusion over excision alone (5-year survival: combined therapy 72% versus excision 23%; $p < 0.05$); notably, the results of this approach in blacks compared favorably with the 5-year survival in Caucasians treated with the same regimen.[12] Another study ($n = 185$) in U.S. blacks and whites reported a 5-year survival rate of 61% using adjuvant immunotherapy with irradiated melanoma cells, suggesting comparable efficacy with isolated limb perfusion.[27] The potential benefit of adjuvant interferon-α in metastatic melanoma is promising, but conflicting results in randomized studies suggest that its exact role remains to be elucidated.[67,68]

Similar to acral melanoma, treatment recommendations for subungual melanoma rely on the experience of large referral centers. Most of these studies have been conducted in white populations, however, which raises the issue of whether they may be generalizeable to persons of color. In the case of subungual melanoma, wide local excision is best achieved by amputation, with or without SLND and adjuvant therapy. For melanoma in situ, resection with 0.5- to 1.0-cm margins including the nail matrix and nailbed may be adequate; this approach may allow salvage of the digit.[50]

The precise level of amputation in subungual melanoma remains an area of contention because it highlights the tradeoff between preserving hand and foot function and ensuring local disease control. One retrospective study ($n = 38$) compared "functional" versus "ablative" amputation for subungual melanoma in a white population.[54] This study defined *functional amputation* as one that retained finger contribution to hand function [e.g., amputation distal to the neck of the proximal phalanx of the thumb or to the proximal interphalangeal (PIP) joint of the finger], whereas *ablative amputation* was defined as amputation proximal to these points and resulted in a digit unable to contribute to hand function. Recurrence analysis showed no difference between these options; therefore, these authors recommend amputation at the neck of the proximal phalanx of the thumb and at the level of the PIP joint of the finger to maximize hand function.[54] In advanced lesions extending to the proximal phalynx of the fingers or toes, ray amputation may be necessary.[39]

Whether choice of amputation level ultimately influences patient outcome, however, is unclear. In fact, one series ($n = 53$) reported no difference in overall survival between subungual melanoma treated with or without amputation given that a large number of subungual melanomas present with metastatic disease.[27] It is reasonable to assume that the outcomes of adjuvant therapies, including isolated limb perfusion, immunotherapy, interferon-α, and node dissection, should be comparable with those observed with acral melanoma; however, a precise estimate of outcome is unclear because most studies did not consider subungual melanoma in a subgroup analysis.[12,17,27,39,67,68]

PROGNOSIS

When compared with nonacral lesions, acral melanomas are associated with higher overall mortality presumably because they occur in an area often overlooked by patients and physicians, leading to diagnostic delay and advanced stage at presentation.[13,27] Histologic subtype has no bearing on survival.[14] Acral melanoma in minority populations, however, carries an even graver prognosis when compared with white populations.

Analysis of the California Cancer Registry noted that blacks, Asians, and Hispanics were significantly more likely to be diagnosed with metastatic disease at presentation compared to whites. Among men, 15% of Hispanics, 13% of Asians, and 12% of blacks had metastatic disease at diagnosis compared with only 6% of whites. Among women, 7% of Hispanics, 21% of Asians, and 19% of blacks had metastatic disease at diagnosis compared with only 4% of whites. These differences are statistically and clinically signficant.[7] Among U.S. blacks, SEER data (1986–1991) similarly report a threefold increase in the proportion of blacks diagnosed with distant disease compared with whites (12% of blacks versus 4% of whites).[1]

Results of large case series involving acral melanoma speak to an analogous experience among blacks, Hispanics, and Asians internationally, characterized by advanced stage at presentation and poor overall survival. The aggregate experience among U.S. and African blacks is that acral melanoma typically presents as a thick lesion (mean Breslow thickness range 2.75–7.10 mm) with a high proportion of histologic ulceration and regional and distant metastases and a dismal 20–30% 5-year survival.[12,17,18,20,30,39,40] By contrast, 5-year survival among contemporaneous whites ranges from 60–85%, a distinction that attained statistical significance in numerous studies.[20,24,27,30,40]

Among U.S. and South American Hispanics, acral melanoma similarly presents as a thick tumor (mean Breslow thickness 5.5 mm)[32] with a high proportion of regional and distant metastases (approximate range 20–40%) and a 23–66% 3-year survival rate.[29,32,56] It is of interest that one series in the southeast United States ($n = 54$) reported a survival advantage of Hispanics over non-Hispanic whites for both local and regional/distant metastatic disease; these authors suggested that the overall younger age of Hispanic patients may explain this finding.[31] The 5-year survival in acral melanoma among eastern Chinese, Japanese, and Indians is similar to that of blacks, ranging from 25–35%.[26,33–35,38,69] One Japanese study ($n = 20$), however, reported a 70% 5-year survival rate for acral melanoma.[36]

There is a paucity of data on the comparative survival of ethnic compared with white populations with subungual melanoma, and most studies considering prognosis in darker-pigmented races consider that of subungual and acral melanoma in aggregate. Owing largely to diagnostic delay, subungual melanoma in whites is associated with a poor prognosis. Mean delay ranges from 9–23 months in approximately 50% in reported series[53] and is complicated by the high proportion of amelanotic lesions (40% in the Sydney Melanoma Unit database).[54] In white populations, subungual melanoma is associated with a 55% overall 5-year survival rate (reported range 16–76%).[54] Lesions present at an advanced stage (median thickness 3.05 mm), with only 20% of subungual tumors presenting at stage I.[54] Nonetheless, one study (n = 3) in native Puerto Ricans reported a median Breslow thickness of 8.0 mm with a mortality rate of 66% at 2 years.[32] All lesions in a Taiwanese study (n = 2) presented at Clark level III–IV and exhibited 100% mortality at 6 years.[35] A U.S. comparative study (n = 11) reported that U.S. blacks with subungual melanoma have a 3.5 times higher mortality rate than Caucasians, which remained significant even after controlling for stage and Clark's level (suggesting that race may be an independent prognostic factor).[47]

The question of whether melanoma is a biologically more aggressive tumor in ethnic populations or whether ethnicity in fact serves as a proxy for social, cultural, and economic factors culminating in diagnostic delay and advanced tumor stage is unclear. Conflicting results arise within the U.S. black experience, with some studies suggesting that race influences prognosis independent of tumor thickness and stage[24,27] and others reporting that the prognostic importance of race becomes immaterial in the face of regression analyses considering established prognostic indicators, such as Breslow thickness, ulceration, and stage.[20,30]

One retrospective study in U.S. blacks (n = 79) examined melanoma outcome over three decades and reported a 35% 5-year survival rate in cohorts diagnosed before 1980 compared with a 49% 5-year survival rate in cohorts diagnosed between 1980 and 1989, reflecting increasing early patient presentation.[30] Earlier melanoma diagnosis and improved survival in more recent decades (1980s and 1990s) similarly was observed in population-based Japanese and Hispanic studies.[29,36] Another study involving 96 U.S. blacks reported that aggressive surgical and adjuvant therapy in stage I black patients amounted to a 78% 5-year survival, which is comparable with the outcome in white patients.[12] These studies provide encouraging evidence that the poor prognosis historically observed in persons of color may be a greater reflection of diagnostic delay and undertreatment rather than intrinsic tumor aggression and suggest that increased public and clinical awareness of melanoma in ethnic skin may continue this trend of improved prognosis.

CONCLUSION

As outlined herein, the melanoma experience in persons of color is distinct from that in Caucasians and is characterized by decreased incidence, a characteristic anatomic distribution on the acral extremities, advanced stage at presentation, and overall poorer prognosis. Perhaps the most concerning of these features are the advanced presentation and poor survival in these populations from a tumor that is plainly visible and eminently curable in its early stages.

Questioning why this occurs is fundamental to any effort to understand and dismantle racial disparities in health care. In relation to dermatology, the concept of "ethnicity" encompasses both skin type and sociocultural beliefs and practices. Although evidence that race may be an independent prognosticator in acral and subungual melanoma exists,[24,27,47] other studies,[20,30] as well as improving survival rates reported in more recent cohorts,[29,36] suggest that the poor prognosis historically observed in persons of color may be a greater reflection of diagnostic delay than intrinsic tumor aggression.

In fact, the American Anthropological Association argues in its "Statement on Race" that modern humans are a relatively homogeneous species and that genetic data suggest as much variability between two people of the same "racial" group as between two people from any two different "racial" groups.[70] Thus few biologic differences should exist between large populations that are of explanatory relevance.[71,72]

Understanding race as a purely biologic variable, divorced from its social and historical context, may oversimplify a public health issue that requires a broad perspective. Access to health care is one consideration in a society where the poor are often persons of color.

One study (n = 28,237) examining the effects of health insurance on early cancer detection reported a significant positive association between lack of health insurance and Medicaid insurance with late-stage melanoma diagnosis.[73] Socioeconomic variables alone, however, do not account for all racial health disparities; indeed, health inequalities exist even when universal access to health care is ensured.[72]

Public awareness campaigns that convey the unique features of melanoma in ethnic populations are necessary. Recent studies suggest a deficiency in the knowledge of U.S. blacks and Hispanics regarding melanoma. According to a nationwide survey conducted by the American Academy of Dermatology, 75% of blacks did not know the meaning of the word *melanoma* compared with only 35% of whites ($p < 0.05$).[74]

A recent study in U.S. Hispanics further demonstrated less awareness of melanoma and skin cancer risk factors and a decreased risk perception relative to non-Hispanic whites.[75] Shared beliefs, attitudes, and behaviors may manifest in particular health practices and illness profiles characteristic of a racial or cultural group. One study noted that cultural in addition to socioeconomic factors were able to account for the discrepancy in breast cancer mortality between U.S. black and white women, where neither was sufficient alone.[72] Perspective on such broad determinants of melanoma outcome in persons of color, alongside attention to their unique clinical expression, is necessary to improve the prognosis for these patients.

REFERENCES

1. Ries L, Eisner M, Kosary C, et al. *SEER Cancer Statistics Review, 1975-2001.* Bethesda, MD, National Cancer Institute, 2004.
2. Anonymous. *US Interim Projections by Age, Sex, Race, and Hispanic Origin.* Washington, US Census Bureau, 2004.
3. Armstrong B, Kricker A. How much melanoma is caused by sun exposure. *Melanoma Res* 1993;3:395-401.
4. Crombie I. Racial differences in melanoma incidence. *Br J Cancer* 1979; 40: 185-193.
5. Elder D. Melanoma and other specific nonmelanoma skin cancers. *Cancer* 1995;75:245-256.
6. Hu S, Ma F, Collado-Mesa F, Kirsner R. UV radiation, latitude, and melanoma in Hispanics and blacks. *Arch Dermatol* 2004;140:819-824.
7. Cress R, Holly E. Incidence of cutaneous melanoma among non-Hispanic whites, Hispanics, Asians and blacks: An analysis of the California Cancer Registry data, 1988-1993. *Cancer Causes Control* 1997;8:246-252.
8. Bergfelt L, Newell G, Sider J. Incidence and anatomic distribution of cutaneous melanoma among United States Hispanics. *J Surg Oncol* 1989;40:222-226.
9. Saxe N, Hoffman M, Krige J, et al. Malignant melanoma in Cape Town, South Africa. *Br J Dermatol* 1998; 138: 998-1002.

10. Weinstock M. Death from skin cancer among the elderly. *Arch Dermatol* 1997; 133:1207-1209.
11. Pennelo G, Devesa S, Gail M. Association of surface ultraviolet B radiation levels with melanoma and nonmelanoma skin cancer in United States Blacks. *Cancer Epidemiol Biomarkers Prev* 2000;9:291-297.
12. Krementz E, Sutherland C, Carter R, Ryan R. Malignant melanoma in the American Black. *Ann Surg* 1976;1976: 533-542.
13. Bennett D, Wasson D, MacArthur J, McMillen M. The effect of misdiagnosis and delay in diagnosis on clinical outcome in melanoma of the foot. *J Am Coll Surg* 1994;179:279-284.
14. Ridgeway C, Hieken T, Ronan S, et al. Acral lentiginous melanoma. *Arch Surg* 1995;130.88-92.
15. Metzger S, Ellwanger U, Stroebel W, et al. Extent and consequences of physician delay in the diagnosis of acral melanoma. *Melanoma Res* 1998;8:181-186.
16. Kuchelmeister C, Schaumburg-Lever G, Garbe C. Acral cutaneous melanoma in caucasians: Clinical features, histopathology and prognosis in 112 patients. *Br J Dermatol* 2000; 143:275-280.
17. Hudson D, Krige J, Subbings H. Plantar melanoma: Results of treatment in three populations. *Surgery* 1998;124: 877-882.
18. Hudson D, Krige J. Plantar melanoma in black South Africans. *Br J Surg* 1993; 80:992-994.
19. Kukita A, Ishihara K. Clinical features and distribution of malignant melanoma and pigmented nevi on the soles of the feet in Japan. *J Invest Dermatol* 1989;92: 210-213S.
20. Bellows C, Belafsky P, Fortgang I, Beech D. Melanoma in African-Americans: Trends in biological behavior and clinical characteristics over two decades. *J Surg Oncol* 2001;78:10-16.
21. Reed R. *Acral Lentiginous Melanoma*. New York, Wile, 1976.
22. Wong T, Ohara K, Kawashima M, et al. Acral lentiginous melanolma (including in situ melanoam) arising in association with naevocellular nevi. *Melanoma Res* 1996;6:241-246.
23. Dwyer P, Mackie R, Watt D, Aitchison T. Plantar malignant melanoma in a white Caucasian population. *Br J Dermatol* 1993; 128:115-120.
24. Reintgen D, McCarty K, Cox E, Seigler H. Malignant melanoma in black American and white American populations. *JAMA* 1982;248:1856-1859.
25. Muchmore J, Mizuguchi R, Lee C. Malignant melanoma in American black females: An unusual distribution of primary sites. *J Am Coll Surg* 1996;183: 457-465.
26. Seiji M, Takematsu H, Hosokawa M, et al. Acral melanoma in Japan. *J Invest Dermatol* 1983;80:56-60S.
27. Slingluff C, Vollmer R, Seigler H. Acral melanoma: A review of 185 patients with identification of prognostic variables. *J Surg Oncol* 1990;45:91-98.
28. Vayer A, Lefor A. Cutaneous melanoma in African-Americans. *South Med J* 1993; 86:181-182.
29. Black W, Goldhahn R, Wiggins C. Melanoma within a southwestern Hispanic population. *Arch Dermatol* 1987;123:1331-1334.
30. Crowley N, Dodge R, Vollmer R, Seigler H. Malignant melanoma in black Americans: A trend toward improved survival. *Arch Surg* 1991;126:1359-1365.
31. Feun L, Raub W, Duncan R, et al. Melanoma in a southeastern hispanic population. *Cancer Detect Prev* 1994; 18:145-152.
32. Vaszqez M, Ramos F, Sanchez J. Melanomas of volar and subungual skin in Puerto Ricans. *J Am Acad Dermatol* 1984;10:39-45.
33. Collins R. Melanoma in the Chinese of Hong Kong: Emphasis on volar and subungual sites. *Cancer* 1984;54:1482-1488.
34. Chen Y-J, Wu C-Y, Chen J-T, et al. Clinicopathologic analysis of malignant melanoma in Taiwan. *J Am Acad Dermatol* 1999;41:945-949.
35. Lin C-S, Wang W-J, Wong C-K. Acral melanoma: A clinicopathologic study of 28 patients. *Int J Dermatol* 1990;29: 107-112.
36. Kuno Y, Ishihara K, Yamazaki N, Mukai K. Clinical and pathological features of cutaneous malignant melanoma: A retrospective analysis of 124 Japanese patients. *Jpn J Clin Oncol* 1996;26:144-151.
37. Swan M, Hudson D. Malignant melanoma in South Africans of mixed ancestry: A retrospective analysis. *Melanoma Res* 2003;13:415-419.
38. Nair M, Varghese C, Mahadevan S, et al. Cutaneous melanoma: Clinical epidemiology and survival. *J Indian Med Assoc* 1998;96:19-20, 28.
39. Krementz E, Reed R, Coleman W, et al. Acral lentiginous melanoma: A clinicopathologic entity. *Ann Surg* 1982; 195: 632-644.
40. Byrd K, Wilson D, Hoyler S, Peck G. Advanced presentation of melanoma in African-Americans. *J Am Acad Dermatol* 2004;50:21-24.
41. Garsaud P, Boisseau-Garsaud A, Ossondo M, et al. Epidemiology of cutaneous melanoma in French West Indies (Martinique). *Am J Epidemiol* 1998;247: 66-68.
42. Stevens N, Liff J, Weiss N. Plantar melanoma: Is the incidence of melanoma of the sole of the foot really higher in blacks than whites? *Int J Cancer* 1990; 45:691-693.
43. Koh D, Wang H, Lee J, et al. Basal cell carcinoma, squamous cell carcinoma and melanoma of the skin: Analysis of the Singapore Cancer Registry data 1968-1997. *Br J Dermatol* 2003;148:1161-1166.
44. Lewis M. Malignant melanoma in Uganda. *Br J Cancer* 1967;21:483.
45. Lewis M, Johnson K. The incidence and distribution of pigmented naevi in Ugandan Africans. *Br J Dermatol* 1968; 80:362-366.
46. Baran R, Kechijian P. Longitudinal melanonychia (melanonychia striata): Diagnosis and management. *J Am Acad Dermatol* 1989;21:1165-1175.
47. O'Leary J, Berend K, Johnson J, et al. Subungual melanoma: A review of 93 cases with identification of prognostic variables. *Clin Orthop* 2000;378:206-212.
48. Finley R, Driscoll D, Blumenson L, Karakousis C. Subungual melanoma: An eighteen year review. *Surgery* 1994; 116:96-100.
49. Kato T, Suetake T, Tabata N, Tagami H. Epidemiology and prognosis of subungual melanoma in 34 Japanese patients. *Br J Dermatol* 1996;134:383-387.
50. Saida T, Oshima Y. Clinical and histopathological characteristics of the early lesions of subungual melanoma. *Cancer* 1989;63:556-560.
51. Takematsu H, Obata M, Tomita Y, et al. Subungual melanoma. *Cancer* 1985; 55:2725-2731.
52. Black W, Wiggins C. Melanoma among southwestern Indians. *Cancer* 1985; 55:2899-2902.
53. Levit E, Kagen M, Scher R, et al. The ABC rule for clinical detection of subungual melanoma. *J Am Acad Dermatol* 2000;42:269-274.
54. Quinn M, Thompson J, Crotty K, et al. Subungual melanoma of the hand. *J Hand Surg* 1996;1996:506-511.
55. Rahman Z, Taylor S. Malignant melanoma in African-Americans. *Cutis* 2001;67:403-404.
56. Panjota E, Llobet R, Roswit B. Melanoms of the lower extremity among native Puerto Ricans. *Cancer* 1976;38:1420-1423.
57. Coleman W, Gately L, Krementz A, et al. Nevi, lentigines, melanomas in blacks. *Arch Dermatol* 1980;116: 548-551.
58. Saida T, Ishihara K, Tokuda Y. Effective detection of plantar malignant melanoma. *Int J Dermatol* 1993;32:722-725.
59. Soon S, Solomon A, McAlpine B, et al. Acral melanoma mimicking benign disease: The Emory experience. *J Am Acad Dermatol* 2003;48:183-188.
60. Fortin P, Freiberg A, Rees R, et al. Malignant melanoma of the foot and ankle. *J Bone Joint Surg* 1995;77A:1396-1403.
61. Blessing K, Kernohan N, Park K. Subungual malignant melanoma: Clinicopathological features of 100 cases. *Histopathology* 1991;19:425-429.
62. Kawamura T, Nishihara K, Kawasakiya S, et al. Pigmentatio longitudinalis striata unguium and the pigmentation of the nail in Addison's disease (abstract). *Jpn J Dermatol* 1958;68:10.
63. Hughes L, Horgan K, Taylor B, Laidler P. Malignant melanoma of the hand and foot: Diagnosis and management. *Br J Surg* 1985;72:811-815.
64. Balch C. Excising melanoma: How wide is enough? and how to reconstruct. *J Surg Oncol* 1990;44:135-136.
65. Shaw J, Koea J. Acral (volar-subungual) melanoma in Auckland, New Zealand. *Br J Surg* 1988;75:69-72.
66. Krige J, King H, Strover R. Prophylactic hyperthermic limb perfusion in stage I melanoma. *Eur J Surg Oncol* 1988; 14: 321-326.
67. Kirkwood J, Strawderman M, Ernstoff M, et al. Interferon alfa-2b adjuvant therapy of high-risk resected cutaneous melanoma: The Eastern Cooperative Oncology Group Trial EST 1684. *J Clin Oncol* 1996;14:1-3.
68. Kirkwood J, Ibrahim J, Sondak V, et al. High- and low-dose interferon alfa-2b in high-risk melanoma: First analysis of intergroup trial E1690/S9111/C9190. *J Clin Oncol* 2000;18:2444-2458.

69. Seiji M, Takahashi M. Acral melanoma in Japan. *Hum Pathol* 1982;13:607-609.
70. Overbey M. AAA tells feds to eliminate "race." *Anthropol Newslett* 1997; 38:1-5.
71. Dressler W. Health in the African-American community: Accounting for health inequalities. *Med Anthropol Q* 1993;7:325-345.
72. Lannin D, Mathews H, Mitchell J, et al. Influence of socioeconomic and cultural factors on racial differences in late-stage presentation of breast cancer. *JAMA* 1998;279:1801-1807.
73. Roetzheim R, Pal N, Tennant C, et al. Effects of health insurance and race on early detection of cancer. *J Natl Cancer Inst* 1999;91:1409-1415.
74. Anonymous. Survey of knowledge of and awareness about melanoma—United States, 1995. *MMWR* 1996; 45: 346-349.
75. Pipitone M, Robinson J, Camara C, et al. Skin cancer awareness in suburban employees: A Hispanic perspective. *J Am Acad Dermatol* 2002;47:118-123.

CHAPTER 42

Squamous Cell Carcinoma

Algin B. Garrett

Key Points

- Primary carcinoma of the skin is the most common form of cancer diagnosed in the United States, but the incidence in people of color is reported as rare.
- Most squamous cell carcinomas (SCCs) in people of color occur in non-sun-exposed areas; however, when SCC does occur in a sun-exposed area, the anatomic distribution is similar to that in Caucasians.
- SCC that occurs in sun-exposed skin has its origin in loss of the organized control of epidermal keratinocyte differentiation secondary to DNA damage as a direct result of ultraviolet light.
- The factors that are responsible for developing skin cancers in non-sun-exposed areas are unknown.
- Areas of chronic inflammation, chronic ulceration, and scarring are predisposed to the development of SCC.

Most of the information regarding nonmelanoma skin cancer reported in the U.S. literature about people of color focuses on disease incidence primarily in the African-American (AA) population. The information is reported in the context of case reports or incidence studies from small groups. Information regarding the incidence of nonmelanoma skin cancer in other ethnic groups, including Native Americans, Asians, and Hispanics, is sparse. The groups of people that constitute people of color have grown considerably. Considering the changing demographics of the United States, in order to keep meaningful and accurate data, prospective research should recognize the population changes that are occurring. Larger population studies should be performed involving people of color, which represents multiple ethnic and racial groups. U.S. Census information predicts that by the year 2050, the white population will be reduced to just over 50% of the total population. This figure will continue to decline during the ensuing decades of continued immigration and assimilation in the United States.

MELANIN AND PHOTOPROTECTION

The reduced incidence of skin cancer in people of color has been attributed to various factors. Montagna and Carlisle[1] have studied racial differences in melanin activity, fibroblast activity, and hair distribution on skin that may help to account for the reduced frequency of skin cancer in people of color. Melanin, which is synthesized in melanosomes, is a known photoprotector in both animals and humans. It essentially creates a shield from the sun by absorbing and deflecting ultraviolet light.[2] The basal cell layer melanocyte and its associated keratinocytes are responsible for the production of melanin. There is no racial difference in the number of melanocytes.[3] The number of melanocytes may vary from one individual to the other and in different anatomic regions.[4] The variations in color that can be seen in people of color are attributed to the size and aggregation of melanosomes in the melanocyte and keratinocyte. The increased number and dispersion of stage IV melanosomes provide a measure of photoprotection.[2] Both racial and ethnic differences, as well as sun exposure, can affect the melanosome grouping. In African-Americans with dark skin, melanosomes are large and nonaggregated, whereas in light-skinned African-Americans, melanosomes are both large and nonaggregated and smaller and aggregated. Sun exposure also has been shown to change the pattern of melanosome distribution in Asian and Caucasian skin.[4,5] In addition to the role of melanin in photoprotection, the compactness or density of the keratinocyte layers also provides a measure of photoprotection.[6] The African-American population is composed of a heterogeneous group with various shades of skin color; all the factors listed combine to provide an average sun protection factor of approximately 13.4.

The relative safety from some of the effects of the sun is demonstrated by the comparatively low incidence of skin cancer in African-Americans. However, there are changes that occur in melanin-laden skin that suggest that the skin in people of color is not immune to photodamage. Kotrajaras and Kligman[7] demonstrated epidermal atypia and atrophy and both dermal collagen and elastin damage. The presence of these changes, which may be consistent with either damage from long-wavelength ultraviolet light or infrared radiation, demonstrates that melanin may be an efficient filter for shorter-wavelength ultraviolet light.

SQUAMOUS CELL CARCINOMA

Incidence

Primary carcinoma of the skin is the most common form of cancer diagnosed in the United States. Even though skin cancer is considered the most common form of cancer, the incidence in people of color is reported as rare. McCalland Chen[8] reported a surprisingly high incidence of squamous cell carcinoma (SCC) in older African-American females and suggest that the incidence may be higher than previously reported. The incidence of SCC involving the skin in white patients has been reported to be approximately 100 per 100,000 in women and 150 per 100,000 in men.[9] The incidence in African-Americans is reported to be approximately 3.4 per 100,000.[10] There are very few incidence reports of skin cancer among other ethnic groups. Koh and colleagues[11] report on the trends and ethnic differences of skin cancers in Chinese, Malays, and Indians living in Singapore. The incidence rate for SCC was 3.2 per 100,000 in men and 1.8 per 100,000 in women. The incidence rate for basal cell carcinoma (BCC) was 6.4 per 100,000 in men and 5.8 per 100,000 in women. Ichihashi and colleagues[12] reported on age-adjusted incidence rates of BCC and solar keratosis in 4736 people in Kasai City. Two BCCs, 36 solar keratoses, and no SCCs were diagnosed in the group. It appears at least in the Asian population that BCCs are more common than SCCs.

BCC is the most commonly diagnosed skin cancer in the United States and is diagnosed most often in whites. BCCs account for approximately 75% of the nonmelanoma skin cancers diagnosed in the United States.[13] However, SCC is the most commonly diagnosed skin cancer in African-Americans.[14] Bang and colleagues[15] reported that 34.1% of 126 African-American patients were diagnosed with SCC, whereas 30.2% of the group was diagnosed with BCC. Fleming and colleagues[16] reported on a small series of 58 African-Americans with skin cancer. Thirty-eight cases of SCC and seven cases of BCC were diagnosed. Unlike BCCs, which occur commonly on sun-exposed skin, most SCCs in people of color develop in non-sun-exposed areas. In a series reported by Howard University in 1988, 65% of the patients diagnosed with SCC had leg involvement, and 15% were diagnosed with anal SCC.[14] SCC involvement of the penis and scrotum also has been reported to occur in African-Americans.[17–19]

Pathogenesis

The pathogenesis of SCC that occurs in sun-exposed skin has its origin in loss of the organized control of epidermal keratinocyte differentiation secondary to DNA damage as a direct result of ultraviolet (UV) light. The factors that are responsible for developing skin cancers in non-sun-exposed areas are unknown. Areas of chronic inflammation, chronic ulceration, and scarring are predisposed to the development of SCC. In these settings, normal cell differentiation and apoptosis of abnormal cells are altered, eventually producing the clonal expansion of a malignant cell line. The altered role of the *p53* gene in its response to cytotoxic stress may imperil the normal keratinocyte and predispose high-risk lesions to develop SCC.[20,21]

Risk Factors

The development of SCC has been linked to natural UV light exposure. UVB radiation is known to cause skin cancer. Phototherapy used to treat chronic skin diseases such as psoriasis has been shown to increase the risk of nonmelanoma skin cancer.[22] As mentioned previously, most SCCs in people of color occur in non-sun-exposed areas, however, when SCC does occur in a sun-exposed area, the anatomic distribution is similar to that in Caucasians (Figure 42-1). SCC develops in the following clinical settings in African-Americans: chronic inflammation or scarring, burns, chronic infections, leg ulcers, albinism (Figure 42-2), lesions of chronic discoid lupus erythematosus (Figure 42-3), chronic radiation exposure (Figure 42-4), and vitiligo[14,23] (Table 42-1). Other predisposing factors include cutaneous horns and scrotal ulcers. Chronic scars represent a significant risk for SCC and result in a higher rate of mortality.[24] Hubbell and colleagues[25] reported on 175 cases of SCC involving the penis in black patients. These authors reported a 15.4% overall mortality.

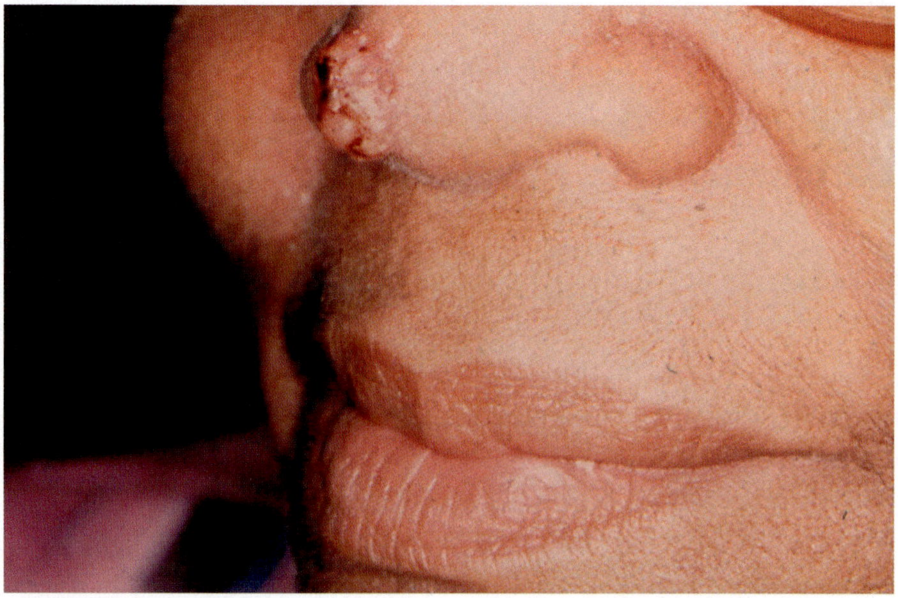

▲ **FIGURE 42-1** Squamous cell carcinoma of the nose in an African-American woman.

Actinic keratoses (AKs) are diagnosed more commonly in fair-skinned people and represent the most common precursor lesion for SCC on sun-exposed skin. AKs are rarely seen in African-Americans and are diagnosed not infrequently in fair-skinned Asians.[11] In individuals who develop AKs, there is up to a 10% risk of developing SCC.[20]

SCC in African-Americans is generally considered to be a more aggressive disease with a poorer prognosis. Mora and colleagues[24] reported an 18.4% mortality in 163 African-Americans diagnosed with SCC of the skin. In their series, the face and leg were the most common sites of involvement. Fleming reported a mortality rate of 29% in his series of African-Americans with SCC. Weintstock reported SCC as the skin cancer that is the major cause of death in African-Americans.[26] Not all reported series regarding SCC in AKs demonstrate comparatively decreased survival rates. Singh and colleagues[27] reported on a series of 215 patients in a case-control study in which the presentation, course, and outcome of head and neck skin cancer in African-Americans

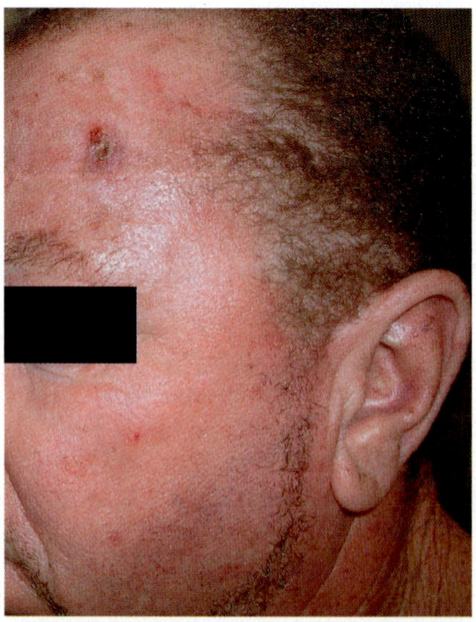

▲ **FIGURE 42-2** Squamous cell carcinoma of the forehead in an African-American albino.

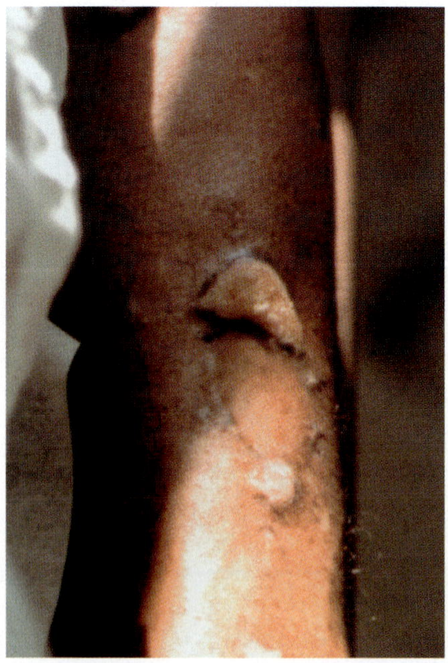

▲ **FIGURE 42-3** Squamous cell carcinoma developing in a chronic lupus erythematosus lesion.

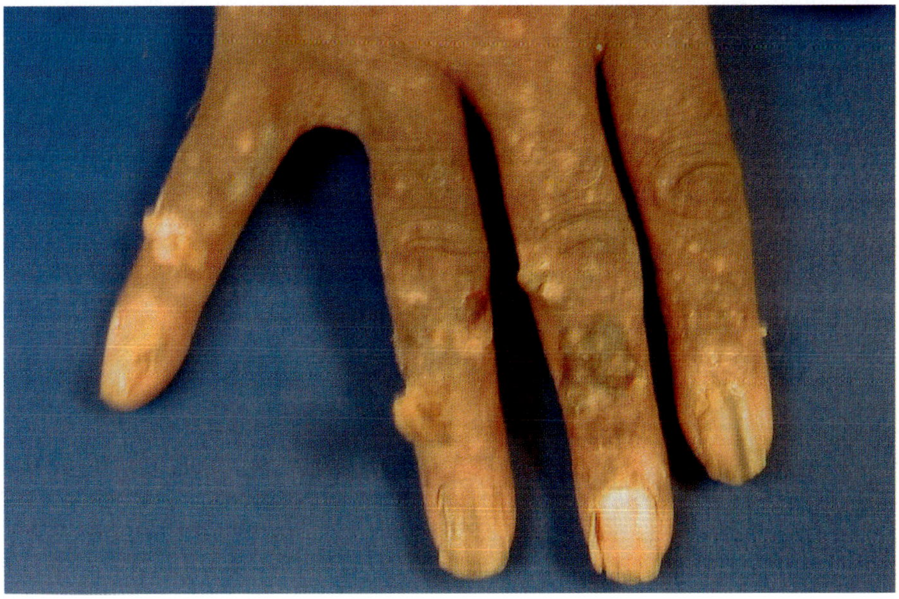

▲ **FIGURE 42-4** Squamous cell carcinoma secondary to chronic radiation exposure.

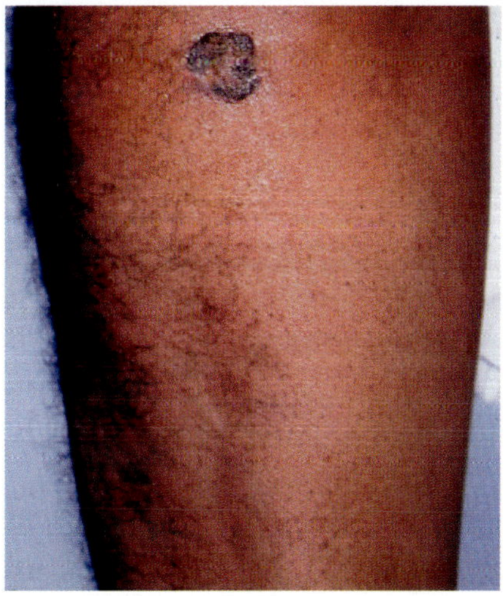

▲ **FIGURE 42-5** Bowen disease on the forearm of an African-American man.

were studied. They showed that head and neck skin cancer is similar with regard to presentation and distribution in white, Latin-American, and African-American patients. The study also showed that the cancers may be less aggressive in African-Americans with appropriate treatment.

Several factors may contribute to the overall poor mortality and morbidity related to SCC in people of color. The diagnosis is usually made at an advanced stage, possibly because of decreased accessibility to the health care system. In some instances, for unknown reasons, SCC has a more aggressive course in African-Americans than in white patients with comparable disease. Often when the diagnosis of SCC is made, other associated diseases coexist and may make management of the advanced skin cancer more difficult.

TABLE 42-1
Risks Factors for Developing Squamous Cell Carcinoma

- Chronic leg ulcers
- Chronic nonhealing wounds
- Discoid lupus erythematosus
- Lichen planus
- Ultraviolet light
- Vitiligo
- Ionizing radiation
- Oculocutaneous albinism
- Nevoid basal cell nevus syndrome
- Organ transplantation
- AIDS
- Scrotal ulcers

ACTINIC KERATOSIS

As stated previously, an AK is a precursor lesion for SCC. The lesion usually occurs in a sun-exposed area and is usually rough in texture. The color may range from pale pink to erythematous, and occasionally, AKs may be pigmented. AKs are not found often in people of color. They can be seen in Asians, Hispanics, and African-Americans who have fair skin and are exposed to risk factors. A similar lesion can be seen in lesions of vitiligo or albinism and areas of depigmentation from a preexisting dermatitis, such as mycosis fungoides and discoid lupus erythematosus.

KERATOACANTHOMA

Keratoacanthoma (KA) is indistinguishable histologically from SCC. Generally it represents an epithelial tumor that grows rapidly over a period of approximately 6 weeks. The lesion may last for several weeks and then involute spontaneously. It usually appears as a solitary lesion and generally presents as a nodule with a crater-like center with a keratin plug. The lesion is rarely reported in people of color.[28]

SQUAMOUS CELL CARCINOMA IN SITU (SCCIS)

SCCIS histologically represents involvement of the entire epidermal thickness with pleomorphic keratinocytes, which is seen in diseases such as Bowen disease and erythroplasia of Queyrat. Bowen disease is less commonly diagnosed in AA than in other cutaneous malignancies.[14] Bowen disease presents as an erythematous solitary patch or plaque that may resemble eczema or psoriasis[29] (Figures 42-5 and 42-6). Even though pigmented lesions are felt to be rare in white patients, the presence of pigment in lesions of Bowen disease in AA is common.

PROGNOSIS

Invasive SCC arising in areas of sun exposure has a better prognosis than SCC that arises in non-sun-exposed areas. Aggressive behavior and local metastases occur more frequently in SCC arising in non-sun-exposed areas.[16,18] SCC of the nail bed has developed in AA and may be more common in females (Figure 42-7). Bowen disease of the digits resembles verrucae or chronic paronychia and has been associated with human papillomavirus (HPV) types 16 and 18.[29,30] SCC involving the mucosal skin has a greater tendency to metastasize and recur. Perianal SCC can arise in preexisting lesions such as perianal warts (Figure 42-8). Anogenital lesions also can develop de novo (Figure 42-9).

SCC that presents in preexisting areas of disease such as a chronic leg ulcers or hidradenitis suppurativa or in areas of chronic scars may resemble the underlying disease. Such areas may appear not to respond to therapy or develop nonhealing ulcers or erosions. Invasive SCC can present as plaques, papules, and ulcers with induration. SCC should be excluded in the appropriate setting in which any of the preceding circumstances exist.

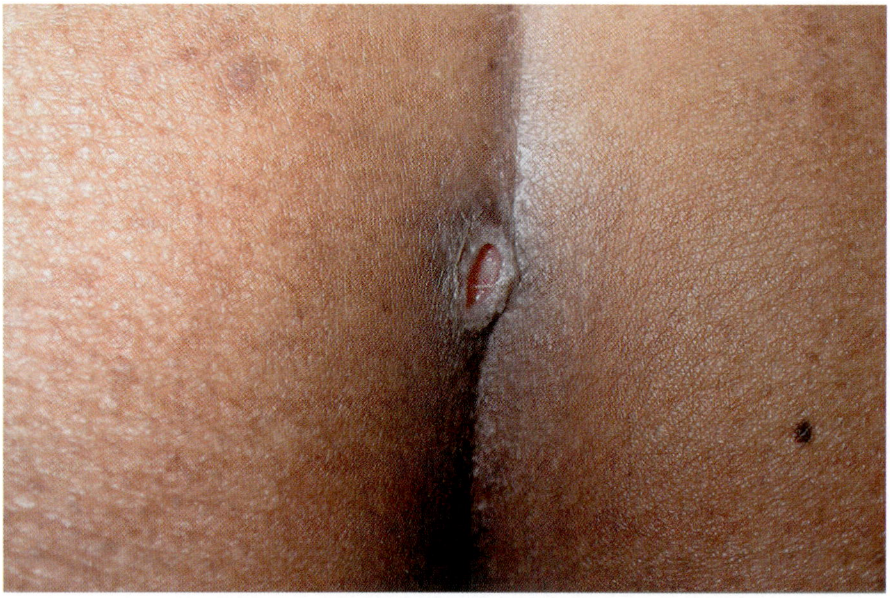

▲ **FIGURE 42-6** Bowen disease in an ulcerated plaque of the presacral area.

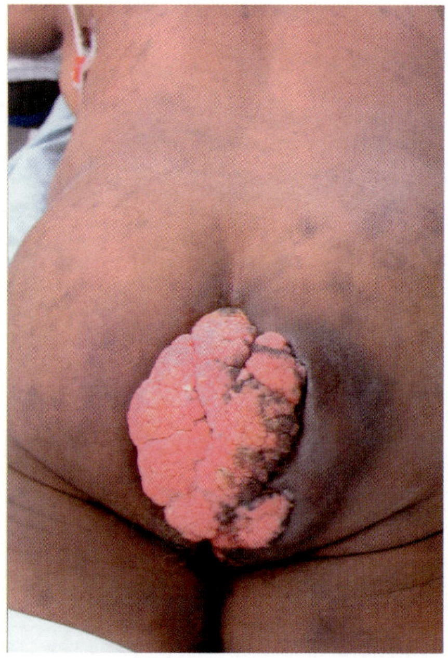

▲ **FIGURE 42-8** Squamous cell carcinoma developing in preexisting lesions such as perianal warts.

DIAGNOSIS AND THERAPY

SCC in an AA is potentially very aggressive and raises the possibility of an associated disease. Therefore, a detailed history and physical examination should be undertaken, and a biopsy of the suspicious lesion should be performed. The history should assess the duration of the lesion and history of prior treatment for preexisting skin cancer or preexisting skin disease. If indicated clinically, any evidence for immune deficiency should be evaluated. A physical examination should be performed for local evaluation of the tumor and to assess the patient for the presence of lymphadenopthy.

The type of biopsy performed should be determined by the characteristics of the lesion. A shave biopsy can be performed on a relatively thin or superficial lesion. Thicker, more indurated plaques or tumors require a deeper punch or excisional biopsy.

The type of therapeutic intervention is determined by the histologic type of SCC, size of the tumor, location of the tumor, and presence or absence of metastatic disease (Table 42-2). In thin lesions such as Bowen disease, a number of therapeutic options could be considered. The CO_2 laser has shown efficacy in the management of severe actinic cheilitis and in the treatment of superficial BCC, Bowen disease, and thin SCCs.[31,32] Both photodynamic therapy and topical 5-fluorouracil have proven to

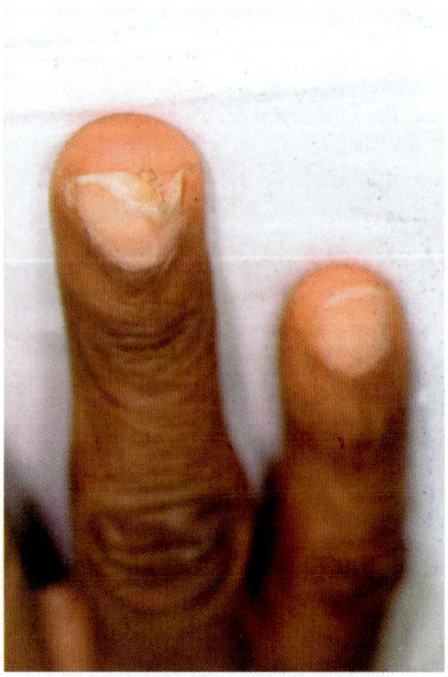

▲ **FIGURE 42-7** Squamous cell carcinoma of nail bed in an African-American man.

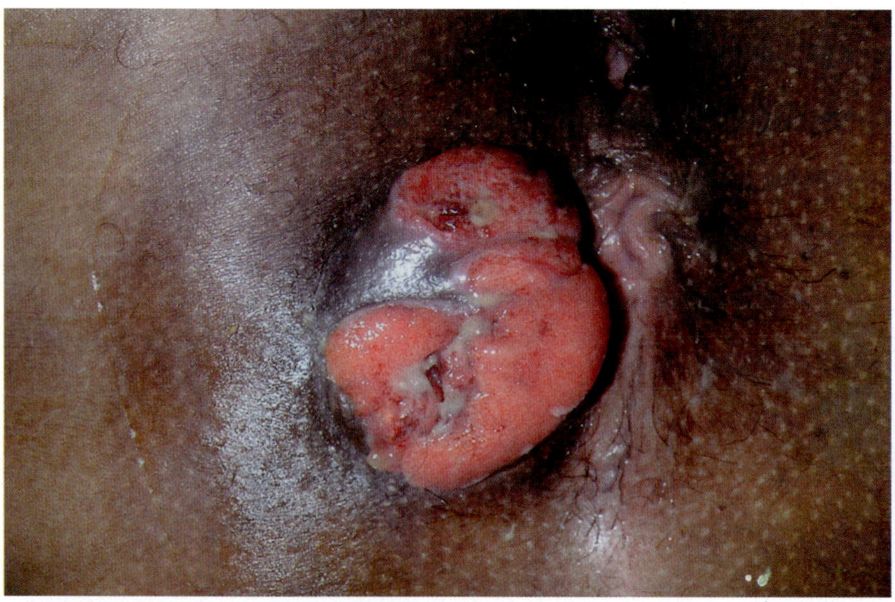

▲ **FIGURE 42-9** Anogenital squamous cell carcinoma also can develop de novo.

TABLE 42-2
Treatments Available for SCC

MEDICAL	SURGICAL
5-Fluorouracil	Cryosurgery
Photodynamic therapy	Electrodesiccation and curettage
Imiquimod	Carbon dioxide laser
Interferon	Excision
Radiation therapy	Mohs micrographic surgery

be efficacious in thin or superficial SCC.[33,34] Interferon-α and imiquimod both have been used in the management of SCCs. Intralesional interferon has been used to treat both SCC and BCC and has shown approximately an 80% cure rate in selected BCCs.[34] The use of imiquimod in the management of BCCs has been approved recently. Its use in the treatment of SCC is currently under study, and its appears in selected lesions to be as effective as it is in the treatment of BCC.[35]

For patients who have localized disease, excisional surgery and Mohs micrographic surgery are the primary forms of treatment. Aggressive management of the tumor is indicated because of the potential for SCC in people of color to be more aggressive and have a higher rate of recurrence. If excisional surgery is undertaken, the tumor should be removed with adequate margins. The margins of the excision should be examined completely for evidence of residual disease. For tumors that are in cosmetically sensitive areas and that are considered high risk, Mohs micrographic surgery may be indicated. Large tumors involving the perianal region or tumors in areas of scarring or chronic ulceration require a wide local excision, often with complex repair.

Radiation therapy is used both as a primary form of therapy and as adjuvant therapy in the management of SCC, particularly of the head and neck. As adjuvant therapy, it is used when lymph nodes are positive, if perineural disease is detected, and if residual disease is suspected after an excision or margin control is not possible.

REFERENCES

1. Montagna W, Carlisle K. The architecture of black and white facial skin. *J Am Acad Dermatol* 1991;24:929-937
2. Kaidbey KH, Agin PP, Sayre RM, et al. Photoprotection by melanin: A comparison of black and Caucasian skin. *J Am Acad Dermatol* 1979;249-260.
3. Starkco RS, Pinkush. Quantitative and qualitative data on the pigment cell of adult human epidermis. *J Invest Dermatol* 1957;28:33.
4. Toda K, Patnak MA, Parrrish A, et al. Alteration of racial differences in melanosome distribution in human epidermis after exposure to ultraviolet light. *Nat New Biol* 1972;236:143-144.
5. Olson RL, Gaylor J, Everett MA. Skin color, melanin, and erythema. *Arch Dermatol* 1973;108:541-144.
6. Freeman RG, Cockerell EG, Armstrong J. Sunlight as a factor influencing the thickness of epidermis. *J Invest Dermatol* 1962; 39:295-298.
7. Kotrajaras R, Kligman AM. The effect of topical tretinoin on photodamaged facial: The Thai experience. *Br J Dermatol* 1993; 129:302-309.
8. McCall CO, Chen SC. Squamous cell carcinoma of the legs in African-Americans. *J Am Acad Dermatol* 2002;47: 524-529.
9. Gray DT, Suman VJ, Su WPD, et al. Trends in the population-based incidence of squamous cell carcinoma of the skin first diagnosed between 1984 and 1992. *Arch Dermatol* 1997;133:735-740.
10. Scotto J, Fears TR, Fraumeni JF Jr. *Incidence of Nonmelanoma Skin Cancer in the United States.* NIH Report No. 83-243. Washington, US Government Printing Office, 1983.
11. Koh D, Wang H, Lee J, et al. Basal cell carcinoma, squamous cell carcinoma and melanoma of the skin: Analysis of Singapore Cancer Registry data 1968–1997. *Br J Dermatol* 2003;148: 1161-1166.
12. Ichihashi M, Naruse K, Harada S, et al. Trends in nonmelanoma skin cancer in Japan. *Recent Results Cancer Res* 1995;139: 126-173.
13. Roenigk RK, Ratz JL, Bailin PL, et al. Trends in the presentation and treatment of basal cell carcinoma. *J Dermatol Surg Oncol* 1986;12:860-865.
14. Halder RM, Bang KM. Skin cancer in African-Americans in the United States. *Dermatol Clin* 1988;6:397-407.
15. Bang KM, Halder RM White JE, et al. Skin cancer in black Americans: A review of 126 cases. *J Natl Med Assoc* 1987;79: 51-58.
16. Fleming ID, Barnawell JR, Burlison PE, et al. Skin cancer in black patients. *Cancer* 1975;33:600-605.
17. Rippentrop JM, Joslyn SA, Konety BR. Squamous cell carcinoma of the penis. *Cancer* 2004;101:1357.
18. Hubbell CR, Rabin VR, Mora RG. Cancer of the skin in blacks: V. A review of 175 black patients with squamous cell carcinoma of the penis. *J Am Acad Dermatol* 1988;18:292-298.
19. McDonald MW. Carcinoma of scrotum. *Urology* 1982;19:269-274.
20. Salasche SJ. Epidemiology of actinic keratoses and squamous cell carcinoma. *J Am Acad Dermatol* 2000;42:S4-7.
21. Glogau RG. The risk of progression to invasive disease. *J Am Acad Dermatol* 2000;42:S23-24.
22. Nijsten TEC, Stern RS. The increased risk of skin cancer is persistent after discontinuation of psoralen plus ultraviolet A: A cohort study. *J Invest Dermatol* 2003;121: 252-258.
23. Halder RM, Bridgeman-Shah S. Skin cancer in African-Americans. *Cancer* 1995; 75:667-673.
24. Mora RG, Perniciaro C, Lee B. Cancer of the skin in blacks: A review of 163 patients with cutaneous squamous cell carcinoma. *J Am Acad Dermatol* 1981;5: 535-543.
25. Hubbell CR, Rabin VR, Mora RG. Cancer of the skin in blacks: V. A review of 175 black patients with squamous cell carcinoma of the penis. *J Am Acad Dermatol* 1988;18:292-298.
26. Weinstock MA. Nonmelanoma skin cancer mortality in the United States, 1969 through 1988. *Arch Dermatol* 1993;129: 1286-1290.
27. Singh B, Bhaya M, Shaha A, et al. Presentation, course and outcome of head and neck skin cancer in African-Americans: A case-control study. *Laryngoscope* 1998;108:1159-1163.
28. Heyl T, Morrison JG. Keratoacanthoma in a Bantu. *Br J Dermatol* 1975;93:699-700.
29. Preston DS, Stern RS. Nonmelanoma cancers of the skin. *N Engl J Med* 1992; 327:1649-1662.
30. Alam M, Ratner D. Cutaneous squamous cell carcinoma. *N Engl J Med* 2001;344: 975-983.
31. Karrer S, Szeimies RM, Hohenleutner U, et al. Role of laser and photodynamic therapy in the treatment of cutaneous malignancy. *Am J Clin Dermatol* 2001;2: 220-237.
32. Tantikun N. Treatment of Bowen's disease of the digit with carbon dioxide laser. *J Am Acad Dermatol* 2000;43: 10801083.
33. Morton CA, Whitehurst C, McColl JH, et al. Photodynamic therapy for large or multiple patches of Bowen disease and basal cell carcinoma. *Arch Dermatol* 2001; 137:319-324.
34. Miller SJ, Maloney ME (eds). *Cutaneous Oncology: Pathophysiology, Diagnosis, and management.* Malden, MA, Blackwell Science, 1998, pp 578-580.
35. Mackenzie-Wood A, Kossard S, de Launey J, et al. Imiquimod 5% cream in the treatment of Bowen's disease. *J Am Acad Dermatol* 2001;44:462-470.

CHAPTER 43

Basal Cell Carcinoma

Seth B. Forman
Algin B. Garrett

Key Points

- Basal cell carcinomas (BCCs) may present with a rolled border, telangiectasia, and erosions, which may cause them to bleed. However, pigmented lesions are seen more often in skin of color.
- Since BCCs are often pigmented, they can be mistaken for seborrheic keratoses, nevocellular nevi, or malignant melanoma.
- BCCs commonly present on the head and neck, but they also can appear in very unusual locations. BCCs have been diagnosed in the groin, on the scrotum, in the perianal region, and on the feet.
- It is important to do a complete skin examination in people of color to ensure that a BCC is not overlooked.
- The approach to treating skin cancers in people of color should be no different from treating patients with light skin.

SYNONYMS

- Basal cell epithelioma
- Nevoid basal cell carcinoma syndrome

Basal cell carcinomas (BCCs) are uncommon but not rare in people of color. The medical literature implies that people of color are individuals of African-American descent. However, Taylor remarked that physicians must consider people of color as a heterogeneous group.[1] Patients of Hispanic, Native American, Asian, African-American, and mixed descent must be recognized. McDonald suggests that classification of patients by skin type may only be of epidemiologic value. He comments that one must use the same diagnostic and therapeutic techniques as one would use for people of lighter skin types.[2]

The incidence of the three most common skin cancers—BCCs, squamous cell carcinomas (SCCs) and malignant melanomas—is less in people of darker skin types. There is the suggestion from prior studies that the aforementioned skin cancers are influenced by ultraviolet (UV) light. All skin types have a similar number and anatomic distribution of melanocytes. Taylor remarks that darker skin has larger melanosomes, more melanosomes, and a different aggregation pattern of melanosomes.[1]

There is the suggestion that melanin protects the skin from UV light. Some support the notion that variation in skin color is an evolutionary advantage. Taylor further suggests that individuals near the equator, people of color, need the darker skin with increased melanin as protection from the harmful effects of UV light. And lighter-skinned people who are further from the equator require less melanin to better absorb vitamin D, which is less plentiful with increased distance from the equator.[1]

While the issue of sun exposure is paramount in the discussion of BCCs, one also must consider the genetic syndromes that occur in both people of color and Caucasians. Gorlin syndrome (nevoid basal cell carcinoma syndrome), oculocutaneous albinism, and xeroderma pigmentosum occur in the populations of people of color.[3,4] These syndromes are associated with an increased incidence of all types of skin cancers, including BCCs.

EPIDEMIOLOGY

BCCs are the most common skin malignancies. But they are not the most common malignancies in people of color. Data suggest that BCCs are 60–65% of skin cancers in the general population.[5,6] Beckenstein and Windle, in a series from 1995, found that 1.8% (5 of 276) of skin cancers in African-Americans were BCCs.[7] Fleming's series noted that 12% (7 of 58) of all skin cancers in African-Americans were BCCs.[5] Halder's series from Howard University showed that 28.8% (38 of 103) of African-American patients with skin cancer had a BCC.[8] Altman and colleagues comment that 2.5% of all skin cancers in African-Americans are BCCs.[9] Even though the data are limited, they do support the decreased incidence of BCC in people of color.

There is debate as to whether BCCs occur more often in sun-exposed versus non-sun-exposed areas in people of color. Bang and Halder suggest that BCCs occur more often in sun-exposed areas, such as the head and neck[10] (Figures 43-1 and 43-2). But Lesher and colleagues note in their series that 10% of BCCs in white patients occurred in covered, non-sun-exposed areas, whereas 24% of BCCs in African-

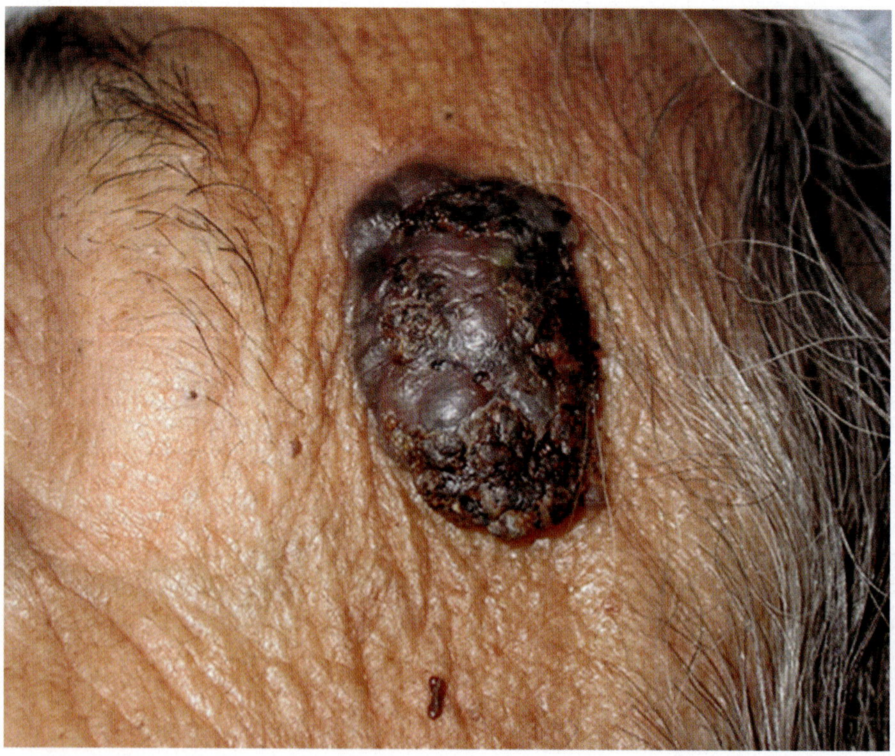

▲ **FIGURE 43-1** Basal cell carcinoma involving the left temple of an African-American woman.

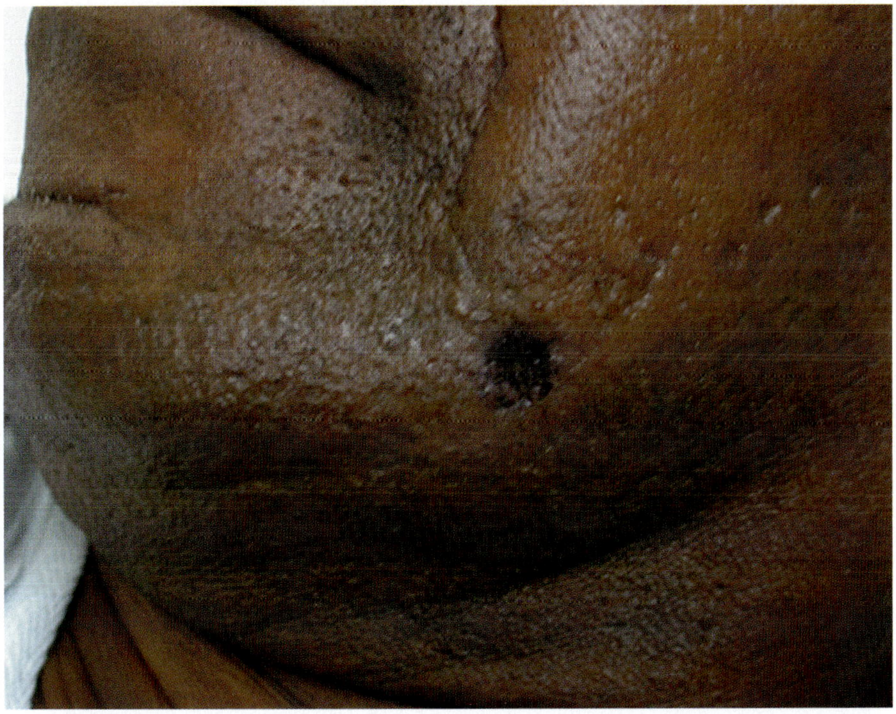

▲ **FIGURE 43-2** Darkly pigmented basal cell carcinoma involving the cheek of an African-American man.

American patients occurred in the covered, non-sun-exposed areas.[11] Abreo and Sanusi found that 88% (38 of 43) of BCCs occurred in the head and neck region of African-American patients.[12] In Fleming's series, 85.7% (6 of 7) of the tumors were in sun-exposed areas.[5] A series by White and colleagues found that 54.5% (6 of 11) of BCCs diagnosed in African-American patients were on covered, non-sun-exposed areas.[13] The data suggest that BCCs occur in a greater frequency in the sun-exposed areas in people of color. However, there is also evidence that a tumor may arise in covered, non-sun-exposed areas as well.

BCCs have appeared in unusual locations in both Caucasians and people of color[9,14–20] (Table 43-1). A complete history and physical examination undoubtedly will aid in the diagnosis and management of the patient with BCCs in these unusual locations. There are reports of BCCs developing in areas of chronic discoid lupus erythematosus lesions, areas previously treated with radiation, and stasis ulcers.[8,21,22]

TABLE 43-1
Unusual Locations of Basal Cell Carcinomas[9,27–33]

- Ankle
- Buttock
- Cervix
- Groin
- Nipple
- Plantar surface of the foot
- Scrotum
- Vulva

The histologic types of BCC in people of color are similar to those seen in people of light skin. Various reports confirm the occurrence of nodular, morpheaform, superficial, adenoid, nodulocystic, and sclerosing types of BCC.[9,11,12,23] (Figures 43-3 and 43-4). The ulcerative type is discussed in many of the series and case reports concerning BCC in people of color and is suggestive of a more aggressive course.[7,10,11] Altman and colleagues and Halder and colleagues, in two distinct series, commented that almost all BCCs are pigmented in people of color.[9,20] Hispanics, even those with fair skin, have a high incidence pigmented BCC (Figure 43-5).

DIAGNOSIS

The diagnosis of BCCs in people of color is made on clinical and pathologic grounds. Reports suggest that a clinical diagnosis of a BCC is more difficult than a histopatholologic one. Altman and colleagues commented that a BCC in people of color may be misdiagnosed clinically as seborrheic keratosis, nevocellular nevus, or a malignant melanoma.[9] Halder and colleagues also remarked that a BCC may be confused for a nevus sebaceous.[20] Beckenstein and Windle reported a BCC being initially (mis)diagnosed as a fungal infection.[7] A

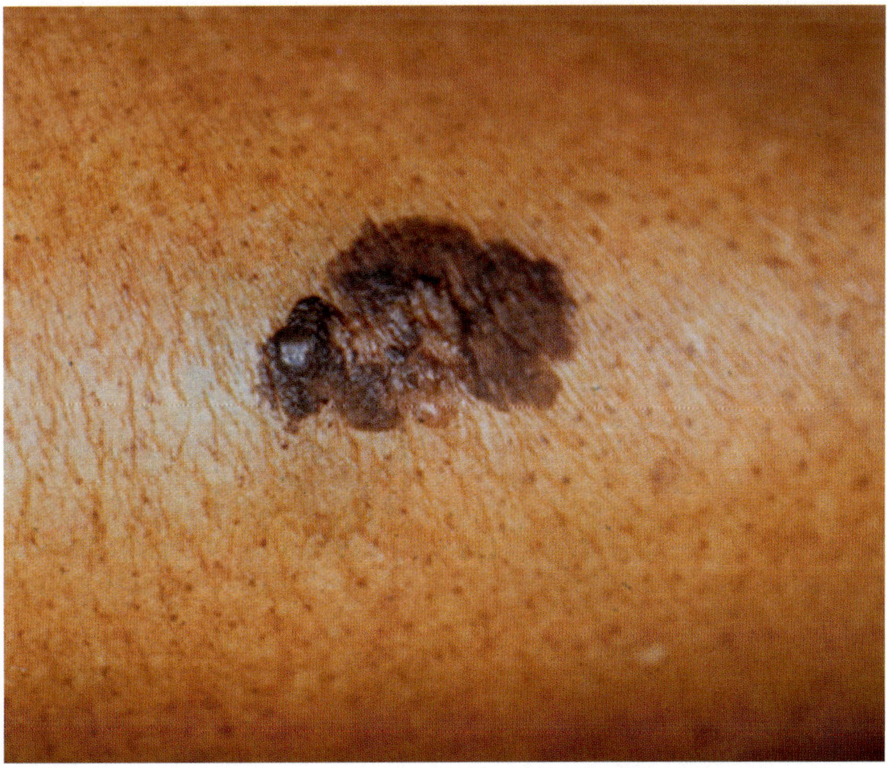

▲ **FIGURE 43-3** Pigmented basal cell carcinoma on the leg of an African-American man.

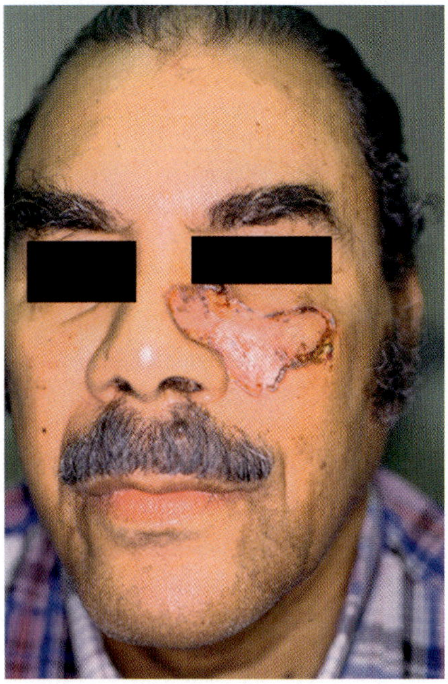

▲ **FIGURE 43-4** Sclerosing basal cell carcinoma on the left cheek of an African-American man.

biopsy is the best and most definitive diagnostic test for a presumed BCC.

PROGNOSIS

A BCC excised with clear surgical margins provides an excellent prognosis. Complications arise when there is delay in diagnosis, resulting in locally aggressive tumor expansion or even metastasis. Itayemi and colleagues in Nigeria reported that BCCs are most aggressive in people of color. They reported two cases of tumors that were locally aggressive and destructive to the underlying bony structures.[24] In the case report of Beckenstein and Windle, a BCC was described as arising within a giant ulcer and spreading locally to the underlying vasculature.[15]

Distant metastasis from BCCs of the scalp to cervical lymph nodes has been reported by Itayemi and colleagues.[24] And Lanehart and colleagues have reported a metastasis to the ipsilateral upper thigh from a primary tumor in a stasis ulcer.[22] Recurrence of BCC in people of color has not been widely reported in the literature. But Walther and colleagues have reported one case that recurred after excision with negative margins and a split-thickness skin graft.[21]

SPECIAL CONSIDERATIONS

The occurrence of a BCC or even multiple BCCs in a person of color should be reason for pause. Mora and Burris noted in their series of 128 patients that 16.8% of patients with a BCC had a second primary malignancy elsewhere.[25] Altman and colleagues found that one patient in their five-patient series had a second primary malignancy.[9] Table 43-2 lists the types of concurrent malignancies reported. SCC of the lung is the most frequently reported second primary malignancy in the series by Mora and Burris.[25] Therefore, it may be appropriate to perform an age-appropriate cancer screening on any patient who has at least one BCC.

TABLE 43-2
Concurrent Second Primary Malignancies[9,25]

Squamous cell carcinoma of the lung
Breast cancer
Cervical cancer
Prostate cancer
Uterine cancer

Other reasons for pause include investigation into whether the patient of color has a genetic predisposition for skin cancers, including BCC. People of color with oculocutaneous albinism (OCA) are most likely to have type II OCA, which is the expression of a mutation in the *P* gene.[26] Abreo and Sanusi reported of an albino patient with 12 separate primary BCCs.[12] Itayemo and colleagues discussed an albino patient with a BCC metastasis to the cervical lymph nodes in their series.[24]

Gorlin syndrome, also known as *nevoid basal cell carcinoma syndrome,* can occur in people of color.[3,27,28] Hall and colleagues commented that fewer than 5% of cases of Gorlin syndrome occur in people of color. And they further stated that initial suspicion of the diagnosis may be made on routine dental examinations that show the odontogenic cysts.[3] Martin and Waisman reported a case of an African-American man with Gorlin syndrome who presented with his first BCC at age 77.[28] Therefore, it may be prudent to look for other diagnostic criteria if one suspects Gorlin syndrome in a person of color, that is, palmar pits, frontal bossing, and odontogenic cysts. One also must consider other conditions predisposing a patient for developing BCC[29] (Table 43-3).

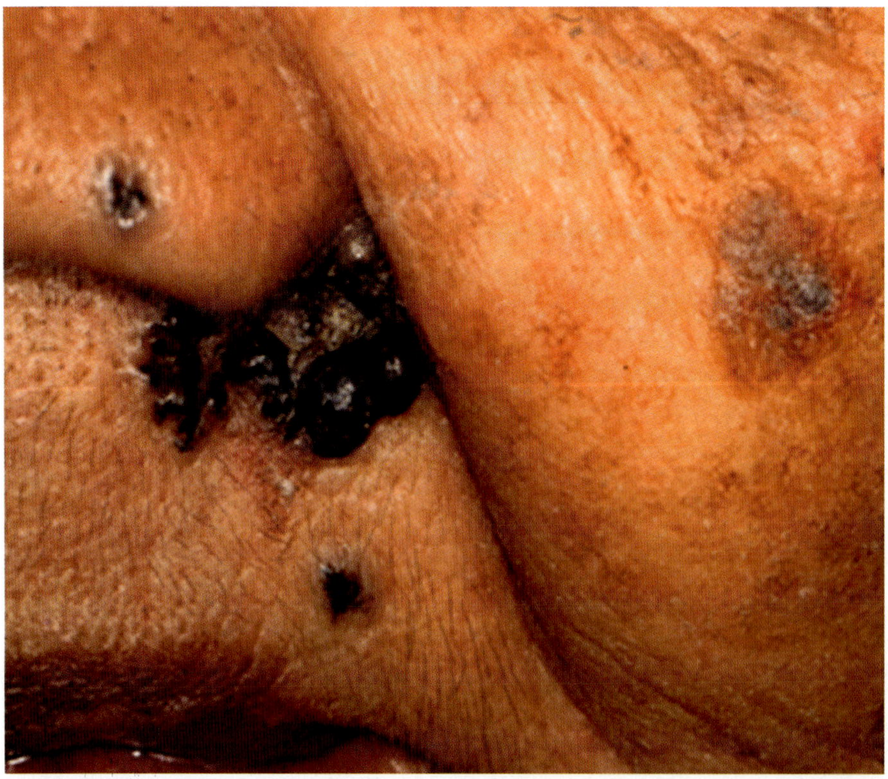

▲ **FIGURE 43-5** Basal cell carcinoma involving the left upper lip and nasal labial fold of a Hispanic woman.

TABLE 43-3
Syndrome with Genetic Predisposition for Developing Basal Cell Carcinoma[3,27–29]

Nevoid basal cell carcinoma syndrome (Gorlin syndrome)
Oculocutaneous albinism
Xeroderma pigmentosum

TREATMENT

The approach to a person of color should not be different from that for a patient with light skin.[30] Management of a BCC should focus on complete extirpation of the tumor. Surgical techniques available to the practitioner include electrodesiccation and curettage, cryosurgery, excisional surgery with clear surgical margins, and Mohs micrographic surgery.[11,15,23,31] Newer modalities in the treatment of BCC include photodynamic therapy, topical imiquimod, and laser surgery.[32] Continued monitoring is essential because recurrence has been reported in up to 37.5% of patients in a series by Ademiluyi and Ijaduola.[4]

REFERENCES

1. Taylor SC. Skin of color: Biology, structure, function and implication for dermatologic disease. *J Am Acad Dermatol* 2002;46(2):S41-62.
2. McDonald CJ. Structure and function of the skin: Are there differences between black and white skin? *Dermatol Clin* 1988; 6:343-347.
3. Hall J, Johnston KA, McPhillips JP, et al. Nevoid basal cell carcinoma syndrome in a black patient. *J Am Acad Dermatol* 1998; 38(2):363-365.
4. Ademiluyi SA, Ijaduola GT. Occurrence and recurrence of basal cell carcinoma of the head and neck in Negroid and albinoid Africans. *J Laryngol Otol* 1987;101: 1324-1328.
5. Fleming ID, Barnwell JR, Burlison PE, et al. Skin cancer in black patients. *Cancer* 1975;3:600-605.
6. Freeman RG Knox JM. Recent experience with skin cancer. *Arch Dermatol* 1970;101: 403-408.
7. Beckenstein MS, Windle BH. Basal cell carcinoma in black patients: The need to include it in the differential diagnosis. *Ann Plast Surg* 1995;35:546-548.
8. Halder RM, Bang KM. Skin cancer in blacks in the United States. *Dermatol Clin* 1988;6:397-405.
9. Altman A, Rosen T, Tschen JA, et al. Basal cell epithelioma in black patients. *J Am Acad Dermatol* 1987;17:741-745.
10. Bang KM, Halder RM. Skin cancer in black Americans: A review of 126 cases. *J Mater Med Assoc* 1987;79:51-58.
11. Lesher JL Jr, d'Aubermont PC, Brown VM. Morpheaform basal cell carcinoma in a young black woman. *J Dermatol. Surg. Oncol* 1988;14:2.
12. Abreo F, Sanusi ID. Basal cell carcinoma in North American blacks. *J Am Acad Dermatol* 1991;25:1005-1006.
13. White, JE, Strudwick WJ, Ricketts WN, et al. Cancer of the skin in Negroes: A review of 31 cases. *JAMA* 1961;178:845-847.
14. Galinski AW. Plantar basal cell carcinoma: A case report. *J Foot Surg* 1980;19:34-35.
15. Beckenstein MS, Windle BH. Basal cell carcinoma in the groin of a black patient with femoral vessel invasion and a second primary malignancy. *Plast Reconstr Surg* 1996;98:872-875.
16. Woods SG. Basal cell carcinoma in the black population. *Int J Dermatol* 1995; 34(7):517-518.
17. McDonald MW. Carcinoma of the scrotum. *Urology* 1982;19:269-274.
18. Powers CN, Stastny JF, Frable WJ. Adenoid basal cell carcinoma of the cervix: A potential pitfall in cervicovaginal cytology. *Diagn Cytopathol* 1996;14: 172-177.
19. Morimoto SS, Gurevitch AW. Residents' corner: Pedunculated pigmented basal-cell carcinoma on the buttock of a black man. *J Dermatol Surg Oncol* 1985;11:115-117.
20. Halder RM, Bridgeman-Shah S. Skin cancer in African-Americans. *Cancer Suppl* 1995;75:667-673.
21. Walther RR, Grossman ME, Troy JL. Basal cell carcinomas on the scalp of a black patient many years after epilation with x-rays. *J Dermatol Surg Oncol* 1981; 7:570-571.
22. Lanehart WH, Sanusi ID, Misra RP, et al. Metastasizing basal cell carcinoma originating in a stasis ulcer in a black woman. *Arch Dermatol* 1983;119: 587-591.
23. Schwartz, RA. Mutilating sclerosing basal cell epithelioma. *J Surg Oncol* 1979;12: 131-135.
24. Itayemi SO, Abioye AA, Ogan O, et al. Aggressive basal cell carcinoma in Nigerians. *Br J Dermatol* 1979;101: 465-468.
25. Mora R, Burris RG. Cancer in the skin of blacks: A review of 128 patients with basal cell carcinoma. *Cancer* 1981;47: 1436-1438.
26. Centurion SA, Schwartz RA. Oculocutaneous albinism type 2. *Acta Dermatol Venereol* 2003;12:32-36.
27. Kulkarni P, Brashear R, Chuang TY. Nevoid basal cell carcinoma syndrome in a person with dark skin. *J Am Acad Dermatol* 2003;49:332-335.
28. Martin S, Waisman M. Basal cell nevus syndrome in a black patient. *Arch Dermatol* 1978;114:1356-1357.
29. Frank W, Morris D. Large basal cell carcinoma in a black patient. *Plast Reconstr Surg* 1995;96:493-494.
30. McDonald, CJ. Some thoughts on differences in black and white skin. *Int J Dermatol* 1976;15:427-430.
31. Singh B, Bhaya M, Shaha A, et al. Presentation, course and outcome of head and neck skin cancer in African-Americans: A case-control study. *Layngoscope* 1998;108: 1159-1163.
32. Geisse J, Lindholm J, Golitz L, et al. Imiquimod 5% cream for the treatment of superficial basal cell carcinoma: Results from two phase III, randomized, vehicle-controlled studies. *J Am Acad Dermatol* 2004;50:722-733.

CHAPTER 44

Cutaneous T-Cell Lymphoma

Halliday Craige McDonald
Amit G. Pandya

Key Points

- Cutaneous T-cell lymphoma (CTCL) refers to a group of non-Hodgkin lymphomas that primarily involve the skin.
- Mycosis fungoides (MF) represent the most common form of CTCL.
- The incidence and mortality rate of MF are higher in African-Americans than in Caucasians.
- Hypopigmented patches and plaques are often the presenting signs in patients with skin of color.
- The age of onset is lower in patients with hypopigmented MF.
- Treatment of CTCL includes topical nitrogen mustard, phototherapy, oral and systemic chemotherapy, and radiation therapy.

Patients with skin of color comprise an important subset of those affected with cutaneous T-cell lymphoma (CTCL). CTCL refers to a group of non-Hodgkin lymphomas that primarily involve the skin and may later involve the lymph nodes, peripheral blood, and other organs. This group of lymphomas includes mycosis fungoides (MF) and Sézary syndrome. MF was first described in 1806 by the French dermatologist Alibert, who named the cutaneous nodules according to their mushroom-like appearance, even though fungi are not involved in etiopathogenesis. MF usually presents with erythematous patches and scaly plaques, sometimes with an affinity for follicles.[1] Less common presentations include hypopigmented macules, pustules, bullae, keratoderma, granulomatous papules and nodules, and subcutaneous plaques.[2,3] Hypopigmented lesions are often the presenting sign of CTCL in patients with skin of color. Malignant cells have an affinity for the epidermis, allowing skin-directed therapy for most patients. More advanced stages of the disease are characterized by loss of this epidermal affinity. Sézary syndrome is the leukemic form of MF, characterized by generalized erythroderma, lymphadenopathy, and atypical T cells located in the peripheral blood.

EPIDEMIOLOGY

According to Weinstock and colleagues,[4–6] the incidence of MF is 0.29 cases per 100,000 per year, comprising 2.2% of all reported lymphomas. There was an estimated 3.2-fold rise in incidence of MF between 1969–1971 and 1984 but no further increase from 1984–1992. The cause of this increased incidence is unknown but may be the result of advances in diagnosis and improved reporting of new cases. Unlike other lymphomas, MF is more common in blacks than in whites, with an incidence 1.7 times higher in blacks than in whites.[5] In addition, the rate ratio for mortality is 2.4 times higher among blacks than among whites. On the other hand, the incidence in Asians and Hispanics is only 0.6 that of whites. The male-to-female incidence ratio is 2.2, and the peak age at presentation is 55–60 years old. However, MF can occur in younger patients as well.

ETIOLOGY

The cause of MF is unknown, but much research has been devoted to determining the mechanisms of disease progression. Normal lymphocytes that express the skin-homing protein cutaneous lymphoid antigen (CLA) are present in inflammatory infiltrates of the skin but not in other tissues. During lymphocyte activation in lymph nodes, the lymphocyte gains the ability to express CLA. The lymphocytes with CLA bind to endothelial cells that express E-selectin 1 on their cell surfaces to facilitate their extravasation into inflamed skin. Expression of CLA by malignant T cells in CTCL helps to explain the skin localization of the disease.[7]

There have been a number of immunologic abnormalities associated with CTCL, including eosinophilia, increased IgE and IgA, decreased natural killer cell activity, and decreased T-cell response to mitogens. These changes have been attributed to an associated increase in Th2-associated cytokines, including interleukin 4 (IL-4), IL-5, IL-6, and IL-10.[8] In addition, patients with CTCL have abnormally high levels of soluble IL-2 receptors, thus decreasing the ability of IL-2 to drive a Th1-mediated response against tumor cells.[9]

It has been suggested that CD8 lymphocytes are important in the survival of CTCL patients. According to Hoppe and colleagues,[10] both T_1 and T_3 stage CTCL patients had a threefold increase in mortality if they had only 0–15% CD8 T cells in their skin biopsies compared with biopsies with more than 20% CD8 T cells after a 6-year follow-up period. In addition, it has been observed that patients who responded favorably to treatment with extracorporeal photochemotherapy had lower CD4-to-CD8 T-cell ratios and high numbers of CD8 T cells at the start of treatment.[11]

Since the advent of immunophenotyping, MF has been shown to consist primarily of epidermotropic malignant CD4 helper T cells, with reactive CD8 and CD4 T cells located mainly in the papillary dermis.[12,13] Occasionally, MF may have a predominant CD8 phenotype, especially in patients with hypopigmented lesions.[12,14]

CLINICAL PRESENTATION

The effect of external factors and infection on the development of MF and Sézary syndrome remains unknown. Environmental and occupational exposure to chemicals was once thought to play a role in MF, but this is not supported by data from a large, case-controlled study reported by Whittemore and colleagues.[15] A viral etiology has been proposed, and human T-lymphotrophic virus I (HTLV-I) has been found in the blood and skin lesions of some MF patients. However, other studies have failed to find such an association.[16,17]

Clinically, MF may present with nonspecific, slightly scaly skin lesions with nondiagnostic biopsies for months or years before a definitive diagnosis can be made, which is known as the *premycotic phase,* or *pre-MF.*[18,19] The eczematous form presents as a persistent, flat, red, pruritic lesion that is fixed in size. *Parapsoriasis en plaque* refers to small oval lesions with an erythematous to yellowish tint, fine scale, and a slightly wrinkled surface, found most often on the buttocks and thighs and ranging from 1–5 cm in diameter. *Poikiloderma vasculare atrophicans* is a term that refers to lesions with "cigarette paper" skin, telangiectasia, atrophy, and a mottled color. Patients with long-standing parapsoriasis-like lesions or poikiloderma vasculare atrophicans are more likely to develop MF. Even when the initial biopsies are negative, repeated

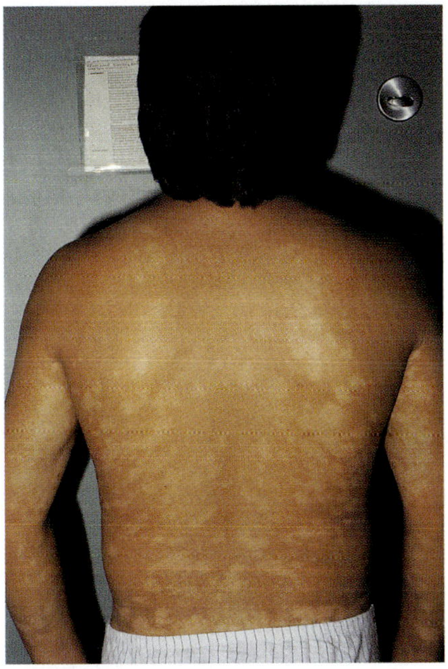

▲ **FIGURE 44-1** Hypopigmented mycosis fungoides in a Latin-American patient.

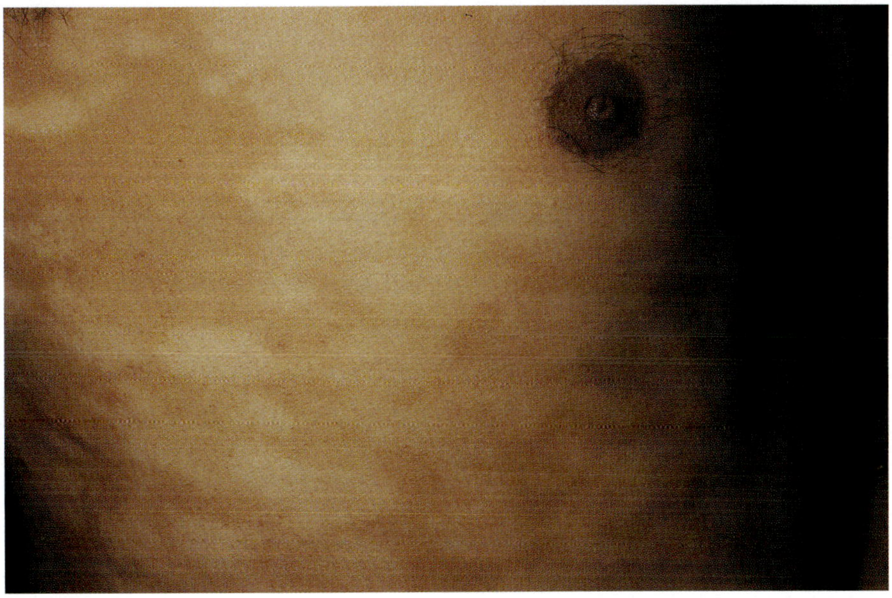

▲ **FIGURE 44-2** Close-up of patient in Figure 44-1 showing multiple oval-shaped hypopigmented macules

biopsies should be performed in patients suspected of having MF. The *patch stage* of MF also presents as erythematous macules, sometimes with hyper- or hypopigmentation and slight scale (Figures 44-1 and 44-2). Plaques are dusky red and scaly and may be round, oval, serpiginous, or arciform in shape. *Plaque-stage* lesions are usually more erythematous than patch-stage lesions. Itching is variable and occasionally severe. If plaques occur in hair-bearing skin, alopecia may result and can be associated with follicular mucinosis on biopsy. The distribution ranges from solitary, isolated lesions to generalized involvement covering the majority of the skin surface area. Plaques can regress spontaneously, remain the same, or occasionally evolve into thicker tumors.[1,18,19]

Tumors of MF may arise from a preformed plaque or from erythematous or uninvolved skin (Figure 44-3). When the tumors arise in plaques, they represent loss of epidermotropism with extension into the deep dermis. These tumors can ulcerate and may become secondarily infected, a common cause of morbidity in MF patients.

Generalized erythroderma in MF is usually accompanied by extreme pruritus and scaling (Figures 44-4 and 44-5). The skin may be lichenified or atrophic, and plaques and tumors of MF also may be present on the background erythema. Lymphadenopathy is common in this form of CTCL. More advanced stages of CTCL are defined by involvement of the lymph nodes, peripheral blood, bone marrow, or other organs (Figures 44-6 through 44-8). Extensive skin involvement is a risk factor for developing

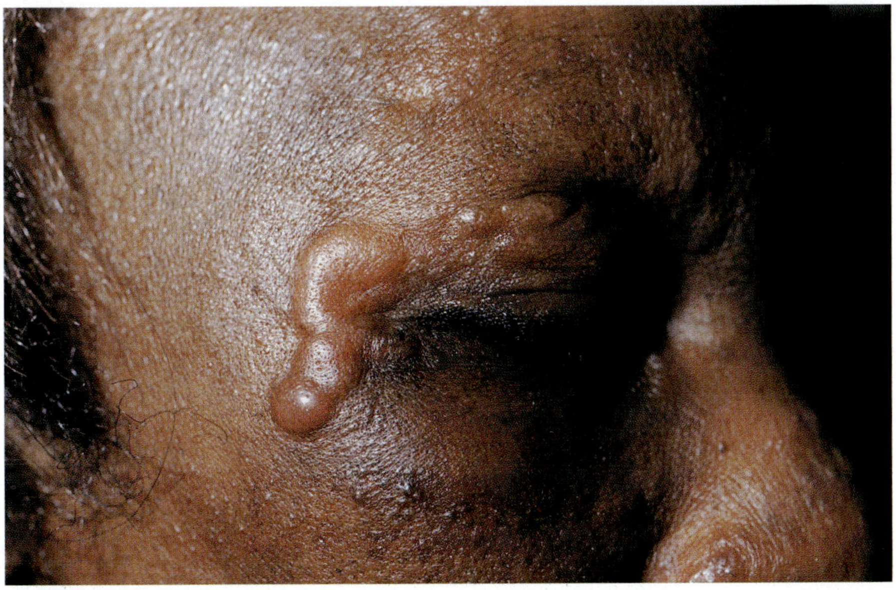

▲ **FIGURE 44-3** Tumor-stage CTCL (stage 2B) in an African-American patient showing infiltrating tumor, erythema, and alopecia of the face.

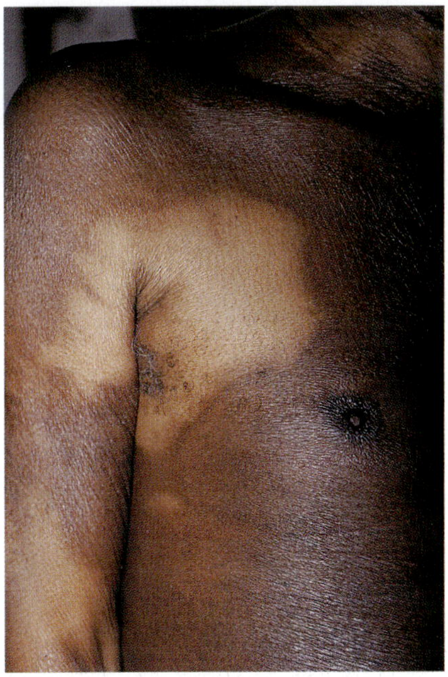

▲ **FIGURE 44-4** Erythrodermic (stage 3) mycosis fungoides in an African-American patient; note contrast between normal skin on lateral chest with involved skin on the remainder of the trunk.

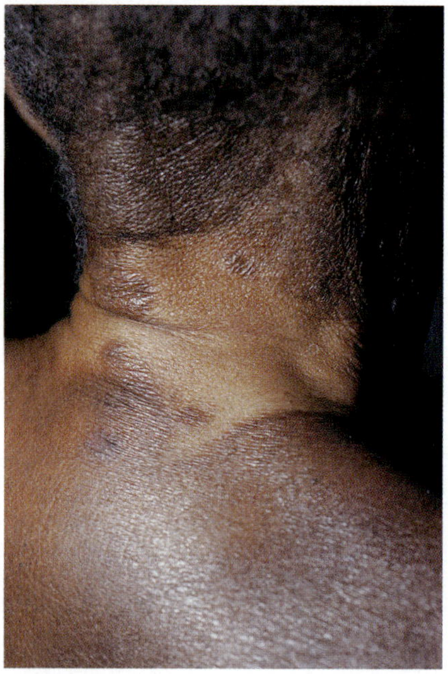

▲ **FIGURE 44-5** Close-up of posterior neck of patient in Figure 44-3.

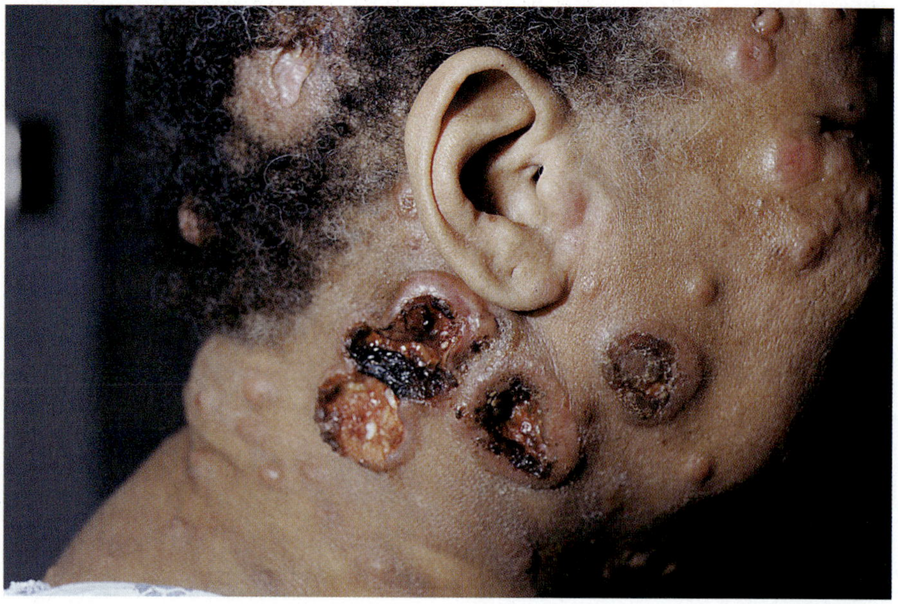

▲ **FIGURE 44-6** Ulcerating tumors in an African-American patient with nodal disease (stage IVA).

extracutaneous skin disease. Whereas localized patch or plaque MF is unlikely to involve extracutaneous tissues, tumor or erythrodermic stages are often accompanied by lymphadenopathy. Visceral involvement is rare and may be a late finding, with the most commonly affected organs being the lungs, liver, spleen, and gastrointestinal tract.

The clinical picture of *Sézary syndrome* includes generalized erythroderma, lymphadenopathy, and circulating abnormal hyperconvoluted lymphoid cells (Sézary cells) in the peripheral blood. The number of cells that must be present to make a diagnosis varies between 5% and 20% of the total lymphocytes.[1] Patients can have all three components, or they may start with generalized erythroderma and then develop lymphadenopathy and peripheral blood involvement. Sézary syndrome has a worse prognosis than erythrodermic MF.

DIFFERENTIAL DIAGNOSIS

MF can imitate many different skin diseases. The differential diagnosis includes atopic dermatitis, psoriasis, drug reactions, photodermatitis, parapsoriasis, neurodermatitis, nummular dermatitis, and tinea corporis. Less common mimickers include acanthosis nigricans, alopecia areata, dyshidrosis, erythema multiforme, perioral dermatitis, pigmented purpuric dermatitis, pityriasis alba, porokeratosis, palmoplantar pustulosis, sarcoidosis, and vitiligo. In patients who present with erythroderma, the differential diagnosis includes atopic dermatitis, contact dermatitis, drug eruption, and erythrodermic psoriasis.[20]

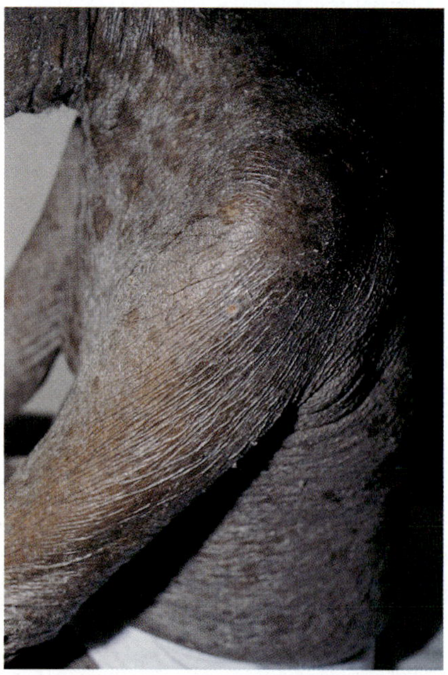

▲ **FIGURE 44-7** An African-American patient with advanced, stage IVB disease with erythroderma, weight loss, and slack skin.

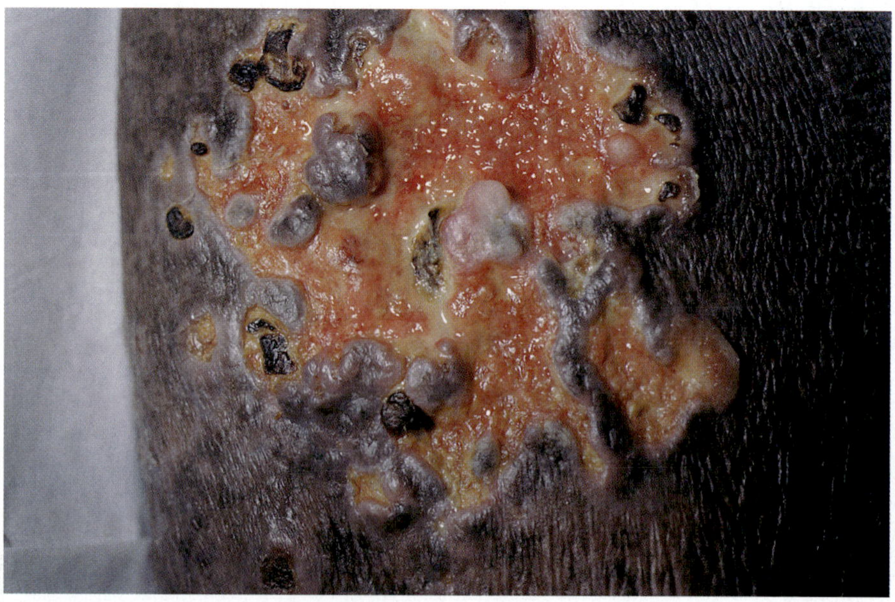

▲ **FIGURE 44-8** Close-up of ulcerated plaque from patient in Figure 44-6.

DIAGNOSIS

The single most important diagnostic tool for MF is the skin biopsy. A biopsy especially may be indicated in patients with skin of color who present with unusual areas of hypopigmentation. Classically, skin biopsy reveals a band-like infiltrate involving the papillary dermis that consists of mononuclear cells with hyperchromatic, cerebriform nuclei without spongiosis. There is an infiltrate of atypical mononuclear cells in the epidermis (epidermotropism) that can form an intraepithelial aggregate known as a *Pautrier microabscess* (Figure 44-9). Often, nonmalignant inflammatory cells are found in the dermis, presumably reacting to the malignant epidermal cells. Using electron microscopy, one can determine the nuclear contour index, which can be used to analyze the degree of lymphocyte nuclear folding and may be helpful to distinguish between MF and benign infiltrates.

Some patients with CTCL may develop nodal disease. In early stages of involvement, histologic examination of a lymph node affected by MF usually reveals small clusters of atypical cells with preserved nodal architecture. With more advanced disease, the clusters of atypical cells in the paracortical regions enlarge and can result in total effacement of the node.

Routine imaging in patients with small lesions or localized MF without lymphadenopathy is of low diagnostic yield and is usually not performed. Patients with lymphadenopathy should have a lymph node biopsy. Physical examination and screening blood tests may reveal abnormalities that warrant further tests, such as computed tomographic scanning or magnetic resonance imaging and bone marrow biopsy.

TABLE 44-1
Tumor-Node-Metastasis (TNM) Classification for MF/Sézary Syndrome

T_1	Limited patch/plaque (<10% of skin surface)
T_2	Generalized patch/plaque (>10% of skin surface)
T_3	Tumors
T_4	Generalized erythroderma
M_0	No visceral metastases
M_1	Visceral metastases
B_0	Atypical circulating cells not present (<5%)
B_1	Atypical circulating cells present (>5%)
N_0	No clinically abnormal peripheral lymph nodes
N_1	Clinically abnormal peripheral lymph nodes
NP_0	Biopsy performed, not CTCL
NP_1	Biopsy performed, CTCL
LN_0	Uninvolved
LN_1	Reactive node
LN_2	Dermatopathic node, small clusters of convoluted cells (<6 cells per cluster)
LN_3	Dermatopathic node with large clusters of convoluted cells (>6 cells per cluster)
LN_4	Lymph node effacement

CLASSIFICATION

Formal staging of MF uses the tumor-node-metastasis (TNM) classification system (Tables 44-1 and 44-2). The extent and type of skin involvement and the presence of extracutaneous disease are the most important prognostic factors in MF. Patients with stage IA disease have an excellent prognosis, with life expectancy comparable with that of age-matched controls.[1] Patients with generalized patch and plaque disease without extracutaneous involvement (stage IB and IIA) have a median survival of over 11 years. They have an increased risk of progression, but only about 20% of patients die of causes related to MF. When patients have tumors or generalized erythroderma (stage IIB or III) without extracutaneous disease, they have a median survival of 3.2 and 4.6 years, respectively. Patients with extracutaneous involvement in lymph nodes or viscera (stage IVA or IVB) have a median survival of only 13 months from the date of first treatment. Transformation of MF or Sézary syndrome to a large cell lymphoma is a poor prognostic sign.[1] Median survival from transformation is only 19 months, and transformation usually occurs less than 2 years from initial diagnosis of MF.

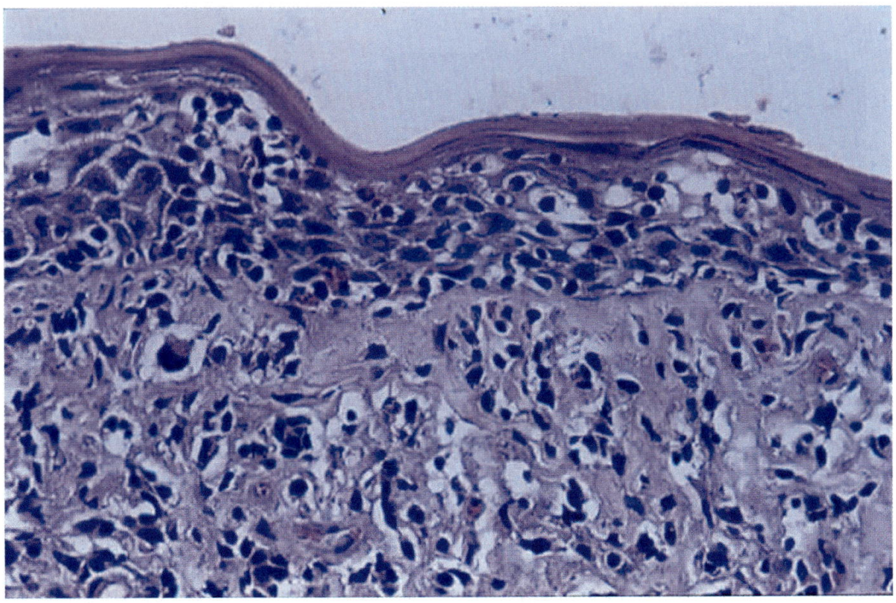

▲ **FIGURE 44-9** Histopathology of patch/ plaque-stage mycosis fungoides showing multiple lymphocytes in the papillary dermis and epidermotropism. Note the small aggregates of lymphocytes in epidermis (Pautrier's microabscesses).

TABLE 44-2
Stage Classification for MF/Sézary Syndrome

Stage	Classification
IA	T_1, N_0NP_0, M_0
IB	T_2, N_0NP_0, M_0
IIA	$T_{1,2}$, N_1NP_0, M_0
IIB	T_3, N_0NP_0, M_0
III	T_4, N_0NP_0, M_0
IVA	$T_{1\text{-}4}$, $N_{0,1}NP_1$, M_0
IVB	T_{1-4}, $N_{0,1}NP_{0,1}$,

TREATMENT

Treatment for MF and Sézary syndrome can be divided into two categories: skin-directed and systemic therapies. Skin-directed therapy includes psoralens plus ultraviolet light (PUVA), UVB light, topical chemotherapy, and radiation therapy. PUVA therapy is administered by taking oral 8-methoxypsoralens, which become activated when exposed to UV light in the 330- to 340-nm range. This drug can inhibit DNA and RNA synthesis by the formation of thymine adducts, gene mutations, or sister chromatid exchanges in the presence of light. During the clearing phase, treatment is given three times per week, followed by a maintenance phase that ranges from once a week to once a month. PUVA therapy is generally restricted to patients with stage I and IIA disease. Side effects include nausea and actinic damage from UVA exposure, but it is generally well tolerated.

Topical chemotherapy includes nitrogen mustard (mechlorethamine) and carmustine. Topical nitrogen mustard therapy is applied daily in solution or ointment form. Major side effects include irritant and contact dermatitis, squamous cell carcinomas, and basal cell carcinomas. Topical carmustine has efficacy similar to nitrogen mustard but is associated with bone marrow suppression in some patients.

Radiation therapy is effective in treating CTCL, particularly electron-beam radiation. Myelosuppression generally does not occur because less than 5% of the dose is delivered beyond 2 cm of the surface. Electron-beam therapy has response rates of 56–96% for stage IA to IIA disease, but it has a high relapse rate if no adjuvant therapy is given subsequently.[1] This therapy is used most often in MF patients with diffuse skin involvement, consisting of thick plaques and tumors, and patients with Sézary syndrome. Side effects include erythema, pain, swelling, hair and nail loss, and loss of sweat gland function. Most of these are reversible, but telangiectasias and xerosis are the most common chronic adverse effects.

Photophoresis is a systemic therapy for CTCL in which patients undergo leukapheresis with isolation of mononuclear cells. These cells are then exposed to 8-methooxypsoralen and UVA light and then returned to the patient. The reinfused cells stimulate a selective immune response against the malignant cells. This therapy is performed on two consecutive days every 2–4 weeks, after which maintenance therapy is given less often. Patients with peripheral blood involvement, particularly with Sézary syndrome with near-normal CD8 counts, and a short duration of advanced disease are the most likely to respond.

Systemic chemotherapy can be used in patients with refractory disease. Single-agent therapy can induce remission, but relapses are common. Agents showing the best results include methotrexate, cyclophosphamide, cisplatin, etoposide, fludarabine deoxycoformycin, bleomycin, doxorubicin, vincristine, and vinblastine. Combination chemotherapy also can be used for refractory disease but does not alter mortality when compared with skin-directed therapy or single-agent chemotherapy.[21]

Interferon-((INF-α) is one of the most active agents in treating MF. In previously untreated patients in all stages of MF and Sézary syndrome, there is an overall response rate of 79%.[1] Adverse effects include fever, chills, myalgias, weight loss, and depression. Leukopenia, thrombocytopenia, and abnormal liver function tests also can occur.

HYPOPIGMENTED MF

Several unique observations have been reported in patients with skin of color who have MF. As mentioned previously, the incidence and mortality rate of MF are higher in African-Americans compared with Caucasians. Protection of the skin by melanin may allow tumor cells to avoid the therapeutic effects of natural UV light from the sun, which may be responsible for MF usually sparing sun-exposed areas. Unchecked, these cells may advance to tumors, which are more common in African-Americans.

Hypopigmented MF is a unique clinical entity that is distinct from the hypopigmentation observed in resolving MF or MF associated with poikiloderma. Although early phases of MF most often present as erythematous, scaly plaques, it also can present with hypopigmented macules with sharp borders and no erythema or scale, particularly in patients with skin of color.[22,23,28] Hypopigmented lesions can be the only manifestation of MF, or they can be associated with erythematous plaques or tumors. The age of onset is lower in patients with hypopigmented MF than in those who present with typical erythematous, scaly plaques. In addition, these patients tend to have a slower progression of their disease.

Histologically, the most consistent features of hypopigmented MF are reduced melanin granules in basal keratinocytes and melanocytes and lymphocytic epidermotropism.[13] Other features include Pautrier's microabscesses and atypical cells.

The pathogenesis of hypopigmented MF remains unclear. In patients who possess a CD8+ phenotype, hypopigmentation may be due to the cytotoxic effect of atypical T cells on melanocytes. Using electron microscopy, Breathnach and colleagues[3] found abnormalities in the melanocytes, including swelling of cytoplasmic organelles, loss of mitochondrial christae, dilatation of the rough endoplasmic reticulum, and cytoplasmic vacuolation. They found evidence of disordered melanogenesis, including the production of spherical, incompletely melanized melanosomes. These changes appeared to be a nonspecific response to cell injury associated with inflammation and may be due to ischemia secondary to disruption of epidermal architecture by edema.

The differential diagnosis of hypopigmented MF includes vitiligo, tinea versicolor, postinflammatory hypopigmentation, leprosy, pityriasis lichenoides chronica, and pityriasis alba. Biopsy is needed to correctly diagnose hypopigmented MF.

Hypopigmented MF usually responds well to PUVA therapy,[24,28] but topical nitrogen mustard and carmustine also can induce complete remission and repigmentation.[23,25] Poor prognostic factors include association of hypopigmented macules with erythematous plaques or tumors and extensive body surface area involvement.[24] These patients tend to relapse after PUVA therapy. Because most reported patients with hypopigmented MF have stage I disease without lymph node involvement, prognosis is generally good.

REFERENCES

1. Siegel RS, Pandolfino T, Guitart J, et al. Primary cutaneous T-cell lymphoma: Review and current concepts. *J Clin Oncol* 2000;18:2908-2925.
2. Price NM, Fuks ZY, Hoffman TE. Hyperkeratotic and verrucous features of mycosis fungoides. *Arch Dermatol* 1977;113:57.
3. Breathnach SM, McKee PH, Smith NP. Hypopigmented mycosis fungoides: Report of five cases with ultrastructural observations. *Br J Dermatol* 1982;106:643-649.
4. Weinstock MA, Horm JW. Mycosis fungoides in the United States: Increasing incidence and descriptive epidemiology. *JAMA* 1988;260:42-46.
5. Weinstock MA, Gardstein B. Twenty-year trends in the reported incidence of

mycosis fungoides and associated mortality. *Am J Public Health* 1999;89:12401244.
6. Weinstock MA, Reynes JF. The changing survival of patients with mycosis fungoides: A population-based assessment of trends in the United States. *Cancer* 1999;85:208-212.
7. Herrick C, Heald P. Advances in clinical research: The dynamic interplay of malignant and benign T cells in cutaneous T-cell lymphoma. *Dermatol Clin* 1997;15:149-157.
8. Rook A, Heald P. The immunopathogenesis of cutaneous T-cell lymphoma. *Hematol Oncol Clin* 1995;9:997-1010.
9. Hoppe RT, Medeiros LJ, Warnke RA, et al. CD8-positive tumor infiltrating lymphocytes influence the long-term survival of patients with mycosis fungoides. *J Am Acad Dermatol* 1995;32:448-455.
10. Drummer R, Posseckert G, Nestle F, et al. Soluble interleukin 2 receptors inhibit interleukin 2-dependent proliferation and cytotoxicity: Explanation for diminished natural killer cell activity in cutaneous T-cell lymphomas in vivo? *J Invest Dermatol* 1992;98:50-54.
11. Heald PW, Rook A, Perez M, et al. Treatment of erythrodermic cutaneous T-cell lymphoma patients with photopheresis. *J Am Acad Dermatol* 1992;27:427-433.
12. Izban KF, Hsi ED, Alkan S. Immunohistochemical analysis of mycosis fungoides on paraffin-embedded tissue sections. *Mod Pathol* 1998;11:978-982.
13. Ralfkiaer E, Wolff-Sneedorff A, Thomsen K, et al. Immunophenotypic studies in cutaneous T-cell lymphomas: Clinical implications. *Br J Dermatol* 1993;129:655-659.
14. El Shabrawi-Caelen L, Cerroni L, Medeiros LJ, et al. Hypopigmented mycosis fungoides: Frequent expression of a CD8+ T-cell phenotype. *Am J Surg Pathol* 26: 450-457, 2002.
15. Whittemore AS, Holly EA, Lee IM, et al. Mycosis fungoides in relation to environmental exposures and immune response: A case-control study. *J Natl Cancer Inst* 1989;81:1560.
16. Hall WW, Liu CR, Schneewind O, et al. Deleted HTLV-I provirus in blood and cutaneous lesions of patients with mycosis fungoides. *Science* 1991;253:317.
17. Wood GS, Salvekar A, Schaffer J, et al. Evidence against a role for human T-cell lymphotrophic virus type I (HTLV-I) in the pathogenesis of American cutaneous T-cell lymphoma. *J Invest Dermatol* 1996;107:301.
18. Hoppe RT, Wood GS, Abel EA. Mycosis fungoides and the Sézary syndrome: Pathology, staging, and treatment. *Curr Prob Cancer* 1990;14:293.
19. Habif TP, *Clinical Dermatology*, 4th ed. St Louis, Mo, Mosby, 2004.
20. Zackheim HS, McCalmont TH. Mycosis fungoides: The great imitator. *J Am Acad Dermatol* 2002;47:914-918.
21. Kaye FJ, Bunn PA Jr, Steinberg SM, et al. A randomized trial comparing combination electron-beam radiation and chemotherapy with topical therapy in the initial treatment of mycosis fungoides. *N Engl J Med* 1989;321:1784-1790.
22. Ryan EA, Sanderson KV, Bartak P, et al. Can mycosis fungoides begin in the epidermis? A hypothesis. *Br J Dermatol* 1973;88:419.
23. Stone ML, Styles AR, Cockerell CJ, et al. Hypopigmented mycosis fungoides: A report of 7 cases and review of the literature. *Cutis* 2001;67:133-138.
24. Ratnam KV, Pang BK. Clinicopathological study and five-year follow-up of 10 cases of hypopigmented mycosis fungoides. *J Eur Acad Dermatol Venereol* 1994;3: 505-510.
25. Zackheim HS, Epstein EH, Grekin DA, et al. Mycosis fungoides presenting as areas of hypopigmentation: A report of three cases. *J Am Acad Dermatol* 1982;6: 340-345.
26. Ardigo M, Borroni G, Muscardin L, et al. Hypopigmented mycosis fungoides in Caucasian patients: A clinicopathologic study of 7 cases. *J Am Acad Dermatol* 2003;49:264-270, 2003.
27. Dabski K, Stoll HL, Milgrom H. Unusual clinical presentation of epidermotropic cutaneous lymphoma: Small hypopigmented macules. *Int J Dermatol* 1985;24: 108-115.
28. Lambroza E, Cohen SR, Phelps R, et al. Hypopigmented variant of mycosis fungoides: Demography, histopathology, and treatment of seven cases. *J Am Acad Dermatol* 1995;32:987-993.

CHAPTER 45

Disorders of Hypopigmentation

Justine H. Park
Doris Hexsel

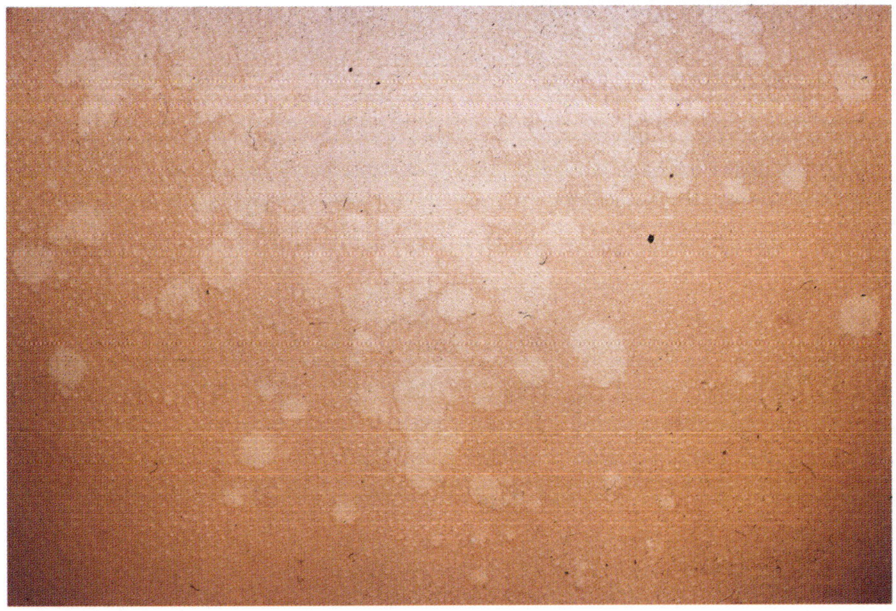

▲ **FIGURE 45-1** Tinea versicolor on trunk.

Key Points

- Disorders of hypopigmentation are the third most common reason for patients with skin of color to seek dermatologic treatment. Dermatologists should know how to recognize and treat these conditions, with special sensitivity to their psychological aspects.
- The causes of hypopigmentation can be divided into two categories based on pathogenesis: melanopenic versus melanocytopenic. They also can be congenital or acquired.
- Hypopigmentation disorders often can be treated successfully with medical, physical, and surgical techniques alone or in association.

This chapter focuses on the conditions in which hypopigmentation or depigmentation of the skin is a hallmark feature. Examples of these conditions include vitiligo, pityriasis alba, idiopathic guttate hypomelanosis, and tinea versicolor. The incidence of some of these conditions, such as pityriasis alba, is increased in individuals of color, whereas others occur equally in Caucasians and ethnic individuals.

Disorders of hypopigmentation are the third most common reason for patients with skin of color to seek dermatologic treatment.[1] The primary complaint of patients is the appearance of the lesions. Hypopigmented skin disorders are more prominent in persons with deeper skin pigment owing to a greater apparent difference in color. Therefore, these individuals are more likely to become distressed and psychologically disturbed, as well as more motivated to seek help for their skin condition than persons with lighter skin tones. Dermatologists should know how to recognize and treat these conditions, with special sensitivity to their psychological aspects. In some patients, disorders of hypopigmentation can be a source of social stigma, depression, and/or anxiety.

Although the many causes of hypopigmentation are protean, they can be divided into two categories based on pathogenesis: melanopenic versus melanocytopenic. The *melanopenic* category refers to disorders of melanin pigment production by the melanocytes, whereas the *melanocytopenic* category refers to disorders leading to a reduction in the numbers of or absence of melanocytes. Clinically, melanocytopenic macules are "dead" or milk white owing to the reflection of incident light. Under the Wood's lamp, they appear stark white in contrast to the surrounding skin. Melanopenic processes can be various degrees lighter than normal skin.

TINEA VERSICOLOR (PITYRIASIS VERSICOLOR)

Clinical Features

Tinea versicolor (TV), caused by the fungus *Pityrosporum ovale* (aka *Microsporum furfur, Malassezia furfur,* or *Pityrosporum orbiculare*), is a superficial infection with a distinctive clinical appearance. Manifesting as hypopigmented or hyperpigmented, ivory to tan, slightly scaly macules and patches that are up to several centimeters in diameter, the lesions predominantly affect the sebaceous areas of the trunk, arms, neck, and face (Figure 45-1). The patients also may present with follicular hypopigmentation (Figure 45-2). Although there is no racial predilection,[2] the dyschromia that results from the infection is often more apparent in persons of color because of greater contrast between the dyschromia and the patient's dark skin. If the diagnosis is in question, a potassium hydroxide (KOH) preparation showing a "spaghetti and meatballs" appearance, representing hyphae and spores, is confirmatory. One also can perform a Wood's lamp examination in which the

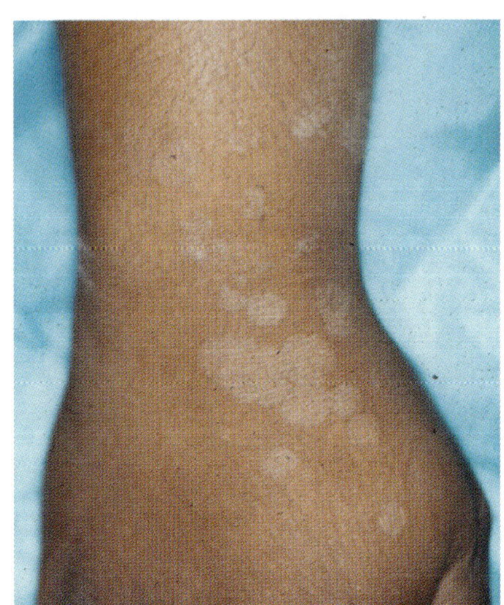

▲ **FIGURE 45-2** Tinea versicolor with follicular hypopigmentation.

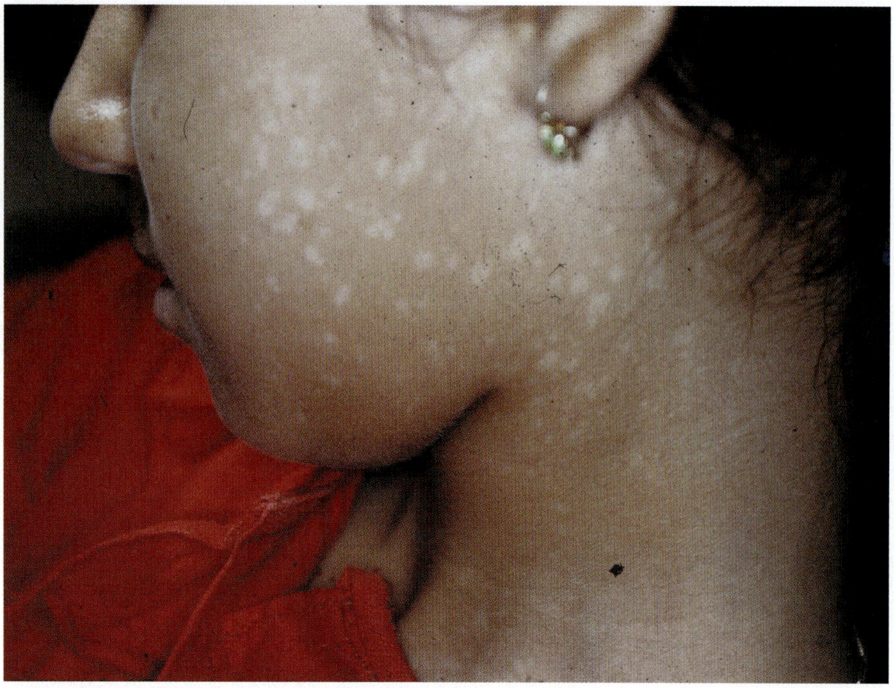

▲ **FIGURE 45-3** Wood's lamp green fluorescence of tinea versicolor.

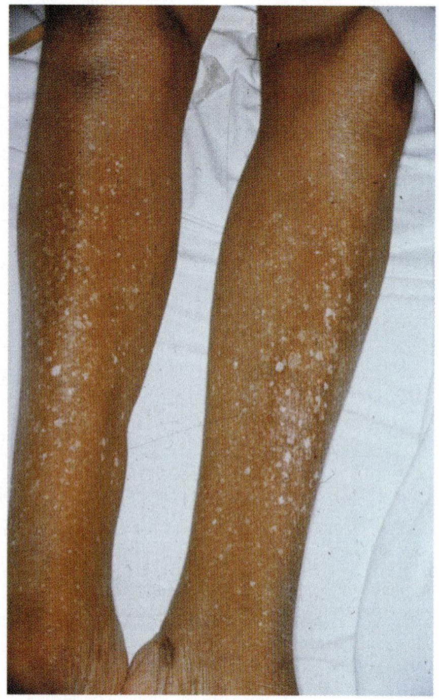

▲ **FIGURE 45-4** Idiopathic guttate hypomelanosis on legs.

hypopigmented skin will have a greenish hue (Figure 45-3).

Pathogenesis

TV is classified as a melanocytopenic disorder. *P. ovale* is known to produce lipoxygenases that act on surface lipids, leading to the oxidization of oleic acid to azelaic acid. This dicarboxylic acid has been shown to inhibit tyrosinase and damage melanocytes in tissue cultures.[3] It is also known that *P. ovale* acts on unsaturated fatty acids to produce lipoperoxidases. It is theorized that these lipoperoxidases are toxic to melanocytes, leading to depigmentation. In addition, ultrastructural studies have shown that the melanosomes in TV lesions are abnormally small,[4–6] and still others postulate that the dispersion of ultraviolet (UV) light by a lipid-like material in the stratum corneum is responsible for the hypopigmentation.[7] Although the exact mechanism by which hypopigmentation occurs is unknown, it is certain that the effect is a result of infection with *P. ovale* because eradication of the organism results in repigmentation, albeit at times gradual, in some patients taking weeks to months.

Treatment

Treatment can be initiated as topical antifungal shampoos, creams, or lotions, including selenium sulfide, terbinafine, or imidazoles, or pulsed systemic antifungal therapy with oral ketoconazole, fluconazole, or itraconazole. Oral terbinafine is not effective. Inform the patient that recurrences are common and that repigmentation can be slow. Once-a-month prophylactic doses may be helpful in cases of relapse. A common regimen is the use of 2.5% selenium sulfide lotion or 2% ketoconazole shampoo to the affected area for 10–15 minutes before rinsing daily for a week, followed by once-weekly maintenance applications for a month. Thereafter, once-a-month maintenance application is often successful. Persistent postinflammatory hypopigmentation can be treated with topical or oral psoralen plus UVA (PUVA) or tar emulsion therapy.

IDIOPATHIC GUTTATE HYPOMELANOSIS

Clinical Features

A very common disorder affecting older persons of all races, idiopathic guttate hypomelanosis (IGH) is an acquired leukoderma of unknown etiology. As with all disorders of hypopigmentation, the lesions are more obvious in persons of color. Typically, the lesions are small, symmetric, and multiple, discrete, depigmented macules usually 2–5 mm in diameter on the extensor aspects of the arms and legs (Figures 45-4 and 45-5). They rarely occur on the face or trunk and appear more often in women than in men. The lesions increase in size and number with advancing age but rarely exceed 1cm in diameter. They are never atrophic or hyperkeratotic. In some cases, they may involve non-sun-exposed areas. As a rule, the lesions are asymptomatic.

Pathogenesis

Although the pathogenesis is unknown, IGH is classified as a melanopenic process in which there is a decreased activity of tyrosinase and decreased staining of melanin.[8–10] However, there is also evidence of a decreased number of melanocytes in lesions of IGH. This has been demonstrated by electronic microscopy.[9] Therefore, one may view IGH as a melanocytopenic as well as a melanopenic disorder. There seems to be two types: (1) actinic IGH, in which sunlight is thought to play a role because the lesions are most commonly distributed over sun-exposed areas of the body, and (2) hereditary IGH, which affects darker-skinned individuals on sun-protected areas like the trunk. Age also may be a contributing factor because the incidence increases with age, and the lesions are quite common in persons over 70 years of age. Fifty percent of African-Americans over the age of 50 years have IGH.

Treatment

Treatment is not necessary, but appearance is a common concern.

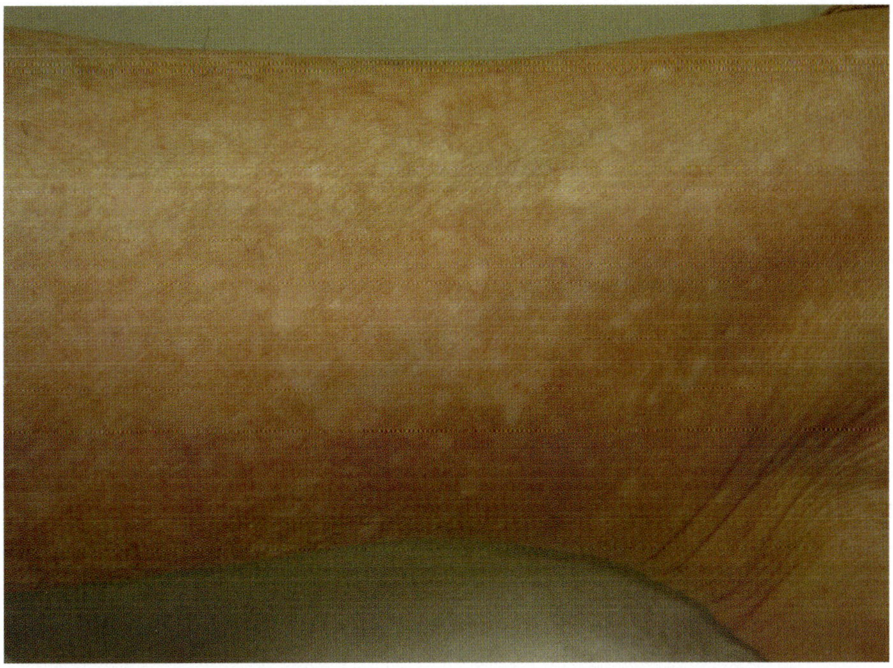

▲ **FIGURE 45-5** Idiopathic guttate hypomelanosis on the ankle. Courtesy Marcia Ramos-e-silva.

Although the changes are usually considered irreversible, intralesional triamcinolone[11,12] and topical tacrolimus and pimecrolimus can be tried with some success. Hexsel and colleagues showed that localized dermabrasion was an effective and safe method.[13] Sun avoidance is strongly encouraged to minimize the contrast in pigment and to avoid potentially worsening the condition. Cosmetic camouflage products also can be used to conceal the lesions.

PITYRIASIS ALBA

Clinical Features

A common self-limited eczematous disorder affecting mostly young children, pityriasis alba (PA) is characterized by multiple, discrete, white-tan macules and patches with indistinct margins and a fine white scale (Figures 45-6 and 45-7). There may be a mild associated pruritus. Sites of predilection include the face, neck, trunk, or arms, and follicular accentuation, especially on the arms, is often present. There is an increased incidence in children of color.[14–16] Whereas the general incidence of this condition in children is anywhere from 1–5% , there are reports of incidences as high as 35% in Hispanic children and 25% in African-American children. The disorder is frequently associated with an atopic diasthesis, although the mechanism of association has not been elucidated.

Pathogenesis

The pathogenesis is not known, but pityriasis alba may be classified best as a melanopenic disorder. Zaynoun has shown a reduction in the number of melanocytes in these lesions.[17] Histologically, the appearance is nonspecific: a chronic spongiotic dermatitis with disruption of melanin pigmentation in the basal layer.[18]

Treatment

Treatment involves gentle skin care, emollients such as petrolatum or 12%

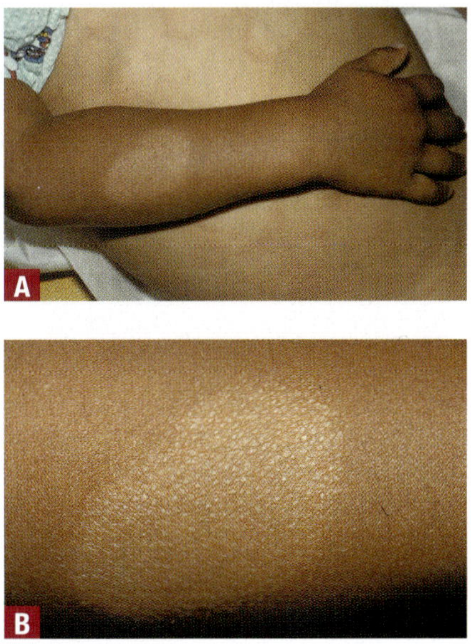

▲ **FIGURE 45-6** Pityriasis alba on arm.

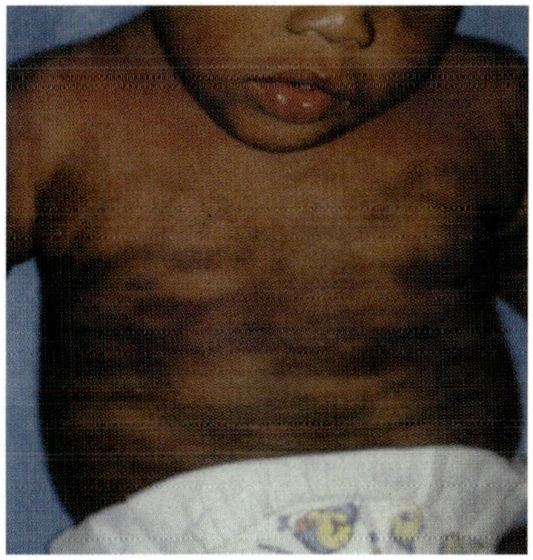

▲ **FIGURE 45-7** Pityriasis alba on body.

ammonium lactate lotion , and sun protection to minimize the disparity between the color of affected and non-affected skin. Other reportedly effective modalities include those used to stimulate melanogenesis, such as tar emulsions, topical steroids, and topical or oral PUVA. Topical tacrolimus and pimecrolimus have been used off-label for this condition. The effectiveness of these steroid-sparing agents is not fully known at this time. Overall, however, the prognosis is good, with lesions typically resolving over a time course of years. As always, one must weigh the risks and benefits of any therapy before initiating treatment, keeping in mind that children are more susceptible to the effects of topical medications.

POSTINFLAMMATORY HYPOMELANOSIS

Clinical Features

Postinflammatory hypomelanosis (aka postinflammatory hypopigmentation) can be the end result of any inflammation. Many conditions—including papulosquamous diseases such as atopic dermatitis, seborrheic dermatitis, and psoriasis; vesiculobullous disorders; inflammatory diseases such as acne and lichen planus; connective tissue disease such as lupus erythematosus; and mycosis fungoides—can lead to it (Figures 45-8 and 45-9). Postinflammatory hypopigmentation is also seen commonly after liquid nitrogen and laser therapies (Figure 45-10). Compared with postinflammatory hyperpigmentation, hypomelanosis is psychologically more devastating in persons of color, and the prognosis for recovery of normal pigmentation is worse.

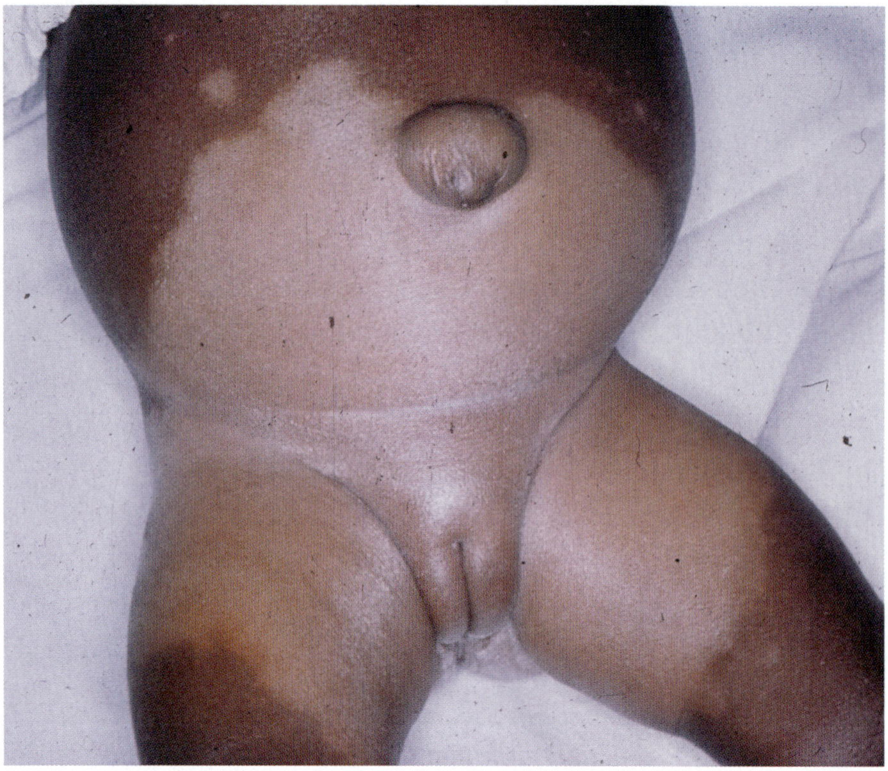

▲ **FIGURE 45-8** Postinflammatory hypomelanosis secondary to diaper dermatitis.

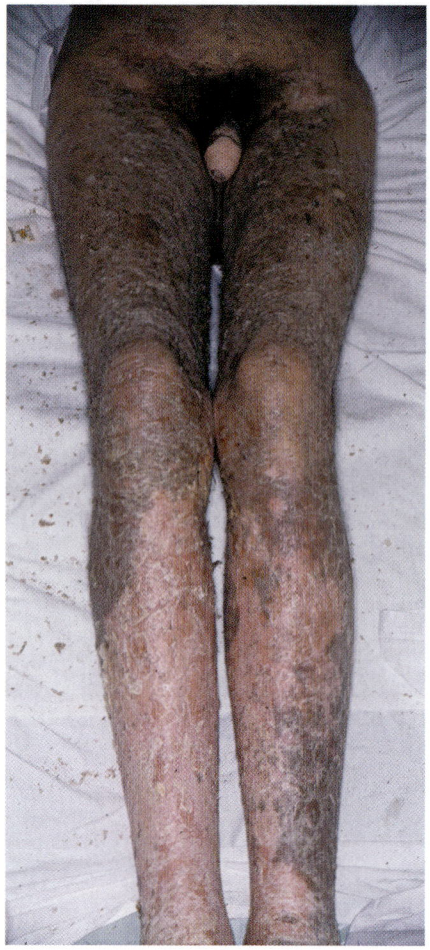

▲ **FIGURE 45-10** Postinflammatory hypomelanosis secondary to proriasis.

Pathogenesis

The pathogenesis of this condition is secondary to a melanopenic process in which the transfer of melanosomes to keratinocytes is blocked.[19] The melanosome-congested melanocytes within the basal cell layer result in the dilution of normal skin color. Inflammatory mediators such as interferon-γ (IFN-γ), tumor necrosis factor-α (TNF-α), and interleukin 6 (IL-6) are thought to play a role. Other proposed theories for the loss or blockage of transfer of melanosomes include edema and rapid cell turnover.

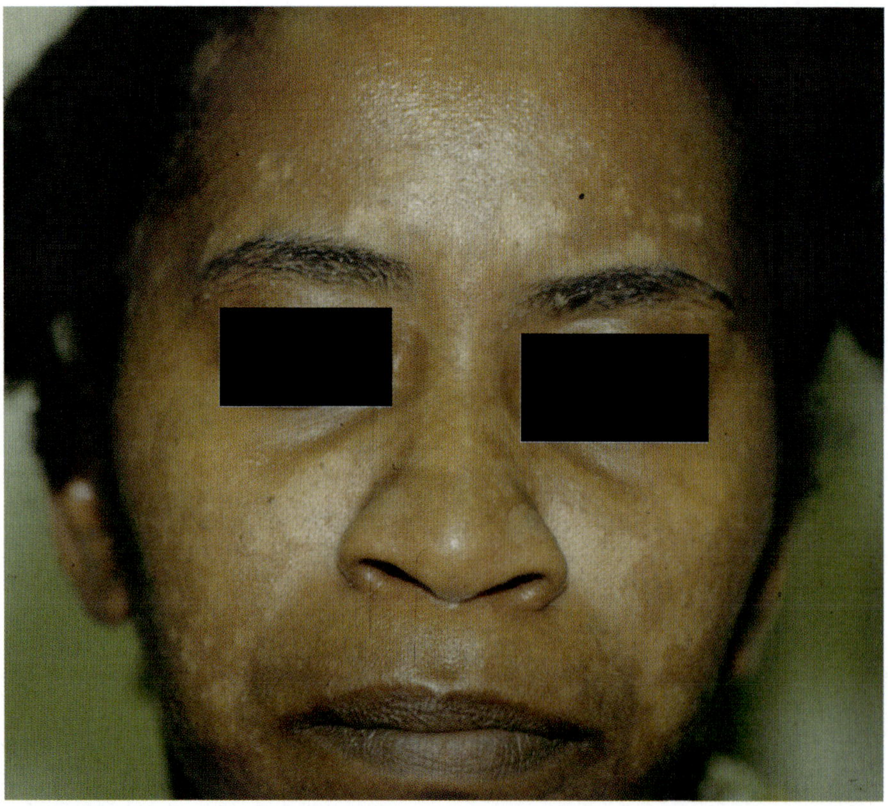

▲ **FIGURE 45-9** Postinflammatory hypomelanosis secondary to seborrheic dermatitis.

Diagnosis

The diagnosis generally is made based on history and physical examination. For example, one might find linear, slightly atrophic hypomelanotic macules at the site of a previous linear excoriation. Postinflammatory hypomelanosis is quite common in African-Americans with atopic eczema. Wood's lamp is not useful.

Treatment

Treatment involves identifying and treating the underlying causative disorder. As long as inflammation persists, repigmentation is not possible. Once the process is controlled, stimulation of melanogenesis with topical or oral PUVA, narrow-band UVB phototherapy, topical steroids, tacrolimus, and skin grafts can be tried. However, no treatment options have good efficacy. Cosmetic blends can be used to mask affected areas.

VITILIGO

See Chapter 46 for an in-depth discussion of vitiligo.

PIEBALDISM

Clinical Features

A rare genodermatosis with an autosomal dominant inheritance pattern, piebaldism affects 1 in 20,000 people worldwide. The distinctive appearance of a white forelock and an amelanotic patch extending from the abdomen to the flanks, sparing the midback, present at birth suggests the diagnosis (Figure 45-11). Other areas that may be involved include the face, arms, and legs; in contrast to vitiligo, the hands and feet are often spared. There may be hyperpigmented macules within the areas of leukoderma and elsewhere on the skin. Generally patients are otherwise normal, but there may be associated heterochronicity of the irides or deafness.

Pathogenesis

The clinical features of piebaldism can be explained by a genetic mutation in the *KIT* gene on c4q12, which encodes a receptor for stem cell factor on melanoblasts in the neural crest.[20,21] When mutated, these melanoblasts fail to migrate to their residence in the skin,[22] leading to an absence of melanocytes on histology and the clinicopathologic correlate—the depigmented lesions characteristic of piebaldism.

Diagnosis

Diagnosis can be made on the basis of autosomal dominant inheritance pattern and congenital presence of characteristic skin findings. Vitiligo is the main differential diagnosis.

Treatment

Treatment is similar to that of vitiligo.

SARCOIDOSIS

Clinical Features

Sarcoidosis is mentioned here to emphasize that hypopigmented lesions of sarcoidosis have been described (Figure 45-12). Sarcoidosis may be slightly more common in women than in men and usually presents between the ages of 20 and 40 years.[23] Interestingly, and for reasons unknown, the incidence of sarcoidosis in blacks is 10 times more common than in whites. In addition, hypopigmented sarcoid is more common in persons of color than in whites.[24,25]

Pathogenesis

The pathogenesis of hypopigmentation in cutaneous sarcoidosis is largely unknown.

Diagnosis and Differential Diagnosis

The diagnosis of sarcoidosis is established by the histologic confirmation of noncaseating granulomas from biopsy specimens taken from two or more different organs or from one biopsy specimen plus a positive Kveim-Siltzbach reaction.[26]

Lupus erythematous can be differentiated by cutaneous biopsy and serologic studies. Papular forms of secondary syphilis are distinguished by the course and associated features of this disease. Occasionally, acne agminata presents difficulties.[27]

Treatment

For cutaneous sarcoidosis, treatment may be difficult and should be tailored to each individual's need, taking into account the severity and presence of systemic disease. In limited cutaneous disease, high-potency topical corticosteroids sometimes may prove helpful, as may intralesional triamcinolone injection. Tacrolimus was reported to be beneficial when used topically in cutaneous sarcoidosis. Cryotherapy and radiotherapy also have been used. PUVA therapy has

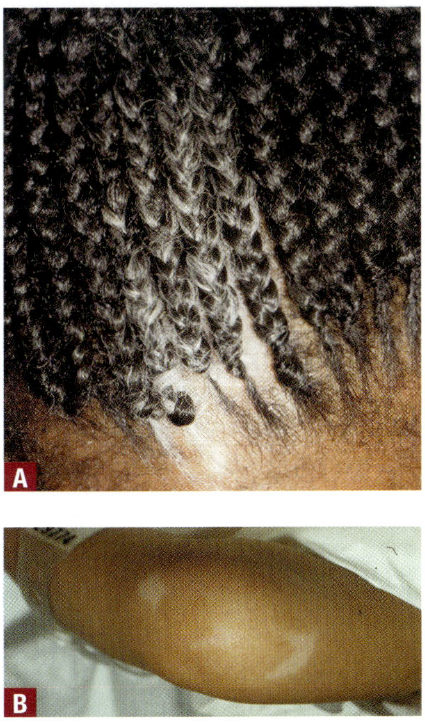

▲ **FIGURE 45-11** Piebaldism forelock and skin.

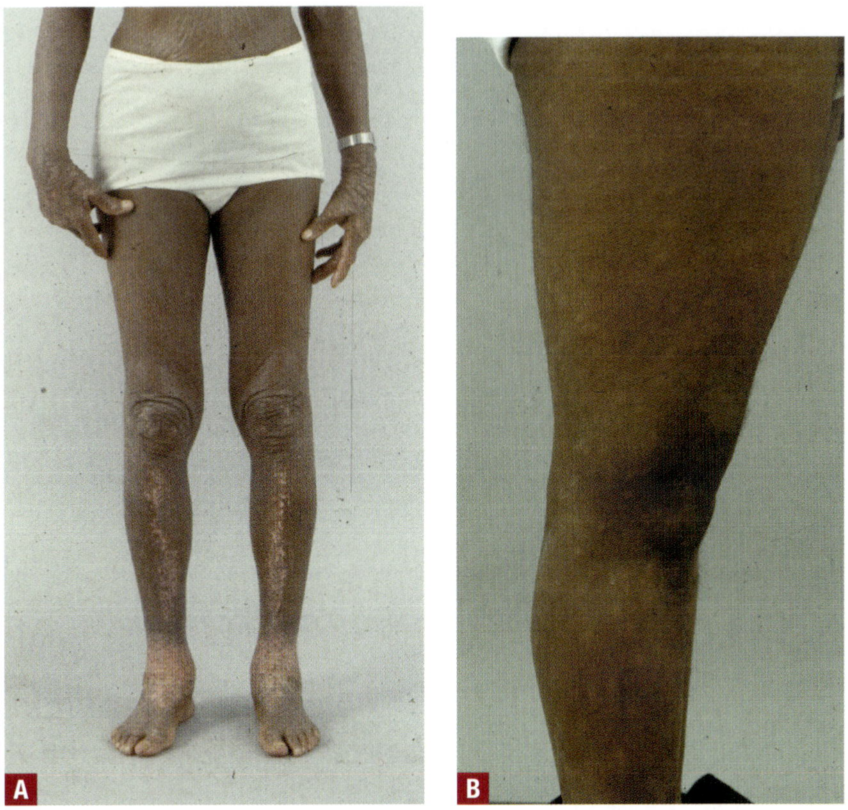

▲ **FIGURE 45-12** Hypopigmented sarcoid.

been successful in hypopigmented and erythrodermic sarcoidosis. In patients with more extensive involvement, systemic therapy with corticosteroids is often effective. In the case that corticosteroids fail or are contraindicated, cytostatic drugs such as methotrexate or other immunomodulating therapies such as infliximab may be tried.[26]

MYCOSIS FUNGOIDES

Clinical Features

Mycosis fungoides (MF) is the most common variant of primary cutaneous T-cell lymphoma (CTCL), generally associated with an indolent clinical course and characterized by well-defined clinicopathologic features. Most cases are diagnosed in the fifth and sixth decades, but individuals can develop this disease in childhood and adolescence. There are different stages in the evolution of the disease, such as patches, plaques, and tumors.[27]

Lesions of MF may present as the typical scaly plaque, but in darker-skinned individuals, presentation as a hypopigmented patch is seen occasionally[28–31] (Figure 45-13). Also, those with dark skin may have multihued lesions (Figure 45-14). The presentation may vary from an eruption of many macules to the presence of one large patch. Often the distribution is central rather than acral. There may be associated scale, resembling pityriasis alba, especially in children. The lesions also may be indurated or erythematous.

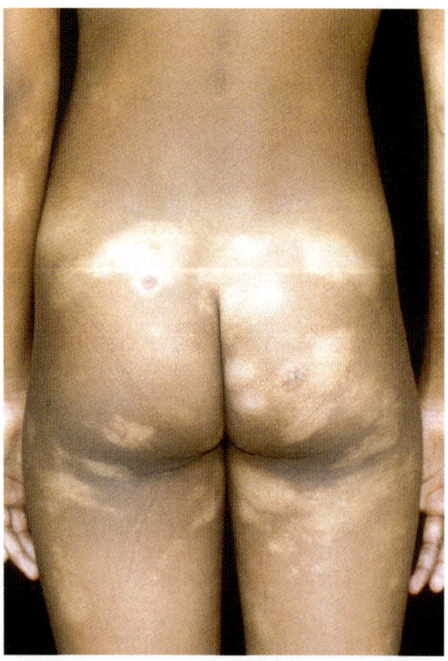

▲ **FIGURE 45-13** Hypopigmented mycosis fungoides. Courtesy Sueli Carneiro and Marcia Ramos-e-Silva.

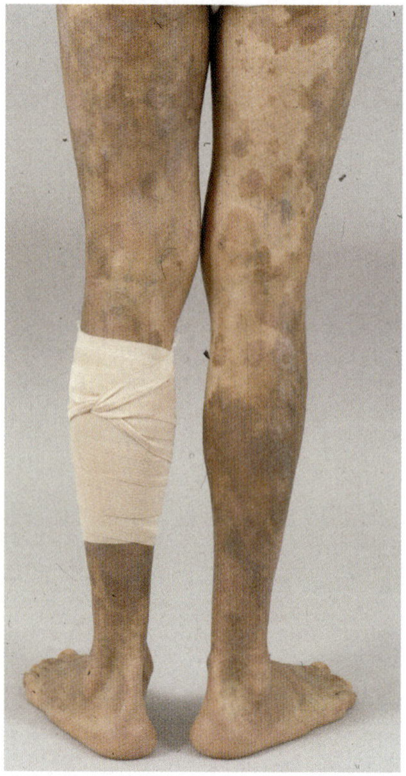

▲ **FIGURE 45-14** Multihued mycosis fungoides.

Pathogenesis

CTCL likely is a melanopenic process with blockage of melanosome transfer.[27]

Diagnosis and Differential Diagnosis

A skin biopsy with histologic confirmation of the disease should be performed in any patient with persistent polymorphic plaques. The earliest pathologic feature is the presence of a predominantly lymphocytic infiltrate in the papillary dermis. As the disease progresses, prominent epidermotropism are seen, leading to clusters of atypical lymphocytes in the epidermis (Pautrier microabcesses).[27]

The differential diagnosis includes pityriasis alba, tinea versicolor, vitiligo, or postinflammatory hypomelanosis.

Treatment

The choice of initial treatment will depend on the stage of the disease as well as the general condition and age of the patient. There is no special treatment protocol for hypopigmented MF.

For patients with limited early-stage MF, topical corticosteroids can produce a clinical response. There is good success of PUVA in the treatment of early-stage MF, but no response in tumor-stage disease.[27] In addition, topical tazarotene and/or imiquimod can be used. Other options in refractory cases include combination bexarotene and PUVA, topical nitrogen mustard, and carmustine.[32,33]

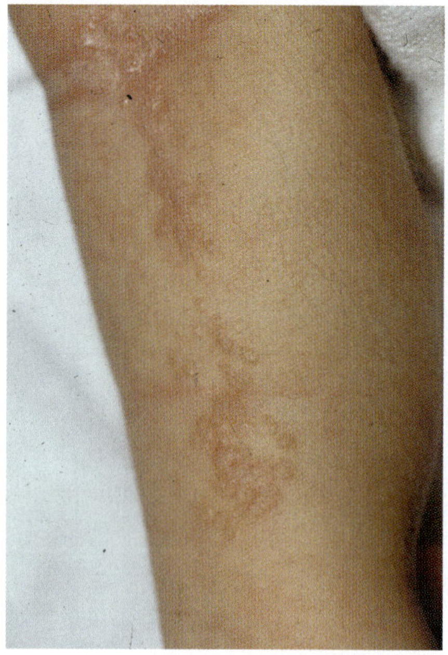

▲ **FIGURE 45-15** Classic lichen striatus.

Prognosis is generally favorable, especially if recognized early.

LICHEN STRIATUS (BLAISE—BLASCHKO LINEAR ACQUIRED INFLAMMATORY SKIN ERUPTION)

Clinical Features

A benign, acquired, self-limited inflammatory dermatosis, lichen striatus typically presents in children between the ages of 5 and 15 years.[34] At present, there is no consensus on gender preference. Some studies have shown an increased incidence in girls,[35] whereas others show an equal incidence in boys and girls. There is no known racial predilection or any basis in heredity.

The lesion is typically an erythematous, scaly, linear plaque following Blaschko's lines (Figure 45-15). The plaque may be only a few centimeters in length or may extend along an entire limb. Lichen striatus occurs most commonly on one arm or leg or on the neck, but other sites may be involved. Usually, there are no symptoms, but pruritus may occur occasionally.[3]

In dark-skinned individuals, the eruption is usually first noted because the papules may be hypopigmented.[37] In addition, in dark-skinned individuals, the resolution of lichen striatus may be followed by temporary hypopigmentation[38–40] (Figure 45-16). Wu and colleagues reported a series of 27 cases in which they described a new entity termed *lichen striatus–like leukoderma*. The

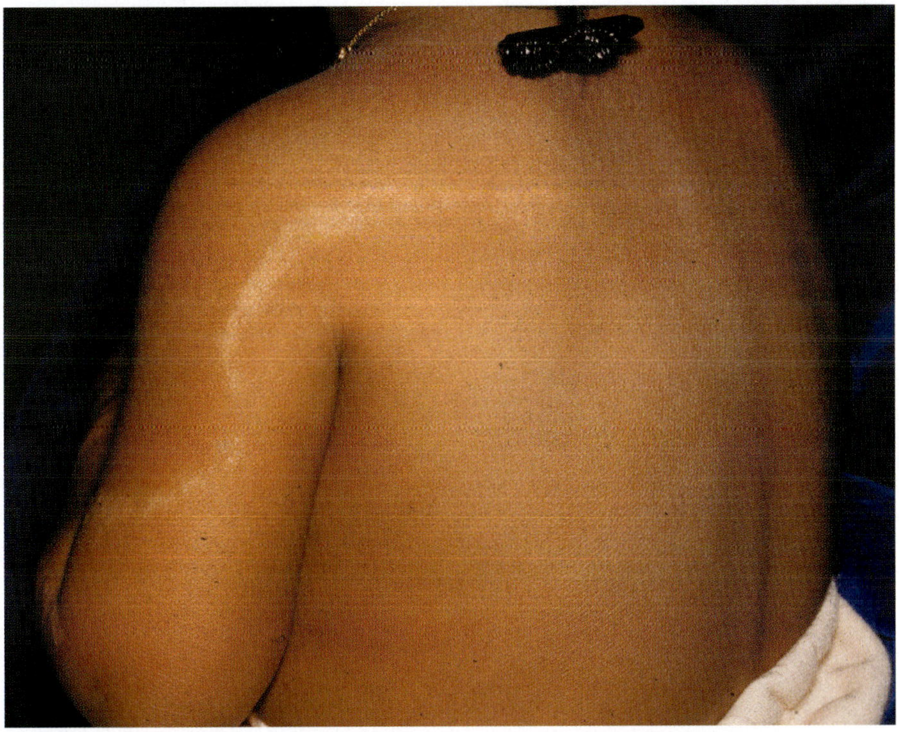

▲ **FIGURE 45-16** Hypopigmented lichen striatus.

main differentiating feature of lichen striatus–like leukoderma from lichen striatus is its strictly macular form.[41]

Pathogenesis

The pathogenesis of the hypopigmentation seen in lichen striatus is not known but is likely due to a melanopenic process because the number of melanocytes is normal.

Diagnosis

The diagnosis generally can be made based on the clinical history and examination of the patient. On histologic examination, the features of lichen striatus are variable, which may be explained by the evolution of the disease process at which the biopsy was performed.[42] Linear forms of lichen planus and psoriasis usually can be differentiated clinically, even in the absence of typical lesions in others sites, which always should be sought. Linear porokeratosis also must considered.[43]

Treatment

Lichen striatus has a self-limited course, generally resolving after a few years untreated. For those who prefer treatment, topical corticosteroids may hasten resolution.[42] In the unusual persistent case, infiltration with steroids may be effective.[43] It is discussed here because in persons of color it often resolves with hypopigmented macules as in postinflammatory hypomelanosis.[38-40]

PROGRESSIVE MACULAR HYPOMELANOSIS

Clinical Features

Progressive macular hypomelanosis (PMH) is a pigmentary skin disorder that occurs mostly on the trunk but can occur on the face, neck, or proximal extremities. It is characterized by ill-defined, nummular, symmetrically localized hypopigmented macules. In the majority of patients, a hypopigmented area that seems to originate from a confluence of the macules is present on the front and back of the trunk[44] (Figure 45-17).

According to Guillet and colleagues, this disorder is caused by mixed racial origin.[45] Borelli suggests that PMH is a genodermatosis.[46]

Pathogenesis

The pathogenesis of PMH is unknown, although a melanopenic process is proposed. Westerhof and Relyveld hypothesized that a factor produced by strains of *P. acnes* interferes with melanogenesis and subsequently causes hypopigmentation. These hypopigmented macules are located on parts of the skin that provide favorable growth conditions for *P. acnes*.[47,48]

Diagnosis and Differential Diagnosis

Diagnosis rests on careful clinical examination and performance of a potassium hydroxide (KOH) test on skin scrapings to exclude the major differential diagnosis: tinea versicolor.[36] In addition, Wood's light examination for red follicular fluorescence in involved areas can be a helpful diagnostic finding.

Treatment

Several treatment modalities have been attempted, including topical and systemic antifungal agents and topical

▲ **FIGURE 45-17** Progressive macular hypomelanosis. Courtesy Dr Marcia Ramos-e-Silva

corticosteroids, but none has been successful. Relyveld and colleagues observed successful treatment with psoralen plus UVA (PUVA) therapy; however, after cessation of the therapy, recurrence of the hypopigmented lesions was seen immediately. The temporary success of PUVA therapy probably can be explained by the temporary inhibition of *P. acnes* by PUVA while stimulating melanogenesis.[44] In 2006, these authors showed that antimicrobial therapy (i.e., benzoyl peroxide 5% hydrogel and clindamycin 1% lotion) in conjunction with UVA irradiation was more effective in repigmentation in patients with PMH than a combination of anti-inflammatory therapy (fluticasone 0.05% cream) and UVA irradiation.[44]

REFERENCES

1. Halder RM, Nootheti PK. Ethnic skin disorders overview. *J Am Acad Dermatol* 2003; 48:S143-148.
2. Halder RM, Nandedkar MA, Neal KW. Pigmentary disorders in ethnic skin. *Dermatol Clin* 2003;21:617-628.
3. Nazzaro-Porro M, Passi S. Identification of tyrosinase inhibitor in culture of *Pityrosporum*. *J Invest Dermatol* 1978;71: 389-402.
4. Odom RB, James WD, Berger TG (eds). Disorders resulting from fungi and yeast, in *Diseases of the Skin,* 9th ed. Philadelphia, Saunders, 2000, p 388
5. Charles CR, Sire DJ, Johnson BL, Beidler JG. Hypopigmentation in tinea versicolor: A histochemical and electron microscopic study. *Int J Dermatol* 1973;12: 48-58.
6. Karaoui R, Bou-Resli M, Alzaid NS, Mousa A. Tinea versicolor: Ultrastructural studies on hypopigmented and hyperpigmented skin. *Dermatologica* 1981;162:69-73.
7. Borgers M, Cauwenbergh G, Van De M, Hernanz AP, Degreef H. Pityriasis versicolor and *Pityrosporum ovale*: Morphogenetic and ultrastructural considerations. *Int J Dermatol* 1987;26: 586-589.
8. Savall R, Ferrandiz C, Ferrer I, Peyri J. Idiopathic guttate hypomelanosis. *Br J Dermatol* 1980;103:635.
9. Ortonne J-P. Idiopathic guttate hypomelanosis: Ultrastructural study. *Arch Dermatol* 1980;116:664.
10. Wilson PD, Lavker RM, Kligman AM. On the nature of idiopathic guttate hypomelanosis. *Acta Dermatol Venereol* 1982; 62:301.
11. Falabella R, Escobar C, Giraldo N, et al. On the pathogenesis of idiopathic guttate hypomelanosis. *J Am Acad Dermatol* 1987;16:35-44.
12. Falabella R. Idiopathic guttate hypomelanosis. *Dermatol Clin* 1988;6:241-247.
13. Hexsel DM. Treatment of idiopathic guttate hypomelanosis by localized superficial dermabrasion. *Dermatol Surg* 1999; 25:917-918.
14. Nanda A, Al-Hasawi F, Alsaleh QA. A prospective survey of pediatric dermatology clinic patients in Kuwait: An analysis of 10,000 cases. *Pediatr Dermatol* 1999;16: 6-11.
15. Dogra S, Kumar B. Epidemiology of skin diseases in school children: A study from northern India. *Pediatr Dermatol* 2003;20: 470-473.
16. Blessmann WM, Sponchiado de Avila LG, Albaneze R. Pityriasis alba: A study of pathogenic factors. *J Eur Acad Dermatol Venereol* 2002;16:463-468.
17. Zaynoun ST, Aftimos BG, Tenekjian KK, Bahuth N, Kurban AK. Extensive pityriasis alba: A histological, histochemical, and ultrastructural study. *Br J Dermatol* 1983;108:83-90.
18. Vargas-Ocampo F. Pityriasis alba: A histologic study. *Int J Dermatol* 1993;32:870-873.
19. Ortonne JP, Bahadoran P, Fitzpatrick TB, Mosher DB, Hori-Y. Hypomelanoses and hypermelanoses, in Freedberg IM, Eisen AZ, Wolff K, et al (eds), *Fitzpatrick's Dermatology in General Medicine,* 6th ed. New York, McGraw-Hill, 2003, p 857.
20. Giebel LB, Strunk KM, Holmes SA, Spritz RA. Organization and nucleotide sequence of the human *KIT* (mast/stem cell growth factor receptor) proto-oncogene. *Oncogene* 1992;7:2207-2217.
21. Boissy RE, Nordlund JJ. Molecular basis of congenital hypopigmentary disorders in humans: A review. *Pigment Cell Res* 1997;10:2-24.
22. Syrris P, Heathcote K, Carrozzo R, et al. Human piebaldism: Six novel mutations of the proto-oncogene *KIT. Hum Mutat* 2002;20:234.
23. Gawkrodger DJ. Sarcoidosis, in Burns T, Breathnach S, Cox N, Griffiths C (eds), *Rook's Textbook of Dermatology,* Vol 3, 7th ed. Oxford, England, Blackwell, 2004, p 581.
24. Jacyk W. Cutaneous sarcoidosis in black South Africans. *Int J Dermatol* 1999;38: 841-845.
25. Johnson BL Jr. Sarcoidosis, in Johnson BL, Moy RL, White GM (eds), *Ethnic Skin, Medical and Surgical.* St Louis, Mosby, 1998, p 177.
26. Kirsner RS, Kerdel FA. Sarcoidosis, in Arndt KA, Leboit PE, Robinson JK, Wintroub BU (eds), *Cutaneous Medicine and Surgery: An Integrated Program in Dermatology,* Vol 1. London, Saunders, 1996, pp 433-437.
27. Whittaker SJ, MacKie RM. Cutaneous lymphomas and lymphocytic infiltrates, in Burns T, Breathnach S, Cox N, Griffiths C (eds), *Rook's Textbook of Dermatology,* Vol 3, 7th ed. Oxford, England, Blackwell, 2004, pp 51-53.
28. Tang M, Tan SH, Lim LC. Leukoderma associated with Sézary syndrome: A rare presentation. *J Am Acad Dermatol* 2003;49: S247-249.
29. Petit T, Cribier B, Bagot M, Wechsler J. Inflammatory vitiligo-like macules that simulate hypopigmented mycosis fungoides. *Eur J Dermatol* 2003;13:410-412.
30. Stone ML, Styles AR, Cockerell CJ, Pandya AG. Hypopigmented mycosis fungoides: A report of 7 cases and review of the literature. *Cutis* 2001;67: 133-138.
31. Whitmore SE, E. Simmons-O'Brien, Rotler FS. Hypopigmented mycosis fungoides. *Arch Dermatol* 1994;130:476-480.
32. Singh F, Lebwohl MG. Cutaneous T-cell lymphoma treatment using bexarotene and PUVA: A case series. *J Am Acad Dermatol* 2004;51:570-573.
33. Knobler E. Current management strategies for cutaneous T-cell lymphoma. *Clin Dermatol* 2004;22:197-208.
34. Gianotti R, Restano L, Grimalt R, Berti E, Alessi E, Caputo R. Lichen striatus—a chameleon: An histopathological and immunohistological study of forty-one cases. *J Cutan Pathol* 1995;22:18-22.
35. Staricco RG. Lichen striatus: A study of fifteen new cases with special emphasis on the histopathological changes and a review of the literature. *AMA Arch Dermatol* 1959;79:311-324.
36. Holden CA, Berth-Jones J. Eczema, lichenification, prurigo and erythroderma, in Burns T, Breathnach S, Cox N, Griffiths C (eds), *Rook's Textbook of Dermatology,* Vol 1, 7th ed. Oxford, England, Blackwell, 2004, pp 17-55.
37. Rook A, Wilkinson DS. Eczema, lichen simplex and prurigo, in Rook A et al (eds), *Textbook of Dermatology,* Vol 1, 3rd ed. Oxford, England, Blackwell, 1979, pp 337-348.
38. Arnold HL, Odom RB, James WD. *Diseases of the Skin,* 8th ed. Philadelphia, Saunders, 2000, pp 199-249.
39. Patrizi A, Neri I, Fiorentini C, Bonci A, Ricci G. Lichen striatus: Clinical and laboratory features of 115 children. *Pediatr Dermatol* 2004;21:197-204.
40. Hauber K, Rose C, Brocker EB, Hamm H. Lichen striatus: Clinical features and follow-up in 12 patients. *Eur J Dermatol* 2000;10:536-539.
41. Wu T. Lichen striatus-like leukoderma. *J Eur Acad Dermatol Venereol* 1998;10: 152-154.
42. Toda K, Okamoto H, Horio T. Lichen striatus. *Int J Dermatol* 1986;25:584-585.
43. Tilly JJ, Drolet BA, Esterly NB. Lichenoid eruptions in children. *J Am Acad Dermatol* 2004;51:606-624.
44. Relyveld GN, Kingswijk MM, Reitsma JB, Menke HE, Bos JD, Westerhof W. Benzoyl peroxide/clindamycin/ UVA is more effective than fluticasone/UVA in progressive macular hypomelanosis: A randomized study. *J Am Acad Dermatol* 2006;55:836-843.
45. Guillet G, Helenon R, Gauthier Y, Surleve-Bazeille JE, Plantin P, Sassolas B. Progressive macular hypomelanosis of the trunk: Primary acquired hypopigmentation. *J Cutan Pathol* 1988;15:286-289.
46. Borelli D. Cutis trunci variata: Nueva genodermatosis. *Med Cutan Ibero Lat Am* 1987;15:317-319.
47. Westerhof W, et al. *Propionibacterium acnes* and the pathogenesis of progressive macular hypomelanosis. *Arch Dermatol* 2004;140:210-214.
48. Relyveld GN, Menke HE, Westerhof W. Progressive macular hypomelanosis: An overview. *Am J Clin Dermatol* 2007;8:13-19.

CHAPTER 46

Vitiligo

Pearl E Grimes

Key Points

- Vitiligo has an equal incidence in all racial and ethnic groups.
- Given the contrast between the depigmented patched and normal skin tones, the disease is most disfiguring in darker racial and ethnic groups.
- Between 20% and 30% of patients report the disease in first- and second-degree relatives.
- The predominant histologic change is an absence of melanocytes.
- Popular pathogenetic mechanisms for vitiligo include autoimmune, genetic, neural, biochemical, and autocytotoxic causes.
- Vitiligo patients have an increased frequency of other autoimmune disorders, including Hashimoto's thyroiditis, Graves' disease, pernicious anemia, and Addison's disease.
- Baseline laboratory tests should include a comprehensive metabolic panel, thyroid function tests, antinuclear antibody tests, and thyroid peroxidase antibodies.
- Therapeutic objectives should include both stabilization and repigmentation of vitiliginous lesions
- Therapies for limited areas of involvement include topical steroids, topical immunomodulators, calcipotriol, and targeted phototherapy.
- Maximal results are achieved with narrow-band ultraviolet B (UVB) phototherapy for patients with greater than 15–20% body surface areas affected by vitiligo.

DEFINITION

Vitiligo is a relatively common acquired pigmentary disorder characterized by areas of depigmented skin resulting from loss of epidermal melanocytes. Given the stark contrast between the white patches and normal skin, the disease is most disfiguring in darker racial and ethnic groups (Figure 46-1). Vitiligo is one of the most psychologically devastating skin diseases. The psychological effects of this disorder are influenced and exacerbated by societal perceptions of skin disfigurement and irregularities in skin color.[1,2] Patients with vitiligo experience low self esteem, isolation, job discrimination, stigmatization, depression, and embarrassment in social and sexual relationships.[3]

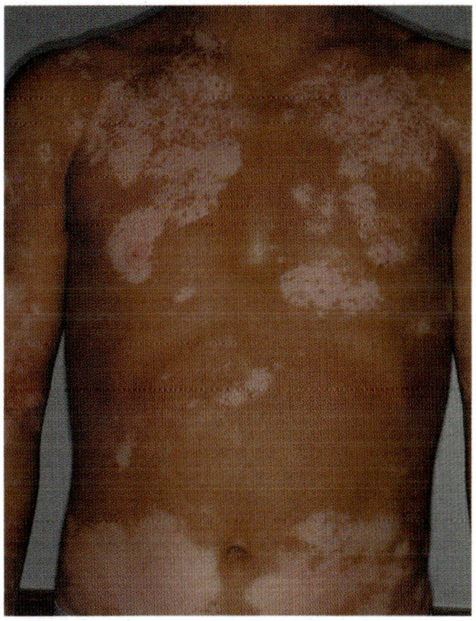

▲ **FIGURE 46-1** Patient with generalized areas of depigmentation. Courtesy of Pearl E Grimes, MD.

EPIDEMIOLOGY AND CLINICAL MANIFESTATIONS

The prevalence of vitiligo varies from 0.1-3% of global populations.[4] Onset may occur at any age, with peak incidence during the second and third decades of life. One-fourth of patients with vitiligo are children. Although females are affected more often than males, the disease shows no racial, ethnic, or socioeconomic predilection. Vitiligo lesions typically are asymptomatic depigmented macules and patches without clinical signs of inflammation, although inflammatory vitiligo with erythematous borders has been reported. Hypopigmented and depigmented lesions may coexist in a vitiligo patient. Occasionally, the depigmented patches are pruritic. Macules of vitiligo frequently begin on sun-exposed or periorificial facial skin and either remain localized or develop on other cutaneous sites. Areas of depigmentation vary in size from a few millimeters to many centimeters, and their borders are usually distinct. Trichome lesions are observed most often in darker-complexioned persons. These lesions are characterized by zones of white, light-brown, and normal skin color. Depigmented hairs are often present in lesional skin and do not always preclude repigmentation of a lesion. In addition, there is a high incidence of premature graying of scalp hair in patients with vitiligo and in their families. Vitiliginous lesions can remain stable or can progress slowly for years. Rarely, patients undergo almost complete spontaneous depigmentation in just a few years.

Vitiligo is classified into different subtypes based on the distribution of skin lesions (Figures 46-1 through 46-3). These subtypes include generalized (vulgaris), acral or acrofacial, localized, and segmental. The generalized pattern is characterized by symmetric depigmented macules or patches occurring in a random distribution. Acral or acrofacial vitiligo consists of depigmented macules confined to the extremities or the face and extremities,

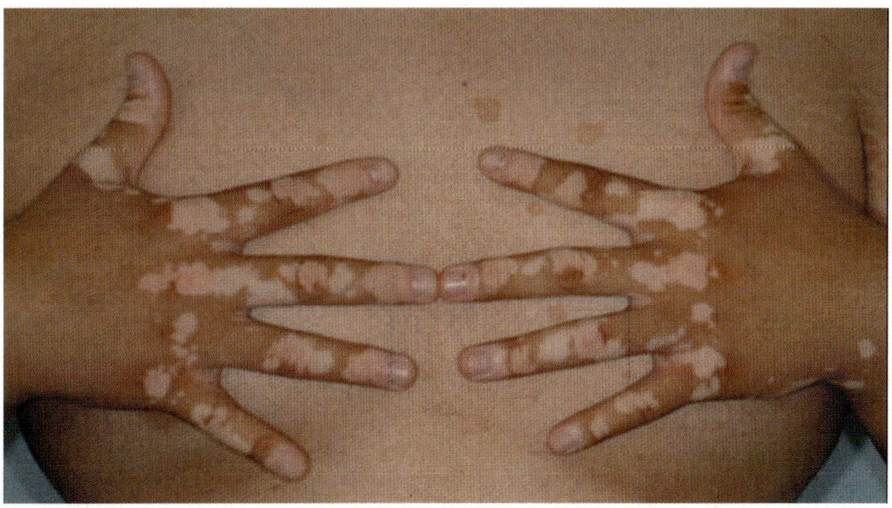

▲ **FIGURE 46-2** Patient with severe involvement of the hands. Courtesy of Pearl E Grimes, MD.

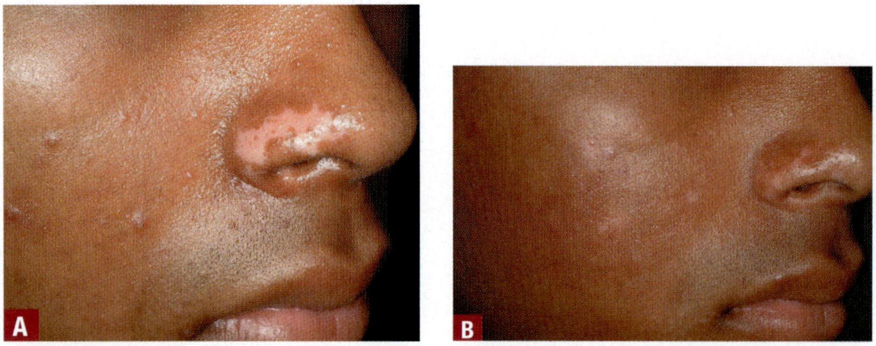

▲ **FIGURE 46-3** *A.* Areas of facial depigmentation. *B.* After 3 months of treatment with tacrolimus. Courtesy of Pearl E Grimes, MD.

respectively. A subcategory of the acrofacial type is the lip-tip variety, in which lesions are confined to the cutaneous lips and distal tips of the digits. The generalized and acrofacial varieties are the most common. Segmental vitiligo occurs in a dermatomal or quasi-dermatomal distribution, most frequently along the distribution of the trigeminal nerve. The areas of depigmentation usually stabilize within a year and rarely spread beyond the affected dermatome. It is the least common subtype of vitiligo. In contrast to other types, it commonly begins in childhood.[5]

Melanocytes of the eye, ear, and leptomeninges also may be involved in vitiligo.

Depigmented areas of the retinal pigment epithelium and choroid have been reported in 39% of patients studied.[6] These asymptomatic lesions did not interfere with visual acuity. However, other studies have reported a significantly lower incidence of ocular abnormalities.[7] Vitiligo is also a manifestation of the Vogt-Koyanagi-Harada syndrome, which is characterized by chronic uveitis, poliosis, alopecia, dysacausia, vitiligo, and signs of meningeal irritation. This syndrome usually begins in the third decade of life, and although no race is spared, the disease tends to be more severe in darker races, especially Asians.

PATHOGENESIS

The predominant finding in the depigmented areas of vitiligo is an absence of epidermal melanocytes.[8] The precise cause of the loss of these epidermal melanocytes is unknown. Light microscopic and ultrastructural studies have revealed vacuolar degeneration of basal and parabasal keratinocytes and dermal lymphohistiocytic infiltrates.[9,10] Genetic, autoimmune, neural, biochemical, oxidative stress, autocytotoxic, viral infection, and melanocyte detachment mechanisms have been proposed to explain the pathogenesis of vitiligo. However, the autoimmune hypothesis remains the most well supported by current data.[8]

Genetic studies support a non-mendelian inheritance pattern for vitiligo and suggest that vitiligo is a multifactorial, polygenic disorder.[11–13] Between 20% and 30% of patients report vitiligo in first- and second-degree relatives. The disease has been associated with specific genetic polymorphisms, such as HLA-DR4, -Dw7, -DR7, -DR1, -B13, -Cw6, -DR53, and -A19; however, haplotypes may vary considerably within the population studied.[11,12] Recently, a genome-wide linkage scan was performed in 71 white multiplex families with vitiligo.[13] Linkage was assessed by a multipoint nonparametric linkage analysis. *AIS1* located on chromosome 1p31 showed highly significant linkage, suggesting that it is a major susceptibility locus in Caucasians. Additional signals on chromosomes 1, 7, 8, 11, 19, and 22 have met genome criteria for suggestive linkage. Genetic studies also vary with the population being evaluated. Studies in Chinese families show linkage evidence to chromosome 4q13-q21, in contrast to data in Caucasian families.[14] These findings support significant genetic heterogeneity for vitiligo in different racial and ethnic populations. Other candidate genes reported to affect vitiligo susceptibility include the catalase gene, *VIT1*, chromosome 2p16, and the guanosine triphosphate cyclohydrolase I gene.[8,11,12] Recently, the *NALP1* gene on chromosome 17p13 was identified as the principal regulator of the innate immune system. The *NALP1* gene encodes the NACHT leucine-rich repeat protein 1, which contributes to a group of epidemiologically associated autoimmune diseases, including vitiligo.[15]

Cytomegalovirus DNA has been demonstrated in the involved and uninvolved skin of patients with vitiligo. No viral DNA was detected in the normal skin for matched control subjects.[16] Herpes simplex viral infection has been reported to trigger vitiligo in the Smith chicken animal model for vitiligo.[17] These findings suggest that in some cases vitiligo may be triggered by a viral infection.

The neural theory is supported by several clinical, biochemical, and ultrastructural observations.[18] These observations include the occurrence of segmental vitiligo; the demonstration of lesional autonomic dysfunction, such as increased sweating; and the demonstration of nerve ending-melanocyte contact. The last observation is rare in normal skin.

Several studies suggest that oxidative stress may be the initial event in the destruction of melanocytes.[19,20] Defective recycling of tetrahydrobiopterin, increased production of hydrogen peroxide, and decreased catalase have been demonstrated in the affected skin of patients with vitiligo.[19,20] In addition, lesional catecholamine biosynthesis and release are increased. Peripheral blood studies of patients with vitiligo have shown low catalase and glutathione levels, whereas superoxide dismutase and xanthine oxidase are elevated.[21] Oxidative stress may contribute to melanocyte destruction in susceptible individuals.

The self-destruction hypothesis proposes that melanocytes may be destroyed by phenolic compounds formed during the synthesis of melanin.[18] In vivo and in vitro studies have demonstrated the destruction of melanocytes by phenols and catechols. In addition, industrial workers who are exposed to catechols and phenols may develop depigmented patches.

A number of environmentally ubiquitious compounds containing catechols, phenols, and sulfhydryls can induce hypopigmentation, depigmentation, or both. These compounds are encountered most often in industrial chemicals and cleaning agents. Possible mechanisms for altered pigment production by these compounds include melanocyte destruction via free-radical formation, inhibition of tyrosinase activity, and interference with the production or transfer of melanosomes.[21]

Substantial new data further implicate immune mechanisms in the pathogenesis of vitiligo and suggest that vitiligo shares common linkages with other autoimmune diseases. Historically, vitiligo has been reported in association with a number of autoimmune endocrinopathies and diseases. Thyroid disorders, in particular Hashimoto's thyroiditis and Graves' disease, are associated most commonly with vitiligo.[5] Other associated disorders include diabetes mellitus, alopecia areata, pernicious anemia, rheumatoid arthritis, autoimmune polyglandular syndrome, and psoriasis.[22–24] In a recent survey of 2624 vitiligo probands in North America and the United Kingdom, a significant increase in six autoimmune diseases was reported in vitiligo probands and first-degree relatives.[5] These diseases included vitiligo, thyroid disease (predominantly hypothyroidism), pernicious anemia, Addison's disease, systemic lupus erythematosus, and inflammatory bowel disease.

Many humoral and cell-mediated immune aberrations have been reported in vitiligo patients. Numerous studies have documented an increased frequency of organ-specific autoantibodies in these patients.[25,26] Antithyroid (thyroglobulin, thyroid microsomal, and thyroid peroxidase), gastric parietal cell, and antinuclear antibodies are the most commonly associated autoantibodies that have been documented. Vitiligo patients with organ-specific autoantibodies, unassociated with overt autoimmune disease, have an increased risk of developing subclinical or overt autoimmune disease.[25] The presence of antibodies to surface and cytoplasmic melanocyte antigens in the sera of vitiligo patients lends additional support for the autoimmune pathogenesis for this disease.[27–29] These antibodies can induce the destruction of melanocytes grown in culture by complement-mediated lysis and antibody-dependent cellular cytotoxicity.[27,28] In addition, melanocyte antibodies, when passively administered to nude mice grafted with human skin, have a destructive effect on melanocytes within the skin graft.[30] Less commonly, antibodies targeting tyrosinase, tyrosinase-related proteins 1 and 2, Pmel17 (glycoprotein 100), and melanin-concentrating hormone 1 (MCHR1) also have been reported in vitiligo patients.[29] The transcription factors SOX9 and SOX10 have been identified as melanocytic autoantigens in autoimmune polyendocrine syndrome and idiopathic vitiligo.[31]

Recent studies provide additional insights into the role of cell-mediated immunity in the destruction of melanocytes, suggesting that cytotoxic T-lymphocytes may play a significant role in melanocyte destruction in vitiligo.[32] Numerous activated cytotoxic T-lymphocytes have been reported in the perilesional area of the vitiliginous skin, often in apposition to disappearing melanocytes.[33] These infiltrating lymphocytes are predominantly cytotoxic CD8+ lymphocytes that express skin homing receptors (i.e., CLA+). In addition, other studies have demonstrated the presence of increased numbers of circulating CD8+ cytotoxic lymphocytes that are reactive to the melanosomal proteins melanA/MART-1, gp100, and tyrosinase in HLA-A2-positive patients with vitiligo.[34–36]

Several investigations also have addressed the role of peripheral blood and lesional cytokine expression in the pathogenesis of vitiligo. Elevated levels of serum soluble interleukin 2 (IL-2) receptor, IL-6, IL-8, and elevated lesional tissue levels of IL-2 have been reported in vitiligo patients.[37–39] These findings correlate with an increased level of T-cell activation. In biopsies of lesional, perilesional, and healthy skin, significantly lower levels of expression of granulocyte colony-stimulating factor and stem cell factor were reported in vitiliginous skin, whereas the expression of IL-6 and tumor necrosis factor α (TNF-α) were increased in lesional skin.[40] Granulocyte colony-stimulating factor, basic fibroblast growth factor, and stem cell factor are paracrine cytokines secreted by keratinocytes. These paracrine cytokines stimulate melanogenesis and melanocyte proliferation, whereas IL-6 and TNF-α inhibit melanocyte proliferation and melanogenesis.[41] Together these findings suggest that keratinocyte function is also impaired in vitiliginous skin.

A subsequent report demonstrated increased expression of TNF-α and interferon-γ in the lesional and adjacent healthy skin of patients with vitiligo compared with the skin of matched controls.[42] After 6 months of treatment with twice-daily application of tacrolimus, a topical immunomodulator, there was a significant depression in the level of TNF-α expression in the lesional and adjacent healthy skin compared with baseline. This observation suggests that suppression of TNF-α may be associated with repigmentation of vitiliginous lesions.[42]

Whether these immunologic aberrations are primary or secondary events in the destruction of melanocytes in vitiligo remains controversial. However, regardless of which event is primary, many of the most effective therapies for vitiligo work via suppression or modulation of the immune response.

DIFFERENTIAL DIAGNOSIS

Other disorders characterized by depigmentation occasionally may mimic vitiligo clinically.[3] These include piebaldism, nevus depigmentosus, nevus anemicus, postinflammatory depigmentation or hypopigmentation, pityriasis alba, tinea versicolor, discoid lupus erythematosus, scleroderma, hypopigmented mycosis fungoides, and sarcoidosis. Therefore, in some instances, a skin biopsy may be necessary to substantiate a diagnosis of vitiligo.

LABORATORY EVALUATION

In view of the association of vitiligo with myriad other autoimmune diseases, the routine baseline evaluation of a patient should include a thorough history and physical examination. Recommended laboratory tests include a complete blood count, erythrocyte sedimentation rate, comprehensive metabolic panel (including liver function tests), and autoantibody tests (e.g., antinuclear antibody, thyroid peroxidase, and parietal cell antibodies).

TREATMENT

Therapeutic objectives for vitiligo should include both stabilization of the disease and repigementation of vitiliginous skin lesions. Repigmentation can be accomplished medically or, in patients with localized stable lesions, surgically. The choice of repigmentation therapies should be predicated on the age of the patient, body surface area affected (severity), and activity or progression of the disease. Many studies document enhanced repigmentation in darker racial and ethnic groups. The disease can be divided into four stages: limited (<10% involvement), moderate (10–25% involvement), moderately severe (26–50% involvement), and severe (>50% involvement).[3]

Commonly used medical therapies for vitiligo include topical and systemic steroids, narrow-band ultraviolet phototherapy, psoralen with ultraviolet A (PUVA), targeted phototherapy, nutritional vitamin supplementation, immunomodulators, and calcipotriol[22,23,43] (Table 46-1). Given the low side-effect profile of narrow-band UVB and targeted

TABLE 46-1
Therapeutic Approaches for Vitiligo

LOCALIZED/LIMITED	MODERATE /SEVERE	RECALCITRANT
Topical steroids	Narrow-band UVB	*Severe*
Topical PUVA	Oral PUVA	Depigmentation
PUVAsol	Systemic steroids	Monobenzone
Topical immunomodulators	Antioxidants/vitamins	
Tacrolimus		*Localized*
Pimecrolimus		Surgical
Targeted phototherapy		Sheet grafts
Calcipotriol		Autologous punch grafts
Antioxidants/vitamins		Split-thickness grafts
		Melanocyte transplants
		Cocultured epidermis

phototherapy, topical and systemic psoralen photochemotherapy is used less commonly.[44]

Steroids

Middle- to high-potency steroids are indicated in patients with limited involvement.[3,22,43] Low-potency topical steroids are usually ineffective. Topical middle- to high-potency steroids can be used safely for 2–3 months and then interrupted for 1 month or tapered to low-potency preparations. Patients must be monitored closely for topical steroid side effects, which include skin atrophy, telangiectasias, hypertrichosis, and acneiform eruptions. Since the introduction of topical immunomodulators (e.g., tacrolimus and pimecrolimus), topical steroids are used less often in vitiligo patients.

A short course of oral prednisone for 1–2 weeks or intramuscular triamcinolone acetonide injections, 40 mg/month for 2–3 months, is often extremely helpful for stabilizing rapidly progressive vitiligo. However, prolonged use of systemic steroids is not indicated.

Topical Immunomodulators

Topical immunomodulatory agents such as tacrolimus and pimecrolimus offer several advantages in treating vitiligo. These agents are extremely well tolerated in children and adults, and they can be used for longer periods without evidence of atrophy or telangiectasias, the common complications associated with long-term steroid use. This is a significant advantage in treating a chronic disease such as vitiligo. Tacrolimus is a topical immunomodulatory agent that affects T-cell and mast cell functions by binding to cytoplasmic immunophilins and by inactivating calcineurin.[45,46] Tacrolimus inhibits the synthesis and release of proinflammatory cytokines and vasoactive mediators from basophils and mast cells.[46] Multiple studies have demonstrated its efficacy and safety for the treatment of atopic dermatitis. The efficacy of tacrolimus for repigmentation of vitiligo was reported initially in a series of six patients with generalized vitiligo.[47] Five of the six patients in this study achieved 50–100% repigmentation of their affected sites (Figure 46-4). A subsequent 24-week study assessed the efficacy and safety of tacrolimus ointment in 23 patients with generalized vitiligo.[42] Nineteen patients completed the study. At 24 weeks, 89% of patients achieved varying levels of repigmentation, and there was a statistically significant decrease in overall disease severity scores. Maximal repigmentation was observed on the face and neck areas (the areas with greater sun exposure), with 68% of patients achieving greater than 75% repigmentation. Adverse events were minimal throughout the study. Other studies have corroborated these results.[48–51]

Another double-blind randomized trial compared the efficacy of tacrolimus versus clobetasol, a topical steroid, for the treatment of childhood vitiligo.[49] Two symmetric lesions were treated on each of the 20 patients, one with tacrolimus 0.1% and the other with 0.05% clobetasol ointment. The mean percentage repigmentation for the tacrolimus-treated lesions was 41% versus 49% for the clobetasol-treated lesions. However, three patients experienced steroid-induced atrophy at their sites treated with clobetasol.

Pimecrolimus, which has a mechanism of action similar to tacrolimus, also can induce repigmentation of vitiliginous skin lesions.[51] The efficacy of pimecrolimus and clobetasol was compared in a right/left prospective study treating symmetric lesions. The two agents had comparable rates of repigmentation.[52] As with tacrolimus, pimecrolimus induces maximal repigmentation in sun-exposed areas.

An increased risk for skin cancer among transplant recipients treated with cyclosporine[53] or systemically administered tacrolimus is well recognized given the immunosuppresssion induced by such agents.[54] The use of topical tacrolimus, however, has not been associated with systemic immunosuppression or an increased risk for skin and other malignancies in clinical studies.[55,56] However, in light of reports documenting an increase in skin cancers and lymphomas in animal models, tacrolimus and pimecrolimus currently have black box labels.[57] These animal studies should be interpreted with caution, given the massive dosing of drug used in animal protocols. Labeling recommends that these agents should not be used in combination with ultraviolet light therapy. Appropriate photoprotective precautions should be taken by patients.

Narrow-Band UVB

Historically, topical and systemic psoralen photochemotherapy with UVA (PUVA) was the "gold standard" for repigmenting vitiliginous skin lesions, but PUVA-induced repigmentation rates varied considerably.[43,44] In addition, adverse effects could be substantial,

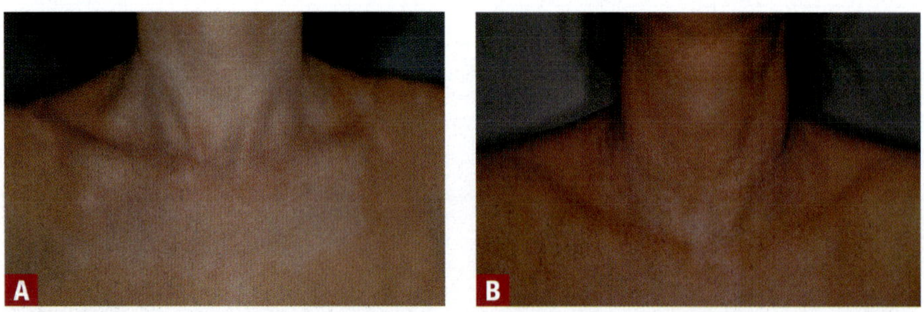

▲ **FIGURE 46-4** ***A.*** A patient with depigmented patches of the neck and chest. ***B.*** After 30 narrow-band UV phototherapy treatments. Courtesy of Pearl E Grimes, MD.

including phototoxicity and gastrointestinal irritation. Oral PUVA also required ocular protection for 12–24 hours following treatment.

Given the comparable efficacy of narrow-band UVB phototherapy and its lack of systemic adverse effects, it has emerged as the initial treatment of choice for patients with moderate to severe disease. Narrow-band UVB involves the use of UV lamps with a peak emission around 311 nm.[58] These shorter wavelengths provide higher energy fluences and induce less cutaneous erythema. Narrow-band UVB induces local immunosuppression, stimulates the production of melanocyte-stimulating hormone, and increases melanocyte proliferation and melanogenesis. The first major study of narrow-band UVB in patients with vitiligo compared the efficacy of narrow-band UVB with that of topical PUVA.[59] Significantly enhanced repigmentation was achieved in patients treated with narrow-band UVB compared with those treated with topical PUVA. Adverse effects were minimal in the group of patients treated with narrow-band UVB in contrast with the increased phototoxicity observed in the patients treated with topical PUVA.

Subsequent studies have further confirmed the efficacy of narrow-band UVB phototherapy for vitiligo[60–64] (Figure 46-5). The efficacy of narrow-band UVB was assessed recently in 60 Asian patients with recalcitrant vitiligo.[63] Forty-two percent of the patients achieved greater than 50% repigmentation of lesions on the face, trunk, arms, and legs. Narrow-band UVB also was used in an open-label study to treat 51 children with generalized vitilgo. Fifty-three percent of the participants achieved greater than 75% repigmentation, and 18% had less than 25% repigmentation. Recent studies document enhanced repigmentation with narrow-ban UVB compared with PUVA.[65]

The major advantages of narrow-band UVB include an established safety profile in both children and adults and lack of systemic toxicity. Narrow-band UVB does not require eye protection beyond treatment exposure time. No studies have documented an increase in squamous cell carcinomas, basal cell cancers, or malignant melanomas in vitiligo patients treated with either PUVA or narrow-band UVB. This contrasts with reports documenting an increase in squamous cell carcinomas and melanomas in psoriasis patients treated with PUVA.[66]

Recently, a functional color yeast assay demonstrated overexpression of a functioning wild-type p53 protein in both the depigmented and healthy pigmented epidermis of patients with vitiligo compared with healthy controls.[67] This wild-type p53 overexpression may explain the possible low risk of skin cancers in patients with vitiligo. However, long-term follow-up studies are needed to fully assess the risks of narrow-band UVB.

Targeted Phototherapy

Targeted phototherapy systems also have demonstrated improved efficacy for the treatment of localized vitiligo.[68] These units deliver high-intensity light only to the affected areas while avoiding exposure of the healthy skin and lowering the cumulative UVB dose. In 1999, the effectiveness of UVB radiation microtherapy was first reported for repigmentation of segmental vitiligo in a small series of eight patients.[69] Five of these patients achieved greater than 75% repigmentation.

Subsequent investigations also have documented the benefits of excimer laser systems and targeted phototherapy units.[70–73] The excimer laser produces monochromatic radiation at a wavelength of 308 nm. An open-label pilot investigation used the excimer laser to treat 29 affected areas of vitiligo in 18 patients.[70] In this study, lesions were treated three times weekly for a maximum of 12 treatments. Twenty-three vitiliginous areas on 12 patients received at least six treatments. Varying degrees of repigmentation were reported in 57% of the treated areas. Of the 11 affected areas that received all 12 treatments, 87% demonstrated some repigmentation. A newly developed unit with a larger irradiation field was used recently on 37 patients.[74] Compared with other targeted units with small irradiation fields (<3 cm), this unit has an irradiation field of 36 by 14 cm, allowing treatment of larger areas. Forty-three percent of patients treated with this unit had 50-75% repigmentation of their lesions, and 49% of patients had 76–100% repigmentation.

Targeted phototherapy systems also can work synergistically with topical therapies. Several studies have assessed the efficacy of combination treatment with an excimer laser and tacrolimus ointment. In a study of eight patients with vitiligo, 24 symmetric vitiliginous areas were treated with the excimer laser three times per week for a total of 24 treatments.[72] Topical tacrolimus ointment or placebo was applied to randomized affected areas twice daily throughout the length of the trial. Fifty percent of the areas treated with the combination excimer laser and topical tacrolimus achieved 75% or greater repigmentation compared with 20% for the placebo group. Subsequently, a randomized, prospective right/left comparison study was performed in 14 patients with similar results.[73] The efficacy of excimer laser monotherapy also has been compared with treatment with the excimer laser in combination with topical methoxsalen. Nine patients were treated with the excimer laser as monotherapy compared with 11 patients who were treated with the excimer laser in combination with topical 8-methoxypsoralen 0.001%.[68] A greater degree of repigmentation occurred in the patients treated

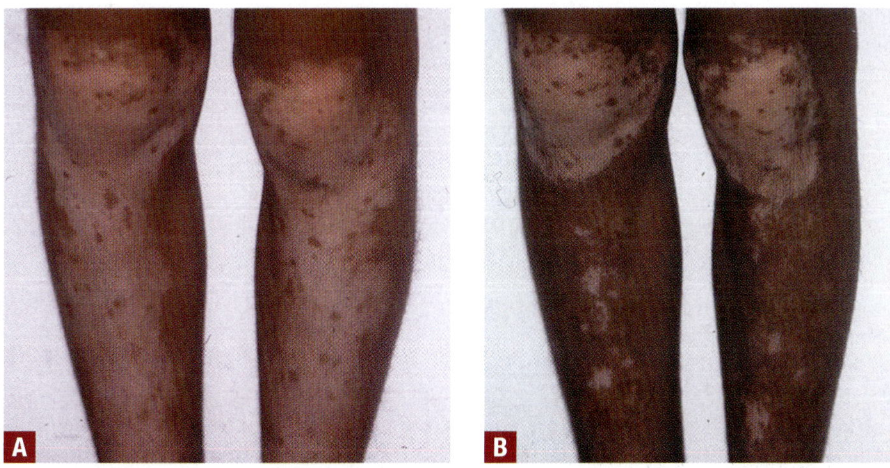

▲ **FIGURE 46-5** A child with depigmented lesions of the lower extremities. ***A.*** Before treatment with narrow-band UVB. ***B.*** After 26 treatments. Courtesy of Pearl E Grimes, MD.

with the combination regimen compared with excimer laser monotherapy. This difference was statistically significant.

Maximal results are achieved with the excimer laser when patients are treated two or three times weekly. Optimal repigmentation is achieved on the face, neck, and trunk areas.[75,76]

Vitamins

Preliminary open-label studies have documented stabilization and repigmentation in vitiligo patients treated with high-dose vitamin supplementation, including daily doses of ascorbic acid (1000 mg), vitamin B_{12} (1000 μg), and folic acid (1–5 mg).

CALCIPOTRIOL Calcipotriol is a synthetic analogue of vitamin D_3. Vitamin D_3 binds to vitamin D receptors in the skin, affecting melanocyte and keratinocyte growth and differentiation. It also inhibits T-cell activation.[77] Melanocytes are thought to express 1-α-dihydroxy vitamin D_3 receptors, which may have a role in stimulating melanogenesis. Several studies have assessed the efficacy of calcipotriol in combination with UV light therapy in patients with vitiligo.[77–82] Some have shown that when used in combination with UV light exposure, calcipotriol is well tolerated and efficacious in treating both children and adults with vitiligo.[45,66] Recently, the efficacy of calcipotriol 0.05% ointment was reported in combination with clobetasol in a series of 12 patients with vitiligo.[80] Clobetasol was used in the morning, and calcipotriene was used in the evening.[70] Eighty-three percent of patients responded to treatment with an average 95% repigmentation of affected areas.

Depigmentation

Since the 1950s, monobenzylether of hydroquinone (MBEH, or monobenzene) has been used as a depigmenting agent for patients with extensive vitiligo. In general, MBEH causes permanent destruction of melanocytes and induces depigmentation locally and remotely from the sites of application. Hence the use of MBEH for other disorders of pigmentation is contraindicated.

Depigmentation is a viable therapeutic alternative in patients with greater than 50% cutaneous depigmentation who have demonstrated recalcitrance to repigmentation or in patients with extensive vitiligo who have no desire to undergo repigmentation therapies.[3] The major side effects of MBEH therapy are dermatitis and pruritus, which usually respond to topical and systemic steroids. Other side effects include severe xerosis, alopecia, and premature graying.

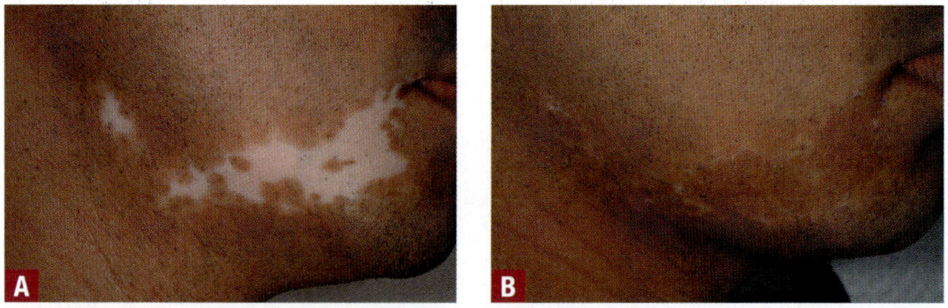

▲ **FIGURE 46-6** A young man with segmental vitiligo. ***A.*** Before grafting. ***B.*** Three months after autologous 1-mm punch grafting. Courtesy of Pearl E Grimes, MD.

Surgery

Surgical therapies have been used for vitiligo for the past 25 years. Recently, substantial advances have been made in the techniques and protocols for harvesting and transplanting melanocytes. Surgical therapies remain viable options for patients with localized areas that have failed medical intervention.[83-86] The major advantage of transplantation procedures is the transfer of a reservoir of healthy melanocytes to vitiliginous skin for proliferation and migration into areas of depigmentation. Transplantation procedures are contraindicated for patients with a history of hypertrophic scars or keloids.

Surgical therapies include autologous suction-blister grafts, punch grafts, split-thickness grafts, autologous melanocyte cultures, cultured epidermal suspensions, and single-hair grafts (Figure 46-6). A systematic review of autologous transplantation methods for vitiligo involved data synthesis of 39 patient series[83] and concluded that maximal repigmentation occurred in patients treated with split-thickness grafting and epidermal blister grafting. Both treatment groups achieved success rates of 90% repigmentation. Other studies have reported the benefits of transplantation of autologous melanocyte cultures and epidermal suspensions containing both melanocytes and keratinocytes.[84,85]

One hundred and seventeen patients were included in a study assessing the influences of age, site of lesion, and type of disease on transplantation outcomes.[86] In this series, the best results were achieved for patients younger than age 20 years and patients with segmental vitiligo. The grafting site did not significantly affect outcome. In most instances, tattooing or micropigmentation should be avoided given the risk of koebnerization and oxidation of tattoo pigment causing further dyschromia.

REFERENCES

1. Robins A. *Biological Perspectives on Human Pigmentation*. Cambridge, England, Cambridge University Press, 1991.
2. Grimes PE. Disorders of pigmentation, in Dale DC, Federman DD (eds), *ACP Medicine*. New York, WebMD Scientific American Medicine, 2003, pp 526-534.
3. Porter J. The psychological effects of vitiligo: Response to impaired appearance, in Hann SK, Nordlund JJ (eds), *Vitiligo*. Oxford, England, Blackwell Science, 2000, pp 97-100.
4. Alkhateeb A, Fain PR, Thody A, et al. Epidemiology of vitiligo and associated autoimmune diseases in Caucasian probands and their families. *Pigment Cell Res* 2003;16:208-214.
5. Grimes PE, Billips M. Childhood vitiligo: Clinical spectrum and therapeutic approaches, in Hann SK, Nordlund JJ (eds), *Vitiligo*. Oxford, England, Blackwell Science, 2000, pp 61-70.
6. Albert DM, Wagoner MD, Pruett RC, et al. Vitiligo and disorders of the retinal pigment epithelium. *Br J Ophthalmol* 1983; 67:153-156.
7. Cowan CL, Halder RM, Grimes PE, et al. Ocular disturbances in vitiligo. *J Am Acad Dermatol* 1986;15:17-24.
8. Grimes PE. New insights and new therapies in vitiligo. *JAMA* 2005;293:730-735.
9. Montes LF, Abulafia J, Wilborn WH, et al. Value of histopathology in vitiligo. *Int J Dermatol* 2003;42:57-61.
10. Le Poole CI, Das PK. Microscopic changes in vitiligo. *Clin Dermatol* 1997;15: 863-873.
11. Majumder PP, Das SK, Li CC. A genetical model for vitiligo. *Am J Hum Genet* 1998; 43:119-125.
12. Nath SK, Majumder PP, Nordlund JJ. Genetic epidemiology of vitiligo: Multilocus recessivity cross-validated. *Am J Hum Genet* 1994;55:981-990.
13. Fain PR, Gowan K, LaBerge GS, et al. A genomewide screen for generalized vitiligo. *Pigment Cell Res* 2003;72:1560-1564.

14. Chen JJ, Huang W, Gui JP, et al. A novel linkage to generalized vitiligo on 4q13-q21 identified in a genomewide linkage analysis of Chinese families. *Am J Hum Genet* 2005;76:1057-1056.
15. Jin Y, Mailoux CM, Gowan K, et al. *NALP1* in vitiligo-associated multiple autoimmune disease. *N Engl J Med*. 2007; 356:1216-1225.
16. Grimes PE, Sevall JS, Vojdani A. Cytomegalovirus DNA identified in skin biopsy specimens of patients with vitiligo. *J Am Acd Dermatol* 1996;35:21-26.
17. Erf GF, Bersi TK, Wang X, et al. Herpes virus connection in the expression of autoimmune vitiligo in Smyth line chickens. *Pigment Cell Res* 2001;14: 40-46.
18. Gauthier Y, Andre MC, Taieb A. A critical appraisal of vitiligo etiologic theories: Is melanocyte loss a melanocytorrhagy? *Pigment Cell Res* 2003;16:322-332.
19. Dell'Anna M, Maresca V, Briganti S, et al. Mitochondrial impairment in peripheral blood mononuclear cells during the active phase of vitiligo. *J Invest Dermatol* 2001;117:908.
20. Picardo M, Grammatico P, Roccella F, et al. Imbalance in the antioxidant pool in melanoma cells and normal melanocytes from patients with melanoma. *J Invest Dermatol* 1996;107:322.
21. Dell'Anna ML, Picardo M. A review and a new hypothesis for non-immunological pathogenetic mechanisms in vitiligo. *Pigment Cell Res* 2006;10:1-6.
22. Njoo MD, Westerhof W. Vitiligo: pathogenesis and treatment. *Am J Clin Dermatol* 2001;2:167-181.
23. Kovacs SO. Vitiligo. *J Am Acad Dermatol* 1998;38:647-666.
24. Boissy RE, Nordlund JJ. Molecular basis of congenital hypopigmentary disorders in humans: A review. *Pigment Cell Res* 1997; 10:12-24.
25. Betterle C, Caretto A, de Zio A, et al. Incidence and significance of organ-specific autoimmune disorders (clinical, latent, or only autoantibodies) in patients with vitiligo. *Dermatologica* 1985;171: 419-423.
26. Grimes PE, Halder RM, Jones C, et al. Autoantibodies and their clinical significance in a black vitiligo population. *Arch Dermatol*1983;119:300-303.
27. Naughton Gk, Eisinger M, Bystryn JC. Detection of antibodies to melanocytes in vitiligo by specific immunoprecipitation. *J Invest Dermatol* 1983;81:540-542.
28. Norris DA, Kissinger RM, Naughton GM, Bystryn JC. Evidence for immunologic mechanisms in human vitiligo. *J Invest Dermatol* 1988;90:783-789.
29. Ongenae K, Van Geel N, Naeyaert JM. Evidence for an autoimmune pathogenesis of vitiligo. *Pigment Cell Res* 2003;16: 90-100.
30. Gilhar A, Pillar T, Eidelman S, Etzioni A. Vitiligo and idiopathic guttate hypomelanosis. *Arch Dermatol* 1989;125:1363-1366.
31. Hedstrand H, Ekwall O, Olsson MJ, et al. The transcription factors SOX9 and SOX10 are vitiligo autoantigens in autoimmune polyendocrine syndrome type I. *J Biol Chem* 2001;276:35390-35395.
32. Ghoneum M, Grimes PE, Gill G, Kelly AP. Natural cell-mediated cytotoxicity in vitiligo. *J Am Acad Dermatol* 1987;17: 600-605.
33. Ogg GS, Rod Dunbar P, Romero P, et al. High frequency of skin-homing melanocyte specific cytotoxic T lympho cytes in autoimmune vitiligo. *J Exp Med* 1998;188:1203-1208.
34. Lang KS, Caroli CC, Muhm A, et al. HLA-A2 restricted, melanocyte-specific CD8(+) T lymphocytes detected in vitiligo patients are related to disease activity and are predominantly directed against melanA/MART1. *J Invest Dermatol* 2001;116:891-897.
35. Palmero B, Campanelli R, Garbelli S, et al. Specific cytotoxic T lymphocyte responses against melan-A/MART1, tyrosinase and gp100 in vitiligo by the use of major histocompatibility complex/peptide tetramers: The role of cellular immunity in the etiopathogenesis of vitiligo. *J Invest Dermatol* 2001;117:326-332.
36. Mandelcorn-Monson RL, Shear NH, Yau E, et al. Cytotoxic T lymphocyte reactivity to gp100, melanA/MART1, and tyrosinase, in HLA-A2-positive vitiligo patients. *J Invest Dermatol* 2003;121:550-556.
37. Yu HS, Chang KL, Yu CL, et al. Alterations in IL-6, IL-8, GM-CSF, TNF-α, and IFN-λ release by peripheral mononuclear cells in patients with active vitiligo. *J Invest Dermatol* 1997;108:527-529.
38. Honda Y, Okubo Y, Koga M. Relationship between levels of soluble interleukin-2 receptors and the types of activity of vitiligo. *J Dermatol* 1997,24.561-563.
39. Caixa T, Hongwen F, Xiran L. Levels of soluble interleukin-2-receptor in the sera and skin tissue fluids of patients with vitiligo. *J Dermatol Sci* 1999;21: 59-62.
40. Moretti S, Spallanzani A, Amato L, et al. New insights into the pathogenesis of vitiligo: Imbalance of epidermal cytokines at sites of lesions. *Pigment Cell Res* 2002;15: 87-92.
41. Imokawa G. Autocrine and paracrine regulation of melanocytes in human skin and in pigmentary disoders. *Pigment Cell Res* 2004;17:96-100.
42. Grimes PE, Morris R, Avaniss-Aghajani E, et al. Topical tacrolimus therapy for vitiligo: Therapeutic responses and skin messenger RNA expression of proinflammatory cytokines. *J Am Acad Dermatol* 2004;51:51-62.
43. Grime PE. Vitiligo: An overview of therapeutic approaches. *Dermatol Clin* 1993;11: 325-338.
44. Grimes PE. Psoralen for photochemotherapy for vitiligo. *Clin Dermatol* 1997;15:921.
45. Tharp MD. Calcineurin inhibitors. *Dermatol Ther* 2002;15:325-332.
46. Kang S, Lucky AW, Pariser D, et al. Tacrolimus ointment study group: Long-term safety and efficacy of tacrolimus ointment for the treatment of atopic dermatitis in children. *J Am Acad Dermatol* 2001;44:S58-S64.
47. Grimes PE, Soriano T, Dytoc MT. topical tacrolimus for repigmentation of vitiligo. *J Am Acad Dermatol* 2002;47:789-791.
48. Tanghetti EA. Tacrolimus ointment 0.1% produces repigmentation in patients with vitiligo: Results of a prospective patient series. *Cutis* 2003;71:158-162.
49. Lepe V, Moncada B, Castanedo-Cazares JP, et al. A double-blind randomized trial of 0.1% tacrolimus vs 0.05% clobetasol for the treatment of childhood vitiligo. *Arch Dermatol* 2003;139:581-585.
50. Travis LB, Weinberg JM, Silverberg NB. Succesful treatment of vitiligo with 0.1% tacrolimus ointment. *Arch Dermatol* 2003; 139:571-574.
51. Mayoral FA, Gonzalez C, Shah NS, Arciniegas C. Repigmentation of vitiligo with pimecrolimus cream: A case report. *Dermatology* 2003;207:322-323.
52. Coskun B, Saral Y, Turgut D. Topical 0.05% clobetasol propionate versus 1% pimecrolimus ointment in vitiligo. *Eur J Dermatol* 2005;15:88-91.
53. Tremblay F, Fernandes M, Habbab F, et al. Malignancy after renal transplantation: Incidence and role of type of immunosuppression. *Ann Surg Oncol* 2002; 9:785-788.
54. Woodle ES, Thistlethwaite JR, Gordon JH, et al. A multicenter trial of FK506 (tacrolimus) therapy in refractory acute renal allograft rejection. *Transplantation* 1996;62:594-599.
55. Arellano FM, Wentworth CE, Arana A, et al. Risk of lymphoma following exposure to calcineurin inhibitors and topical steroids in patients with atopic dermatitis. *J Invest Dermatol* 2007;127:8-16
56. Thaci D, Salgo R. The topical calcineurin inhibitor pimecrolimus in atopic dermatitis: A safety update. *Acta Dermatolvenerol Alp Paronica Adriat* 2007;16:60-62.
57. Ormerod AD. Topical tacrolimus and pimecrolimus and the risk of cancer: How much cause for concern. *Br J Dermatol* 2005;153:701-705.
58. Parrish JA, Jaenicke KF. Action spectrum for phototherapy of psoriasis. *J Invest Dermatol* 1981;76:359-362.
59. Westerhof W, Nieuweboer-Krobotova L. Treatment of vitiligo with UV-B radiation vs topical psoralen plus UV-A. *Arch Dermatol* 1997;133:1525-1528.
60. Njoo MD, Spuls PL, Bos JD, et al. Nonsurgical repigmentation therapies in vitiligo: Meta-anlaysis of the literature. *Arch Dermatol* 1998;134:1532-1540.
61. Njoo MD, Bos JD, Westerhof W. Treatment of generalized vitiligo in children with narrow-band (TL-01) UVB radiation therapy. *J Am Acad Dermatol* 2000;42:245-253.
62. Tijoe MJ, Gerritsen MJD, Juhlin L, van de Kerkhof PC. Treatment of vitiligo vulgaris with narrow band UVB (311 nm) for one year and the effect of addition of folic acid and vitamin B_{12}. *Acta Dermatol Venereol* 2002;82:369-372.
63. Natta R, Somsak T, Wisuttida T, Laor L. Narrowband ultraviolet B radiation therapy for recalcitrant vitiligo in Asians. *J Am Acad Dermatol* 2003;49:473-476.
64. Chen GY, Hsu M, Tai HK, et al. Narrowband UVB treatment of vitiligo in Chinese. *J Dermatol* 2005;32:793-800.
65. Bhatnagar A, Kanwar AJ, Parsad D, De D. Psoralen and ultraviolet A and narrow-band ultraviolet B in inducing stability in vitiligo, assessed by vitiligo disease activity score: An open prospective comparative study. *J Eur Acad Dermatol Venereol* 2007;21:1381-1385.
66. Nijsten TE, Stern RS. The increased risk of skin cancer is persistent after discontinuation of psoralen + ultraviolet A: A cohort study. *J Invest Dermatol* 2003;121: 252-258.
67. Schallreuter KU, Behrens-Williams S, Khaliq TP, et al. Increased epidermal functioning wild-type p53 expression

in vitiligo. *Exp Dermatol* 2003;12: 268-277.
68. Grimes PE. Advances in the treatment of vitiligo: targeted phototherapy. *Cosmet Dermatol* 2003;16:18-22.
69. Lotti TM, Menchini G, Andreassi L. UVB radiation microphototherapy: An elective treatment for segmental vitiligo. *J Eur Acad Dermatol Venereol* 1999;13:102-108.
70. Spencer JM, Nossa R, Ajmeri J. Treatment of vitiligo with the 308-nm excimer laser: A pilot study. *J Am Acad Dermatol* 2002;46: 727-731.
71. Taneja A, Trehan M, Taylor C. 308-nm excimer laser for the treatment of localized vitiligo. *Int J Dermatol* 2003;42: 658-662.
72. Passeron T, Ostovari N, Zakaria W, et al. Topical tacrolimus and the 308 nm excimer laser. *Arch Dermatol* 2004;140: 1065-1069.
73. Kawalek AZ, Spencer JM, Phelps RG. Combined excimer laser and topical tacrolimus for the treatment of vitiligo: A pilot study. *Dermatol Surg* 2004;30: 130-135.
74. Leone G, Iaconelli P, Para Vidalin A, Picardo M. Monochromatic excimer light 308 nm in the treatment of vitiligo: A pilot study. *J Eur Acad Dermatol Venereol* 2003;42:658-662.
75. Hofer A, Hassan H, Legar FJ, et al. Optimal weekly frequency of 308 nm excimer laser treatment in vitiligo patients. *Br J Dermatol* 2005;152:981-985.
76. Hadi S, Tinio P, Al-Ghaithi K, et al. Treatment of vitiligo using the 308-nm excimer laser. *Photomed Laser Surg* 2006; 24:354-357.
77. Parsad D, Saini R, Verma N. Combination of PUVAsol and topical calcipotriol in vitiligo. *Dermatology* 1998;197: 167-170.
78. Ermis O, Alpsoy E, Cetin L, Yilmaz E. Is the efficacy of psoralen plus ultraviolet A therapy for vitiligo enhanced by concurrent topical calcipotriol? A placebo-controlled, double blind study. *Br J Dermatol* 2001;145:472-475.
79. Baysal V, Yildirim M, Erel A, Kesici D. Is the combination of calcipotirol and PUVA effective in vitiligo? *J Eur Acad Dermatol Venereol* 2003;17:299-302.
80. Travis LB, Silverberg NB. Calcipotriene and corticosteroid combination therapy for vitiligo. *Pediatr Dermatol* 2004;21: 495-498.
81. Goktas EO, Aydin F, Senturk N, et al. Combination of narrowband UVB and topical calcipotriol for the treatment of vitiligo. *J Eur Acad Dermatol Venerol* 2006; 20:553-557.
82. Kullavanijaya P, Lim HW. Topical calcipotriene and narrowband ultraviolet B in the treatment of vitiligo. *Photodermatol Photoimmunol Photmed* 2004;20:248-251.
83. Njoo MD, Westerhof W, Bos JD, Bossuyt PM. A systematic review of autologous transplantation methods in vitiligo. *Arch Dermatol* 1998;134:1543-1549.
84. Van Geel N, Ongenae K, De M, et al. Double-blind placebo-controlled study of autologous transplanted controlled study of autologous transplanted epidermal cell suspensions for repigmenting vitiligo. *Arch Dermatol* 2004;140:1203-1208.
85. Chen YF, Yang PY, Hu DN, et al. Treatment of vitiligo by transplantation of cultured pure melanocyte suspension: Analysis of 120 cases. *J Am Acad Dermatol* 2004;51:68-74.
86. Gupta S, Kumar B. Epidermal grafting in vitiligo: Influence of age, site of lesion, and type of disease on outcome. *J Am Acad Dermatol* 2003;49:99-104.

CHAPTER 47

Albinism

Anezi N. Okoro

Key Points

- Albinism is a heterogeneous group of genetically determined disorders of the melanin pigment system in which the synthesis and processing of melanin are reduced or absent.
- Albinism is characterized in humans by congenital hypopigmentation of the skin, hair, and eyes.
- Albinism is found in every racial group but stands out most strikingly among people of darker color.
- Ocular features are the most constant in all types of albinism. These includes photophobia, nystagmus, strabismus, reduced visual acuity, reduced iris and retinal pigment, iris translucency, and foveal hypoplasia.

Albinism refers to a heterogeneous group of genetically determined disorders of the melanin pigment system in which there is a normal number of melanocytes, but the synthesis and processing of melanin are reduced or absent. Albinism is characterized in humans by congenital hypopigmentation of the skin, hair, and eyes. Albinism is also found in the animal kingdom in mammals, birds, reptiles, amphibians, and fish.

In humans, albinism is found in every racial group but stands out most strikingly among people of darker color. References to albinism were made by Plinius in the first century AD.[1] The term *albino* to refer to a person with this pigmentary disorder is now unacceptable on account of its stigmatization. The term was used in the seventeenth century (1660) by Bathazar Tellez, the Portuguese explorer, to describe "white Negroes" seen in Africa.

Despite this early recognition of albinism among Negroes, less research has been done on them and on other people of color than on Caucasians, a reflection of the intensity of medical research in the developed world.

Ocular features are the most constant in all types of albinism. These include photophobia (i.e., sensitivity to bright light and glare), nystagmus (i.e., rhythmic involuntary eye movements), strabismus (i.e., squint with both vertical and horizontal deviations), reduced visual acuity, reduced iris and retinal pigment, iris translucency, foveal hypoplasia, and abnormal routing of the neural connections between the retina and the visual cortex.

CLASSIFICATION OF ALBINISM

This has remained in the phenotypic realm for most of its history. Albinism was recognized as genetic in origin and thought at first to be a single-gene disorder. An early classification recognized oculocutaneous albinism (OCA) as being autosomal recessive, presenting with characteristic clinical features in the skin, hair, and eyes; and ocular albinism (OA) as sex-linked (X-linked), presenting with clinical features in the eyes.

The hair bulb incubation test introduced in the 1960s (Witkop and King) subdivided OCA into tyrosinase-negative (OCA1) and tyrosinase-positive (OCA2) types, based on their inability or ability to form pigment on incubation with tyrosinase. Biochemical tests developed in the next two decades further subdivided OCA into tyrosinase-negative, yellow mutant, platinum, minimal pigment, temperature-sensitive, tyrosinase-positive, brown, rufous, Hermansky-Pudlak syndrome (HPS), and Chediak- Higashi syndrome (CHS). An autosomal recessive ocular albinism (AROA) also was delineated.

Molecular studies in the 1990s separated OCA into OCA1, OCA2, OCA3, and OCA4, whereas HPS has been separated into HPS1 through HPS6. Today's classification of albinism is outlined in Table 47-1.

Far from albinism being a single-gene disorder, the complexity of the problem has been confirmed by the identification of 12 different genes whose mutations result in various types of albinism. So far, over 100 mutations associated with albinism have been identified. This shows that the complexity of the disorder has not been completely uncovered.

TABLE 47-1
Today's Classification of Albinism

OCA1: Tyrosinase-related oculocutaneous albinism:
- OCA1A
- OCA1B
- Autosomal recessive ocular albinism

OCA2: *P*-gene-related oculocutaneous albinism
- Brown OCA

Prader-Willi and Angelman syndrome

OCA3: *TRP1*-Related OCA
- Hermansky-Pudlak syndrome (HPS)
- Chediak-Higashi syndrome (CHS)
- OA1 X-linked ocular albinism
- Autosomal recessive ocular albinism (AROA)

MELANOCYTES AND MELANOGENESIS

Melanocytes are dendritic cells that derive from two different embryonic tissues: the neural crest and the optic cup. Melanocytes that originate in the neural crest migrate to three main locations: the basal layer of the epidermis, the hair follicles, and the eyes (the choroid and iris stroma). Melanocytes that originate in the outer layer of the optic cup migrate to the retinal pigment epithelium. The development process of melanocytes is covered in Table 47-2.

Melanogenesis, the production of melanin, takes place in the melanocytes, in specific subcellular membrane-bound organelles called *melanosomes,* which have four stages of development (Table 47-3). The process of melanogenesis is regulated by various factors: ultraviolet light, hormones, growth factors, cytokines, and other modulators in the skin. Epidermal melanocytes synthesize melanin throughout life, and hair bulbs undergo a regular cycle of melanogenesis. Melanogenesis in the retinal pigment epithelium starts early in fetal life and is usually completed

Table 47-2
Steps in Melanocyte Development

- Melanoblast development in the neural crest and optic cup
- Melanoblast migration to specific sites in the skin, hair, and eyes
- Survival in sites of normal metabolism
- Proliferation, differentiation, and performance of normal functions
- Barrier against actinic or ionizing radiation
- Participant in developmental processes in the skin, hair, and eyes
- Cosmetic/aesthetic values
- Potential scavenger of cytotoxic radicals and intermediates

Table 47-3
Stages of Melanogenesis

1. Eumelanosomes with a membrane-bound organelle containing microvesicles and filaments.
2. Melanosomes become elongated and oval, the filaments parallel to the long axis of the organelle.
3. Melanin is deposited in an even pattern within the melanosomes.
4. A homogeneous ellipsoidal dark body is produced.

soon after birth. Melanogenesis takes place within the melanocytes. It starts with the substrate L-tyrosine. The copper-containing enzyme tyrosinase is critical to the process of melanogenesis. It catalyzes the hydroxylation of L-tyrosine to L-3,4-dihydroxyphenylalanine (L-dopa) and then converts to L-dopa to dopaquinone.

The third step is the production of either red-yellow pheomelanin or brown-black eumelanin. A second enzyme, dopachrome oxidoreductase, converts dopachrome to 5,6-dihydroxyindole. Tyrosinase next acts to convert 5,6-dihydroxyindole to indole-5,6-quinone. Beyond the actions of tyrosinase, other melanogenic enzymes and melanogenic inhibitors can modify the chemical and physical properties of melanins.

Cysteine is needed for the biosynthesis of the pheomelanins, which are low-molecular-weight heterogeneous polymer compounds. Eumelanin is a high-molecular-weight copolymer of tyrosine intermediates with a chromophore covalently bound to protein. Eumelanin and pheomelanin differ in their color, solubility, and ultraviolet absorption.

FUNDAMENTAL DEFECTS IN ALBINISM

Melanogenesis is regulated at various levels and is influenced directly or indirectly by various genes. Mutations of these genes can alter melanin pigmentation at distinct genetic loci and produce clinical conditions of hypopigmentation in various types of albinism.

There is congenital reduction in melanin synthesis in the melanocytes of the skin, hair, and eyes in tyrosinase-related OCA. It is produced by loss of function of the melanocytic enzyme tyrosinase that results from mutations of the tyrosinase gene. In OA, a sex-linked disorder, there is congenital reduction of melanin synthesis mainly in the retinal pigment epithelium of the eyes.

Reduction of melanin in the skin is associated with sensitivity to ultraviolet rays and a predisposition to sunburn, degenerative changes in the skin, actinic keratoses, and skin cancer. Eye changes are found in all types of albinism. Reduced melanin during development is associated with reduced retinal pigment, nystagmus, foveal hypoplasia with reduced visual acuity, and misrouting of the optic fibers from the retina to the visual cortex. Reduction of melanin in the iris stroma and the posterior epithelial layer results in a translucent iris that transmits light on globe transillumination.

OCA had been recognized as exhibiting wide phenotypic expression and therefore was thought not to be due to a single-gene defect. The hair bulb incubation test, which demonstrates the presence or absence of tyrosinase activity, led to biochemical tests that provided evidence of heterogeneity in OCA.

Witkop and colleagues[2] discovered an albino family that had earlier been reported by Trevor-Roper. They found that the mother was tyrosinase-negative OCA, whereas the father was tyrosinase-positive OCA. This confirmed that these two forms of OCA were nonallelic. This was further confirmed when an African-American couple, father tyrosinase-negative and mother tyrosinase-positive, had a normally pigmented daughter.[3] Since then, much wider heterogeneity in OCA has been demonstrated, amounting to over 10 different disorders with phenotypic features of OCA (Table 47-4).

TABLE 47-4
Heterogeneity in Oculocutaneous Albinism (OCA)

Type of OCA	Main Features	Distinguishing Features	Biochemical Tests
Tyrosinase-negative	Pink skin, white hair, gray to blue irides, photophobia, nystagmus, poor visual acuity	Sunsensitivity, inability to tan	Hair bulb tyrosinase test negative
Tyrosinase-positive	Yellow-brown skin, light yellow blond hair, pigmented irides, nystagmus	Freckles, lentigines, actinic keratoses on exposed parts	Hair bulb tyrosinase test positive
Yellow mutant	Cream skin, yellow to light red hair	Pigmented nevi	Hair bulb tyrosinase test variable
Platinum (minimum pigment)	Resembles tyrosinase-negative OCA in infancy	Skin and hair darken in middle or late childhood	Hair bulb tyrosinase test variable
Hermansky-Pudlak syndrome	Skin and hair resemble tyrosinase-positive OCA	Haemorrhagic diathesis, storage-pool-deficient platelets	Hair bulb tyrosinase test positive
Chediak-Higashi syndrome	Skin cream, hair brown, nystagmus, photophobia	Proneness to infections, lymphoreticular infiltrations, malignancies	Hair bulb tyrosinase test positive
Brown	Skin and hair darker than tyrosinase-positive OCA, brown or hazel irides, nystagmus	Lentigines on sun-exposed parts	Hair bulb tyrosinase test positive
Rufous	Skin mahogany brown, hair brown to red	Mild photophobia and nystagmus	Hair bulb tyrosinase test positive
Cross (rare) syndrome	Pale skin, blond hair	Severe retardation	Hair bulb tyrosinase test positive
Autosomal dominant OCA (rare)	Hypopigmentation of skin and hair	Nystagmus, reduced visual acuity	Hair bulb tyrosinase test positive
OCA with black lock (rare)	Pale skin with brown patches, white hair with black patches	Nystagmus, photophobia, profound hearing loss	Hair bulb tyrosinase test positive

THE ROLE OF GENES

Molecular (genetic) studies have further shown the profound complexity of hypopigmentation in albinism, clarified the heterogeneity of the disorder, and assisted with more accurate classification. As the critical factor in melanogenesis, the tyrosinase gene family has three members: tyrosinase (*TYR*), tyrosinase-related protein 1 (*TRP1*) and tyrosinase-related protein 2 (*TRP2*). The *TYR* locus has been mapped to chromosome 11q, the *TRP1* to chromosome 9p, and *TRP2* to chromosome 13q.

The various genes encode proteins with similar amino acid sequences but bind different divalent metal cations, giving them distinct catalytic properties in the process of melanogenesis. Gene mutations produce different types of albinism.

In oculocutaneous albinism type 1 (OCA1), the tyrosinase gene on chromosome 11q acts as a melagenic enzyme. In OCA2, P protein on chromosome 15q acts as a melanosomal membrane protein. In HPS, membrane protein on chromosome 10q acts as a lysosome, affecting melanosome structure and function. OCA, OA, and other types of albinism are defined by the gene locus involved in the mutation (Table 47-5).

TABLE 47-5
Genetic Defects in Various Types of Albinism

Type of Albinism	Distinctive Features	Genetic Defect	Gene Map (Chromosome)	Gene Mutation
OCA1 (OCA1A and OCA1B)	Tyrosinase-negative	Autosomal recessive	11q	Tyrosinase gene
OCA2	Tyrosinase-positive	Autosomal recessive		*P* gene
Brown OCA	Tyrosinase-positive	Autosomal recessive		*P* gene
Rufous	Tyrosinase-positive	Autosomal recessive		*TRP1* gene
Hermansky-Pudlak syndrome	Tyrosinase-positive	Autosomal recessive	10q	*HPS1–HPS6* genes
Chediak-Higashi syndrome	Tyrosinase-positive	Autosomal recessive	1q	*CHS1* gene
Ocular (OA1)	Ocular features only	X-linked	Xp22	*OA1* gene
OCA3	Tyrosinase-positive	Autosomal recessive		*TRP1* gene
OCA4	Tyrosinase-positive	Autosomal recessive		Membrane-associated transport protein
Piebladism	Tyrosinase-positive	Autosomal recessive		Tyrosine kinase receptor gene

PREVALENCE OF ALBINISM IN PEOPLE OF COLOR

Because of its obvious phenotype, congenital reduction in melanin pigment in the skin, hair, and eyes, albinism in humans has attracted research interest for at least two millennia, from Pliny the Elder (23–79 AD) to the current mapping of the human genome. The disorder is seen in every racial stock: Caucasoid, Mongoloid, Negroid, Australoid, and each racial stock with subdivisions and admixtures. People with albinism stand out most strikingly among races of darker color. Historical milestones in studies on albinism would include Pliny the Elder in the first century AD; Balthazar Tellez with his description of "white Negroes" in 1660; Archibald Garrod with his listing of the inborn errors of metabolism in 1908[4]; Pearson, Nettleship, and Usher with their monograph on albinism in 1911–1913[5]; and Clyde Keeler with his decades of study of the Cuna Moonchild Indians in Panama[6]; Kugelman and Van Scott with their hair bulb incubation in tyrosinase[7]; Witkop Jr. with his work on HPS[8]; and Guillery, Okoro, and Witkop Jr. with their demonstration of abnormal visual pathways in the brain of a human albino.[9]

Work on the prevalence of albinism in people of color is understandably multfocal and sporadic, with the group scattered on all six continents and various continental islands. Through the ages, attitudes toward albinism in various parts of the world varied from curiosity to concern, from revulsion to reverence, from benign neglect to overprotection, and from passive documentation to empathy and active management.

The closeness of figures from the studies by Witkop Jr.[8] and King and colleagues[11] confirms the higher, sometimes very much higher prevalence of OCA among people of color compared with the world survey (Table 47-6). Clyde Keeler's prevalence of 1 in 160 among Cuna Moonchild Indians on San Blas Island in Panama ranks among the highest prevalence rates in the world.[6]

Following Okoro's 1974 report of 1000 people with albinism in Nigeria,[10] Witkop Jr. led a team (Witkop Jr, Cervenka, King, and Creel) to Enugu, Nigeria, to expand Okoro's work in the 1970s and 1980s. This collaborative work confirmed the high prevalence of albinism and an alarming rate of squamous cell carcinoma in albinos in the region.[11] It also yielded the demonstration of abnormal visual pathways in the brain of a human albino,[9] visual system anomalies in human albinos,[9] and the absence of chromosome breaks and sister chromatid exchanges in albinos,[12] and it delineated *brown albinism,* a new autosomal recessive oculocutaneous type.[11]

GENERAL CLINICAL FEATURES IN PEOPLE OF COLOR

Ocular

REDUCED VISUAL ACUITY This is related to the degree of ocular pigmentation and varies with the type of albinism. In tyrosinase-negative OCA1, there is very poor visual acuity. In tyrosinase-positive OCA2, brown albinism, and rufous albinism, visual acuity is only slightly reduced. Near vision is usually better than equivalent distance vision.

NYSTAGMUS Spasmodic movement of the eyes may be side to side or rotatory. In tyrosinase-negative OCA1, there is marked nystagmus, but in tyrosinase-positive OCA, brown albinism, and rufous albinism, nystagmus is mild. Factors responsible for nystagmus include foveal hypoplasia with reduced visual acuity, poor fixation, misrouting of the optic fibers at the chiasma, and refractory errors.

TABLE 47-6
Comparison of Figures from Witkop Jr. (1985) and King and Colleagues (2002)

Country/Group	Type, Witkop 1985(A)	Type, King 2002(B)	Source A	Source B
World survey	All types, 1:20,000	All types, 1:10,000–20,000	Pearson et al., 1911	Pearson et al., 1911
African-American	Tyrosinase-negative, 1:28,000; tyrosinase-positive, 1:15,000	All OCA, 1:10,000; OCA1, 1:28,000; OCA2, 1:10,000	Witkop et al., 1974	Witkop et al., 1989
Igbo, Nigeria	Tyrosinase-positive, 1:1100, 1:10,000	—	Witkop et al., 1977	—
Bamileke, Cameroun	All types, 1:3800	—	—	—
Transkei, South Africa	All types, 1:3000	OCA1, rare; OCA2, 1:3900; OCA3, 1:8500	—	Kromberg, 1982; Manga, 1997
Cuna, Panama	Tyrosinase-positive, 1:143	—	—	—
SJemez, US; Hopi, US; Zuni, US	Tyrosinase-positive, 1:140; tyrosinase-positive, 1:227; tyrosinase-positive,1:240	OCA2, 1:227; OCA2, 1:240	—	Woolf, 1965; Witkop, 1972
Maya, Guatemala	Tyrosinase-positive, 1:6500	—	—	—
Tanzania	—	OCA2, 1:1429	—	Spritz, 1995
Zimbabwe	—	OCA2, 1:2833	—	Puri, 1997
Puerto Rico (west)	HPS, 1:2000	—	—	—

HYPOPLASIA OF THE FOVEA This is present in OCA1, OCA2, and X-linked OA. Normal foveal light reflex and normal hyperpigmentation of the macular pigment epithelium are absent.

HYPOPIGMENTATION OF THE OPTIC FUNDUS In OCA1, pigment epithelium of the retina and the choroid lack pigment, and there is hypopigmentation of the fundus. Varying degrees of pigmentation of the fundus are seen in other forms of OCA.

TRANSLUCENCY OF THE IRIS In OCA1, there is marked translucency of the iris. This is demonstrated by applying a penlight to the lower eyelid.

STRABISMUS (SQUINT) There is a higher incidence of strabismus in tyrosinase-negative OCA than in other types of albinism.

ABNORMAL HEAD POSTURE AND HEAD NODDING These are compensatory moves during reading to lessen the disability from nystagmus.

HIGH REFRACTORY ERRORS People with various types of albinism are prone to astigmatism with myopia or hypermetropia. Since these errors are not due only to ocular lens defects, they are not readily amenable to correction.

ABNORMAL DECUSSATION AND MISROUTING OF THE OPTIC FIBERS AT THE OPTIC CHIASM In eyes that are normally pigmented during development, the proportion of nasal retinal optic fibers that decussate (cross over) at the optic chiasm to end in the contralateral geniculate nucleus is about 55%. In albinism, the proportion of fibers that cross at the chiasm is about 90%, resulting in a virtual loss of stereoscopic vision. This misrouting of the optic fibers at the chiasm can be demonstrated by recording monocular visual evoked responses or anatomically.[9]

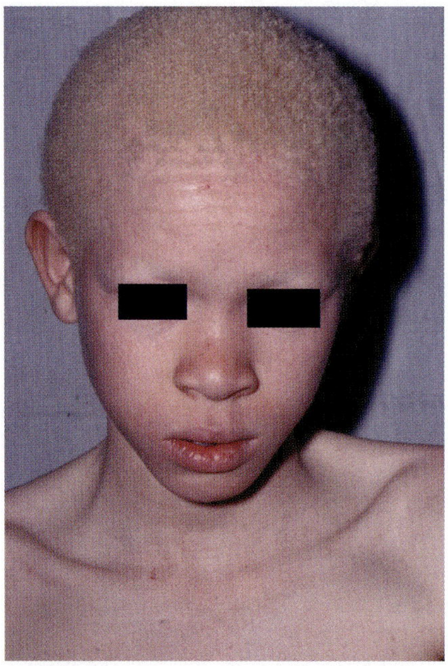

▲ **FIGURE 47-1** A 13-year-old albino boy. Note white skin, blonde hair, hazel eyes, and mild cheilitis of the lower lip. Courtesy of Barbara Leppard, M.D.

Cutaneous Features

TYROSINASE-NEGATIVE OCA This is inherited as an autosomal recessive trait. The skin is pink with no freckles or lentigines. It is very sensitive to sunlight, burns readily, but does not tan (Figure 47-1). Repeated exposure to sunlight leads to pachydermia, collagen degeneration, elastosis (Figure 47-2), solar keratoses (Figure 47-3), and squamous cell carcinoma. The hair is white but may become yellowish in adult life. Anagen hair bulbs incubated in L-tyrosine or L-dopa fails to form pigment. Assay for tyrosinase is zero.

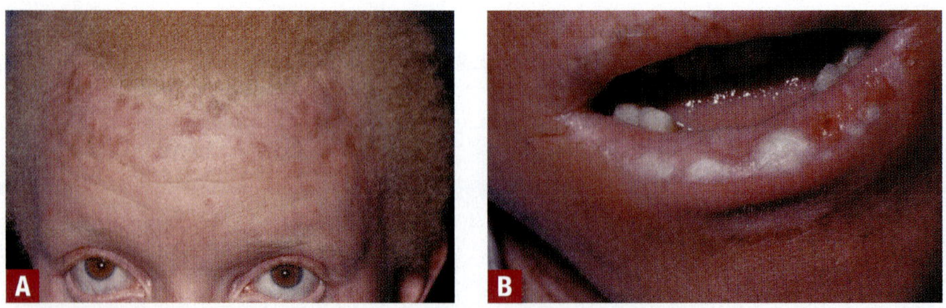

▲ **FIGURE 47-2** *A.* Solar keratoses on the forehead of a 22-year-old man. *B.* Severe actinic cheilitis of the lips in a 37-year-old man. Courtesy of Barbara Leppard, M.D.

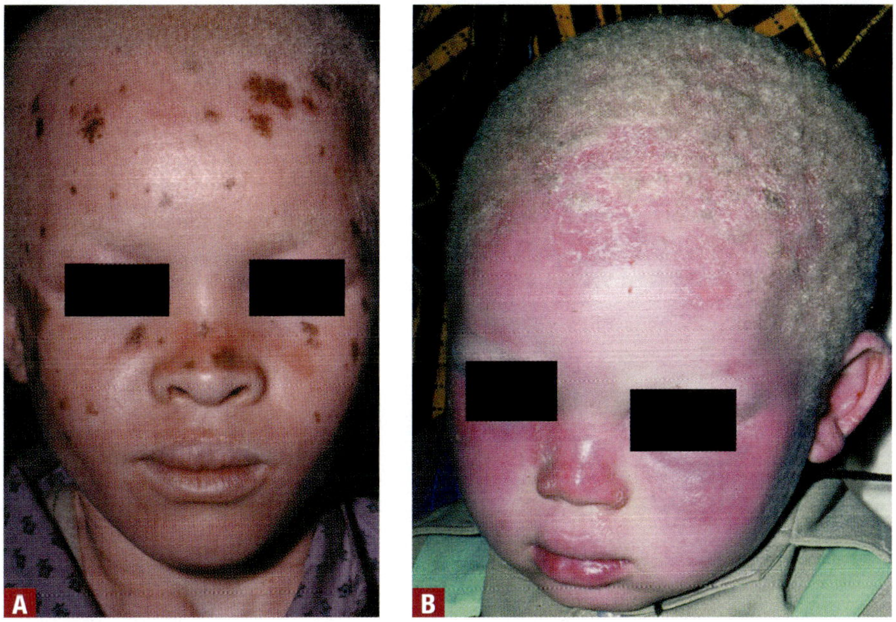

▲ **FIGURE 47-3** *A.* A 10-year-old albino boy with multiple lentigoes on the face. *B.* Sunburn in a 4-year-old boy. Courtesy of Barbara Leppard, M.D.

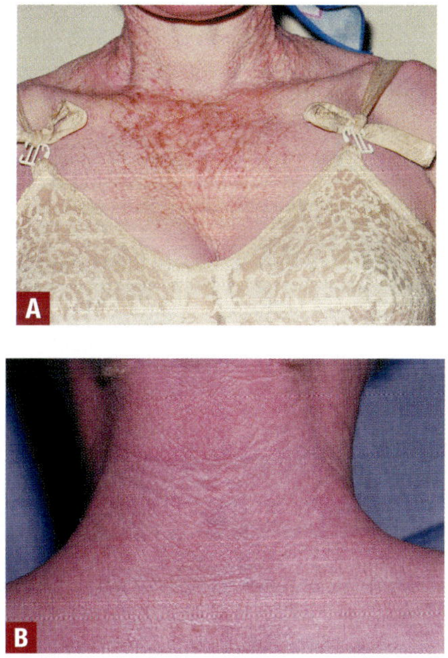

▲ **FIGURE 47-4** *A.* Solar elastosis on the V of the neck of a 37-year-old woman. *B.* Solar elastosis on the back of the neck of a 12-year-old girl. Courtesy of Barbara Leppard, M.D.

Prenatal diagnosis can be made by obtaining scalp biopsy at 20 weeks' gestation and conducting the hair bulb incubation test, a tyrosinase assay, and histopathologic studies.

TYROSINASE-POSITIVE OCA This is inherited as an autosomal recessive trait. The skin is pale or light brown and sun sensitive. It burns on sun exposure but may tan. It develops freckles, pigmented nevi, and lentigines (Figure 47-3). It is also prone to pachydermia, elastosis (Figure 47-4), basal cell carcinoma (Figure 47-5), keratoacanthoma (Figure 47-6), solar keratoses (Figure 47-7), and squamous cell carcinoma (Figure 47-8). Some of the squamous cell carcinoma may ulcerate as they develop (Figure 47-9). The hair is light yellow or blond and gradually acquires more pigment with age.

Epilated anagen hair bulbs contain a few faint melanin granules. Incubation of hair bulbs in L-tyrosine or L-dopa shows definite melanin formation. Assay for tyrosinase is positive.

YELLOW MUTANT OCA This is inherited as an autosomal recessive trait, The skin resembles that of tyrosinase-negative OCA in infancy but becomes dark cream, yellow, or light red with age. It then develops pigmented nevi and can tan on sun exposure. The hair is light reddish brown. Epilated anagen hair bulbs show golden yellow or red pigment. Ultrastructurally, small round stage 3 prepheomelanosomes are seen. On incubation of the hair bulbs in L-tyrosine, yellow-red pigment is formed.

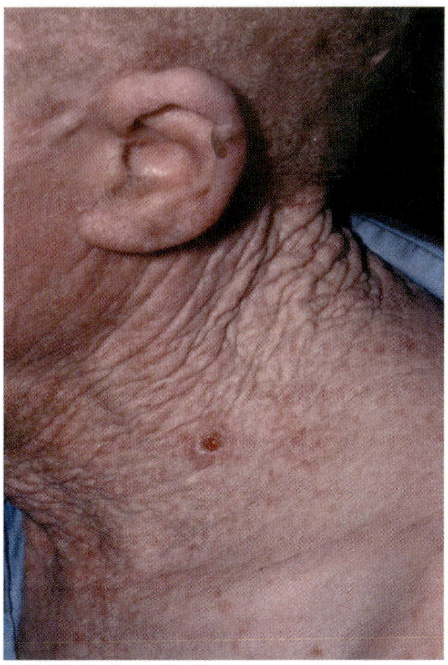

▲ **FIGURE 47-5** Basal cell carcinoma on the left side of the neck of a 53-year-old man. Note the marked solar elastosis on his neck and the solar keratosis on his ear. Courtesy of Barbara Leppard, M.D.

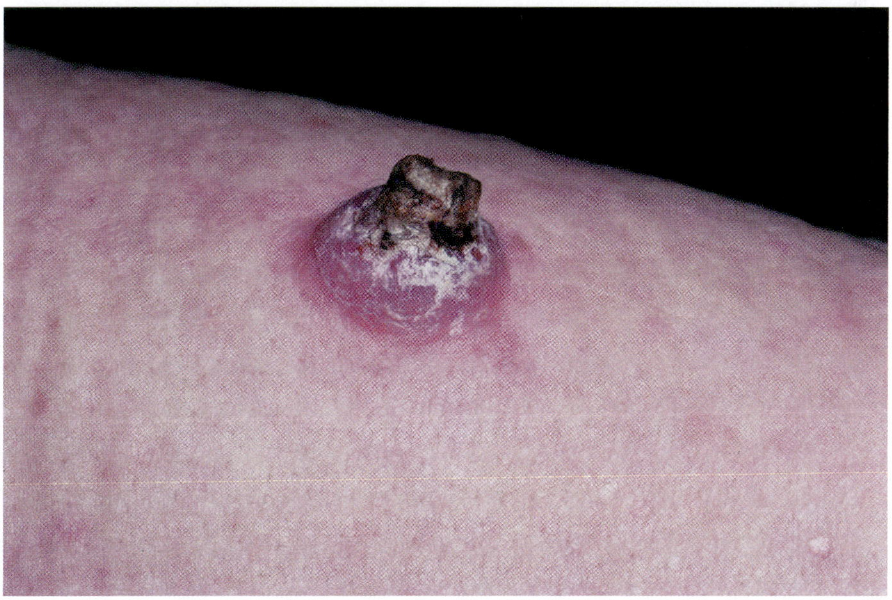

▲ **FIGURE 47-6** Keratoacanthoma on the upper arm of a 74-year-old man. Courtesy of Barbara Leppard, M.D.

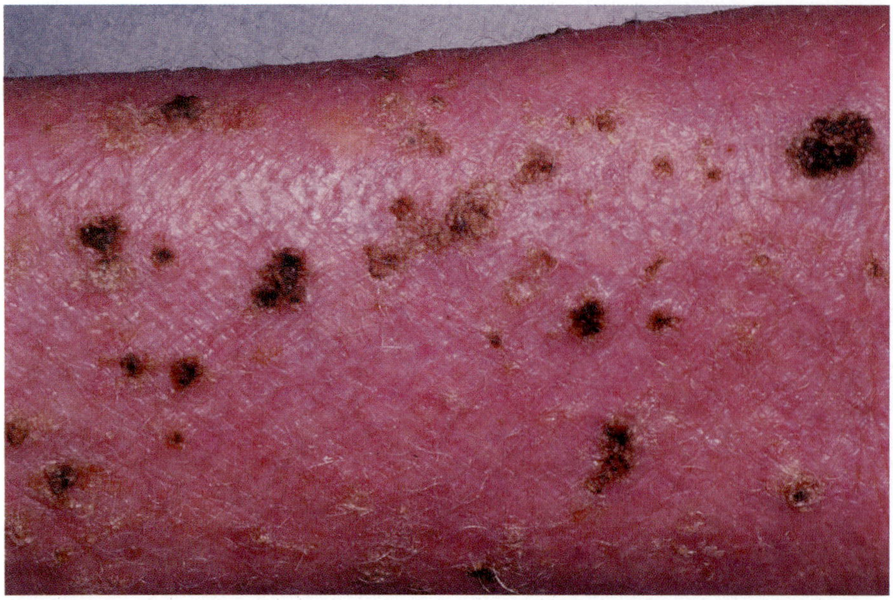

▲ **FIGURE 47-7** Solar keratoses on the leg of a 39-year-old woman. Courtesy of Barbara Leppard, M.D.

PLATINUM OCA This is inherited as an autosomal recessive trait and is rare in people of color. Patients resemble tyrosinase-negative OCA patients.

BROWN OCA This is inherited as an autosomal recessive trait. Patients are generally darker than those with tyrosinase-positive OCA. Brown albinism was recently well delineated among Nigerians,[11] in natives of New Guinea, in South Africans, and in African-Americans. The skin is light brown to olive in color, darker than in tyrosinase-positive OCA but lighter than in unaffected siblings. The skin is less sun sensitive than tyrosinase-positive OCA skin. It does not burn on sun exposure, it does tan, and it does not develop lentigines. It is prone to develop pachydermia and solar keratoses, but squamous cell carcinoma rarely develops.

RUFOUS OCA This is inherited as an autosomal recessive trait. It had been termed *red* and *xanthous* and was described in Africans by Stannus,[13] in New Guineans by Walsh,[14] and in African-Americans by Witkop Jr. The skin is mahogany brown with a red tinge and is not markedly sun sensitive. The hair color is variable, mahogany brown to sandy red or black. Epilated anagen hair bulbs form pigment when incubated in L-tyrosine.

HERMANSKY-PUDLAK SYNDROME (HPS) This is a form of OCA seen almost exclusively in Puerto Ricans.[15] It is inherited as an autosomal recessive trait. The disorder consists of tyrosinase-positive OCA, hemorrhagic diathesis owing to storage-pool-deficient platelets, and accumulation of a ceroid-like substance in tissues and urine. The disorder also has been reported in Holland, India, and Switzerland.

The most extensive work on HPS was carried out in Puerto Rico by Witkop Jr., who described other associated conditions: pulmonary, cardiac, gastrointestinal, renal, and bone marrow disorders. The disorder presents with petechial haemorrhage, easy bruising, and prolonged bleeding after dental extraction. The hair is blond, brown, or reddish. The hair bulb tyrosinase test is positive.

CHEDIAK-HIGASHI SYNDROME (CHS) This is inherited as an autosomal recessive trait. It is characterized by susceptibility to infection in infancy or childhood and by lymphoreticular infiltration of tissues in adult life. The skin varies in color from cream to gray, is sun sensitive, and tends to burn on sun exposure. The hair ranges in color from fair to light brown to gray. Anagen hair bulbs incubated in L-tyrosine produce pigment. Ultrastructurally, melanocytes

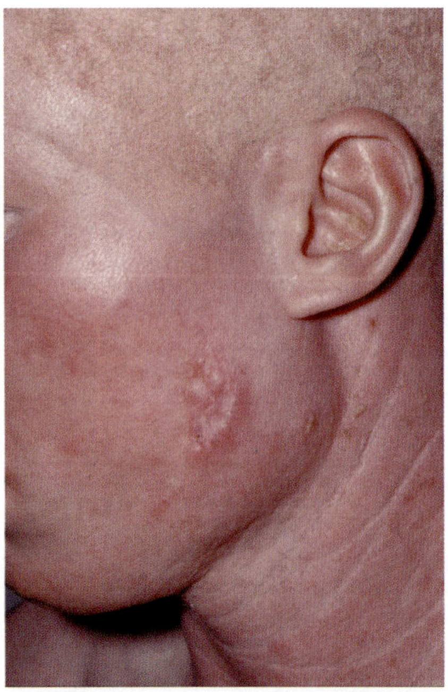

▲ **FIGURE 47-8** Squamous cell carcinoma on the left cheek of a 26-year-old man. Courtesy of Barbara Leppard, M.D.

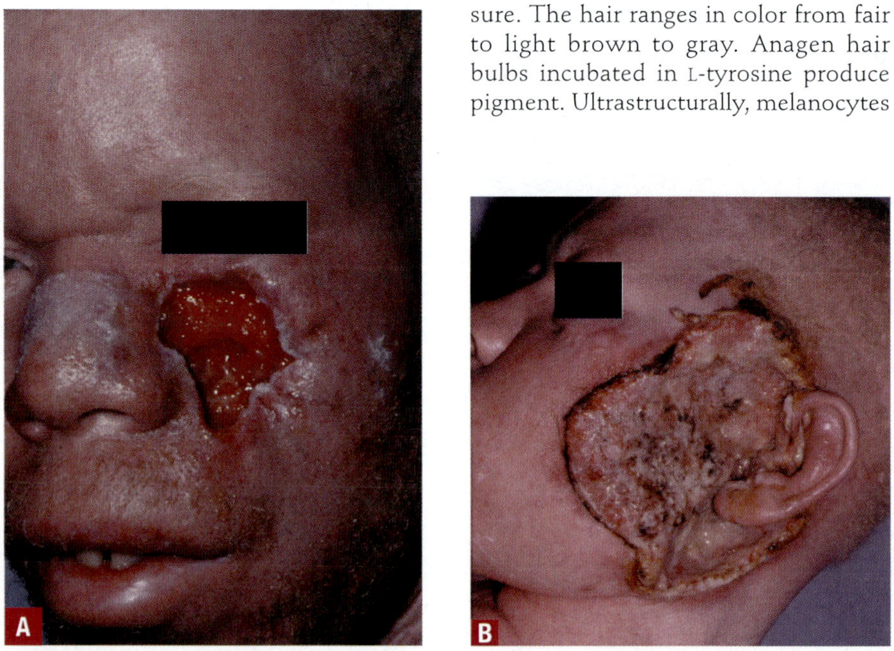

▲ **FIGURE 47-9** *A.* Ulcerating squamous cell carcinoma on the left cheek of a 39-year-old man. *B.* Ulcerating squamous cell carcinoma on the face of a 27-year-old man. Courtesy of Barbara Leppard, M.D.

contain melanosomes at all stages of development. Histologically, CHS is distinguished by the presence of giant melanosomes within melanocytes.

OCULAR ALBINISM (OA) Patients with OA usually have the range of skin and hair color consistent with their racial or ethnic group but may show more hypopigmentation than their siblings. Their distinguishing features are the ocular features, malformations, and disabilities.

In X-linked ocular albinism (OA1), affected males have photophobia, nystagmus, and reduced visual acuity.[16,17] Obligate heterozygotes show a mosaic pattern of pigmentation in their fundi. In Africans and African-American males, the irides are brown, and there is little iris translucency. In affected Japanese males, the irides are brown, and there is no iris translucency. There is lack of hyperpigmentation in the foveal area, and there may be patches of hypopigmentation on the skin. Visual acuity is variable and usually better than in people of color. In OA1, melanocytes in the skin, hair follicles, irides, and retinas contain normal-sized melanosomes and giant melanosomes or macromelanosomes.

AUTOSOMAL RECESSIVE OA In this type of albinism, males and females in some families are equally affected, but without evidence of X-linked inheritance. The hypopigmented skin patches seen in X-linked OA are not seen. Hair bulb incubation activity is within the normal range. Macromelanosomes are not seen in skin, hair follicles, or irides.

Rarer types of albinism that more molecular studies may elucidate include

- *Autosomal dominant OCA.* Generations of kindreds with features of OCA transmitted as an autosomal dominant trait have been described. All affected members had hypopigmentation, nystagmus, and reduced visual acuity.
- *Cross syndrome.* Hypopigmentation with microphthalmos, mental retardation, growth retardation, and spasticity.
- *Oculocutaneous albinism with black lock and congenital sensorneural deafness.* Black-locks-albinism-deafness syndrome (BADS).
- *Forsius-Eriksson syndrome (Aland eye disease).* Males have a high prevalence of color blindness, astigmatism, axial myopia, nystagmus, and foveal hypoplasia.
- *Ocular-albinism-lentigines-deafness syndrome.*
- *Albinoidism.* Generalized hypopigmentation of the skin, hair, and eyes without photophobia, nystagmus, and reduced visual acuity:
  - Autosomal dominant albinoidism
  - Punctate oculocutaneous albinoidism
  - Autosomal dominant albinoidism and deafness
  - Ocular depigmentation and Apert syndrome (acrocephalosyndactylia)
  - Waardenburg-like syndrome—lack of dystopia of the inner canthus
  - Marked fundus hypopigmentation, iris translucency, foveal hypoplasia, reduced visual acuity
  - Hypopigmentation-immunodeficiency disease
  - Menkes syndrome—X-linked inheritance. Growth retardation, cerebral and cerebellar degeneration, deficient copper absorption, and negative hair bulb test
  - Piebaldism—autosomal dominant congenital stable leukoderma, characterized by vitiligo-like amelanotic macules and a white forelock

Eumelanosomes of the skin, hair, and uveal tract are ellipsoidal. Those of the pigment epithelium are larger and spherical in the iris and ellipsoidal in the retina.

The dendrites of epidermal and hair bulb melanocytes contact adjacent keratinocytes, forming epidermal melanin units. Mature melanosomes are transferred from the melanocytes via dendrites to the keratinocytes as melanin granules. Melanosomes of the uveal tract and retinal pigment are not so transferred.

TABLE 47-7
The Comparative Incidence of Various Types of Albinism

Type of Albinism	Number in Population
OCA type 1	1:40,000 population
OCA type 2	1:15,000 population
OCA type 3	Not known
OCA type 4	In Japan, 24% of OCA individuals have this type
OA	1:50,000 population
Chediak-Higashi syndrome	Very rare
Hermansky-Pudlak syndrome	Rare; most common in Puerto Rico with 1:1800 population
Griscelli syndrome	Very rare

CONCLUSION

As stated earlier, albinism occurs in all racial groups, but the actual incidence depends on gene pools, marriage customs, and other social and environmental factors (Table 47-7).

REFERENCES

1. Rackman H (ed). *Pliius Secunduc the Edler in the natural history of Pliny,* Book 7. London, William Heineman, 1942.
2. Witkop CJ Jr, Nance WE, Rawls RF, White JG. Autosomal recessive oculocutaneous albinism in man: Evidence for genetic heterogeneity. *Am J Hum Genet* 1970;22:55-74.
3. Nance WE, Witkop CJ Jr., Rawls RF. Genetic and biochemical evidence for two forms of oculocutaneous albinism in man. *Birth Defects* 1971;7:125-128.
4. Garrod AF. Inborn errors of metabolism. Croonian Lectures. Lecture 1. *Lancet* 1908; 2:1-7.
5. Peason K, Nettleship E, Usher CH. A monograph on albinism in man, in *Draper's Company Research Memoirs.* Biometric Series VI. London, Dulan, 1991, p 1.
6. Cuna Moonchild albinism, 1950-1970. *J Hered* 1970;61:273-277.
7. Kugelman TP, Van Scott EJ. Tyrosinase activity in melanocytes of human albinos. *J Invest Dermatol* 1961;37:73-76.
8. Witkop CJ Jr. Albinism: Hematologic storage disease, susceptibility to skin cancer and optic neuronal defects shared in all types of oculocutaneous and ocular albinisim. *Ala J Med Sci* 1979;16:327-330.
9. Guillery RW, Okoro AN, Witkop CJ Jr. Abnormal visual pathways in the brain of a human albino. *Brain Res* 1975;96: 373-377.
10. Okoro AN. Albinism in Nigeri. *Br J Dermatol* 1975;92:485-492.
11. King RA, Creel D, Cervenka J, Okoro AN. Albinism in Nigeria with delineation of a new recessive oculocutaneous type. *Clin Genet* 1980;17:259-270.
12. Cervenka J, Witkop CJ Jr, Okoro AN, King RA. Chromosome breaks and sister chromatid exchanges in albinos in Nigeria. *Clin Genet* 1979;15:17-21.
13. Stannus HS. Anomalies among natives of Nyasaland: A condition to the study of albinism. *Biometrika* 1913;9:333-365.
14. Walsh RJ. A distinctive pigment of the skin in New Guinea indigenes. *Am J Hum Genet* 1971;34:379-385.
15. Hermansky R, Pudlak P. Albinism associated with hemorrhagic diathesis and unusual pigmented reticular cells in the bone marrow: Report of new cases with histochemical studies. *Blood* 1959;14:162-169.
16. Nettleship E. On some hereditary diseases of the eye. *Ophthalmol Soc UK* 1909;29: 57-198.
17. Falls HF. Sex-linked ocular albinism displaying typical fundus changes in female heterozygote. *Am J Ophthalmol* 1951;34: 41-50.

CHAPTER 48

Melasma

Wendy E. Roberts

Key Points

- Melasma is a chronic, acquired, relapsing hypermelanosis.
- Melasma should not be dismissed as simply a cosmetic entity because it adversely affects quality of life.
- Women with darker skin types, those of Latina, African-American, African-Caribbean, and Asian ancestry have a higher incidence of melasma.
- Although the exact cause of melasma is unknown, it is strongly associated with three factors: hormonal influences, ultraviolet radiation, and genetic predisposition.
- Melasma therapy is based on four mechanisms of actions: minimizing ultraviolet exposure, minimizing contributing hormonal influences, preventing melanin production, and the removal of melanin.
- Sun protection and avoidance in combination with topical lightening agents are the cornerstones of therapy.
- Physical modalities, including chemical peels, microdermabrasions, and laser and intense pulse light therapy, may be used cautiously in skin of color patients.

Melasma is a chronic, acquired cutaneous hypermelanosis characterized by hyperpigmented patches on sun-exposed areas of the face, neck, and forearms (Figures 48-1 and 48-2). Also referred to as *chloasma* and the *mask of pregnancy,* the most accepted terminology to describe this entity is *melasma.* Symmetric lesions are a consistent finding of melasma and can be used to differentiate it from other cutaneous disorders of hyperpigmentation. While there are several clinical presentations, the most common is symmetrical irregularly shaped areas of hyperpigmentation on both cheeks (Figures 48-3 and 48-4). In the United States, melasma affects approximately 5–6 million individuals, primarily but not exclusively women. In one study, the cited male incidence was 5–10%.[1] Melasma should not be dismissed as simply a cosmetic entity because it often evokes emotional distress. Additionally, stigma may be associated with melasma, particularly in Asian cultures.

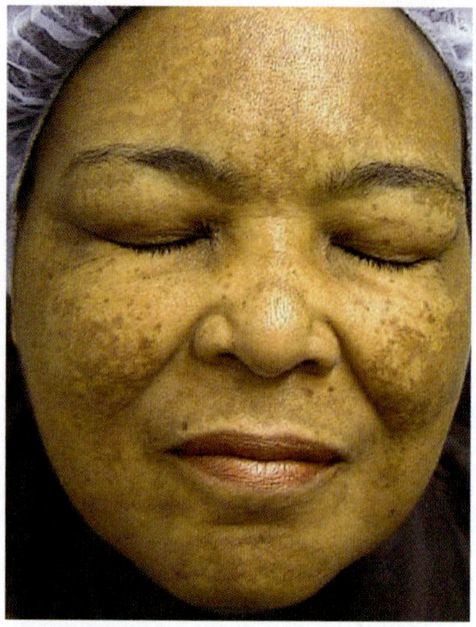

▲ **FIGURE 48-1** Melasma of the face (frontal view).

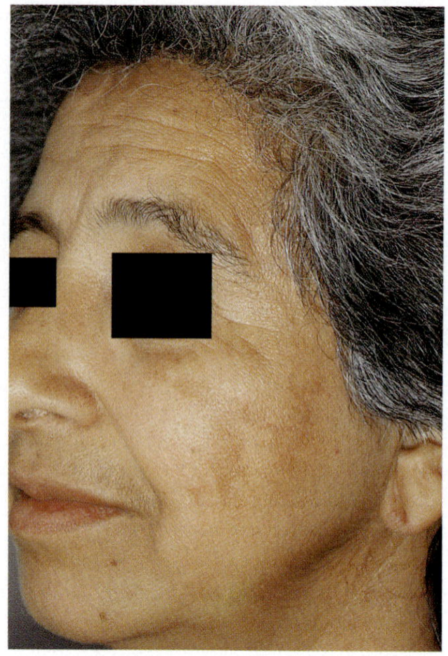

▲ **FIGURE 48-2** Melasma of the face (side view).

SYNONYMS

- Melasma
- Chloasma
- Mask of pregnancy

PATHOGENESIS

Although the exact cause of melasma is unknown, it is strongly associated with three factors: hormonal influences, ultraviolet (UV) radiation, and genetic predisposition.

Hormonal Influences

Melasma occurs commonly during pregnancy, with data suggesting an incidence of 50–70% in pregnant women.[2] It occurs frequently in women using oral contraceptives.[3] Women taking unopposed estrogen rarely manifest melasma, but women taking hormone-replacement therapy (HRT) that includes progestational hormones may develop melasma.[4] Menopausal and postmenopausal women receiving HRT

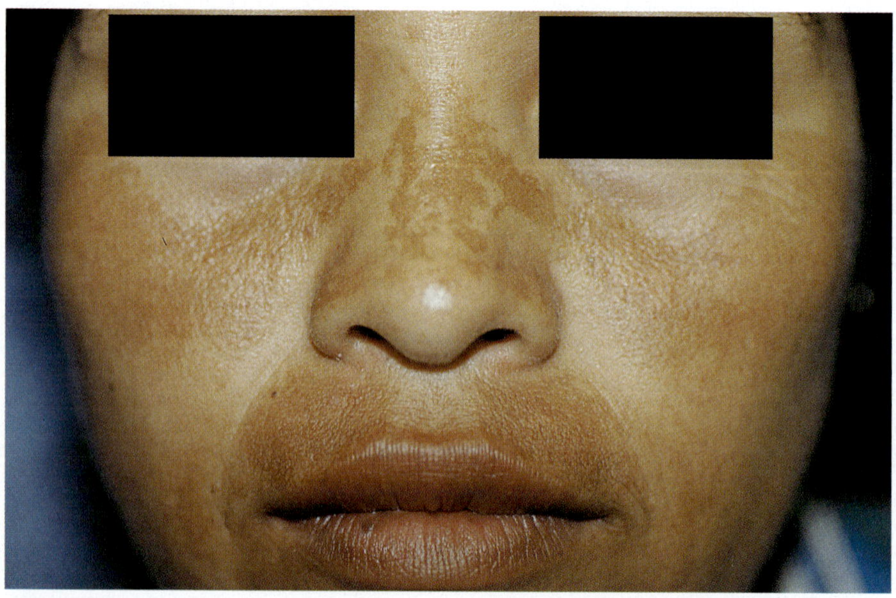

FIGURE 48-3 Melasma involving the cheeks symmetrically with prominent upper lip and nasal involvement.

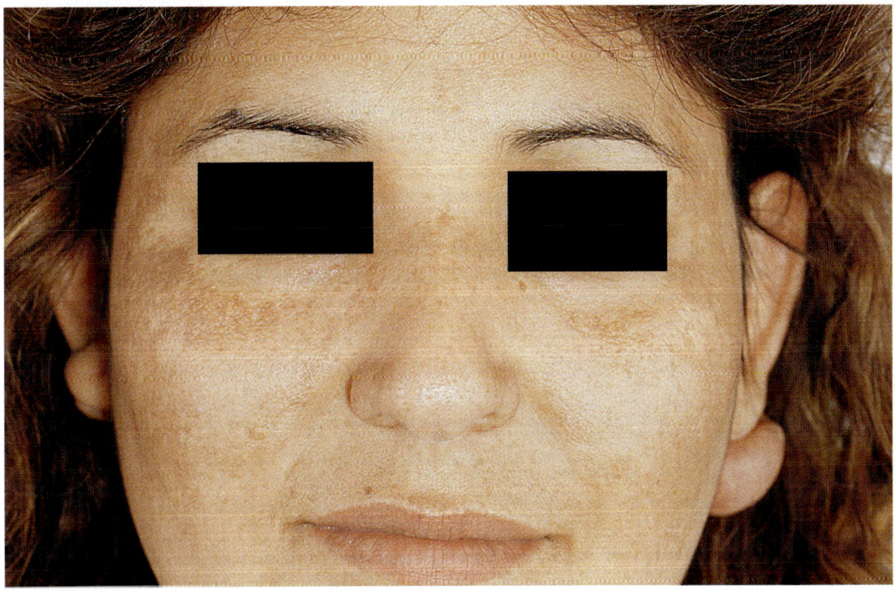

▲ **FIGURE 48-4** Melasma involving the cheeks symmetrically.

reportedly have had lesions on the forearms.[5] Additionally, melasma may be triggered by nutritional supplements, especially those that have estrogen- and progesterone-like properties. Although progesterone, estrogen, melanocyte-stimulating hormone (MSH), and luteinizing hormone have been implicated as a trigger of melasma, levels have not been consistently elevated in these patients.

Ultraviolet Radiation

Exposure to UV radiation is believed to be the leading factor in the development of melasma. Supporting this observation is the predominance of melasma observed in geographic areas with high levels of UV light. Furthermore, patients whose melasma has improved or nearly resolved may relapse completely or develop darkening of existing lesions from one episode of UV exposure. In addition, melasma lesions tend to improve or fade during winter months with less UV exposure. It is well known that skin darkening is a result of UVA exposure and to a lesser extent UVB, which trigger increased melanocyte activity and melanogenesis. Kang and colleagues examined skin biopsies of 56 Korean patients and reported that increased solar radiation induced dermal changes in the cohort with the diagnosis of melasma.[6]

Genetic Predisposition

The common occurrence of melasma in families supports a hereditary component to this disorder.[7] It has been suggested that the increase in pigmentation following exposure to UV radiation is a consequence of DNA repair.[4]

CLINICAL FEATURES

Women with darker skin types, those of Latina, African-American, African-Caribbean, Native American, and Asian ancestry, have a higher incidence of melasma.[8–10] Although the mean age of diagnosis of melasma is 32 years, it is seen routinely in women in their childbearing years and those in menopause.[5] It has been cited rarely in premenstrual girls.

The primary lesions of melasma are bilateral, symmetric, hyperpigmented macules and patches that may vary in color from tan to blue-gray. The color variations are attributed to several factors, including the amounts of melanin pigment produced, the size of the melanosomes, and the location of melanin and melanophages within the epidermis and dermis. Melasma occurs most often on the upper lip, nose, cheeks, forehead, chin, mandible, neck, chest, and forearm areas. Three patterns of facial melasma have been described:

1. Central facial with lesions involving the cheeks, forehead, upper lip, nose, and chin (Figure 48-5A). This pattern was seen in the majority of patients (63%). Melasma on the upper lip typically occurs in women taking oral contraceptives.
2. Malar with lesions involving the cheeks and nose only, which is seen in 21% of patients (Figure 48-5B).
3. Mandibular with involvement of the ramus of the mandible, which is seen in 16%.

While associated with sun-exposed skin, melasma also has been observed on the nipples and external genitalia.[11]

HISTOPATHOLOGY OF MELASMA

With the use of a Wood's lamp and light microscopy, Sanchez and colleagues classified melasma into three histopathologic categories with the following features[12]:

1. *Epidermal type* (70–90% of all melasma cases)
   - *Location of pigmentation.* Melanin deposition in the basal and suprabasal layers through the stratum corneum.
   - *Woods lamp.* Pigment is intensified (Fitzpatrick I–IV skin types).
2. *Dermal type*
   - *Location of pigmentation.* Melanin-laden macrophages and melanosomes within the superficial dermis and perivascularly in the middermis. May impart a blue-gray color to the overlying skin via the Tyndall phenomenon.

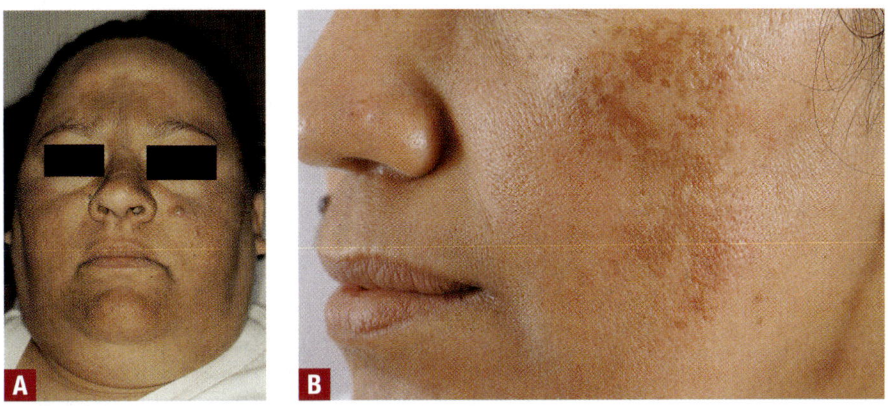

▲ **FIGURE 48-5** *A.* Central facial melasma. *B.* Malar melasma.

TABLE 48-1
Ultrastructural Features of Melasma

- Increased number of melanocytes
- Increased melanocyte activity
- Increased melanosome size
- Increased melanosome formation
- High percentage of melanosomes individually dispersed within the keratinocyte
- Increase of melanosome transfer

- *Woods lamp.* Pigment is not intensified under Wood's lamp (Fitzpatrick I–IV skin types)

3. *Compound (mixed) type*
   - Features of both epidermal and dermal types (recently reported at 24% of all cases).

Twenty-one patients were included in a study by Grimes and colleagues of light microscopic, immunohistochemical, and ultrastructural changes in melasma as compared with normal skin.[13] Although there were no quantitative increases in melanocytes in lesional skin, there was increased deposition of melanin in the epidermis and dermis. However, the melanocytes were larger, intensely stained cells with very prominent dendrites. Electron microscopy revealed more melanosomes within keratinocytes, melanocytes, and dendrites in lesional versus normal skin (Table 48-1). Mild lymphohistiocytic infiltrates were present in 75% of the hyperpigmented areas.

DIFFERENTIAL DIAGNOSIS

The differential diagnosis of melasma includes a variety of pigmentary disorders (Table 48-2). However, the diagnosis of melasma is often based on clinical presentation as well as medical history. Additionally, the bilateral and symmetric nature of the disorder typically sets it apart from other disorders of pigmentation.

TREATMENT

Melasma is a chronic, relapsing disorder that can be managed effectively but not cured. Effective treatment of melasma often has a prolonged course, and the patient must be aware of the "long-term commitment" necessary to achieve a successful outcome. Melasma therapy is based on four mechanisms of action:

- Minimizing UV exposure
- Minimizing contributing hormonal influences
- Preventing melanin production
- Removing melanin

Each therapeutic mechanism and appropriate agents and maneuvers will be discussed below.

TABLE 48-2
The Differential Diagnosis of Melasma

Riehl's melanosis. Histopathology demonstrates an inflammatory infiltrate at the epidermal-dermal junction and a perivascular lymphocytic infiltrate consistent with an inflammatory disorder.
Hori's macules. Dermal pigment that presents as speckled or confluent brown-blue or slate-gray facial pigmentation in women of Asian ancestry.[14]
Bilateral nevus of Ota. May be associated with ocular and mucosal melanosis.
Postinflammatory hyperpigmentation (PIH). Usually lacks the symmetric component, and history reveals a preceding inflammatory or traumatic event such as acne vulgaris or contact dermatitis.
Eythema dyschromicum perstans (ashy dermatosis). Ashy dermatosis begins in the first or second decade and occurs on sun-protected as well as sun-exposed areas.
Minocycline pigmentation. Dermal macrophages contain iron-staining pigment (siderophages).
Centrofacial neurodysraphic lentiginosis. Malar lentigines that manifest as part of a syndrome associated with CNS defects such as seizures and mental retardation.

Minimizing UV Exposure

SUN AVOIDANCE Geographic location often places a patient at risk for UV exposure from ordinary daily activities. Avoidance of peak times of UV exposure, especially between the hours of 10 a.m. and 3 p.m., should be emphasized. Sunbathing is contraindicated, as are sporting activities without sun-protective clothing and hats, as well as sunblock. Because many Latin and African-American women of color believe they have "built-in" sun protection, studies point to infrequent and improper use of sunscreen.

SUN PROTECTION Broad-spectrum sunblock with UVA and UVB protection and a skin protection factor (SPF) of 30 or higher is a critically important adjunct to first-line melasma therapy. Additionally, sunblock must be reapplied every 2–3 hours, particularly when in broad daylight. Mineral powdered cosmetics that contain physicial blockers and hence a high SPF are excellent for reapplying SPF over other moisturizers and foundation makeup. Avoidance of possibly sensitizing sunblock preparations that can worsen melasma in an allergic individual is important. Sun-protective clothing, especially broad-brimmed hats, high-collared shirts, and sunglasses, add additional coverage for melasma patients.

AVOID PHOTOSENSITIZERS Medications and supplements that have photosensitization characteristics should be avoided (Table 48-3). Even seemingly benign

TABLE 48-3
Drugs which may cause Photosensitivity*

Acetominophen
Acitretin
Acyclovir
Allopurinol
Alprazolam
Amantadine
Amiodarone
Azithromycin
Bupropion
Captopril
Chloroquine
Chlorothiazide
Doxycycline
Estrogens
Flurouracil
Gentamicin
Glyburide
Griseofulvin
Heroin
Hydralazine
Hydrochlorothiazide
Ibuprofen
Interferon
Isotretinoin
Ketoconazole
Ketoprofen
Lisinopril
Loratidine
Minocycline
Minoxidil
Naproxen
Oral Contraceptives
St. Johns Wort
Sulfamethoxazole
Trimethoprim
Vitamin A
Zolpidem

*Abbreviated list from Litt JZ Drug Eruption Reference Manual 9th Edition Parthenon 2003

medications such as ibuprofen and St. John's wort may induce photosensitivity reactions that will trigger melasma and/or darken existing lesions.

Minimizing Contributing Hormonal Influences

Both oral contraceptive pills and HRT have roles in the development of melasma. In addition, a review of medications is necessary to identify any substances that may have hormone-like activity such as "antiaging" supplements and pharmacy-compounded creams used to reduce the symptoms of menopause. It is important to remove the hormonal stimulus in consultation with the patient's other health care professionals. Failure to eliminate the hormonal agent may make treatment of melasma refractory.

Preventing Melanin Production

Prevention of melanin production can be achieved by inhibiting melanocyte activity and inhibiting the transfer of melanosomes from melanocytes into keratinocytes.

Removing Melanin

Treatments for melasma may use the strategy of removing melanin contained in melanosomes from the epidermis. Both topical and physical modalities have been used individually and in combination for the treatment of melasma (Table 48-4).

Topical preparations of lightening agents for the treatment of melasma are numerous and constitute first-line therapy either as monotherapy or as combination therapy.[15] Hydroquinone remains the "gold standard" of melasma treatment either as monotherapy or combined with other agents. Amer and colleagues studied the effect of hydroquinone 4% cream used with a sunscreen in 50 melasma patients.[16] a good to excellent response was achieved in 89.5% of subjects with melasma. The combination of hydroquinone with other agents was pioneered by Kligman and Willis with a formula containing hydroquinone 5%, tretinoin 0.1%, and dexamethasone 21-acetate 0.1% and was found to be effective in the treatment of melasma.[17]

Taylor and colleagues, using 4% hydroquinone in combination with tretinoin 0.05% [retinoic acid (RA)] and fluocinolone acetonide 0.01% (FA); (Tri-Luma) in 641 patients, found after 8 weeks that significantly more (77%) of the patients treated with the combination had "complete" or "near complete" clearing of their melasma.[18]

Topical tretinoin either as monotherapy or in combination may be used effectively in the treatment of melasma when applied in the evening. A study by Griffiths and colleagues demonstrated statistically significant improvement in facial melasma in 50 women treated with topical tretinoin 0.1% versus vehicle for 40 weeks.[19] Kimbrough-Green and colleagues also demonstrated improvement in moderate to severe melasma in 30 black patients after using tretinoin 0.1% for 40 weeks.[20]

TABLE 48-4
Treatments for Melasma

	Topical	Systemic	Physical	Note
First line	SPF in a.m. Triple combination in p.m. or dual combination or monotherapeutic skin-lightening agent bid (topical vitamin C, Kojic acid)			
Second line	SPF in a.m. and hydroquinone in p.m.		Microdermabrasion every other week for 6 sessions Salicylic acid peels every 2–4 weeks for 3–6 peels	May use as hydroquinone as monotherapy or triple-combination agent (Triluma) after pigmentation is clear not during
Third line	SPF in a.m.		Fractional laser resurfacing effects in skintypes I–IV	IPL (effective in some Asian skin types)

Other topical agents used for the treatment of melasma include azelaic acid, kojic acid, arbutin, 4-isopropylcatechol, *N*-acetyl-4-*S*-cysteaminylphenol, adapalene and licorice extracts.[15]

In second-line therapy, topical bleaching preparations may be used in combination with physical modalities such as chemical peels or microdermabrasion. Sarkar and colleagues performed six glycolic acid peels (30% and 40%) in combination with a modified Kligman's hydroquinone formula on 40 Indian melasma patients. They had a statistically significantly better response to therapy than the group that only used the topical formula.[22] Grimes reported improvement in melasma with a series of five salicylic acid peels (20% and 30%) in six melasma patients.[23] Roberts reported that microdermabrasion followed by a combination skin-lightening agent containing hydroquinone, tretinoin, and fluocinolone was efficacious in melasma patients.[24]

As a third line and reserved for melasma refractory to first- and second-line treatments is the laser. Lasers and intense pulsed light (IPL) traditionally have been unpredictable when used for the treatment of melasma in darker skin types owing to postinflammatory hyperpigmentation.[25] A spot test should be performed when performing laser therapy for melasma prior to the actual treatment. The pathogenesis of the postinflammatory hyperpigmentation has not been completely elucidated but is thought to be due to increased activity of melanogenic enzymes overlying solar radiation–induced dermal changes.[25] Sublethal laser damage of melanocytes by a pigment laser may increase melanin production because it stimulates rather than kills the melanocyte.[26] The photomechanical effect of the Q-switched (QS) laser also may contribute to post-laser hyperpigmentation by leading to melanosome disruption. When comparing the QS laser with the long-pulsed 532-nm Nd:YAG laser in the treatment of melasma, the 532-nm Nd:YAG laser is associated with less postinflammatory hyperpigmentation because it lacks the photomechanical effects of the QS laser. The 510-nm pulsed-dye laser may lead to purpura and subsequent hyperpigmentation after melasma treatment and should be avoided in darker skin tones. IPL has been demonstrated to be safe and effective for the treatment of melasma in Asian skin but should be used at low energy settings. Wang and colleagues treated 17 patients with IPL in 16 sessions with a 39.8% improvement in melasma compared with baseline.[27]

Thirty-five percent of IPL patients received an excellent or good improvement level. There were two cases of postinflammatory hyperpigmentation. Lasers that have been proven safe and efficacious in ethnic skin types IV–VI are the long-pulsed 532-nm QS laser and, more recently, fractional laser resurfacing using the nonablative 1540-nm CO_2 laser. They have shown efficacy in the epidermal subtype of melasma. Risk factors for hyperpigmentation after laser treatments include high fluence, small spot sizes, and mixed-type melasma versus epidermal melasma.

REFERENCES

1. Sialy R, Hasan I, Kaur I, et al. Melasma in men: A hormonal profile. *J Dermatol* 2000; 27:64-65.
2. Pandya AG, Guevara IL. Disorders of pigmentation. *Dermatol Clin* 2000: 18:91-98.
3. Resnik S. Melasma induced by oral contraceptive drugs. *JAMA* 1967;199: 95-99.
4. Ponzio HA, Favaretto AL, Rivitti EA. Proposal of a quantitative method to describe melasma distribution in women. *J Cosmet Dermatol* 2007; 20:103-111.
5. Abdel- Malek Z. Regulation of human pigmentation by ultraviolet light and by endocrine, paracrine and autocrine hormones, in *Ftizpatrick's Dermatology in General Medicine,* 4th ed. New York, McGraw-Hill, 1999.
6. Kang WH, Yoon KH, Lee ES, et al. Melasma: Histopathological characteristics in 56 Korean patients. *Br J Dermatol* 2002;146:228-237.
7. Sanchez NP, Pathak MA, Sato S, et al. Melasma: A clinical, light microscopic, ultrastructural, and immunofluorescence study. *J Am Acad Dermatol* 1981;4: 698-710.
8. Grimes PE. Melasma: Etiologic and therapeutic considerations. *Arch Dermatol* 1995; 131:1453-1457.
9. Taylor SC. Epidemiology of skin diseases in people of color. *Cutis* 2003;71:271.
10. Pandya AG, Guevara IL. Disorders of hyperpigmentation. *Dermatol Clin* 2000; 18:91-98.
11. Baran R, Maibach HL (eds). *Textbook of Cosmetic Dermatology,* 2nd ed. London, Martin Dunitz, 1998.
12. Sanchez NP, Pathak MA, Sato S, et al. Melasma: A clinical, light microscopic, ultrastructural and immunofluorescence study. *J Am Acad Dermatol* 1981;4:698.
13. Grimes PE, Yamada N, Bhawan J. Light microscopic, immunohistochemical, and ultrastructural alterations in patients with melasma. *Am J Dermatopathol* 2005; 27:96-101.
14. Hori Y, Kawashima M, Oohara K. Acquired bilateral nevus of Ota-like macules. *J Am Acad Dermatol* 1984;10:961-964.
15. Gupta AK, Gover MD, Nouri K, Taylor SC. The treatment of melasma: A review of clinical trials. *J Am Acad Dermatol* 2006; 55:1048-1065.
16. Amer M, Metwalli M. Topical hydroquinone in the treatment of some hyperpigmentary disorders. *Int J Dermatol* 1998; 37:449-450.
17. Kligman AM, Willis I. A new formula for depigmenting human skin. *Arch Dermatol* 1975;111:40-48.
18. Taylor SC, Torok H, Jones T, et al. Efficacy and safety of a new triple-combination agent for the treatment of facial melasma. *Cutis* 2003;72:67-72.
19. Griffiths CE, Finkel LJ, Ditre CM, et al. Topical tretinoin (retinoic acid) improves melasma: A vehicle-controlled clinical trial. *Br J Dermatol* 1993;129:415-421.
20. Kimbrough-Green CK, Griffiths CE, Finkel LJ, et al. Topical retinoic acid (tretinoin) for melasma in black patients: A vehicle-controlled clinical trial. *Arch Dermatol* 1994;130:727-733.
21. Gupta AK, Gover MD, Nouri K, Taylor SC. The treatment of melasma: A review of clinical trials. *J Am Acad Dermatol* 2006;55:1048-1065.
22. Sarkar R, Kaur C, Bhalla M, Kanwar AJ. The combination of glycolic acid peels with a topical regimen in the treatment of melasma in dark-skinned patients: A comparative study. *Dermatol Surg* 2002; 28:828-832.
23. Grimes PE. The safety and efficacy of salicylic acid chemical peels in darker racial-ethnic groups. *Dermatol Surg* 1999;25: 18-22.
24. Roberts WE. Microdermabrasion Dual Therapy. *Microdermabrasion Skin and Allergy News* 2002;33:42.
25. Chan HL. The use of lasers and intense pulsed light for treating melasma. *J Cosmet Dermatol* 2007;20:81-84.
26. Chan H. The use of lasers and intense pulsed light sources for the treatment of acquired pigmentary lesions in Asians. *J Cosmet Laser Ther* 2003;5:198-200.
27. Chan H, Alam M, Kono, et al. Clinical applications of lasers in Asians. *Dermatol Surg* 2002;28:556-563.
28. Wang CC, Hui CY, Sue YM, et al. Intense pulsed light for the treatment of refractory melasma in Asian persons. *Dermatol Surg* 2004;30:1196-1200.

CHAPTER 49

Postinflammatory Hyperpigmentation

Candrice R. Heath
Susan C. Taylor

Key Points

- Postinflammatory hyperpigmentation (PIH) is a common disorder affecting individuals with skin of color.
- PIH presents with tan, brown, or gray macules or patches occurring at the site of a previous inflammatory stimulus.
- Although PIH is not a life-threatening disorder, it negatively affects quality of life.
- Diagnosis of PIH does not require complicated or extensive testing but is usually clinical.
- The cornerstone of treatment is hydroquinone in combination with sun protection.
- Physical modalities such as chemical peels, microdermabrasion, and laser therapy also may be effective in treatment.

Postinflammatory hyperpigmentation (PIH) is a common disorder that occurs in just about all individuals with skin of color (Figure 49-1). This acquired pigmentation involves areas of prior inflammatory disease, infection, allergic contact or irritant reactions, injury from prior procedures or trauma, sites of papulosquamous or vesiculobullous disease, and medication reactions[1–3] (Figure 49-2). It commonly appears on the skin as brown to gray macules or patches. PIH can be emotionally distressing for patients, affecting all aspects of their personal and professional lives.[4]

EPIDEMIOLOGY, ETIOLOGY, AND PATHOGENESIS

PIH affects women and men with equal incidence and may occur at any age. Although PIH may be more apparent in Fitzpatrick skin types III–VI, all skin types have the potential to develop PIH lesions (see Figures 49-1 and 49-2). The PIH in Fitzpatrick skin types III–VI patients may last longer and sometimes never completely fades.[1,2,5,6] Some authors have concluded that people with skin of color are more likely to develop PIH owing to the large amount of melanin contained in melanosomes within the epidermis.[1,2] Other investigators have theorized that a person's tendency to develop PIH is related to the specific type of melanocyte present: weak, strong, or normal. After an inflammatory event or skin trauma, weak melanocytes result in hypopigmenatation owing to the decreased production of melanin, whereas strong melanocytes produce excess pigment, leading to hyperpigmentation.[2] Although melanin production may be increased in PIH, the number of melanocytes is normal.[1] Normal melanocytes continually produce appropriate quantities of melanin, resulting in normochromia.[2]

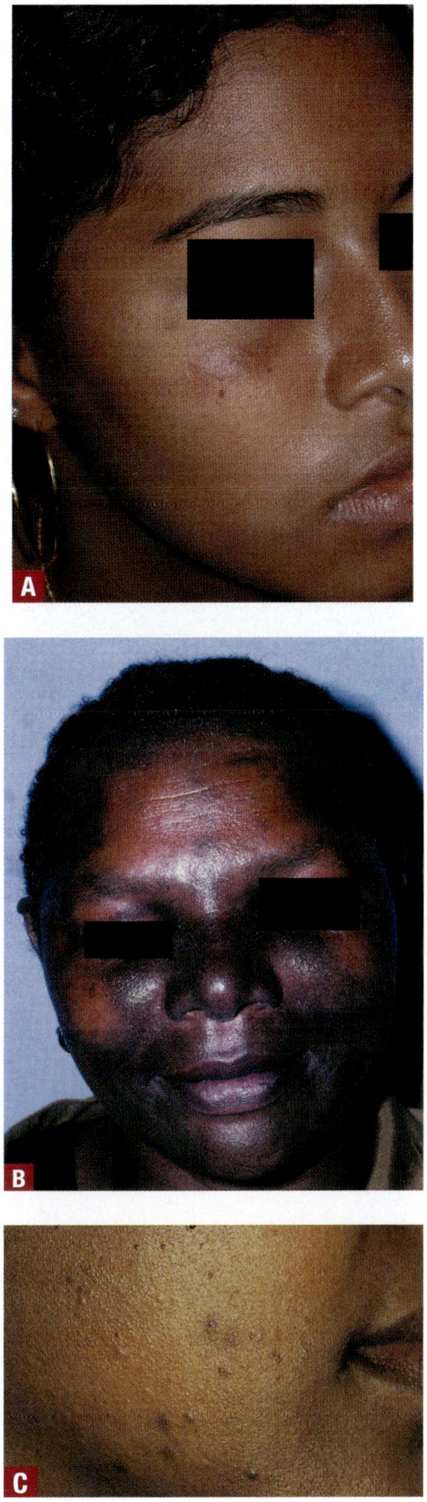

▲ **FIGURE 49-1** Hyperpigmentation on the face. **A.** Postinflammatory hyperpigmentation from acne in a skin type V woman. **B.** Hyperpigmentation on the face of a skin type VI woman. **C.** Hyperpigmenation on the cheek of a skin type IV Latina woman.

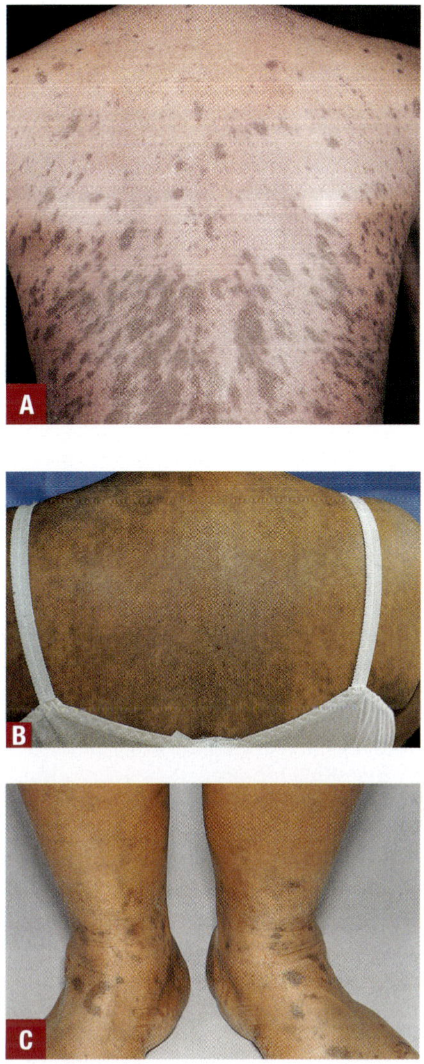

▲ **FIGURE 49-2** Postinflammatory hyperpigmentation may occur after drug eruption, lichen planus, psoriasis, tinea versicolor, or eczema. **A.** Postinflammatory hyperpigmentation on the back of a skin type IV East Indian woman. From *Fitzpatrick's Color Atlas of Dermatology,* 5th ed. New York, McGraw-Hill, 2005, Fig. 13-10. **B.** Postinflammatory hyperpigmentation on the back of a skin type V African-American woman. **C.** Postinflammatory hyperpigmentation from lichen planus on the ankles and feet of a skin type V woman.

TABLE 49-1
Stimuli Producing PIH

- Dermatologic diseases
  - Acneiform
  - Papulosquamous
  - Lichenoid
  - Psoriasiform
  - Vesiculobullous
- Infections
- Dermatologic therapy
  - Topical agents
  - Drug eruptions
- Cosmetic procedures
  - Chemical peels
  - Microdermabrasion
  - Cryosurgery
  - Laser therapy
  - Intense pulse light therapy
  - Fillers
- Trauma

There are a myriad of stimuli that may result in PIH (Table 49-1). The hyperpigmented macules and patches seen in PIH result from mechanisms occurring in both the epidermal and the dermal layers of the skin. Inflammatory cells release mediators and cytokines that play a role in PIH.[3] In response to inflammation, arachidonic acid mediators such as prostaglandins and leukotrienes stimulate increased melanin synthesis and transport to keratinocytes.[5,7] Oleic acid and stem cell factor also have been implicated in the pathogenesis of PIH.[8,9] Inflammation may cause the disruption of melanocytes and the release of pigment into the dermis, a phenomenon called *pigment incontinence*.[2,5]

CLINICAL FINDINGS

History

The chief complaint of the patient with PIH includes dark marks, dark spots, uneven skin tone, discolorations, and blemishes. Patients with PIH have underlying cutaneous inflammatory conditions that may be clinical or subclinical or a history of trauma.

Physical Findings

The morphology of the macules and patches of PIH is variable, but the borders are often hazy and are distributed in areas of prior inflammation. When melanin is deposited in the epidermis, the lesions tend to be brown, but melanin in the dermis causes lesions to have a dark gray or gray-blue hue.[1,2]

Laboratory and Other Tests

The diagnosis of PIH does not require a biopsy. However, if the diagnosis is unclear, a biopsy may be helpful in elucidating this disorder. Evidence of PIH may be found in the epidermis, dermis, or both. In a study of PIH as a result of acne, biopsies were taken and screened for numerous inflammatory and pigmentary mediators. However, compared with normal skin, there were no significant differences in the endothelin-1, interleukin-1, α-melanocyte-stimulating hormone, basic fibroblast growth factor, or CD1α, a Langerhans cell marker.[10] Some authors suggest using a Wood's lamp to distinguish between epidermal and dermal melanin. Under the Wood's lamp, lesions with increased epidermal pigment appear darker.[11]

DIFFERENTIAL DIAGNOSIS (FIGURES 49-3 THROUGH 49-5)

Most Likely

- Melasma

Consider

- Exogenous ochronosis
- Amyloidosis (lichenoid/macular)
- Tinea versicolor
- Lichen planus
- Acanthosis nigricans
- Erythema dyschromicum perstans (ashy dermatosis)
- Morphea

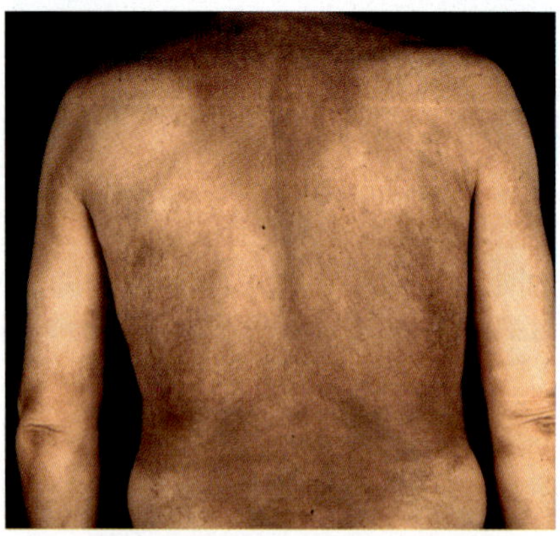

▲ **FIGURE 49-3** Macular amyloidosis on the back of an Arabian man. From *Fitzpatrick's Color Atlas of Dermatology,* 5th ed. New York, McGraw-Hill, 2005, Figure 14-4.

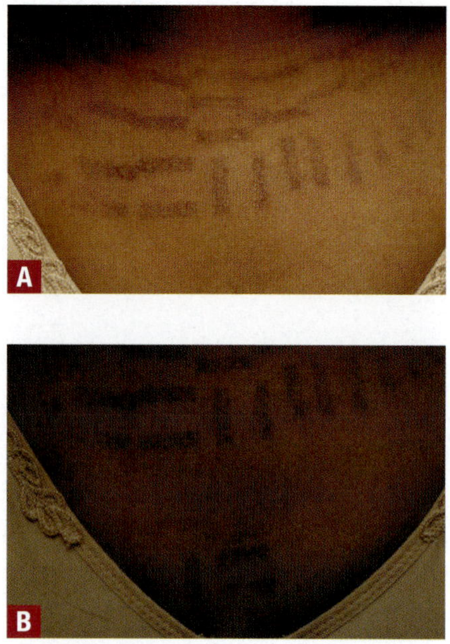

▲ **FIGURE 49-4 A, B.** Laser hair removal induced postinflammatory hyperpigmentation in a skin type V African-American woman.

Always Rule Out

- Addison disease
- Systemic lupus erythematosus

COMPLICATIONS

Complications may occur owing to irritation associated with therapy. An unfortunate treatment complication is further hyperpigmentation.

PROGNOSIS/CLINICAL COURSE

Epidermal pigment may take 6–12 months to fade, whereas dermal pigment may be present for years.[12] Underlying inflammatory conditions, if

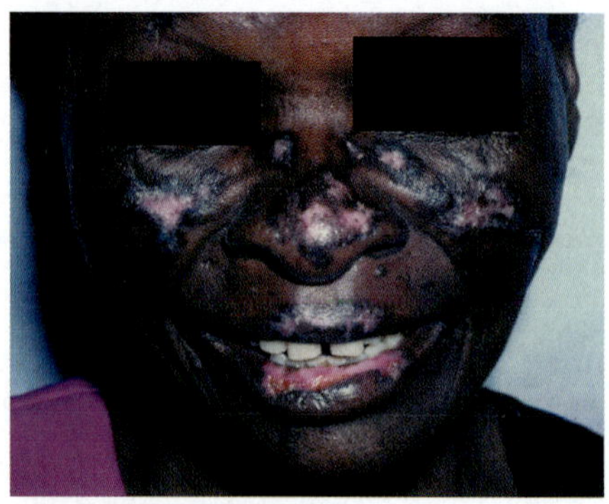

▲ **FIGURE 49-5** Hyperpigmentation secondary to discoid lupus on the face of a skin type VI woman.

left untreated, could result in new areas of PIH.[12] Treating PIH is challenging, but many viable options are available, particularly for epidermal hyperpigmentation.

PREVENTION

The cornerstone of preventing or reducing PIH is to treat the underlying inflammatory condition. In addition, photoprotection with the use of a broad-spectrum sunscreen with a skin protection factor (SPF) of at least 30, coupled with protective clothing, hats, and sunglasses, is essential.[1,13] With that said, the location of the pigment plays a role in how helpful photoprotection may be. It is less likely to be helpful when the pigment is in the dermis, in which case the hyperpigmentation has a slate-blue to brown color.[13]

TREATMENT

There are several factors that influence the success of PIH treatment, including the location of the pigment, epidermal or dermal; adequate treatment of any underlying inflammatory disease affecting the skin; patient compliance; and the patient's response to available treatments. Resolution may be spontaneous, obviating the need for therapy).

Topical skin-lightening agents and physical modalities such as chemical peels, microdermabrasion, and laser treatments also may be used to treat PIH.[1] However, these treatments may induce hyperpigmentation owing to irritation and inflammation.[1]

Hydroquinone (HQ) has been considered the "gold standard" for treating all forms of hyperpigmentation.[1,14] It prevents the conversion of tyrosine to dopa, in turn inhibiting the synthesis of melanin.[14] HQ is also thought to cause injury to existing melanocytes.[11] Although HQ is used in the treatment of most patients with PIH, there is a paucity of clinical studies demonstrating its effectiveness in treating hyperpigmentation.[15–17] Additionally, adverse events have been reported. HQ may induce irritation, erythema, and scaling.[1] In patients using HQ as a spot treatment, halo hypopigmentation may occur around the treated hyperpigmented patch.[1] Additionally, exogenous ochronosis may occur after long-term HQ use.[18–20]

Ultraviolet (UV) light stimulates melanogenesis, whereas retinoic acid inhibits melanin production.[21] Retinoids may induce skin lightening owing to the epidermal melanin redistribution or dispersion.[22] Retinoids may be used to treat various types of hyperpigmentation, including PIH.[22–24] Tretinoin 0.1%, adapalene 0.1% gel, and tazarotene 0.1% cream all have demonstrated efficacy in improving PIH induced by acne vulgaris after 12–40 weeks of therapy.

The tyrosinase inhibitors azelaic acid and kojic acid also have been used in the treatment of PIH with varied efficacy and tolerability. They are generally considered second-line therapy and are used in situations where HQ and/or retinoids cannot be used.[25,26]

Recently, several combination therapies for PIH have been reported, including[1]

- Hydroquinone 4% and retinol 0.3%
- Mequinol 2% and tretinoin 0.01%
- Fluocinolone acetonide 0.01% and hydroquinone 4% and tretinoin 0.05%

Chemical peels, specifically glycolic acid peels, have been very helpful in the treatment of PIH.[27,28] However, there is a risk of trauma to the skin and hence further hyperpigmentation.[28] Microdermabrasion alone or in addition with chemical peels and dermabrasion has been effective in treating PIH.[29,30] Cryotherapy is not used for the treatment of PIH owing to the unpredictability of results. Finally, various lasers, including the Q-switched ruby laser and the pulseddye laser, have been used, although the adverse events outweigh the benefit of the therapy (See Figure 49-6).[31,32]

CONCLUSION

PIH is one of the most common cutaneous disorders occurring in individuals with skin of color. It is the result of a wide range of cutaneous disorders, trauma, or medications, to name just a few. Several treatments are available for PIH, although topical hydroquinone remains the cornerstone of therapy.

Treatment	Clinical Research Studies demonstrating efficacy for the treatment of hyperpigmentation disorders
Hydroquinone 4%	-Amer M, Metwalli M. Topical Hydroquinone in the treatment of some hyperpigmentary disorders. *Int J Dermatol* 1998; 37:449-450 -Haddad AL, Matos LF, Brunstein F, Ferreira LM, Silva A, Costa D Jr. A clinical trial, prospective, randomized, double-blind trial comparing skin whitening complex with hydroquinone vs placebo in the treatment of melasma. *Int J Dermatol* 2003; 42: 153-156
Retinoids (ex. Tretinoin, Tazarotene)	-Griffiths CE, Finkel LJ, Ditre CM, Hamilton TA, Ellis CN, Voorhees JJ. Topical tretinoin (retinoic acid) improves melasma: a vehicle-controlled, clinical trial. *Br J Dermatol* 1993; 129: 415-421 -Kimbrough-Green CK, Griffiths CE, Finkel LJ, Hamilton TA, Bulengo-Ransby SM, Ellis CN, et al. Topical retinoic acid (tretinoin) for melasma in black patients: a vehicle-controlled clinical trial. *Arch Dermatol* 1994; 130: 727-733 -Grimes P, Callender V. Tazarotene Cream for Postinflammatory Hyperpigmentation and Acne Vulgaris in Darker Skin: A Double-Blind, Randomized, Vehicle-Controlled Study. *Cutis* 2006; 77: 45-50
Corticosteroids (ex. Betamethasone 17-valerate 0.2%)	-Neering H. Treatment of melasma (cholasma) by local application of a steroid cream. *Dermatologica* 1975; 151: 349-353
Combination (Hydroquinone 4% + Tretinoin 0.05% + Flucinolone Acetonide) (Hydroquinone 4% + Retinol 0.15% + Antioxidants) (Hydroquinone 4% + Retinol 0.15%)	-Taylor SC, Torok H, Jones T, Lowe N, Rich P, Tschen E, et al. Efficacy and safety of a new triple-combination agent for the treatment of facial melasma. *Cutis* 2003; 72: 67-72 -Cook-Bolden FE, Hamilton SE. An open-label study of the efficacy and tolerability of microencapsulated hydroquinone 4% and retinol 0.15% with antioxidants for the treatment of hyperpigmenation. *Cutis* 2008; 81: 365-371 -Grimes PE. A microsponge formulation of hydroquinone 4% and retinol in the treatment of melasma and postinflammatory hyperpigmentation. *Cutis* 2004; 74: 362-368
Azelaic Acid	-Lowe NJ, Rizk D, Grimes P, Billips M, Pincus S. Azelaic acid 20% cream in the treatment of facial hyperpigmenation in darker-skinned patients. Clin *Ther* 1998; 20:945-959 -Verallo-Rowell VM, Verallo V, Graupe K, Lopez-Villafuerte L, Garcia-Lopez M. Double-blind comparison of azelaic acid and hydroquinone in the treatment of melasma. *Acta Derm Venereol* Suppl (Stockh) 1989; 143: 58-61

▲ **FIGURE 49-6** Topical modalities for the treatment of hyperpigmentation.(*Continued*)

	-Balina LM, Graupe K. The treatment of melasma: 20% azelaic acid versus 4% hydroquinone cream. *Int J Dermatol* 1991; 30: 893-895 -Kakita LS, Lowe NJ. Azelaic acid and glycolic acid combination therapy for facial hyperpigmentation in darker-skinned patients: a clinical comparison with hydroquinone. *Clin Ther* 1998; 20:960-970
Kojic Acid	-Lim JT. Treatment of melasma using kojic acid in a gel containing hydroquinone and glycolic acid. *Dermatol Surg* 1999; 25:282-284 -Garcia A, Fulton JE Jr. The combination of glycolic acid and hydroquinoe or kojic acid for the treatment of melasma and related conditions. *Dermatol Surg* 1996; 22:443-447
Glycolic Acid	-Hurley MD, Guevara IL, Gonzalez RM, Pandya AG. Efficacy of glycolic acid peels in the treatment of melasma. *Arch Dermatol* 2002; 138: 1578-1582 -Sarkar R, Kaur C, Bhalla M, Kanwar AJ. The combination of glycolic acid peels with a topical regimen in the treatment of melasma in dark-skinned patients: a comparative study. *Dermatol Surg* 2002; 28: 828-832 -Javaheri SM, Handa S, Kaur I, Kumar B. Safety and efficacy of glycolic acid facial peel in Indian women with melasma. *Int J Dermatol* 2001; 40: 354-357 -Lim JT, Tham SN. Glycolic acid peels in the treatment of melasma among Asian women. *Dermatol Surg* 1997; 23: 177-179
Salicylic acid	-Grimes PE. The safety and efficacy of salicylic acid chemical peels in darker racial-ethnic groups. *Dermatol Surg* 1999; 25: 18-22
Trichloroacetic acid	-Chun EY, Lee JB, Lee KH. Focal trichloroacetic acid peel method for benign pigmented lesions in dark-skinned patients. *Dermatol Surg* 2004; 30: 512-516

▲ **FIGURE 49-6** *Continued*

REFERENCES

1. Taylor SC, Burgess C, Callendar V, et al. Postinflammatory hyperpigmentation: Evolving combination treatment strategies. *Cutis* 2006;78:1-25.
2. Ruiz-Maldonado R, de la Luz Orozco-Covarrubias M. Postinflammatory hypopigmentation and hyperpigmentation. *Semin Cutan Med Surg* 1996; 16:36-43.
3. Halder R, Nootheti P. Ethnic skin disorders overview. *J Am Acad Dermatol* 2003; 48:S143-148.
4. Chadurvedi SK, Singh G, Gupta N. Stigma experience in skin disorders: An Indian perspective. *Dermatol Clin* 2005; 23:635-642.
5. Bose SK, Ortonne JP. Pigmentation: dyschromia, in Baran R, Maibach HI (eds), *Cosmetic Dermatology*. London, Martin Dunitz, 1994, pp 277-298.
6. Stulberg DL, Clark N, Tovey D. Common hyperpigmentation disorders in adults: II. Melanoma, seborrheic keratoses, acanthosis nigricans, melasma, diabetic dermopathy, tinea versicolor, and postinflammatory hyperpigmentation. *Am Fam Physician* 2003;68:1963-1968.
7. Tomita Y, Maeda K, Tagami H. Melanocyte-stimulating properties of arachidonic acid metabolites: Possible role in postinflammatory pigmentation. *Pigment Cell Res* 1992;5:357-361.
8. Kitawaki A, Tanaka Y, Takada K. New findings on the mechanism of post-inflammatory pigmentation. *Pigment Cell Res* 2003;16:603.
9. Maurer M, Galli SJ. Lack of significant skin inflammation during elimination by apoptosis of large numbers of mouse cutaneous mast cells after cessation of treatment with stem cell factor. *Lab Invest* 2004;84:1593-1602.
10. Grimes PE, Bhawan J, Kim J. An assessment of the histopathological features of post-inflammatory hyperpigmentation. Poster, American Academy of Dermatology, 2005.
11. Paraskevas PR, Halpern AC, Marghoob AA. Utility of the Wood's light: Five cases from a pigmented lesion clinic. *Br J Dermatol* 2005;152:1039-1044.
12. Lacz N, Vafaie J, Kihiczak N, et al. Postinflammatory hyperpigmenatation: A common but not troubling condition. *Int J Dermatol* 2004;43:362-365.
13. Epstein J. Postinflammatory hyperpigmentation. *Clin Dermatol* 1989;7:55-65.
14. Halder R, Richards GM. Topical agents used in the management of hyperpigmentation. *Skin Ther Lett* 2004;9:45-50.
15. Cook-Bolden F. The efficacy and tolerability of a combination cream containing 4% hydroquinone in the treatment of postinflammatory hyperpigmentation in skin types IV-VI. *Cosmet Dermatol* 2004; 17:149-155.
16. Swinyer LJ, Wortzman M. Study of hydroquinone USP 4%, 0.05% tretinoin, and in combination in UV-induced dyschromia with actinic photodamage. *Cosmet Dermatol* 2000;3:13-18.
17. Grimes PE. A microsponge formulation of hydroquinone 4% and retinol 0.15% in the treatment of melasma and postinflammatory hyperpigmentation. *Cutis* 2004; 74:362-368.
18. Lawrence N, Bligard CA, Reed R, Perret WJ. Exogenous ochronosis in the United Stated. *J Am Acad Dermatol* 1988; 18:1207-1211.
19. Levin CY, Maibach H. Exogenous ochronosis: An update on clinical features, causative agents and treatment options. *Am J Clin Dermatol* 2001; 2:213-217.
20. Olumide Y, Akinkugbe A, Altraide D, et al. Complications of chronic use of skin lightening cosmetics. *Int J Dermatol* 2008; 47:344-353.
21. Romero C, Aberdam E, Larnier C, et al. Retinoic acid as modulator of UVB-induced melanocyte differentiation. *J Cell Sci* 1994; 107:1095-1103.
22. Bulengo-Ransby SM, Griffiths CEM, Kimbrough-Green CK. Topical tretinoin (retinoic acid) therapy for hyperpigmented lesions caused by inflammation of the skin in black patients. *N Eng J Med* 1993; 328:1438-1443.
23. Jacyk WK, Mpofu P. Adapalene gel 0.1% for topical treatment of acne vulgaris in African patients. *Cutis* 2001;68:48-54S.
24. Grimes P, Callender V. Tazarotene cream for postinflammatory hyperpigmentation and acne vulgaris in darker skin: A double-blind, randomized, vehicle-controlled study. *Cutis* 2006;77:45-50.
25. Lowe NJ, Rizk D, Grimes P, et al. Azelaic acid 20% cream in the treatment of facial hyperpigmentation in darker-skinned patients. *Clin Ther* 1998; 20:945-959.
26. Nakagawa M, Kawai K, Kawai K. Contact allergy to kojic acid in skin care products. *Contact Dermatitis* 1995;32:9-13.
27. Burns RL, Prevost-Blank PL, Lawry MA, et al. Glycolic acid peels for postinflammatory hyperpigmentation in black patients: A comparative study. *Dermatol Surg* 1997; 23:171-174.
28. Roberts W. Chemical peeling in ethnic/dark Skin. *Dermatol Ther* 2004; 17: 196-205.
29. Cotellessa C, Peris K, Fargnoli MC, et al. Microabrasion versus microabrasion followed by 15% trichloracetic acid for treatment of cutaneous hyperpigmentations in adult females. *Dermatol Surg* 2003; 23:352-356.
30. Kunachak S, Leelaudomlipi P, Wongwaisayawan S. Dermabrasion: A curative treatment for melasma. *Aesthet Plast Surg* 2001;25:114-117.
31. Taylor CR, Anderson RR. Ineffective treatment of refractory melasma and postinflammatory hyperpigmentation by Q-switched ruby laser. *J Dermatol Surg Oncol* 1994;20:592-597.
32. Dierickx C, Goldman MP, Fitzpatrick RE. Laser treatment of erythematous/hypertrophic and pigmented scars in 26 patients. *Plast Reconstr Surg* 1955;95: 84-90.

CHAPTER 50

Periorbital Hypermelanosis

Raechele Cochran Gathers

Key Points

- Colloquially referred to as dark circles, characterized by bilateral homogeneous hyperchromia involving primarily the upper and lower eyelid regions.
- Generally benign, occurs very often although the exact prevalence is unclear.
- May be secondary to excessive epidermal or dermal melanin deposition, excessive or superficial vasculature or skin laxity, and periorbital fat pseudoherniation.
- Infrequently may be associated with systemic disease, drugs, or allergy.
- Treatment, which should be directed toward the primary etiology, includes sunscreens, topical bleaching agents, chemical peels, lasers, dermal fillers, and surgical intervention.

EPIDEMIOLOGY, ETIOLOGY AND PATHOGENESIS

Periorbital hyperpigmentation, often colloquially referred to as *dark circles,* is defined as bilateral, homogeneous hyperchromic macules and patches primarily involving the upper and lower eyelids but also sometimes extending toward the eyebrows, malar regions, and lateral nasal root.[1,2] Periorbital hyperpigmentation can be much more noticeable in ethnic populations[3] and is often a significant cosmetic concern because it can portend a fatigued, sad, or aged appearance. Despite the perceived prevalence of periorbital hyperpigmentation, there are few comprehensive epidemiologic data. Although not rare in males, owing to hormonal factors, females may be affected more frequently.[4,5]

Many causal factors have been implicated in the development of periorbital hyperpigmentation (Table 50-1). Genetics,[2,6,7] fatigue, stress and emotional lability, exhaustion of the periorbital muscles, and aging all may play a significant role. Lifestyle factors associated with periorbital hyperpigmentation may include alcohol overuse, smoking, and excessive intake of caffeinated beverages.[4] Various systemic etiologies also have been associated with periorbital hyperpigmentation, including cachexia, biliary disease, hyperthyroidism,[8] vitamin K deficiency, Addison disease, heart and kidney disease, and other circulatory conditions that may cause excessive fluid retention.[4] Periorbital hyperpigmentation also may be seen in ectodermal dysplasia,[9] erythema dyschromicum perstans,[10] and acanthosis nigricans. A rare autosomally dominant pattern of periorbital hyperpigmentation also may be seen.[6,7]

TABLE 50-1
Etiology of Periorbital Hyperpigmentation

Most Likely

- Fatigue/stress
- Hereditary factors
- Aging/photodamage
- Lifestyle factors (alcohol, smoking, caffeine)

Consider

- Postinflammatory
- Atopy
- Eye strain
- Hormonal
- Medications (oral contraceptives, antipsychotics, chemotherapeutics, etc.)

Always Rule Out

- Hepatic/renal disease
- Thyroid disease
- Addison disease
- Carcinoma
- Ecchymoses
- Vitamin K deficiency
- Hereditary blood disorder

Patients with atopic dermatitis, contact dermatitis, or any airborne or food allergy may experience periorbital itching and irritation with ensuing periorbital hyperpigmentation.[4] Atopic individuals also may develop inferior lid discoloration (allergic shiners) resulting from mucosal edema and venous stasis of the paranasal sinuses.[10,11] Periorbital ecchymoses (raccoon's eyes) resulting from anterior fossa fracture may lead to periorbital hyperpigmentation. Additionally, neoplasms must be considered. Eyelid melanoma and, in children, neuroblastoma metastatic to the orbits may lead to periorbital hyperpigmentation. Finally, chronic use of some drugs, including oral contraceptives, hormone-replacement therapy, antipsychotics, iron-containing compounds, gold, and chemotherapeutic agents, can lead to periorbital hyperpigmentation.[10] When assessing the patient with periorbital hyperpigmentation, a comprehensive history and directed review of systems should be performed. A complete medical evaluation may be necessary in cases of sudden onset, rapid progression, or unexplained symptomatology.

Histologic characteristics of periorbital hyperpigmentation suggest that it may be caused by a number of pathogenetic factors, including epidermal and dermal hypermelanosis, excessive or superficial vasculature and periorbital edema, and shadowing of the skin secondary to anatomic factors such as skin laxity and pseudoherniation of periorbital fat.[1,4]

CLINICAL FINDINGS

The clinical presentation of periorbital hyperpigmentation is related to its pathogenesis. Periorbital hyperpigmentation secondary to excessive epidermal melanin may appear brown in color (Figure 50-1). Pigmentation secondary to excessive dermal melanin may appear blue-gray in color. A Wood's light examination has been proposed to help distinguish between epidermal and dermal melanin but may not be useful in darker skin types.[12]

Periorbital hyperpigmentation related to hypervascularity often has a violaceous or bluish color owing to visibility of the dermal capillary network.[13] Applying pressure or stretching the affected skin often will lessen the appearance of the pigmentation. Periorbital hyperpigmentation owing to periorbital edema is often characterized by variability, a purplish hue, and is often worse in the morning or after a salty meal.[1]

Pseudoherniation of the periorbital fat and skin laxity can result in the creation of dark shadows. Facial movements may cause repositioning of the muscles and skin, thus altering the pattern of light on the face and emphasizing the appearance of hyperpigmentation.[4] While history and physical examination are usually sufficient to determine the primary cause of periorbital hyperpigmentation, confirmation by histologic examination may rarely be necessary.

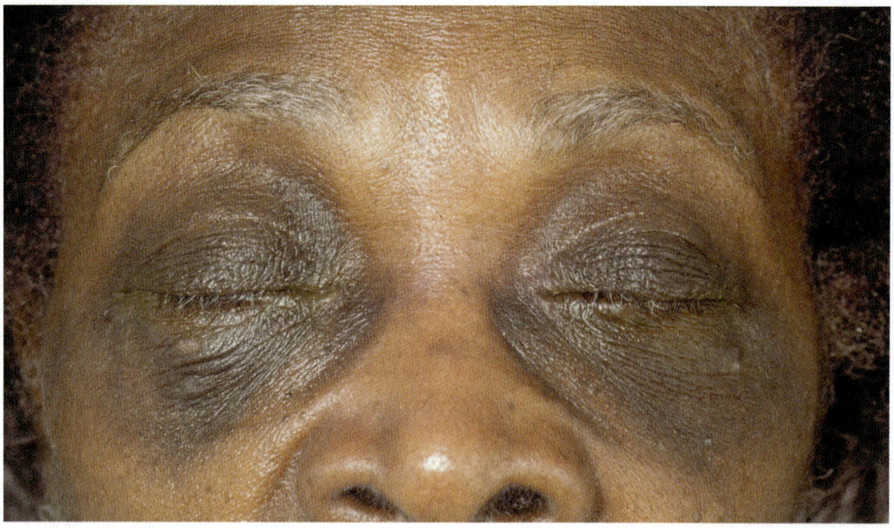

▲ **FIGURE 50-1** Woman with periorbital hyperpigmentation.

DIFFERENTIAL DIAGNOSIS

The differential diagnosis or periorbital hyperpigmentation includes inflammatory dermatoses, pigmentary disorders, vascular lesions, and skin cancer (Table 50-2).

COMPLICATIONS

Although periorbital hyperpigmentation may indicate more serious systemic disease, it is in and of itself a benign physical finding. Nevertheless, many patients may be considerably frustrated by their cosmetic appearance. Further, the injudicious use of medicated and cosmetic creams may result in many side effects, including acne, dermatitis, skin fragility, and worsening hyperpigmentation.[5]

PROGNOSIS/CLINICAL COURSE

Periorbital hyperpigmentation is often resistant to treatment. Clinical relapse is also fairly common. Skin of color, owing to its propensity toward hyperpigmentation, necessitates special therapeutic considerations. Prognosis depends on identification and management of the primary causes of hyperpigmentation.[4] Unfortunately, even with a thorough understanding of etiologic factors, periorbital hyperpigmentation may remain variably recalcitrant to therapeutic intervention. Proper management of patient expectations therefore is paramount.

TABLE 50-2
Differential Diagnosis of Periorbital Hyperpigmentation

Most Likely

- Postinflammatory hyperpigmentation
- Irritant/allergic contact dermatitis

Consider

- Nevus of Ota
- Acanthosis nigricans
- Erythema dyschromicum perstans
- Fixed drug eruption

Always Rule Out

- Ecchymoses
- Melanoma

TREATMENT

The treatment of periorbital hyperpigmentation should be directed toward the primary cause of the hyperpigmentation (Table 50-3). Often, several treatment modalities will need to be used for optimal response. Because of the lengthy treatment course, patients should be actively involved in the planning of any therapeutic regimen. Treatment options include sunscreens, various lightening agents, chemical peels, laser therapy, botulinum toxin, soft tissue fillers, and surgical intervention. Over-the-counter cosmetics may play a valuable role in camouflage.

Sunscreens

Since periorbital hyperpigmentation is often caused by excessive melanin deposition, the first line of therapy is often the use of a broad-spectrum (UVA/UVB) sunscreen. For optimal ultraviolet A (UVA) coverage, products containing Helioplex or Mexoryl (ecamsule) are preferable. In addition, all-weather UV coated sunglasses that block 99–100% of UVA/UVB are recommended.[4]

Skin-Lightening Agents

A wide range of phenolic and nonphenolic lightening agents exist. Topical hydroquinone, a phenolic lightening agent, has been the "gold standard" for treating hyperpigmentation for more than a half century.[14] Commonly available in 3% and 4% prescription strengths, hydroquinones are most effective in the treatment of epidermal hyperpigmentation. Often, antioxidants such as vitamin C, retinoids, and α-hydroxyacids may be added to improve the efficacy of hydroquinone. Other agents include *N*-acetyl-4-cysteaminylphenol (NCAP), another phenolic agent not yet available in North America. As with hydroquinone, NCAP inhibits tyrosinase activity but also stimulates the production of pheomelanin rather than eumelanin.[15] NCAP may be more stable and less irritating than hydroquinone. Tretinoin, a vitamin A derivative, has been used in the treatment of hyperpigmentation, particularly epidermal melanin.[16] Topical steroids and hydroquinone may be added to tretinoin to improve its efficacy. Other retinoids, including tazarotene and adapalene, have been found to be comparable in efficacy to tretinoin for the treatment of hyperpigmentation, but with

TABLE 50-3
Etiology and Treatment of Periorbital Hyperpigmentation

Etiology	Treatment
Epidermal/dermal melanin	Sun protection Topical bleaching agents Chemical peels Laser
Superficial or excessive vasculature	Topical vitamin K preparations Laser
Skin laxity/fat pseudoherniation	Dermal fillers Botox Surgical intervention (blepharoplasty)

the added benefit of greater tolerability for adapalene.[17]

Topical azelaic acid, a naturally occurring nonphenolic dicarboxylic acid, has been used for its selective effect on abnormal melanocytes. Kojic acid, a naturally occurring hydrophilic fungal derivative, popular in Asia, is similar to hydroquinone in its mechanism of action but may cause contact dermatitis and erythema. Arbutin, another agent popular in Asia, is an extract of the bearberry plant. It is effective in higher concentrations but also may cause paradoxical hyperpigmentation. Finally, glycyrrhetinic acid, an extract from licorice (*Glycyrrhiza glabra*), may inhibit both inflammation and pigmentation.

Chemical Peels

Chemical peels may be useful in the treatment of periorbital hyperpigmentation. Superficial salicylic acid peels have proven efficacy in darker skin types.[18] Glycolic acid peels also have been found to be effective. Although not commonly used in darker skin types, phenol peels, along with transconjunctival blepharoplasty, have been reported as therapeutic in skin type V.[19] Nonetheless, with this method, significant pigment irregularity is a possible adverse event. Despite their possible risks, when performed by a properly trained provider skilled in the treatment of ethnic skin, chemical peels are a useful therapeutic adjunct.[3] It should be noted that when periorbital hyperpigmentation is caused primarily by hypervascularity, chemical peels are contraindicated because they may worsen the clinical appearance.[4]

Laser Therapy

Lasers that target pigment and vascularity are now a viable treatment option for darker skin types. Longer wavelengths and cooling devices have made laser therapy a valuable therapeutic alternative for ethnic skin. The Q-switched ruby laser has been described in the treatment of periorbital hyperpigmentation.[20] Emitting a red light, it causes the selective destruction of melanized melanosomes.[21] When using lasers, physicians must be aware that darker skin types may require more frequent visits and necessitate longer therapeutic time requirements, and as with other modalities, the pigment may not be completely cleared.

Botulinum Toxin and Soft Tissue Fillers

Botulinum toxin type A may help to lessen the appearance of periorbital hyperpigmentation in cases where active musculature alters the pattern of light on the face and emphasizes dark shadows.[4] Restylane (hyaluronic acid) is the most popular filler for ethnic skin[3] and may be used to fill periorbital hollows and to restore volume, thus decreasing shadowing. Other fillers, including Sculptra (poly-L-lactic acid), which acts to stimulate collagen fiber production, are gaining popularity.

Surgery

Blepharoplasty, either alone or in conjunction with other procedures, may be useful in eliminating periorbital hyperpigmentation caused by shadows cast by fat deposits and skin laxity.[4] Transconjunctival blepharoplasty, coupled with phenol peels, has been reported to be effective in darker skin types.[19]

Cosmeceuticals

Although response may be modest, over-the-counter cosmetics can improve the appearance of periorbital hyperpigmentation temporarily by helping to restore moisture and tone. A topical product containing growth factors obtained from cultured human foreskin fibroblasts, TNS (Skin Medica Co.), may help to diminish periorbital pigmentation.[3] Topical preparations containing vitamin K may be of some benefit because of their effect on the clotting mechanism. There are also many highly effective cosmetic concealers that can more than adequately mask the appearance of periorbital hyperpigmentation.

PREVENTION

While diligent use of sunscreens, proper nutritional and lifestyle choices, and avoidance of environmental triggers may help to decrease the incidence of periorbital hyperpigmentation, genetics and the normal aging process make it unlikely that periorbital hyperpigmentation can be avoided in all patients. Proper understanding of the causes of periorbital hyperpigmentation, judicious selection of treatment modalities, and management of patient expectations are key.

REFERENCES

1. Freitag FM, Cestari TF. What causes dark circles under the eyes. *J Cosmet Dermatol* 2007;6:211.
2. Maruri CA, Diaz LA. Dark circles around the eyes. *Cutis* 1969;5:979.
3. Downie JB. Esthetic considerations for ethnic skin. *Semin Cutan Med Surg* 2006; 25:158.
4. Gendler EC. Treatment of periorbital hyperpigmentation. *Aesthet Surg J* 2005; 25:618.
5. Mashhood AA. Treatment of hyperpigmentation disorders. *J Pakistan Assoc Dermatol* 2006;16:65.
6. Goodman RM, Belcher RW. Periorbital hyperpigmentation. *Arch Dermatol* 1969; 100:169.
7. Haddock N, Wilkin JK. Periorbital hyperpigmentation. *JAMA* 1981;246:835.
8. Jeghers H. Pigmemtation of the skin. *N Engl J Med* 1944;23:122.
9. Lelis J. Autosomal recessive ectodermal dysplasia. *Cutis* 1992;49:435.
10. Ing EB, Buncic JR, Weiser BA, et al. Periorbital hyperpigmentation and erythema dyschromicum perstans. *Can J Ophthalmol* 1992;27:353.
11. Carlson R, Hering P. Allergic shiners. *JAMA* 1981;246:835.
12. Gilchrest BA, Fitzpatrick TB, Anderson RR, et al. Localization of melanin pigmentation in the skin with Wood's lamp. *Br J Dermatol* 1977;96:245.
13. Manuskiatti W, Fitzpatrick RE, Goldman MP. Treatment of facial skin using combinations of CO2, Q-switched alexandrite, flashlamp-pumped pulsed dye and Er:YAG lasers in the same treatment session. *Dermatol Surg* 2000;26:114.
14. Halder RM, Richards GM. Topical agents used in the management of hyperpigmentation. *Skin Therapy Letter;* available at *www.skintherapyletter.com/2004/9.6/1. html.*
15. Alena F, Dixon W, Thomas P, et al. Glutathione plays a key role in the depigmenting and melanocytotoxic action of *N*-acetyl-4-cysteaminylphenol in black and yellow hair follicles. *J Invest Dermatol* 1995;104:792.
16. Kimbrough-Green CK, Griffiths CE, Finkel LJ, et al. Topical retinoic acid (tretinoin) for melasma in black patients: A vehicle-controlled clinical trial. *Arch Dermatol* 1994;130:727.
17. Dogra S, Kanwar AJ, Parsad D. Adapalene in the treatment of melasma: A preliminary report. *J Dermatol* 2002; 29:539.
18. Grimes PE. The safety and efficacy of salicylic acid chemical peels in darker racial-ethnic groups. *Dermatol Surg* 1999;25:18.
19. Epstein JS. Management of infraorbital dark circles: A significant concern. *Arch Facial Plast Surg* 1999;1:303.
20. Watanabe S, Nakai K, Ohnishi T. Condition known as dark rings under the eyes in the japanese population is a kind of dermal melanocytosis which can be successfully treated by Q-switched ruby laser. *Dermatol Surg* 2006;32:785.
21. Halder RM, Nootheti PK. Ethnic skin disorders overview. *J Am Acad Dermatol* 2003;48:143.

CHAPTER 51

Maturational Hyperpigmentation

A. Melvin Alexander

Key Points

- Maturational hyperpigmentation (MH) is a previously unrecognized, common entity seen among African-Americans and other people of color who have various allergies and a diabetic diathesis.
- MH occurs almost exclusively (if not exclusively) in overweight/obese adult males and females of color.
- Physical pressure or friction (e.g., sleeping on a pillow, etc.) may contribute to its presentation (proposed by Janet Sloane, DC).
- MH may have pathogenic similarities to acanthosis nigricans seen in overweight individuals with hyperinsulinism and abnormal glucose metabolism.
- Allergies may be a factor in the development of MH.
- Evaluations of MH patients over time should help clarify whether MH improves with weight loss, as does acanthosis nigricans associated with obesity.
- Studies are needed to assess whether there are topical medications or other modalities that are safe and effective in treating MH on a short- and long-term basis.

Maturational hyperpigmentation (MH) is a mysterious yet common dermatosis among African-Americans and other people of color. It was described initially by this author during a presentation at the L'Oreal Institute for Ethnic Hair and Skin Research's 3rd International Symposium in 2006. At the time of publication, this disorder had not been described in dermatology journals or textbooks.

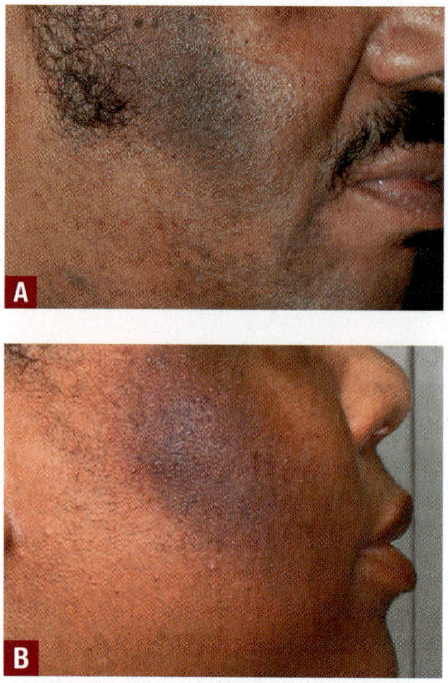

▲ **FIGURE 51-1** Maturational hyperpigmentation in (**A**) an African-American man and (**B**) and African-American woman.

Clinically, MH appears on the cheeks, especially the malar eminences, as a diffuse melasma-like hyperpigmentation (Figure 51-1). However, unlike melasma, it has ill-defined borders that fade into the person's normal skin color. Melasma usually has a medium brown color, whereas MH has a dark brown to black color. It may be unilateral or bilateral.

The etiopathogenesis seems to be excessive weight gain over a variable time span. All of the 20 adult patients who were evaluated by this author (16 females and 4 males, ranging from 26 to 61 years of age) denied precipitating trauma, or change in medications. However, 75% had various allergies. Ninety percent claimed the hyperpigmentation was more prominent on the side where they usually slept.

Several patients had biopsies, and the findings were minimal inflammation in the dermis; increased pigmentation in the basal and squamous layers; and increased melanocytes in the basal layer. Other hyperpigmented dermatoses may show increased pigmentation in the basal or squamous layer but typically do not show increased melanocytes (indicative of melanocyte proliferation).

Fourteen of the twenty patients had several laboratory tests obtained. Of this group, seven (50%) had hyperglycemia and five (36%) showed hyperinsulinism. Additionally, of the seven patients who had melanocyte-stimulating hormone (MSH) measured, six (86%) showed low levels of this hormone, which is surprising considering the clinical hyperpigmentation and the melanocyte proliferation seen in the biopsies. On the other hand, MSH has been shown to suppress appetite, and the low levels found may be related to the excessive weight exhibited by all the patients. Taken collectively, these findings suggest that MH may, in a manner similar to a recognized type of acanthosis nigricans, be a "new" cutaneous marker for diabetes or prediabetes.

Therapy has not been consistently successful using hydroquinones, topical retinoids, and/or mild corticosteroids or microdermabrasion.

CHAPTER 52

Solar Lentigines

Doris Hexsel

Key Points

- Solar lentigines are hyperpigmented macules that are round or oval in shape with slightly irregular edges.
- They are common in skin of color populations except with skin of color Asian populations.
- Ultraviolet (UV) light sources and genetic predisposition are the most important factors in the development of solarlentigines.
- Treatment may include physical modalities and depigmenting agents.
- Sun avoidance, protective clothing, sunscreen, and blocking agents are indicated to prevent solar lentigines.

Solar lentigines (SLs) are benign, hyperpigmented macules that occur in sun-exposed areas of the skin.[1–4] They are induced by natural or artificial sources of ultraviolet (UV) radiation and are also called *sun-induced freckles, sunburn freckles, freckles in adulthood, age spots, actinic lentigines,* and *senile lentigines.*[5,6]

EPIDEMIOLOGY, ETIOLOGY, PATHOGENESIS, AND HISTOPATHOLOGY

This benign pigmentary disorder is prevalent among fair-skinned patients, classified as Fitzpatrick's skin types I and II (who always burn and who tan a little or not at all).[5,7] The incidence increases with age, affecting more than 90% of white people older than age 50 years.[2–4,8] Solar lentigines are also a clinical features of photoaging in East and Southeast Asian populations. In this skin of color population, discrete pigmentary changes including solar lentigines and mottled hyperpigmentation are seen frequently.[9] In a study by Chung and colleagues of Koreans aged 30–92 years, hyperpigmented macules were the major pigmentary lesion associated with photoaging in women. As is the case with the Caucasian population, the number of hyperpigmented macules increased with each decade of age.[10]

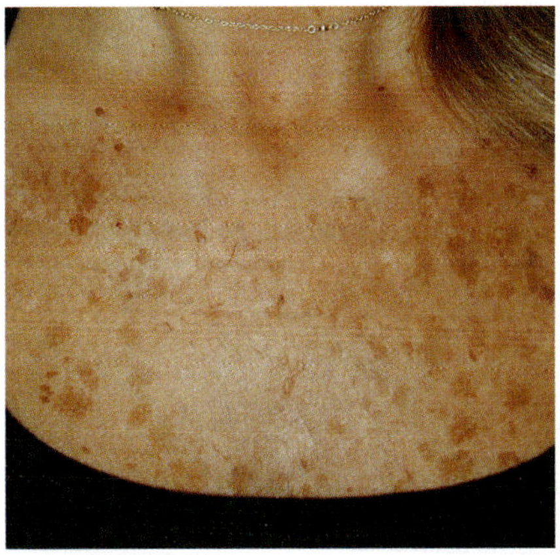

▲ **FIGURE 52-1** Solar lentigines on the chest of a patient who had early and intense sun exposure.

Bastiaens and colleagues demonstrated that SLs have a positive association with cumulative lifetime sun exposure and early sun exposure[6] (Figure 52-1). There is also a possible genetic susceptibility to the development of SLs in response to acute or chronic UV exposure.[5] Aoki and colleagues demonstrated that SLs are induced by the mutagenic effect of repeated UV exposure in the past, leading to the characteristic enhancement of melanin production, together with decreased proliferation and differentiation of lesional keratinocytes, against a background of chronic inflammation.[11]

SLs may appear after chronic photochemotherapy (6–8 months). However, individual susceptibility factors such as race, age, and tanning and burning response to sunlight are important to determine the prevalence and density of SLs.[5]

The histopathology of SLs shows a linear increase in melanocytes along the dermal-epidermal junction.[12] There is more melanin than normal in the adjacent epidermis and stratum corneum, but no atypicality or pigment incontinence is seen.[2,4,5,13] Moreover, melanocytes display increased activity, as manifested by marked dopa reactivity, elongated dendrites, numerous normal-appearing melanosomes, enlarged perikarya with developed rough endoplasmatic reticula, numerous mitochondria, and hypertrophic Golgi complexes.[5]

CLINICAL FINDINGS

SLs are macular hyperpigmented lesions that range in color from pale yellow to

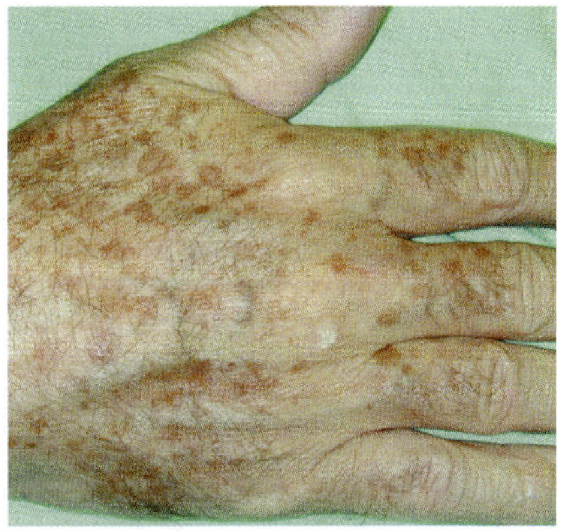

▲ **FIGURE 52-2** Solar lentigines on the back of the hands.

dark brown and vary in size from a few millimeters to 2 cm (Figure 52-2). Lesions are round or oval with slightly irregular edges.[1,2,7] They are more common in fair-skinned patients, such as those presenting Fitzpatrick's skin phototypes I–III, and are less frequent in dark-skinned subjects.[2,3] A previous history of acute sunburn followed by the sudden appearance of large numbers of macular lesions is often found.[13] Usually, similar lesions appear in the same area, such as the face, arms, hands, chest, and back.[1–4,7] SLs are diagnosed by clinical examination.[12] Other methods, such as dermoscopy[9,15,16] and confocal microscopy (CM)[17–19] also may be used in the diagnosis of SLs and for differential diagnoses (Figure 52-3). CM obtains images from deep inside the skin without interference from scattered or out-of-focus light.[17] Langley and colleagues evaluated SLs using CM and demonstrated an absence of atypical melanocytes.[18] Yamashita diagnosed SLs using CM and showed numerous aggregated melanosomes.[19]

▲ **FIGURE 52-3** Dermoscopy of solar lentigines (50×).

DIFFERENTIAL DIAGNOSIS

SLs can be distinguished from ephelides, lentigo simplex, pigmented actinic keratosis, flat seborrheic keratosis, melanocytic nevus, and malignant melanoma by their clinical appearance. Other lesions that may be misdiagnosed are "flat" varieties of junctional melanocytic nevi, pigmented actinic keratoses, large cell acanthomas, and benign pigmented keratoses.[5,20]

Dalton and colleagues studied 147 patients with facial lentigo maligna (LM). In 44 patients (30%), there was the presence of SLs in the biopsy specimen. The presence of an associated SL can make the diagnosis of LM more difficult, leading to misdiagnosis.[20]

Dermoscopy is helpful in the differential diagnoses of a number of skin lesions, such as seborrheic keratosis, lentigo simplex, melanoma in situ, lichen planus–like keratosis, and pigmented actinic keratosis.[9,15,16]

PROGNOSIS/CLINICAL COURSE

SLs may appear at any time in life, but most of the cases occur in people older

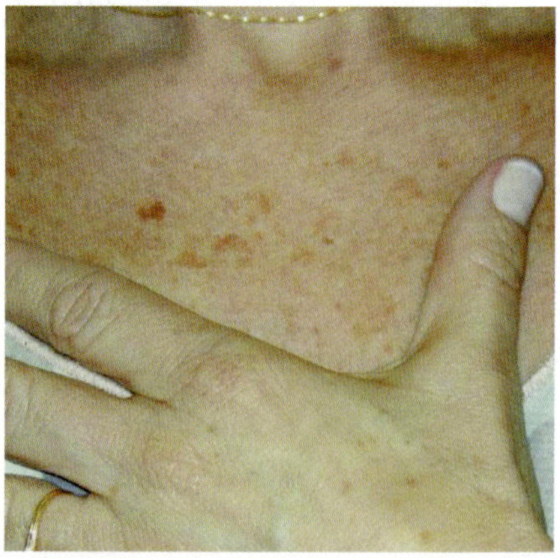

▲ **FIGURE 52-4** A 40-year-old patient showing SLs on the chest and back of the hands. Lesions are more numerous in area of acute sun exposure than in area of chronic sun exposure.

than 50 years of age[2] (Figure 52-4). Once formed, it is possible that SLs may fade slightly or persist indefinitely. During the clinical course, SLs may enlarge, darken, and become more irregular and "fixed" over time, similar to the progression of LM.[5] It is possible that SLs evolve into varieties of intraepidermal melanocytic dysplasia, similar to LM, in some individuals.[5] Recurrence after treatment also may take place.[21]

PREVENTION

Sun avoidance, protective clothing, and sunscreens are recommended for the prevention of SLs. These protective measures must be initiated in childhood and continued throughout life.[5]

TREATMENT

There are a number of treatment options for SLs. They can be divided into two categories: physical modalities and topical therapy.[22] Physical modalities includes cryotherapy, chemical peels, lasers, pulsed light, and dermabrasion, whereas topical therapy involves the use of hypopigmenting agents such as hydroquinone, tretinoin, tazarotene, adapalene, and some combinations of these agents. These treatments are categorized according to the quality and level of evidence from clinical studies published in the literature in Tables 52-1 and 52-2. Table 52-1 refers to the commonly used procedures, and

TABLE 52-1
Summary of Physical Therapy Studies

Study/Source	Quality of Evidence	Level of Evidence	Number of Subjects	Outcome and Follow-up
Cryotherapy				
Raziee et al.,[24] 2007	I	A	25	Cryotherapy was more likely to produce substantial lightening of SLs than trichloroacetic acid (TCA) 33% ($p = 0.025$).
Lugo-Janer et al.,[25] 2003	I	A	25	Liquid nitrogen (LN) was more likely to produce significant lightening of SLs than 30% TCA solution ($p < 0.05$).
Chemical peels				
Chun et al.,[26] 2004	IIa	B	49	86% of the subjects showed a good clinical response with TCA 10–65%. These clinical results were maintained for 12 months after the treatment.
Cook and Cook,[27] 2000	IIa	A	3100	There is a significant decrease with 40% TCA–70% glycolic peel in irregular pigmentation of nonfacial skin, including SLs.
Laser therapy				
Rashid et al.,[28] 2002	IIa	C	6	All patients showed improvement of 50% with Nd:YAG laser (532 nm), and no recurrence was reported after 24-month follow-up.
Kopera et al.,[29] 1997	IIa	A	8	A single course of Q-switched ruby laser resulted in fading of the lesions without scarring and no recurrence within a 6- to 8-week follow-up period.

continued

TABLE 52-1 *(Continued)*
Summary of Physical Therapy Studies

Rosenbach et al.,[30] 2002	IIa	B	11	There was a significant improvement with alexandrite laser among the treated lentigines: 2 lesions were graded as "good," 14 as "excellent," and 5 as "clear" compared with untreated areas at 4 weeks ($p < 0.001$).
Intense pulsed light therapy (IPL)				
Kawada et al.,[31] 2000	III	B	45	There was more than a 50% improvement in SLs in 40% of the patients after four treatments.
Kawana et al.,[32] 2007	IIc	C	18	IPL was considered effective in 12 of 18 patients (66.6% improvement).
Kligman et al.,[33] 2004	IIc	C	23	There was a decrease in SLs after three treatments with IPL.
Microdermabrasion				
Cotellessa et al.,[34] 2003	III	D	40	The combination of microdermabrasion with 15% TCA resulted in complete remission in 50% of patients.
Lasers + cryotherapy				
Stern et al.,[35] 1994	IIa	C	13	Good results were reported in 61%, 62%, and 75% of patients treated with the CO_2 laser, argon laser, and cryotherapy, respectively.
Todd et al.,[1] 2000	IIa	B	27	After 12 weeks, the frequency-doubled Q-switched Nd:YAG laser provided significant lightening compared with the krypton laser ($p = 0.001$), the 532-nm diode-pumped vanadate laser ($p = 0.001$), and liquid nitrogen ($p = 0.001$).
Laser therapy + chemical peels				
Li and Yang,[36] 1999	IIa	A	20	The frequency-doubled Q-switched Nd:YAG laser proved to be significantly more effective than 35% TCA ($p = 0.0004$).
Dermabrasion + cryotherapy				
Hexsel et al.,[2] 2000	IIa	B	10	Localized dermabrasion is an efficacious and effective technique comparable with liquid nitrogen. Moreover, dermabrasion was associated with fewer side effects, such as hypochromia, than liquid nitrogen.

Table 52-2 refers to topical agents for the treatment of SLs. Quality of evidence was graded according to a six-point scale as follows:

I. Evidence obtained from at least one properly designed randomized, controlled trial

IIa. Evidence obtained from well-designed controlled trials without randomization

IIb. Evidence obtained from well-designed cohort or case-control analytic studies, preferably from more than one center or research group

IIc. Evidence obtained from multiple time series with or without the intervention (Dramatic results in uncontrolled experiments also could be regarded as this type of evidence.)

III. Opinions of respected authorities based on clinical experience, descriptive studies, or reports from expert committees

IV. Inadequate evidence owing to problems of methodology (e.g., sample size or length or comprehensiveness of follow-up or conflicts in evidence)[23]

Level of evidence was classified on a five-point scale as follows:

A. There is good evidence to support the use of this procedure.

B. There is fair evidence to support the use of this procedure.

C. There is poor evidence to support the use of the procedure.

D. There is fair evidence to support the rejection of the use of the procedure.

E. There is good evidence to support the rejection of the use of this procedure.[23]

TABLE 52-2
Summary of Topical Therapy Studies

Study/Source	Quality of Evidence	Level of Evidence	Number of Subjects	Outcome
Hydroquinone				
Petit and Piérard,[37] 2003	I	A	30	Reflectance spectrophotometric measurements showed a significant decrease in the differential melanin index by 3.5% and 8.7% after 1 and 2 months, respectively ($P < 0.05$). Video image analysis showed a 17% decrease in the areas of SLs at 2 months ($P < 0.01$). Melanin density in the stratum corneum was reduced by 4.9% ($p < 0.01$) and 18.6% ($p < 0.001$) after 1 and 2 months, respectively.
Tretinoin				
Weiss et al.,[38] 2006	I	B	45	Tretinoin microsphere gel 0.1% was superior to placebo in improving photodamage, including SLs after 6 months ($p = 0.0054$).
Kang et al.,[39] 2005	I	B	204	Tretinoin cream 0.05% resulted in significantly greater improvement in clinical signs of photodamage, including SLs, compared with placebo ($p < 0.05$).
Weinstein et al.,[40] 1991	I	B	251	Overall improvement of photodamaged skin, including SLs, was reported in 79% of patients at 0.05% dose compared with improvement in 57% of patients at 0.01% dose and 48% of the patients with the vehicle.
Rafal et al.,[41] 1992	I	B	58	After 10 months, 83% of the patients with facial lesions treated with retinoic acid (RA) had lightening of these lesions compared with 29%of the patients treated with placebo.
Tazarotene				
Kang et al.,[42] 2005	I	B	568	Tazarotene cream was significantly more effective than vehicle in reducing SLs (59% versus 28%, $p < 0.001$) at week 24.
Phillips et al.,[43] 2002	I	B	563	The application of 0.1% tazarotene produced clinical improvement in SLs compared with placebo (55% versus 15%; $p < 0.001$).
Adapalene				
Kang et al.,[44] 2003	I	B	90	At 9 months, 57% and 59% of patients had lighter lesions in the 0.1% and 0.3% adapalene gel groups, respectively, compared with 36% in the control group ($p < 0.05$).
Hydroquinone-tretinoin				
Yoshimura et al.,[45] 2000	IIc	B	90	At 8 weeks, successful lightening of lesions was achieved in 82.2% of patients (excellent or good benefits).
Mequinol(4HA)-tretinoin				
Jarratt,[46] 2004	I	A	216	Mequinol 2%/tretinoin 0.01% solution is a highly effective and well-tolerated treatment for SLs and related hyperpigmented lesions, being superior to HQ 3%

continued

TABLE 52-2 *(Continued)*
Summary of Topical Therapy Studies

Fleischer et al.,[47] 2000	I	A	1175	Mequinol 2%–tretinoin 0.01% demonstrated significant superiority over 4HA and vehicle ($p = 0.0001$).
Draelos,[48] 2006	IIc	C	259	Over 80% of all subjects responded to 4HA 2%–tretinoin 0.01% therapy and maintained clinical benefit at 4 weeks posttreatment.
Ortonne,[49] 2004	IIc	C	378	80% and 88% of the target lesions of the arm and face, respectively, treated with 4HA-RA were clear or almost clear after 4 weeks of follow-up.

CONCLUSION

SLs are commonly found among patients with skin phototypes I–III and most common in people older than 50 years of age. These lesions are induced by natural or artificial sources of UV radiation. Therefore, protective measures must be initiated in childhood to prevent their appearance later in life.

A number of physical and topical therapies, either alone or in various combinations, have been demonstrated to be efficacious and safe. However, the results are often not permanent, and recurrence is frequent. Thus management remains a challenge for dermatologists. Finally, additional double-blind studies are in order to identify better treatments for SLs.

REFERENCES

1. Todd MM, Rallis TM, Gerwels JW, et al. A comparison of three lasers and liquid nitrogen in the treatment of solar lentigines: A randomized, controlled comparative trial. *Arch Dermatol* 2000;136:841.
2. Hexsel DM, Mazzuco R, Bohn J, et al. Clinical comparative study between cryotherapy and local dermabrasion for the treatment of solar lentigo on the back of the hands. *Dermatol Surg* 2000; 26:457.
3. Grimes PE. Cosmetic issues of concern for potential surgical patients, in Soriano T, Hexsel DM, Kim J (eds), *Aesthetic and Cosmetic Surgery for Darker Skin Types.* Philadelphia, Lippincott Williams & Wilkins, 2008, p 49.
4. Baumann L. Disorders of pigmentation, in Weisberg E (ed), *Cosmetic Dermatology: Principles and Pratice.* New York, McGraw-Hill, 2002, p 67.
5. Freedberg IM, Eisen AZ, Wolff K, et al (eds). *Fitzpatrick's Dermatology in General Medicine.* New York, McGraw-Hill, 1999, p 1047.
6. Bastiaens M, Hoefnagel J, Westendorp R, et al. Solar lentigines are strongly related to sun exposure in contrast to ephelides. *Pigment Cell Res* 2004;17:225.
7. Baran R, Maibach HI. Pigmentation: Dyschromia, in Baran R, Maibach HI (eds), *Cosmetic Dermatology*. London, Martin Dunitz, 1994, p 282.
8. Sampaio SAP. in Discromia, Sampaio SAP, Rivitti, EA (eds), *Dermatologia*. São Paulo, Artes Medicas, 1998, p 277.
9. Goh SH. The treatment of visible signs of senescence: The Asian experience. *Br J Dermatol* 1990;122:S105-109.
10. Chung JH, Lee SH, Youn CS, et al. Cutaneous photodamage in Koreans. *Arch Dermatol* 2001;137:1043-1051.
11. Aoki H, Moro O, Tagami H, et al. Gene expression profiling analysis of solar lentigo in relation to immunohistochemical characteristics. *Br J Dermatol* 2007; 156:1214.
12. Champion RH, Burton JL, Burns DA, et al (eds). *Rook's Textbook of Dermatology,* Vol 2. Oxford, England, Blackwell Science, 2004, p 1719.
13. Baran R, Maibach HI. in Pigmentation: Dyschromia, in Baran R. Maibbach HI (eds). *Textbook of Cosmetic Dermatology,* 3rd ed. London, Taylor & Francis, 2005, p 396.
14. Rassner G, Steinert U (eds). *Dermatologia: Tratado e Atlas.* São Paulo, Livraria Editora Santos, 1994, p 203.
15. Wang SQ, Katz B, Rabinovitz H, et al. Lessons on dermoscopy 11: Solar lentigo. *Dermatol Surg* 2000;26:1173.
16. Braun RP, Rabinovitz HS, Oliviero M, et al. Dermoscopy of pigmented skin lesions. *J Am Acad Dermatol* 2005; 52: 109.
17. Nicholas A, Egerton IB, Lim AC, et al. Imaging the skin. *Australas J Dermatol* 2003;44:19.
18. Langley RG, Burton E, Walsh N, et al. In vivo confocal scanning laser microscopy of benign lentigines: Comparison to conventional histology and in vivo characteristics of lentigo maligna. *J Am Acad Dermatol* 2006;55:88.
19. Yamashita T, Negishi K, Hariya T, et al. Intense pulsed light therapy for superficial pigmented lesions evaluated by reflectance-mode confocal microscopy and optical coherence tomography. *J Invest Dermatol* 2006;126:2281.
20. Dalton SR, Gardner TL, Libow LF, et al. Contiguous lesions in lentigo maligna. *J Am Acad Dermatol* 2005;52:859.
21. Kede MPV, Sabatovich O (eds). *Dermatologia Estética.* São Paulo, Editora Atheneu, 2003, p 656.
22. Ortonne JP, Pandya AG, Hexsel DM, et al. Treatment of solar lentigines. *J Am Acad Dermatol* 2006;54:262.
23. Williams HC. Health care needs assessment, second series, in Stevens A, Raftery J (eds), *Dermatology.* Oxford, England, Radcliffe Medical Press, 1997, p 340.
24. Raziee M, Balighi K, Shabanzadeh-Dehkordi H, et al. Efficacy and safety of cryotherapy vs trichloroacetic acid in the treatment of solar lentigo. *J Eur Acad Dermatol Venereol* 2008;22:316-319.
25. Lugo-Janer A, Lugo-Somolinos A, Sanchez JL. Comparison of trichloroacetic acid solution and cryosurgery in the treatment of solar lentigines. *Int J Dermatol* 2003; 42:829.
26. Chun EY, Lee JB, Lee KH. Focal trichloroacetic acid peel method for benign pigmented lesions in dark-skinned patients. *Dermatol Surg* 2004; 30:512.
27. Cook KK, Cook WR Jr. Chemical peel of nonfacial skin using glycolic acid gel augmented with TCA and neutralized based on visual staging. *Dermatol Surg* 2000; 26:994.
28. Rashid T, Hussain I, Haider M, et al. Laser therapy of freckles and lentigines with quasi-continuous, frequency-doubled, Nd:YAG (532 nm) laser in Fitzpatrick skin type IV: A 24-month follow-up. *J Cosmet Laser Ther* 2002;4:81.
29. Kopera D, Hohenleutner U, Landthaler M. Quality-switched ruby laser treatment of solar lentigines and Becker's nevus: A histopathological and immunohistochemical study. *Dermatology* 1997;194:338.
30. Rosenbach A, Lee SJ, John RH. Treatment of medium-brown solar lentigines using an alexandrite laser designed for hair reduction. *Arch Dermatol* 2002;138:547.
31. Kawada A, Shiraishi H, Asai M. Clinical improvement of solar lentigines and ephelides with an intense pulsed light source. *Dermatol Surg* 2002;28:504.
32. Kawana S, Ochiai H, Tachihara R. Objective evaluation of the effect of intense pulsed light on rosacea and solar lentigines by spectrophotometric analysis of skin color. *Dermatol Surg* 2007;33:449.
33. Kligman DE, Zhen Y. Intense pulsed light treatment of photoaged facial skin. *Dermatol Surg* 2004;30:1085.

34. Cotellessa C, Peris K, Fargnoli MC. Microabrasion versus microabrasion followed by 15% trichloroacetic acid for treatment of cutaneous hyperpigmentations in adult females. *Dermatol Surg* 2003;29:352.
35. Stern RS, Dover JS, Levin JA, et al. Laser therapy versus cryotherapy of lentigines: A comparative trial. *J Am Acad Dermatol* 1994;30:985.
36. Li YT, Yang KC. Comparison of the frequency-doubled Q-switched Nd:YAG laser and 35% trichloroacetic acid for the treatment of face lentigines. *Dermatol Surg* 1999;25:202.
37. Petit L, Piérard GE. Analytic quantification of solar lentigines lightening by a 2% hydroquinone-cyclodextrin formulation. *J Eur Acad Dermatol Venereol* 2003; 17:546.
38. Weiss JS, Shavin JS, Nighland M. Tretinoin microsphere gel 0.1% for photodamaged facial skin: A placebo-controlled trial. *Cutis* 2006;78:426.
39. Kang S, Bergfeld W, Gottlieb AB. Long-term efficacy and safety of tretinoin emollient cream 0.05% in the treatment of photodamaged facial skin: A two-year randomized, placebo-controlled trial. *Am J Clin Dermatol* 2005;6:245.
40. Weinstein GD, Nigra TP, Pochi PE. Topical tretinoin for treatment of photodamaged skin: A multicenter study. *Arch Dermatol* 1991;127:659.
41. Rafal ES, Griffiths CE, Ditre CM, et al. Topical tretinoin (retinoic acid) treatment for liver spots associated with photodamage. *N Engl J Med* 1992;326: 368.
42. Kang S, Krueger GG, Tanghetti EA, et al. A multicenter, randomized, double-blind trial of tazarotene 0.1% cream in the treatment of photodamage. *J Am Acad Dermatol* 2005;52:268.
43. Phillips TJ, Gottlieb AB, Leyden JJ, et al. Efficacy of 0.1% tazarotene cream for the treatment of photodamage: A 12-month multicenter, randomized trial. *Arch Dermatol* 2002;138:1486.
44. Kang S, Goldfarb MT, Weiss JS, et al. Assessment of adapalene gel for the treatment of actinic keratoses and lentigines: A randomized trial. *J Am Acad Dermatol* 2003;49:83.
45. Yoshimura K, Harii K, Aoyama T, et al. Experience with a strong bleaching treatment for skin hyperpigmentation in Orientals. *Plast Reconstr Surg* 2000;105:1097.
46. Jarratt M. Mequinol 2%/tretinoin 0.01% solution: An effective and safe alternative to hydroquinone 3% in the treatment of solar lentigines. *Cutis* 2004; 74:319.
47. Fleischer AB, Schwartzel EH, Colby SI, et al. The combination of 2% 4-hydroxyanisole (Mequinol) and 0.01% tretinoin is effective in improving the appearance of solar lentigines and related hyperpigmented lesions in two double-blind multicenter clinical studies. *J Am Acad Dermatol* 2000;42:459.
48. Draelos ZD. The combination of 2% 4-hydroxyanisole (Mequinol) and 0.01% tretinoin effectively improves the appearance of solar lentigines in ethnic groups. *J Cosmet Dermatol* 2006;5:239.
49. Ortonne JP, Camacho F, Wainwright N, et al. Safety and efficacy of combined use of 4-hydroxyanisole (Mequinol) 2%/ tretinoin 0.01% solution and sunscreen in solar lentigines. *Cutis* 2004;74:261.

CHAPTER 53

Nevus of Ito/Ota

Marvi Iqbal

Key Points

- Nevus of Ota is a dermal melanocytic hamartoma that is unilaterally distributed along the first and second branches of the trigeminal nerve.
- It presents clinically as a bluish gray hyperpigmentation of the skin.
- Nevus of Ito is a similar melanocytic condition, but the distribution is along the shoulder.
- It is felt that these melanocytic disorders represent melanocytes that did not migrate completely from the neural crest to the epidermis during the embryonic period.
- Nevus of Ota and nevus of Ito occur more frequently in Asian populations and are rare in Caucasians.

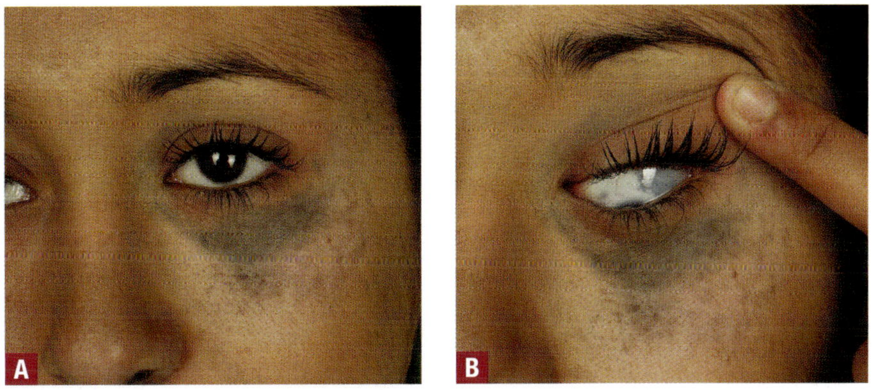

▲ **FIGURE 53-2** **A** Nevus of OTA with infra orbital hyperpigmentation and **B** infra orbital and scleral hyperpigmentation.

Oculodermal melanosis was first described by Hulke in 1861[1]. The entity *nevus of Ota* became known after it was described by Ota in 1939 as a bluish gray hyperpigmentation along the first and second divisions of the trigeminal nerve with occasional mucosal involvement[2] (Figure 53-1; Figure 53-2A and B). *Nevus of Ito,* described by Minor Ito in 1954, is a similar melanocytic condition, but the distribution is along the shoulder[3] (Figure 53-3A and B).

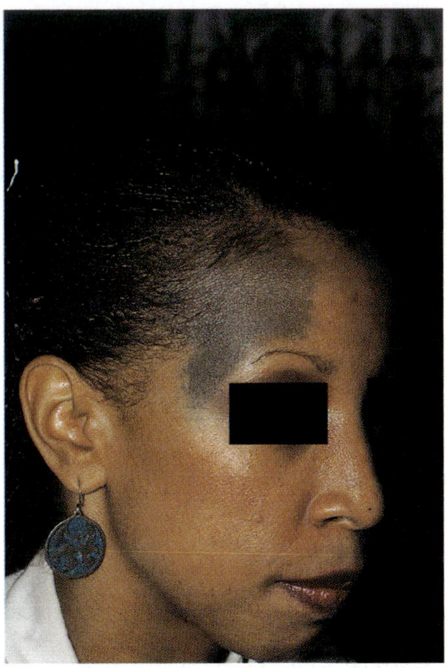

▲ **FIGURE 53-1** Nevus of Ota on the right forehead of an Afican-America woman with type V skin.

The etiology of nevus of Ota/Ito is unknown. It is possible that these melanocytic disorders represent melanocytes that did not migrate completely from the neural crest to the epidermis during the embryonic period.[4,5] It is also possible that hormones play a role in the development of nevus of Ota because the two peaks of onset are infancy and puberty. Other factors, such as ultraviolet (UV) light, infection, and trauma, also may play a role.[6,7]

Nevi of Ota and Ito occur more frequently in Asian populations and are rare in Caucasians. Some studies have shown the incidence to be from 0.014–1.1%.[8,9] Nevus of Ota is more prevalent in women, with the male-to-female ratio being 1:4.8; the ratio for nevus of Ito is unknown. Most patients with nevi of Ota or Ito do not have a family history.

Nevus of Ota is considered to be a dermal melanocytic hamartoma that is unilaterally distributed along the first and second branches of the trigeminal nerve. It appears as a blue-black or slate-gray macule. It may be classified according to the distribution of cutaneous involvement,[9] histologically based on the depth of melanocytic dermal involvement, and according to laser response.

Histologically, the nevus of Ota has a normal epidermis; the dentrictic melanocytes are distributed in the papillary and midreticular dermis, surrounded by fibrous sheaths. Based on their location, there are five histologic groups: superficial, superficial dominant, diffuse, deep dominant, and deep. Superficial lesions tend to be in the cheek area, whereas deep lesions are found more in the periorbital areas, temple, and forehead[3] (Table 53-1).

Classification based on laser response is a novel approach, most likely developed since punch biopsy is rarely performed to diagnose this condition. The classification is as follows[10]:

1. Nevus of Ota without periorbital involvement, other birthmarks, and extracutaneous involvement
2. Nevus of Ota with periorbital involvement but without other birthmarks and extracutaneous involvement
3. Nevus of Ota with another birthmarkmark but without extracutaneous involvement
4. Nevus of Ota with extracutaneous involvement

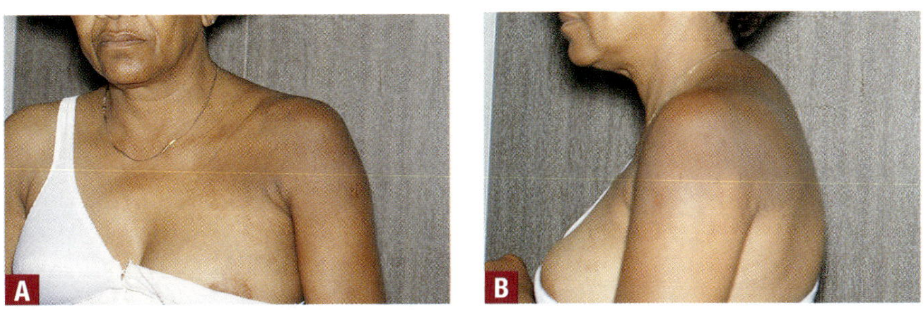

▲ **FIGURE 53-3** **A** Hyperpigmentation along the shoulder and **B** hyperpigmentation of the left shoulder and upper back.

TABLE 53-1
Nevi of Ota and Ito

Ota = oculodermal melanosis
Ito = shoulder melanosis
Both = peaks of onset during infancy, puberty
Both = more frequent in Asians
Ota = higher prevalence in woman
Ota = deep (periorbital area and temple)
Ota = superficial (cheeks)

A similar classification for nevus of Ito does not exist but histologically, nevi of Ito and Ota are described in the same way.

Nevus of Ota at times may be associated with extracutaneous involvement. One type is known as *phakomatosis pigmentovascularis,* which is a congential generalized hemangioma associated with nevus of Ota. This may present with systemic involvement such as ocular and nuerologic disorders (e.g., Strug-Webber and Klippel-Trenaunay syndromes), and intracranial arteriovenous malformations.[11–14] Nevus of Ota also may be associated with ocular complications such as increased ocular pressure with or without glaucoma (10.3%), asymmetric cupping of the optic nerve head not associated with glaucoma (9.8%), uveitis (2.6%), cararacts (1%), and orbital melanoma (0.5%). Although it is rare, nevus of Ota has been reported to be associated with malignant melanoma; most cases are orbital melanoma, but involvement of skin and meninges have also been reported. In most of the reported cases, the patients are Caucasian, but other groups have been reported as well. Only one case of melanoma has been reported with nevus of Ito. In terms of extracutaneous manifestations, although rare, nevus of Ito has been reported to occur simultaneously with nevus of Ota. Nevus of Ito also can be associated with sensory changes in the involved skin.[3]

TABLE 53-2
Laser Therapy

QS ruby laser
QS 1069-Ndyag
QS Alexandrite
Recurrence (0.6–1.2%) after complete clearance

With the introduction of laser surgery, the treatment of nevus of Ota has improved significantly. Before laser surgery, therapy was limited to cryotherapy, dermabrasion, and surgical excision, all of which had significant risk of scarring and/or were unreliable. A study of 114 nevus of Ota patients treated with the Q-swiched ruby laser found that most patients had an excellent response with four to five treatments, and no patient in the study had atrophic or hypertophic scarring. The Q-swiched ruby laser (694.3 nm, 6 J/cm^2, 30-ns pulse) has been shown to interact selectively with cells that contain pigment, such as dermal melanocytes.[15] The Q-switched alexandrite and Q-switched 1064-nm neodymium:yttrium-aluminum-garnet (QS 1064-nm Nd:YAG) lasers also have been shown to be effective in the treatment of nevus of Ota. The Nd:YAG laser was shown to be more effective than the QS alexandrite laser in lightening the nevus of Ota, although the QS alexandrite laser was better tolerated.[16,17] It is important to keep in mind that there is a risk of recurrence 0.6–1.2% after complete clearing with laser treatment. This is a special consideration in children when weighing the risks and benefits of multiple laser surgery treatments (Table 53-2).

REFERENCES

1. Chan HH, Kono T. Nevus of Ota: Clinical aspects and management. *Skinmed* 2003; 59:200-210.
2. Bhattacharya SK, Girgla HS, Singh G. Naevus of Ota. *Int J Dermatol* 1973;12: 344-347.
3. Lui H, Zhou Y. Nevi of Ota and Ito. *www.e-medince.com.*
4. Kopf AW, Weidman AI. Naevus of Ota. *Arch Dermatol* 1962;85:195-208.
5. Mishima Y, Mevorah B. Nevus of Ota and nevus of Ito in American Negroes. *J Invest Dermatol* 1961;36:133-154.
6. Hidano A, Kajama H, Ikeda S, et al. Natural history of naevus of Ota. *Arch Dermatol* 1967; 95:187-195.
7. Stuart C. Naevus of Ota. *Br J Dermatol* 1955;67:317.
8. Gonder JR, Ezell PC, Sheilds JA, et al. Ocular melanocytosis: A study to determine the prevalence rate of ocular melanocytosis. *Ophthalmology* 1982;89: 950-952.
9. Tanino H. Uber eine in Japan haufig vorkommende Navusform: "Naevus fusco-caeruleus opthalmo-maxillaris Ota": I. Mitteilung:beobachtunguber lokalisation, verfarbung, anordnung and histologische veranderung. *Jpn J Dermatol* 1939;46:435-451.
10. Chan HH, Lam LK, Wong DS, et al. Nevus of Ota: A new classification based upon the response to laser treatment. *Lasers Surg Med* 2001;28:267-272.
11. Hasegawa Y, Yasuhara M. Phakomatosis pigmentovascularis type IVa. *Arch Dermatol* 1985;121:651-655.
12. Massey EW, Brannon WL, Moreland M. Nevus of Ota and intracranial arteriovenus malformation. *Neurology* 1979;29: 1626-1627.
13. Ota M, Kawamura T, Ito N. Phakomatosis pigmentovascularis. *Jpn J Dermatol* 1947; 52:1-3.
14. Kumar A, Singh J. Naevus of Ota with primary retinitis pigmentosa: A syndrome. *Can J Ophthalmol* 1985;20:261-263.
15. Watanabe S, Takahashi H. Treatment of nevus of Ota with the Q-switched ruby laser. *N Engl J Med* 1994;331:1745-1750.
16. Chan HH, King WWK, Chan ESY, et al. In vivo trial comparing patients' tolerance of Q-switched alexandrite and Q-switched neodymium:yttrium-aluminum- garnet lasers in the treatment of nevus of Ota. *Lasers Surg Med* 1999; 24:24-28.
17. Chan HH, Ying SY, Ho WS, et al. An in vivo trial comparing the clinical efficacy and complications of Q-swithced 755-nm alexandrite and Q-switched 1064-nm (Nd-YAG) lasers in the treatment of nevus of Ota. *Dermatol Surg* 2000;26: 919-922.

SECTION 8

Mucosal Disorders

CHAPTER 54

Biology and Pathology of the Oral Mucosa

Diana V. Messadi
Ahn Le
Ginat W. Mirowski
Heddie O. Sedano

Key Points

- Leukoedema is the most common benign oral condition related to dark-skinned individuals.
- No treatment is necessary for leukoedema.
- The oral cancer incidence rate is similar among African-Americans and Caucasians, but the mortality rate is higher in African-Americans owing to late diagnosis.
- Early detection of oral cancer is important to decrease the high mortality and morbidity rates seen in African-Americans.
- Physiologic oral pigmentation is due to greater melanocytic activity rather than a higher number of meloncytes.

Workup of the patient with oral complaints requires an organized approach that consists of obtaining a complete medical, dental, dermatologic, family, and social and medication history. Also important are the use of medications, herbs, and vitamins, as well as a history of all possible allergic reactions, a physical examination, and evaluation of any available laboratory studies.

The physical examination includes evaluation of the musculoskeletal and soft tissues of the head and neck, including lymph nodes, thyroid and salivary gland palpation, and a complete mucocutaneous examination. Intraoral examination requires proper visualization and a bimanual palpation of the soft and hard tissues of the head and neck, including the lips, the tempomandibular joint, the neck, and the tongue. A complete evaluation requires the use of gauze to dry the mucosa and to facilitate visual inspection and palpation of the lips and the tongue. Evaluation of the teeth and periodontal status is necessary as well.

Laboratory studies, scrapings, cytology, serum studies, cultures, and biopsies should be performed when indicated. This chapter focuses on the mucocutaneous findings of the oral cavity, particularly in African-Americans and other people of color.

INTRAORAL EXAMINATION

The external margin of the lips, that is, the transition zone between skin and mucous membrane, is known as the *vermilion.* It is pink to brown in color, hairless, and covered by a thin, dry epithelium; at the junction of the vermilion and the lips, the vermilion is slightly palpable except in advanced age or with chronic sun exposure (Figure 54-1).

Intraorally, the oral cavity is divided into the vestibule and the oral cavity proper. The vestibule is limited by the gingiva and the teeth medially and by the labial and buccal mucosae laterally. The superior and inferior aspect to the vestibule are called *vestibular sulci.* Anterior and lateral ferula traverse the vestibular sulci from the lip and buccal mucosae to the gingival mucosa. The lateral ferula are seen bilaterally at the maxillary and mandibular premolars.

The labial and buccal mucosae are normally pale pink in color, shiny, and kept moist by minor salivary glands that secrete myxoid saliva directly onto the mucosae. On the buccal mucosa, a horizontal line called the *linea alba,* of varying prominence, may be seen bilaterally reflecting the occlusal plane of the teeth. Stensen's papilla, a papule that protects the opening of *Stensen's duct* (main excretory duct of the parotid gland), can be seen above the linea alba. Clear aqueous saliva is easily expressed from Stensen's duct by gently applying manual pressure over the parotid gland. Both the labial and buccal mucosae contain numerous minor salivary glands that occasionally may produce a pebbly appearance. Fordyce granules appear as yellow to white, 1–2 mm, and are ectopic sebaceous glands that are present in the buccal mucosa in around 85% of the general population. These granules also may be seen on the vermilion and labial mucosa.

The mucosa of the hard palate is firmly attached to the underlying bone, rendering it slightly paler than the rest of the oral mucosae. The hard palate mucosa is covered by a layer of keratin. The incisive papilla is located in the anterior portion of the hard palate immediately behind the two central maxillary incisors. Adjacent and posterior to the incisive papilla, ridges called *palatal rugae* radiate laterally. The distribution and shape of these rugae are particular to each individual. The palatine raphe is a slightly elevated ridge that runs, in the palatal midline, from the incisive papilla to the soft palate.

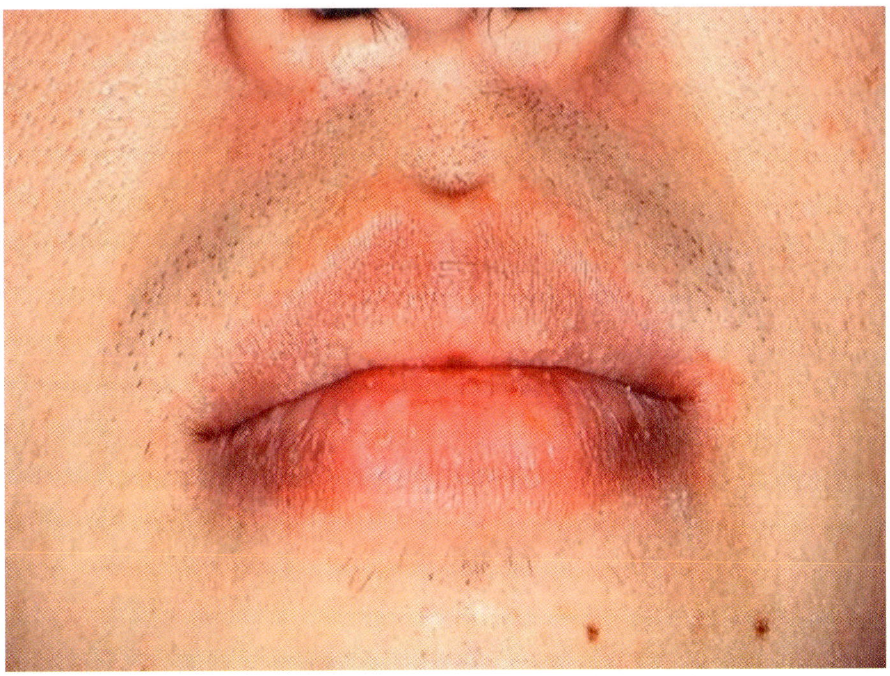

▲ **FIGURE 54-1** Lips showing the vermilion border, junction between skin and oral mucosa, in an Asian man.

Some individuals present a bony exostosis in the center of the hard palate of variable degree and shape known as *torus palatinus.* This bony exostosis is inherited in an autosomal dominant fashion, and generally, it makes itself evident around puberty.

Minor, mostly mucous salivary glands are also found bilaterally and off the midline in the posterior third of the hard palate. The excretory ducts of these glands appear as small 1-mm erythematous umbilicated papules.

Separating the hard from the soft palate is a vibrating line that is visible when saying "Ahh." The soft palate is rich in blood vessels; hence it is redder than the hard palate, and it extends toward the fauces, or folds. The palatoglossal folds are seen laterally and represent the fusion of the soft palate with the pharyngeal wall. The uvula is an extension of soft tissue located in the midline of the free border of the soft palate. Minor salivary glands are also found in the soft palatal mucosa.

The anterior two-thirds of the dorsal surface of the tongue are derived from the ectoderm, and this is the functional, or tasting, portion of the tongue. The posterior third is derived from the endoderm and is the lymphatic portion because it contains the lingual tonsils. This posterior portion is characterized by a laterally irregular nodular surface with cryptic openings, the *foveate papillae*. The division of these two tongue areas is established by the lingual V, which is actually formed by 10–12 round and flat vallate or circumvallate papillae converging at the angle of the V at the site of the foramen cecum, which represents the embryonal site of origin of parts of the thyroid gland.

The anterior two-thirds of the lingual dorsum is covered by papillae, giving this area a rough, white appearance. The filiform papillae are elongated and white in color owing to keratinization of their end portions. In the vicinity of the lingual V, they also have a V arrangement, but closer to the lingual tip, they acquire a horizontal arrangement. The fungiform papillae are small and red and are evenly distributed throughout the anterior dorsal tongue surface. Brown or black accumulation of melanin pigmentation can be seen in the fungiform papillae in African-Americans and other people of color in general (Figure 54-2). In some patients, the posterolateral borders of the tongue present small lymphoid aggregates. The center of the lingual dorsum is occupied by a fissure of variable depth. Horizontal fissures can be seen in 5% of the population (fissure, scrotal tongue). The ventral surface of the tongue is shiny, smooth, and reddish and characteristically shows the ranine veins that become varicose with age. The ventral surface is continuous with the oral floor. The lingual frenulum is located in the midline of the oral floor, extending from the mandibular gingiva to the ventral surface of the tongue.

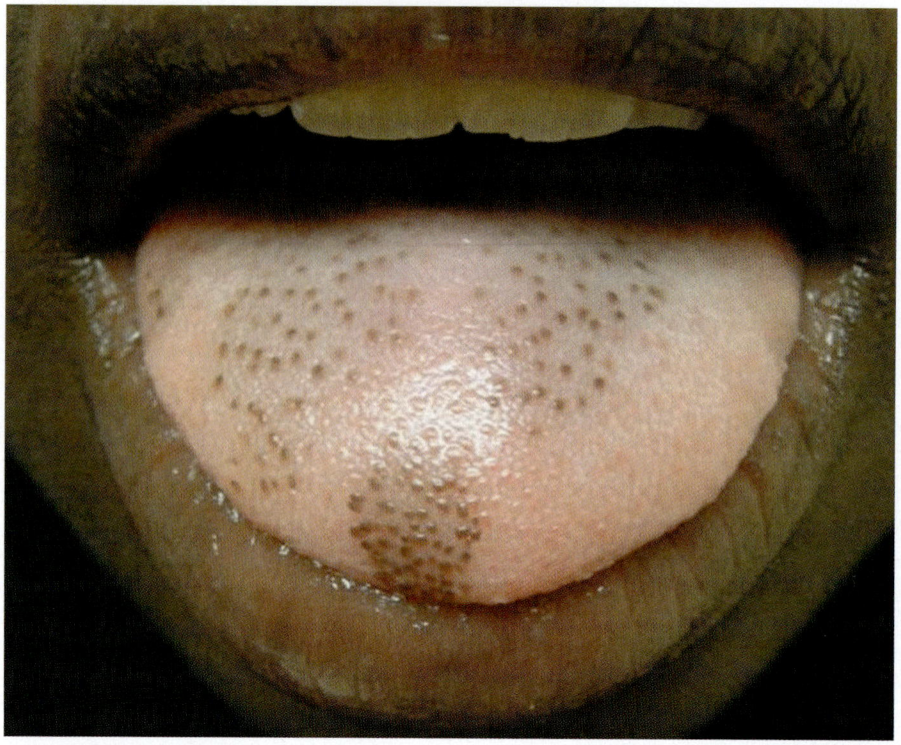

▲ **FIGURE 54-2** Well-delineated pigmentation on the fungiform papillae on the dorsal tongue of an African-American woman.

The floor of the mouth is a continuation of the ventral lingual mucosa on one side, and on the other side it is reflected onto the gingiva. The openings of the submandibular and sublingual glands are seen as elevated, crater-like structures (sublingual caruncles) at each side of the lingual frenum. The sublingual folds are elevations seen at each side of the midline produced by the sublingual glands.

The gingiva is divided into free marginal gingiva and attached gingiva by the free marginal groove. The free marginal gingiva has an undulating or scalloped contour, and from its upper border emerge the interdental papillae with their characteristic triangular shape occupying the spaces between the teeth. The marginal end of the gingiva bends over the tooth surface and attaches itself to the tooth below the gingival border. The gingival sulcus, or crevice, is the space found between tooth and gingiva. The depth of the sulcus varies from 0.1–0.3 cm. The attached gingiva extends from the free gingival groove to the beginning of the alveolar crest and is continuous with the alveolar mucosa. Vestibular and lingual gingivae are essentially identical in clinical appearance, presenting a whiter color owing to surface keratinization that is absent in the alveolar mucosa. An undulating band of melanin pigmentation of variable width and intensity of color can be seen in the gingiva of individuals of African ancestry and people of color (as further explained below). The geniohyoid processes are located bilaterally at each side of the mandibular midline on the lingual attached gingiva.

COMMON ORAL DISEASES

White Lesions

LEUKOEDEMA Leukoedema is an asymptomatic, symmetric gray-white diffuse film on the oral mucosa that occurs most commonly bilaterally on the buccal mucosa; it also may be noted on the floor of the mouth and palantopharyngeal tissues (Figure 54-3). It is a common oral condition of unknown etiology. There may be an association between the development of leukoedema, poor oral hygiene, and abnormal biting patterns. Leukoedema has a greater prevalence in dark-skinned individuals, especially African-Americans and Hispanics. It has

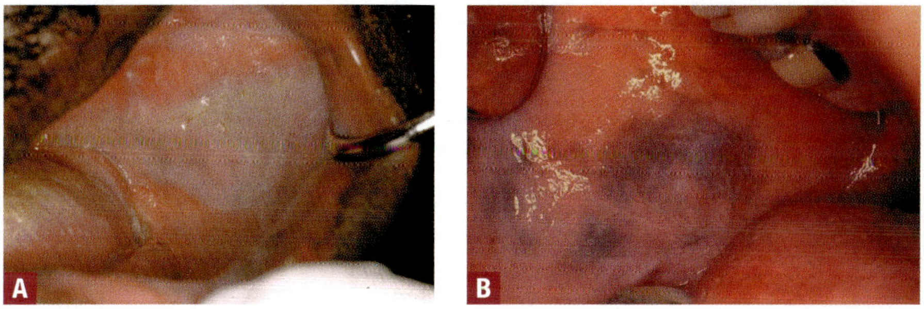

▲ **FIGURE 54-3** **A.** Leukoedema of the buccal mucosa of an African-American man. Lesions appear opalescent, whitish gray, and are usually bilateral. Lesions disappear when mucosa is stretched. **B.** Some leukoedema lesions are accompanied by physiologic pigmentations.

been reported that it is present in 70–90% of African-American adults.[1] Because of this high prevalence, it has been speculated to be a variant of normal versus a pathologic process. However, some reports have shown that leukoedema is more severe in smokers and lessens with smoking cessation. Diagnosis is made by stretching of the oral mucosa. The white, opaque character of the lesion diminishes or disappears with the stretching and eversion of the oral mucosa. Any diffuse white lesions of the oral mucosa always should be stretched out to rule out any other underlying lesions. Histologically, oral lesions show parakeratosis and an increase in thickness of the oral mucosal epithelium with intracellular edema of the spinous layer. The cells of the spinous layer are large with pyknotic nuclei. Rete ridges may be elongated. No dysplasia or hypergranulosis is noted. No treatment is necessary for this benign condition. Leukoedema has no malignant potential.[2]

SUBMUCOUS FIBROSIS Oral submucous fibrosis (OSF) is a unique premalignant condition that presents as a generalized white discoloration of the oral mucosa of individuals in India and Southeast Asia who chew betel quid (a blend of tobacco, slaked lime, areca nut and its constitutes, mainly arecoline, and betel leaves). Reports have shown that chemicals such as arecoline appear to interfere with the molecular processes of deposition and/or degradation of extracellular matrix molecules such as collagen, causing imbalance in the normal process. The most likely events that take place with regard to this imbalance may be reduced phagocytosis of collagen by fibroblasts and up- or downregulation of key enzymes such as lysyl oxidase, matrix metalloproteinases, and tissue inhibitors of matrix metalloproteinases. The process also may be influenced by increased secretion of inflammatory cytokines and growth factors and decreased production of antifibrotic cytokines.[3,4] Reports have shown that the prevalence of OSF in India and Southeast Asia ranges from 0.04–24.4%. The highest rate of 24.4% was reported from a study collected from an aboriginal community of southern Taiwan, with a 69.5% areca quid chewing prevalence rate. The malignant transformation rate of OSF is reported as 2.3–7.6%. Other possible etiologic factors include capsaicin in chilies and micronutrient deficiencies of iron, zinc, and essential vitamins. In addition, a possible autoimmune basis to the disease with demonstration of various autoantibodies and an association with specific human leukocyte antigens (HLAs) has been proposed. This raises the possibility of a genetic predisposition of some individuals to develop OSF. However, from the available scientific literature, it is clear that the regular use of areca nut is the major etiologic factor.[5]

Clinically, it presents as a chronic progressive disease leading to marked limitation of mouth opening and is characterized by the oral mucosa becoming stiff owing to fibroelastic transformation of the juxtaepithelial and deeper connective tissue; ultimately, trismus, masticatory difficulty, dysphagia, and severe xerostomia predominate. Progressive fibrosis results in the development of painful mucosal atrophy and restrictive fibrotic bands (Figures 54-4). Histologically, it is characterized by submucosal deposition of dense avascular connective tissue fibers with a number of inflammatory cell infiltrates (Figure 54-5). The epithelium is hyperkeratotic, and some epithelial atrophy is seen in elder patients. It is an irreversible condition with no effective treatment. Frequent monitoring for malignant transformation is essential, and surgical interventions may be necessary in more advanced cases to release fibrotic bands and improve trismus.[6]

SQUAMOUS CELL CARCINOMA (SCC) Oral cancer is a global health problem with increasing incidence and mortality rates; around 400,000 patients annually are estimated to have oral cancer worldwide.[7] In the United States, around 30,000 oral cancer cases are diagnosed every year; of these, oral cancer will claim approximately 8000 lives a year.[8] During 2000–2004, the annual incidence rate among black men in the United States was not a lot higher than the rate among whites (10.3 versus 9.9 new cases per 100,000). The annual mortality rate among black men was 1.5 times higher (3.9 versus 2.4 deaths per 100,000). The average age of diagnosis of oral and pharyngeal cancer for black men is approximately 10 years younger than that for whites. Among these diagnosed cancer lesions, only 19% are at the early stage compared with 38% in white men.[9] The 5-year survival rate for blacks is 40% and for whites is 55%. This discrepancy in the morbidity and mortality rates has been attributed mainly to the more advanced or later stage at which the cancer was diagnosed in black men. Oral cancer occurs mostly on the lips, tongue, floor of the mouth, palate, gingiva, alveolar and buccal mucosae, and oropharynx. SCC accounts for 96% of all oral cancers; sarcomas and salivary gland tumors account for the remainder.[10]

The major risk factors are smoking and alcohol consumption. A number of oncogenic viruses may be associated with the development of SCC, especially HPV-16; tumor suppressor genes *p53* also has been implicated in the pathogenesis of SCC. Other major risk factors include age, ultraviolet (UV) radiation exposure, immunosuppression, nutritional deficiency, and intraoral infection with syphilis, *Candida* (chronic), or human papillomavirus.[11]

Clinically, oral SCC may present as leukoplakia, erythroplakia, erythroleukoplakia, irregular endophytic masses with ulceration (Figure 54-6), or exophytic nodules (Figure 54-7). High-risk anatomic sites for development of SCC are the ventrolateral tongue, floor of the mouth, and vermilion border of the lip. Gingival lesions are more common in women. Any persistent oral lesion should be biopsied . High-risk lesions (including persistent ulcer) in high-risk sites (e.g., floor of mouth, site of previous SCC, or site of previous radiation) have a high probability of being malignant. A second primary lesion of the aerodigestive tract is found in up to one-fourth of patients with oral SCCs. Oral SCCs in

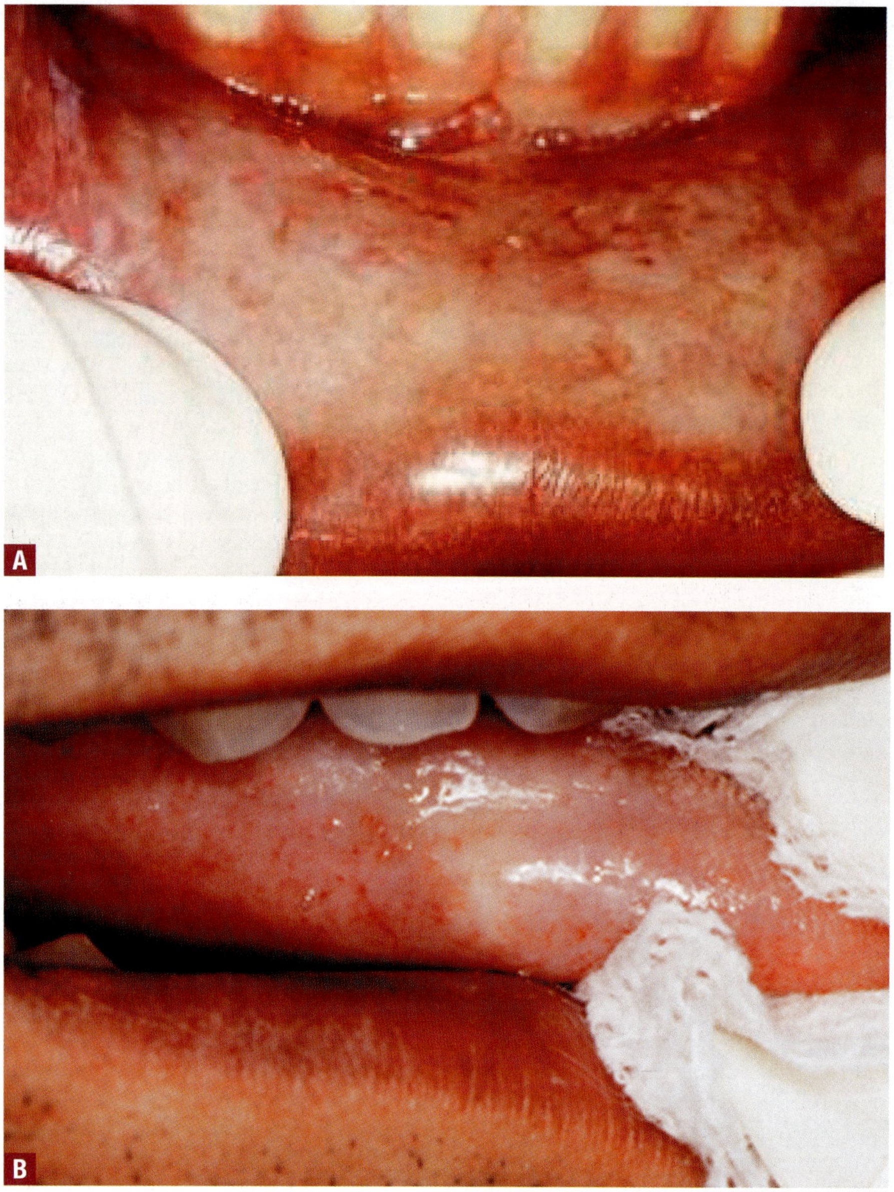

▲ **FIGURE 54-4** Submucous fibrosis: **A.** Mucosal atrophy: Lower lip mucosa of a Pakistani man who practiced the habit of chewing betel nut mixed with tobacco (PAAN). Note the white, marble-like appearance of the mucosa. The patient had limited mouth opening and complained of mouth dryness. **B.** Local fibrosis of the lateral tongue border of the same patient showing similar clinical findings.

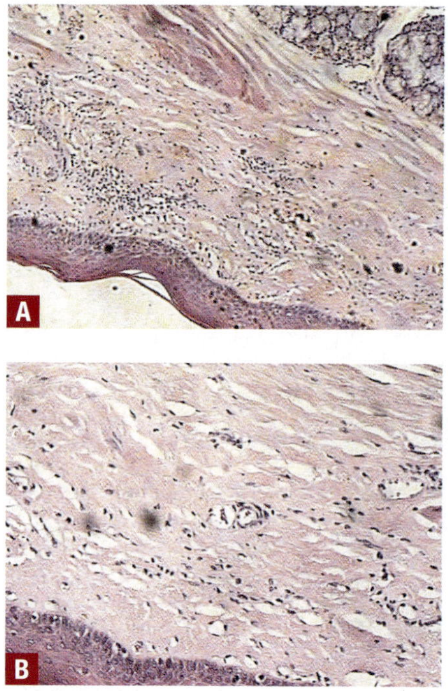

▲ **FIGURE 54-5** **A.** This biopsy from the lip of the patient shown in Figure 54-4 shows marked fibrosis of the collagenic connective tissue with a moderate, mostly lymphocytic inflammatory infiltrate. The epithelium is atrophic and is covered by a thin layer of parakeratin. These are typical findings in submcuous fibrosis. **B.** This higher magnification of another field of the same biopsy shows similar findings.

general have a high rate of metastasis, but the incidence depends on the site of involvement, duration of the lesion, and histologic grade. Overall, more posterior SCCs demonstrate higher rates of metastasis to regional lymph nodes. Distant metastases do occur and typically involve the lungs, liver, and bone. Ultimately, prognosis is best determined by clinical staging. Tobacco-cessation measures should be initiated.[12]

Histologically, oral SCC encompasses a wide range from well-differentiated (low-grade) lesions, in which the tumors resemble normal epithelium, to poorly differentiated or anaplastic (high-grade) lesions, where the tumor cells lose their resemblance to the epithelial tissues.

Depending on the stage of the disease, the treatment of choice is aggressive surgical intervention. Patients with lymph node involvement typically require surgery followed by external-beam radiation. Adjuvant therapy with chemotherapeutic agents or epidermal growth factor receptor inhibitors may be employed in recurrent or metastatic cases. Additionally, systemic retinoids and antioxidants may serve a chemopreventive role in high-risk patients.[13]

ACTINIC PRURIGO Actinic prurigo (AP) is a frequent idiopathic photodermatosis mainly affecting Native Americans and Mestizos, mostly from Latin America. AP also has been reported in the Inuit and occasionally in Caucasians and individuals of African descent. AP starts early in life with a slight predilection for women and children younger than 10 years of age.[14–18] AP affects the exposed areas of the skin as well as the lip.

The pathogenetic mechanisms of AP are unknown, although an association with several HLA alleles has been reported.[19] It has been shown that there is a strong association between AP and the HLA allele DR4, specifically with the DRB1*0407 allele, which has been reported to be present in over 60% of patients with AP.[20–23] This finding has been confirmed in different populations, and is most likely an important pathogenetic factor.[24]

AP affects the sun-exposed areas of the skin, manifesting as erythematous papules and lichenoid plaques that follow the initial presentation of a severe and persistent chronic pruritus. Occasionally, areas not exposed to the sun also can be affected. Cheilitis is found in over 80% of patients with skin lesions and is characterized by severe pruritus, pain, and tingling mostly of the vermilion border of the lips, especially the lower lip (Figure 54-8). AP

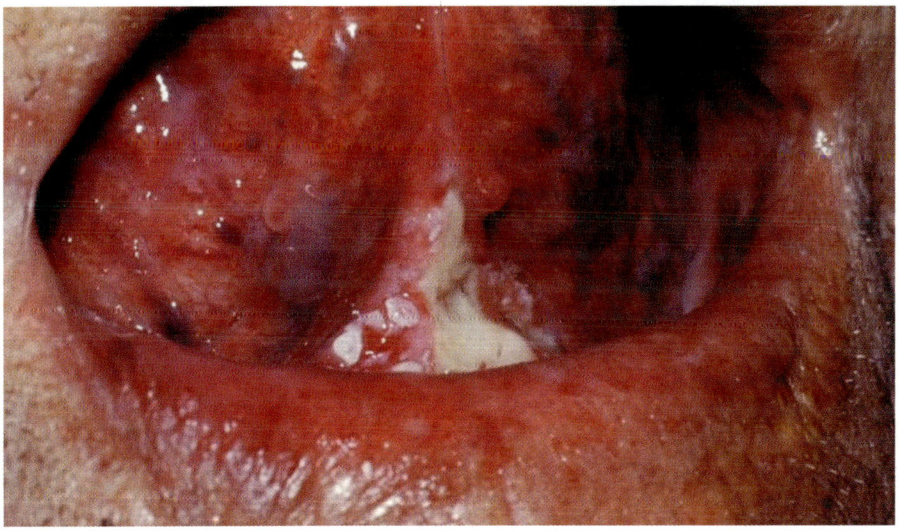

▲ **FIGURE 54-6** Squamous cell carcinoma of the floor of the mouth and ventral surface of the tongue.

cheilitis also has been reported as an isolated example in patients free of the dermatologic manifestations.[18] The appearance of the lips is disfiguring owing to areas of ulceration eventuating in crust formation.[17]

The histopathologic findings mostly consist of acanthosis, spongiosis, basal cell vacuolation, and edema of the lamina propria. The surface is generally ulcerated and covered by a serohematic crust.[18] The underlying connective tissue presents a profuse lymphocytic inflammatory infiltrate and the typical presence of well-defined lymphoid follicles. Additionally, melanophages and eosinophils can be identified.[17,18,24]

AP cheilitis is best treated with a combination of protection from the sun by means of hats and/or sunblocking creams, topical steroids, and thalidomide.[16]

HEREDITARY POLYMORPHIC LIGHT ERUPTION (HPLE) This condition is prevalent in South, Central and North American natives.[25,26] Clinically, it is essentially identical to actinic prurigo; the main distinguishing feature is the fact that over 75% of affected individuals have other family members similarly affected. HPLE is inherited as an autosomal dominant condition. Fusaro and Johnson[25] have reported that 28% of their Caucasian patients and 53% of their African-American patients with HPLE had a definite family history of Native American heritage. Patients with HPLE also develop cheilitis that persists into adulthood and which presents the same clinical findings, that is, pruritus, papular eruption, and excoriation of the lips. The possibility that AP and HPLE represent manifestations of a single spectrum with a shared etiology in antigenic and genetic factors should be explored in detail.

MULTIFOCAL PAPILLOMAVIRUS EPITHELIAL HYPERPLASIA Carlos and Sedano proposed the name *multifocal papillomavirus epithelial hyperplasia* (MPVEH) based on the viral nature and clinical multifocality typical of this disease.[27] MPVEH is a benign, proliferative, wartlike disease of the oral mucosa, sometimes affecting the anal/genital mucosa with a rare skin involvement. It shows an unusual racial and geographic distribution frequently seen in Inuit's and native peoples from North, Central, and South America, Eskimos, and Africans.[28,29] Most authors report a sex distribution of 2:1 women to men, and over 90% of cases are observed in patients in the first and second decades of life.[27,30,31] The first reports in the North American literature were those of Archard and colleagues,[28,32] who independently proposed the name *focal epithelial hyperplasia* and the eponym *Heck disease.* Praetorius demonstrated evidence of viral infection in biopsies of this lesion, and Pfister and colleagues identified the presence of human papillomavirus type 13. Beaudenon and colleagues isolated another virus from lesions of this disease, which they named *human papilomavirus type 32.*[33–35]

Immunohistochemical studies and in situ hybridization have shown that the majority of cases of MPVEH demonstrate the presence of human papillomavirus (i.e., HPV-13 or HPV-32). Even if HPV-13 and HPV-32 are considered the causative agents, other factors such as genetic predisposition, malnutrition, hygiene, and living conditions of affected individuals should be considered of etiologic importance.[36–39]

Clinically, MPVEH is characterized by multiple papulonodular eruptions located mostly on the buccal and lower lip mucosa, followed by the lateral border of the tongue. Rarely, lesions will be found in the palatal mucosa and on the ventral surface of the tongue. These lesions mostly have a smooth surface that can have the normal mucosal color,

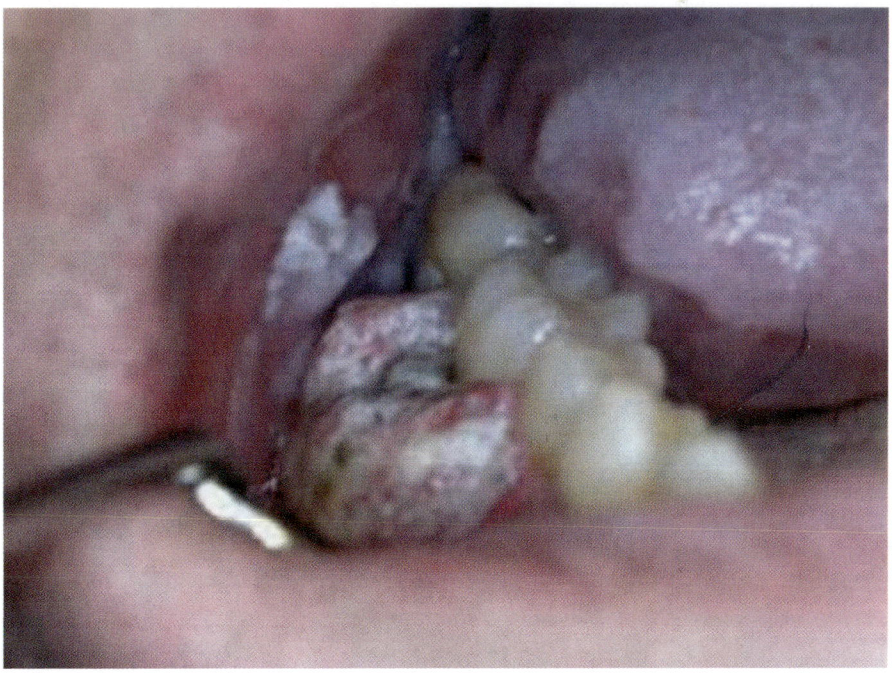

▲ **FIGURE 54-7** Squamous cell carcinoma of the posterior lower gingival tissues.

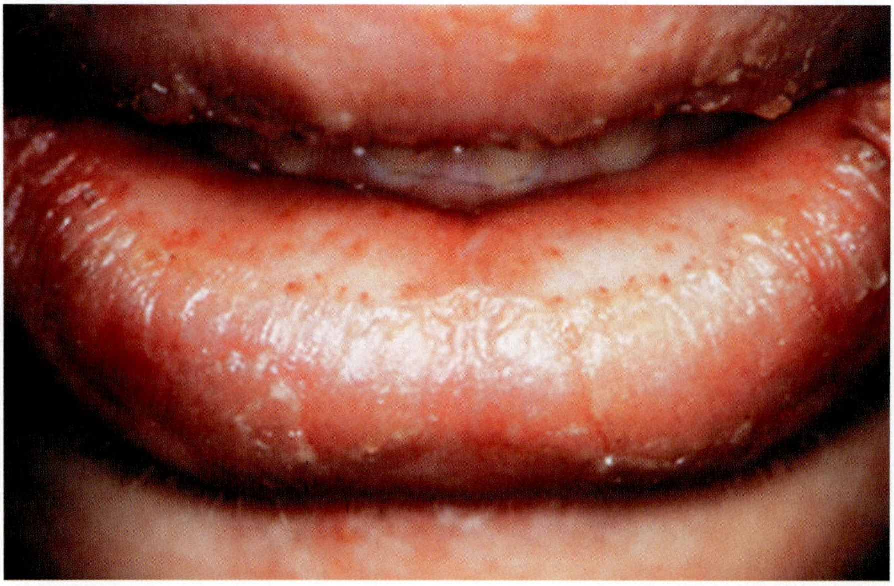

▲ **FIGURE 54-8** In actinic prurigo, the lower lip shows marked denudation of the superficial epithelial layers as well as pinpoint areas of ulceration. Also note the crust formation, especially on the upper lip.

but in some patients they can be corrugated and have a whitish color (Figure 54-9). A small number of patients will present with additional lesions having a definite papilloma-like or papillated appearance[27] (Figure 54-10). Familial incidence has been noted by several authors, and it can be explained by the viral contagious nature of the disease and a possible genetic predisposition.[40] MPVEH has been reported almost exclusively in children and youngsters who live in extreme poverty.[30] Some cases have been documented in human immunodeficiency virus (HIV)–positive and acquired immune deficiency syndrome (AIDS) patients.[41]

Histologically, biopsies of MPVEH present acanthosis of the superficial epithelium, and deeper epithelial layers present swollen cells, ballooning cellular degeneration, and individual cell keratinization. The epithelium at the connective tissue interface shows anastomosing rete ridges. The epithelial cellular appearance produced by nuclear abnormalities, which have been classically described as "mitosoid," or cell within a cell, is the typical distinguishing histologic feature of MPVEH[27,30,33,40] (Figure 54-11).

Surgical or laser ablation can be used to treat large lesions that interfere with mastication or that bleed when bitten. Most cases disappear with time. The use of podophyllin to treat these lesions is not recommended. Cimetidine has been used, especially in HIV-positive patients, with mixed results. Interferon-β has been used to treat some patients with positive results.[42]

Oral Pigmented Lesions

Oral pigmented lesions are frequently noted on physical examination and must be differentiated from signs of a malignant process or a systemic condition.

PHYSIOLOGIC (RACIAL) PIGMENTATION The color of clinically normal gingiva is usually described as pale or coral pink; the color also depends on vascularity, keratinization, and the presence or absence of inflammation. There is in fact considerable variation in the color of normal gingiva that results from differences in the amount of melanin pigment. The color of the gingiva varies depending on the complexion of the individual. Pigmentation is prominent in the normal gingiva of Africans, Orientals, Native Americans, South Americans, and Mediterraneans.[43] Physiologic pigmentation, which is due to greater melanocytic activity rather than a greater number of melanocytes, develops during the first two decades of life but may not come to the patient's attention until later. The color ranges from light to dark brown. The attached gingiva is the most common intraoral site of such pigmentation, where it appears as a bilateral, well-demarcated, ribbonlike dark brown band that usually spares the marginal gingiva.[44] People worldwide have various degrees of physiologic pigmentation, and the color varies from brown to black. The involvement may be in isolated patches or a diffuse speckling (Figure 54-12). Pigmentation of the buccal mucosa, hard palate, and lips also may be seen as brown patches with less well-defined borders. The fungiform papillae on the dorsal surface of the tongue can show pigmentations (see Figure 54-2). The pigmentation is asymptomatic, and no treatment is required.[45]

LENTIGINES Lentigines are common oral melanocytic lesions that appear as brown macules on the palate, gingiva, or lips. Microscopically, melanocytic hyperplasia with elongation of the rete ridges is observed. Labial melanotic macules (focal melanosis) present as asymptomatic, well-circumscribed, 2- to 5-mm blue, black, or brown macules on the vermilion, with no malignant potential.

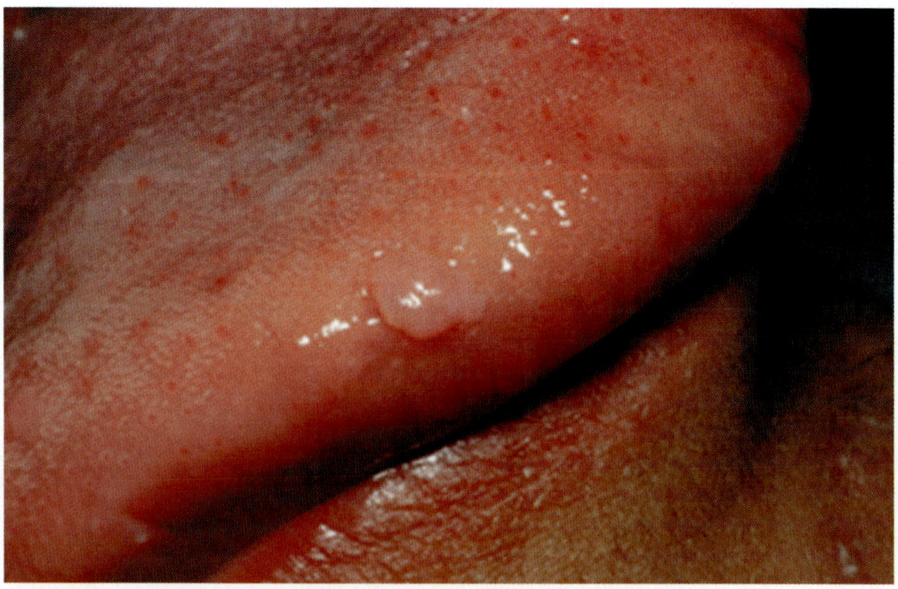

▲ **FIGURE 54-9** Note the small nodules on the lateral border of the tongue on Native American child with multifocal papillomavirus epithelial hyperplasia (MPVEH).

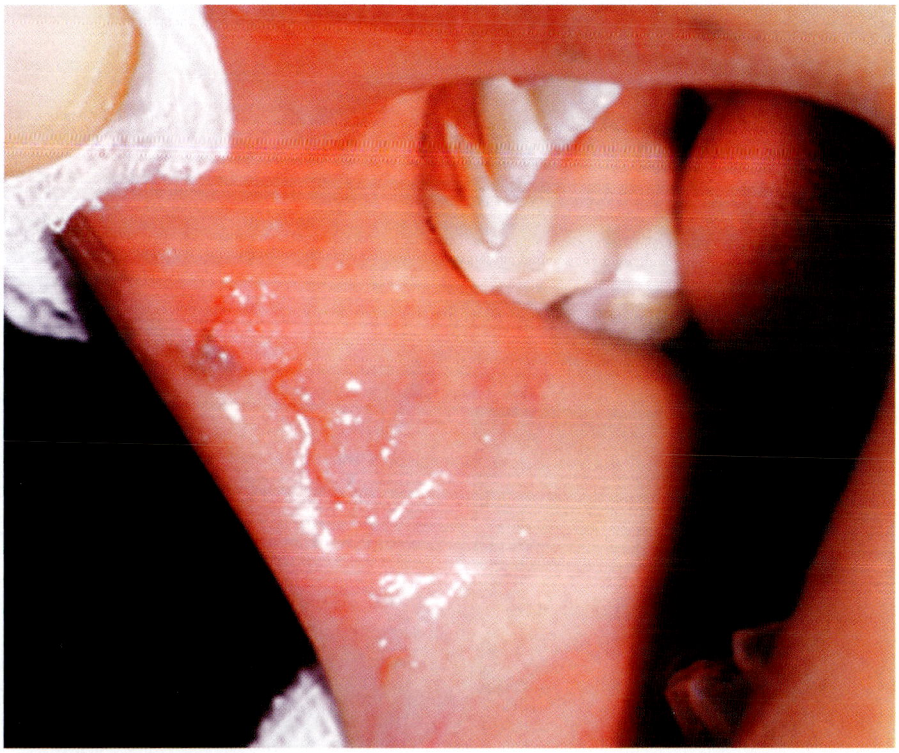

▲ **FIGURE 54-10** Left buccal mucosa of another child of Native American ancestry showing multiple hyperplastic nodes with a smooth surface typical of MPVEH.

The lower lip is affected more commonly, with less frequent involvement in the buccal mucosa, the gingiva, the palate, and the tongue. The presence of pigmentation may be of cosmetic concern. Surgical excision is the most common treatment, but scarring may result. Cryosurgery is effective but is limited owing to the absence of tissue verification.[46] Histologically, increased basal layer melanin without rete ridge elongation is observed with a focal increase in melanin in the basal cell layer, lamina propria, or both.

Both lentigines and melanotic macules tend to be solitary and are more common in women. Solitary lesions may resemble an early malignant melanoma but are negative for human melanoma black-45 (HMB-45) reactivity. When multiple labial macules are observed, one must consider a number of conditions, including Peutz-Jeghers syndrome, Carney complex (NAME, LAMB, or LEOPARD syndrome), Laugier-Hunziker syndrome, and Addison disease.

LAUGIER-HUNZIKER SYNDROME This is a benign syndrome of unknown etiology that is characterized by macular hyperpigmentation on the oral and genital mucosa, conjunctiva, palms, and soles and longitudinal melanonychia. This entity was first described in 1970. Most patients are middle-aged Caucasian woman. Laugier-Hunziker syndrome is seen only rarely in African-Americans or in men but appears to be more common in France and Italy. Patients present with a variable number of gray to brown pigmented macules on the lips, hard palate, fingertips, labial commissures, gingiva, and floor of mouth (Figure 54-13). In contrast to Peutz-Jergers syndrome, there are no associated systemic or internal manifestations.[47,48] Dermoscopic findings show a parallel pattern on mucosa of longitudinal homogeneous pigmentation on toenails parallel furrow on palms and the soles. Histology is consistent with mucosal melanosis.[49]

PEUTZ-JEGHERS SYNDROME This is an autosomal dominant condition characterized by mucocutaneous hyperpigmentation, multiple gastrointestinal hamartomas, and visceral malignant tumors that was first described in 1921.[50,51]

This syndrome is due to a mutation in the serine/threonine kinase STK11 gene mapped to 19p13.3. Patients present in infancy and early childhood with anal and mucocutaneous pigmentation (Figure 54-14). With time, mucosal pigmentation, particularly on the lips (95%) and the buccal mucosa (85%) will persist; cutaneous pigmentation fades and decreases in diameter, particularly on the face, in the periorbital region. Polyps may occur in any part of the gastrointestinal tract, but jejunal polyps are a consistent feature. Malignant degeneration of the small intestinal polyps is rare but does occur in the colon. Intussusceptions and gastrointestinal bleeding are well described. An increase in breast carcinoma, benign ovarian tumors, testicular tumors, and pancreatic cancer has been documented, while extragastrointestinal polyps, namely, ureteral, bladder, renal pelvis, bronchial, and nasal polyps, also have been noted. Gynecomastia with testis tumors also may be seen.[52]

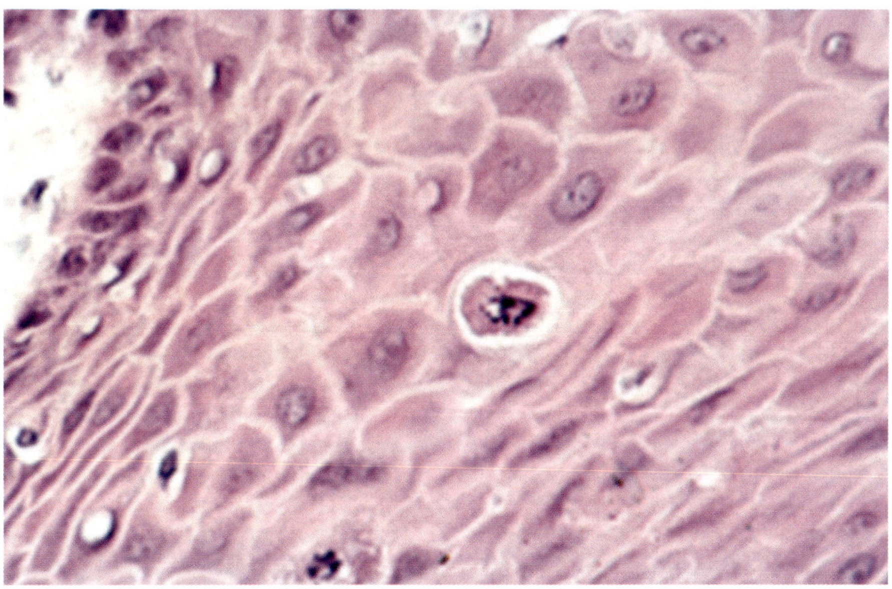

▲ **FIGURE 54-11** Microscopy of a lip lesion of MPVEH showing the characteristic cell-within-a-cell or mitosoid appearance of some epithelial cells as well as cytoplasmic vacuolization.

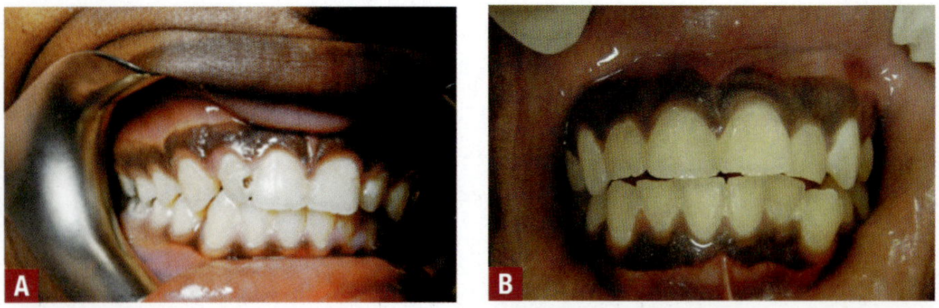

▲ **FIGURE 54-12** Well-delineated marginal gingival pigmentation with a chevron appearance in an African-American man.

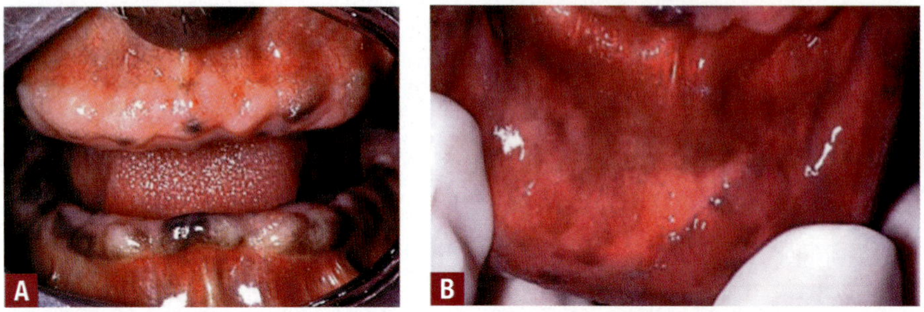

▲ **FIGURE 54-13** Laughier Hunziker syndrome is characterized by mucosal pigmented macules, as seen here on the gingiva of an edentulous African-American man **(A)** and involving the labial mucosa of this same individual **(B)**.

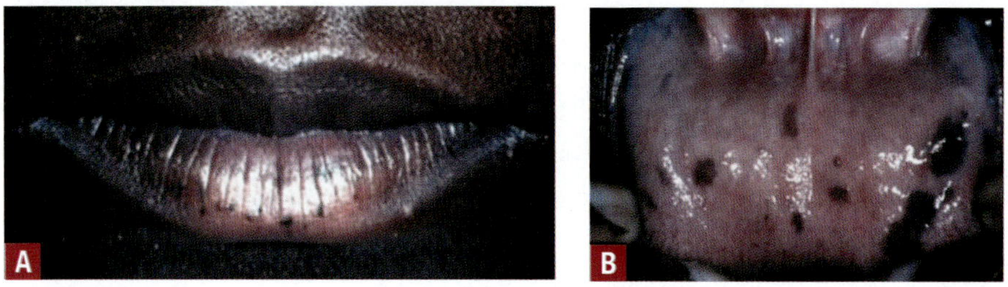

▲ **FIGURE 54-14 A.** PEUTZ-Jegers syndrome is characterized by pigmented macules on the vermilion of this African-American woman. **B.** Note that the intraoral macules are significantly larger in diameter.

POSTINFLAMMATORY HYPERPIGMENTATION Postinflammatory hyperpigmentation (PIH) is the most common complications of laser surgery among dark-skinned patients. This undesirable adverse effect is a major reason why laser resurfacing is much less popular among patients with darker skin. Dermatologic diseases, including lichenoid dermatitides such as erythema multiforme and lichen planus, are known to be associated with PIH of any skin type, but patients with darker skin have more prominent PIH. In lichenoid dermatitis, the inflammatory zone between the epidermal and dermal junction contributes to the pigmentary incontinence that could lead to a great degree of PIH. New methods in facial rejuvenation using fractional laser resurfacing with modified density and energy have been reported to improve the risk of PIH in individual patients.[53]

MELANOACANTHOMA Intraoral melanoacanthoma, a rapidly progressive phenomenon, arises in response to a traumatic stimulus. Melanoacanthomas arise suddenly on the buccal mucosa in black women in the third decade of life and are reported to reach a diameter of several centimeters in just a few weeks. Melanoacanthomas are darkly pigmented, well-demarcated irregular plaques. A biopsy must be performed to exclude malignant melanoma. Dendritic melanocytes are seen throughout the mucosal epithelium, accompanied by acanthosis and spongiosis. Importantly, no pleomorphism or mitoses are observed. Often, melanoacanthomas regress spontaneously after removal of any ongoing trauma.

SMOKER'S MELANOSIS This benign pigmentation develops in the anterior mandibular region, with less prominent pigmentation on the palate and buccal mucosa. Its prevalence varies from 15–31% of smokers, and it may reverse over months to years when smoking stops. Pipe smoking contributes to this even more than cigarettes. It is hypothesized that a component in tobacco stimulates melanocytes, although female hormones (e.g., birth control pills) also may play a role. The intensity of the pigmentation is directly related to the duration and dose (Figures 54-15 and 54-16). Histologically an increase in melanin production is noted. Although pigmentation is most pronounced in individuals of color, even Caucasians such as the Swedish population can develop smoker's melanosis.

ORAL MELANOMA Oral mucosal malignant melanoma is a rare tumor that may evolve within or at the mucocutaneous junction. Contrary to popular belief, mucosal melanomas are often amelanotic. In contrast to cutaneous melanoma, oral melanoma is equally prevalent in African-Americans as in Caucasians. Intraoral melanoma presents as an irregular, pigmented macule, patch, or papule on the hard palate or maxillary gingiva in patients over age 50 (Figure 54-17). While often asymptomatic, advanced lesions may ulcerate or bleed. The clinical differential diagnosis includes lymphoma and angiosarcoma. The histology reveals nested and single atypical melanocytes, with angioinvasion and multicentric metastatic disease noted early on. Oral melanoma is positive for S-100, HMB-45, melanocyte antigen (Melan-A), and melanoma antigen recognized by T-cells (MART 1) reactivity. The growth pattern resembles a nodular pattern. The prognosis is poor if the lesion is larger than 2 mm. Clinical staging is based on local disease, regional lymph node disease, or disseminated disease at the time of diagnosis. Clinical workup should include a total body skin examination, baseline computed tomographic (CT) scanning, or magnetic resonance imaging (MRI) and a basic metabolic workup.

ORAL INFECTIOUS DISEASES

Syphilis

Infective syphilis is caused by the anaerobic filamentous spirochete, *Treponema pallidum*. In the past decade, there has been a significant rise in the prevalence of infective syphilis in the developed countries, including eastern Europe and

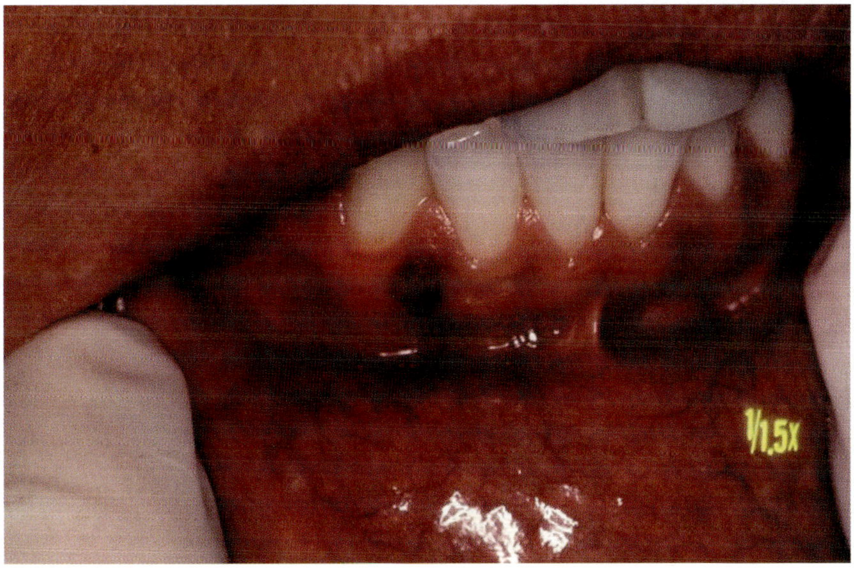

▲ **FIGURE 54-15** Well-circumscribed pigmented lesion of the lower gingiva in a heavy smoker.

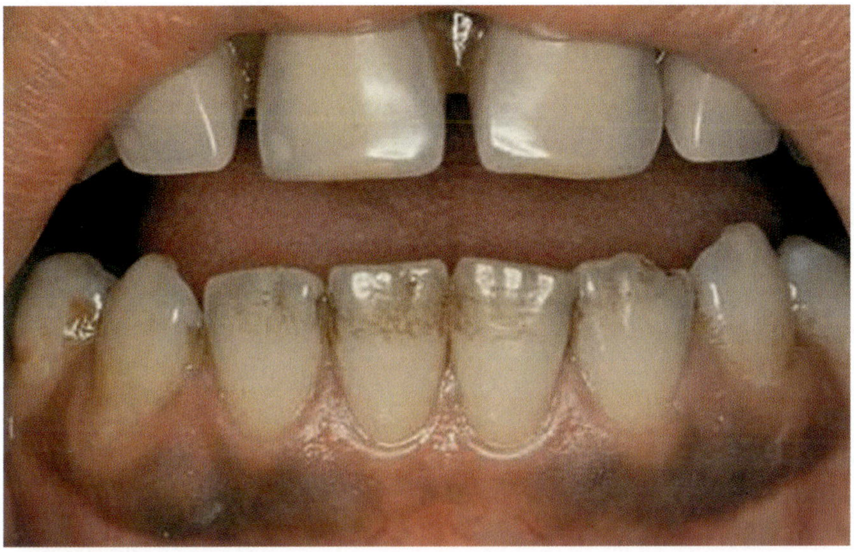

▲ **FIGURE 54-16** Diffuse pigmented lesion on the lower gingiva owing to heavy smoking.

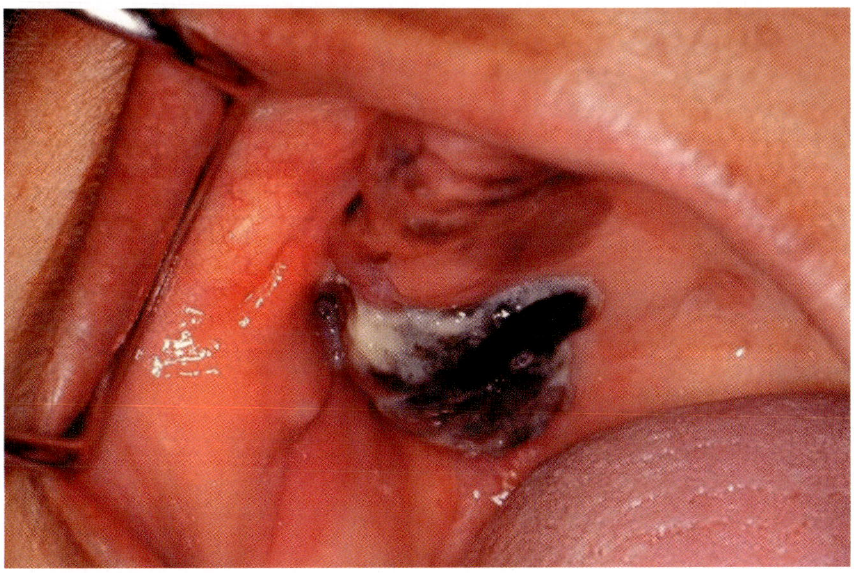

▲ **FIGURE 54-17** Oral melanoma of the palate in a 53-year-old Hispanic woman.

to a small extent western Europe and the United States. In eastern Europe, the increased frequency of syphilis has been predominantly in heterosexuals, whereas in the United Kingdom and the United States, the outbreaks are among heterosexuals and homosexuals.[54,55]

From 2000–2004, the incidence of primary and secondary syphilis in the United States increased from 2.2–2.7 cases per 100,000 population.[56] Among the U.S. metropolitan centers, San Francisco has experienced a striking increase from an estimate of 5 cases in 1998 to 320 cases in 2004. Additionally, the rates of primary and secondary syphilis among blacks were estimated to be 5.1 times higher in 2003 and 5.6 times higher in 2004 than those in whites.[57]

The clinical presentation of syphilis varies depending on the disease stage.[58,59] The first stage, known as *primary syphilis*, is clinically evident 2–3 weeks after inoculation, followed by the second stage, or *secondary* (disseminated) *syphilis*. Infected patients are highly contagious during the first two stages. Oral syphilis lesions are rare but may occur at any stage. Primary syphilis is manifested orally as a chancre at the site of inoculation on the lips, tongue, palate, gingiva, and tonsils. The oral lesions usually present as a deep ulceration with a red, purple, or brown base and an irregular, raised border, accompanied by regional lymphadenopathy. The ulceration of primary syphilis sometimes may be confused with other solitary ulcerative disorders, most notably traumatic ulceration. The diagnosis of primary syphilis may be difficult and relies on a detailed history of the sexual and/or social lifestyles of the patient and the involved sexual partner(s). In the early disease stage, infected patients may not show a positive nonspecific reaginic test, that is, rapid plasma reagin (RPR) or venereal disease reference laboratory (VDRL) test, and these should be supplemented with specific tests for IgG antibodies to *T. pallidum*. Definite diagnosis of early syphilis is made through visualization of *T. pallidum* spirochetes on dark-field microscopy, with direct fluorescent antibody tests, or with polymerase chain reaction assay. However, these tests are usually impractical and time-consuming.[60]

The oral manifestations of secondary syphilis vary and can be more extensive than those of primary disease. Oral lesions usually arise in at least 30% of patients with secondary syphilis, manifested primarily as mucous patches and maculopapular lesions and, to a lesser extent, nodular lesions. *Macular syphilides* are macular lesions that arise on the hard palate and manifest as flat to slightly raised, firm red lesions. *Papular syphilides* are rare and present as red, raised, firm round nodules with a gray, ulcerated center. These papules usually arise on the buccal mucosa or commissures. *Mucous patches* are oval to crescenteric erosions or shallow ulcers covered by a gray mucoid exudate with an erythematous border. These patches usually arise bilaterally on the mobile surfaces of the oral cavity. Another rarer form, ulceronodular disease, also known as *Lues maligna,* is an explosive generalized form of secondary syphilis characterized by fever, headache, and myalgia followed by a papulopustular eruption that rapidly transforms into necrotic, sharply demarcated ulcers bordered by hemorrhagic brown crusts. Lues maligna can arise on the gingivae, palate, or buccal mucosa, tongue, and lower lip. Lesions may occur on the vermilion, mimicking SCC or keratoacanthoma.

After the second stage, patients may enter a period free of lesions or symptoms known as *latent syphilis* or may progress further to *tertiary syphilis.* In addition to serious complications involving the vascular system and central nervous system, less significant but more characteristic oral presentations are the foci of granulomatous inflammation known as *gumma* seen frequently on the palate or tongue. Diffuse atrophy of the dorsal tongue papillae can give rise to a condition known as *luetic glossitis.* Pregnant women may transmit the infection to the fetus during any stages of the disease, with the greatest developmental effect at the fourth month of gestation. The clinical changes secondary to fetal infection are known as *congenital syphilis.* Congenital syphilis was defined initially to consist of three pathognomonic diagnostic features known as *Hutchinson's triad*—Hutchinson's teeth, interstitial keratitis, and eighth nerve deafness. However, few patients exhibit all three features.

Concurrent HIV infection and syphilis is not uncommon, particularly in young adults and homosexuals. The recent increase in the incidence of primary and secondary syphilis among hetero- and homosexuals has been correlated with high rates of HIV coinfection, high-risk sexual behavior, Internet partner recruitment, and drug use.[61] There have been some reports of prolonged primary and secondary disease in patients coinfected with HIV as compared with those not infected.[62] The 2006 guideline by the Centers for Disease Control and Prevention (CDC) on sexually transmitted diseases[63] has recommended cerebrospinal fluid (CSF) evaluation in any suspected high-risk patient (HIV-positive or HIV-negative) at any stage of disease who has clinical evidence of neurologic involvement with syphilis (e.g., cognitive dysfunction, motor or sensory deficits, cranial nerve palsies, ophthalmic or auditory symptoms, or signs of meningitis) and/or uveitis or other ocular manifestation associated with syphilis (e.g., iritis, neuroretinitis, or optic neuritis).

Treatment of syphilis-infected patients and their sexual contacts remains an important public health challenge. Standard therapy as recommended by the CDC[63] for treating syphilis is intramuscular injection of benzathine penicillin G or oral doxycycline in penicillin-allergic patients. Other alternatives include oral azithromycin as single-dose therapy, which has proven to be as effective in the treatment of syphilis in the developing countries, in which intramuscular administration of penicillin may be more problematic.[64]

Paracoccidioidomycosis (Blastomycosis)

Paracoccidioidomycosis (PCM) is a subacute or chronic systemic mycosis that is endemic to certain regions in South America and therefore also known as *South American blastomycosis.* The causative agent is *Paracoccidioides brasiliensis,* a thermal dimorphic fungus. The primary mode of infection is respiratory, but all organs and mucous membranes can be affected by lymphatic dissemination. Oropharyngeal lesions were the most common sign on physical examination, followed by lymphadenopathy, dysphonia, and skin lesions. The diagnosis can be carried out by biopsy or wet mounts of sputum, bronchoalveolar lavage products, or mucous membrane samples that are positive for *P. brasiliensis.* Antifungal agents such as the sulfamethoxazole-trimethoprime combination, amphotericin B, and especially azole derivatives are used in the therapeutic management of patients.[65] Antigen detection assay for the gp43 and gp70 molecules of *P. brasiliensis* is useful in early diagnosis and follow-up of patients with PCM.[66] Without treatment, the natural evolution of the disease is typically death. In patients with immunosuppression, such as AIDS patients, the infection can progress to full-blown disseminated disease.[67]

REFERENCES

1. Martin JL. Leukoedema: An epidemiological study in white and African-Americans. *J Tenn Dental Assoc* 1997; 77:18-21.
2. Neville BD, Damm DD, Allen CM, Bouquot JE. Developmental defects of the oral and maxillofacial region, in *Oral and Maxillofacial Pathology.* Philadelphia, Saunders, 2002, pp 7-8.
3. Jeng JH, Chang MC, Hahn LJ. Role of areca nut in betel quid-associated chemical carcinogenesis: Current awareness and future perspectives. *Oral Oncol* 2002; 37:477.
4. Rajendran R. Oral submucous fibrosis: Etiology, pathogenesis, and future research. *Bull WHO* 1994;72:985.
5. Tilakaratne WM, Klinikowski MF, Takashi S, et al. Oral submucous fibrosis: Review on etiology and pathogenesis. *Oral Oncol* 2006;42:561-568.
6. Pei-Shan Ho, Yi-Hsin Yang A, Shieh T-Y, et al. Consumption of areca quid, cigarettes, and alcohol related to the comorbidity of oral submucous fibrosis and oral cancer. *Oral Surg Oral Med Oral Pathol Oral Radiol Endod* 2007;104: 647-652.
7. 2003 Incidence and Mortality Report. United States Cancer Statistics. Available at *www.cdc.gov/cancer/npcr/npcrpdfs/US_Cancer_Statistics_2003_Incidence_and_Mortality.pdf.*
8. Surveillance Epidemiology and End Results (SEER) Cancer Statistical Review 1975-2004. Available at *http://seer.cancer.gov/csr/1975_2004/.*
9. Surveillance Epidemiology and End Results (SEER) Cancer Stat Fact Sheets. Available at *http://seer.cancer.gov/statfacts/html/all.html.*
10. Rodu B, Cole P. Oral cavity and pharynx-throat cancer in the United States, 1973-2003. *Oral Surg Oral Med Oral Pathol Oral Radiol Endod* 2007;104:653-658.
11. Rhodus NL. Oral cancer: Leukoplakia and squamous cell carcinoma. *Dent Clin North Am* 2005;49:143.
12. Noonan VL, Kabani S. Diagnosis and management of suspicious lesions of the oral cavity. *Otolaryngol Clin North Am* 2005;38:21.
13. Sciubba JJ. Oral cancer: The importance of early diagnosis and treatment. *Am J Clin Dermatol* 2001;2:239.
14. Cornelison RL Jr. Cutaneous diseases in Native Americans. *Dermatol Clin* 2003; 21:699-702.
15. Gómez A, Umana A, Trespalacios AA. Immune responses to isolated human skin antigens in actinic prurigo. *Med Sci Monit* 2006;12:BR106-113.
16. Magaña M, Cervantes M. Histopathology of sun prurigo. *Rev Invest Clin* 2000;52:391-396.
17. Mounsdon T, Kratochvil F, Auclair P, et al. Actinic prurigo of the lower lip: Review of the literature and report of five cases. *Oral Surg Oral Med Oral Pathol* 1988;65:327-332.
18. Vega-Memije ME, Mosqueda-Taylor A, Irigoyen-Camacho ME, et al. Actinic prurigo cheilitis: Clinicopathologic analysis and therapeutic results in 116 cases. *Oral Surg Oral Med Oral Pathol Oral Radiol Endod* 2002;94:83-91.

19. Hojyo-Tomoka MT, Vega-Memije ME, Cortes-Franco R, et al. Diagnosis and treatment of actinic prurigo. *Dermatol Ther* 2003;16:40-44.
20. Grabczynska SA, Hawk JL.What is actinic prurigo in Britain? *Photodermatol Photoimmunol Photomed* 1997;13:85-86.
21. Grabczynska SA, McGregor JM, Kondeatis E, et al. Actinic prurigo and polymorphic light eruption: Common pathogenesis and the importance of HLA-DR4/DRB1*0407. *Br J Dermatol* 1999;140:232-236.
22. Millard TP, Kondeatis E, Cox A, et al. A candidate gene analysis of three related photosensitivity disorders: Cutaneous lupus erythematosus, polymorphic light eruption and actinic prurigo. *Br J Dermatol* 2001;145:229-236.
23. Zuloaga-Salcedo S, Castillo-Vazquez M, Vega-Memije E, et al. Class I and class II major histocompatibility complex genes in Mexican patients with actinic prurigo. *Br J Dermatol* 2007; 156:1074-1075.
24. Herrera-Geopfert R, Magaña M. Follicular cheilitis: A distinctive histopathologic finding in actinic prurigo. *Am J Dermatopathol* 1995; 17: 357-361.
25. Fusaro RM, Johnson JA. Hereditary polymorphic light eruption of American Indians: Occurrence in non-Indians with polymorphic light eruption. *J Am Acad Dermatol* 1996;34:612-617.
26. Birt AR, Hogg GR. The actinic cheilitis of hereditary polymorphic light eruption. *Arch Dermatol* 1979;115:699-702.
27. Carlos BR, Sedano HO. Multifocal papillomavirus epithelial hyperplasia. *Oral Surg Oral Med Oral Pathol* 1994;77: 631-635.
28. Archard HO, Heck JW, Stanley JR. Focal epithelial hyperplasia: An unusual oral mucosal lesion found in Indian children. *Oral Surg Oral Med Oral Pathol* 1965; 20:201-212.
29. Praetorius-Clausen F. Geographical aspects of oral focal epithelial hyperplasia. *Pathol Microbiol* 1973;39:204-213.
30. Gonzalez LV, Gaviria AM, Sanclemente G, et al. Clinical, histopathological and virological findings in patients with focal epithelial hyperplasia from Colombia. *Int J Dermatol* 2005;44:274-279.
31. Harris AMP, van Wyk CW. Heck's disease (focal epithelial hyperplasia): A longitudinal study. *Commun Dent Oral Epidemiol* 1993;21:82-85.
32. Witkop CJ, Niswander JD. Focal epithelial hyperplasia in Central and South American Indians and Latinos. *Oral Surg Oral Med Oral Pathol* 1965;20:213-217.
33. Praetorius-Clausen F. Histopathology of focal epithelial hyperplasia: Evidence of viral infection. *Tandlaegebladet* 1969; 73:1013-1022.
34. Pfister H, Heltich J, Runne U, Chilf GN. Characterization of human papillomavirus type 13 from focal epithelial Heck lesions. *J Virol* 1983;47:363-366.
35. Beaudenon S, Praetorius F, Kremsdorf D, et al. A new type of human papillomavirus associated with oral focal epithelial hyperplasia. *J Invest Dermatol* 1987; 88:130-135.
36. Garlick JA, Calderon S, Buchner A, Mitrani-Rosenbaum S. Detection of human papillomavirus (HPV) DNA in focal epithelial hyperplasia. *J Oral Pathol Med* 1989;18:172-177.
37. Henke RP, Guèrin-Reverchon I, Milde-Langosch K, et al. *In situ* detection of human papillomavirus types 13 and 32 in focal epithelial hyperplasia of the oral mucosa. *J Oral Pathol Med* 1989;18: 419-421.
38. Padayachee A, van Wyk CW. Human papillomavirus (HPV) DNA in focal epithelial hyperplasia by in situ hybridization. *J Oral Pathol Med* 1991; 20:210-214.
39. Garlick JA, Taichman LB. Human papillomavirus infection of the oral mucosa. *Am J Dermatopathol* 1991;13:386-395.
40. Ledesma-Montes C, Garces-Ortiz M, Hernandez-Guerrero JC. Clinicopathological and immunocytochemical study of multifocal epithelial hyperplasia. J Oral Maxillofac Surg 2007; 65:2211-2217.
41. Moerman M, Danielides VG, Nousia CS, et al. Recurrent focal epithelial hyperplasia due to HPV-13 in an HIV-positive patient. *Dermatology* 2001; 203: 339-341.
42. Steinhoff M, Metze D, Stockfleth E, Luger TA. Successful topical treatment of focal epithelial hyperplasia (Heck's disease) with interferon-β. *Br J Dermatol* 2001;144:1067-1069.
43. Kauzman A, Pavone M, Blanas P, Bradley G. Pigmented lesions of the oral cavity: Review, differential diagnosis, and case presentations. *J Can Dent Assoc* 2004;70:682-683.
44. Eisen D. Disorders of pigmentation in the oral cavity. *Clin Dermatol* 2000; 18: 579-587.
45. Yeh C-J. Simple cryosurgical treatment of the oral melanotic macule. *Oral Surg Oral Med Oral Pathol Oral Radiol Endod* 2000;90:12-13.
46. Gaeta GM, Satriano RA, Baroni A. Oral pigmented lesions. *Clin Dermatol* 2002; 20:286-288.
47. Lampe AK, Hampton PJ, Woodford-Richens K, et al. Hunziker syndrome: An important differential diagnosis for Peutz-Jeghers syndrome. *J Med Genet* 2003;40:e77; available at *www.jmedgenet.com/cgi/content/full/40/6/e77*.
48. Ayoub N, Barete S, Bouaziz J-D, Le Pelletier F. Additional conjuctival and penile pigmentation in Laugier-Hunziker syndrome: A report of two cases. *Int J Dermatol* 2000;43:571-574.
49. Gencoglan G, Gerceker-Turk B, Kilinc-Karaarslan I, et al. Dermoscopic findings in Laugier-Hunziker syndrome. *Arch Dermatol* 2007;143:631-633.
50. Peutz JLA. Very remarkable case of familial polyposis of mucous membrane of intestinal tract and nasopharynx accompanied by peculiar pigmentations of skin and mucous membrane (in Dutch). *Nederl Maandschr Geneesk* 1921;10:134-146.
51. Jeghers H, McKusick VA, Katz KH. Generalized intestinal polyposis and melanin spots of the oral mucosa, lips and digits. *N Engl J Med* 1949;241:993-1005, 1031-1036.
52. *www.ncbi.nlm.nih.gov/entrez/dispomim.cgi? id=175200.*
53. Chan HH, Manstein D, Yu CS, et al. The prevalence and risk factors of postinflammatory hyperpigmentation after fractional resurfacing in Asians. *Lasers Surg Med* 2007;39:381-385.
54. Ashton M, Sopwith W, Clark P, et al. An outbreak no longer: Factors contributing to the return of syphilis in Greater Manchester. *Sex Transm Infect* 2003; 79:-291-293.
55. Hughes G, Paine T, Thomas D. Surveillance of sexually transmitted infections in England and Wales. *Eur Surveill* 2001; 6:71-80.
56. Centers for Disease Control and Prevention. Primary and secondary syphilis—United States, 2002. *MMWR* 2003;52:1117-1120.
57. Primary and secondary syphilis—United States, 2003-2004. *MMWR* 2006; 55: 269-273.
58. Centers for Disease Control and Prevention. *Sexually Transmitted Disease Surveillance, 2003*. Atlanta: US Department of Health and Human Services, 2004.
59. Leão JC, Gueiros LA, Porter SR. Oral manifestations of syphilis. *Clin Dermatol* 2006;61:161-166.
60. Augenbraun M, Rolfs R, Johnson R, et al. Treponemal-specific tests for the serodiagnosis of syphilis. Syphilis and HIV Study Group. *Sex Transm Dis* 1998; 25:549-552.
61. Wong W, Chaw JK, Kent CK, Klausner JD. Risk factors for early syphilis among gay and bisexual men seen in an STD clinic: San Francisco, 2002-2003. *Sex Transm Dis* 2005;32:458-463.
62. Kumar B, Muralidhar S. Malignant syphilis: A review. *AIDS Patient Care STDs*. 2001;12:921.
63. Workowski KA, Berman SM. Sexually transmitted diseases treatment guidelines, 2006. *MMWR* 2006;55:1-94.
64. Riedner G, Rusizoka M, Todd J, et al. Single-dose azithromycin versus penicillin G benzathine for the treatment of early syphilis. *N Engl J Med* 2005; 353: 1236-1244.
65. Queiroz-Telles F, Goldani LZ, Schlamm HT, et al. An open-label comparative pilot study of oral voriconazole and itraconazole for long-term treatment of paracoccidioidomycosis. *Clin Infect Dis* 2007;45:1462-1469.
66. Marques-da-Silva SH, Colombo AL, Blotta MH, et al. Diagnosis of paracoccidioidomycosis by detection of antigen and antibody in bronchoalveolar lavage fluids. *Clin Vaccine Immunol* 2006; 13: 1363-1366.
67. Blotta MH, Mamoni RL, Oliveira SJ, et al. Endemic regions of paracoccidioidomycosis in Brazil: A clinical and epidemiologic study of 584 cases in the southeast region. *Am J Trop Med Hyg* 1999;61:390-394.

CHAPTER 55

Genital Lesions in Men

Sean D. Doherty
Ted Rosen

Key Points

- Genital lesions are difficult to diagnose based solely on morphology.
- The physician may need to perform additional studies, including biopsies, when evaluating genital lesions.
- Genital dermatoses may occur only on the genitalia or may occur anywhere on the body, and lesions may have a different appearance when found on genital skin compared with other anatomic sites.
- Genital lesions may have a unique appearance in skin of color, and both the frequency and the appearance may vary between men and women.

Genital dermatoses include a wide variety of diagnoses, and lesions may occur only on the genitalia or also may occur elsewhere on the body. When lesions appear on genital skin, they may have a unique morphology. The thin, moist skin typically found in the genital region is at least partially responsible for the different characteristics of lesions in this region.[1] For example, the dry scale that may be a prominent manifestation of lesions elsewhere may not be present in the genital region. Furthermore, genital lesions in skin of color may manifest a somewhat markedly different appearance than those in white skin, and there may be variation in both statistical frequency and clinical characteristics of selected lesions between men and women.

Genital lesions and the concern over the possibility of a sexually transmitted infection (STI) may cause significant anxiety for the patient. Genital lesions may result from a variety of etiologies, however, including non-STI agents, inflammatory cutaneous disorders, multisystem diseases, benign and malignant neoplasms, and exogenous factors.

It is often difficult to distinguish between one genital disorder and similar entities based solely on morphology. In various published studies, physicians have had an accuracy of only 33–80% in diagnosing genital lesions based solely on appearance.[2] The physician should not hesitate to perform additional diagnostic testing, including serologic studies, bacterial and viral cultures, cytologic studies, colposcopic examination, incisional and excisional biopsies, and other appropriate studies. Additionally, a full body skin check, comprehensive physical examination, and a detailed review of systems may be necessary when evaluating a patient with genital lesions.

INFECTIOUS DISEASES

Sexually Transmitted Infections

SYPHILIS

Epidemiology, Etiology, and Pathogenesis

Syphilis is caused by the spirochete *Treponema pallidum,* with an incubation period of 9–90 days. The organism is transferred between individuals by direct sexual contact. Infection is most likely to occur through microbreaks in normal skin occurring during sexual activity but may occur though intact mucus membranes.[3]

In 2000, the rate of primary and secondary syphilis in the United States was the lowest since reporting began in 1941. From 2001–2004, the rate increased 30% to 2.7 cases per 100,000 population. The increased rate was primarily due to increases in cases in men who have sex with men. Cumulative data from the Centers for Disease Control and Prevention (CDC) also have shown that rates of primary and secondary syphilis are higher in African-Americans and Hispanics than in other groups.[4]

There is a notable association between syphilis and human immunodeficiency virus (HIV) infection. The diseases affect similar patient groups, and coinfection is common.[5] Additionally, syphilis increases sexual transmission of HIV by six- to sevenfold, likely secondary to increased incidence of genital ulcers.[6]

Clinical Findings Syphilis presents initially with a solitary, painless, indurated ulceration (chancre) about 3 weeks (actual range 9–90 days) after contact with an infected partner (Figure 55-1). In men, the primary lesion is most commonly located on the distal penis and usually is accompanied by unilateral lymphadenopathy. This lesion of primary syphilis remits spontaneously and is followed in 1–2 months by secondary syphilis, a papulosquamous eruption that may involve the palms and soles, trunk, face, and genitalia. Secondary syphilis may be associated with exudative anogenital plaques (condyloma lata), which appear to be more common in blacks[7] (Figure 55-2). Atypical presentations of primary and

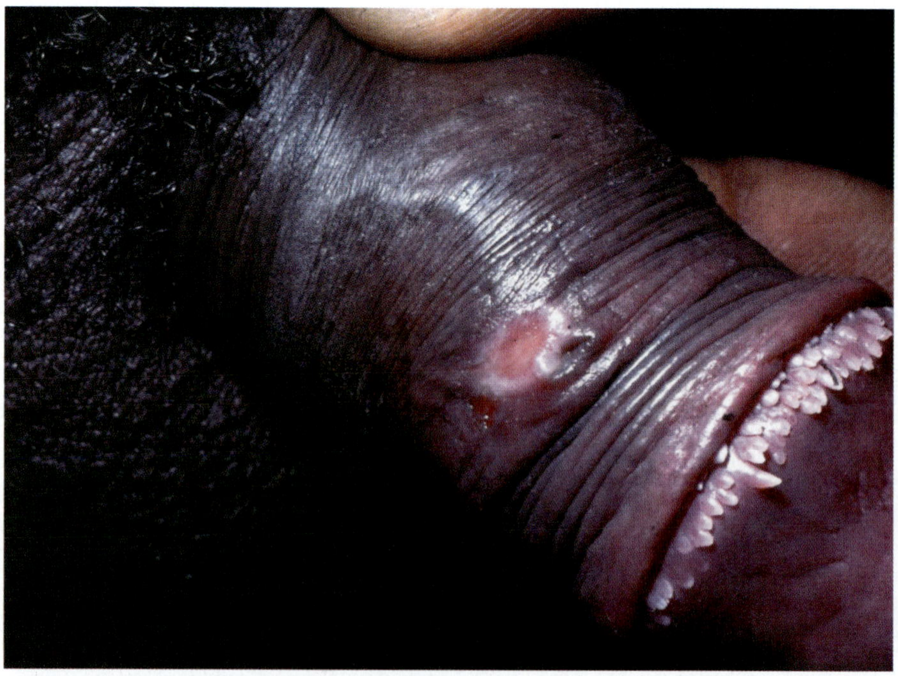

▲ **FIGURE 55-1** Reepithelializing chancre at midshaft. Incidental pearly penile papules on corona.

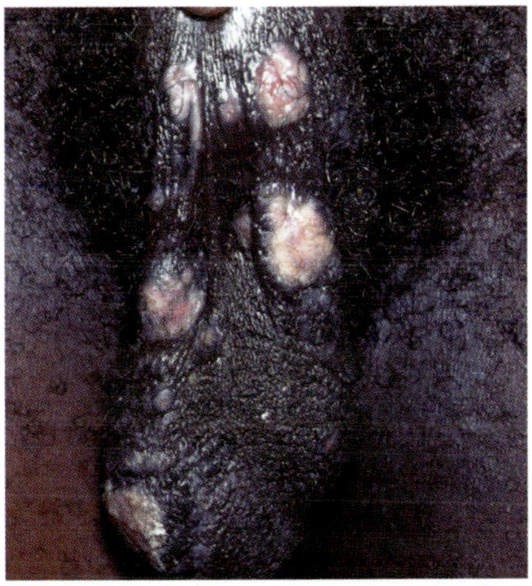

▲ **FIGURE 55-2** Exophytic nodules typify condyloma lata.

secondary syphilis may occur in individuals who are coinfected with HIV or in individuals who have been infected with syphilis previously.[6]

Serologic testing is the most commonly used diagnostic technique. Nontreponemal antigen tests, including the rapid plasma reagin (RPR) and the Venereal Disease Research Laboratory (VDRL) tests, are used for screening, and treponemal-specific tests, including the *T. pallidum* particle agglutination (TPPA) and fluorescent treponemal antibodies (FTA-abs) tests, are used to confirm the diagnosis. *T. pallidum* cannot be cultured, but it can be demonstrated directly by dark-field microscopy. The organism also can be detected in biopsy specimens using specific treponemal fluorescent antibody stains or silver stains such as the Warthin-Starry stain.[6] However, the latter stain also reacts with melanin, which may make diagnosis difficult in skin of color.[7] All individuals testing positive for syphilis also should be counseled and evaluated for HIV infection.

Differential Diagnosis of Primary and Secondary Syphilis

- Chancroid
- Condyloma acuminata (external genital warts)
- Fixed drug eruption
- Genital aphthosis, including Behçet syndrome
- Granuloma inguinale
- Herpes progenitalis
- Lymphogranuloma venereum
- Papulosquamous diseases (e.g., psoriasis, seborrhea)
- Traumatic ulceration (e.g., bite wound, vacuum erection device)

Complications The complications of syphilis occur years after primary infection in the tertiary stage. These include cardiovascular syphilis, gummatous disease, and the late manifestations of neurosyphilis, including tabes dorsalis and general paresis. All the late complications are rare, occurring in fewer than 15% of untreated individuals. Early neurosyphilis occurs in 5% of individuals before the tertiary stage and may result in meningitis, cranial neuritis, ocular involvement, and meningovascular disease.[6]

Prognosis/Clinical Course Untreated syphilis passes through four stages: primary, secondary, latent, and tertiary. Treatment of primary syphilis results in rapid disappearance of the chancre. Secondary syphilis occurs only in untreated or inadequately treated individuals. Since the primary chancre will resolve spontaneously without treatment within a month or two, the RPR titer should be followed in patients to confirm adequate treatment.

Treatment Therapy of choice for syphilis infection of less than 1 year duration (primary, secondary, or early latent infectious) consists of 2.4 million units of benzathine penicillin G intramuscularly. Tetracycline drugs are second-line agents. RPR titers should be followed to confirm successful treatment. Individuals with a clear-cut diagnosis of syphilis who fail to respond should be retested for HIV infection and treated with weekly benzathine penicillin G 2.4 million units intramuscularly for 3 weeks (Table 55-1).

Prevention ***T. pallidum*** is spread through direct sexual contact. Condoms will prevent transmission of the organism if they cover the primary chancre. Ideally, sexual contact should be avoided with affected individuals.

CHANCROID

Epidemiology, Etiology, and Pathogenesis Chancroid is a sexually transmitted infection caused by the gram-negative coccobacillus *Haemophilus ducreyi*. The bacterium initiates an infective process within genital skin after epidermal microabrasions occur during sexual intercourse.[8] Like syphilis, chancroid is a genital ulceration associated with both increased occurrence and transmission rates of HIV.

H. ducreyi is the most common pathogen isolated in genital ulcer disease in Africa. In the United States, reported cases generally occur in urban epidemics and are most common in black men. The increased incidence in males is due to spread from infected commercial sex workers and the more rapid resolution of the infection in females.[9]

Clinical Findings After a 3- to 14-day incubation period, a pustule develops at the site of inoculation that rapidly evolves into a shallow, ragged, painful erosion. In men, the ulcers are found (in decreasing order of frequency) on the prepuce, coronal sulcus, glans, frenulum, and penile shaft. Autoinoculation frequently leads to the presentation of multiple ulcers (Figure 55-3). Painful inguinal lymphadenopathy occurs in up to 50% of patients and is more common in men.[8] Percutaneous rupture with purulent drainage (bubo formation) is frequent (Figure 55-4).

Diagnosis of clinically suspicious lesions typically is confirmed with culture on enriched and vancomycin-impregnated gonococcal and Mueller-Hinton agars under conditions of high humidity and high CO_2 tension.[10] Gram-stained ulcer material should not be used to diagnose chancroid owing to the low specificity and sensitivity of this test.[8] The most sensitive and specific modality for diagnosis is mutiplex polymerase chain reaction (PCR), which has a resolved sensitivity and specificity for *H. ducreyi* of 98.4% and 99.6%, respectively.[9] Infected patients should be tested for HIV infection.

DIFFERENTIAL DIAGNOSIS

- Aphthous ulcers and Behçet disease
- Factitious ulceration

TABLE 55-1
Treat of Syphilis (Systemic)

First line	Benzathine penicillin G	Duration < 1 year: 50,000 units/kg IM up to 2.4 million units (adults) Duration >1 year or unknown: 50,000 units/kg IM up to 2.4 million units (adults), weekly for 3 weeks
Second line (penicillin allergy)	Doxycycline Tetracycline Erythromycin	100 mg PO bid for 14 days 500 mg PO qid for 14 days 500 mg PO qid for 14 days

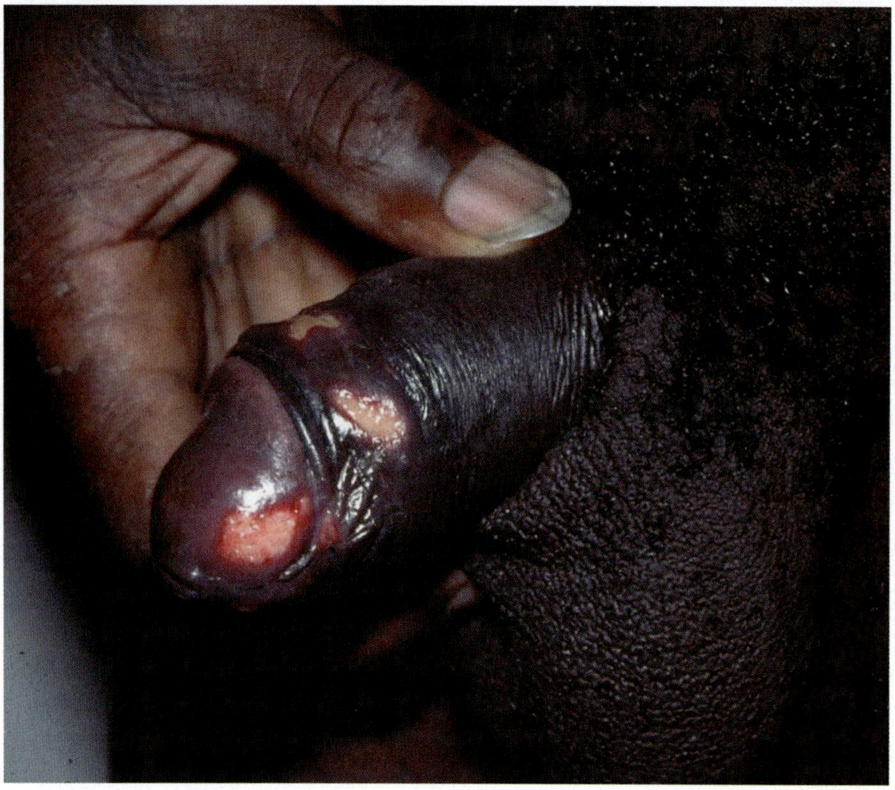

▲ **FIGURE 55-3** Multiple ulcers of chancroid.

- Granuloma inguinale
- Herpes progenitalis
- Lymphogranuloma venereum
- Metastatic (extraintestinal) Crohn disease
- Squamous cell carcinoma
- Syphilis
- Traumatic ulceration

Complications Aside from HIV acquisition, complications that occur in conjunction with chancroid include phimosis and additional destructive ulceration owing to secondary bacterial infection.

Prognosis/Clinical Course If untreated, ulcers will persist for roughly 2–3 months before healing spontaneously with significant scar formation. Adequately treated chancroid resolves in approximately 10 days.[3]

Treatment Currently accepted treatments of equal efficacy include erythromycin, azithromycin, and ceftriaxone. Large, fluctuant nodes should be aspirated for symptomatic relief and to avoid rupture. Incision and drainage with subsequent wound packing also may be performed (Table 55-2).

Prevention Condom use will prevent the spread of *H. ducreyi* if the infectious lesion is covered. Empiric treatment of high-risk individuals, such as commercial sex workers, in endemic areas has helped to control the spread of the disease in those regions.

GRANULOMA INGUINALE

Epidemiology, Etiology, and Pathogenesis Granuloma inguinale, also called *donovanosis,* is caused by *Calymmatobacterium granulomatis,* an intracellular gram-negative encapsulated bacillus. Although sexual contact is the likely method of spread, there is some controversy regarding the mode of transmission.[11]

Endemic foci of granuloma inguinale are seen in New Guinea, Africa, Australia, and parts of India and China. Worldwide, the disease is more common in males than in females and is more common in men who have sex with men than in other groups. There have been fewer than 10 cases per year in the United States since 1989. There was a higher incidence in blacks in these cases. As with other genital ulcerative diseases, granuloma inguinale can increase the transmission rate of HIV infection.

Clinical Findings After an incubation period of 8–90 days (usually 2–3 weeks), a papule or nodule appears on the anogenital region. Erosion through the skin occurs rapidly, yielding a clean-based remarkably painless ulceration that bleeds readily to the touch and demonstrates a rolled border[12] (Figure 55-5). The most common locations of lesions in men are the coronal sulcus, the subpreputial region, and the anus.[13] True adenopathy is rare, but involvement of nearby tissue may produce a periadenitis that may be mistaken for a lymph node, giving rise to the term *pseudobubo.*[14]

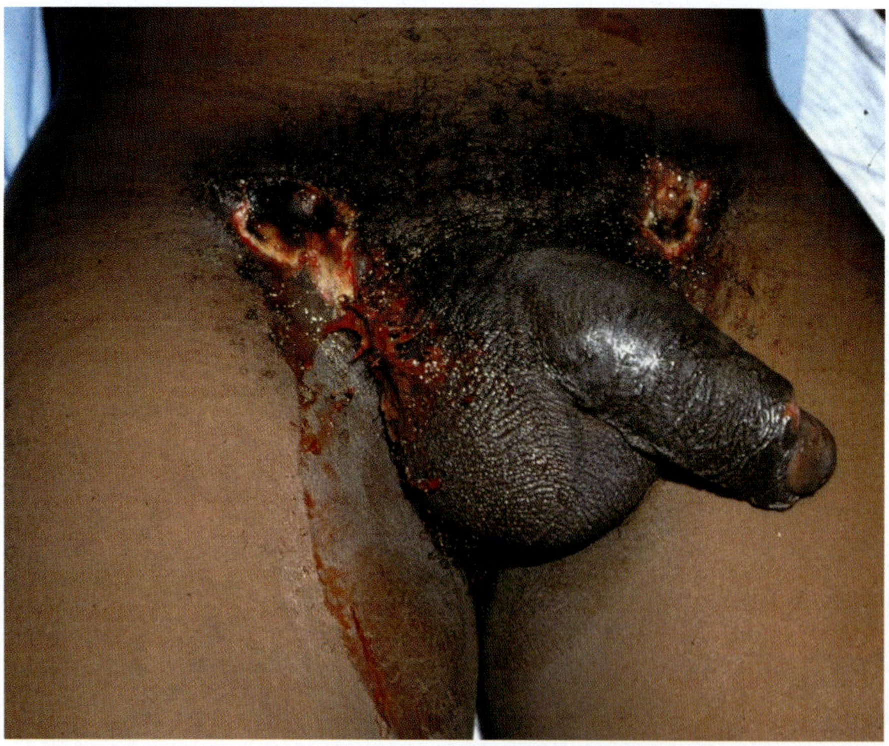

▲ **FIGURE 55-4** Ruptured inguinal lymph nodes (bubo formation) in untreated chancroid.

TABLE 55-2
Treatments for Chancroid

	Physical	Systemic	
First line	Aspirate large, fluctuant nodes	Erythromycin	500 mg orally four times per day × 7 days
Second line		Azithromycin	1 g orally single dose
		Ceftriaxone	250 mg IM single dose
		Ciprofloxacin	500 mg PO bid × 3 days

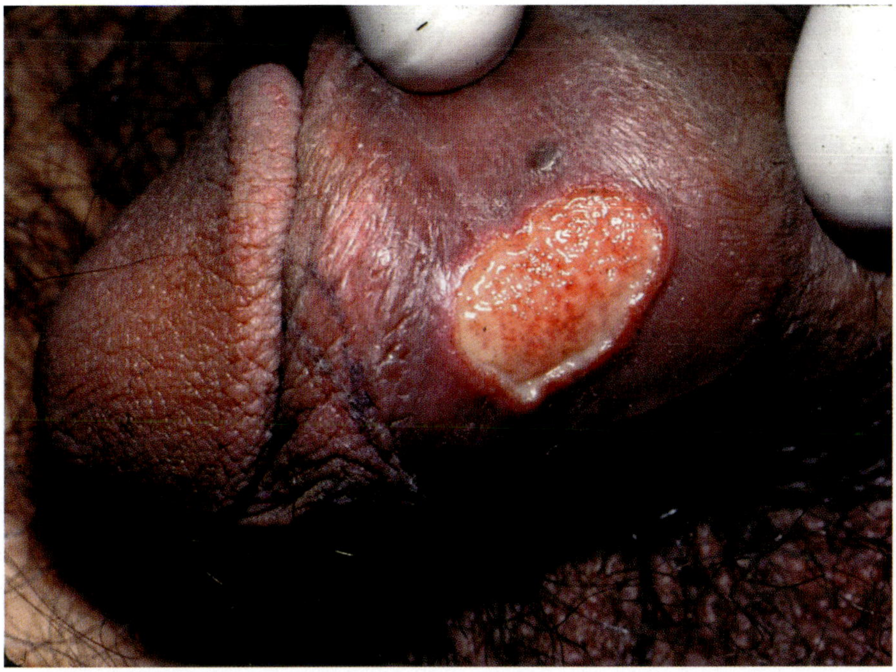

▲ **FIGURE 55-5** Rolled border and friable base typical of granuloma inguinale in a Hispanic patient from the Caribbean.

Diagnosis of granuloma inguinale may be made clinically in endemic areas with some confidence. In nonendemic areas, such as the United States, laboratory diagnosis requires a crush specimen from a punch biopsy stained with Wright or Giemsa stain. The biopsy specimen should be taken before cleaning the lesion or removing any necrotic tissue. Diagnosis is made by the visualization of Donovan bodies, deeply staining rods in the cytoplasm of macrophages. Ultrathin histologic sections may be necessary for good visualization of the causative organism.[14]

Differential Diagnosis

- Cutaneous amebiasis
- Behçet syndrome
- Chancroid
- Condyloma acuminata
- Condyloma lata
- Deep mycosis (in endemic areas)
- Herpes progenitalis (severe)
- Leishmaniasis (in endemic areas)
- Scrofuloderma
- Squamous cell carcinoma
- Syphilis (primary)
- Tuberculosis (cutaneous)

Complications The disease process can lead to fibrosis and keloid formation, causing genital deformation, paraphimosis, and lymphatic obstruction with localized elephantiasis. The lesions also may become infected secondarily. Extensive ulceration of the soft tissues can lead to fistula formation and genital mutilation. Additionally, there is an increased incidence of squamous cell carcinoma occurring in long-standing lesions.[14]

Prognosis/Clinical Course If left untreated, granuloma inguinale will not remit spontaneously, although lesions may be stable for long periods of time. Hematogenous and lymphatic spread, along with autoinoculation, can lead to lesions in extragenital locations.[14] Proper treatment will halt lesion progression, but prolonged therapy may be required to allow complete healing.[15]

Treatment Several antimicrobial regimens are effective to treat granuloma inguinale. Few controlled trials have been published, and recommended regimens vary between the CDC and the World Health Organization (WHO). The CDC recommends doxycycline and trimethoprim-sulfamethoxazole as first-line therapy, whereas the WHO guidelines recommend azithromycin.[13–15] All therapies should be continued for at least 3 weeks or until all lesions are healed. If improvement does not occur during the first few days of therapy, an intravenously administered aminoglycoside such as gentamicin may need to be added to the treatment regimen[15] (Table 55-3).

Prevention In endemic areas, house-to-house visits with medical examinations and treatment of suspected cases has decreased disease incidence. Larger epidemics have been controlled by annual examination and population registration, with compulsory treatment and forced hospital admission. Education and improvement in overall hygienic standards also can prevent disease spread. Barrier protection is presumably effective for individuals.

TABLE 55-3
Treatments for Granuloma Inguinale (Systemic)

First line	Doxycycline	100 mg orally twice a day for at least 3 weeks
	Trimethoprim-sulfamethoxazole	800 mg/160 mg orally twice a day for at least 3 weeks
	Azithromycin	1 g orally once a week for 3 weeks
Second line	Ciprofloxacin	750 mg orally twice a day for at least 3 weeks
	Erythromycin	500 mg orally four times daily for at least 3 weeks

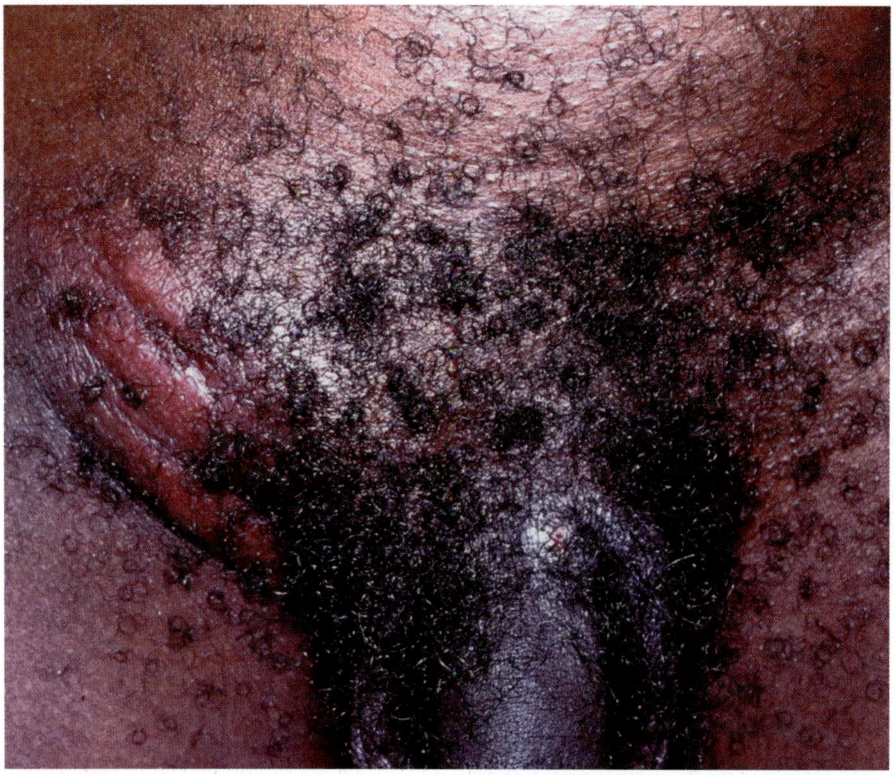

▲ **FIGURE 55-6** Pathognomonic pattern of inguinal adenopathy in LGV.

LYMPHOGRANULOMA VENEREUM

Epidemiology, Etiology, and Pathogenesis

Lymphogranuloma venereum (LGV) is a sexually transmitted disease caused by *Chlamydia trachomatis* (serotypes L1, L2, and L3), a gram-negative intracellular parasite. LGV is most common in tropical regions but does occur with a low incidence in the Western world. Fewer than 100 cases are reported annually in the United States, and the disease is 5–10 times more common in men than in women. This ratio may be due in part to decreased diagnosis in female patients, but recent outbreaks of LGV proctitis have been associated with groups of men who have sex with men.

Clinical Findings After a 1- to 2-week incubation period, LGV begins with a painless papule or shallow ulcer. The most common locations for the primary lesion in men are the coronal sulcus and the glans penis. The primary lesion lasts only 2–3 days and goes unnoticed in approximately 75% of patients. After 1–3 weeks, tender unilateral adenopathy develops. The lymphadenopathy involves the inguinal nodes more frequently than the femoral nodes but may involve both, giving rise to the groove sign of Greenblatt (corresponding to the inguinal ligament) (Figure 55-6). Unfortunately, this nearly pathognomonic sign appears in only about 20% of LGV patients.[16] The lymph nodes become tender and fluctuant and are referred to as *buboes.* The nodes may develop multiple fistulas that drain purulent material. Systemic symptoms, including fever, malaise, headache, and arthralgia, are common.[3] Diagnosis is made by culturing pus aspirated from enlarged nodes. A Giemsa stain also may be performed on a smear to look for intracellular corpuscles of Gamma-Migawa.[14]

Differential Diagnosis

- Chancroid
- Genital herpes
- Hodgkin disease
- Syphilis
- Ganglionic tuberculosis

Complications Late complications include fibrosis and tissue destruction. Fibrosis may lead to elephantiasis of the penis and scrotum.[14]

Prognosis/Clinical Course If left untreated, LGV will persist for years and may result in the complications listed earlier. Treatment prevents these sequelae.

Treatment Multiple antibiotics successfully treat LGV. Additionally, fluctuant nodes should be aspirated as often as necessary. Nodes should not be incised because fistulas may develop[3] (Table 55-4).

Prevention Barrier protection, such as condoms, can prevent the spread of the *Chlamydia* serotypes that lead to LGV.

TABLE 55-4
Treatments for Lymphogranuloma Venereum

	Physical	Systemic	
First line	Aspirate fluctuant nodes	Doxycycline	100 mg orally two times per day for 3 weeks
Second line		Tetracycline	500 mg orally four times per day for 3 weeks
		Erythromycin	500 mg orally four times per day for 3 weeks

GENITAL HERPES

Epidemiology, Etiology, and Pathogenesis

Genital herpes is a very prevalent disease, with at least 50 million people in the United States infected and an estimated 500,000–700,000 new cases occurring each year.[17] Genital herpes generally is caused by herpes simplex virus type 2 (HSV-2), although a minority of these lesions may be caused by HSV-1, the usual etiologic agent of herpes labialis.[18] Black individuals have a lower prevalence of HSV-1-induced lesions (1.3%) than the general population.[19] HSV is a double-stranded DNA virus that enters the body via direct skin-to-skin contact, mucosal contact, or contact with infected secretions. The virus multiplies in the epidermis before ascending sensory nerve roots to the dorsal root ganglion, where it becomes latent. When the virus reactivates, it travels back down the sensory root, leading to a mucocutaneous outbreak.

Clinical Findings Primary lesions appear in an individual approximately 6 days after infection. The primary lesion consists of painful, grouped vesicles on an erythematous base that may rupture, leading to erosion or ulcer formation (Figure 55-7). The lesion is found most commonly on the shaft or glans of the penis in men but may be located in the perianal area, thighs, or buttocks.

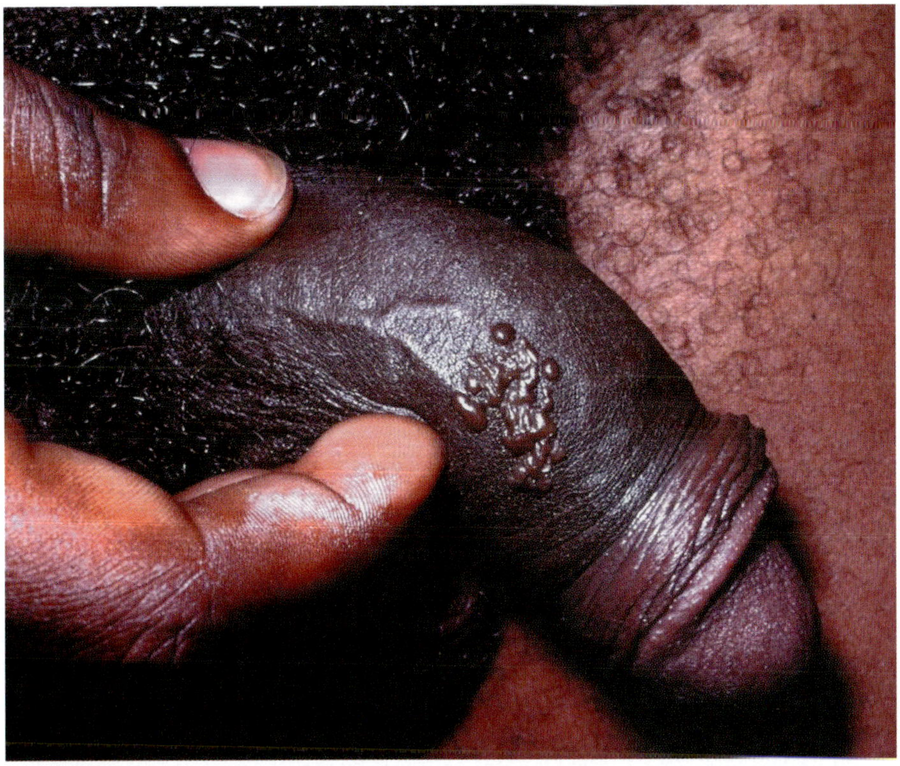

▲ **FIGURE 55-7** Grouped vesicles characteristic of herpes progenitalis.

Perianal lesions, including persistent large ulcerations, may be seen in conjunction with receptive anal intercourse in homosexual men (Figure 55-8). During the initial event, the patient may complain of fever, headache, or malaise. Recurrent HSV outbreaks are usually less severe than the initial episode and typically are preceded by a prodrome of local pain or tingling.[17] The diagnosis of genital herpes usually can be made based on clinical appearance. If the diagnosis is in question, a Tzank smear (showing viral acantholytic giant cells), a viral culture, a skin biopsy, or the PCR test for HSV DNA may be performed.

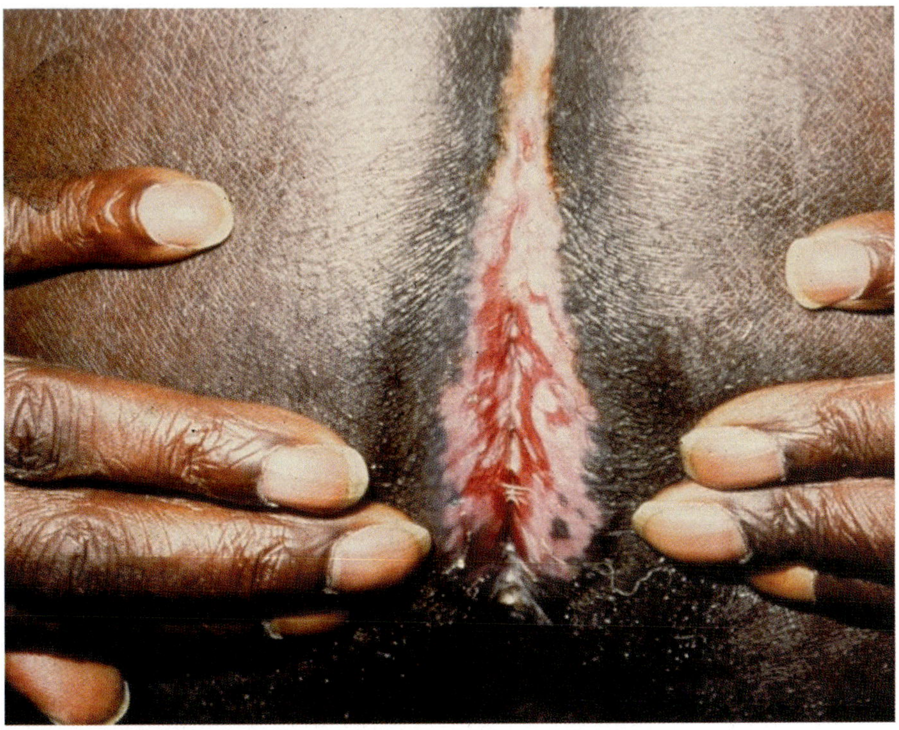

▲ **FIGURE 55-8** Persistent ulceration owing to HSV with HIV coinfection.

Differential Diagnosis

- Aphthous ulcers
- Behçet disease
- Chancroid
- Granuloma inguinale
- Lymphogranuloma venereum
- Pemphigus vulgaris
- Syphilis
- Traumatic ulceration

Complications Rarely, men may develop urinary retention symptoms from urethral lesions. Perianal infection with proctitis is common in men who have sex with men.[17]

Prognosis/Clinical Course There is no cure for genital herpes. The recurrence rate for untreated genital herpes is variable, with a median of four episodes per year. HSV-1 recurs less frequently than HSV-2, and men tend to have more recurrences than women. Recurrences are most often spontaneous and unpredictable, but emotional stress, hormonal changes, or other factors may trigger them. Over time, recurrent episodes become less frequent. It should be noted that asymptomatic viral shedding may occur at any time, and it is estimated that some 70% of genital herpes is acquired when an uninfected individual has genital contact with an infected person who is shedding virus without knowing this. Male-to-female transmission is more efficient than the converse.

Treatment Since there is no cure for genital herpes, treatment is aimed at decreasing the duration of outbreaks, decreasing the frequency of outbreaks, and decreasing the number of asymptomatic shedding episodes.[20] Oral antiviral medications, including acyclovir, valacyclovir, and famciclovir, are used for initial infections, recurrences, and suppressive therapy. All are effective if they are taken during the prodrome or during the first sign of recurrence. Topical therapies are not recommended. Alternative and complementary remedies have little scientific validation (Table 55-5).

Prevention The use of condoms has been shown to prevent transmission of HSV to susceptible women if the condom completely covers the lesions of an infected man. Condom use does not

TABLE 55-5
Treatments for Genital Herpes (Systemic)

First line	Acyclovir	Initial infect.	400 mg three times daily for 7–10 days
		Recurrence	400 mg three times daily for 5 days
		Suppressive	400 mg twice daily
	Famciclovir	Initial infect.	250 mg three times daily for 7–10 days
		Recurrence	125 mg twice daily for 5 days
		Suppressive	250 mg twice daily
	Valacyclovir	Initial infect.	1 g twice daily for 7–10 days
		Recurrence	500 mg twice daily for 3–5 days
		Suppressive	500 mg daily

significantly reduce transmission rates to men. Education is very important to reduce the spread of HSV. Individuals should understand the chronic nature of their disease and should abstain from sexual activity when lesions or prodromal symptoms are present. Suppression therapy reduces asymptomatic shedding of viral particles but does not totally prevent it. Nonetheless, chronic suppressive therapy appears to reduce transmission from infected to uninfected partners.[21]

GENITAL WARTS

Epidemiology, Etiology, and Pathogenesis

Genital warts, or condyloma acuminata, are a sexually transmitted infection caused by human papillomavirus (HPV) infection. HPV is a DNA virus with more than 100 different types. Types 6 and 11 are most commonly associated (90%) with genital warts.[22] It is likely that more than half of sexually active adults in the United States have been infected with at least one type of genital HPV, but only about 1% of them have clinically apparent warts.[23]

Clinical Findings Visible lesions develop after an average interval of 2–3 months following sexual exposure to HPV.[24] Lesions occur most commonly on the penile shaft and glans in men. Genital warts can have variable appearances, but the most common appearance is that of mildly elevated, flat-topped papules. The classic wart (true condyloma acuminatum) is a filiform papilloma that is 3- to 10-mm high and 2- to 3-mm in diameter with a brushlike terminal end (Figure 55-9). Genital warts usually can be diagnosed clinically, although biopsy rarely may be required to differentiate genital warts from neoplastic growths.[25] Viral typing is not routine.[26]

Differential Diagnosis

- Condyloma lata (secondary syphilis)
- Enlarged sebaceous glands (variation of normal)
- Fibroepitheliomas (skin tags)
- Lichen planus
- Molluscum contagiosum
- Pearly penile papules
- Squamous cell carcinoma in situ (Bowen disease)

Complications The HPV types 6 and 11 that cause genital warts are not oncogenic and do not carry a high risk of malignancy, like some other types of HPV. Rarely, long-standing genital warts theoretically have caused invasive squamous cell carcinoma.[26] However, in this situation, the initial lesion may well have been an unrecognized malignant neoplasm from inception.

Prognosis/Clinical Course The course of HPV infections is variable, with lesions regressing spontaneously, persisting, resolving with therapy, or appearing after a prolonged latency.[24] Most clinical manifestations of HPV infections are transient and become clinically undetectable within several years.[22]

Treatment Treatment of genital warts includes patient-applied treatments, physician-applied treatments, and procedures. An important aspect of treatment is patient counseling because genital warts can cause significant patient distress, including concern about future malignancy. Most patients prefer treatments that they can perform at home without coming into the office. Immunomodulation (imiquimod) has been associated with the lowest recurrence rate of all modalities, but it is more effective in women (~75% clearance rate) than in men (~33% clearance rate).[27] One potential drawback to the use of imiquimod on skin of color is its capacity to induce local vitiligo-like depigmentation[28] (Table 55-6).

Prevention Condoms may offer some protection against HPV spread. A recently Food and Drug Administration (FDA)–approved quadrivalent vaccine (HPV types 6, 11, 16, and 18) has proven dramatically effective in the prevention of all genital manifestations of HPV infection in women.[29] This vaccine may prevent most genital warts when administered to individuals before their first HPV exposure. Trials in men are underway.

MOLLUSCUM CONTAGIOSUM

Epidemiology, Etiology, and Pathogenesis

Molluscum contagiosum is caused by the poxvirus molluscum contagiosum virus (MCV). This DNA virus is spread through sexual contact in adults. MCV occurs most commonly in underdeveloped areas and tropical climates.[30] The

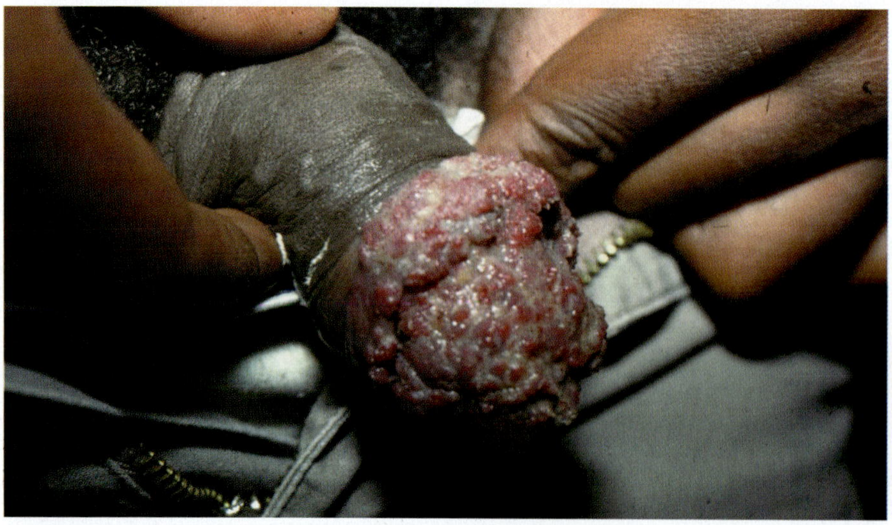

▲ **FIGURE 55-9** Neglected genital warts forming large verrucous mass.

TABLE 55-6
Treatments for Genital Warts

	Patient-Applied		Physician-Applied		Physical
First line	Imiquimod 5% cream	Apply at bedtime 3 times per week for up to 16 weeks			
Second line	Podofilox	Apply twice daily for 3 days and then rest for 4 days; may repeat for 4 cycles	Podophyllin resin	Apply once a week	Cryotherapy Laser therapy
			Trichloroacetic acid	Apply once a week	Surgical excision

incidence of molluscum contagiosum has increased over the last 30 years owing to sexual spread. The worldwide prevalence of molluscum contagiosum is from 2–8%.[31]

Clinical Findings After an incubation period of 2–7 weeks or more, a papular eruption of multiple umbilicated lesions develops. The lesions are dome-shaped and opalescent in color (Figure 55-10). The central umbilication is present 25% of the time and, if present, is pathognomonic for the disease. The papules may become inflamed, leading to an atypical appearance. In men, the lesions are found most commonly on the penile shaft but may be located anywhere in the groin, thighs, or lower abdomen when the infection is acquired sexually.[32] The diagnosis of molluscum contagiosum usually can be made from clinical appearance. If there is any uncertainty, a biopsy can be performed that will reveal intracytoplasmic inclusion bodies known as *molluscum bodies* or *Henderson-Paterson bodies.*

Differential Diagnosis

- Condyloma acuminata
- Cutaneous cryptococcus (in HIV+)
- Epidermal inclusion cyst (or milium)
- Herpes simplex or herpes zoster
- Lichen planus
- Papular granuloma annulare
- Sebaceous glands (variation of normal)

Complications If lesions become inflamed or are picked, they can lead to scarring. Immunocompromised individuals can develop generalized cutaneous infection.

Prognosis/Clinical Course In immunocompetent patients, the infection follows a self-limited course marked by spontaneous clearing within a few months. In patients with HIV infection, immunosuppressive therapy, or atopic dermatitis, lesions can be atypical, widespread, or resistant to clearing even with therapy.[30]

Treatment Although the lesions usually will resolve on their own, treatment will reduce the duration of lesions and their infectivity. Therapy consists of mechanical treatments that remove the molluscum core or topical or systemic treatments. The value of the latter is questionable (Table 55-7).

Prevention The only way to prevent spread of the lesions is to avoid the close skin-to-skin contact that occurs during sexual contact. Condoms likely prevent the spread of the lesion.

SCLEROSING LYMPHANGITIS

Epidemiology, Etiology, and Pathogenesis Sclerosing lymphangitis occurs in men following vigorous sexual activity. It has an unknown etiology but may be related to trauma. The disease usually occurs in 20- to 40-year-old men of any ethnic background.[33]

Clinical Findings Sclerosing lymphangitis is characterized by the acute onset of a flesh-colored, firm, cordlike lesion of the coronal sulcus (Figure 55-11) that may extend onto the penile shaft.[34] The lesion is normally painless but may be associated with some discomfort, especially with erection. The diagnosis can

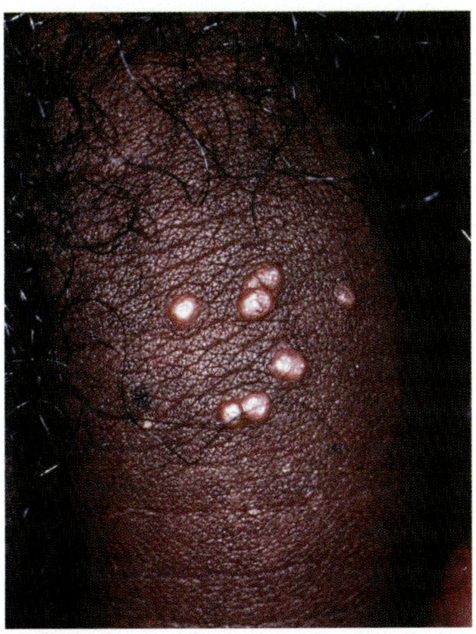

▲ **FIGURE 55-10** Many small, dome-shaped papules typical of molluscum contagiosum.

TABLE 55-7
Treatments for Molluscum Contagiosum

	Topical		Physical	Systemic	
First line	Trichloroacetic acid	Apply once in office	Curettage		
	Cantharadin	Apply once a week	Cryotherapy CO_2 laser		
	Podophyllin	Apply once a week			
	Potassium hydroxide	Twice daily until inflammation develops	Electrodesiccation		
Second line	Tretinoin 0.1% cream	Apply once a week		Cimetidine	40 mg/kg/day in two divided doses for 2 months
	KOH 10% aqueous solution	Apply twice daily			
	Imiquimod	Apply daily for 2-6 weeks			

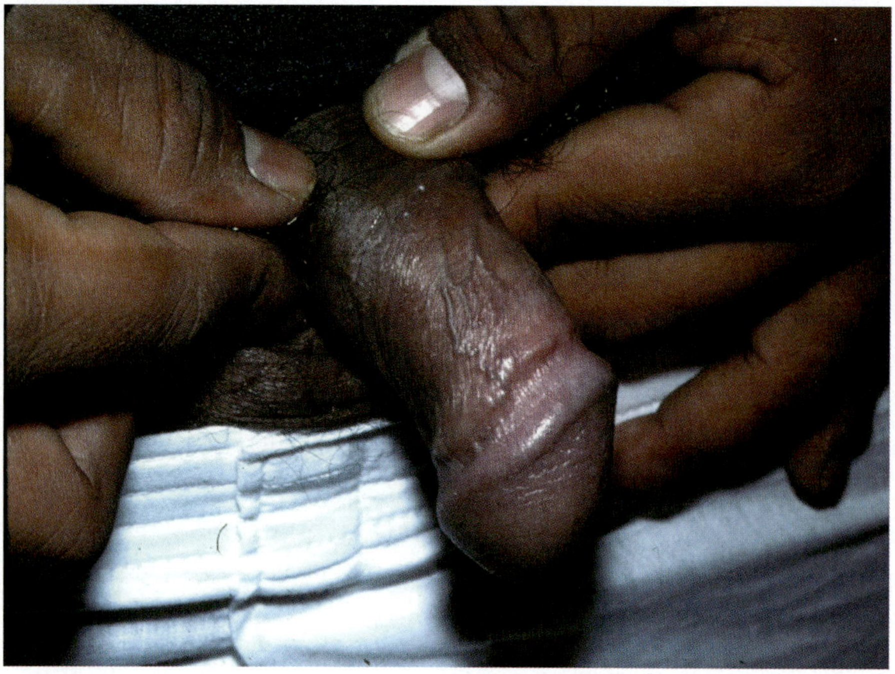

▲ **FIGURE 55-11** Cordlike induration seen in sclerosing lymphangitis.

be made clinically. Sexually transmitted infections, particularly gonococcal and nongonococcal urethritis, frequently occur in association with this condition. Patients thus should have a full workup for sexually transmitted infections.[34]

Differential Diagnosis Lesions are essentially pathognomonic, and there is no substantial differential.

Complications In rare instances, tenderness may persist for a long period of time.

Prognosis/Clinical Course The lesions usually resolve spontaneously within 1–2 months.[34]

Treatment A cessation or reduction in sexual activity is recommended while the lesion resolves. Very rarely, persistently tender lesions may require surgical removal of the indurated tissue (Table 55-8).

Prevention A cessation of vigorous sexual practices may prevent the lesion from occurring.

TABLE 55-8
Treatments for Sclerosing Lymphangitis (Physical)

First line	Decrease or abstain from sexual activity while lesion resolves
Second line	Surgical removal

Non-Sexually-Transmitted Infections

TINEA CRURIS

Epidemiology, Etiology, and Pathogenesis Tinea cruris is a common dermatophyte infection of the genital skin that occurs most commonly in postpubertal men of any ethnic background. The most common etiologic agent is *Trichophyton rubrum,* and the cutaneous infection is frequently secondary to concomitant toenail onychomycosis.

Clinical Findings Tinea cruris is classically characterized as erythematous, scaly, sharply demarcated plaques over the inner thighs to the crural crease, but black patients may present with striking hyperpigmentation rather than erythema, and genital skin may not have scale (Figure 55-12). The eruption may have an annular appearance and is often pruritic. Individuals with coarse hair may have papules within the leading edge of the eruption. In men, the infection usually spares the scrotum and shaft of the penis. The diagnosis of tinea cruris generally can be made clinically, especially if the individual has other dermatophyte fungal infections such as tinea pedis or onychomycosis. If the diagnosis of tinea cruris is unclear, a potassium hydroxide (KOH) examination or culture of the peripheral scale may be performed.

Differential Diagnosis

- Candidiasis
- Contact dermatitis
- Erythrasma
- Neurodermatitis
- Psoriasis
- Tinea versicolor (rarely affects genital skin)

Complications The condition may become extensive or may involve follicles, making it harder to clear.

Prognosis/Clinical Course Tinea cruris generally can be eradicated with therapy, although recurrences are not uncommon, and patients may require intermittent treatment. Some susceptible patients may require chronic suppressive therapy.

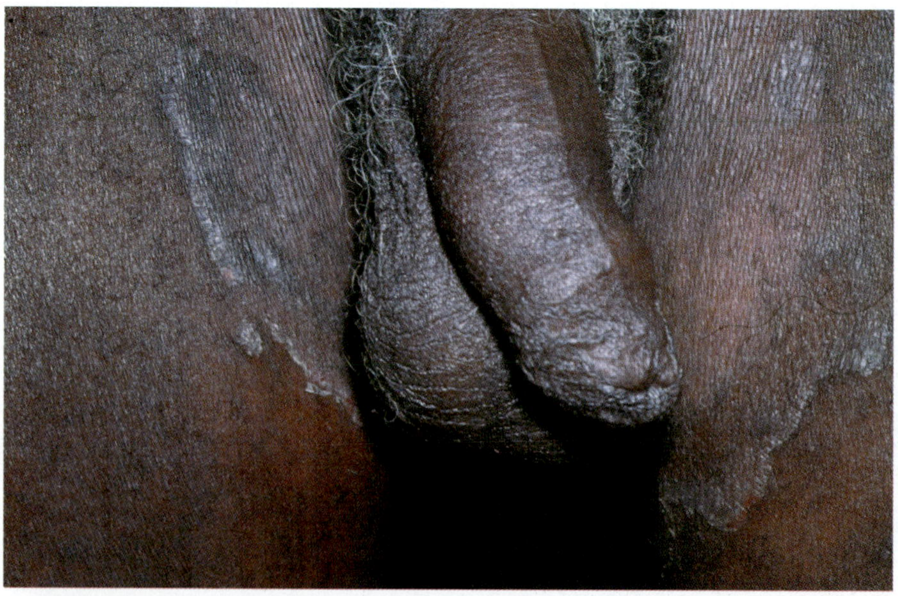

▲ **FIGURE 55-12** Tinea cruris characterized by annular scaling and erythema in the groin.

TABLE 55-9
Treatments for Tinea Cruris

	Topical (Daily)	Systemic	
First line	Terbinafine 1% cream	Terbinafine	250 mg orally daily for 2 weeks
	Naftifine 1% cream/gel		
Second line	Clotrimazole 1% cream	Itraconazole	100 mg orally daily for 2–4 weeks or 200 mg orally daily for one week
	Econazole 1% cream		
	Ketoconazole 2% cream		
	Miconazole 2% cream	Fluconazole	150 mg once weekly for 2–4 weeks
	Oxiconazole 1% cream/lotion	Ketoconazole	200 mg daily for 1–2 months
	Sulconazole 1% cream	Griseofulvin	500 mg orally daily for 2–4 weeks
	Butenafine 1% cream		
	Ciclopirox 0.77% cream/gel		
	Honey-olive oil-beeswax 1:1:1		

Treatment Multiple topical antifungals may be used to effectively clear tinea cruris. The two main classes are allylamines, including terbinafine and naftifine, and azoles, including clotrimazole, econazole, ketoconazole, miconazole, oxiconazole, sertaconazole, and sulconazole; alternative topical therapies include topical butenafine and ciclopirox creams.[35] It is very important to treat onychomycosis, if present, with appropriate systemic therapy. Patients also may require systemic therapy for extensive or refractory tinea cruris or for suppression (Table 55-9).

Prevention Individuals who are prone to fungal infections may require suppressive antifungal therapy. Excessive moisture and perspiration commonly predispose to tinea cruris, so patient education about hygiene may help to prevent some infections. This may include keeping the skin dry and cool as much as feasible and avoiding sharing towels or articles of clothing.[36,37]

CANDIDA

Epidemiology, Etiology, and Pathogenesis

Cutaneous candidiasis is extremely common. The disorder is caused by *Candida* species, a family of yeasts that normally colonizes human hosts. *Candida albicans* is the most common cause of cutaneous candidiasis (~90%), and infection frequently occurs in individuals who have poorly controlled diabetes, are immunosuppressed, or are taking broad-spectrum antibiotics. Men are affected in the genital region less frequently than women.

Clinical Findings Genital candidiasis in men takes two forms. It can present either as balanitis in uncircumcised men or as the more common flat erythema that begins in the inguinal-scrotal fold. The surface of the erythema may appear white owing to the mild scaling that may occur. The disease can spread to the scrotum and upper thigh and may be associated with papules and pustules. Erythematous satellite lesions are characteristic. The diagnosis of candidiasis can be made clinically, or KOH preparations or culture may be performed for verification.

Differential Diagnosis

- Contact dermatitis
- Darier disease
- Eczema
- Hailey-Hailey disease
- Intertrigo
- Lichen simplex chronicus
- Psoriasis
- Seborrheic dermatitis
- Tinea cruris

Complications The lesions of cutaneous candidiasis are frequently pruritic, and an itch-scratch cycle may lead to the development of lichen simplex chronicus.

Prognosis/Clinical Course Cutaneous candidiasis may clear spontaneously, but treatment is usually required to resolve the condition. Additionally, owing to the fact that *Candida* is a normal commensal, relapses are common and may require additional treatment.

Treatment The treatment of cutaneous *Candida* infections must involve resolving or limiting any predisposing conditions such as immobility, diabetes, or immunosuppressive disorders. Treatment of *Candida* infections involves application of the topical polyene nystatin or topical or systemic treatment with azoles (e.g., clotrimazole, miconazole, ketoconazole, itraconazole, fluconazole, or voriconazole).[38] Because of its inherent anti-inflammatory properties, topical ciclopirox is a good choice for treatment of severely symptomatic cutaneous candidiasis[39,40] (Table 55-10).

Prevention Optimal control of blood sugar and limited use of antibiotics and steroids, along with wearing nonocclusive cotton clothing, may help to prevent infection.

AMEBIASIS

Epidemiology, Etiology, and Pathogenesis

Amebiasis is a worldwide disease but is most common in the tropics. The etiologic agent of amebiasis is *Entamoeba histolytica*. As much as 10% of the world's population is infected with *E. histolytica*.[41] Genital amebiasis is rare and even less common in men than in women. In the United States, the disease is most common in immigrant populations from tropical and subtropical areas. The dis-

TABLE 55-10
Treatments for Cutaneous *Candida*

	Topical		Systemic	
First line	Clotrimazole 1%	Apply bid for 7–10 days	Itraconazole	200 mg per day for 3–5 days
	Miconazole 2%	Apply bid for 7–10 days		
	Nystatin 100,000 units/g	Apply bid for 7–10 days	Fluconazole	150 mg per day for 1–3 day
	Ketoconazole 2%	Apply bid for 7–10 days		
	Ciclopirox 0.77%	Apply bid for 7–14 days		

ease is most encountered in men who have sex with men, presumably owing to infection from an individual with intestinal amebiasis.[42] It also can be spread following coitus with a woman with vulvovaginal amebiasis.[41]

Clinical Findings Penile amebiasis begins as a vesicle on the foreskin or glans that evolves into a painful ulcer several days later. The ulcers are rapidly progressive and may have foul-smelling exudate. In endemic areas, amebiasis should be suspected in any individuals with erosive balanitis who do not respond to antibiotic therapy.[41,42] Diagnosis can be made by biopsy demonstrating superficial necrosis with trophozoites present, although direct examination of the Papanicolaou smear of necrotic debris may be diagnostic. Biopsy is helpful to rule out squamous cell carcinoma.

Differential Diagnosis

- Chancroid
- Granuloma inguinale
- Genital leishmaniasis
- Primary syphilis
- Squamous cell carcinoma

Complications The disease is rapidly progressive, and severe disease may cause genital mutilation or even penile loss. Genital amebiasis also may increase the risk for genital cancer.[42]

Prognosis/Clinical Course Genital amebiasis is rapidly progressive and, without treatment, will progress to severe genital mutilation. Individuals who receive prompt treatment have a good prognosis for recovery.

Treatment The treatment of choice for genital amebiasis is metronidazole. More severe cases may require combination with another systemic agent. Patients with severe deformity may require surgical reconstruction. Topical therapy is ineffective (Table 55-11).

Prevention Risk factors for genital amebiasis include sex with infected partners, poor genital hygiene, and intestinal amebiasis. Limiting the number of sexual partners, condom use, education about sexual hygiene, and prevention of intestinal amebiasis through improved sanitation help to prevent the infection.

LEISHMANIASIS

Epidemiology, Etiology, and Pathogenesis Cutaneous leishmaniasis is a parasitic disease caused by various species of the *Leishmania* protozoan. The disease affects 1–2 million people each year, mainly in tropical and subtropical areas. Genital manifestations of leishmaniasis are quite rare because the cutaneous manifestations usually occur on exposed skin. Genital lesions have been described in farmers, miners, nude sunbathers, and individuals who normally sleep naked.[43] The disease is spread by the bite of the sandfly of genus *Lutzomyia* in the new world and *Phlebotomus* in the old world. The parasite is able to survive within macrophages in the host.[44] Clinical lesions develop secondary to continued release of cytokines as part of the host immune response.[45]

Clinical Findings After a 2- to 8-week or longer incubation, an erythematous papule develops at the site of the sandfly bite. The papule enlarges into a nodule that promptly ulcerates (Figure 55-13). The ulcer is usually painless unless secondarily infected. When the disease occurs on the genitalia of men, the ulcers usually occur on the glans or scrotum.[43] The most common test to diagnose cutaneous leishmaniasis is a scraping from the center of the lesion following cleaning. Giemsa stain should reveal Leishman-Donovan bodies, amastigotes within monocytes. A biopsy of the lesion also can be performed to identify amastigotes. Newer tests, including culture on selective media and PCR assay, may enhance detection.[45]

Differential Diagnosis

- Amebiasis
- Chancroid
- Granuloma inguinale
- Primary syphilis (chancre)
- Squamous cell carcinoma

Complications Cutaneous lesions can become disseminated, especially in immunosuppressed patients. The lesions also can become secondarily infected with bacteria and fungi. Untreated lesions may result in genital deformity.

Prognosis/Clinical Course Old world leishmaniasis tends to heal spontaneously in months, whereas new world lesions may take years to do so. Scarring usually results after involution.

Treatment The treatment of choice for cutaneous leishmaniasis is pentavalent antimony. The antimonial agent used in the United States, sodium stibogluconate, must be obtained from the CDC, which can counsel the physician in its use. Antimonials have a high incidence of reversible side effects. Other treatments for leishmaniasis have been reported.[46] Azole antifungals may prove particularly useful for leishmaniasis acquired in the Middle East by contractors and service personnel serving in war zones (Table 55-12).

Prevention Avoiding sandflies is important to prevent leishmaniasis. Sandflies are small enough to pass through mosquito nets. Use of repellants, insecticides, and fine-weave pyrethroid-impregnated bed nets has helped to prevent spread of the disease in endemic areas.[44]

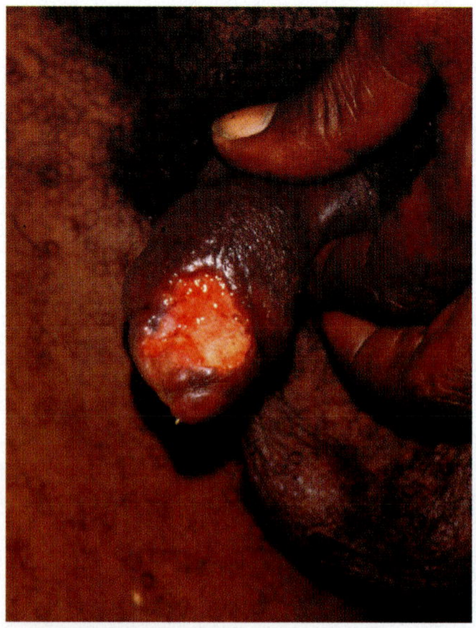

▲ **FIGURE 55-13** Persistent painless ulcer of genital leishmaniasis.

TABLE 55-11
Treatments for Amebiasis

		Systemic
First Line	Metronidazole	800 mg orally three times per day for 5 days
Second Line	Iodoquinol	650 mg orally three times per day for 20 days
	Hydrochloric emetine	1 mg/kg/day (max 60 mg) IM for 5 days

TABLE 55-12
Treatments for Leishmaniasis

	Topical		Physical	Systemic	
First line	Leshcutan ointment (15% paromomycin sulfate and 12% methylbenzethonium chloride in soft white paraffin)	Twice daily for 10 days	Cryotherapy Thermotherapy (difficult for genital lesions)	Sodium stibogluconate	20 mg/kg/day for 20 days (IM)
Second line				Amphotericin B	0.5–1.0 mg/kg every other day for up to 8 weeks
				Fluconazole	200 mg/day for 6 weeks
				Allopurinol	Various regimens
				Dapsone	
				Itraconazole	
				Ketoconazole	
				Pentamidine	

INFLAMMATORY DISEASES

Papulosquamous

PSORIASIS

Epidemiology, Etiology, and Pathogenesis Psoriasis is a T-cell-mediated autoimmune disorder wherein keratinocyte proliferation follows aberrant cytokine elaboration and secretion.[47] Psoriasis occurs less commonly in black Americans (0.1%) than in white Americans (1%); however, in East Africa, psoriasis occurs in 1.4% of the black population.[48] Psoriasis has a genetic basis, with 30% of affected individuals having an affected first-degree relative, but environmental factors also may play a role in the disease process.

Clinical Findings The typical lesions of psoriasis consist of erythematous plaques with an overlying silvery scale (Figure 55-14). However, in skin of color, psoriasis may present as bluish black, minimally scaly, flattened plaques. Psoriatic lesions occur most frequently over the scalp, elbows, and knees, although genital involvement does occur with some regularity. The lesions commonly occur over the elbows and knees because of Koebner's phenomenon, in which lesions occur at sites of injury or irritation. This phenomennon may have an effect on genital lesions as well because heat and friction produce mild irritation. When psoriasis occurs on genital skin, it may appear less thickened and has less scale owing to the occluded, damp nature of genital skin. Psoriasis is common in the inguinal crease, upper inner thighs, perineum, scrotum, and penile shaft and glans. Although the diagnosis of psoriasis usually can be made based on clinical appearance, lesions in black individuals may possess an atypical morphology and thus may require biopsy confirmation. Additionally, black individuals are less likely to have associated psoriatic features such as nail dystrophy that could assist in the diagnosis.[48] Genital psoriasis may be identical in clinical morphology to Reiter disease, although the latter is uncommon in African-Americans.

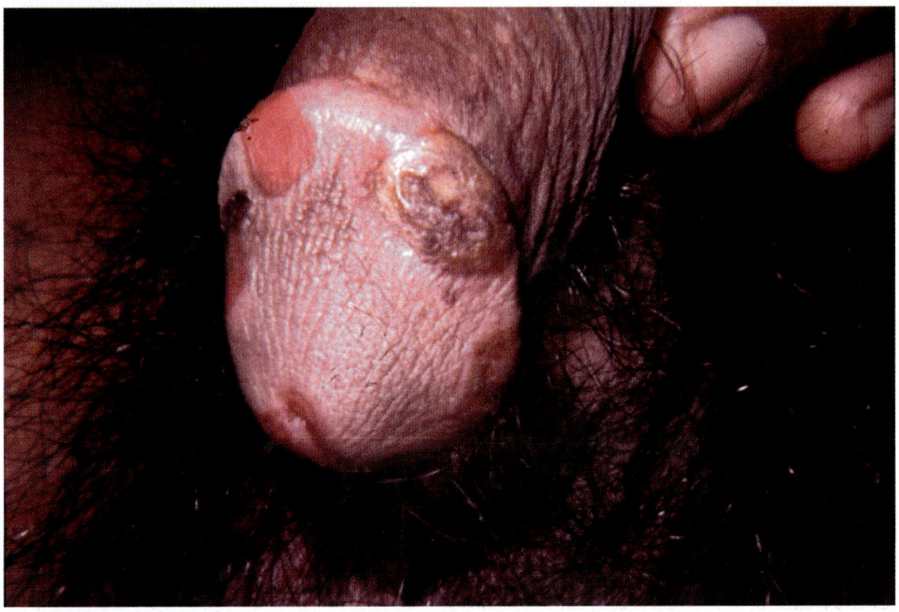

▲ **FIGURE 55-14** Plaques, some with and some without scale, of psoriasis.

Differential Diagnosis

- Bowen disease
- Candidiasis
- Contact dermatitis
- Drug eruption
- Eczema, including lichenified eczema
- Lichen planus
- Paget disease (extramammary)
- Reiter disease
- Seborrheic dermatitis
- Tinea cruris
- Zoon balanitis plasmacellularis

Complications Psoriasis may be associated with several comorbidities, including emotional distress, arthritis, and an increased risk of lymphoma and nonmelanoma skin cancers. The local maceration that can occur in psoriasis, along with the use of topical corticosteroids, can increase the risk of infection with *Candida* or dermatophytes.

Prognosis/Clinical Course Psoriasis is a chronic disease with a waxing and waning clinical course. There is no cure for psoriasis, and treatments are aimed at managing the disease.

TABLE 55-13
Treatments for Psoriasis

	Topical		Physical		Systemic	
First line	Hydrocortisone 1–2.5%	Apply qd	UVB	TIW	Methotrexate	10–25 mg PO/IM weekly
	Calcipotriene 0.005%	Apply bid	UVB Narrow band	TIW	Cyclosporine	2.5–4.0 mg/kg/day bid in divided dose
					Acitretin	25–50 mg qd
Second line	Anthralin 0.1%	All are applied daily	PUVA	TIW	Alefacept	15 mg IM weekly
	Coal tar 2%					
	Tazarotene 0.05%				Efalizumab	Initial dose: 0.7 mg/kg SC; then 1 mg/kg SC weekly
	Tacrolimus 0.1%				Etanercept	50 mg SC twice weekly ×12, then 50 mg SC weekly
	Pimecrolimus 1%				Infliximab	3 to 10 mg per kg IV infusions at weeks zero, 2, 6, and q8wks

Treatment The first-line treatment for psoriasis, topical corticosteroid therapy, is more effective on the genitalia than elsewhere because the skin is thin and occluded by clothing. High-potency topical steroids should be avoided on the genitalia. Topical vitamin D derivatives may be used alone or in conjunction with corticosteroids. Topical calcineurin inhibitors appear promising, especially for treatment of anogenital psoriasis.[49] Other topical treatments, such as coal tar, anthralin, and topical retinoids, may be associated with prohibitive irritation when applied to genital skin. UV light is logistically difficult. The systemic agents used for severe psoriasis generally are not required for genital lesions (Table 55-13).

Prevention Psoriasis cannot be prevented, but known risk/trigger factors can be avoided or minimized, namely, psychological stress, medications (e.g., lithium, beta blockers, antimalarial drugs, nonsteroidal anti-inflammatory drugs, and oral/parenteral steroid withdrawl), tightly fitting undergarments, and infections.[50]

LICHEN PLANUS

Epidemiology, Etiology, and Pathogenesis Lichen planus, like psoriasis, is probably related to errant T-cell autoimmunity.[51] Approximately 25% of men demonstrate genital involvement, usually of the glans.[2]

Clinical Findings Although the lesions of lichen planus typically appear as polygonal papules with a violaceous hue (Figure 55-15), variations are very common in skin of color. Lesions are usually deeper in color, and annular lesions are more common.[52] Erosive lichen planus can occur on the penis but is much more common in females; this is discussed in Chapter 56. Although classic lichen planus is diagnosed clinically, genital lesions may require a biopsy for diagnosis.[51]

Differential Diagnosis

- Bowen disease and bowenoid papulosis
- Candidiasis
- Condyloma acuminata (external genital warts)
- Erythema multiforme
- Fixed drug reaction
- Granuloma annulare
- Lichen simplex chronicus

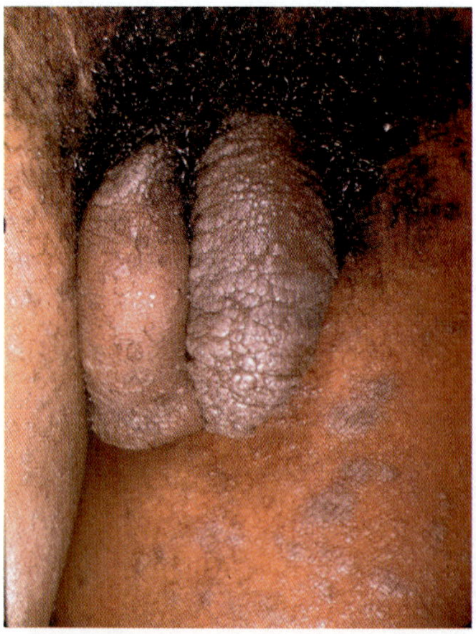

▲ **FIGURE 55-15** Numerous flat-topped violaceous papules of lichen planus.

- Psoriasis
- Scabies
- Syphilis (secondary)

Complications Lichen planus is associated with systemic illnesses such as myasthenia gravis, ulcerative colitis, primary biliary cirrhosis, and chronic active hepatitis C (HCV). Chronic ulcerative lichen planus may degenerate into squamous cell carcinoma. Phimosis may develop in uncircumcised men.[50] Lichen planus therapy is immunosuppressive, thereby increasing the risk of superimposed *Candida* and dermatophyte infections.

Prognosis/Clinical Course The course of lichen planus is variable. Some lesions remit spontaneously, whereas others persist. Nonerosive lesions, typical in men, are usually well controlled with therapy.

Treatment The papular disease that occurs on the genitalia of men is much easier to treat than the erosive variant, which is more common in women. First-line therapy consists of topical steroids or topical calcineurin inhibitors.[53] Systemic therapy should be considered only after failure of these topical modalities and, even then, only for as short a time as possible (Table 55-14).

Prevention Lichen planus is not a preventable disease.

Non-Papulosquamous

LICHEN SCLEROSUS ET ATROPHICUS

Epidemiology, Etiology, and Pathogenesis The etiology of lichen sclerosus et atrophicus (LSA) is unknown. There is

TABLE 55-14
Treatments for Lichen Planus

	Topical		Systemic	
First Line	Hydrocortisone 1% to Clobetasol propionate 0.05%	Applied once to twice daily Potency as response dictates		
	Pimecrolimus 1% or Tacrolimus 0.1%	Applied once to twice daily, as response dictates		
Second Line			Prednisone	40–60 mg daily for 2–4 weeks
			Isotretinoin	1 mg/kg/d (controversial)

evidence that it is genetic, autoimmune, or associated with infectious agents. The condition is 6–10 times more common in women than in men but shows no ethnic predilection.[54] Like psoriasis, LSA can be precipitated by trauma, and this may explain the predilection for the genitalia.

Clinical Findings The most common clinical appearance in men is hypochromic, atrophic, and sclerotic plaques over the glans, sulcus, or penile shaft. Lesions are often associated with pruritus and/or tenderness. Long-standing LSA also may cause poor urinary stream and difficulty retracting the foreskin. When the condition occurs in boys, they present with phimosis, and it typically resolves completely with circumcision.[54] The diagnosis of lichen sclerosis is made by biopsy, the latter helping to exclude other similar-appearing disorders (see below).

Differential Diagnosis

- Morphea
- Postinflammatory dyschromia
- Squamous cell carcinoma in situ
- Vitiligo (the closest clinical mimic)

Complications Patients with genital LSA have a considerable risk of developing squamous cell carcinoma. In one series of patients with penile disease, 5.8% of patients developed malignant changes.[55] Additionally, advanced lichen sclerosus may result in meatal stenosis that requires surgical correction.[55]

Prognosis/Clinical Course Lichen sclerosus is a chronic disease, but individuals who are properly treated generally have good control of symptoms. If malignancy ensues, it usually accompanies LSA that has been present 10 or more years.

Treatment The treatment of choice for lichen sclerosus is topical corticosteroids. Although high-potency topical steroids generally are avoided on the genitalia, clobetasol has been employed most successfully to manage LSA. Circumcision is indicated as a first-line treatment for phimosis in men. Topical hormonal therapy, although once quite popular, has been demonstrated to generally be ineffective and is used rarely at present. After the disease is controlled, surgery may be required to reverse meatal stenosis. Systemic retinoids have been used in women with LSA gas mentioned in Chapter 56. Similarly, topical tacrolimus and pimecrolimus have been used more widely in women, although a few cases of success in men have been reported[56] (Table 55-15).

Prevention Since lichen sclerosus can occur at sites of trauma or injury (koebnerization), it is important to wear loose-fitting clothing, avoid elective surgery, and protect against preventable injury. The disease is progressive, and there is debate as to whether asymptomatic children and adults should be treated to prevent disease progression.

ZOON BALANITIS

Epidemiology, Etiology, and Pathogenesis Zoon balanitis, or plasma cell balanitis, has an unknown etiology but generally occurs in older uncircumcised men of any ethnic background. It is thought that inflammation may be an inciting event in the disease process.[57]

Clinical Findings Zoon balanitis presents as a sharply demarcated, shiny, erythematous and geographic shallow erosion affecting the glans penis and/or the inner surface of the prepuce (Figure 55-16). The lesion is usually asymptomatic. The diagnosis is established by biopsy, which must be performed to rule out squamous cell carcinoma in situ.[58]

Differential Diagnosis

- Squamous cell carcinoma in situ
- Squamous cell carcinoma (invasive)
- *Candida* and *Pseudomonas* balanitis
- Contact dermatitis
- Psoriasis
- Lichen planus

Complications Zoon balanitis does not usually lead to any complications.

Prognosis/Clinical Course Zoon balanitis may be well controlled or even eradicated with treatment. It is unclear if untreated disease resolves, persists

TABLE 55-15
Treatments for LS&A

	Topical		Physical	Systemic
First Line	Triamcinolone 0.01% or Clobetasol 0.05%	Apply daily to twice daily for 2–3 months	Circumcision	See next chapter
Second Line	Pimecrolimus 1.0% or Tacrolimus 0.1%		Daily to twice daily	

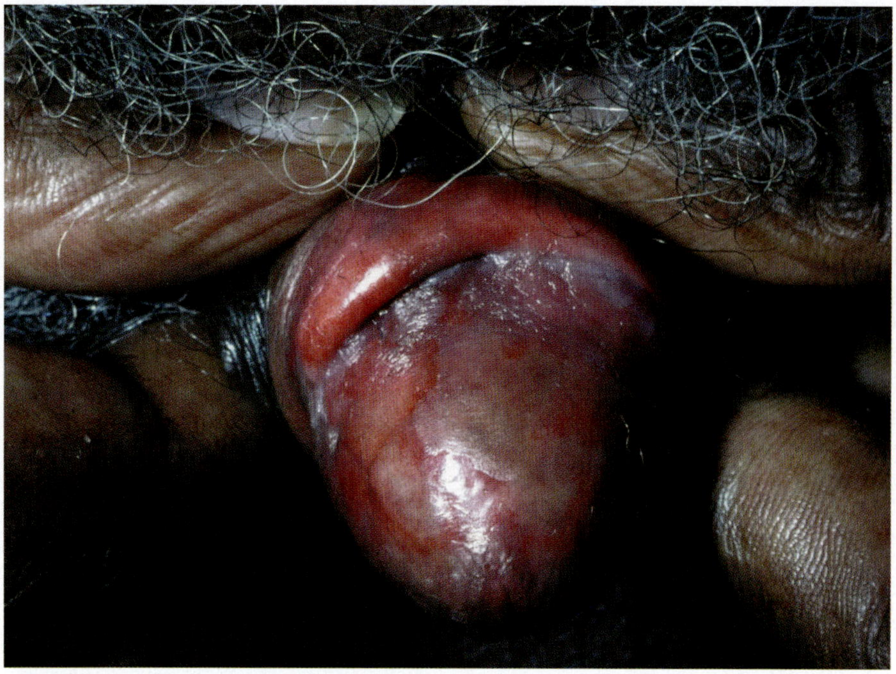

▲ **FIGURE 55-16** Shallow asymptomatic erosion (Zoon balanitis).

indefinitely, or evolves into a more recognizable disease such as lichen planus. Rare cases of squamous cell carcinoma have been reported to develop within this otherwise benign lesion.[59]

Treatment The treatment of choice for Zoon balanitis is circumcision, which may result in cure. Other less well-documented treatments include topical corticosteroids, topical retinoids, and topical tacrolimus. Although laser ablation (e.g., carbon dioxide, erbium:YAG) has been suggested as a therapeutic option,[60,61] the risk of permanent dyschromia in skin of color militates against this maneuver (Table 55-16).

Prevention It has been suggested that factors such as infection and the presence of a foreskin may lead to the inflammation that is the inciting event for this disease process. Although circumcision may prevent the disease, this may not be feasible owing to some ethnic groups' cultural standards.

TABLE 55-16
Treatments for Zoon Balanitis

	Topical		Physical
First line	Hydrocortisone 1% (or higher-potency steroids)	Apply daily	Circumcision
Second line	Tretinoin 0.025%	Apply daily	Laser ablation
	Tacrolimus 0.1% qd	Apply daily	

VITILIGO

Epidemiology, Etiology, and Pathogenesis Vitiligo is an autoimmune disease of uncertain etiology that results in destruction of melanocytes; there are predisposing genetic loci explaining a familial predilection.[62] While there is no ethnic predilection, the disease is so obvious (and cosmetically distressing) in patients with skin of color that more patients who fall into this category may seek medical attention. Most vitiligo patients relate an onset before age 40; men and women are at equal risk.

Clinical Findings Areas of absolute depigmentation are apparent (Figure 55-17). The periorificial regions of the face and the dorsum of the hands and feet are frequent sites of initial involvement. The glans penis is another favored area.

Differential Diagnosis

- Discoid lupus erythematosus
- Hansen disease (tuberculoid)
- Lichen sclerosus et atrophicus (most important)
- Postinflammatory dyschromia
- Seborrhea
- Tinea versicolor (rare on genital skin)

Complications Vitiligo itself poses no serious medical threat. However, thyroid dysfunction, pernicious anemia, and diabetes mellitus should be sought as potential comorbid conditions.[63]

Prognosis/Clinical Course The disease may resolve, persist, or expand. It is highly unpredictable.

Treatment A number of therapeutic modalities have been touted to induce repigmentation, but none is assured to succeed.[64] The likelihood of success is always better in recent-onset, limited disease occurring in younger patients compared with widespread vitiligo of long duration in older individuals. Genital skin is particularly difficult to approach surgically (e.g., epidermal grafts and laser therapy) owing to the risk of scar induction.[65] Genital skin is also a suboptimal area for phototherapy owing to concern about induction of neoplasia. Standard therapy for genital vitiligo consists of application of topical steroids and/or topical calcineurin inhibitors.[64,66]

Vitiliginous genital skin has been restored recently following transfer of noncultured keratinocyte-melanocyte cell suspensions.[67] When therapy is unsuccessful, careful camouflage techniques may be considered, including a therapeutic tattoo (Table 55-17).

Prevention Vitiligo is not a preventable disorder.

MULTISYSTEM DISEASES

REITER SYNDROME

Epidemiology, Etiology, and Pathogenesis Reiter syndrome is a reactive multisystem disorder that occurs in genetically susceptible individuals; it is often associated with an infection. Many microorganisms have been implicated, most prominently *Chlamydia, Ureaplasma, Shigella, Salmonella, Yersinia,* and *Campylobacter* species.[68] Reiter syndrome occurs almost exclusively in men and has the well-known clinical triad of urethritis, conjunctivitis, and arthritis. Twenty percent of affected individuals develop genital lesions.[69] Reiter syndrome is associated with HLA-B27 antigen positivity; both the disease and HLA-B27 are less common in African-Americans.[70]

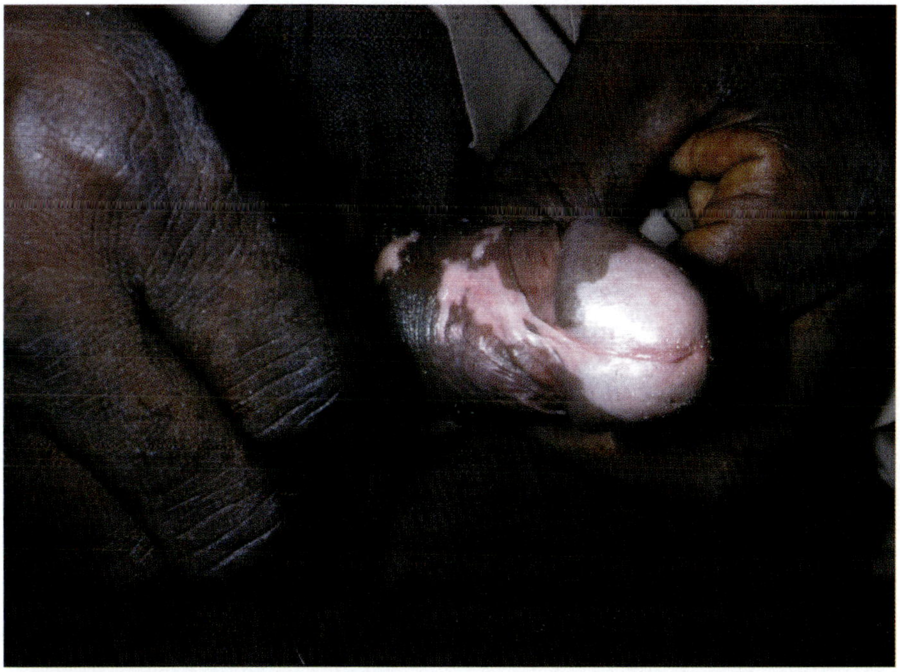

▲ **FIGURE 55-17** Depigmentation of vitiligo.

Clinical Findings The genital lesions, termed *balanitis circinata,* occur most commonly on the glans and corona and resemble those of pustular psoriasis. The lesions are erythematous, well demarcated, and exhibit thick, adherent scaling. In black skin, the lesions often appear hyperpigmented rather than red. The lesions on the glans may appear as white annular plaques in uncircumcised individuals. The diagnosis of Reiter syndrome is made by a constellation of clinical findings. A biopsy may be performed, but the biopsy cannot differentiate the disease from pustular psoriasis.[69]

Differential Diagnosis

- Psoriasis (including pustular)

Complications Disabling arthritis can occur but usually can be managed with systemic therapy.

Prognosis/Clinical Course Although the severity of Reiter syndrome may decrease after several months, many symptoms are chronic or intermittent, thereby requiring ongoing therapy.

Treatment Topical corticosteroids are the mainstay of treatment for skin disease, although topical calcineurin inhibitors appear promising.[71] Generally, systemic therapy is required to control other manifestations. Antibiotic therapy has been used to attempt to control the disease because of the presumed underlying bacterial etiology, but antibiotics have not been uniformly effective in trials (Table 55-18).

Prevention Reiter syndrome is not a preventable disease.

TABLE 55-17
Treatments for Vitiligo

	Topical		Physical	Camouflage
First line	Triamcinolone 0.01% or clobetasol 0.05%	Apply daily to twice daily for 2–3 months	Keratinocyte-melanocyte transfer	Cosmetic coverup
Second line	Pimecrolimus 1.0% or tacrolimus 0.1%	Daily to twice daily	Epidermal grafts Excimer laser	Therapeutic tattoo

TABLE 55-18
Treatments for Reiter Syndrome

	Topical		Systemic	
First line	Hydrocortisone 0.1% Triamcinolone 0.1% Clobetasol 0.05%	All are applied daily to twice daily	Indomethacin	75 mg PO bid
Second line	Tacrolimus 0.1% Pimecrolimus 1%	Daily to twice daily	Doxycycline	100 mg PO bid × 3 months
			Methotrexate	7.5–25 mg/week

BEHÇET SYNDROME

Epidemiology, Etiology, and Pathogenesis Behçet syndrome is a relatively uncommon disease that consists of a triad of oral ulcers, genital ulcers, and ocular inflammation. Anogenital ulcerations are found in roughly 90% of patients with Behçet syndrome and may be the presenting manifestation. Although common in the Middle East and Japan, this disorder is rare in both black Africans and Americans.[72]

Clinical Findings In men, the genital lesions of Behçet syndrome present as extremely painful, small, "punched out" ulcers over the scrotum (Figure 55-18) and, less commonly, the penile shaft.[73] The diagnosis of Behçet syndrome is made clinically. The diagnostic criteria include the presence of oral apthae plus any two of the following: genital ulceration, eye disease, other skin lesions, or skin pathergy (the formation of a pustule at the site of intracutaneously injected saline).

Differential Diagnosis

- Chancroid
- Crohn disease (extraintestinal)
- Granuloma inguinale
- Herpes progenitalis
- Syphilis
- Traumatic ulceration

Complications Behçet syndrome may be associated with gastrointestinal symptoms, arthritis, thrombophlebitis, psychiatric problems, or neurologic defects. Patients also may manifest other cutaneous problems, including erythema nodosum and erythema multiforme. Ocular disease may be severe enough to lead to blindness.

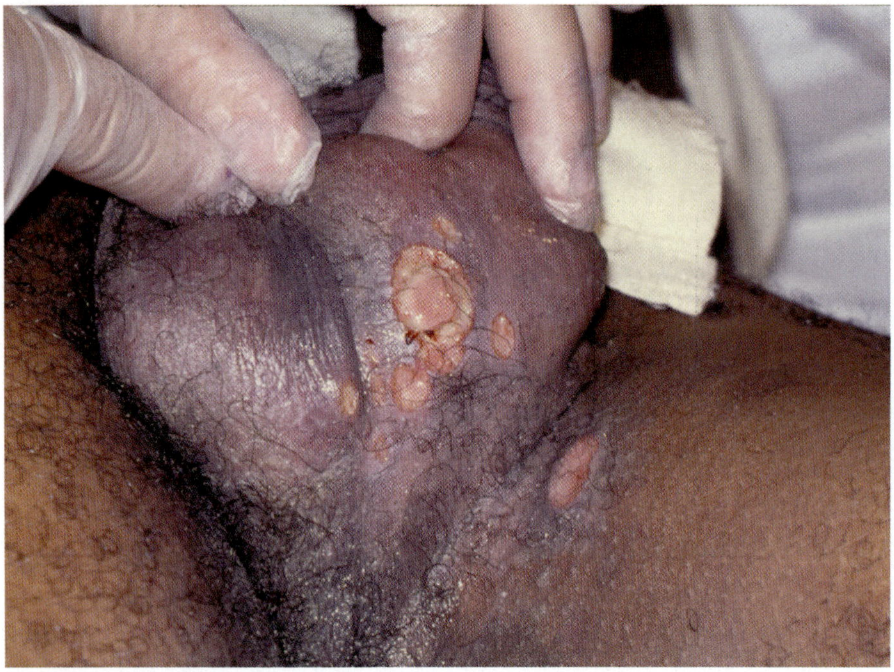

▲ **FIGURE 55-18** Multiple painful scrotal ulcers of Behçet syndrome.

Prognosis/Clinical Course The genital lesions follow a variable course. Some lesions will heal while other lesions will form. The systemic manifestations of the disease are more progressive.

Treatment Traditional systemic treatment for Behçet syndrome consists of steroids (with or without various cytotoxic agents), dapsone, and colchicine.[74] Thalidomide has proven beneficial in a handful of cases. Recent reports suggest the utility of anti–tumor necrosis factor-alpha biologic drugs[75–77] (Table 55-19).

Prevention Behçet syndrome is not a preventable disease.

METASTATIC CROHN DISEASE

Epidemiology, Etiology, and Pathogenesis Crohn disease is a systemic inflammatory disease of unknown etiology postulated to be related to infectious etiologies, autoimmune conditions, or genetic susceptibility. The disease can involve the gastrointestinal tract anywhere from the mouth to the anus. Extraintestinal manifestations of the disease can occur, and there is cutaneous involvement in 22–44% of patients. The skin can be involved by direct extension from the gastrointestinal tract or via involvement away from the gastrointestinal tract, so-called metastatic Crohn disease.[78] Genital involvement in Crohn disease is less frequent in men than in women. Among those with inflammatory bowel disease seen in the United States, Caucasians and African-Americans are equally likely to manifest Crohn disease, whereas those of Hispanic origin more often have ulcerative colitis.[79]

TABLE 55-19
Treatments for Behçet Syndrome (Systemic)

First line	Prednisone	5–60 mg PO daily (combined with immunosuppressive)
Second line	Dapsone	100 mg daily
	Colchicine	0.6 mg PO bid-tid
	Cyclosporine	4–5 mg/kg PO bid
	Methotrexate	7.5–25 mg weekly
Third line	Azathioprine	50–150 mg PO daily
	Cyclophosphamide	500–1000 mg IV bolus per month
	Thalidomide	100 mg PO daily
Uncertain efficacy	Etanercept	50–100 mg/week SC
	Infliximab	5 mg/kg IV at 0, 2, and 6 weeks; then every 8 weeks

Clinical Findings Both males and females may develop characteristic linear fissures in the intertriginous folds, termed the *knife cut sign,* but males also may present with either ulcers in or near the coronal sulcus or swelling of the penis or scrotum.[80]. These lesions may occur in the presence of or exclusive of active gastrointestinal involvement.[78]. If the patient has had gastrointestinal manifestations previously, the diagnosis is not difficult to make. Conversely, a biopsy can help to confirm the diagnosis if the patient has not had prior bowel symptoms.[81]

Differential Diagnosis

- Actinomycosis
- Angioedema
- Chancroid
- Extramammary Paget disease
- Factitious dermatitis (foreign-body reaction following penile injection)
- Filariasis
- Fixed drug eruption
- Granuloma inguinale
- Hidradenitis suppurativa

Complications Patients with Crohn disease may develop fistulas, migratory arthritis, uveitis and iritis, or other systemic manifestations. About 15% of Crohn disease patients also manifest erythema nodosum or pyoderma gangrenosum.[82]

Prognosis/Clinical Course Anogenital lesions are chronic but most often will improve if the gastrointestinal manifestations of the disease are well controlled.

Treatment The treatment of the anogenital lesions is directed at controlling the gastrointestinal manifestations of the disease. There are few treatments directed primarily at the genital lesions (Table 55-20).

Prevention Crohn disease has an unknown etiology and is not preventable.

TUMORS

Benign

SEBORRHEIC KERATOSIS

Epidemiology, Etiology, and Pathogenesis Seborrheic keratoses are benign neoplasms that have an unknown etiology. The generally occur in individuals who have relatives with similar lesions, begin in midlife, and become more numerous

TABLE 55-20
Treatments for Metastatic Crohn Disease

	Topical		Physical	Systemic	
First line	Ultrapotent topical steroids	Daily to twice daily		Sulfasalazine	1–2 g PO tid-qid
				Mesalamine	3–4 g PO daily
				Prednisone	5–60 mg PO daily
				Budesonide	9 mg daily × 8 weeks
Second line			Excision and skin graft	Azathioprine	2 mg/kg PO daily
				6-Mercaptopurine	1.5 mg/kg PO daily
				Infliximab	5 mg/kg IV every 8 weeks

and larger with age. There is no ethnic predilection.

Clinical Findings. Seborrheic keratoses classically appear as brown-black, sharply marginated plaques or papules with a characteristic "stuck on" appearance. A rough keratotic surface is usually present on the lesions, but lesions may appear and feel smooth when they are found on genital skin. If the diagnosis of the lesion is uncertain, a biopsy can be performed to differentiate it from other lesions, as listed below.

Differential Diagnosis

- Bowen disease and bowenoid papulosis
- Genital warts
- Melanoma
- Nevi

Complications Seborrheic keratoses can become irritated, but this is generally self-limited.

Prognosis/Clinical Course Seborrheic keratoses become larger and more numerous with age.

Treatment No treatment is necessary for seborrheic keratoses unless they are bothersome cosmetically. The lesions are easily removed by a variety of destructive techniques (Table 55-21).

TABLE 55-21
Treatments for Seborrheic Keratosis (Physical)

First line	Horizontal shave excision Cryotherapy Electrodesiccation

Prevention Seborrheic keratoses cannot be prevented.

ANGIOKERATOMA OF FORDYCE

Epidemiology, Etiology, and Pathogenesis Angiokeratomas are small benign vascular tumors with overlying keratotic epithelium commonly found on the scrotum. The lesions affect older men of all ethnic backgrounds. There are two theories regarding their pathogenesis. The first is that angiokeratomas are congenital lesions that become visible with advancing age. The second is that angiokeratomas occur following injury to local capillaries from direct trauma or local venous hypertension.[83]

Clinical Findings Angiokeratomas of Fordyce present as multiple purple-black, keratotic papules located over the scrotum or penis. The lesions are usually asymptomatic, although pruritus, pain, or bleeding rarely may be complaints.[83] The diagnosis usually can be made clinically, but a biopsy is confirmatory.

Differential Diagnosis

- Condyloma acuminata
- Condyloma lata
- Kaposi sarcoma
- Molluscum contagiosum
- Nevi
- Pyogenic granuloma
- Seborrheic keratosis

Complications Occasionally, the lesions may become irritated, itch, or bleed.

TABLE 55-22
Treatments for Angiokeratoma of Fordyce (Physical)

First line	Excision Cryotherapy Electrodesiccation Laser ablation

Confluence of the lesions may lead to "red scrotum" or "strawberry glans penis."

Prognosis/Clinical Course Although angiokeratomas of Fordyce generally have an asymptomatic course, they do become more numerous throughout life.

Treatment Treatment is not necessary but may be performed for bleeding, discomfort, or cosmetic concerns. Individual lesions can be destroyed, but conditions predisposing to increased scrotal venous pressure, including varicocele and inguinal hernia, should be investigated and treated[84] (Table 55-22).

Prevention Angiokeratomas may be prevented by treating conditions that lead to local increases in scrotal venous pressure, when such conditions exist.

EPIDERMAL INCLUSION CYST

Epidemiology, Etiology, and Pathogenesis The most common genital cysts are epidermal inclusion cysts (EICs). The cysts usually occur when a hair follicle becomes obstructed, leading to a spherical accumulation of keratinous debris.

Clinical Findings EICs are yellow-white to flesh-colored. They are commonly found over the scrotum but occasionally may be seen on the penis. An overlying puncta is frequently present and is pathognomonic. Diagnosis almost always can be made clinically.

Differential Diagnosis

- Lipoma
- Neurofibroma

Complications Cysts may become inflamed or may rupture, leading to a painful foreign-body inflammatory response.

Prognosis/Clinical Course Individuals who develop EICs tend to develop more over time. Bothersome lesions can be removed surgically with ease.

TABLE 55-23 Treatments for Epidermal Inclusion Cyst (Physical)	
First line	Surgical excision

Treatment EICs do not require therapy except for cosmetic reasons or if they are inflamed. Definitive therapy involves surgical removal of the cyst sac (Table 55-23).

Prevention EICs cannot be prevented.

Malignant

SQUAMOUS CELL CARCINOMA

Epidemiology, Etiology, and Pathogenesis Squamous cell carcinoma (SCC) is the most common tumor of the penis, accounting for more than 95% of malignant genital neoplasms. In the Western world, penile carcinoma accounts for less than 1% of adult male cancers, but in some developing areas in Africa, Asia, and South America, the disease can constitute up to 17% of malignancies in men. The disease is seen most commonly in 50- to 70-year-old individuals. In the United States, African-American men tend to present with genital SCC at a younger age and at a more advanced state than Caucasians.[85] A high mortality from genital SCC also has been reported in the past among black patients, both in the United States and in Africa.[86] Risk factors for the disease include not being circumcised as a child, human papillomavirus infection (subtypes 16, 18, 31, 33, 35, 51, and 52), tobacco use, ionizing radiation, chemical agents, and immunosuppression. SCC in situ is a precursor of invasive SCC, but only 10% of these lesions will transform.[87] Carcinoma in situ of the penis is often referred to as *erythroplasia of Queyrat* when it occurs on the glans and *Bowen disease* when it occurs on the shaft.

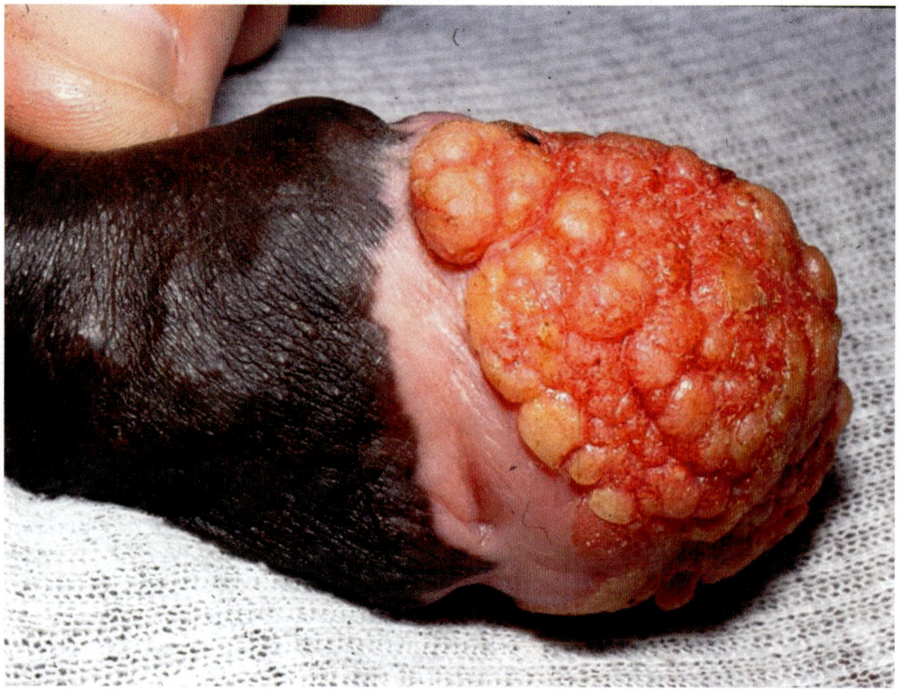

▲ **FIGURE 55-20** Verrucous, nonulcerating squamous cell carcinoma that required partial penectomy.

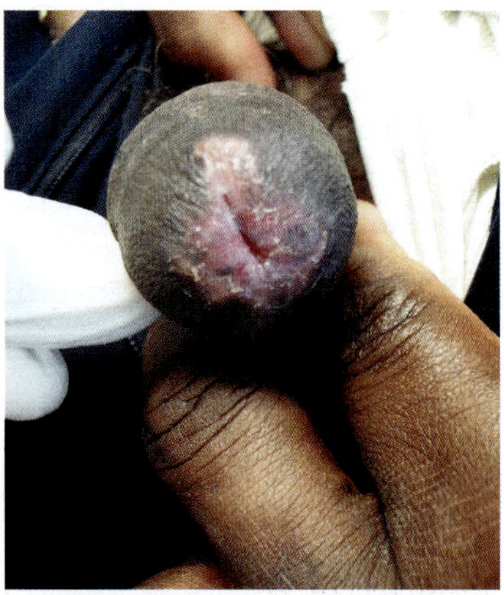

▲ **FIGURE 55-19** Velvety, erythematous erosion of squamous cell carcinoma in situ.

Clinical Findings In situ SCC presents as velvety papules and plaques or shallow nonhealing erosions on the glans or shaft of the penis (Figure 55-19). Invasive SCC can occur on the penis or scrotum. The lesions may have variable clinical morphology but typically appear as friable and/or ulcerated nodules and plaques. They also may appear as red or brown flat-topped papules or plaques that are identical to the appearance to in situ lesions. Alternatively, they may appear as a rock-hard, verrucous or hyperkeratotic nodules without evidence of ulceration (Figure 55-20). The diagnosis of SCC is established with a biopsy.

Differential Diagnosis

- Condyloma acuminata
- Condyloma lata
- Extrammary Paget disease
- Lichen planus (SCC in situ)
- Psoriasis (SCC in situ)
- Seborrhea (SCC in situ)
- Zoon balanitis (SCC in situ)

Complications Invasive lesions that have persisted for many years can lead to significant destruction of tissue (Figure 55-21). Destructive ulceration, "rodent ulcers," can lead to autoamputation of

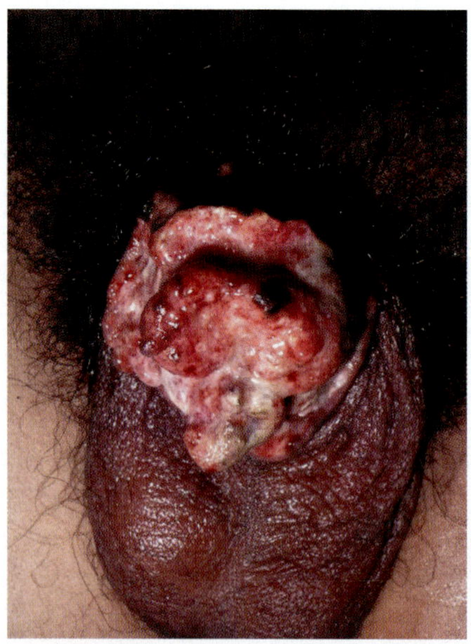

▲ **FIGURE 55-21** Advanced tissue destruction with invasive squamous cell carcinoma in a Hispanic patient from Panama.

TABLE 55-24
Treatments for Squamous Cell Carcinoma

	Topical		Physical
First line	Imiquimod 5% (SCC in situ only)	Apply 5 times per week × 6–12 weeks	Surgical resection
	5-Fluorouracil 5% (SCC in situ only)	Apply twice daily × 3–6 weeks	Mohs micrographic surgery
Second line			Laser ablation—CO_2 laser
			Radiation therapy

TABLE 55-25
Treatments for Melanoma (Physical)

First line	Surgical resection, with or without inguinal node dissection
Second line	Local radiation, chemotherapy

the distal penis. There is a risk of metastatic spread and death associated with invasive SCC.

Prognosis/Clinical Course Untreated invasive penile SCC will metastasize to local lymph nodes and result in death, usually within a few years.

Treatment Treatment of invasive SCC involves resection of the tumor or ablation of the tumor if it is small. Mohs micrographic surgery is an increasingly used tissue-sparing alternative to traditional surgery. Laser ablation and radiation therapy also have been used. Patients with lymph node metastasis must undergo lymphadenectomy. Courses of topical 5-fluorouracil or imiquimod may be attempted for in situ lesions before surgical extirpation or laser ablation is entertained[88] (Table 55-24).

Prevention Neonatal circumcision reduces the incidence of penile carcinoma by at least a factor of 10. This may be secondary to eliminating the chronic irritative effects of smegma. Changes in industrial practices that limit worker exposure to carcinogenic chemicals has decreased the incidence of scrotal carcinoma dramatically in these fields.[89] Limiting or eliminating medical or industrial exposure to ionizing radiation has had a similar effect. Although only a small number of precancerous and in situ lesions develop into invasive carcinoma, properly treating these lesions can decrease the incidence of invasive disease.

MALIGNANT MELANOMA

Epidemiology, Etiology, and Pathogenesis

The etiology and pathogenesis of malignant melanoma are poorly understood, especially for melanomas occurring in non-sun-exposed areas. Melanoma of the genitalia is rare, accounting for less than 2% of all primary penile malignancies. Melanomas of the penis, scrotum, and urethra have been reported and occur most commonly in the sixth and seventh decades of life.[90] Nodular melanomas are most common in this anatomic region.

Clinical Findings Penile melanoma is located most frequently on the glans penis, followed by the prepuce, the penile shaft, and the urethral meatus. Penile melanoma usually presents as a bleeding nodule, but the appearance can be quite variable. Any pigmented lesion that appears suspicious should undergo biopsy.

Differential Diagnosis

- Benign penile melanosis
- Nevoid lesions
- Seborrheic keratosis
- Squamous cell carcinoma

Complications Melanomas will metastasize, eventually causing the patient's death.

Prognosis/Clinical Course All other factors being equal, genital melanomas carry a higher risk of distant metastasis and a much lower 5-year survival rate than melanomas located on sun-exposed skin. Most patients will die within a few years of presentation.[90]

Treatment The treatment of melanoma of the genitalia traditionally has been wide local resection or amputation when the lesion occurs on the penis.[91] Lymph node dissection is indicated for thick melanomas or when palpable inguinal adenopathy is present. Some melanomas are radiosensitive, and this may play a role in palliation. Chemotherapy has not shown significant effects in melanoma (Table 55-25).

Prevention There is no known prevention for melanoma.

EXTRAMAMMARY PAGET DISEASE

Epidemiolog, Etiology, and Pathogenesis

Extramammary Paget disease (EMPD) is a rare neoplastic condition that usually affects the anogenital skin of older individuals.[92] The condition is less common in men than in women. EMPD either arises from the malignant transformation of multipotent germinal epidermal cells that are precursors of the apocrine gland or eccrine gland or arises from the epidermotropic spread of carcinoma from other organs.[93]

Clinical Findings EMPD typically presents as well-demarcated, erythematous plaques with a moist, eczematous appearance.[92] The lesions typically are associated with pruritus, but patients may experience burning, irritation, pain, tenderness, bleeding, or swelling.[94] The lesions are located most commonly on the penoscrotal junction but may be located on the glans, scrotum, inguinal area, or suprapubic region.[92,93] The diagnosis of EMPD is confirmed by the histologic presence of Paget cells.[95] It is important to rule out associated internal gastrointestinal or genitourinary malignancies in these patients.

Differential Diagnosis

- Contact dermatitis
- *Candida* infection
- Psoriasis
- SCC in situ
- Tinea

Complications Invasive adnexal carcinoma has been reported in roughly one-fourth of patients with EMPD, and roughly 10% of patients with penile or scrotal EMPD have been reported to have internal malignancies of the genitourinary system.[93]

Prognosis/Clinical Course The lesions of EMPD develop slowly and enlarge over many years. Owing to the slow development of lesions, patients are frequently unconcerned about the lesions and present with advanced disease. The

TABLE 55-26
Treatments for Extramammary Paget Disease

	Topical		Physical
First line	Imiquimod 5%	3 times per week for 8–16 weeks	Surgical excision using the Mohs micrographic technique with or without prior 5-fluorouracil application
Second line			Electrodesiccation and curettage Laser surgery Radiotherapy Photodynamic therapy with aminolevulinic acid

overall mortality rate as a result of either invasive adnexal carcinoma or internal genitourinary carcinoma at distant sites is 25%; however, owing to the insidious nature of the disease process, the 5-year survival of these patients is high.

Treatment The treatment of choice for EMPD has been surgical excision, preferably using the Mohs micrographic technique. The condition is often multifocal with skip areas, and 5-fluorouracil has been used to enhance the subclinical delineation of the disease. Recently, there have been multiple reports of success in treating EMPD with topical imiquimod[94,95] (Table 55-26).

Prevention There is no known prevention for EMPD.

KAPOSI SARCOMA

Epidemiology, Etiology, and Pathogenesis Kaposi sarcoma (KS) is a multicentric malignant tumor of lymphatic origin that can be one of four types: classic KS, endemic African KS, AIDS-related KS, and transplant-related KS. The etiologic agent of all types of KS is human herpes virus type 8.[96] The incidence of KS in the United States has decreased dramatically with the advent of highly active antiretroviral therapy (HAART) for HIV infection.[97] There is no sex predilection in the United States. In Africa, KS is very common, accounting for up to 10% of all malignancies in some areas; men are affected 20–30 times more frequently than women in these areas.[98]

Clinical Findings Lesions that involve the genitalia can be either primary lesions or part of generalized disease. The lesional morphology is similar in all forms of KS, starting as soft, spongy macules and plaques that enlarge into hard, violaceous nodules and tumors (Figure 55-22). In primary penile KS, lesions usually present as a violaceous nodule on the glans but may involve the foreskin, coronal sulcus, meatus, or rarely, the shaft. The lesions may be associated with significant edema.[99] The diagnosis of KS is confirmed with biopsy. Primary penile lesions are most commonly associated with HIV infection, and all patients should be tested for HIV.[100]

Differential Diagnosis

- Acral angiodermatitis
- Angiokeratoma
- Atypical acid-fast bacilli infection
- Deep fungal infection
- Lichen planus
- Metastatic tumor from visceral malignancy
- Soft tissue sarcoma

Complications KS can metastasize to the lymph nodes, the gastrointestinal tract, the pulmonary system, or the oral cavity.[100]

Prognosis/Clinical Course In most classic and African endemic cases, progression of the disease is slow. Individuals with HIV-associated KS and some individuals with other forms of KS have a rapidly progressive course with rapid dissemination. Complete cure is attained rarely in individuals with disseminated disease. In transplant-associated KS, diminution of immunosuppression may lead to lesional involution.[100]

Treatment For penile lesions, surgical excision is recommended for small solitary lesions, whereas conservative radiation therapy may be useful for larger lesions. Intralesional chemotherapy may be used for isolated lesions. Adjuvant α or β interferon is used in some patients, but systemic chemotherapy is reserved for patients with visceral involvement or generalized lesions[99] (Table 55-27).

Prevention Decreasing the spread of human herpes virus type 8 may decrease the incidence of KS. Optimal control of HIV with HAART also may prevent development of KS.

EXOGENOUS DISEASES

LICHEN SIMPLEX CHRONICUS

Epidemiology, Etiology, and Pathogenesis Lichen simplex chronicus (LSC) is an eczematous disease caused by unremit-

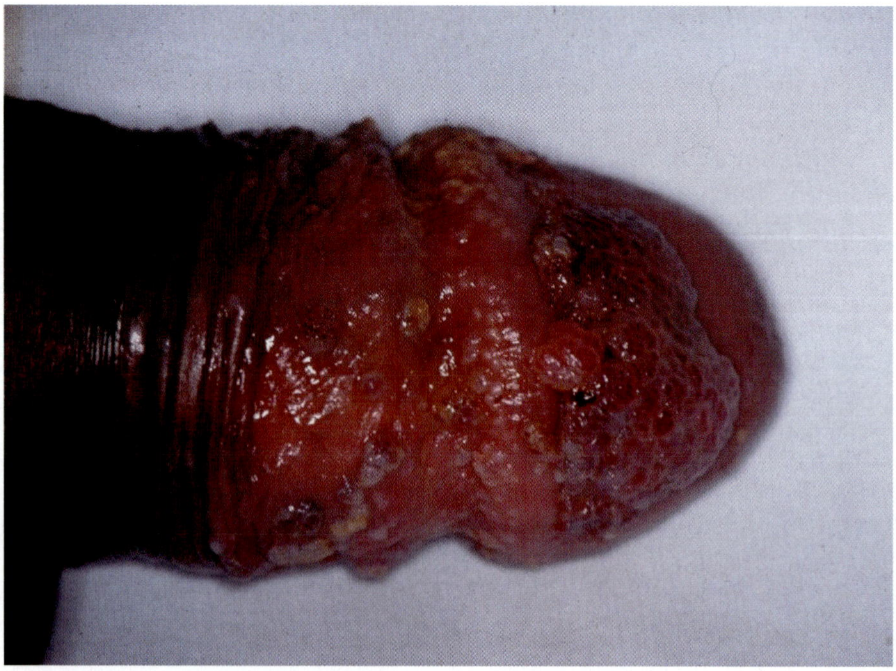

▲ **FIGURE 55-22** Purple-colored papules and nodules of Kaposi sarcoma.

TABLE 55-27
Treatments for Kaposi Sarcoma

	Topical		Physical	Systemic	
First line	Alitretinoin gel	Apply bid-qid × 2–14 weeks	Surgical excision	Interferon-α	36 million units SC/IM 3×/week
			Extended-field radiotherapy	HAART	Per protocol (HIV+)
			Laser therapy		
			Cryotherapy	Decrease immunosuppression	Transplant KS
Second line				Vincristine	
				Vinblastine	

ting itching and scratching. Primary LSC arises de novo on normal-appearing tissue and has been called "the itch that rashes." Secondary LSC develops in the presence of a preexisting dermatologic disease. The triggers of primary LSC are psychological and environmental factors, and primary LSC often occurs in the presence of atopy, whereas, the trigger of secondary LSC is the underlying dermatologic condition. The itch-scratch cycle is responsible for the condition in all types.[101]

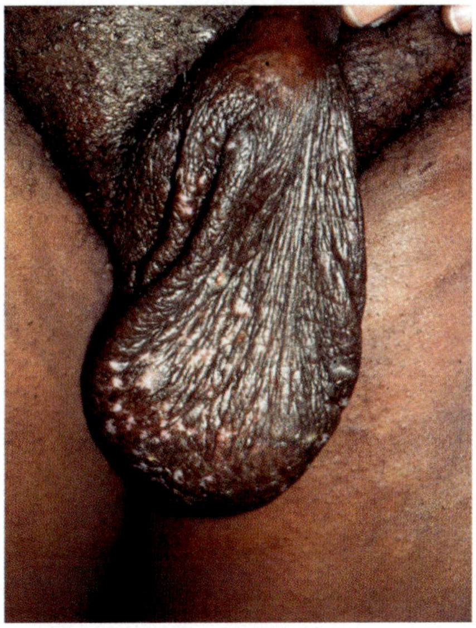

▲ **FIGURE 55-23** Thickened, scaly skin of lichen simplex chronicus.

Black skin is more prone to developing and resistant to clearing lichenification than white skin.

Clinical Findings LSC presents as thickened, hyperpigmented plaque with accentuated skin markings and overlying scale that may be associated with discrete hyperkeratotic nodules (prurigo nodularis) (Figure 55-23). In men, the scrotum is the most commonly involved site, but lesions also can occur on the proximal penis or the upper, inner thighs. In genital skin, the lesions may appear white and wrinkled instead of thickened and scaly secondary to the high moisture content of the area.[101] A variant of lichen simplex common in older black men exists in which thickening and hypo- and hyperpigmentation of the scrotum coexist. The diagnosis of LSC is made clinically with a compatible history of excessive itching that may be subconscious or occur at night. Biopsy finding are nonspecific.

Differential Diagnosis

- Atopic dermatitis
- Bowen disease
- Candidiasis
- Contact dermatitis (chronic)
- Psoriasis
- Pubic lice
- Scabies
- Tinea cruris

Complications Scratching of the area may be so vigorous that genital distortion, fibrosis, and scarring may occur. The condition may mask other premalignant and malignant conditions (e.g., lichen sclerosus or SCC in situ). In individuals with dark skin, postinflammatory hyper- and hypopigmentation can occur even if the condition is well controlled.[101]

Prognosis/Clinical Course LSC is a chronic disease that will persist indefinitely without treatment, although the disease severity will wax and wane. Even following successful treatment, the condition likely will recur.

Treatment The treatment of LSC involves identification of underlying disease, repair of barrier layer function, reduction of inflammation, and disruption of the itch-scratch cycle[101] (Table 55-28).

Prevention Individuals with atopic diathesis are predisposed to developing LSC, and a number of triggers are associated with the disease process. These include heat, sweating, irritation, and psychological distress. Minimizing these triggers may help to prevent the disease process.

TABLE 55-28
Treatments for Lichen Simplex Chronicus

	Topical		Physical	Systemic	
First line	Triamcinolone 0.1%	Apply qd-qid	Sitz baths	Hydroxyzine	10–25 mg PO at bedtime
			Lubricating creams and ointments	Other antihistamines as indicated	Dosed per drug chosen
Second line				Prednisone	40 mg qd for 7 days followed by 20 mg qd for 7 days
				Triamcinolone	40–80 mg IM once

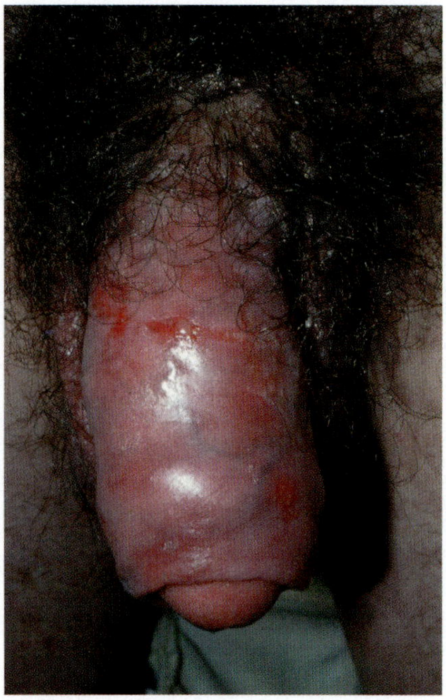

▲ **FIGURE 55-24** Marked pruritic erythema and edema; contact allergy to vaginal lubricant in a Hispanic male from Guatemala.

TABLE 55-29
Treatments for Contact Dermatitis

	Topical		Systemic	
First line	Triamcinolone 0.1%	Apply qd-qid	Hydroxyzine	10–25 mg PO at bedtime
Second line			Prednisone	up to 40–80 mg daily for 7–14 days

CONTACT DERMATITIS

Epidemiology, Etiology, and Pathogenesis

Contact dermatitis (CD) is a common inflammatory skin reaction to external agents. Allergic contact dermatitis (ACD) is a delayed-type hypersensitivity reaction and requires a prior antigen sensitization, but irritant contact dermatitis (ICD) is a nonimmunologic skin response to direct damage from a skin irritant. In both cases, the offending agent may be transferred to the genitalia by the hand or by the mucosa of sexual partners. To date, many offending agents have been described for both ACD and ICD, but most genital ACD results from topical cosmetic products, medications, latex condoms, or local anesthetic agents used to delay ejaculation by dulling sensation.[102–104]

Clinical Findings ACD of the genitalia presents as pruritic erythema and edema (Figure 55-24) that may have associated vesicles or bullae. The lesion may be painful as well. More chronic irritation shows scaly skin with accentuated skin markings. The high moisture content and friction of genital skin may spread the offending substance, making a geometric distribution less obvious than in other skin areas. The diagnosis of both ICD and ACD generally is made with a careful history because the clinical appearance and even biopsy may be nonspecific. Biopsy can be performed to rule out other possible diagnoses. Patch testing may be useful in some patients if the clinical findings suggest ACD but no offending agent can be determined by the history.[104]

Differential Diagnosis

- Bowen disease
- Candidiasis
- Extramammary Paget disease
- Lichen simplex chronicus
- Psoriasis
- Seborrheic dermatitis

Complications Severely irritating chemicals may cause erosions of the penis. Additionally, severe inflammation may damage melanocytes, leading to permanent dyschromia.

Prognosis/Clinical Course Patients allergic to one substance generally have a good prognosis once the offending agent is removed and anti-inflammatory treatment is initiated. Patients with more chronic symptoms and no obvious single etiology generally have a prolonged course with chronic management requirements.

Treatment Treatment involves removal of the offending agents and topical anti-inflammatory treatment. Oral steroids are reserved for patients with severe disease. Patients with significant pruritus or pain may be helped by sedating antihistamines at night (Table 55-29).

Prevention If the offending agent or agents can be identified and avoided, the condition usually can be prevented in the future.

GENITAL BITE WOUND

Epidemiology, Etiology, and Pathogenesis

Human genital bites usually result from sexual activity and are reported infrequently secondary to embarrassment. Bites may be deliberate or accidental, and penile bites may cause serious damage that leads to disfigurement and sexual dysfunction. Genital bites may transmit many possible communicable infectious diseases, especially if the person inflicting the bite is at high risk for having infectious diseases, such as prostitutes, men who have sex with men, intravenous drug abusers, or anyone receiving multiple blood transfusions prior to 1985. Rapidly progressive, necrotic genital infections following a bite generally are caused by oral flora such as *Eikenella corrodens,* a gram-negative facultative anaerobe.[105,106]

Clinical Findings Genital bite wounds can present as lacerations, ulcers, cellulitis, or balanoposthitis. Diagnosis is made based on a careful history, which must include health status of the biter, time elapsed since the injury, and the victim's medical condition, including his immune status. A wound culture for aerobic and anaerobic organism always should be performed on these lesions. Baseline and follow-up tests for syphilis, hepatitis, and HIV should be obtained.

Differential Diagnosis

- Chancroid
- Granuloma inguinale
- Herpes progenitalis (severe)
- Primary syphilis

Complications Localized infection secondary to microorganisms carried in the saliva can be a very serious complication. Infections can lead to erosion and ulceration, cellulitis, abscess formation, lymphadenitis or lymphangitis, and infrequently, seeding of prosthetic joints or artificial heart valves (Figure 55-25). Rarely, sepsis may occur.[106]

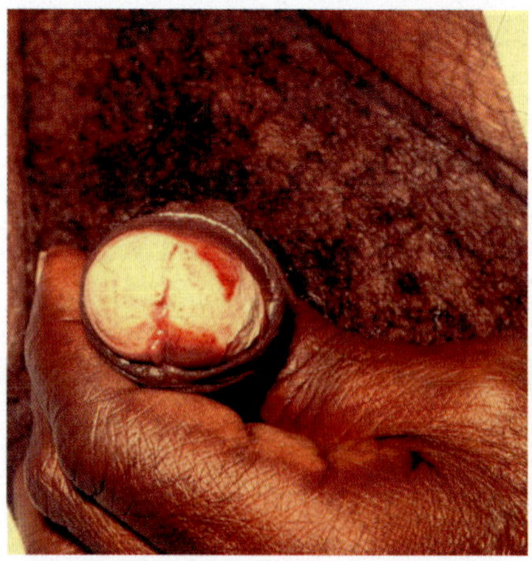

▲ **FIGURE 55-25** Necrotic ulceration characterizes a genital bite wound.

TABLE 55-30
Treatments for Bite Wound

	Physical	Systemic	
First line	1% Povodone-iodine irrigation Debride necrotic areas	Amoxicillin-clavulanate	875 mg/125 mg PO every 12 hours until lesions heal
Second line		Cefuroxime Dicloxacillin + penicillin V	0.75–1.5 g IV/IM every 8 hours 250 mg PO every 6 hours 250–500 mg PO every 6–8 hours × 10 days

Prognosis/Clinical Course If the bite did not cause anatomic damage to the penis and the wound does not become infected, the prognosis is good. Infections caught early and treated appropriately also have a good prognosis.

Treatment Prompt treatment of human bite wounds should be initiated at presentation to avoid complications. The wound should be irrigated with a bactericidal and virucidal solution. Tetanus boosters need to be given if immunizations are not current. Broad-spectrum antibiotic treatment should be instituted empirically before culture results return because copious amounts of subcutaneous tissue in the genital area allow bacterial spread. The genital area carries a high risk for infection, so bite wounds are not closed[105,106] (Table 55-30).

Prevention Genital bite wounds can be prevented with safer sexual practices.

REFERENCES

1. Goldman BD. Common dermatoses of the male genitalia. *Postgrad Med* 2000;108:89-91.
2. Rosen T. Update on genital lesions. *JAMA* 2003;290:1001-1005.
3. Lynch PJ, Edwards L. Infectious primary ulcers, in Lynch PJ, Edwards L (eds), *Genital Dermatology.* New York, Churchill-Livingstone, 1994, pp 205-212.
4. Primary and secondary syphilis—United States, 2003-2004. *MMWR* 2005;55: 269-273.
5. Lynn WA, Lightman S. Syphilis and HIV: A dangerous combination. *Lancet Infect Dis* 2004;4:456-466.
6. Zeltser R, Kurban AK. Syphilis. *Clin Dermatol* 2004;22:461-468.
7. Rosen T. Diseases with unusual features: Syphilis, in *Clinical Dermatology in Black Patients.* Bari, Italy, PiGreco Press, 1995, pp 59-63.
8. Lewis DA. Chancroid: Clinical manifestations, diagnosis, and management. *Sex Transm Infect* 2003;79:68-71.
9. Bong CTH, Bauer ME, Spinola SM. *Haemophilus ducreyi*: Clinical features, epidemiology, and prospects for disease control. *Microbes Infect* 2002;4:1141-1148.
10. Jones CC, Rosen T. Cultural diagnosis of chancroid. *Arch Dermatol* 1991;127: 1823-1827.
11. Rosen T, Tschen JA, Ramsdell W, et al. Granuloma inguinale. *J Am Acad Dermatol* 1984;11:433-437.
12. Rosen T. Tropical infections: Granuloma Inguinale, in *Clinical Dermatology in Black Patients.* Bari, Italy, PiGreco Press, 1995, pp 169-170.
13. O'Farrell N. Donovanosis. *Sex Transm Infect* 2002;78:452-457.
14. Lupi O, Madkan V, Tyring SK. Tropical dermatology: Bacterial tropical diseases. *J Am Acad Dermatol* 2006;54:559-578.
15. Sexually transmitted diseases treatment guidelines 2002. *MMWR* 2002;51: 1-78.
16. Rosen T, Brown TJ. Genital ulcers: Evaluation and treatment. *Dermatol Clin* 1998;16:673-685.
17. Beauman JG. Genital herpes: A review. *Am Fam Physician* 2005;72:1527-1534.
18. Lynch PJ, Edwards L. Vesicular disease, in Lynch PJ, Edwards L (eds), *Genital Dermatology.* New York, Churchill-Livingstone, 1994, pp 181-186.
19. Solomon J, Cannon MJ, Reyes M, et al. Epidemiology of recurrent genital herpes simplex virus types 1 and 2. *Sex Transm Infect* 2003;79:456-459.
20. Gupta R, Wald A. Genital herpes: Antiviral therapy for symptom relief and prevention of transmission. *Expert Opin Pharmacother* 2006;7:665-675.
21. Corey L, Wald A, Patel R, et al. Once-daily valacyclovir to reduce the risk of transmission of genital herpes. *N Engl J Med* 2004;350:11-20.
22. Dupin N. Genital warts. *Clin Dermatol* 2004;22:481-486.
23. Koutsky L. Epidemiology of genital human papillomavirus infection. *Am J Med* 1997;102:3-8.
24. Handsfield HH. Clinical presentation and natural course of anogenital warts. *Am J Med* 1997;102:16-20.
25. Tyring S. Introduction: perspectives on human papillomavirus infection. *Am J Med* 1997;102:1-2.
26. Kodner CM, Nasraty S. Management of genital warts. *Am Fam Physician* 2004;70: 2335-2342.
27. Scheinfeld N, Lehman DS. An evidence-based review of medical and surgical treatments of genital warts. *Dermatol Online J* 2006;12:5.
28. Brown T, Zirvi M, Cotsarelis G, Gelfand JM. Vitiligo-like hypopigmentation associated with imiquimod treatment of genital warts *J Am Acad Dermatol* 2005;52:715-716.
29. Villa LL, Costa RL, Petta CA, et al. Prophylactic quadrivalent human papillomavirus (types 6, 11, 16, and 18) L1 virus-like particle vaccine in young women: A randomised, double-blind, placebo-controlled multicentre phase II efficacy trial. *Lancet Oncol* 2005;6: 271-278.
30. Smith KJ, Skelton H. Molluscum contagiosum: Recent advances in pathogenic mechanisms, and new therapies. *Am J Clin Dermatol* 2002;3:535-545.
31. Hanson D, Diven DG. Molluscum contagiosum. *Dermatol Online J* 2003;9:2.
32. Lynch PJ, Edwards L. Skin-colored nodules, in Lynch PJ, Edwards L (eds), *Genital Dermatology.* New York, Churchill-Livingstone, 1994, pp 137-148.
33. Kumar B, Narang T, Radotra BD, Gupta S. Mondor's disease of the penis: A forgotten disease. *Sex Transm Infect* 2005;81:480-482.
34. Rosen T, Hwong H. Sclerosing lymphangitis of the penis. *J Am Acad Dermatol* 2003;49:916-918.
35. Gupta AK, Ryder JE, Chow M, Cooper EA: Dermatophytosis: The management of fungal infections. *Skinmed* 2005;4:305-310.
36. Nadalo D, Montoya C. What is the best way to treat tinea cruris? *J Fam Pract* 2006;55:256-258.
37. Gupta AK, Chaudhry M, Elewski B. Tinea corporis, tinea cruris, tinea nigra and piedra. *Dermatol Clin* 2003;21: 395-400.
38. Huang DB, Ostrosky-Zeichner L, Wu JJ, et al. Therapy of common superficial fungal infections. *Dermatol Ther* 2004;17: 517-522.
39. Rosen T, Schell BJ, Orengo I. Anti-inflammatory activity of anti-fungal preparations. *Int J Dermatol* 1997;36: 788-792.
40. Gupta AK, Skinner AR. Ciclopirox for the treatment of superficial fungal infections. *Int J Dermatol* 2003;42:3-9S.
41. Hejase MJ, Bihrle R, Castillo G, Coogan CL. Amebiasis of the penis. *Urology* 1996;48:151-154.
42. Antony SJ, Lopez-Po P. Genital amebiasis: Historical perspective of an unusual disease presentation. *Urology* 1999;54: 952-955.
43. Grunwald MH, Amichai B, Trau H. Cutaneous leishmaniasis on an unusual site: The glans penis. *Br J Urol* 1998;82:928.
44. Markle WH, Makhoul K. Cutaneous leishmaniasis: Recognition and treatment. *Am Fam Physician* 2004;69: 455-460.
45. Richens J. Genital manifestations of tropical diseases. *Sex Transm Infect* 2004;80:12-17.
46. Lee SA, Hasbun R. Therapy of cutaneous leishmaniasis. *Int J Infect Dis* 2003;7:86-93.
47. Krueger G, Ellis CN. Psoriasis: Recent advances in understanding its pathogenesis and treatment. *J Am Acad Dermatol* 2005;53:S94-100.
48. Rosen T. Diseases with unusual features: Psoriasis, in *Clinical Dermatology in Black Patients.* Bari, Italy, PiGreco Press, 1995, pp 51-54.
49. Martin Ezquerra G, Sanchez Regana M, Herrera Acosta E, Umbert Millet P. Topical tacrolimus for the treatment of

psoriasis on the face, genitalia, intertriginous areas and corporal plaques. *J Drugs Dermatol* 2006;5:334-336.
50. Farber EM, Nall L. Genital psoriasis. *Cutis* 1992;50:263-266.
51. Moyal-Barracco M, Edwards L. Diagnosis and therapy of anogenital lichen planus. *Dermatol Ther* 2004;17:38-46.
52. Rosen T. Diseases with unusual features: Lichen planus, in *Clinical Dermatology in Black Patients.* Bari, Italy, PiGreco Press, 1995, pp 36-40.
53. Lonsdale-Eccles AA, Velangi S. Topical pimecrolimus in the treatment of genital lichen planus: A prospective case series. *Br J Dermatol* 2005;153:390-394.
54. Powell JJ, Wojnarowska F. Lichen sclerosus. *Lancet* 1999;353:1777-1783.
55. Nasca MR, Innocenzi D, Micali G. Penile cancer among patients with genital lichen sclerosus. *J Am Acad Dermatol* 1999;41:911-914.
56. Bohm M, Frieling U, Luger TA, Bonsmann G. Successful treatment of anogenital lichen sclerosus with topical tacrolimus. *Arch Dermatol* 2003;139: 922-924.
57. Moreno-Arias GA, Camos-Fresneda A, Llaberia C, Palou-Almerich J. Plasma cell balanitis treated with tacrolimus 0.1%. *Br J Dermatol* 2005;153: 1204-1206.
58. Stern JK, Rosen T. Balanitis plasmacellularis circumscripta (Zoon's balanitis plasmacellularis). *Cutis* 1980;25:57-60.
59. Davis-Daneshfar A, Trueb RM. Bowen's disease of the glans penis (erythroplasia of Queyrat) in plasma cell balanitis. *Cutis* 2000;65:95-98.
60. Retamar RA, Kien MC, Chouela EN. Zoon's balanitis: Presentation of 15 patients, five treated with a carbon dioxide laser. *Int J Dermatol* 2003;42:305-307.
61. Albertini JG, Holck DE, Farley MF. Zoon's balanitis treated with erbium: YAG laser ablation. *Lasers Surg Med* 2002;30:123-126.
62. Passeron T, Ortonne JP. Pathophysiology and genetics of vitiligo. *J Autoimmun Dis* 2005;25:63-68S.
63. Handa S, Kaur I. Vitiligo: Clinical findings in 1436 patients. *J Dermatol* 1999; 26:653-657.
64. Grimes PE. New insights and new therapies for vitiligo. *JAMA* 2005;293:730-735.
65. Falabella R. Surgical approaches for stable vitiligo. *Dermatol Surg* 2005;31: 1277-1284.
66. Kostovic K, Pasic A. New treatment modalities for vitiligo: Focus on topical immunomodulators. *Drugs* 2005;65: 447-459.
67. Mulekar SV, Al Issa A, AL Eisa A, Asaad M. Genital vitiligo treated by autologous, noncultured melanocyte-keratinocyte cell transplantation. *Dermatol Surg* 2005;31:1737-1739.
68. Kataria RK, Brent LH. Spondyloarthropathies. *Am Fam Physician* 2004;69: 2853-2860.
69. Schneider JM, Matthews JH, Graham BS. Reiter's syndrome. *Cutis* 2003;71: 198-200.
70. Kahn MA, Askari AD, Braun WE, Aponte CJ. Low association of HLA-B27 with Reiter's syndrome in blacks. *Ann Intern Med* 1979;90:202-203.
71. de Almeida HL Jr, de Oliveira Filho UL. Topical pimecrolimus is an effective treatment for balanitis circinata erosiva. *Int J Dermatol* 2005;44:888-889.
72. Jacyk WK. Behçet's disease in South African blacks: Report of five cases. *J Am Acad Dermatol* 1994;30:869-873.
73. Fisher BK, Margesson LJ. Inflammatory lesions of the penis, in *Genital Skin Disorders: Diagnosis and Treatment.* St Louis, MO, Mosby, 1998, pp 40-64.
74. Barnes CG. Treatment of Behçet's syndrome. *Rheumatology (Oxf)* 2006;45: 245-247.
75. Atenzi F, Sarzi-Puttini P, Capsoni F, et al. Successful treatment of resistant Behçet's disease with etanercept. *Clin Exp Rheumatol* 2005;23:729.
76. Connolly M, Armstrong JS, Buckley DS. Infliximab treatment for severe orogenital ulceration in Behçet's disease. *Br J Dermatol* 2005;153:1073-1075.
77. Haugeberg G, Velken M, Johnsen V. Successful treatment of genital ulcers with infliximab in Behçet's disease. *Ann Rheum Dis* 2004;63:744-745.
78. Acker SM, Sahn EE, Rogers HC, et al. Genital cutaneous Crohn disease. *Am J Dermatopathol* 2000;22:443-436.
79. Basu D, Lopez I, Kulkarni A, Sellin JH. Impact of race and ethnicity on inflammatory bowel disease. *Am J Gastroenterol* 2005;100:2254-2261.
80. Zelhof B, Biyani CS, Anathhanam AJ, et al. Severe penile edema: An unusual presentation of metastatic Crohn disease. *Int J Urol* 2006;13:189-191.
81. Martinez-Salamanca JI, Jara J, Miralles P, et al. Metastatic Crohn's disease. *Scand J Urol Nephrol* 2004;38:436-437.
82. Knutson D, Greenberg G, Cronau H. Management of Crohn's disease: Practical approach. *Am Fam Physician* 2003;68:707-714, 717-718.
83. Erkek E, Basar MM, Bagci Y, et al. Fordyce angiokeratomas as clues to local venous hypertension. *Arch Dermatol* 2005;141:1325-1326.
84. Jansen T, Bechara FG, Stucker M, Altmeyer P. Angiokeratoma of the scrotum (Fordyce type) associated with angiokeratoma of the oral cavity. *Acta Dermatol Venereol* 2002;82:208-210.
85. Rippentrop JM, Joslyn SA, Konety BR. Squamous cell carcinoma of the penis: Evaluation of data from the surveillance, epidemiology, and end results program. *Cancer* 2004;101:1357-1363.
86. Hubbell CR, Rabin VR, Mora RG. Cancer of the skin in blacks: V. A review of 175 black patients with squamous cell carcinoma of the penis. *J Am Acad Dermatol* 1988;18:292-298.
87. Kroon BK, Horenblas S, Nieweg OE. Contemporary management of penile squamous cell carcinoma. *J Surg Oncol* 2005;89:43-50.
88. Orengo I, Rosen T, Guill CK. Treatment of squamous cell carcinoma in situ of the penis with 5% imiquimod cream: A case report. *J Am Acad Dermatol* 2002;47:S225-228.
89. Alam M, Ratner D. Cutaneous squamous cell carcinoma. *N Engl J Med* 2001;344:975-983.
90. Demitsu T, Nagato H, Nishimaki K, et al. Melanoma in situ of the penis. *J Am Acad Dermatol* 2000;42:386-388.
91. Sanchez-Ortiz R, Huang SF, Tamboli P, et al. Melanoma of the penis, scrotum and male urethra: A 40-year single institution experience. *J Urol* 2005;173: 1958-1965.
92. Henning JS. Extramammary Paget's disease of the penis and scrotum. *J Drugs Dermatol* 2006;5:652-654.
93. Yang WJ, Kim DS, Im YJ, et al. Extramammary Paget's disease of the penis and scrotum. *Urology* 2005;65: 972-975.
94. Badgwell C, Rosen T. Treatment of limited extent extramammary Paget's disease with 5% imiquimod cream. *Dermatol Online J* 2006;12:22.
95. Cohen PR, Schulze KE, Tschen JA, et al. Treatment of extramammary Paget's disease with topical imiquimod cream: Case report and literature review. *South Med J* 2006;99:396-402.
96. Pantanowitz L, Dezube BJ. Advances in the pathobiology and treatment of Kaposi sarcoma. *Curr Opin Oncol* 2004; 16:443-449.
97. Noy A. Update in Kaposi sarcoma. *Curr Opin Oncol* 2003;15:379-381.
98. Rosen T. Diseases more often seen in blacks: Kaposi's sarcoma, in *Clinical Dermatology in Black Patients.* Bari, Italy, PiGreco Press,1995, pp 90-92.
99. Micali G, Nasca MR, Pasquale RD, Innocenzi D. Primary classic Kaposi's sarcoma of the penis: Report of a case and review. *J Eur Acad Dermatol Venereol* 2003;17:320-323.
100. Rosen T, Hoffman J, Jones A. Penile Kaposi's sarcoma. *J Eur Acad Dermatol Venereol* 1999;13:71-73.
101. Lynch PJ. Lichen simplex chronicus (atopic/neurodermatitis) of the anogenital region. *Dermatol Ther* 2004;17:8-19.
102. Bircher AJ, Hirsbrunner P, Langauer S. Allergic contact dermatitis of the genitals from rubber additives in condoms. *Contact Dermatitis* 1993;28:125-126.
103. Foti C, Bonamonte D, Antelmi A, et al. Allergic contact dermatitis to condoms: Description of a clinical case and analytical review of current literature. *Immunopharmacol Immunotoxicol* 2004;26: 481-485.
104. Kugler K, Brinkmeier T, Frosch PJ, Uter W. Anogenital dermatoses: Allergic and irritative causative factors. Analysis of IVDK data and review of the literature. *J Dtsch Dermatol Ges* 2005;3: 979-986.
105. Rosen T, Conrad N. Genital ulcer caused by human bite to the penis. *Sex Transm Dis* 1999;26:527-530.
106. Rosen T. Penile ulcer from traumatic orogenital contact. *Dermatol Online J* 2005;11:18.

CHAPTER 56

Genital Lesions in Women

Christy B. Doherty
Ted Rosen

Key Points

- Genital lesions are difficult to diagnose based solely on morphology.
- The physician may need to perform additional studies including biopsies when evaluating genital lesions.
- Genital dermatoses may occur only on the genitals or may occur anywhere on the body, and lesions may have a different appearance when found on genital skin than when seen elsewhere on the body.
- Genital lesions may have a unique appearance in skin of color, and the appearance may vary between men and women.

INFECTIOUS DISEASES

Sexually Transmitted Infections

SYPHILIS

Epidemiology, Etiology, and Pathogenesis
Syphilis primarily affects young adults of both sexes. After the rate of syphilis dropped to the lowest reported rate of 2.1 cases per 100,000 population in 2000, the primary and secondary syphilis rate increased to 2.7 between 2001 and 2004.[1] From 2000–2004, overall rates of primary and secondary syphilis were higher among blacks and Hispanics than among whites, although rates decreased among black females.[1] Syphilis is caused by the bacterial spirochete *Treponema pallidum* and is transmitted via sexual contact, likely by inoculation into tiny abrasions from sexual trauma.[2] After spread to the regional lymph nodes, treponemes spread via a hematogenous route to other parts of the body.

Clinical Findings The primary lesion of syphilis is a solitary, painless ulcer (chancre) that develops in the genital area approximately 9–90 days after sexual contact with an infected individual.[3] The labia major and the perineal skin just adjacent to the vaginal orifice are the most frequent sites affected (Figure 56-1). Most women are unaware of the primary chancre.[4] Cervical, anal, and oral lesions are possible, although extragenital chancres are apparently less common in black patients.[3] One to two months after the chancre disappears, secondary syphilis presents with a generalized papulosquamous rash involving the palms, soles, trunk, face, and genitalia with or without concomitant lymphadenopathy, patchy alopecia, condyloma lata (exudative anogenital plaques), and/or mucous patches in the form of grayish white round papules and thin plaques in the mouth and on the vulvar and perineal area. Black patients, especially black women, are reportedly more likely to develop condyloma lata in secondary syphilis than whites.[3] The annular syphilid (round facial lesions located near orifices) is nearly unique to black patients[3] (Figure 56-2).

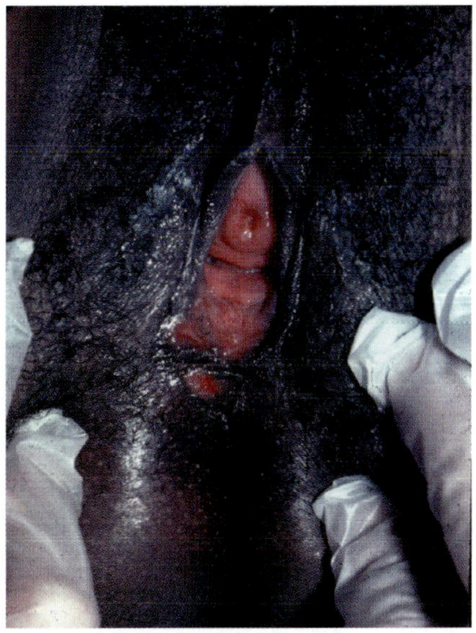

▲ **FIGURE 56-1** Solitary chancre of primary syphilis.

Diagnosis may be made by identification of treponemes using dark-field microscopy of samples from primary chancre, condyloma lata, genital mucosal lesions, skin papules, or lymph node aspirate.[2] Using specific treponemal fluorescent antibody stains or silver stains (i.e., Warthin-Starry stain), organisms may be detectable in biopsy specimens. However, silver also stains melanin, complicating interpretation of black skin biopsies.[3] Serologic tests available for confirmation are nontreponemal cardiolipin–based, such as the rapid plasma reagin (RPR) and the Venereal Disease Research Laboratory

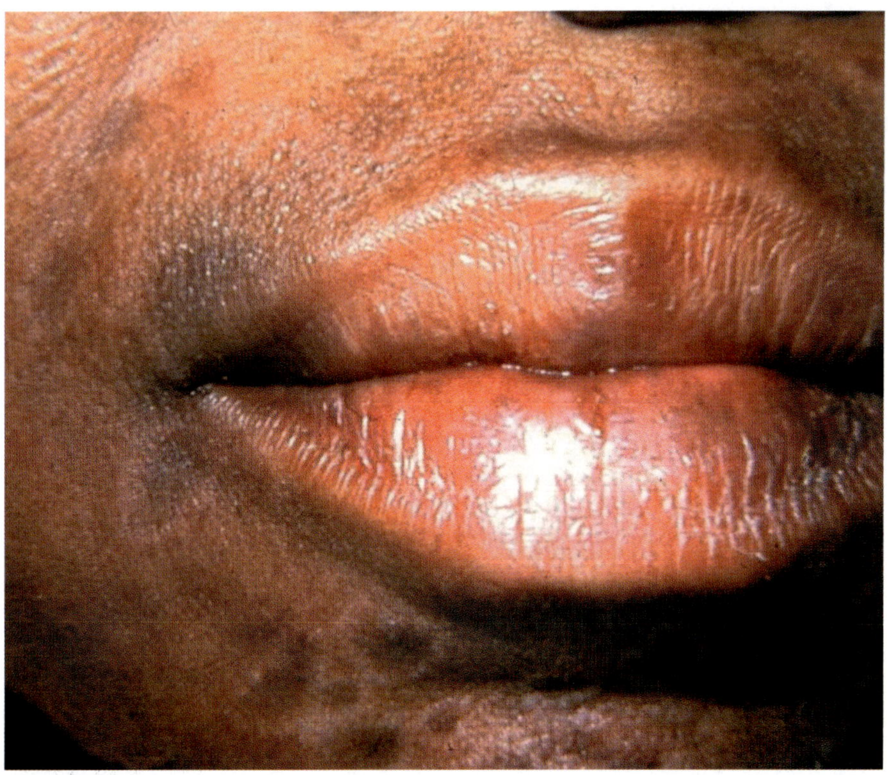

▲ **FIGURE 56-2** Perioral annular syphilids (secondary lues).

TABLE 56-1
Treatments for Syphilis (Systemic)

First line	Benzathine penicillin G	Duration <1 year: 50,000 units/kg IM up to 2.4 million units Duration >1 year or unknown: 50,000 units/kg IM up to 2.4 million units weekly for 3 weeks
Second line (penicillin allergy)	Doxycycline	100 mg PO bid for 14 days
	Tetracycline	500 mg qd for 14 days
	Erythromycin	500 mg qd for 14 days

(VDRL) test, or treponemal antigen–based such as the *T. pallidum* particle agglutination (TPPA) or hemaglutination (TPHA) and fluorescent antibody absorption (FTA-abs) tests. A new diagnosis of syphilis mandates investigation for concomitant human immunodeficiency virus (HIV) infection.

Differential Diagnosis

- Behçet syndrome
- Chancroid
- Condyloma acuminata (external genital warts)
- Fixed drug eruption (secondary syphilis)
- Granuloma inguinale
- Herpes progenitalis (genital herpes)
- Lichen planus (secondary syphilis)
- Lymphogranuloma venereum
- Psoriasis (secondary syphilis)
- Traumatic ulcer

Complications Tertiary syphilis is characterized by destructive gummas, manifesting dermatologically as heavily crusted granulomatous lesions of the skin. Neurologic and cardiovascular structures are vulnerable to gummatous syphilis as well.

Prognosis/Clinical Course Failure to receive adequate treatment at any stage of syphilis may result in the development of subsequent stages of the disease. However, adequate treatment of primary, secondary, or early latent infectious syphilis should result in disappearance of the clinical manifestations of active disease, although residual postinflammatory hyperpigmentation is possible in dark skin. The titer of RPR or VLDL and the clinical symptoms must be followed after treatment to verify therapeutic efficacy. The treatments for syphilis are outlined in Table 56-1.

Prevention Syphilis is spread via sexual contact. Avoidance of sex with infected individuals or the use of barrier protection (e.g., condoms) that cover the primary chancre should prevent transmission.

CHANCROID

Epidemiology, Etiology, and Pathogenesis

Hacinophilus ducreyl, the causative organism of chancroid, likely gains entry into the host skin via epidermal microabrasions that accompany sexual intercourse.[5] *H. ducreyi* is endemic in regions of Africa, Asia, and Latin America, but infection is limited primarily to sporadic outbreaks in industrialized nations.[6] In the United States, *H. ducreyi* infection is reportedly more common among African-American and Hispanic men than in other ethnic groups. Reported male-to-female ratios range from 3:1 to 50:1.[7] Undetected lesions within the vagina or on the cervix of women in part may explain the discrepancy in prevalence between men and women. It also has been proposed that women resolve their initial lesions more frequently than men.[6]

Clinical Findings The first sign of chancroid is a papule on the vulva, posterior commissure, cervix, or perianal area that develops 3–14 days after contact with an infected individual. The papule evolves into a pustule that ultimately ulcerates. The subsequent ulcer is painful with a ragged border and a grayish surface. Multiple ulcers may develop as a result of autoinoculation.[8] Although more prevalent in men, a painful unilateral inguinal lymphadenitis may occur 1–2 weeks later, and the lymph nodes may develop into draining buboes.[5]

Diagnosis is made primarily by clinical presentation, but confirmation is achieved with the culturing recovery of causative organisms on enriched gonococcal agar and Mueller-Hinton agar (under conditions of high humidity and low oxygen tension).[9] The most sensitive and specific modality is multiplex polymerase chain reaction (PCR).[6] Chancroid is associated with an increased occurrence and transmission rate of HIV.

Differential Diagnosis

- Aphthous ulcers
- Behçet disease
- Factitial ulceration
- Granuloma inguinale
- Herpes progenitalis
- Lymphogranuloma venereum
- Metastatic (extraintestinal) Crohn disease
- Squamous cell carcinoma
- Syphilis
- Traumatic ulceration

Complications Further ulceration secondary to bacterial superinfection is possible.[5] Additionally, incision and drainage of fluctuant, enlarged lymph nodes may result in chronic sinus formation. Therefore, needle aspiration is the preferred treatment for fluctuant or enlarged nodes.

Prognosis/Clinical Course If left untreated, chancroid ulcers heal spontaneously after 2 or more months, typically with scar formation. With appropriate antibiotic management, ulcers resolve in approximately 10 days without scarring. Reinfection with *H. ducreyi* occurs easily because prior infection produces no protective immunity.[4] Table 56-2 outlines the treatments for chancroid.

Prevention As with other ulcerative genital lesions transmitted through sexual contact, condom use should prevent

TABLE 56-2
Treatments for Chancroid

	Physical	Systemic
First line	Aspirate large, fluctuant nodes	Erythromycin 500 mg PO qid × 7 days
Second line		Azithromycin 1 g PO, single dose Ceftriaxone 250 mg IM, single dose Ciprofloxazcin 500 mg PO bid × 3 days

transmission if the infectious lesion is covered. Distributing condoms, educating the public, and giving empirical treatment to high-risk individuals have helped to decrease chancroid rates in endemic areas that have employed such measures.[6]

GRANULOMA INGUINALE

Epidemiology, Etiology, and Pathogenesis

Granuloma inguinale, also known as *donovanosis,* is caused by infection with an encapsulated gram-negative rod called *Calymmatobacterium granulomatosis*. Transmission is most likely due to sexual contact,[10] and infection is seen predominately in sexually active individuals aged 18 to 40 with a 3:1 male predominance.[11] This infection is endemic in New Guinea, Africa, Australia, and areas of India, China, and the Caribbean basin but rare in the United States.[12] Owing to the natural geographic distribution of donovanosis, it is more likely to be encountered among those who fall into the skin of color category.

Clinical Findings After a variable incubation period from 2 weeks to 6 months, granuloma inguinale begins as single or multiple nodules that erode to become well-defined, painless, friable ulcerations with a rolled border.[10] As lesions extend to involve normal surrounding skin, the ulcer base develops a beefy red color that resembles granulation tissue.[11] Despite ulceration, the lesions tend to be painless, and regional adenopathy is not a feature of this disorder. The most commonly affected sites in females are the labia minora and perigenital area, although infection also may involve the cervix, uterus, and adnexa (Figure 56-3). Diagnosis is based on the demonstration of *Donovan bodies* (intracellular bipolar-staining bacteria within histiocytes) with Giemsa, Wright's, or silver stains performed on tissue crush preparations or biopsy specimens obtained from the leading edge of the ulcer. Culture is impractical.

Differential Diagnosis

- Behçet syndrome
- Chancroid
- Condyloma acuminatum (external genital warts)
- Condyloma lata
- Deep mycosis
- Herpes progenitalis
- Leishmaniasis (rare on genitalia)
- Lymphogranuloma venereum
- Squamous cell carcinoma

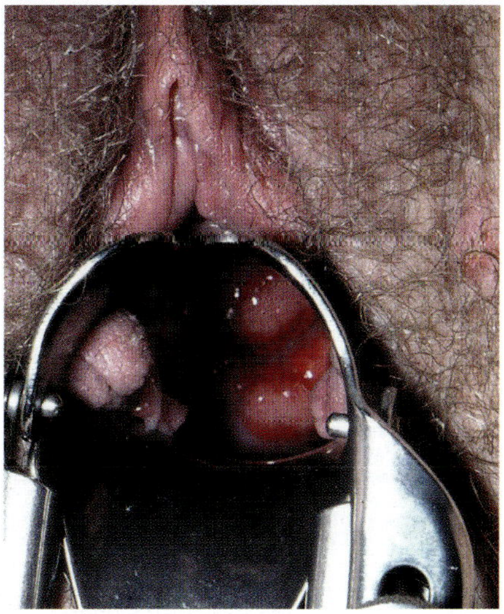

▲ **FIGURE 56-3** Cervical lesions of donovanosis.

- Syphilis
- Tuberculosis of the skin

Complications With extensive and deep ulceration and necrosis of soft tissues, fistulas may form.[10] Mutilating genital destruction may eventuate in untreated disease. There is a small but real increased incidence of squamous cell carcinoma of affected genital skin.

Prognosis/Clinical Course Lesions may stabilize but will not remit independent of treatment. Prolonged therapy may be necessary to allow for complete healing.[12] Table 56-3 lists treatment options.

Prevention Improved screening and treatment campaigns in endemic areas have helped to decrease disease incidence. To help prevent disease spread, education regarding safe sex practices is recommended.[13]

LYMPHOGRANULOMA VENEREUM

Epidemiology, Etiology, and Pathogenesis

Lymphogranuloma venereum (LGV), a sexually transmitted infection caused by *Chlamydia trachomatis* (serotypes L1, L2, and L3), is more common in tropical and subtropical regions but does occur in low incidence throughout the Western world.[12] The vast majority of new cases reportedly occur among men.

Clinical Findings The primary stage of LGV may go unnoticed by the infected individual and consists of a relatively small, painless ulcer or abrasion in the genital area. Physical examination during this stage may reveal small erosions or ulcers around the clitoris, vulvar introitus, or vaginal wall. From 1–4 weeks later, the secondary stage occurs and consists of cervicitis or salpingitis with tender lymphadenopathy, accompanied by fever, malaise, headache, arthralgia, and nausea. Pelvic or abdominal pain may mimic an intraabdominal abscess, endometriosis, or a ruptured ovarian cyst. Enlarged lymph nodes are more commonly perirectal or pelvic in women, as opposed to inguinal as in men. In women, LGV typically results in genital edema and elephantiasis-like enlargement owing to lymphatic disruption.

Culturing purulent aspirate from enlarged nodes should be diagnostic. Smears stained with Giemsa or fuchsin stain may reveal the intracellular corpuscles of Gamma-Miyasaki.[10] Both of these diagnostic maneuvers are easier in men. Serologic tests may confirm the diagnosis because an LGV complement-fixation test should demonstrate a titer of greater than 1:64 in active disease.[4]

Differential Diagnosis

- Chancroid
- Herpes simplex
- Hodgkin disease
- Syphilis
- Ganglionic tuberculosis

Complications If enlarged perirectal lymph nodes break down or rupture, individuals may develop rectovaginal fistulas, rectitis, tenesmus, and mucosanguineous rectal discharge.[4,10] Fluctuant nodes should not be incised

TABLE 56-3
Treatments for Granuloma Inguinale (Systemic)

First line	Doxycycline	100 mg orally twice a day for at least 3 weeks
	Trimethoprim-sulfamethoxazole	800 mg/160 mg orally twice a day for at least 3 weeks
	Azithromycin	1 g orally once a week for 3 weeks
Second line	Ciprofloxacin	750 mg orally twice a day for at least 3 weeks
	Erythromycin (pregnancy)	500 mg orally four times daily for at least 3 weeks

TABLE 56-4
Treatments for Lymphogranuloma Venereum

	Physical	Systemic	
First line	Aspirate fluctuant nodes	Doxycycline	100 mg orally two times a day for 3 weeks
Second line		Tetracycline	500 mg orally four times a day for 3 weeks
		Erythromycin	500 mg orally four times a day for 3 weeks

because incision may result in fistula formation.

Prognosis/Clinical Course In the absence of treatment, LGV likely *will* pass through all stages of disease and may result in any of the complications discussed earlier. Table 56-4 discusses treatment modalities.

Prevention The transmission of *Chlamydia* serotypes that result in LGV may be prevented though use of condoms.

HERPES

Epidemiology, Etiology, and Pathogenesis

Herpes simplex virus (HSV) is a sexually transmitted infection that enters the body through the skin or mucous membranes via direct sexual contact with the secretions or mucosal surfaces of an infected individual.[14] After multiplying initially in the epithelial layer, the virus travels in the sensory nerve roots to the dorsal root ganglion, where it becomes latent. Mucocutaneous outbreaks of HSV are triggered by the reactivation of latent virus, which subsequently travels back down the nerve root. HSV type 2 (HSV-2) is more commonly causative in cases of genital herpes, as opposed to HSV type 1 (HSV-1), which is more closely associated with herpes labialis.

Genital herpes is a prevalent infection, with approximately 50 million Americans infected and 500,000–700,000 new infections per year.[14] HSV-2 seropositivity appears to be higher among black individuals in the United States than among whites and more prevalent among women than among men, reflecting the greater ease of transmission from men to their female partners.[15,16]

Clinical Findings After an incubation period of 2–20 days (average 7 days), primary lesions develop, consisting of painful, grouped vesicles that ultimately rupture to become painful ulcers[4] (Figure 56-4). In women, ulcers may appear on the introitus, urethral meatus, labia, and perineum.[14] Women typically are afflicted with more severe disease, systemic symptoms, and complications than men. Particularly with the initial outbreak, cervical ulcerative lesions are possible. Additionally, women may complain of dysuria and urinary retention secondary to urethral lesions. Recurrent HSV outbreaks typically are milder than the initial outbreak, and women reportedly have fewer recurrences than men.

While the diagnosis of genital herpes is largely clinical, it may be confirmed using viral culture, a Tzanck smear (showing viral acantholytic giant cells), a PCR test for HSV DNA, or characteristic histopathology.

Differential Diagnosis

- Aphthous ulcers
- Behçet disease
- Chancroid
- Granuloma inguinale
- Lymphogranuloma venereum
- Pemphigus vulgaris or vegetans
- Syphilis
- Trauma

Complications Women are more susceptible to systemic complications, such as aseptic meningitis.[14] Perhaps the most dreaded complication is transmission to a neonate owing to viral shedding in the genital tract during normal vaginal delivery. The risk of neonatal herpes is greatest when a woman has acquired the disease during gestation and has active lesions at the time of delivery (risk of neonatal herpes about 50%). Conversely, the risk is lowest when the disease is long-standing and there are no active lesions at the time of delivery (risk of neonatal herpes about 0.04%).

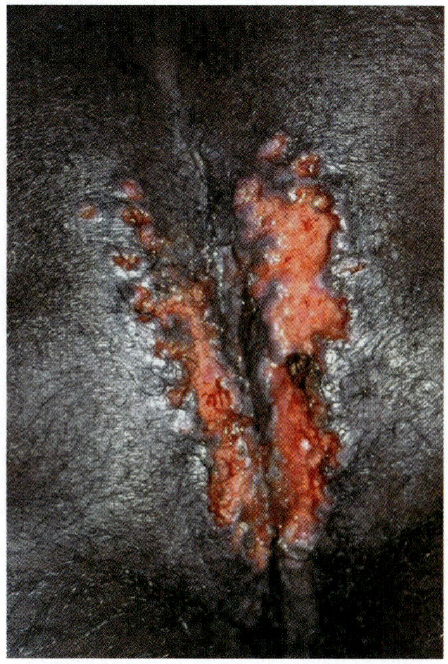

▲ **FIGURE 56-4** Perianal HSV-2-related erosions acquired via receptive anal intercourse.

Prognosis/Clinical Course There is no cure for herpes, and recurrence of lesions is expected with an average of four outbreaks per year. Individuals who experience more severe primary infections appear to have recurrent episodes more frequently. Treatments for systemic genital herpes are outlined in Table 56-5.

Prevention Condom use has been shown to reduce HSV-2 acquisition rates in women but not in men.[14] In discordant couples (one partner with known genital herpes and the other without), chronic suppression with valacyclovir appears

TABLE 56-5
Treatments for Genital Herpes (Systemic)

First line	Acyclovir	Initial infect.	400 mg three times daily for 7–10 days
		Recurrence	400 mg three times daily for 5 days
		Suppressive	400 mg twice daily
	Famciclovir	Initial infect.	250 mg three times daily for 7–10 days
		Recurrence	125 mg twice daily for 5 days
		Suppressive	250 mg twice daily
	Valacyclovir	Initial infect.	1 g twice daily for 7–10 days
		Recurrence	500 mg twice daily for 3–5 days
		Suppressive	500 mg daily

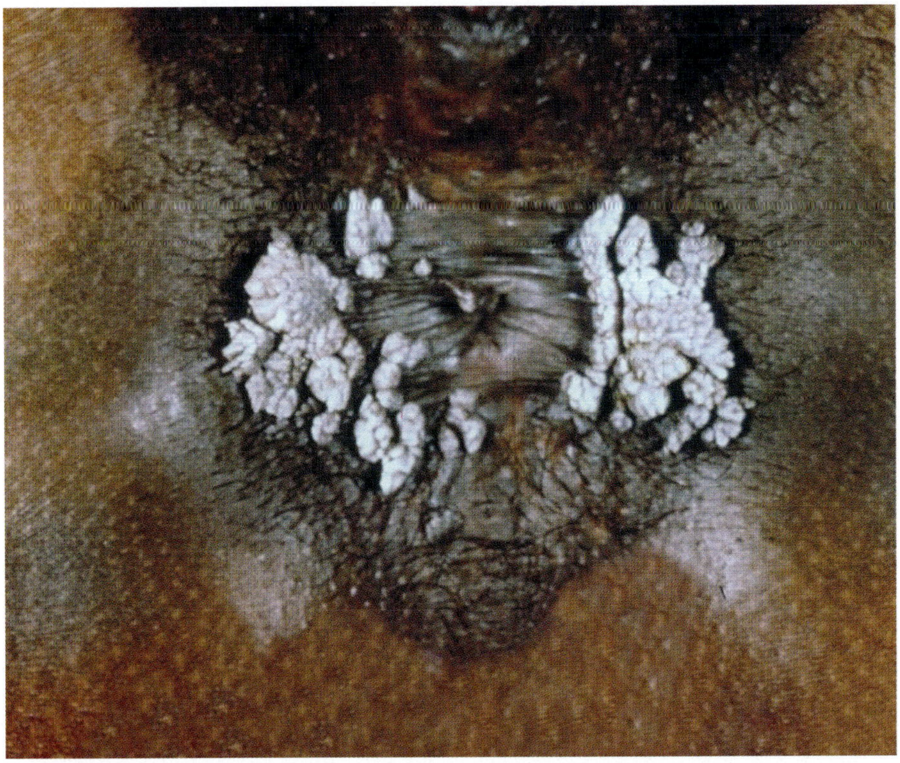

▲ **FIGURE 56-5** Aggregate cauliflower-shaped masses typical of anogenital warts.

beneficial in reduction of herpes transmission to the uninfected individual.[17] The use of suppressive antiviral medication during the third trimester of pregnancy appears to reduce overt active herpes and viral shedding at the time of delivery and therefore reduces the need for cesarean section and the risk of neonatal herpes.[18]

GENITAL WARTS (CONDYLOMA ACUMINATA)

Epidemiology, Etiology, and Pathogenesis Genital warts, or condyloma acuminata, are caused by human papillomavirus (HPV), most commonly types 6 and 11.[19] Transmission of the virus in most adults is primarily sexual. Seroprevalence suggest that 1% of sexually active American adults have visible genital warts, whereas at least 15% have subclinical infection.[20] Sexually active women under the age of 25 have the highest rates of genital HPV infection.

Clinical Findings Lesions typically develop 2–3 months after exposure and begin as small papules that may develop into skin-colored to reddish, filiform, asymptomatic papules. The skin around the vaginal introitus and perianal area is affected most commonly, but the cervix also may have lesions[19] (Figure 56-5). While genital warts are chiefly a clinical diagnosis, confirmation may be achieved though biopsy.

Differential Diagnosis

- Molluscum contagiosum
- Lichen planus
- Enlarged sebaceous glands
- Condyloma lata
- Vulvar intraepithelial neoplasia

Complications Invasive squamous cell carcinoma arising from long-standing genital warts is possible but rare.[21]

Prognosis/Clinical Course HPV infections tend to have a fluctuating clinical course of visible lesions, latency, and recurrence.[22] However, most clinically apparent lesions eventually resolve in several months to years.Treatments are outlined in Table 56-6.

Prevention Condoms may provide some protection against HPV infection, but the ability of condoms to prevent genital warts is not proven. Trials of a recently approved quadrivalent vaccine to HPV types 6, 11, 16, and 18 clearly demonstrate the vaccine's ability to prevent genital warts.[23]

MOLLUSCUM CONTAGIOSUM

Epidemiology, Etiology, and Pathogenesis Molluscum contagiosum, caused by a poxvirus [molluscum contagiosum virus (MCV)], is spread predominately though sexual contact in adults.[24] Infection is more prevalent in underdeveloped or tropical regions. The incidence of molluscum contagiosum, especially as a sexually transmitted disease, has increased over the past 30 years.[24]

Clinical Findings MCV lesions start few in number and then spread 2–7 weeks after initial exposure.[4] Patients may be asymptomatic or complain of mild pruritus. Physical examination reveals small, dome-shaped, umbilicated, discrete or grouped skin-colored papules in the suprapubic area or on upper inner thighs. Molluscum lesions are easily diagnosed by clinical appearance, but histopathogic examination can confirm the diagnosis by demonstrating characteristic large intracytoplasmic inclusion bodies.[24,25]

TABLE 56-6
Treatments for Genital Warts

		Patient-Applied		Physician-Applied		Physical
First line	Imiquimod	Apply at bedtime 3 times a week for up to 16 weeks				
Second line	Podofilox	Apply twice daily for 3 days and then rest for 4 days; may repeat for 4 cycles		Podophyllin resin	Apply once a week if necessary	Cryotherapy Laser ablation Surgical excision Electrodesiccation
				Trichloroacetic acid	Apply once a week if necessary	

TABLE 56-7
Treatments for Molluscum Contagiosum

		Topical	Physical	Systemic	
First line	Trichloroacetic acid	Apply once in office	Curettage Cryotherapy CO_2 laser Electrodesiccation		
	Cantharadin	Apply once a week			
	Podophyllin	Apply once a week			
	Potassium hydroxide	Twice daily until inflammation develops			
Second line	Tretinoin 0.1% cream	Apply once a week		Cimetidine	40 mg/kg per day in 2 divided doses for 2 months
	KOH 10% aqueous solution	Apply twice daily			
	Imiquimod	Apply daily for 4 weeks or until clear			

Differential Diagnosis

- Condyloma acuminata
- Cutaneous cryptococcosis (HIV+)
- Epidermal inclusion cyst
- Herpes simplex or zoster
- Lichen planus
- Papular granuloma annulare
- Vestibular papillomas

Complications The development of eczematous dermatitis around MCV lesions is possible, as is disseminated eruption in patients with a history of atopic dermatitis. HIV-positive patients may present atypically large MCV lesions that are resistant to treatment.

Prognosis/Clinical Course In immune-competent hosts, MCV follows a self-limited course, typically clearing spontaneously within a few months.[25] Table 56-7 outlines the treatment options for molluscum contagiosum.

Prevention Barrier protection may prevent transmission only if all lesions are covered. Close contact with MCV lesions should be avoided.

Non-Sexually-Transmitted Infections

TINEA CRURIS

Epidemiology, Etiology, and Pathogenesis Tinea cruris ("ringworm") is caused most commonly by *Trichophyton umbrum,* the same organism responsible for most cases of tinea corporis.[26] This condition is less common in women than in men and typically affects young adults.[4] Infection can be spread via sexual contact with infected skin or through autoinoculation from tinea pedis by shaving upward toward the bikini line.

Clinical Findings A pruritic, erythematous, scaling rash develops over weeks that involves any area from the proximal inner thigh area to the crural crease. In women, the rash has a propensity to involve the hair-bearing portion of the vulva. Patients with black skin may present with striking hyperpigmentation instead of erythema (Figure 56-6). A peripheral border with overlying scale lends to an annular appearance, but it is not always present. Feet also should be examined because concurrent onychomycosis is often present.

Tinea cruris may be diagnosed clinically, but the diagnosis can be confirmed by potassium hydroxide (KOH) examination or fungal culture of peripheral scale. Care should be taken to distinguish tinea from candidiasis. Whereas tinea cruris tends to have annular lesions with central clearing and no satellite lesions, candidiasis presents with confluent erythema and satellite pustules.

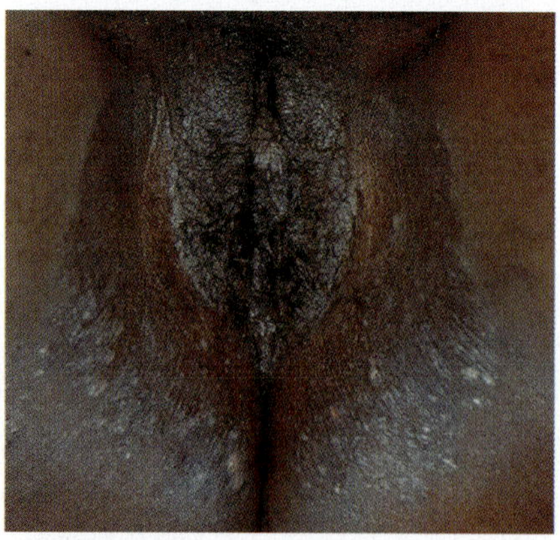

▲ **FIGURE 56-6** Hyperpigmented, scaly patch of tinea cruris.

Differential Diagnosis

- Candidiasis
- Contact dermatitis
- Erythrasma
- Neurodermatitis
- Psoriasis
- Tinea versicolor (rarely affects genital skin)

Complications Follicular or extensive involvement makes the infection more difficult to clear.

Prognosis/Clinical Course Affected individuals are at elevated risk for recurrence, although infections may be eradicated temporarily with therapy. Ongoing intermittent therapy with topical antifungals may be indicated to prevent return of infection.[27] Table 56-8 outlines treatment options.

Prevention To prevent transmission, women should be advised to use separate razors to shave the lower extremities and bikini area. Patient education about hygiene may help to prevent infection because excessive moisture and synthetic clothing may predispose to tinea cruris.[26]

CANDIDA

Epidemiology, Etiology, and Pathogenesis Candidiasis is a mucocutaneous yeast infection found commonly in women, particularly immunocompromised individuals. Most infections are due to *Candida albicans,* an organism found in the vagina and gastrointestinal tract of healthy women, that becomes pathogenic under the influence of factors such as medication (e.g., antibiotics, corticosteroids, and chemotherapy), disease

TABLE 56-8
Treatments for Tinea Cruris

	Topical	Systemic	
First line	Terbinafine 1% cream	Terbinafine	250 mg orally daily for 2 weeks
	Naftifine 1% cream/gel		
Second line	Clotrimazole 1% cream	Itraconazole	100 mg orally daily for 2–4 weeks or
	Econazole 1% cream		200 mg orally daily for 1 week
	Ketoconazole 2% cream	Fluconazole	150 mg orally once weekly for 2–4 weeks
	Miconazole 2% cream		
	Oxiconazole 1% cream	Ketoconazole	200 mg orally daily for 1–2 months
	Sulconazole 1% cream	Griseofulvin	500 mg orally each day for 2–4 weeks
	Butenafine 1% cream		
	Ciclopirox 0.77% cream/gel		

(e.g., diabetes and immunodeficiency), and hormones (e.g., pregnancy and birth control pills). The source of infection may be a sexual partner.

Clinical Finding Women may develop candidal vaginitis, vulvitis, or vulvovaginitis, with presenting symptoms being moderate to severe itching or burning and a varying amount of curd-like vaginal discharge. Inflammation with satellite pustules may be seen within the vestibule, in the interlabial crease, and over the labia minora and majora. If infection is more severe, inflammation may be found in the crural fold and on the upper inner thigh (Figure 56-7). Vulvar edema, at times severe, may be present. Diagnosis is clinical, with confirmation via culture and/or potassium hydroxide wet mount.

Differential Diagnosis

- Contact dermatitis
- Darier disease
- Eczema
- Hailey-Hailey disease
- Lichen simplex chronicus
- Psoriasis
- Seborrheic dermatitis
- Tinea cruris
- Vulvar vestibulitis

Complications In patients with persistent infection, constant scratching may lead to secondary lichenification, excoriation, and chronic swelling that resembles lichen simplex chronicus or chronic contact dermatitis.[4] In severe infections, particularly those seen in immunocompromised patients, erosions may complicate the disease course.

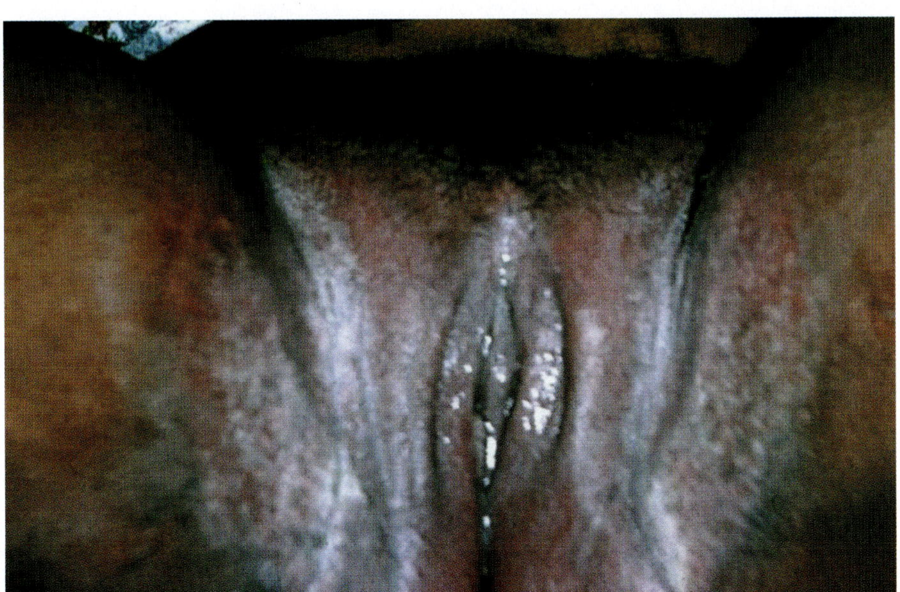

▲ **FIGURE 56-7** Erythema and edema extending from vulva to inner thigh in severe *Candida* infection.

Prognosis/Clinical Course In most cases, treatment is necessary to clear infection. Women with vulvovaginitis are susceptible to recurrence because *Candida* is a normal inhabitant of the gastrointestinal tract and vagina. Frequently recurrent or chronic vaginal candidiasis is a common problem, and there is no simple remedy.[28] Several different treatment strategies have been employed, such as continuous or intermittent suppressive therapy with oral or topical antifungals. However, long-term studies evaluating such protocols are not available. It is important that women with recurrent symptoms be evaluated for bacterial vaginosis, *Trichomonas* infection, and infection with a non-*albicans Candida* species because all mentioned conditions will not respond well to conventional treatment. Table 56-9 outlines treatment options.

Prevention Preventative measures include practicing good hygiene, keeping the skin dry and cool, wearing loose-fitting clothing, and avoiding sharing towels or clothing with infected individuals. If suppressive therapy does not prevent recurrences, removing copper-bearing intrauterine devices (IUDs) may be of assistance.[4,28]

AMEBIASIS

Epidemiology, Etiology, and Pathogenesis Amebiasis is classically a gastrointestinal disease caused by *Entamoeba histolytica* with a worldwide distribution and an increased prevalence in the tropics.[29] In the United States, almost all cases are seen among immigrant populations from Asia, Africa, and Central and South America. Genital amebiasis is a rare manifestation of infection. Genital amebiasis is reportedly more common in women than in men. Transmission to women is proposed to be via anal and vaginal intercourse with partners who have active genital lesions. Additionally in women, genital amebiasis may be due to autoinoculation from an infected gastrointestinal tract.[30]

Clinical Findings Women with genital amebiasis commonly present with foul-smelling bloody vaginal discharge and abdominal pain.[29] Less common clinical manifestations include painful ulcerative genital lesions and weight loss. Diagnosis is made by direct smear (Papanicolaou smear) in the majority of patients or via biopsy of ulcerative lesions, if present.

TABLE 56-9
Treatments for Vulvar/Crural *Candida*

	Topical		Systemic*	
First line	Clotrimazole 1%	Apply bid for 7–10 days	Itraconazole	200 mg daily for 3–5 days
	Miconazole 2%	Apply bid for 7–10 days		
	Nystatin 100,000 units/g	Apply bid for 7–10 days	Fluconazole	150 mg daily for 1–3 days
	Ketoconazole 2%	Apply bid for 7–10 days		
	Ciclopirox 0.77%	Apply bid for 7–14 days		

*Pregnant patients should receive topical therapy only.[4]

Superficial necrosis with trophozoites should be present.

Differential Diagnosis

- Behçet syndrome
- Chancroid
- Granuloma inguinale
- Primary syphilis
- Squamous cell carcinoma

Complications For reasons not completely understood, there appears to be an association between genital amebiasis and genital tract cancer, such as squamous cell carcinoma of the vulva or cervix.[29] It is theorized that *E. histolytica* trophozoites causes disruption of the genital epithelium with subsequent invasion of cancer cells.

Prognosis/Clinical Course Medical treatment is almost completely effective, but disease may progress to produce genital mutilation if left untreated.[29,30] Surgery may be indicated to treat coexistent carcinoma or deformity. Table 56-10 lists treatment options.

Prevention Prevention includes limiting the number of sexual partners, condom use, prompt treatment of intestinal amebiasis, and prevention of intestinal amebiasis though improved sanitation practices.

LEISHMANIASIS

Epidemiology, Etiology, and Pathogenesis Cutaneous leishmaniasis is a disease caused by various species of intracellular parasites transmitted to humans following the bite of a vector female sandfly. The disease occurs throughout the southern portion of the western hemisphere, from Texas to Argentina, and in the old world, particularly the Middle East and North Africa.[31] Each year in the United States, approximately 50–100 cases are diagnosed, although this number has been rising owing to the deployment of civilian and military personnel to the Middle East. Genital leishmaniasis is exceeding rare in women, with one reported case of vulvar involvement.[32] Genital infection is thought to occur from an insect bite on the genitalia, but disease may be transmissible via contact with oozing skin lesions on a sexual partner.

Clinical Findings. Following a sandfly bite, the area of involved skin develops an erythematous papule that increases in size to become a nodule. Eventually, the nodule ulcerates, and the subsequent ulcer becomes crusted with a raised, distinct border. Unless there is secondary bacterial infection, the ulcer is typically painless. A depressed scar remains after lesional healing. Diagnosis is conformed via demonstration of *Leishmania* amastigotes in smear or biopsy material.[33]

Differential Diagnosis

- Behçet syndrome
- Chancroid
- Granuloma inginale
- Primary syphilis
- Squamous cell carcinoma

Complications Genital deformity is possible with large untreated lesions.

Prognosis/Clinical Course *Leishmania tropica, L. major* (the causative organisms for old world leishmaniasis) and *L. mexicana,* which is found in Latin America and the United States, result in lesions that tend to heal spontaneously in months.[31,34] However, *L. braziliensis,* which is also found in Latin America and the United States, may produce ulcerations that take years to heal. Treatment options are listed in Table 56-11.

Prevention The use of insecticides and repellants appears to decrease the transmission rate of leishmaniasis.

INFLAMMATORY DISEASES

Papulosquamous

PSORIASIS

Epidemiology, Etiology, and Pathogenesis Psoriasis is a common hereditary papulosquamous skin eruption whose exact etiology is unknown. It is currently felt that psoriasis is due to an aberrant immune response to an unidentified antigen. Lesions are susceptible to koebnerization because they may appear or worsen as a result of trauma. While psoriasis is less common in blacks, it is seen in about 0.1% of American and West African blacks compared with the 1% incidence among white Americans and 1.5% incidence among Europeans.[35] Interestingly, the incidence among East Africans is about 1.4%.

Clinical Findings While psoriasis is classically characterized by well-defined, reddish plaques and papules with silvery scale, psoriasis in black patients may present as minimally scaly, flattened plaques with a bluish black discoloration.[35] Additionally, psoriasis involving the inguinal or crural areas, called *psoriasis inversus* or *flexural psoriasis,* may be missing the characteristic scale. Inverse psoriasis typically appears bilaterally symmetric with erythema, maceration, and fissuring extending in a linear fashion from the inguinal crease into the gluteal cleft. Vulvar psoriasis is often associated with irritation or pruritus, and lesions may appear without a history of psoriasis in more classic locations (e.g., scalp, extensor surfaces, nails, etc.). Mucosal areas of the vulva are not involved. Secondary changes such as excoriations, lichenification, and bacterial or yeast infection may confuse the

TABLE 56-10
Treatments for Amebiasis (Systemic)

First line	Metronidazole	800 mg orally three times per day for 5 days
Second line	Iodoquinol	650 mg orally three times per day for 20 days
	Hydrochloric emetine	1 mg/kg/day (max 60 mg) IM for 5 days

TABLE 56-11
Treatments for Leishmaniasis

	Topical		Physical	Systemic	
First line	Leshcutan ointment (15% paromomycin sulfate and 12% methylbenzethonium chloride in soft white paraffin)	Twice daily × 10 days	Cryotherapy Thermotherapy	Sodium stibogluconate*	20 mg/kg per day for 20 days
Second line				Amphotericin B	0.5–1.0 mg/kg every other day for up to 8 weeks
				Fluconazole	200 mg/day for 6 weeks
				Allopurinol	Various regimens
				Dapsone	
				Itraconazole	
				Ketoconazole	
				Pentamidine	

*Sodium stibogluconate, the antimonial agent used in the United States, must be obtained from the Centers for Disease Control and Prevention (CDC), which can counsel the physician in its use.

clinical appearance of psoriasis lesions. Diagnosis typically is based on clinical features, but biopsy may be necessary in patients who fall into the skin of color spectrum given the possibility for nondiagnostic lesional morphology.

Differential Diagnosis

- Bowen disease
- Candidiasis
- Contact dermatitis
- Drug eruptions
- Eczema, including atopic disease
- Lichen simplex chronicus
- Lichen planus
- Paget disease
- Seborrheic dermatitis
- Tinea cruris

Complications Areas of maceration where topical corticosteroids are used are susceptible to candidiasis or tinea cruris.[36] Psoriasis may be associated with comorbidities such as arthritis and clinical depression from cosmetic effects or symptomatology of the disease.[37] Additionally, individuals with psoriasis are thought to be at increased risk of lymphoma.

Prognosis/Clinical Course. Treatments for psoriasis are aimed at managing the disease because psoriasis is a chronic disease with no cure. The clinical course is typically waxing and waning in nature. Table 56-12 lists treatment options.

Some treatments are more appropriate for genital psoriasis. For example, delivery of ultraviolet (UV) light therapy would be difficult. Systemic biologic drugs would be reserved for more severe, generalized disease. Tazarotene and tar therapy likely would prove to be too irritating for the genital area.

Prevention Vulvar or surrounding psoriasis may be worsened with stress, heat, humidity, and the use of sanitary napkins, tight synthetic clothing, and irritating soaps. Therefore, avoidance of these triggers may help to prevent psoriatic exacerbations. Additionally, avoiding medications known to worsen psoriasis, such as systemic administration of lithium and beta-blockers, may help to prevent flares.

LICHEN PLANUS

Epidemiology, Etiology, and Pathogenesis Lichen planus (LP) is a papulosquamous

TABLE 56-12
Treatments for Psoriasis

	Topical		Physical		Systemic	
First line	Hydrocortisone 1–2.5%	Apply daily	UVB	TIW*	Methotrexate	10–25 mg PO/IM weekly
	Calcipotriene 0.005%	Apply twice daily	UVB narrow band	TIW	Cyclosporine	2.5–4.0 mg/kg per day bid divided dose
					Acitretin	25–50 mg daily
Second line	Anthralin 0.1% Coal tar 2% Tazarotene 0.05% Tacrolimus 0.1% ointment Pimecrolimus 1% cream	All are applied daily	PUVA	TIW	Alefacept	15 mg IM weekly
					Efalizumab	Initial dose 0.7 mg/kg SC; then 1 mg/ kg SC weekly
					Etanercept	50 mg SC twice per week for 3 months; then decrease to 50 mg SC per week
					Infliximab	3–10 mg/kg IV infusions at weeks 0, 2, 6, and 8

* TIW; Apply three times per week.

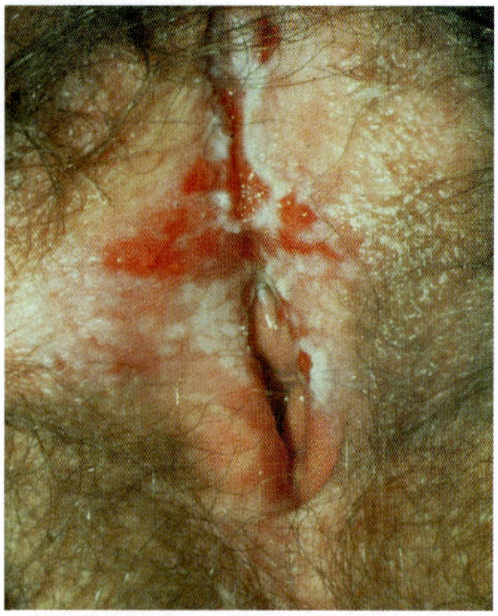

▲ **FIGURE 56-8** Erosive lichen planus resembles genital herpes. Image courtesy of Libby Edwards, M.D.

skin condition thought to be related to T-cell autoimmunity.[38] Vulvovaginal LP most commonly affects women of all ethnic backgrounds aged 30 to 60 years. Once thought to be an uncommon occurrence, genital LP is being diagnosed more frequently, especially in women, because more physicians are familiar with the entity and its wide morphologic range. Approximately 1% of the general population has oral LP; of women with oral LP, 20–25% also have genital disease.[39]

Clinical Findings Patients with genital LP may complain of severe pruritis and, if there is scanning, dyspareunia. Vulvar LP, particularly the erosive variant, typically is associated with inflammatory vaginitis, and patients may bleed during sexual intercourse or gynecologic examination and complain of purulent, irritating vaginal discharge.[38]

Genital LP lesions vary widely in morphology, but the most common and most difficult to treat is the erosive variant (Figure 56-8). Erosive LP occurs more often in women than in men and occurs on the moist skin of the vulva and within the vagina. The most common site to be affected by erosive lesions is the posterior vulvar vestibule, from which lesions extend to involve the labia minora. Patients also may exhibit superficial gingival erosions, termed *vulvovaginal-gingival syndrome.*

Vulvar LP, when associated with generalized LP, resembles the more classic violaceous, polygonal, papular or plaque morphology seen on extragenital skin and involves the labia or mons pubis.[40] In patients with black skin, classic lesions are typically deeper in color owing to the larger amount of melanin displaced from the epidermis.[39]

The least common form of vulvar LP is the hypertrophic variant, which presents with extensive white scarring of the periclitoral area that extends along the interlabial sulcus to the introitus. White hyperkeratotic papules may have classic-appearing reticulate surface markings.

Diagnosis is achieved through biopsy of a noneroded red or white macule or papule.[38] The edge of erosion should be taken when sampling such a lesion. Direct and indirect immunoflourescence can exclude an autoimmune blistering disorder.

Differential Diagnosis

Erosive disease

- Candidiasis
- Cicatricial pemphigoid
- Lichen sclerosus
- Lupus erythematosus
- Pemphigus vulgaris

Papulosquamous form

- Bowen disease
- Condyloma acuminata (genital warts)
- Erythema multiforme
- Fixed drug reaction
- Lichen sclerosus
- Lichen simplex chronicus
- Psoriasis
- Scabies
- Secondary syphilis

Complications With chronic erosive disease, inflamed and eroded surfaces may adhere and result in adhesions and disappearance of the normal external architecture, including loss of the labia minora, agglutination of the clitoral prepuce with covering of the clitoris under scar, and narrowing of the introitus.[40] Although uncommon, erosive LP of the mouth or vulva eventually may develop into squamous cell carcinoma (SCC).[38] SCC should be suspected in a chronic, indurated or granulated ulcer or in a white hyperkeratotic, poorly demarcated papule or plaque.

Prognosis/Clinical Course Nonerosive LP lesions may be well controlled with topical corticosteroids, and disease may remit spontaneously. Erosive disease tends to be chronic, recalcitrant, and scarring. The course of erosive LP is one of exacerbations with slow healing, recurrent secondary infections, and slow response to therapy. Table 56-13 lists treatment options.

TABLE 56-13
Treatments for Lichen Planus

	Topical		Systemic	
First line (nonerosive)	Triamcinolone 0.1%	Apply daily		
First line (erosive)	Fluocinonide 0.05%	Apply daily		
	Clobetasol propionate 0.05%	Apply daily		
	Tacrolimus ointment	Apply twice daily		
	Pimecrolimus cream	Apply twice daily		
First line (vaginal)	Hydrocortisone acetate 25-mg suppository	Insert into vagina daily for 1 month with gradual taper		
Second line			Prednisone	40–60 mg each morning for 2–4 weeks
			Hydroxychloroquine	200 mg bid
			Isotretinoin (?)	1 mg/kg daily

TABLE 56-14
Treatments for Lichen Sclerosus et Atrophicus

	Topical		Physical	Systemic	
First line	Triamcinolone 0.01% or clobetasol 0.05%	Daily to twice daily	Surgical lysis of scarring		
Second line	Tacrolimus 0.1%	Daily to twice daily		Etretinate	1 mg/kg/day
	Pimecrolimus 1%	Twice daily		Pentoxifylline	400 mg tid

Prevention Exacerbations of erosive disease may be mitigated by avoiding irritants and by wearing cool, ventilated clothing.

Nonpapulosquamous

LICHEN SCLEROSUS ET ATROPHICUS

Epidemiology, Etiology, and Pathogenesis Lichen sclerosus is a chronic inflammatory skin condition that most commonly affects middle-aged women.[41] Various studies give a female-to-male ratio that ranges from 6:1 to 10:1.[41] While the etiology is largely unknown, there appears to be a genetic susceptibility and a connection with autoimmune mechanisms. Lichen sclerosus is thought to exhibit the Koebner phenomenon such that trauma and injury may trigger symptoms in vulnerable individuals.

Clinical Findings Genital lesions may appear as a complete or incomplete "figure of eight" pattern of hypopigmentation around the vulva and anus, with patients complaining of intractable pruritus and soreness of the affected areas. Dysuria, dyspareunia, and pain with defecation are not uncommon. Skin changes include the development of areas of pallor ranging from small polygonal patches to large plaques, as well as atrophic, fragile skin with telangiectasias, purpura, erosions, and tender fissures. Biopsy is used to confirm the diagnosis of lichen sclerosus and to rule out malignant degeneration.

Differential Diagnosis

- Lichen planus (chronic)
- Morphea
- Postinflammatory dyschromia
- SCC in situ/vulvar intraepithelial neoplasia
- Vitiligo

Complications Scarring may disrupt the normal architecture of the genitalia.[41] The labia minora may fuse or be entirely resorbed, the clitoris may become buried, and the introitus may narrow. Additionally, approximately 3–5% of vulvar lichen sclerosus lesions progress to SCC.[41]

Prognosis/Clinical Course Individuals treated properly do well, often with cessation of symptoms and no further scarring. However, there is no reversal of existing scarring, and the disease does not remit permanently. Therefore, ongoing topical therapy generally is indicated to maintain control of disease. Surgery may be required to lyse scars that interfere with normal functioning. Based on recent reports, topical calcineurin inhibitors seem to be particularly effective in the management of LSA in women.[42–44] Table 56-14 lists treatment options.

Prevention Exacerbations may be preventable via the use of very mild cleansers, avoidance of strong detergents, use of ventilated cotton clothing, and use of a mild lubricant for sexual intercourse. On the other hand, the disease is quite unpredictable.

VULVITIS PLASMACELLULARIS

Epidemiology, Etiology, and Pathogenesis Vulvar plasmacellularis (VP) or vulvitis circumscripta plasmacellularis is a rare disorder, with fewer than 40 reported cases in the literature.[45] Most reported cases are among postmenopausal women. The etiology is unknown, but viral, hormonal, traumatic, and autoimmune etiologies have been proposed.[46]

Clinical Findings Patients typically present with a long-standing erythematous patch or an ulcerative lesion of the labia minora associated with burning and pruritus.[45] Lesions may appear as glistening (lacquer-like) brick red/orange macules with multiple pinpoint brighter red spots and clearly defined borders (cayenne pepper spots).[46] Symptoms are often present for years prior to presentation. Diagnosis is established via biopsy, with histologic examination revealing dense plasma cell infiltrate without other pathology. Negative syphilis serology should be confirmed.

Differential Diagnosis

- Allergic contact dermatitis
- Behçet syndrome
- Chancroid
- Fixed drug eruption
- Granuloma inguinale
- Herpes simplex
- Lichen planus
- Paget disease
- Pemphigus vulgaris
- Syphilis (primary)
- Trauma

Complications There is evidence for neither malignant degeneration nor other serious sequelae.

Prognosis/Clinical Course Lesions are known for being recalcitrant to treatment, but they typically resolve spontaneously over an extended period of time.[46] Therapy with potent topical steroids, topical cyclosporine, intralesional interferon-α, and imiquimod has been attempted (Table 56-15).

Prevention. Predisposing factors such as poor hygiene, heat, sweating, trauma, and constant friction should be avoided.

TABLE 56-15
Treatments for Vulvitis Plasmacellularis

	Topical		Physical
First line	Imiquimod	Apply TIW*	Surgical excision
	Betamethasone valerate	Apply daily	

*TIW, Three times per week.

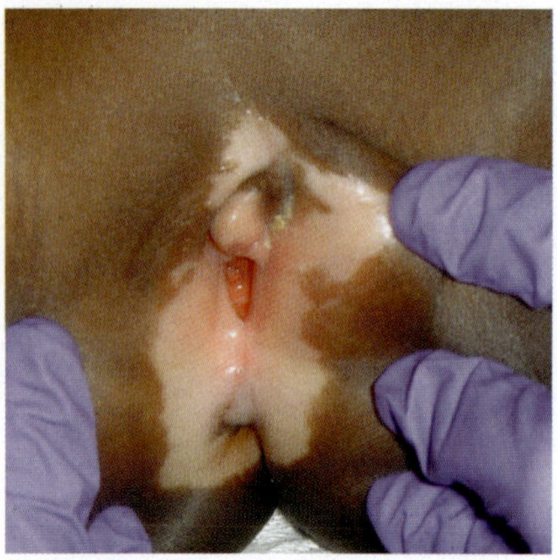

▲ **FIGURE 56-9** Genital vitiligo often begins at an early age, as in this patient. Image courtesy of Noah Scheinfeld, M.D.

VITILIGO

Epidemiology, Etiology, and Pathogenesis Vitiligo is an autoimmune disease of uncertain etiology that results in destruction of melanocytes; there are predisposing genetic loci explaining a familial predilection.[47] While there is no ethnic predilection, the disease is so obvious (and cosmetically distressing) in skin of color that more patients who fall into this category may seek medical attention. The vast majority of vitiligo patients relate on onset before age 40; men and women are at equal risk.

Clinical Findings Areas of depigmentation are apparent. The periorificial regions of the face and the dorsa of the hands and feet are frequent sites of initial involvement. The vulva is another favored area (Figure 56-9).

Differential Diagnosis

- Discoid lupus erythematosus
- Hansen disease (tuberculoid)
- Lichen sclerosus et atrophicus (most important)
- Postinflammatory dyschromia
- Seborrhea
- Tinea versicolor (rare on genital skin)

Complication Vitiligo itself poses no serious medical threat. However, thyroid dysfunction, pernicious anemia, and diabetes mellitus should be sought as potential comorbid conditions.[48]

Prognosis/Clinical Course The disease may resolve, persist, or expand. It is highly unpredictable.

Treatment A number of therapeutic modalities have been touted to induce repigmentation, but none is assured to succeed.[49] The likelihood of success is always better in recent-onset limited disease occurring in younger patients compared with widespread vitiligo of long duration in older individuals. Genital skin is particularly difficult to approach surgically (epidermal grafts and laser therapy) owing to the risk of scar induction.[50] Genital skin is also a suboptimal area for phototherapy owing to the concern about induction of neoplasia. Standard therapy for genital vitiligo consists of application of topical steroids and/or topical calcineurin inhibitors.[49] Vitiliginous genital skin has been restored recently following transfer of noncultured keratinocyte-melanocyte cell suspensions.[51] When therapy is unsuccessful, careful camouflage techniques may be considered, including therapeutic tattoo. The latter would be difficult for genital disease (Table 56-16).

Prevention Vitiligo is not a preventable disorder.

MULTISYSTEM DISEASES

REITER SYNDROME

Epidemiology, Etiology, and Pathogenesis In its classic form, Reiter syndrome consists of a triad of arthritis, urethritis, and conjunctivitis.[52] It is rare in females, in whom presentation may be atypical or incomplete. Reiter syndrome is likely an aberrant immune response to infection in individuals with a hereditary predisposition because the disorder typically presents 1–4 weeks after a urogenital or enteric infection, particularly after chlamydial urethritis.[53] Other causative organisms include *Neisseria gonorrhoeae* and *Ureaplasma, Shigella, Salmonella, Yersinia,* and *Campylobacter* species. HLA antigen B27 positivity is strongly correlated with Reiter syndrome and is found in 70–90% of affected individuals.

Clinical Findings Vulvar lesions associated with Reiter syndrome may appear as red crusted plaques, circinate erosions, linear ulcers, verrucous lesions, or pustules.[52] There may be accompanying psoriasiform skin lesions, oral ulcers, cervicitis, keratoderma, and nail dystrophy in addition to the classic symptoms of arthritis, urethritis, and conjunctivitis. Urethritis may be asymptomatic. Reiter syndrome is a clinical diagnosis, but supportive evidence may be obtained via histologic examination. Additionally, positive cultures or serology for *Chlamydia* or enteric organisms may contribute to a diagnosis of Reiter syndrome.

Differential Diagnosis

- Pustular psoriasis with psoriatic arthritis

Complications Reactive arthritis associated with Reiter syndrome may persist chronically, causing long-term disability.

Prognosis/Clinical Course Many symptoms are chronic and require ongoing therapy, although the severity of Reiter syndrome may decrease after months to years.

Treatment Topical and systemic therapy is available for Reiter syndrome. Individual lesions are best managed topically, whereas systemic medication is indicated for other manifestations of the disorder (Table 56-17).

Prevention Safe sex practices and improved general sanitation may prevent transmission of presumed causative organisms.

BEHÇET SYNDROME

Epidemiology, Etiology, and Pathogenesis Behçet syndrome is a systemic vasculitis

TABLE 56-16
Treatments for Vitiligo

	Topical		Surgical	Camouflage
First line	Triamcinolone 0.01% or clobetasol 0.05%	Apply daily to twice daily for 2–3 months	Keratinocyte-melanocyte transfer Epidermal grafts	Cosmetic coverup Therapeutic tattoo
Second line	Pimecrolimus 1.0% or tacrolimus 0.1%	Both applied daily to twice daily	Excimer laser	

TABLE 56-17
Treatments for Reiter Syndrome

	Topical		Systemic	
First line	Hydrocortisone 1% Triamcinolone 0.1% Clobotacol 0.05%	All applied daily to twice daily	Indomethacin	75 mg PO bid
Second line	Tacrolimus 0.1%	Daily to twice daily	Doxycycline Methotrexate	100 mg PO bid 7.5–25 mg weekly

of small and large vessels that may involve almost any organ system.[54] The condition is more prevalent in the Middle and Far East, with peak occurrence usually between 30 and 40 years of age. However, this disorder can present in adolescence and may suggest sexual abuse or sexually transmitted infection.[55] The pathogenesis of Behçet syndrome is not entirely clear, but a heritable disposition is suspected.

Clinical Findings Behçet syndrome is a multisystem condition, and patients may present with orogenital ulcerations, uveitis, erythema nodusum, arthritis, thrombophlebitis, gastrointestinal ulcerations, and central nervous system symptoms. With vulvar involvement, the presenting complaint may be dyspareunia associated with recurrent crops of multiple, very tender genital ulcers with a "punched out" appearance. Lesions typically take 2–4 weeks to heal.

The diagnosis of Behçet syndrome is one of exclusion, with criteria being the presence of oral apthae plus any two of the following: genital ulceration, eye disease, other skin lesions, or skin pathergy (the formation of a pustule at the site of intracutaneously injected saline).

Differential Diagnosis

- Chancroid
- Crohn disease (extraintestinal)
- Granuloma inguinale
- Herpes progenitalis
- Syphilis
- Traumatic ulceration

Complications Ulcerations of the vulva often form contiguous lesions that can lead to sinus formation and destruction of the labia. Sight-threatening uveitis, thrombophilia, stroke, paralysis, nerve palsies, and psychosis are possible morbidities.[54]

Prognosis/Clinical Course Women tend to experience more mild overall disease than men.[54] The course of the disorder is variable, with some genital lesions healing while other lesions form. The possible systemic manifestations of the disease are more progressive and continuous.

Treatment Traditional systemic treatment for Behçet syndrome consists of steroids (with or without various cytotoxic agents), dapsone, and colchicine. Thalidomide has proven beneficial in a handful of patients. Recent reports suggest the utility of anti–tumor necrosis factor-α biologic drugs[56–58] (Table 56-18).

Prevention Behçet syndrome is not a preventable disease.

CROHN DISEASE

Epidemiology, Etiology, and Pathogenesis Crohn disease (CD) is a chronic granulomatous disorder that may involve any portion of the gastrointestinal tract.[59] The disease typically begins between the ages of 20 and 30 but can persist into the geriatric years. Cutaneous manifestations occur in 22–44% of patients with CD. The skin can be involved by direct extension from the gastrointestinal tract or via involvement away from the gastrointestinal tract, so-called metastatic CD. Genital involvement in CD is less frequent in men than in women. About 2% of women with CD have vulvar involvement.[59] The etiology of CD is unknown, but proposed causes include an unrecognized infectious agent or a disturbed immunologic reaction to an intestinal organism in genetically vulnerable individuals.

Among those with inflammatory bowel disease seen in the United States, Caucasians and African-Americans are equally likely to manifest CD, whereas those of Hispanic origin more often have ulcerative colitis.[60]

Clinical Findings There are three patterns of anogenital CD involvement. *Contiguous disease* represents direct extension from the involved intestine with the formation of sinuses/fistulas involving the skin. *Metastatic disease,* albeit rare, consists of ulcers and swelling in the vulvar area. There are also *nonspecific mucocutaneous lesions,* including apthous ulcers and pyoderma gangrenosum. Female patients with metastatic CD classically present with painful swelling and ulceration of the vulvar or perianal area. The classic ulcerations are deemed "knife cut" linear fissures and are located along the labiocrural fold (Figure 56-10). Ulcers also may be solitary, deep, and necrotic. The diagnosis of cutaneous CD is based on a biopsy showing the typical granulomatous change.

TABLE 56-18
Treatments for Behçet Syndrome (Systemic)

First line	Prednisone	5–60 mg PO qd (combined with immunosuppressive)
Second line	Dapsone	100 mg daily
	Colchicine	0.6 mg PO bid-tid
	Cyclosporine	4–5 mg/kg PO bid
	Methotrexate	7.5–25 mg weekly
Third line	Azathioprine	50–150 mg PO qd
	Cyclophosphamide	500–1000 mg IV bolus per month
	Thalidomide	100 mg PO qd
Uncertain efficacy	Etanercept	50–100 mg/week SC
	Infliximab	5 mg/kg IV at 0, 2, and 6 weeks; then every 8 weeks

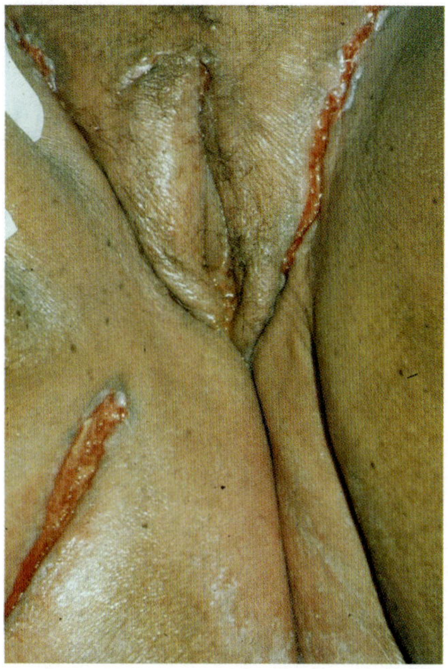

▲ **FIGURE 56-10** Cutlike perigenital erosions characteristic of Crohn disease. Image courtesy of Libby Edwards, M.D.

Differential Diagnosis

- Actinomycosis
- Angioedema
- Behçet disease
- Chancroid
- Extramammary Paget disease
- Factitious dermatitis
- Filariasis
- Fixed drug eruption
- Granuloma inguinale
- Hidradenitis suppurativa

Complications Patients may present with complications directly related to the underlying inflammatory bowel disease such as enteric fistulas, granulomatous salinities and oophoritis, vulvar abscesses, destructive perineal disease, and vulvar granulomas.[59] Complications unrelated to bowel involvement include anemia, dysmenorrhea, Bowen carcinoma of the vulva or vagina, and pyoderma gangrenosum (at any body site).

Prognosis/Clinical Course Anogenital lesions are chronic but should improve if the gastrointestinal manifestations of the disease are controlled.[61]

Treatment Treatment is directed at the underlying gastrointestinal disease. There has not been an effective therapy directed solely at cutaneous manifestations (Table 56-19).

Prevention CD has an unknown etiology and is therefore not preventable.

TABLE 56-19
Treatments for Metastatic Crohn Disease

	Topical		Physical	Systemic	
First line	Ultrapotent topical steroids	Twice daily		Sulfasalazine	1–2 g PO tid-qid
				Mesalamine	3–4 g PO qd
				Prednisone	5–60 mg PO qd
				Budesonide	9 mg PO qd
Second line			Excision and skin graft	Azathioprine	2 mg/kg PO qd
				6-Mercaptopurine	1.5 mg/kg PO qd
				Infliximab	5 mg/kg IV every 8 weeks

TUMORS

Benign

SEBORRHEIC KERATOSIS

Epidemiology, Etiology, and Pathogenesis Seborrheic keratosis is a common benign proliferation of the epidermis that occurs after age 30. This growth is considered a clonal expansion, so seborrheic keratosis qualifies as a neoplasm.[62] There is no predilection for either sex or any ethnic group.

Clinical Findings Seborrheic keratosis usually arises on sun-exposed skin but may be scattered on the lower abdomen, inner thighs, and (rarely) the nonmucosal surface of the vulva.[62,63] Lesions are usually asymptomatic but may be associated with pruritus. The lesions are tan-colored to brownish black with a "stuck on" appearance and a smooth to frankly verrucous surface. Diagnosis is both clinical and histopathologic.

Differential Diagnosis

- Bowen disease
- Condyloma acuminata (genital warts)
- Melanoma
- Nevocellular nevus

TABLE 56-20
Treatments for Seborrheic Keratosis (Physical)

First line	Shave biopsy/excision Curettage Cryotherapy Electrodesiccation, with or without curettage

Complications Seborrheic keratoses can become irritated.

Prognosis/Clinical Course The number and size of seborrheic keratoses increase with age.

Treatment No treatment is necessary for seborrheic keratoses unless they are bothersome to the patient or they are of such a size/position to interefere with function (Table 56-20).

Prevention Seborrheic keratoses are not preventable.

ANGIOKERATOMA

Epidemiology, Etiology, and Pathogenesis Vulvar angiokeratomas are rare benign vascular lesions seen most often in women of childbearing age in any ethnic group.[64] It has been proposed that angiokeratomas are telangiectasias with secondary epithelial proliferation and resulting acanthosis and hyperkeratosis. While the etiology is not entirely understood, lesions may be associated with increased venous pressure. Patients with multiple angiokeratomas may have underlying disorders of glycosphingolipid metabolism.[63]

Clinical Findings Lesions occur most commonly on the labia majora, but they may occur on the clitoris.[64] Angiokeratomas may be solitary or multiple and may have a smooth, hyperkeratotic or verrucous papular appearance with coloration that may range from violet through red to brown or blue-black. Angiokeratomas are typically asymptomatic but may present with intermittent bleeding or pruritus. Diagnosis is largely clinical, but pathologic confirmation may be necessary in rare instances.

Differential Diagnosis

- Condyloma acuminata
- Condyloma lata
- Kaposi sarcoma
- Hidradenoma papilliform

TABLE 56-21
Treatments for Angiokeratoma (Physical)

First line	Local excision Electrodesiccation Laser ablation

- Malignant melanoma
- Molluscum contagiosum
- Nevi
- Pyogenic granuloma
- Seborrheic keratosis

Complications Associated glycosphingolipid metabolism disorders, if present, may lead to severe renal, ophthalmologic, and neurologic changes.

Prognosis/Clinical Course No treatment is indicated for asymptomatic lesions because they have no malignant potential (Table 56-21).

Prevention Angiokeratomas are not preventable.

BENIGN CYSTS

Epidemiology, Etiology, and Pathogenesis

Benign genital cysts are very common, with an estimated prevalence of 1 in 200 women affected; this is thought to be an underestimation because most cysts are not reported.[65] Cyst formation appears to increase with age but has no ethnic predilection.

Epidermal inclusion cysts are the most common genital cyst in women.[63] They develop from buried epithelial fragments, most commonly following episiotomy or other surgical procedures, or from a blockage in the pilosebaceous duct. Bartholin's duct cysts are due to ductal obstruction within one of the two major vulvar vestibular glands, typically from previous infection or inspissated mucus. Vestibular mucous cysts are simple cysts of the vulvar vestibule composed of mucus-secreting epithelium. Skene's duct cysts (uncommon paraurethral duct cysts) are caused by obstruction of the Skene's ducts, most commonly secondary to gonorrheal infection.[66]

Clinical Findings Vaginal cysts are most commonly found incidentally on examination, but patients may complain of mild discomfort, vaginal pressure, or urinary incontinence or retention.

Epidermal inclusion cysts are classically round, firm, smooth, and mobile; overlying skin may have a yellowish color. Bartholin's duct cysts present as round or ovoid cystic lesions at the 5 or 7 o'clock positions on the hymenal ring. Cysts are usually 1–4 cm in diameter, but lesions may cause enough swelling to block the entire introital area. Vestibular mucous cysts range from 0.5–1.5 cm in diameter. There are typically located around the introitus and are mobile, nontender, and yellowish or bluish. Skene's duct cysts are located near the edge of the urethral meatus, are mobile, and are skin-colored or translucent. Diagnosis of cysts is clinical, but biopsy may confirm the diagnosis.

TABLE 56-22
Treatments for Genital Cysts (Physical)

First line	Surgical excision

Differential Diagnosis

- Fibroma
- Furuncle (tender, hot, and red at inception)
- Hidradenitis suppurativa (purulent discharge)
- Lipoma
- Neuroma
- Nevus
- Xanthoma

Complications If cystic lesions continue to grow, they may obstruct the urethral meatus or the vaginal introitus. Cysts may become infected and subsequently tender.

Prognosis/Clinical Course Asymptomatic, small cysts need not be treated and likely will not become problematic. However, cysts causing pain or urinary symptoms should not be expected to remit spontaneously and should be treated by excision (Table 56-22).

Prevention Cysts cannot be prevented.

Malignant

SQUAMOUS CELL CARCINOMA

Epidemiology, Etiology, and Pathogenesis

Squamous cell carcinoma (SCC) accounts for 85–90% of malignant tumors of the vulva, and neoplasms may be classified as either intraepithelial or invasive. Intraepithelial SCC may be referred to as *squamous cell carcinoma in situ* (SCCIS) or *vulvar intraepithelial neoplasia* (VIN) or *squamous intraepithelial lesion* (SIL). SCCIS has been associated with HPV types 16, 18, 31, 33, 35, 51, and 52. Advanced age, immunosuppression, and smoking appear to contribute to the development of VIN.[63,67] Multifocal intraepithelial neoplasia affects women aged 20–50 years of age, whereas women over age 60 are more likely to be afflicted by solitary intraepithelial neoplasia. The risk of developing invasive vulvar cancer increases with age. Studies have shown that among black women, rates of in situ squamous cell tumors have increased by 7.9% per year from 1973 through 1998.[68] Whether this increased incidence is simply related to the enhanced use of biopsy to investigate suspicious vulvar lesions or represents a true population dynamic is not known.

Clinical Findings. Multifocal intraepithelial neoplasia, also called *bowenoid papulosis,* is characterized by papules and plaques of variable color with clearly defined borders that appear scattered on the vestibule, outer labia minora, and labia majora (Figure 56-11). Women tend to have larger lesions than men; lesions may reach 2–3 cm in diameter.[63] Additionally, women may have significantly more lesions than men. Solitary intraepithelial neoplasia, also termed *Bowen disease,* typically presents as a single pink or erythematous, sharply bordered patch or plaque. Plaques may have a velvety appearance. Approximately 50% of women complain of pruritus with solitary lesions. Invasive vulvar cancer typically presents as erythematous or white, unifocal lesions that may ulcerate or become nodular morphologically. Lesions appear on the

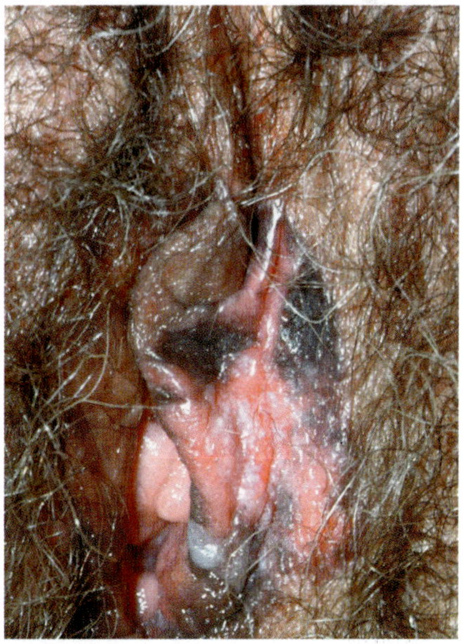

▲ **FIGURE 56-11** Multifocal plaques of variable color typify in situ squamous cell carcinoma (Hispanic woman).

posterior fourchette, labia minora, or interlabial sulcus.[63,67]

Vulvar cancer typically is suspected clinically and confirmed via biopsy. Gross examination of the vulva should be followed by a colposcopic examination of the vulva, vagina, and cervix. Potential areas of active HPV infection can be identified by the use of topically applied diluted acetic acid, with biopsies taken from the acetowhite regions.

Differential Diagnosis

- Acrochordons (skin tags)
- Bartholin's duct obstruction
- Condyloma acuminata (genital warts)
- Epidermal inclusion cyst
- Hemangioma
- Hidrandenomas
- Lentigo
- Lichen sclerosus
- Mucous cysts
- Seborrheic keratoses
- Varicosities
- Verrucae

Complications Large lesions (>2 cm), invasive SCC, and SCC of mucous membranes are associated with a high risk of recurrence and metastasis.[69] Additionally, SCC arising in injured or chronically diseased skin is associated with an approximate risk of metastasis of 40%.[69]

Prognosis/Clinical Course In the absence of metastatic disease, most patients with primary SCC have an excellent prognosis.

Treatment SCCIS may respond to prolonged application of topical immune response modification (imiquimod) or 5-fluorouracil.[70,71] Otherwise, lesions must be extirpated or destroyed surgically (Table 56-23).

Prevention Limiting the number of sexual partners and using barrier protection may decrease the transmission of HPV, one risk factor for developing vulvar cancer. Furthermore, regular gynecologic examinations are indicated to screen for suspicious lesions.

MALIGNANT MELANOMA

Epidemiology, Etiology, and Pathogenesis

While vulvar melanoma is rare, this disease accounts for 8–11% of vulvar neoplasia, making it the second most common vulvar malignancy.[72] Unlike melanomas elsewhere on the body, sunlight exposure is not thought to be an etiopathogenic for genital melanoma. Therefore, the etiology remains elusive. Risk factors include a family history of melanoma, a personal history of atypical nevi elsewhere on the body, and immunosuppression. Women in their fifties or sixties are most commonly affected, but childhood melanoma has been reported. It has been proposed that women of color develop vulvar melanoma less frequently than white women but that the former have a worse prognosis.[73] Vaginal melanoma is less common than vulvar melanoma and is associated with a poorer prognosis given that lesions are often large and deep by the time they are found.

Clinical Findings Primary vulvar melanoma typically presents on the labia major, labia minora, clitoris, or clitoral hood.[72] Presenting symptoms include appearance of a mass or local discoloration, swelling, bleeding, discharge, pruritus, dysuria, or pain. Primary vaginal melanoma typically presents with vaginal discharge or irregular bleeding. Superficial spreading melanomas account for 50% of vulva melanomas, and nodular melanomas account for 35%.[74] Acral lentiginous melanoma accounts for 15% of vulvar melanomas and is more common in Asians. Diagnosis is achieved via clinical and histopathologic examination.

TABLE 56-23
Treatments for Squamous Cell Carcinoma

	Topical		Physical
First line	Imiquimod 5% (SCC in situ only)	Apply 3–5 times per week × 6 weeks	Surgical resection Loop electrosurgical excision (LEEP)
	5-Fluorouracil 5% (SCC in situ only)	Apply twice daily × 3–6 weeks	
Second line			Laser ablation—CO_2 laser Radiation therapy Photodynamic therapy

TABLE 56-24
Treatments for Melanoma (Physical)

First line	Surgical resection
Second line	Local radiation Chemotherapy

Differential Diagnosis

- Angiokeratoma
- Mucosal melanotic macule
- Nevus
- Seborrheic keratosis
- Vulvar intraepithelial neoplasia (VIN)

Complications Melanoma metastatic to distant sites may be fatal.

Prognosis/Clinical Course Proposed poor prognostic factors for vulvar melanoma and cutaneous melanoma are similar and include lymph node involvement, ulceration, higher tumor thickness, higher mitotic rate, advanced age, microsatellitosis, extensive regression, nonwhite race, and low income.[72] The overall 5-year survival for vulvar melanoma ranges from 27–54%.[75] For vaginal melanoma, the 5-year survival is less promising and ranges from 5–19%[73] (Table 56-24).

Prevention Early detection through regular gynecologic examination may improve overall survival.

PAGET DISEASE

Epidemiology, Etiology, and Pathogenesis

Extramammary Paget disease (EMPD) is a rare neoplastic condition of apocrine gland–bearing skin (including genital and perigenital areas) that may be associated with internal malignancy.[76] EMPD is thought to originate either from the intraepithelial cells of apocrine gland ducts or from pluripotent keratinocyte stem cells. The most commonly affected demographic is postmenopausal Caucasian women.[77]

Clinical Findings The pruritic patches and plaques of EMPD are nonspecific, such that there is often a significant time delay between the initial presentation and diagnosis.[78] Lesions most commonly affect the vulvar and perianal regions and appear as well-demarcated, erythematous or leukoplakic patches or plaques with an eczematous appearance. Biopsy demonstrating infiltrating intraepithelial neoplastic cells with glandular differentiation is diagnostic.

TABLE 56-25
Treatments for Extramammary Paget Disease

	Topical		Physical
First line	Imiquimod 5%	3 times per week for 8–16 weeks	Surgical excision using Mohs micrographic technique with or without prior 5-fluorouracil application
Second line			Electrodesiccation and curettage Laser surgery Radiotherapy Photodynamic therapy with aminolevulinic acid

Differential Diagnosis

- Contact dermatitis
- Candidiasis
- Psoriasis
- SCCIS
- Tinea

Complications External genital EMPD may be associated with bladder, urethral, uterine, breast, or cervical cancer, and perianal EMPD may be related to colorectal cancer.[76] Given these associations, a workup of EMPD should include cystoscopy, gastrointestinal endoscopy, pelvic examination with Papanicolaou test, breast examination, and colposcopy.[79]

Prognosis/Clinical Course The overall mortality rate from either locally invasive or internal genitourinary carcinoma at distant sites is 25%.[74] The 5-year survival of these patients is high owing to the slow nature of this disease process.

Treatment Lesions small enough to be surgically excised should undergo such treatment. Involvement of multiple areas may be exposed by preoperative application of either imiquimod or 5-fluorouracil. Limited-extent EMPD may be amenable to monotherapy with imiquimod[79,80] (Table 56-25).

Prevention EMPD cannot be prevented.

KAPOSI SARCOMA

Epidemiology, Etiology, and Pathogenesis Kaposi sarcoma (KS) is a multicentric malignant tumor of lymphatic origin that can be one of four types: classic KS, endemic African KS, acquired immune deficiency syndrome (AIDS)–related KS, and transplant-related KS. The etiologic agent of all types of KS is human herpes virus type 8 (HHV-8).[81] There is no sex predilection in the United States. By contrast, in Africa, KS is very common, accounting for up to 10% of all malignancies in some areas; men are affected 20–30 times more frequently than women in these areas.[82] Risk factors for HHV-8 infection in HIV-positive women include intravenous (IV) drug use, sexual partners with a history of IV drug use, crack cocaine use, previous syphilis infection, and black race.

Clinical Findings KS of female genitalia and surrounding skin may present as red or purple nodules and plaques on the skin or mucocutaneous surfaces.[81] Vulvar KS may be mistaken for benign conditions such as a Bartholin's gland abscess. Diagnosis is histopathologic.

Differential Diagnosis

- Angiokeratoma
- Bartholin's gland abscess
- Deep fungal infection
- Lichen planus
- Metastatic tumor from visceral malignancy
- Soft tissue sarcoma

Complications KS affecting women tends to be more aggressive or perhaps diagnosed in later stages owing to atypical presentations. Therefore, female patients with KS have an increased incidence of lymph node involvement, lymphedema, and metastatic disease.

Prognosis/Clinical Course Women with KS carry a worse prognosis, with a median survival time of approximately 14 months less than men.[81] With metastatic disease, prognosis is poor (Table 56-26).

Prevention Optimal highly active antiretroviral therapy (HAART) control of HIV infection may decrease the risk of developing KS.

EXOGENOUS DISEASES

LICHEN SIMPLEX CHRONICUS

Epidemiology, Etiology, and Pathogenesis Lichen simplex chronicus (LSC) is an eczematous disease characterized by constant pruritus and scratching. Most affected individuals are generally atopic, with common disease triggers being psychological distress, heat, sweating, and excess dryness.[83] Additionally, LSC may be superimposed on other anogenital conditions, such as psoriasis, lichen sclerosus, tinea cruris, and neoplasia. Approximately 0.5% of American are affected by LSC, with the majority of patients being in their middle to late adult life. In adults, LSC is slightly more common in women. There may be a predilection for LSC among men and women of Asian ethnicity.

Clinical Findings Patients report the presence of itching that may be severe

TABLE 56-26
Treatments for Kaposi Sarcoma

	Topical		Physical	Systemic	
First line	Alitretinoin gel	Apply bid-qid × 2–14 weeks	Surgical excision Extended-field radiotherapy Laser therapy Cryotherapy	Interferon-α	36 million units SC/IM 3 times per week
				HAART	Per protocol (HIV+)
				Vincristine	Per protocol
Second line				Vinblastine	

TABLE 56-27
Treatments for Lichen Simplex Chronicus

	Topical		Physical	Systemic	
First line	Triamcinolone 0.1% cream (or more potent steroids)	Apply qd-qid	Sitz baths Lubricating creams and ointments	Hydroxyzine Other antihistamines	10–25 mg PO at bedtime Per standard dose
Second line				Prednisone	40 mg qd for 7 days, followed by 20 mg qd for 7 days
				Triamcinolone	40–80 mg IM once

and intractable, and individuals acknowledge that they respond to this pruritus with scratching or rubbing. Most patients scratch subconsciously during the day or scratch while asleep at night. The labia majora are most likely to be involved, but lesions are also possible on the labia minora, vulvar vestibule, and mons pubis. Erythematous, scaling, lichenified plaques with overlying excoriation typically are seen on physical examination. Because of moisture present in the anogenital area, lesions may be lacking visible scale or surface roughness in this region and instead may appear whitened, wrinkled, and relatively smooth. Chronic disease sufferers, particularly those with dark skin, may develop lesions that are dusky red (early) or show postinflammatory dyschromia late in the course (either hypopigmentation or hyperpigmentation). Diagnosis may be made by identification of lichenification and excoriation as well as a supportive history. Biopsy is neither needed nor desirable in most cases.

Differential Diagnosis

- Atopic dermatitis
- Candidiasis
- Chronic contact dermatitis
- Lice (pubic)
- Lichen sclerosus
- Psoriasis
- Scabies
- Tinea cruris

Complications Genital distortion, fibrosis, and scarring may occur with vigorous scratching. Black skin develops lichenification more readily than white skin, and when present, it appears to be more recalcitrant to therapy.

Prognosis/Clinical Course Without treatment, LSC persists as an itch-scratch cycle with waxing and waning. Avoidance of triggers alone is unlikely to result in disease remission. Patients may achieve long-term relief if therapy successfully repairs the damaged barrier layer, reduces inflammation, and breaks the itch-scratch cycle[83] (Table 56-27).

Prevention Minimizing triggers (e.g., psychological distress, heat, sweating, and excess dryness) may decrease exacerbations of the itch-scratch cycle.

CONTACT DERMATITIS

Epidemiology, Etiology, and Pathogenesis
Contact dermatitis (CD) is an inflammatory reaction to external material. Possible triggers for genital CD include seminal fluid, spermicides, latex condoms, lubricant jelly, perfumes (e.g., feminine hygiene sprays, scented soaps, and scented tampons), self-adhesive feminine napkins, topical antibiotics (e.g., neomycin), and moisturizers (e.g., lanolin).[84] Irritant contact dermatitis (ICD) is caused by prolonged or repeated exposure to irritating substances, whereas allergic contact dermatitis (ACD) is a true allergy to a low dose of a chemical substance. ACD involves a delayed-type hypersensitivity reaction, whereas ICD does not require prior sensitization.

Clinical Findings Vulvar CD may present with edema, vesicles or bullae, erythema, and weeping. Patients with black skin may show hyperpigmentation instead of erythema. Secondary lichenification or excoriation may be present. Compared with more generalized CD, chronic CD in the genital area may have a decreased amount of visible scale owing to the high-moisture environment. CD is a diagnosis based largely on history because clinical appearance and even biopsy may be nonspecific. Biopsy can be performed to rule out other possible diagnoses, and patch testing may be useful to confirm ACD.

Differential Diagnosis

- Atopic dermatitis
- Bowen disease (SCCIS)
- Candidiasis
- Intertrigo (nonspecific)
- Lichen simplex chronicus
- Paget disease
- Psoriasis
- Tinea

Complications Hyper- or hypopigmentation may occur owing to melanocyte damage from severe inflammation.

Prognosis/Clinical Course If patients are able to avoid the offending substance and receive anti-inflammatory therapy, they have a good prognosis. Patients with chronic symptoms and no obvious etiology generally have a prolonged course with long-term management (Table 56-28).

Prevention Avoidance of the offending agent should prevent episodes of CD.

TABLE 56-28
Treatments for Contact Dermatitis

	Topical		Systemic	
First line	Triamcinolone 0.1%	Apply qd-qid	Hydroxyzine	10–25 mg PO at bedtime
Second line			Prednisone	upto 40–80 mg daily for 7–14 days

REFERENCES

1. Primary and secondary syphilis—United States, 2003–2004. *MMWR* 2005;55:269-273.
2. Goh BT. Syphilis in Adults. *Sex Transm Inf* 2005;81:448-452.
3. Rosen T. Diseases with unusual features: Syphilis, in *Clinical Dermatology in Black Patients*. Bari, Italy, PiGreco Press, 1995, pp 59-63.
4. Fisher BK, Margesson LJ. Infectious diseases of the vulva, in *Genital Skin Disorders: Diagnosis and Treatment*. St Louis, MO, Mosby, 1998, pp 128-149.
5. Lewis DA. Chancroid: Clinical manifestations, diagnosis, and management. *Sex Transm Inf* 2003;79:68-71.
6. Bong CTH, Bauer ME, Spinola SM. *Haemophilus ducreyi*: Clinical features, epidemiology, and prospects for disease control. *Microbes Infect* 2002;4:1141-1148.
7. Lynch PJ, Edwards L. Infectious primary ulcers, in Lynch PJ, Edwards L (eds), *Genital Dermatology*. New York, Churchill-Livingstone, 1994, pp 207-209.
8. Rosen T. Tropical infections: Chancroid, in *Clinical Dermatology in Black Patients*. Bari, Italy, PiGreco Press, 1995, pp 164-166.
9. Jones CC, Rosen T. Cultural diagnosis of chancroid. *Arch Dermatol* 1991;127:1823-1827.
10. Lupi O, Madkan V, Tyring SK. Tropical dermatology: Bacterial tropical diseases. *J Am Acad Dermatol* 2006;54:559-578.
11. Rosen T. Tropical infections: Granuloma Inguinale, in *Clinical Dermatology in Black Patients*. Bari, Italy, PiGreco Press, 1995, pp 169-170.
12. Sexually transmitted diseases treatment guidelines 2002. *MMWR* 2002;51:1-78.
13. O'Farrell N. Donovanosis. *Sex Transm Inf* 2002;78:452-457.
14. Beauman JG. Genital herpes: A review. *Am Fam Physician* 2005;72:1527-1534.
15. Solomon J, Cannon MJ, Reyes M, et al. Epidemiology of recurrent genital herpes simplex virus types 1 and 2. *Sex Transm Inf* 2003;79:456-459.
16. Fleming DT, Leone P, Esposito D, et al. Herpes virus type 2 infection and genital symptoms in primary care patients. *Sex Transm Dis* 2006;33:416-421.
17. Corey L, Wald A, Patel R, et al. Once-daily valacyclovir to reduce the risk of transmission of genital herpes. *N Engl J Med* 2004;350:11-20.
18. Sheffield JS, Hill JB, Hollier JM, et al. Valacyclovir prophylaxis to prevent recurrent herpes at delivery: A randomized clinical trial. *Obstet Gynecol* 2006;108:141-147.
19. Dupin N. Genital warts. *Clin Dermatol* 2004;22:481-486.
20. Koutsky L. Epidemiology of genital human papillomavirus infection. *Am J Med* 1997;102:3-8.
21. Kodner CM, Nasraty S. Management of genital warts. *Am Fam Physician* 2004;70:2335-2342.
22. Handsfield HH. Clinical presentation and natural course of anogenital warts. *Am J Med* 1997;102:16-20.
23. Villa LL, Costa RL, Petta CA, et al. Prophylactic quadrivalent human papillomavirus (types 6, 11, 16, and 18) L1 virus-like particle vaccine in young women: A randomised, double-blind, placebo-controlled multicenter phase II efficacy trial. *Lancet Oncol* 2005;6:271-278.
24. Hanson D, Diven DG. Molluscum contagiosum. *Dermatol Online J* 2003;9:2.
25. Smith KJ, Skelton H. Molluscum contagiosum: Recent advances in pathogenic mechanisms and new therapies. *Am J Clin Dermatol* 2002;3:535-545.
26. Nadalo D, Montoya C. What is the best way to treat tinea cruris? *J Fam Pract* 2006;55:256-258.
27. Huang DB, Ostrosky-Zeichner L, Wu JJ, et al. Therapy of common superficial fungal infections. *Dermatol Ther* 2004;17:517-522.
28. Hay RJ. The management of superficial candidiasis. *J Am Acad Dermatol* 1999;40:S35-42.
29. Antony SJ, Lopez-Po P. Genital amebiasis: Historical perspective of an unusual disease presentation. *Urology* 1999;54:952-955.
30. Kenner BM, Rosen T. Cutaneous amebiasis in a child and review of the literature. *Pediatr Dermatol* 2006;23:231-234.
31. Markle WH, Makhoul K. Cutaneous leishmaniasis: Recognition and treatment. *Am Fam Physician* 2004;69:455-460.
32. Blickstein I, Dgani R, Lifscitz-Mercer B. Cutaneous leishmaniasis of the vulva. *Int J Gynaecol Obstet* 1993;42:46-47.
33. Richens J. Genital manifestations of tropical diseases. *Sex Transm Inf* 2004;80:12-17.
34. Cabello I, Carabello A, Millan Y. Leishmaniasis in the genital area. *Rev Inst Med Trop Sao Paulo* 2002;44:105-107.
35. Rosen T. Diseases with unusual features: Psoriasis, in *Clinical Dermatology in Black Patients*. Bari, Italy, PiGreco Press, 1995, pp 51-54.
36. Lynch PJ, Edwards L. Red plaques with papulosquamous features, in Lynch PJ, Edwards L (eds), *Genital Dermatology*. New York, Churchill-Livingstone, 1994, pp. 27-56.
37. Luba KM, Stulberg DL. Chronic plaque psoriasis. *Am Fam Physician* 2006;73:636-644.
38. Moyal-Barracco M, Edwards L. Diagnosis and therapy of anogenital lichen planus. *Dermatol Ther* 2004;17:38-46.
39. Rosen T. Diseases with unusual features: Lichen planus, in *Clinical Dermatology in Black Patients*. Bari, Italy, PiGreco Press, 1995, pp 36-40.
40. Fisher BK, Margesson LJ. Inflammatory diseases of the vulva, in *Genital Skin Disorders: Diagnosis and Treatment*. St Louis, MO, Mosby, 1998, pp 154-176.
41. Powell JJ, Wojnarowska F. Lichen sclerosus: *Lancet* 1999;353:1777-1783.
42. Ginarte M, Toribio J. Vulvar lichen sclerosus successfully treated with topical tacrolimus. *Eur J Obstet Gynecol Reprod Biol* 2005;123:123-124.
43. Luesley DM, Downey GP. Topical tacrolimus in the management of lichen sclerosus. *Br J Obstet Gynaecol* 2006;113:832-834.
44. Goldstein AT, Marinoff SC, Christopher K. Pimecrolimus for the treatment of vulvar lichen sclerosus: A report of 4 cases. *J Reprod Med* 2004;49:778-780.
45. Bhaumik J. Vulvitis circumscripta plasmacellularis: Success with a modified treatment regimen using imiquimod. *J Obstet Gynecol* 2006;26:72-86.
46. Ee HL, Yospovitch G, Chan R, Ong BH. Resolution of vulvitis circumscripta plasmacellularis with topical imiquimod: Two case reports. *Br J Dermatol* 2003;149:638-641.
47. Passeron T, Ortonne JP. Pathophysiology and genetics of vitiligo. *J Autoimmun* 2005;25:63-68S.
48. Handa S, Kaur I. Vitiligo: Clinical findings in 1436 patients. *J Dermatol* 1999;26:653-657.
49. Grimes PE. New insights and new therapies for vitiligo. *JAMA* 2005;293:730-735.
50. Falabella R. Surgical approaches for stable vitiligo. *Dermatol Surg* 2005;31:1277-1284.
51. Mulekar SV, Al Issa A, AL Eisa A, Asaad M. Genital vitiligo treated by autologous, noncultured melanocyte-keratinocyte cell transplantation. *Dermatol Surg* 2005;31:1737-1739.
52. Lotery HE, Galask RP, Stone MS, Sontheimer RD. Ulcerative vulvitis in atypical Reiter's syndrome. *J Am Acad Dermatol* 2003;48:613-616.
53. Kataria RK, Brent LH. Spondyloarthropathies. *Am Fam Physician* 2004;69:2853-2860.
54. Yurdakul S, Hamuryudan V, Yazaci H. Behçet syndrome. *Curr Opin Rheumatol* 2003;16:38-42.
55. Deitch HR, Huppert J, Adams Hillard PJ. Unusual vulvar ulcerations in young adolescent females. *J Pediatr Adolesc Gynecol* 2004;17:13-16.
56. Atenzi F, Sarzi-Puttini P, Capsoni F, et al. Successful treatment of resistant Behçet's disease with etanercept. *Clin Exp Rheumatol* 2005;23:729.
57. Connolly M, Armstrong JS, Buckley DS. Infliximab treatment for severe orogenital ulceration in Behçet's disease. *Br J Dermatol* 2005;153:1073-1075.
58. Haugeberg G, Velken M, Johnsen V. Successful treatment of genital ulcers with infliximab in Behçet's disease. *Ann Rheum Dis* 2004;63:744-745.
59. Feller ER, Ribaudo S, Jackson ND. Gynecologic aspects of Crohn's disease. *Am Fam Physician* 2001;64:1725-1728.
60. Basu D, Lopez I, Kulkarni A, Sellin JH. Impact of race and ethnicity on inflammatory bowel disease. *Am J Gastroenterol* 2005;100:2254-2261.
61. Lynch PJ, Edwards L. Noninfectious primary ulcers, in Lynch PJ, Edwards L (eds), *Genital Dermatology*. New York, Churchill-Livingstone, 1994, pp 213-221.
62. Thompson LD. Seborrheic keratosis. *Ear Nose Throat J* 2006;85:79.
63. Fisher BK, Margesson LJ. Tumors and cysts of the vulva, in *Genital Skin Disorders: Diagnosis and Treatment*. St Louis, MO, Mosby, 1998, pp 154-176.
64. Smith BL, Chu P, Weinburg JM. Angiokeratomas of the vulva: Possible association with radiotherapy. *Skinmed* 2004;3:171-172.
65. Eilber KS, Raz S. Benign cystic lesions of the vagina: A literature review. *J Urol* 2003;170:717-722.
66. Rosen T. Unusual presentation of gonorrhea. *J Am Acad Dermatol* 1982;6:369-372.

67. Tyring SK. Vulvar squamous cell carcinoma: Guidelines for early detection and treatment. *Am J Obstet Gynecol* 2003;189:S17-23.
68. Howe HL, Wingo PA, Thun MJ, et al. Annual report to the nation on the status of cancer (1973-1998), featuring cancers with recent increasing trends. *J Natl Cancer Inst* 2001;93:824-842.
69. Alam M, Ratner D. Cutaneous squamous cell carcinoma. *N Engl J Med* 2001;344:975-983.
70. Le T, Hicks W, Menard C, et al. Preliminary results of 5% imiquimod cream in the primary treatment of vulvar intraepithelial neoplasia grade 2/3. *Am J Obstet Gynecol* 2006;194:377-380.
71. Jayne CJ, Kaufman RJ. Treatment of vulvar intraepithelial neoplasia 2/3 with imiquimod. *J Reprod Med* 2002;47: 395-398.
72. Wechter ME, Gruber SB, Haefner HK. Vulvar melanoma: A report of 20 cases and review of the literature. *J Am Acad Dermatol* 2004;50:554-562.
73. Weinstock MA. Malignant melanoma of the vulva and vagina in the United States. *Am J Obstet Gynecol* 1994; 171:1225-1230.
74. Lynch PJ, Edwards L. Dark-colored papules and nodules, in Lynch PJ, Edwards L (eds), *Genital Dermatology.* New York, Churchill-Livingstone, 1994, pp 63-172.
75. Verschraegen CF, Benjapibal M, Supakarapongkul W, et al. Vulvar melanoma at the MD Anderson Cancer Center: 25 years later. *Int J Gynecol Cancer* 2001;11:359-364.
76. Lloyd J, Flanagan AM. Mammary and extramammary Paget's disease. *J Clin Pathol* 2000;53:742-749.
77. Stapleton JJ. Extramammary Paget's disease of the vulva in a young, black woman: A case report with histogenic confirmation by immunostaining. *J Reprod Med* 1984;29:444-446.
78. Zollo JD, Zeitouni NC. The Roswell Park Cancer Institute experience with extramammary Paget's disease. *Br J Dermatol* 2000;142:59-65.
79. Cohen PR, Schulze KE, Tschen JA, et al. Treatment of extramammary Paget's disease with topical imiquimod cream: Case report and literature review. *South Med J* 2006;99:396-402.
80. Badgwell C, Rosen T. Treatment of limited extent extramammary Paget's disease with 5% imiquimod cream. *Dermatol Online J* 2006;12:22.
81. Laartz BW, Cooper C, Degryse A, Sinnott JT. Wolf in sheep's clothing: Advanced Kaposi sarcoma mimicking vulvar abscess. *South Med J* 2005;98: 475-477.
82. Rosen T. Diseases more often seen in blacks: Kaposi's sarcoma, in *Clinical Dermatology in Black Patients.* Bari, Italy, PiGreco Press,1995, pp 90-92.
83. Lynch PJ. Lichen simplex chronicus (atopic/neurodermatosis) of the anogenital region. *Dermatol Ther* 2004;17: 8-19.
84. Sonnex C. Genital allergy. *Sex Transm Inf* 2004;80:4-7.

SECTION 9

Dermatologic Infections

CHAPTER 57

Bacterial Infections

Micole Tuchman
Jeffrey M. Weinberg

Key Points

- Individuals with skin of color may encounter a wide range of cutaneous infections involving either gram-positive or gram-negative organisms.
- In most cases, these infections do not differ significantly from those that occur in the general population.
- Staphylococcus aureus and Streptococcus pyogenes are the two major gram-positive organisms that are implicated most often in common skin and soft tissue infections.
- Gram-negative infections of the skin are more common in children, patients with diabetes, and immunocompromised patients.
- While empirical antibiotic treatment is an important first step in treating bacterial infections, once the diagnosis is established, treatment then should be dictated by the antibiotic sensitivities of the cultured organism.

Individuals with skin of color may encounter a wide range of cutaneous infections involving either gram-positive or gram-negative organisms. In most cases, these infections do not differ significantly from those that occur in the general population. This chapter describes some of the more common infections that occur in the population as well as preferred treatments.

GRAM-POSITIVE INFECTIONS

Staphylococcus aureus and *Streptococcus pyogenes* are the two major gram-positive organisms that are most often implicated in common skin and soft tissue infections. Infections usually begin and remain contained at the site of a minor wound or skin abrasion, but once skin penetration occurs, risks of systemic conditions such as sepsis, local necrosis, and endocarditis increase. The cutaneous infections listed in Table 57-1 typically are diagnosed clinically and treated empirically.

TABLE 57-1
Common Gram-Positive Bacterial Infections

Erythrasma
Impetigo, ecthyma
Infectious folliculitis
Abscess, furuncle, carbuncle
Paronychia
Cellulitis, erysipelas
Blistering distal dactylitis
Cutaneous anthrax
Staphylococcal scalded skin syndrome
Toxic shock syndrome
Scarlet fever

If antibiotics are indeed required for these infections, one with activity against gram-positive organisms such as a pencillinase-resistant penicillin, a cephalosporin, a macrolide, or a fluoroquinone is selected.[1] While empirical antibiotic treatment is an important first step, once the diagnosis is established, treatment should be dictated by the antibiotic sensitivities of the cultured organism.

Erythrasma

Erythrasma is a chronic bacterial infection caused by *Corynebacterium minutissimum* that affects the intertriginous areas of the axillae, groin, and toes. It is often misdiagnosed as a fungal infection because of the intertriginous predilection of both infections.

CLINICAL DESCRIPTION The skin lesions of erythrasma (Figure 57-1) are typically sharply marginated, reddish brown macules, sometimes with hyperkeratotic white maceration, erosion, or fissures, particularly in the webbing of the toes. The condition may be pruritic with resulting secondary excoriation and lichenification.

TREATMENT For prophylactic measures, looser-fitting clothing is encouraged. An absorbant powder such as Zeasorb AF powder can be used.[2] The treatment of choice is a 14-day course of erythromycin, 250 mg qid. Second-line treatments include tertracycline and chloramphenicol. Clarithromycin also may prove to be effective. In interdigital areas, or if erythromycin treatment fails, a combination of topical clindamycin, Whitefield's ointment, sodium fusidate ointment, or antibacterial soaps may be necessary for both treatment and prophylaxis. Whitefield's ointment has been shown to have greater efficacy than erythromycin for interdigital areas.[2]

Impetigo/Ecthyma

Impetigo may be either bullous or nonbullous in nature. Bullous impetigo is caused by *S. aureus*. In industrialized countries, nonbullous impetigo is also primarily caused by staphylococci, whereas in developing nations, nonbullous impetigo also frequently

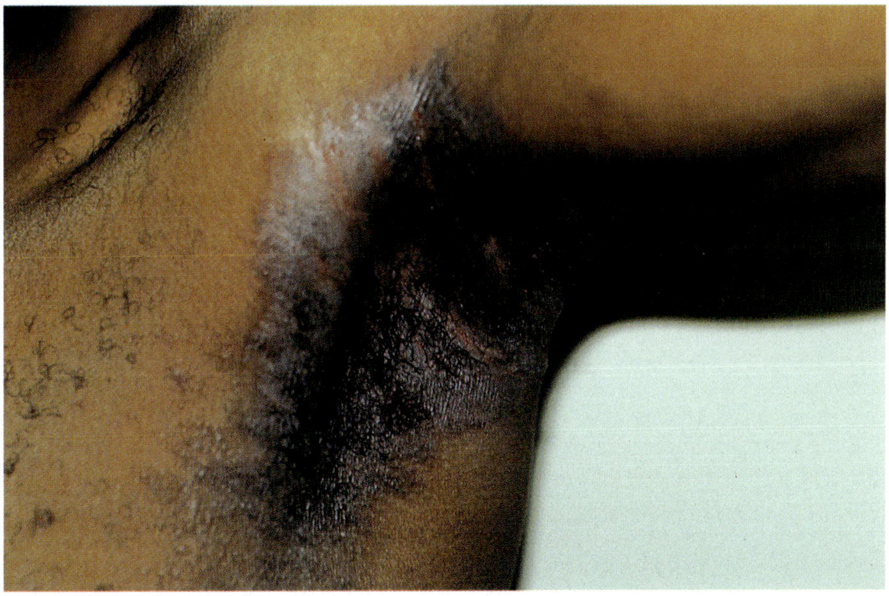

▲ **FIGURE 57-1** Skin lesions of erythrasma typically appear in intertriginous areas such as the axillae.

can be caused by *S. pyogenes,* a group A beta-hemolytic streptococcus, or both organisms. When both bacteria are found, it is thought to be due to primary infection with *Streptococcus* and secondary infection with *Staphylococcus.* The bacteria initially infect the superficial layer of the epidermis. While some lesions will resolve spontaneously, others will extend into the dermis. In this case, the infection is then called an *ecthyma.*

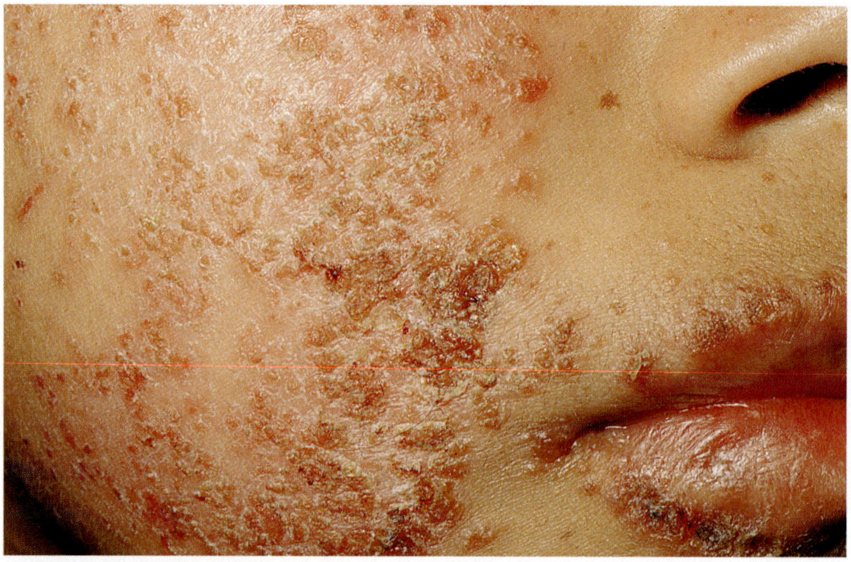

▲ **FIGURE 57-2** Non-bullous impetigo.

CLINICAL DESCRIPTION Nonbullous impetigo, which accounts for more than 70% of cases of impetigo, presents with small superficial pustules or blisters that quickly rupture and evolve into a crusted plaque, often of a honey color that appear "stuck on." (Figure 57-2) Surrounding erythema may be present. Patients lack constitutional symptoms. The most common location for these lesions is the face, but any area may be involved. The lesions are often scattered and discrete but without treatment often will coalesce. Autoinoculation may lead to distant sites of infection. Nonbullous impetigo characteristically heals without scarring.

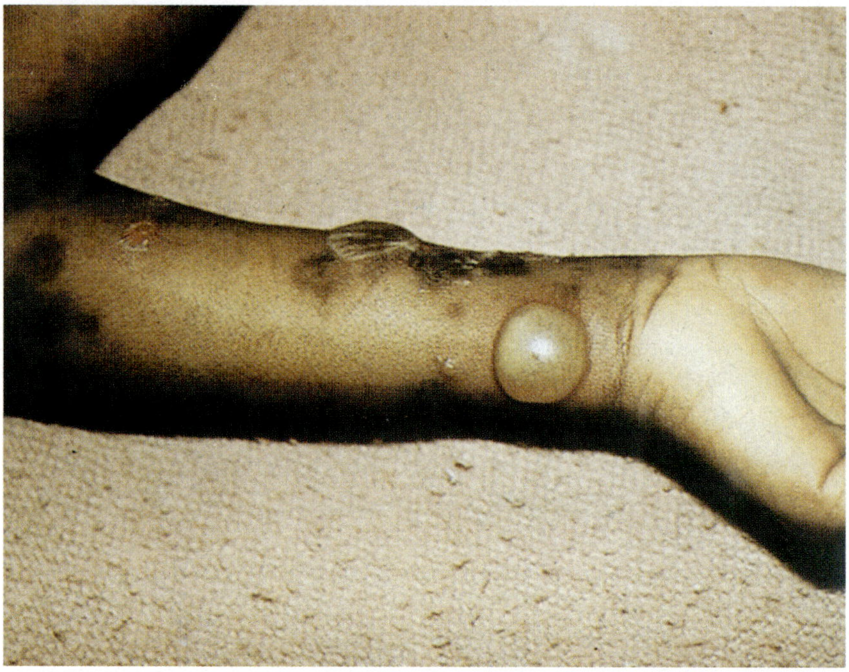

▲ **FIGURE 57-3** Bullous impetigo.

Bullous impetigo is characterized by bullae with cloudy to yellow fluid arising from normal-colored skin and a complete lack of surrounding erythema (Figure 57-3). Bullous impetigo occurs when staphylococci produce toxins (namely, exfoliative toxins A and B), which causes splitting of the epidermis. Both types of impetigo are most common in, but not limited to, intertriginous areas.

Ecthyma, a more severe form of streptococcal impetigo, presents with punched-out ulcerations of the epidermis with a surrounding thick adherent crust (Figure 57-4). There also may be a surrounding area of erythema. Ecthyma may be associated lymphangitis or lymphadenopathy. Unlike nonbullous impetigo, ecthymas are more commonly on the extremities and may heal with scarring.

TREATMENT Topical treatment includes mupirocin applied three times daily to the involved skin, as well as to the nares, where about 25% of people carry and incubate *S. aureus.* To eliminate staphyloccal carriage, rifampin and dicloxacillin are often used in conjunction. For severe infections, oral antibiotics such as dicloxacillin or cephalexin are prescribed, whereas in penicillin-allergic patients, erythromycin is administered.[3] The Swedish Medical Products Agency recommends treating impetigo with soap, water, or oral antibiotics and favors not using mupirocin because mupirocin is the cornerstone in the treatment of methicillin-resistant *S. aureus.*[3] While the authors warn against excessively liberal prescription of mupirocin, they do indicate that the 1- or 2-week course in the treatment of impetigo would be very unlikely to allow enough time for the emergence of resistant strains. On the contrary, they discourage the use of mupirocin for the treatment of more chronic conditions with more prolonged courses of treatment.[3]

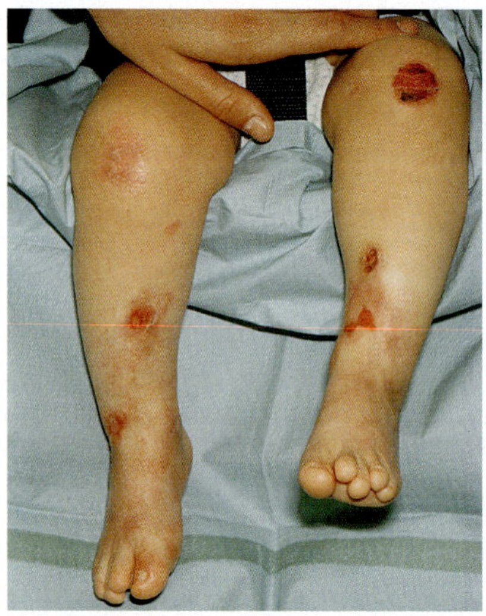

▲ **FIGURE 57-4** Ecthyma

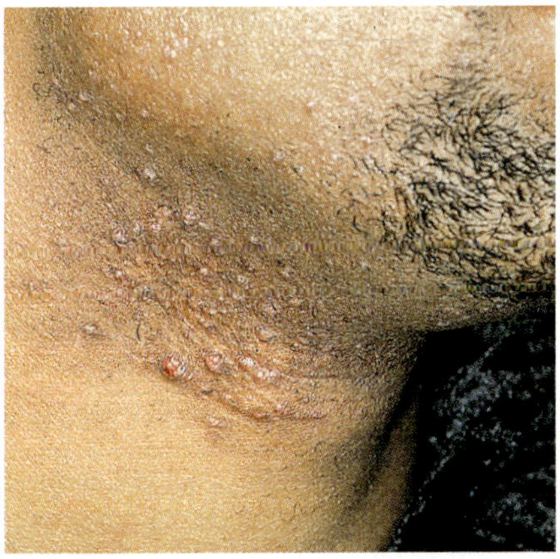

▲ **FIGURE 57-5** Infectious Folliculitis

Infectious Folliculitis

Infectious folliculitis affects the upper portion of the hair follicle. When the infection extends to the entire length of the follicle, it is called *sycosis*. The etiology of folliculitis may include bacterial, fungal, or viral causes. Bacterial agents include *S. aureus* (seen in both superficial and deep folliculitis), *Pseudomonas aeruginosa* (associated with hot tub folliculitis), and gram-negative folliculitis (associated with acne vulgaris and those who have been treated with oral antibiotics).

CLINICAL DESCRIPTION Skin lesions typically show a papule or pustule that is confined to the hair follicle but may exhibit surrounding erythema (Figure 57-5). Pustules can rupture, leading to crusty erosions that can be scattered or more frequently clustered. The superficial infection can progress to an abscess, especially when the causative agent is *S. aureus*. While the superficial infection typically heals without scarring, in skin of color patients, there can be considerable postinflammatory hypo- and/or hyperpigmentation.

Also of note in the skin of color population is pseudofolliculitis barbae (PFB). Although not a primary infectious disorder, pseudofolliculitis barbae is inflammatory in nature and characterized by the formation of papules, pustules, and hyperpigmentation as a result of ingrown hairs. This disorder is often complicated by a *S. aureus* superinfection. Men of color are especially prone to the development of PFB owing to the combination of a curved hair follicle and tightly coiled or curly hair, which is more prone to becoming ingrown and thus secondarily infected. It is estimated that PFB affects 45–83% of black men who shave regularly. In a recent published study, it was found that twice-daily applications of benzoyl peroxide 5%–clindamycin 1% gel produced reductions in papule and pustule counts ranging from 38.2% at week 2 to 63.9% at week 10.[4] Another type of inflammatory folliculitis that especially affects individuals of color is keloidal folliculitis, also termed *acne keloidalis nuchae*. In this condition, chronic papules and pustules at the nape of the neck can lead to extensive hypertrophic scarring and keloid formation, which ultimately can result in significant hair loss. Keloidal folliculitis also can become complicated by bacterial superinfection.

TREATMENT In infectious folliculitis, affected areas should be washed with antibacterial soap or a benzoyl peroxide preparation. Antimicrobial therapy may include oral antibiotics such as ampicillin or sulfamethoxazole-trimethoprim. Gram-negative folliculitis in acne and rosacea patients is best treated with isotretinoin (0.5–1 mg/kg daily for 4–5 months).[5] For treatment of pseudomonal folliculitis, please refer to gram-negative infections below.

Abscess, Furuncle, Carbuncle

Abscesses, furuncles, and carbuncles generally represent more severe infections caused by staphylococcal infection.[1] An *abscess* is a well-circumscribed collection of pus associated with tissue destruction and localized inflammation. A *furuncle* is acute and deeper than an abscess, is tender and erythematous, and develops around a hair follicle. A *carbuncle* is an even deeper and more extensive lesion forming from an abscess. The most common cause is *S. aureus,* and these infections occur mostly in individuals who are nasal carriers of this organism.

CLINICAL DESCRIPTION Cutaneous abscesses present initially as warm, tender red nodules (Figure 57-6). They can occur anywhere on the skin, typically surrounding hair follicles, in areas of trauma or burn, or at sites of insertion of intravenous catheters. Abscesses typically enlarge without treatment and form a pus-filled cavity. Furuncles are firmer, tender nodules, larger than abscesses, that occur in hair-bearing skin, such as the beard, neck, scalp, axillae, and buttocks (Figure 57-7). They may be very painful and associated with constitutional symptoms in severe cases. There may be a surrounding area of cellulitis. After several days, the nodules will rupture and discharge pus and often necrotic tissue. Finally, a carbuncle is comprised of multiple coalesced furuncles and typically is found on the nape of the neck, back, or thighs (Figure 57-8). Constitutional symptoms are often present. The involved area is erythematous and indurated and develops a yellow-colored crater at its center. When the carbuncle heals, there is a permanent scar that is very apparent.

TREATMENT Washing daily with antibacterial soap or benzoyl peroxide is important for patients susceptible to staphylococcal infections. Additionally, mupirocin ointment can be applied daily to the nares or other known carrier sites. Application of heat to the lesion can

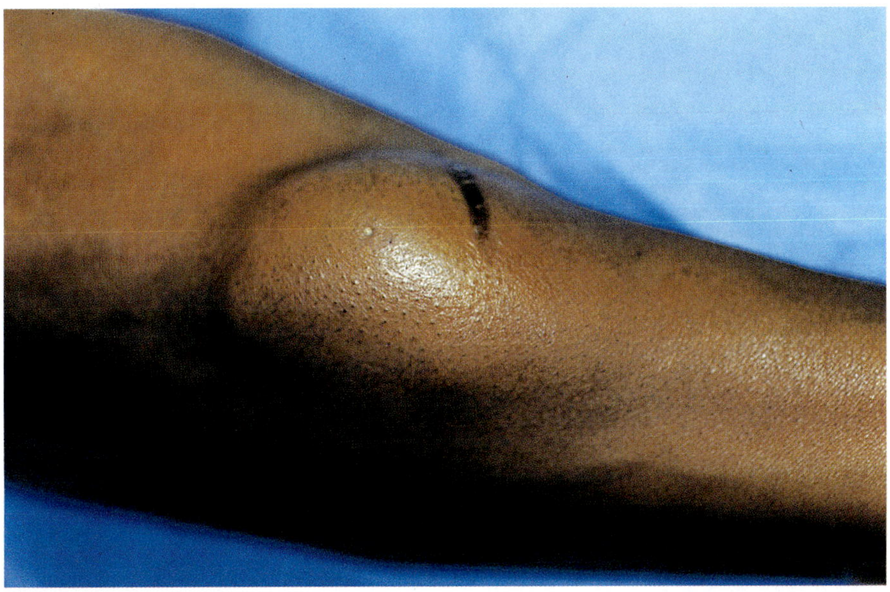

▲ **FIGURE 57-6** Abscess

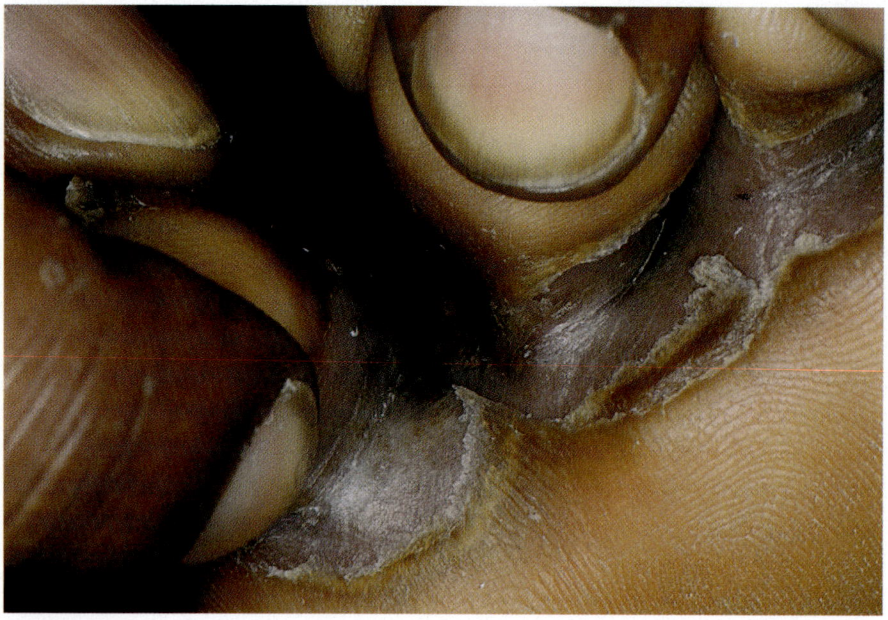

▲ **FIGURE 57-7** Furuncle

promote consolidation and may even aid in spontaneous drainage if done early in the course of the infection. Incision and drainage provide adequate treatment of many lesions, especially in otherwise healthy individuals, but oral antibiotics can hasten resolution and are required in immunosuppressed individuals. To eliminate active infection, oral antibiotics such as dicloxacillin, cephalexin, and erythromycin, as well as intravenous vancomycin in more severe cases, may be used.

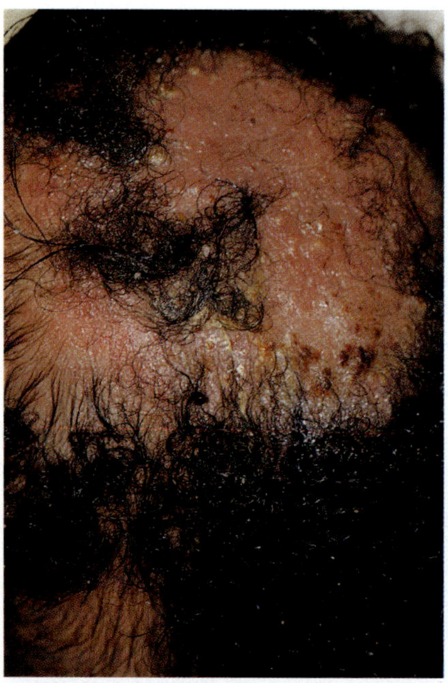

▲ **FIGURE 57-8** Carbuncle

Paronychia

While the chronic form of paronychia is caused by the yeast *Candida albicans,* the acute form is typically caused by *S. aureus* and is seen in people with hand trauma or those chronically exposed to water through hand washing or exposure to moisture.

CLINICAL DESCRIPTION In acute paronychia, the lateral and/or proximal nail folds are erythematous, hot, and tender and, if not treated, will evolve into an abscess.

TREATMENT Treatment includes both oral and topical antibiotics. If there is an abscess present, incision and drainage also will be necessary.[6]

Pitted Keratolysis

Pitted keratolysis, caused by *Micrococcus sedantarius,* is a condition that affects only the feet, specifically the soles of the feet, with lesions being most notable on areas of pressure such as the ball or heel of the foot, as well as the webbing between the toes.[7] Predisposing factors include occlusive footwear and hyperhidrosis.

CLINICAL DESCRIPTION Cutaneous findings show pitting of varying depth within the thickly keratinized skin of the plantar foot. The pits range from 1–8 mm in diameter and can become confluent. There can be involvement of one or both feet.

TREATMENT Less occlusive footwear should be worn, and a moisture-absorbing powder may be applied to shoes. Affected areas should be cleansed with a benzoyl peroxide soap, and either a benzoyl peroxide gel or a topical erythromycin should be applied daily after cleansing the area.

Cellulitis and Erysipelas

Cellulitis is an acute, diffuse, edematous suppurative inflammation of the dermis and subcutaneous tissues and is often associated with systemic symptoms such as fever, malaise, and chills. *S. aureus* and group A *Streptococcus* (GAS) are the most commonly involved bacteria, but others may include group B *Streptococcus* (specifically in the newborn), *Pneumoccocus,* and gram-negative bacilli. *Cellulitis* is a generic term because there are many different types of cellulitis.[8]

CLINICAL DESCRIPTION The lesions of cellulitis are macular and poorly demarcated from uninvolved skin. The tissue often feels hard and is painful on palpation. The overlying epidermis can become necrotic with resulting epidermal sloughing, or in some cases the infection may lead to both dermal and subcutaneous abscess formation. Cellulitis typically is found on the extremities and usually is associated with lymphangitis.

Erysipelas is an acute infection of the dermal and subcutaneous tissues that is typically red, hot, and tender and is most frequently caused by GAS and rarely by *S. aureus.* Streptococcal infection carries with it a high morbidity rate. Risk factors include venous insufficiency, toe webspace intertrigo, lymphedema, and obesity.[9]

CLINICAL DESCRIPTION Erysipelas differs from cellulitis in that it is often a painful, raised, indurated plaque with borders that are markedly distinguishable from the surrounding uninvolved skin. In severe cases, the epidermis can become bullous, pustular, and necrotic. Patients also typically report a prodrome of headache, malaise, and fever. The legs have become the most common areas of infection, with a decrease reported in cases affecting the face.[10]

A more severe form of cellulitis is gangrenous cellulitis or necrotizing fascitis, which is further subcategorized into a number of different diseases. In general, gangrenous cellulitis is characterized by the rapid progression of infection, with necrosis of both subcutaneous tissue and the overlying skin. The clinical picture, as well as the name of the disease, differs depending on the bacterial organism involved, comorbid conditions, and anatomic location of the infection. In general, there is local erythema, heat, and pain in the involved area. Constitutional symptoms typically are present and increase over time. Often there are visible gangrenous changes, including a dusky blue change in color of the affected area, as well as the onset of vesicles, with subsequent rupture of bullae. This is often accompanied by numbness and a black necrotic eschar resembling a third-degree burn. Alternatively, there may be a much more extensive process occurring than the skin changes would suggest. In this case, there can be destruction of small blood vessels and subcutaneous nerves that can lead to an anesthetic area. An immediate diagnosis of gangrenous cellulitis and differentiation from cellulitis is obviously imperative in order to quickly begin therapy. Therapy depends on the extent and severity of disease and can include simple drainage, antibiotics, and surgical debridement of necrotic tissue and amputations. Of special mention is necrotizing fasciitis, generally caused by group A beta-hemolytic streptococci and typically occurring on the leg of an elderly adult with an underlying chronic illness. The patient may present with symptoms similar to toxic shock syndrome (discussed below), and this disorder carries with it a high fatality rate.

TREATMENT The local care of cellulitis involves elevation and immobilization of the involved limb to reduce swelling and cool sterile saline dressings to remove purulent drainage. The approach to antimicrobial therapy selection involves identification of the source. Comorbidities of the patient (such as diabetes or immunosuppression) should be considered in treatment decisions. Streptococci (groups A, G, and B) and *S. aureus* are the most frequently isolated bacterial species.[10]

Identification of the responsible organism is obtained via culture, often performed at the portal of entry. Often the organism is not found because only about 5% of patients will have positive cultures.[10] Initial empirical treatment for mild cellulitis or erysipelas includes oral dicloxacillin, which covers both staphylococci and streptococci. Initial empirical antimicrobial treatment for moderate or severe cellulitis consists of an intravenous cephalosporin (e.g., cefazolin or ceftriaxone) or nafcillin (vancomycin in patients with an allergy to penicillin), followed by dicloxacillin or an oral cephalosporin, generally for a course of 7–14 days. In patients with recurrent cellulitis of the leg, fissures in the interdigital spaces caused by dermatophytosis should be treated with topical antifungal agents to prevent recurrences. Daily prophylaxis with oral penicillin G (or amoxicillin) may be considered for patients who have had more than two episodes of cellulitis at the same site.[10]

Blistering Distal Dactylitis

Blistering distal dactylitis is typically due to GAS but also can be caused by group B organisms. Cases of staphylococcal dactylitis also have been reported presenting with an identical clinical picture. The blisters typically occur in children and adolescents.

CLINICAL DESCRIPTION On physical examination, there is a large, purulent, fluid-filled blister, usually on the skin overlying the distal finger or toe pads, but it may extend either to the proximal aspects of the digits or more distally to the nails. There is often a surrounding erythematous base.

TREATMENT The infection responds readily to incision and drainage, compresses, and a course of an organism-specific oral antibiotic—usually oral penicillin or erythromycin.[11]

Cutaneous Anthrax

Cutaneous anthrax is caused by *Bacillus anthracis.* Under natural conditions, humans acquire anthrax infection (usually the cutaneous form) from contact with infected animals or contaminated animal products, such as hides, wool, hair, and ivory tusks. More than 95% of naturally occurring anthrax is the cutaneous form.[12]

CLINICAL DESCRIPTION The cutaneous manifestations of anthrax evolve over 2–3 weeks. The primary lesion, which is a painless, pruritic papule, appears at the site of inoculation 1–7 days later. Within 1–2 days of the appearance of the primary lesion, small clear or serosanguineous fluid–filled vesicles may develop. As the vesicle enlarges, satellite vesicles may develop. A nonpitting, gelatinous edema surrounds the lesion, and it may become massive, especially when the primary lesion is on the neck or face. Low-grade fever and malaise are frequently present. When the vesicle ruptures, it undergoes necrosis, forming an ulcer covered by a characteristic black eschar. The eschar dries and falls off in 1–2 weeks with little residual scarring. Regional lymphadenopathy is present initially. Secondary infection with streptococci or *S. aureus* is uncommon but would be suggested by the recurrence of fever with lymphangitis, local pain, and purulent drainage. Bacteremia is a rare complication.[12]

TREATMENT Without antibiotic treatment, mortality can be as high as 20%. Incision or debridement of an early-stage lesion should be avoided because it may increase the possibility of bacteremia. For mild cases of cutaneous anthrax in adults, oral treatment with ciprofloxacin (500 mg every 12 hours) is recommended. If the strain is susceptible, oral doxycycline (100 mg every 12 hours) and amoxicillin (500 mg every 8 hours) are suitable alternatives. Treatment should be continued for 7–10 days, unless the infection was acquired in a bioterrorism context, in which case treatment should be continued for 60 days. Severe cutaneous anthrax is treated with the same drugs and dosages as inhalation anthrax. The recommended initial therapy for adults with clinically evident inhalation anthrax is 400 mg ciprofloxacin given intravenously every 12 hours.[12]

Staphylococcal Scalded Skin Syndrome

Staphylococcal scalded skin syndrome (SSSS) is an epidermolytic disease that is caused by two distinct toxins released by a strain of *S. aureus* of phage group II, primarily type 71. The toxins cause erythema with associated detachment of the superficial layers of the epidermis. SSSS occurs primarily in newborns and infants younger than 2 years of age, as well as in immunocompromised adults. The forms of SSSS range in severity from completely localized (bullous impetigo) to more generalized and extensive forms.[13]

CLINICAL DESCRIPTION The localized form is characterized by clusters of intact purulent bullae that rupture and produce erythematous and crusted erosive lesions. The most common sites are the intertriginous areas. The erythema typically deepens in color, and the skin becomes very tender. In addition to the axillae and groin, presentation is also periorificially on the face and neck, becoming more widespread as time progresses. There is often an accompanying fever, and the erythematous eruption can progress rapidly to flaccid bullae that wrinkle and exfoliate, leaving behind a tender denuded epidermis with an oozing erythematous base.

TREATMENT Therapy includes local care with baths and compresses for debridement of the sloughing epidermal layers. Topical antimicrobial agents that may be used include mupirocin, bacitracin, and sulfadiazine ointment. Successful systemic antimicrobial therapy has been found to include intravenous naficillin.[13] In severe cases, fluid and electrolyte loss must be carefully managed.

Toxic Shock Syndrome

Toxic shock syndrome (TSS) is an acute toxin-mediated febrile illness that is caused by the production and release of exotoxins by *S. aureus.* Systemic symptoms include acute onset of fever, hypotension, generalized skin and mucosal erythema, and multisystem failure. TSS has occurred more commonly but not exclusively in women who are using vaginal tampons of high absorbency for extended lengths of time. Nonmenstrual cases associated with localized infections, surgery, or insect bites have increased and now account for approximately one-third of all cases. Patients with nonmenstrual TSS have a higher mortality rate than those with menstrual TSS.[14]

CLINICAL DESCRIPTION Classic cutaneous findings of TSS include a generalized scarlatinform erythroderma with accompanying fever and hypotension. There is often extensive generalized nonpitting, nondependent, and dependent edema. One to two weeks following resolution of the erythema, there is desquamation of the palms and soles. Intense erythema of the bulbar conjunctivae, mouth, tongue, pharynx, vagina, and tympanic membranes may occur, often with ulceration. Strawberry tongue and subconjunctival hemorrhages are also typical. Nonspecific gastrointestinal symptoms also can manifest.

TREATMENT The treatment of TSS generally is supportive.[15] Patients usually are admitted to the intensive care unit for observation and treatment. Management includes fluid replacement for shock, careful organ system monitoring, and antibiotic therapy to eliminate staphylococcal colonization or infection. In severe cases, methylprednisolone has been administered, although this treatment is of uncertain value. In vitro studies have shown that immune globulins may have an important role in the treatment of the TSS.

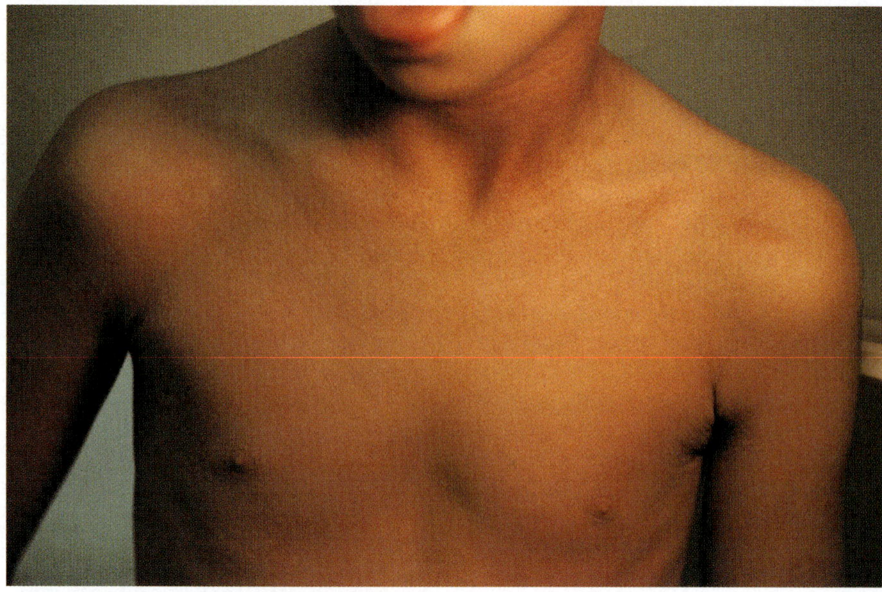

▲ **FIGURE 57-9** Scarlet Fever exanthem

Scarlet Fever

Scarlet fever is an acute infection of the tonsils and skin by an exotoxin-producing strain of GAS that typically occurs in children.[16]

CLINICAL DESCRIPTION The initial site of infection is typically the tonsils or pharynx, with resulting pharyngitis or tonsillitis, although it may begin in the skin or an infected wound. The first signs present with fine erythema on the upper trunk that may be accentuated in skin folds. The palms and soles are typically spared. The face is flushed with perioral pallor. The initial lesions become confluent and scarlitiniform. Scattered petechiae and distant lesions may occur (Figure 57-9). The exanthem usually fades within 4–5 days and is followed by desquamation on the body and extremities and exfoliation of the palms and soles. The tongue is characteristically white with scattered hyperkeratotic red papillae (white strawberry tongue). The hyperkeratotic membrane is sloughed and gives way to a strawberry tongue on day 4 or 5. Erythema and petechiae also may occur on the palate. The patient often appears acutely ill with anterior cervical lymphadenitis present.

TREATMENT Treatment includes acetaminophen for fever or pain. Penicillin is the antibiotic of choice because of its efficacy in preventing rheumatic fever. Clindamycin also can be used. Some recommend antibiotic prophylaxis for all those in close contact with a patient with invasive streptococcal disease. Human immune globulin contains considerable amounts of toxin-neutralizing antibodies and, if given at an early stage of invasive disease, may have a beneficial effect.[16]

GRAM-NEGATIVE INFECTIONS

Gram-negative infections of the skin are more common in children, patients with diabetes, and immunocompromised patients (Table 57-2). These infections typically are treated with a second- or third-generation cephalosporin.[1]

Cat-Scratch Disease

Cat-scratch disease is usually caused by the gram-negative bacillus *Bartonella henselae.*[17] It is a relatively benign, self-limited disease that typically occurs after being scratched by a cat, although cases have been reported after contact with a cat that does not involve a scratch.

TABLE 57-2
Gram-Negative Infections

Cat-scratch disease
Tularemia
Cutaneous P. aeruginosa infections

CLINICAL DESCRIPTION The primary lesion occurs in the area of inoculation as a small papule or pustule that is firm and sometimes tender. Lesions typically occur on exposed skin, but mucous membrane inoculation has been reported. In that case, there is typically a light yellow granulation on the palperbral conjunctivae with associated preauricular or cervical lymphadenopathy. Most patients are afebrile.

TREATMENT The literature is full of conflicting suggestions about the role and selection of antibiotics for cat-scratch disease mostly because it is a disease in which most patients are not seriously ill and spontaneous resolution is very common.[18] The disease is typically self-limiting with a maximum duration of about 2 months, although extended times have been reported. Antimicrobial therapy has not been proven to alter the course of the disease. However, ciprofloxacin, doxycycline, and erythromycin are therapeutic options.[19] Azithromycin may shorten the duration of lymphadenopathy, as was demonstrated in a small prospective, comparative study published recently.[20] In a minority of patients (about 15%) with typical cat-scratch disease, the affected lymph node undergoes suppuration and becomes exquisitely tender. Drainage with a large-bore needle usually results in the almost immediate relief of pain. However, incision and drainage are seldom necessary and may result in the development of a chronic sinus tract.

Tularemia

Tularemia is caused by *Fransiella tularensis,* a gram-negative coccobacillus. Transmission can be through a puncture or abrasion in the skin, autoinoculation, or from ingestion or inhalation. Although accidental exposure can occur through arthropod bites (e.g., ticks or dearflies), handling infected animals (e.g., rabbits and squirrels), or breathing in aerosols, cases usually are isolated and contained. While we will focus on the cutaneous transmission or tularemia, it is noteworthy to remember that a much more devastating transmission via inhalation exists. Its high infectivity makes it a major concern to public health officials as a possible biological weapon.[21]

CLINICAL DESCRIPTION Tularemia has six potential presentations: ulceroglandular, glandular, oculoglandular, oropharyngeal, typhoidal, and pneumonic. The ulceroglandular form is the most common and the one that typically presents with skin lesions. If there is an inoculation site, it is typically an erythematous, tender papule that enlarges with raised, well-demarcated crusted borders, surrounded by an area of cellulitis. There is a depressed center that is covered by a black eschar, evidence of rapid necrosis. Mucous membrane involvement includes the conjunctivae and typically causes a purulent, painful, edematous conjunctivitis with small yellow nodules visible on the conjunctivae. A high fever, chills, headache, and malaise typically accompany the rash, and as the bacteremia ensues, painful regionally lymphadenopathy develops.

TREATMENT Much of management focuses on prevention by ensuring complete protective gear when handling wild rabbits. The drug of choice is streptomycin, 1–2 g/day, until the patient has been afebrile for 7–10 days. Gentamicin, tetracycline, and quinolones are also effective.[22]

Cutaneous *P. aeruginosa* Infections

P. aeruginosa produces a host of bacterial infections and is most concerning because of its propensity for infecting hospitalized and immunocompromised patients.[23] *Pseudomonas* rarely infects healthy people but instead infects hosts when the normal flora has been disrupted, a normal cutaneous barrier has been disrupted by a foreign object, or following an injury or trauma. Once local invasion occurs, ecthyma gangrenosum, a necrotizing soft tissue infection, ensues and is associated with blood vessel invasion, sepsis, vascular occlusion, and infarction of tissue throughout the body.

CLINICAL DESCRIPTION Cutaneous manifestations of pseudomonal infection include colonization on the undersurface of nails in patients with onychomycotic nails, in the hair follicles of healthy patients exposed to hot tubs, and in macerated intertiginous spaces. An outbreak of *Pseudomonas* among people using hot tubs and whirlpools occurs on submerged parts of the skin, which develop erythematous, follicular papules and pustules. The symptoms of this self-limited condition usually last from 7–10 days. *Pseudomonas* hot foot syndrome manifests with tender nodules on the soles of children's feet after using a wading pool. *Pseudomonas* also can cause a primary infection at a break in the skin, a hair follicle, or a secondary infection at a site of trauma or disease.

TREATMENT Treatment of mild cutaneous disease is usually supportive, with antipruritic agents administered orally or topically. Acetic acid 5% compresses applied for 20 minutes twice daily also can be used for symptomatic relief. When systemic manifestations (e.g., fever, chills, and lymphadenopathy) are present, a course of oral ciprofloxacin therapy (500 mg twice daily for a week) may be warranted. Adequate chlorination and control of the pH level of the hot tub can help to prevent hot tub folliculitis.[23] Treatment of more severe cases or cases in immunocompromised patients includes correcting an existing low white blood cell count by giving a colony-stimulating factor, antimicrobial therapy appropriate for the specific sensitivity of the infecting strain, and surgical debridement of areas of skin infarction.[23]

A number of cutaneous infections have the potential of infecting individuals with skin of color. General knowledge of the offending agent, as well as appropriate therapy, is important for physicians caring for this patient population.

REFERENCES

1. Stulberg DL, Penrod MA, Blatny RA. Common bacterial skin infections. *Am Fam Physician* 2002;66:119-124.
2. Holdiness MR. Management of cutaneous erthythrasma. *Drugs* 2002;62: 1131-1141.
3. Axelsson I. Treatment of impetigo: Save mupirocin. *Br Med J* 2004;329:979.
4. Cook-Bolden FE, Barba A, Halder R, Taylor S. Twice-daily applications of benzoyl peroxide 5%/clindamycin 1% gel versus vehicle in the treatment of pseudofolliculitis barbae. *Cutis* 2004;73: 18-24S.
5. Boni R, Nehrhoff B. Treatment of gram-negative folliculitis in patients with acne. *Am J Clin Dermatol* 2003;4:273-276.
6. Scott PM. Drainage for an acute paronychia. *J Am Acad Phys Assist* 2002;15:57-58.
7. Takama H, Tamada Y, Yano K, et al. Pitted keratolysis: Clinical manifestations in 53 cases. *Br J Dermatol* 1997; 137:282-285.
8. Hedrick J. Acute bacterial skin infections in pediatric medicine: Current issues in presentation and treatment. *Paediatr Drugs* 2003;5:35-46S.
9. Bonnetblanc JM, Bedane C. Erysipelas: Recognition and management. *Am J Clin Dermatol* 2003;4:157-163.
10. Swartz MN. Clinical practice: Cellulitis. *N Engl J Med* 2004;350:904-912.
11. McCray MK, Esterly NB. Blistering distal dactylitis. *J Am Acad Dermatol* 1981;5: 592-594.

12. Carucci JA, McGovern TW, Norton SA, et al. Cutaneous anthrax management algorithm. *J Am Acad Dermatol* 2002;47:766-769.
13. Schenfeld LA. Images in clinical medicine: Staphylococcal scalded skin syndrome. *N Engl J Med* 2000;342:1178.
14. Manders SM. Infectious disease update. *Dermatol Clin* 2001;19:749-756.
15. Manders SM. Toxin-mediated streptococcal and staphylococcal disease. *J Am Acad Dermatol* 1998;39:383-398.
16. Bialecki C, Feder HM Jr, Grant-Kels JM. The six classic childhood exanthems: A review and update. *J Am Acad Dermatol* 1989;21:891-903.
17. Lamps LW, Scott MA. Cat-scratch disease: Historic, clinical, and pathologic perspectives. *Am J Clin Pathol* 2004;121:71-80S.
18. Adal KA, Cockerell CJ, Petri WA Jr. Cat scratch disease, bacillary angiomatosis, and other infections due to Rochalimaea. *N Engl J Med* 1994;330:1509-1515.
19. Margileth AM. Cat scratch disease. *Adv Pediatr Infect Dis* 1993;8:1-21.
20. Bass JW, Freitas BC, Freitas AD, et al. Prospective, randomized, double-blind, placebo-controlled evaluation of azithromycin for treatment of cat-scratch disease. *Pediatr Infect Dis J* 1998;17:447-452.
21. Gallagher-Smith M, Kim J, Al-Bawardy R, Josko D. *Francisella tularensis:* Possible agent in bioterrorism. *Clin Lab Sci* 2004;17:35-39.
22. Senol M, Ozcan A, Karincaoglu Y, et al. Tularemia: A case transmitted from a sheep. *Cutis* 1999;63:49-51.
23. Werlinger KD, Moore AY. Therapy of other bacterial infections. *Dermatol Ther* 2004;17:505-512.

CHAPTER 58

Folliculitis

Kim Nichols

Key Points

- Folliculitis is an inflammatory condition of the hair follicle caused by infection, physical injury, or chemical irritation.
- Certain deep follicular disorders, such as pseudofolliculitis barbae and acne keloidalis nuchae, are more common in African-Americans.
- The most common type of folliculitis is infectious usually secondary to *Staphylococcus aureas* which is treated with topical and oral antibiotics.
- Staphylococcal folliculitis is particularly prevalent in the African-American human immunodeficiency virus (HIV)–positive population.
- The noninfectious folliculitides are induced by drugs/chemicals and mechanically.
- Eosinophilic folliculitis is a rare sterile folliculitis encompassing the classic Ofuji disease, HIV-associated eosinophilic folliculitis, and eosinophilic pustular folliculitis of infancy.

SYNONYMS

- Pseudofolliculitis barbae
- Tinea barbae
- Barber's itch

Folliculitis is an inflammatory disorder of the hair follicle caused by infection (most commonly coagulase-positive staphylococci), physical injury, or chemical irritation. These insults result in the disruption or obstruction of individual hair follicles and the associated pilosebaceous units. Folliculitis is classified according to the level of involvement of the hair follicle—superficial or deep—and the microbial etiology. Superficial folliculitis (impetigo of Bockhart) affects the upper portion of the hair follicle, the follicular infundibulum, whereas deep folliculitis (sycosis) extends into the isthmus and deeper portions of the hair follicle. In superficial folliculitis, the follicular inflammation is confined, leading to the formation of the characteristic clustered 1- to 4-mm pustules or crusted nontender eythematous papules that heal without scarring. They are found more often in areas with terminal hairs. Deep folliculitis appears as large tender erythematous papules or nodules that can scar. And when the perifollicular inflammation extends into the surrounding tissues, pus-filled furuncles or carbuncles can form.

Although folliculitis does not have a specific racial predilection, because the condition is more common in economically disadvantaged groups in the United States, it is seen disproportionately in African-Americans and Latinos as compared with Caucasians. And the deep folliculitides pseudofolliculitis barbae and acne keloidalis are particularly more common in African-Americans.

The most common type of folliculitis is infectious, and although most often secondary to *S. aureus* infection, it also can be caused by *Pseudomonas aeruginosa,* gram-negative bacteria, dermatophytes, *Pityrosporum, Candida, Demodex,* and viruses. Secondary infectious folliculitis can be seen in other folliculocentric inflammatory disorders such as acne keloidalis nuchae, pseudofolliculitis barbae, and perifolliculitis capitis absecedens et suffodiens. This secondary infectious folliculitis is also known as *dissecting cellulitis,* which, with hidradenitis suppurativa and acne conglobata, make up the *follicular occlusion triad.* When pilonidal sinus accompanies this triad, it is called the *follicular occlusion tetrad.* Folliculitis also can be noninfectious in origin, as in drug, irritant-, and chemically-induced folliculitis. There are also the sterile eosinophilic folliculitides—eosinophilic pustular folliculitis (Ofuji disease), HIV-associated eosinophilic folliculitis, and eosinophilic pustular folliculitis of infancy—a group of rare, noninfectious follicular inflammatory disorders of unknown etiology.

EPIDEMIOLOGY AND PATHOGENESIS

Folliculitis is a very common disorder that occurs in children and adults and affects males and females equally. As mentioned earlier, it is often seen in association with acne keloidalis nuchae, pseudofolliculitis barbae, and dissecting cellulitis, follicular disorders (but not true folliculitides) that are more common in African-Americans. The overall incidence of folliculitis is increased in the obese and immunocompromised populations, such as those with diabetes mellitus, HIV infection or the acquired immune deficiency syndrome (AIDS), transplant patients, and people with immunologic disorders (e.g., hypogammaglobunemia and chronic granulomatous disease). Predisposing factors to folliculitis include occlusion, friction, maceration, and hyperhidrosis. Manipulation of the hair by shaving, waxing, or plucking can lead to traumatic folliculitis. Use of topical corticosteroids can precipitate folliculitis, particularly when moist lesions are occluded for many hours. In addition, those with preexisting dermatidides such as atopic dermatitis are more prone to develop a concomitant or secondary infection of folliculitis. Folliculitis also may follow skin injuries, arthropod bites, abrasions, and surgical wounds or draining abscesses.

The infectious folliculitides often occur more frequently in particular populations or under specific conditions. For instance, because *S. aureus* is a normal inhabitant of the anterior nares in approximately 20% of adults, nasal carriers are particularly prone to *S. aureus* folliculitis. Staphylococcal outbreaks are also common in team athletes who wear occlusive clothing in hot, humid weather, share fomites such as towels and athletic equipment, and shower in group facilities. Hot tub folliculitis, or *Pseudomonas* folliculitis, is seen most often in people exposed to contaminated water (e.g., whirlpools, swimming pools, water slides, and bathtubs). Gram-negative folliculitis develops in acne patients as a consequence of long-term antibiotic therapy. Tinea barbae is a fungal folliculitis affecting the mustache and beard areas of men (usually farm workers) who are exposed to *Trichophyton*-carrying cattle and dogs. And majocchi's granuloma (caused by *T. rubrum*), herpetic folliculitis, and molluscum folliculitis almost always occur after shaving.

STAPHYLOCOCCAL AND OTHER INFECTIOUS FOLLICULITIDES

Clinical Features

S. aureus superficial folliculitis (impetigo of Bockhart) is characterized by a gridlike grouping of papules or pustules on hair-bearing skin. It can occur on all body surfaces but is found most commonly on the head and neck (especially the perioral, scalp, and beard areas), upper trunk, axillae, groin, and buttocks. Folliculitis involving an eyelash is called a *hordeolum* or *sty.* When found in the pubic area, it may be secondary to sexual transmission. The primary lesions are erythematous papules and fragile yellowish white dome-shaped pustules with central hairs, although the hair shaft is not always seen. Secondary characteristics can include crusting, scale, and excoriations. Although most often asymptomatic, folliculitis lesions can be pruritic, especially in occluded areas. The lesions heal without scarring. And in most cases of common folliculitis, systemic symptoms are absent. In dark-skinned patients, the classic erythema seen in light-skinned patients is often masked.

Deep staphylococcal folliculitis involves the entire hair follicle, causing furuncles or "boils" (walled-off collections of pus around hair follicles), carbuncles, and sycoses (barbae and lupoid). Furuncles usually evolve from a superficial folliculitis in hair-bearing occluded regions of the body. They are deep-seated erythematous nodules that can enlarge to up to 2 cm and become hard, painful, and fluctuant. Over several days, they may undergo abscess formation, discharge pus, and eventually rupture with gradual diminution of pain and erythema (Figure 58-1). Carbuncles, which are seen most often on the neck, back, and thighs, are more extensive types of furuncles characterized by red indurated nodules with multiple draining pustules. They are often exquisitely painful, associated with fever and malaise, and can heal with prominent scarring[1] (Figure 58-2).

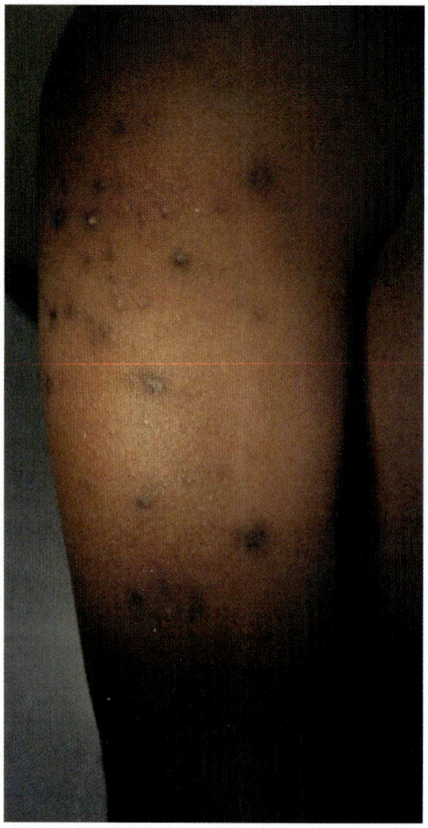

▲ **FIGURE 58-1** Staphylococcal folliculitis, right lateral arm.

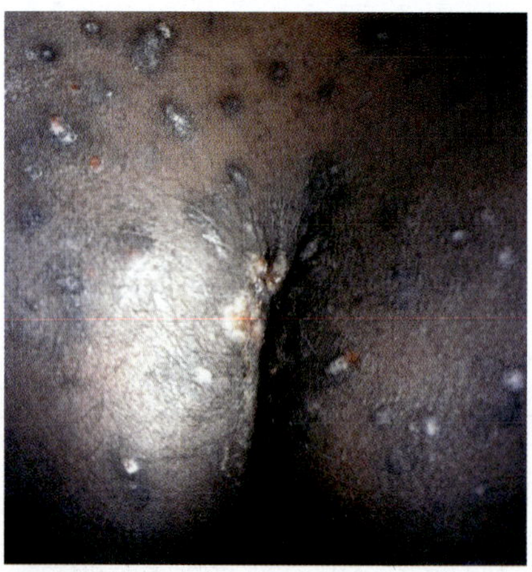

▲ **FIGURE 58-2** Extensive carbuncles, buttocks and intergluteal cleft.

HIV-seropositive patients are especially prone to more serious cases of staphylococcal folliculitis, furunculosis, and carbuncles. *S. aureus* is the most common cutaneous bacterial pathogen because about half of all HIV-positive patients are nasal carriers. In one series, 54% of patients with AIDS experienced clinical symptoms of *S. aureus* cutaneous infection during the course of their illness.[2] In another recent multicenter longitudinal study of HIV infection in women, the prevalence of skin disorders was compared in 2018 HIV-infected women and 557 HIV-uninfected women.[3] Skin abnormalities were reported more frequently among HIV-infected than uninfected women (63% versus 44%, respectively), and infected women were more likely to have more than two skin diagnoses. HIV infection was correlated with several specific skin conditions, including folliculitis, seborrheic dermatitis, herpes zoster, Kaposi sarcoma, and onychomycosis, whereas a significant difference was not found in the prevalence of warts, tinea pedis, nongenital herpes simplex, psoriasis, or xerosis between the HIV-infected and uninfected women. Interestingly, there also was an unexpected increased proportion of skin conditions in African-American HIV-positive women compared with their Caucasian and Hispanic counterparts. The reasons for this racial predilection were unclear, but it was supposed that clinicians may be less likely to identify lesions in the patients with light skin.[3]

Sycosis barbae (also known as *sycosis vulgaris* or *barber's itch*) is a deep folliculitis with perifollicular inflammation occurring in the bearded areas of the face and lip. It is caused by staphylococcal or dermatophytic infection and occurs only in postpubertal men who have begun shaving. It begins with the appearance of a few scattered papules and pustules that later rupture and autoinoculate, creating a pattern of recurrence and chronicity. The deeper, chronic and scarring form of sycosis barbae is termed *lupoid sycosis.*[4] Sycosis barbae is to be distinguished from tinea barbae, pseudofolliculitis barbae (PFB), and herpetic sycosis. Tinea barbae is often unilateral and rarely affects the upper lip. PFB is noninfectious in etiology, occurs mainly in African-American men, and shaving makes PFB worse, whereas it usually improves sycosis barbae.[5] And in herpes folliculitis there are most often vesicles present at some point during the disease course.

The nonstaphylococcal infectious folliculitides may not be clinically distinguishable from both the superficial and deep forms of *S. aureus* folliculitis and thus may require culture, potassium hydroxide (KOH), or even biopsy for diagnosis. However, a complete history and thorough physical examination usually will serve to narrow the microbial etiology. For example, if a patient has been swimming in the community pool and breaks out in erythematous papulopustules sparing the face, the most likely diagnosis is *P. aeruginosa* folliculitis. Table 58-1 summarizes the pathogens, clinical features, and treatments for common nonstaphycoccal infectious folliculitides.

Diagnosis

In practice, folliculitis is usually diagnosed clinically and treated empirically. However, in cases resistant to therapy, a Gram stain, culture, KOH test, or Tzanck smear may be required. A bacterial Gram stain and culture are performed by unroofing a pustular lesion and depositing the material on the cotton swab of a culture medium. Typically, the result shows the gram-positive cocci of *S. aureus,* but it is often

TABLE 58-1
Common Nonstaphycoccal Infectious Folliculitides[1,6]

Type	Clinical Features
Bacterial Folliculitis	
P. aeruginosa folliculitis	Hot tub folliculitis
Gram-negative folliculitis	Occurs at site of acne vulgaris often on the face after long-term antibiotic therapy
Syphilitic folliculitis	Secondary syphilis; acneform
Dermatophyte Folliculitis	
Tinea barbae	Due to *T. mentaprophytes* var. *mentagrophytes* or *T. verrucosum* classically in male farm workers
Majocchi granuloma	Usually due to *T. rubrum*, characteristically develops in women who shave their legs
***Pityrosporum* Folliculitis**	Often occurs in young adults in areas of occlusion and increased sweat production
***Candida* Folliculitis**	
Viral Folliculitis	
Herpes simplex folliculitis	Herpes sycosis barbae is seen in men who shave with a history of recurrent facial herpes simplex infection
Follicular Molluscum Contagiosum	
***Demodex* Folliculitis**	Often seen in association with immune suppression
Drug-Induced Folliculitis	Common offending agents include corticosteroids, androgenic hormones, iodides, bromides, lithium, INH, anticonvulsants and ACTH

Sources: Data from Kelly AP: Folliculitis and the follicular occlusion triad, in Bolognia JL, Jorizzo JL, Rapini RP, et al (eds), *Dermatology*, 1st ed. London, Mosby, 2003, p 554 and Lee PK, Zipoli MT, Weinberg AN, et al. Pyodermas: *Staphylococcus aureus, Streptococcus,* and Other Gram-Positive Bacteria, in Freedberg IM, Eisen AZ, Austen KF, et al (eds), *Fitzpatrick's Dermatology in General Medicine*, 6th ed. New York, McGraw-Hill, 2003, p 1860.[1,6]

falsely negative.[6] In chronic cases of suspected staphylococcal folliculitis, a nasal culture should be performed to identify chronic nasal carriers. Viral cultures and Tzanck smears are performed to diagnose herpetic sycosis, showing the multinucleate giant cells characteristic of herpetic infection. And because bacterial folliculitis can be complicated by concomitant mite infection, skin scrapings can be analyzed microscopically to look for *D. folliculorum;* however, again, false-negative results are common.

Pathology

In rare cases, a biopsy of an acute pustular lesion might be required for a definitive diagnosis. Superficial folliculitis (impetigo of Bockhart) is characterized histologically by a subcorneal pustule at the follicular opening surrounded by a dense inflammatory infiltrate predominated by neutrophils. A furuncle shows an area of perifollicular necrosis containing fibrinoid material and neutrophils. In chronic deep folliculitis (sycosis barbae and lupoid), the perifollicular infiltrate is mixed with neutrophils, lymphocytes, histiocytes, and plasma cells and forms a large abscess that eventually destroys the hair follicle. In older lesions, granulation tissue with foreign-body giant cells is seen surrounding the necrotic follicle. Eventually, as is the case in lupoid sycosis, fibrotic scar tissue can form.[7]

Similar histology is seen in *Pseudomonas* folliculitis with disruption and often rupture of the follicle by a dense polymorphic inflammatory infiltrate. In other infectious folliculitides, the biopsy can help to pinpoint the microbial etiology of lesions that clinically appear very similar. For example, in herpetic sycosis, the pathology often will show ballooning degeneration of the follicular epithelium and sebaceous cells with central eosinophilic inclusion bodies. And in suspected *Pityrosporum* folliculitis, periodic acid–Schiff (PAS) staining often reveals single-budding *Malassezia* yeasts and spores in the central and deep follicles.[8]

Differential Diagnosis

Although the infectious types of folliculitis can present similarly, a detailed history and examination of lesional morphology and body distribution usually can lead to the etiology. For staphylococcal folliculitis, the leading differential diagnoses include the noninfectious folliculitides (e.g., drug-induced, eosinophilic folliculitis, and pseudofolliculitis barbae), acne vulgaris, miliaria, milia, pustular psoriasis, impetigo, steroid acne, intertrigo, tinea cruris, arthropod bites, and all the other many conditions that can present with papulopustular eruptions. Most often in folliculitis, the strictly perifollicular location of the papules and pustules and the lack of other associated primary lesions (i.e., comedones in acne vulgaris, scaly erythematous plaques in tinea cruris, and honey-crusted plaques in impetigo) will lead to the diagnosis.

Treatment

Mild cases of staphylococcal folliculitis are treated initially with antibacterial soaps and washes (e.g., Lever 2000, Hibiclens, and Betadine washes). It is recommended that affected areas be washed at least three times daily. In addition, topical benzoyl peroxide and topical antibiotics such as clindamycin may be used. For more severe cases of superficial folliculitis, and for most cases of sycosis, empirical treatment with penicillinase-resistant oral antibiotics is indicated (e.g., a first-generation cephalosporin, azithromycin, or dicloxacillin). In cases where methicillin-resistant *S. aureus* (MRSA) is cultured, appropriate MRSA antibiotic therapy should be employed. And for recurrent or recalcitrant folliculitis, 2% mupirocin ointment should be applied to the anterior the nares to treat *S. aureus* nasal carriers. The treatments of the nonstaphylococcal folliculitides are discussed in Table 58-1.

For furuncles and carbuncles, treatment consists of local measures such as warm compresses and surgical drainage along with the use of penicillinase-resistant antibiotics (or vancomycin if MRSA is isolated). Prophylaxis against recurrences should include good personal hygiene, use of hexachlorophene soap for bathing, and topical use of mupirocin to the nares to eradicate colonization. In chronic furunculosis, extended courses of oral antibiotics such as low-dose clindamycin or rifampin have been used to eradicate the carrier state.

In all cases, care should be taken to eliminate predisposing factors. Recommendations include the removal of occlusive clothes or dressings; the treatment of hyperhidrosis with frequent clothes changes, Domeboro soaks, and aluminum chloride solution; and the appropriate treatment and/or cure of concomitant preexisting dermatitides and skin injuries.

DRUG-, CHEMICAL-, AND MECHANICALLY-INDUCED FOLLICULITIS

Drug-induced folliculitis can occur in all age groups, but it more common in acne-prone patients. It can develop within 2 weeks of starting a drug, and its appearance and severity usually are dose- and duration-dependent. It can look quite similar to acne with monomorphic erythematous papules and pustules on the chest and back, but comedones are rarely present. Numerous medications have been implicated, including topical and oral corticosteroids, iodides, bromides, isonazid, anticonvulsants, corticotropin, androgenic hormones, and lithium.[9] Lithium, for example, can cause or exacerbate folliculitis, acne, and psoriasis—conditions that are characterized by the pathologic findings of neutrophilic infiltration. In controlled studies, patients treated with lithium developed more cutaneous reactions than patients receiving other psychotropics, with a prevalence as high as 45%.[9] Folliculitis is also often a side effect of chemotherapeutic agents, most commonly dactinomycin, methotrexate, and cisplatin.[10] And case reports have indicated that granulocyte colony-stimulating factor (G-CSF) can cause a folliculitis of the face and torso in healthy individuals.[11] For drug-induced folliculitis, discontinuing the medication, if possible, should be the first course of therapy. In addition, topical and oral antibiotics may facilitate more rapid resolution.

Numerous chemical irritants can cause folliculitis, especially on the job. It is estimated that over 1 million workers in the United States regularly use oils and greases at work.[12] Exposure to these solvents, cutting oils, tars, and crude petroleum oils and subsequent mechanical blockage of the pilosebaceous units can lead to occupational acne and folliculitis. Treatment recommendations include avoidance of occupational irritants, if possible, and frequent cleansing of skin and washing of oil-soaked uniforms.[12]

For other workers, folliculitis occurs as a consequence of mechanical irritation. Wherever there is frictional trauma or occlusion, folliculitis can be seen. For example, truck drivers are prone to folliculitis of the buttocks and back, and football players have a high incidence of folliculitis underneath their padding and on the posterior scalp and neck secondary to helmet irritation. Again, frequent skin washing and changing of tight, moist clothing is advised.

EOSINOPHILIC FOLLICULITIDES

Eosinophilic folliculitis is a sterile type of folliculitis that should be considered in the differential diagnosis of a papulopustular eruption. There are three major types: (1) eosinophilic pustular folliculitis, (2) HIV/AIDS-associated eosinophilic folliculitis, and (3) eosinophilic pustular folliculitis of infancy.

Classic eosinophilic pustular folliculitis (EPF or Ofuji disease) is a rare dermatosis of unknown etiology. It primarily affects young-adult males and is characterized clinically by recurrent pruritic follicular papules and pustules that coalesce to form annular plaques on the face, upper back, and upper extremities. Peripheral blood eosinophilia is also seen. Histologically, infundibular eosinophilic pustules are the characteristic finding. The perifollicular infiltrate is mixed with eosinophils, lymphocytes, histiocytes, and mast cells. These mast cells are believed to be important in the pathogenesis of EPF because they are involved in the production of inflammatory mediators such as prostaglandin. For this reason, recent studies have shown that owing to its antiprostaglandin properties, indomethacin is a directed and effective treatment of EPF. Other therapies tried include ultraviolet B (alone or in conjunction with indomethacin), oral corticosteroids, minocycline, retinoids, and dapsone.[13]

HIV/AIDS-associated eosinophilic pustular folliculitis (AIDS-EF) is a pruritic papular eruption similar to classic EPF histologically but differing clinically. In AIDS-EF, the papules do not coalesce into figurate plaques, and the eruption is more chronic. AIDS-EF most often affects adult men with CD4+ counts of less than 300 cells/mm^3. It is characterized by intensely pruritic perifollicular erythematous papules and pustules found on the head and neck, trunk, and proximal extremities. Although not fully understood, it has been postulated that a shift toward Th2 cells and their related cytokines in the course of HIV infection induces IgE production and eosinophilia, leading to an allergic response that may, in part, explain the pathogenesis of AIDS-EF.[2] There is no definitive treatment for AIDS-EF. However, in addition to appropriate highly active antiretroviral therapy (HAART), topical and oral corticosteroids, permethrin cream, isotretinoin, and ultraviolet B all have been shown to be effective in certain cases.

Eosinophilic pustular folliculitis in infancy is a rare disorder affecting neonates in the first days to weeks of life, many times within the first 24 hours. Clinically, it looks very similar to Ofuji disease, but it usually localizes mainly to the scalp and face. In infants of color, it is important to distinguish EPF from transient neonatal pustular melanosis and infantile acropustulosis, disorders that primarily affect darkly pigmented children.[6] Parents must be reassured that EPF of infancy is a cyclic disease that is self-limiting and usually remits by the first few years of life.

REFERENCES

1. Lee PK, Zipoli MT, Weinberg AN, et al. Pyodermas: *Staphylococcus aureus, Streptococcus,* and other gram-positive bacteria, in Freedberg IM, Eisen AZ, Austen KF, et al (eds), *Fitzpatrick's Dermatology in General Medicine,* 6th ed. New York, McGraw-Hill, 2003, p 1860.
2. Garman ME. The cutaneous manifestations of HIV infection. *Dermatol Clin* 2002;20:193-208.
3. Halder RM. Pseudofolliculitis barbae and related disorders. *Dermatol Clin* 1998;6: 407-412.
4. Böni R. Treatment of gram-negative folliculitis in patients with acne. *Am J Clin Dermatol* 2003;4:273-276.
5. Bonifaz A. Tinea barbae (tinea sycosis): Experience with nine cases. *J Dermatol* 2003;30:898-903.
6. Kelly AP. Folliculitis and the follicular occlusion triad, in Bolongia JL, Jorizzo JL, Rapini RP (eds), *Dermatology,* 1st ed. London, Mosby, 2003, p 554.
7. Lucas S. Bacterial disease, in Elder D, Elenitsas R, Jaworsky C, et al (eds), *Lever's Histopathology of the Skin,* 8th ed. Philadelphia, Lippincott Williams & Wilkins, 1997, p 461.
8. Assaf RR, Weil ML. The superficial mycoses. *Dermatol Clin* 1996;14:57-67.
9. Yeung CK. Cutaneous adverse effects of lithium: Epidemiology and management. *Am J Clin Dermatol* 2004;5:3-8.
10. Epstein EH, Lutzner MH. Folliculitis induced by actinomycin D. *N Engl J Med* 1969;281:1094.
11. Paul C, Giachetti S, Pinquier L et al. Cutaneous effects of granulocyte colony-stimulating factoring healthy volunteers. *Arch Dermatol* 1998; 134:111.
12. Peate WE. Occupational skin disease. *Am Fam Physician* 2002;66:1025-1032.
13. Ishiguro N, Shishido E, Okamato R. Ofuji's disease: A report of 20 patients with clinical and histopathologic analysis. *J Am Acad Dermatol* 2002;46: 827-833.

CHAPTER 59

Fungal and Yeast Infections

Aditya K. Gupta
Lindsay E. Lynch

Key Points

- Although cutaneous fungal infections are common among most races, factors such as socioeconomic status, geographic location, and cultural or religious practices often correlate with ethnicity and may be the true influencers of susceptibility to fungal infections.
- The primary causative agents of superficial fungal infections are dermatophytes, whereas nondermatophyte molds and yeasts occur less frequently and are often associated with a change in immune status.
- Climatic differences affect the growing conditions for fungi; high ambient temperature and humidity provide an ideal setting for fungal proliferation.
- Occlusive clothing and footwear worn in cooler settings may generate suitable microclimates for mycotic activity.
- Underlying immunologic diseases such as human immunodeficiency virus (HIV) infection and the acquired immune deficiency syndrome (AIDS), which are of epidemic proportions in Africa, are associated with the higher incidence of fungal infections on this continent.
- Cultural or religious customs, such as communal bathing, may create opportunities for the transmission of fungi.
- Variations in hygienic practices also may explain increased susceptibility to fungal invasion.

Fungi are ubiquitous worldwide. By and large, the immune system provides adequate defense against fungal invasion; however, keratin has become an adaptive substrate for a group of fungi referred to as *dermatophytes,* the primary causative agents of superficial fungal infections. Nondermatophyte molds and yeasts are also cutaneous pathogens, but these infections are less frequent and are often associated with a change in immune status.

The presence of cutaneous mycoses does not appear to be a reflection of differences in the biologic characteristics of skin color; in fact, cutaneous fungal infections are common among most races.[1] Factors such as socioeconomic status, geographic location, and cultural or religious practices often correlate with ethnicity and may be the true influencers of susceptibility. Underlying immunologic diseases such as human immunodeficiency virus (HIV) infection and acquired immune deficiency syndrome (AIDS) are of epidemic proportions in Africa, and studies in this region have identified higher incidences of associated fungal infections. Climatic differences affect the growing conditions for fungi; high ambient temperature and humidity provide an ideal setting for fungal proliferation. In addition, occlusive clothing and footwear worn in cooler settings may generate suitable microclimates for mycotic activity. Cultural or religious customs, such as communal bathing, may create opportunities for the transmission of fungi. Variation in hygienic practices also may explain increased susceptibility to fungal invasion.

This chapter provides an overview of superficial fungal infections that are common to most skin types, including skin of color. Tinea capitis and seborrheic dermatitis are fungal infections found more frequently in people with skin of color, and these two disorders are covered in detail in Chapters 36 and 37.

MYCOLOGIC EXAMINATION

Accurate diagnosis of a fungal infection is necessary before selecting an appropriate treatment regimen. Mycologic methods are similar for most mycoses, the goal being confirmation of the presence of fungi and identification of the pathogenic species. Light microscopic examination is used to determine whether a fungal organism is present in the tissue sample. Direct examination is performed using 10–20% potassium hydroxide (KOH) to dissolve the surrounding keratin. In addition, calcofluor white or periodic acid–Schiff (PAS) stain may be added to the KOH preparation to enhance visibility of the fungal organism.[3,4] It should be noted that a negative microscopic result is not necessarily indicative of fungus-free tissue; sampling error and nonproliferating fungi that may not be visible on microscopic examination may contribute to false-negative results.[3]

Since antifungal agents have different spectra of activity, species identification is an integral part of disease management.[3,4] If species cannot be identified by microscopy, samples must be cultured to obtain this information. Culture media containing cycloheximide and chloramphenicol are used to deter the growth of nonpathogenic molds that may mask proliferation of the true fungal or yeast pathogen(s).[4] As with microscopy, a number of factors may contribute to false-negative culture results; therefore, the use of both microscopy and culture as diagnostic tools is encouraged.[3,4]

PITYRIASIS VERSICOLOR (TINEA VERSICOLOR)

Definition

Pityriasis versicolor (PV) is a noncontagious chronic benign disorder characterized by scaly hypo- or hyperpigmented superficial lesions on the body. It occurs mainly on the upper trunk, neck, and upper arms,[5,6] and usually involves areas of the skin rich in sebaceous glands.

Epidemiology

PV is distributed worldwide; however, it is more common in tropical climates. The disease affects mainly young adults of both sexes, although in tropical zones it is also common in infancy and even in neonates.[5] PV is generally uncommon before puberty and in old age, possibly owing to alterations in sebum production. Without treatment, PV is a chronic disease, and even after treatment, recurrence is common, affecting 60% of patients 1 year following treatment and 80% 2 years after treatment.[7]

Halder and colleagues, based on the diagnosis of 2000 black patients in Washington, DC, between 1980 and 1982, found that PV occurred in 2.4% of black patients compared with 0.2% of white patients.[8] A more recent epidemiologic report showed that PV in the United States occurs in 2.2% of the black population.[9] In southeast London, England, between January and March 1996, a diagnosis of PV was seen in 3.8% of the patients.[10] Furthermore, in Rwanda on the continent of Africa, PV was one of most commonly reported cutaneous diseases.[11]

Etiology

The lipophilic yeasts *Malassezia* species are the etiologic agents of PV. *M. globosa*[12,13] and *M. sympodialis*[14] may be the most common etiologic agents, whereas *M. furfur* has been isolated in some lesions.[15]

Malassezia yeasts are a part of normal skin flora; however, in individuals who develop PV, the organisms transform from saprophytic, round-celled, or yeast phase to the mycelial phase. A number of factors probably stimulate this conversion. The most important of these factors relates to local conditions on the skin; both high temperature and high humidity promote development of the disease, which may explain why PV is observed more commonly in tropical climates. Genetic susceptibility is also likely.[16] Other factors such as malnutrition, immunodeficiency, use of oral contraceptives, and hyperhidrosis may play a role in the etiology of PV.[16]

The frequent use, in individuals with skin of color, of palm oil or cocoa butter on the face also may promote growth of the yeast. These substances both contain high concentrations of complex lipids (e.g., glycol stearate, squalene, lanolin, mineral oil, and spermaceti), some of which have been proven to enhance growth of *M. furfur* in culture media.[17] In addition, these substances may act to occlude the skin, resulting in an increased carbon dioxide concentration, altered microflora, and altered pH range, leading to a subsequent overgrowth of fungi.[18]

Histopathology

Lesional skin samples show that *Malassezia* is present in all layers of the stratum corneum but least often in the lower part of the horny layer. The normal horizontal direction of the skin cells may be disrupted in the superficial and middle layers of the stratum corneum when the organism enters the keratinocytes.[19,20] The skin cells may swell and split, expelling the cell matrix and organelles, resulting in a "clear zone" around the invading yeast cells. Alternatively, the keratin within the invaded cells may be replaced by lipid-dense material.[21]

Hyperpigmented lesions of PV contain more spores and hyphae than either normal or hypopigmented skin. Merkel cells that contain melanosomes and secretory granules may have increased activity, and melanocytes may appear larger, singly distributed, and hypertrophic. Melanin production may be inhibited by azelaic acid or lipoxygenase produced by *Malassezia*.[22] A perivascular inflammation and lymphocyte infiltration have been reported in both hypopigmented and hyperpigmented skin.[23] In hypopigmented lesions, there may be a decrease in melanosomes in the stratum spinosum, and the horny layer may be hyperkeratotic.[23,24]

Diagnosis and Clinical Appearance

In individuals of color, PV lesions present as flaky round or oval maculae that are either hypo- or hyperpigmented. Some patients experience mild pruritus, but for most, PV is asymptomatic and mainly a cosmetic concern

The diagnosis of PV is confirmed by KOH preparations of skin scrapings that demonstrate pseudohyphae and spores. Wood's light is a useful diagnostic tool for cases of PV in which *M. furfur* is the etiologic agent.[25] The lesions appear bright yellow or gold in color. Culturing the yeast is not necessary for diagnosis.

The differential diagnosis includes vitiligo, chloasma, tinea corporis, pityriasis alba, pityriasis rotunda, pityriasis rosea, secondary syphilis, pinta, and seborrheic dermatitis. The distinguishing feature of PV is a characteristic "spaghetti and meatballs" appearance under the microscope that results from the transformation of the yeast to a mycelial form.

Treatment

Both topical and oral medications have demonstrated efficacy in the treatment of PV. Nonspecific agents, such as selenium sulfide and propylene glycol, physically or chemically remove infected stratum corneum. Modern antifungal medications have fungistatic (azoles) or fungicidal (allylamines) activity against *Malassezia* yeasts.

Patients who suffer from severe or widespread involvement of the skin with PV may prefer oral therapy (Table 59-1). Treatment selection requires a number of

TABLE 59-1
Commonly Used Systemic Treatment Regimens for Cutaneous Fungal Infections

Condition	Drug	Dose	Duration
Pityriasis versicolor	Itraconazole*	200 mg/day	5–7 days
	Fluconazole*	300-mg single dose	Repeated once at 7 days
	Ketoconazole*	200 mg/day	5–10 days
		400-mg single dose	Repeated once at 7 days
Tinea corporis/ cruris	Terbinafine	250 mg/day	2–4 weeks
	Itraconazole	200 mg/day	2 weeks
	Fluconazole	150 mg once weekly	2 weeks
	Griseofulvin	250 mg every 12 hours	Until infection clears
	Ketoconazole	200 mg/day	4–8 weeks
Tinea pedis	Terbinafine	250 mg/day	4 weeks
	Itraconazole	200 mg/day or	2 weeks
		200 mg twice daily	1 week (1 pulse)
	Fluconazole	150 mg once weekly	4–6 weeks
	Griseofulvin Microsize	500 mg every 12 hours	4–8 weeks
	Griseofulvin UltraMicrosize	250–375 mg every 12 hours	4–8 weeks
	Ketoconazole†	200–400 mg/day	1–8 weeks
	Terbinafine	250 mg/day	Fingernails—6 weeks Toenails—12 weeks
	Itraconazole pulse	200 mg twice daily	Fingernails—1 week/ month for 2 months Toenails—1 week/month for 3 months‡
	Itraconazole continuous	200 mg/day	Fingernails—6 weeks Toenails—12 weeks
	Fluconazole*	150 mg once weekly	Fingernails—for up to 9 months

*Regimen not approved by the U.S. Food and Drug Administration for this indication.
†For recalcitrant fungal infections, the prescribing limit is 1 g/day.
‡Not approved for the treatment of toenails in the United States.

considerations: extent and location of lesions, risks and benefits of treatment modality, age of patient, likelihood of compliance, and cost. Relapse of PV is not uncommon, and there is interest in the development of prophylactic treatment.

OTOMYCOSIS

Otomycosis is a subacute or chronic infection of the outer ear canal. Etiologic agents include *Aspergillus fumigatus, A. flavus,* and *A. nigers*.[26,27] Patients present with unilateral inflammation, pruritus, pain, scaling, and itching in the ear canal. Otoscopy reveals greenish or black fuzzy growth or debris in the canal. Compact clusters of branching, densely packed septate hyphae are seen on KOH preparation examination. Treatment may include application of imidazole creams or topical nystatin following careful cleaning of the canal.[26–28]

TINEA NIGRA

Tinea nigra is a rare asymptomatic infection of the stratum corneum affecting the palms, soles, neck, and trunk.[29] This infection is most commonly in tropical/subtropical areas. The causative agent, *Exophiala wernickii,*[30,31] resides in sewage, soil, decaying vegetation, wood, and humid environments. Clinical lesions are slightly scaly, mottled brownish or greenish black velvety macules. Lesions may develop as one or several spots and spread centrifugally, darkening at the border.[29,30,32] Macules may resemble melanoma on silver nitrate and India ink stains. Skin biopsy shows hyperkeratosis without dermal inflammation. KOH preparation examination of scrapings shows brownish or olive-colored branching septate hyphae and budding cells in the upper layers of the stratum corneum.[31,32] Diagnosis can be made readily by KOH preparation examination. The therapy of choice for tinea nigra is topical imidazoles.[32,33]

TINEA PIEDRA

Tinea piedra is an asymptomatic infection of the hair shaft. Two varieties of piedra exist: black piedra and white piedra.[34,35] Black piedra is commonly in the tropical regions of South America, the Far East, and the Pacific Islands and is less frequent in Africa and Asia. White piedra is found in the temperate regions of South America, Europe, Asia, and the southern United States. The causative organism of black piedra is *Piedraia hortae,* whereas white piedra is a result of *Trichosporon beigelii* infection.[34,35] Scalp hair is the most common site of black piedra infection. White piedra more commonly infects the beard, mustache, or pubic hair. KOH preparation examination of black piedra reveals hard, brown-black nodules on the hair shaft that are cemented together and resemble organized tissue. Nodules vary in size and are gritty to touch. White piedra has less firmly adherent nodules that are softer and vary in color from light brown to white and lack the organized appearance of black piedra.[34,35] Microscopic examination distinguishes piedra from nits, hair casts, developmental hair defects, and trichomycosis axillaris. Oral terbinafine is an effective therapy for black piedra. Treatment for white piedra includes imidazoles, ciclopirox olamine, 2% selenium sulfide, 6% precipitated sulfur in petrolatum, chlorhexidine solutions, and zinc pyrithione.[36,37]

TINEA CORPORIS/CRURIS (RING WORM, JOCK ITCH)

Definition

Tinea corporis (ringworm) includes all superficial dermatophyte infections of the glabrous skin, not including the scalp, beard, face, hands, feet, and groin.[37] Tinea cruris (jock itch) includes infections of the genitalia, pubic area, and perineal and perianal skin[37] and often involves the upper thigh.[4]

Etiology and Epidemiology

A number of dermatophytes may cause tinea corporis; however, *Microsporum canis, T. rubrum,* and *T. mentagrophytes* are usually the causative organisms.[38] Tinea corporis is found mainly in children, especially those exposed to animals with ringworm (*M. canis*). Tinea cruris is usually caused by *T. rubrum, T. mentagrophytes,* or *E. flocossum.*[38] A common predisposing factor for these dermatophyte infections in adults is excessive perspiration.[38] Also, occlusive clothing may provide an environment where the organisms can thrive.[38] There is a high incidence of tinea corporis/cruris in hot, humid areas of the world, with males being affected by tinea cruris more often than females.[38]

Pathogenesis

The responsible dermatophytes generally reside in the stratum corneum and do not penetrate below the epidermis.[39] The skin responds to the superficial infection by increasing proliferation, and this results in scale and epidermal thickening.[39]

Clinical Manifestations

Tinea corporis may take several clinical forms and may be mild to severe. In individuals with skin of color, the lesions may not be erythematous but rather brown or gray in color. Likewise, with tinea cruris, the characteristic red scaling plaques may in fact be tan, brown, or gray in color and extend down the sides of the inner thighs, waist area, and buttocks.[40]

Histopathology

Histopathologically, fungal organisms can be seen in the stratum corneum. If compact orthokeratosis is found in a section, there should be a search for fungal hyphae stained with hematoxylin.[38]

Diagnosis and Laboratory Findings

Diagnosis frequently can be established through review of the patient history and physical examination. However, there is greater diagnostic accuracy if the clinical diagnosis is verified by laboratory tests.[39] The affected area should be disinfected with alcohol or cleansed with water, and specimens should be obtained from the active border of the infection.[41]

Treatment

Noninflammatory, less severe cases of tinea corporis and cruris infections can be treated with topical antifungals such as econazole, clotrimazole, ciclopirox, etc. Systemic treatment (e.g., terbinafine, itraconazole, and fluconazole) should be considered when the infection is inflammatory, involves a large surface area of skin, in instances where host immunity is reduced or abnormal, and when there is chronic or recurrent infection with a poor response to topical therapy[41] (see Table 59-1). Other factors that determine the choice of therapy include the immunocompetence of the host, identity of the causative organism, site and extent of the infection, patient preference (oral versus topical treatment), and the cost-effectiveness of the two forms of therapy.[41]

TINEA PEDIS (ATHLETE'S FOOT)

Epidemiology

Tinea pedis (athlete's foot) is one of the most common superficial fungal infections, affecting at least 10% of the world population at any given time.[42] Prevalence rates for Europe and Asia are similar, ranging from 3–27%[43,44] and 4–20%,[45,46] respectively. In the Middle East, approximately 10% of the population is affected.[47] In general, race does not appear to affect the distribution of this disease; however, in South Africa, a higher incidence of tinea pedis et unguium was reported in men attending Muslim mosques, likely owing to religious practices involving barefoot communal washing and prayer.[48]

Tinea pedis is more common in men and the elderly.[43] Predisposing factors include diabetes, obesity, trauma, and immunosuppression.

Etiology

The dermatophytes *T. rubrum* and *T. mentagrophytes* are the most common causal organisms of tinea pedis. *Epidermophyton floccosum*[49,50] and nondermatophyte pathogens such as *Scytalidium dimidiatum* and *Fusarium* species,[45] are also associated with this disease.

Clinical Manifestations

Tinea pedis has three clinical types: interdigital, hyperkeratotic (moccasin), and vesicobullous.[49,51] Interdigital (dermatophytosis simplex), the most prevalent and often chronic form, usually affects toe web space between the fourth and fifth toes, followed by the toe web space between the third and fourth toes. The skin may appear white and macerated with red erosions.[51] The formation of diffuse hyperkeratosis and desquamative erythema on the sole and toes in a chronic and nonseasonal manner is characteristic of hyperkeratotic tinea pedis. This form is often accompanied by tinea unguium and generally is caused by *T. rubrum*.[52] The vesicobullous form, frequently caused by *T. mentagrophytes,* is characterized by inflammatory vesicles or bullous lesions.[42] It is sometimes associated with a secondary infection (dermatophytosis complex), itching, and maceration.[51] Severe cases are difficult to diagnose because secondary bacterial infections causing inflammation can mask the primary condition.[51]

Treatment

Patients should be examined for other fungal infections, especially onychomycosis, because the nails can acts as a reservoir of infection.[42,51] Prophylactic measures include wearing nonocclusive footwear, changing socks and shoes regularly,[42] and using antifungal foot powders.[53] Public baths and pools are major sources of infection by dermatophytes[54] and should be avoided, if possible. Washing the feet with soap and thoroughly drying them also have been found to reduce the presence of dermatophytes.[54]

Oral and topical antifungal agents can be used to treat tinea pedis depending on the presentation. Treatment of dermatophytosis simplex involves topical antifungal agents (e.g., azoles, allylamines, and ciclopirox). Therapy for dermatophytosis complex requires both antibacterial and antifungal activity in addition to a local astringent to dry the affected area, such as ciclopirox gel.[55]

While oral griseofulvin and ketoconazole are currently the only indicated systemic treatment options for tinea pedis in the United States (see Table 59-1), clinical success with modern oral antifungals terbinafine, itraconazole, and fluconazole are now providing physicians with a larger variety of acceptable therapeutic options.[56]

ONYCHOMYCOSIS (TINEA UNGUIUM)

Definition

Onychomycosis is a fungal infection involving the nail unit.

Etiology

Approximately 90% of infections are caused by dermatophytes, with *T. rubrum* being the most commonly isolated etiologic agent.[57,58] Other dermatophyte pathogens include *T. mentagrophytes* and *E. floccosum*.[59] Nondermatophyte molds such as *Scopulariopsis brevicaulis, Acremonium* species, *Aspergillus* species, *Scytalidium* species, *Onychocola canadensis, Alternaria* species, and *Fusarium* species are responsible for 2.1–12.5% of onychomycotic infections depending on geographic location.[60] *Candida* onychomycosis is rare and usually limited to immunocompromised individuals.[60]

Epidemiology

Onychomycosis accounts for nearly 50% of all nail disorders.[59,61] North American epidemiologic studies suggest prevalence rates between 8% and 13.8%.[57,59] Slightly higher prevalence rates were reported for Europe (23–26%) and East Asia (22%).[62] The distribution of onychomycosis does not appear to be directly affected by race,[59] although cultural and socioeconomic factors may play a role. Dermatophytes were isolated from communal ablution areas in several Muslim mosques in a South African study; the incidence of infection reported in males regularly attending these mosques was higher than in non-Muslim males from the same community.[48]

Toenails generally are affected more often than fingernails.[57] Predisposing factors include diabetes mellitus, peripheral arterial disease, compromised immune system, smoking, increasing age, and the male gender.[63]

Pathogenesis and Clinical Manifestations

There are four main routes of entry into the nail unit, each with a corresponding clinical presentation.[64,65] Total dystrophic onychomycosis (TDO) results from the progression of one or more of the four main presentations (secondary infection) or from simultaneous invasion of all nail tissues as a result of immunosuppression (primary infection), as seen in patients with chronic mucocutaneous candidiasis.[64]

Histopathology

Histologic examination reveals fungal elements (spores or hyphae) in the stratum corneum, deep portion of the nail plate, or hyponychium depending on the clinical type.[66]

Diagnosis

Clinical suspicion calls for mycologic examination of the affected nail to rule out psoriasis, chronic onycholysis, lichen planus, yellow nail syndrome, trauma, etc.[61] Samples should be collected from different sites of the nail unit, including proximal nail clippings, curetted subungual debris, and nail plate shavings from the diseased portion of the nail, in order to maximize positive results.[67]

Treatment

Oral antifungal agents are the most effective treatments currently available for onychomycosis (see Table 59-1). The mechanism of action of azole (itraconazole) and allylamine (terbinafine) antifungal agents involves the inhibition of ergosterol biosynthesis, an essential component of the fungal cell membrane. These drugs penetrate the nail unit via the nail bed.

Modern topical antifungal nail lacquers, such as ciclopirox 8% and amorolfine 5%, exploit the use of a concentration gradient that promotes penetration of the active compound to the affected portion of the nail. Topical nail lacquers may provide a safe alternative for patients with onychomycosis of mild to moderate disease severity.

Removal of the affected portion of the nail by chemical or mechanical means may be used as an adjunct to antifungal therapy to reduce the fungal burden. Nail avulsion or debridement without concomitant antifungal therapy has a high potential for relapse.[68]

CUTANEOUS CANDIDOSIS (CANDIDIASIS)

Candida species are part of the normal human cutaneous microflora but may become pathogenic when host factors such as immune status are altered. Lesions may affect several body sites, including nails [see "Onychomycosis (Tinea Unguium)" above], with warm, moist intertriginous areas being affected most frequently. *C. albicans* is the main etiologic agent.

Clinical Manifestations

Cutaneous candidosis occurs in moist, macerated folds of skin. It presents as pruritic, erythematous, macerated areas.[69]

Laboratory Findings/Histopathology

For superficial candidal infections, examination of skin scrapings shows typical budding yeasts with hyphae or pseudohyphae in the stratum corneum. Culture results in whitish, mucoid colonies within 2–5 days.[70]

Treatment

Anticandidal topical therapy includes clotrimazole, econazole, ketoconazole, miconazole, ciclopirox, and nystatin. Oral itraconazole or fluconazole may be considerations if oral therapy is warranted.[71]

REFERENCES

1. Taylor SC. Epidemiology of skin diseases in ethnic populations. *Dermatol Clin* 2003;21:601.
2. Hartshorne ST. Dermatological disorders in Johannesburg, South Africa. *Clin Exp Dermatol* 2003;28:661.
3. Weinberg JM, Koestenblatt EK, Tutrone WD, et al. Comparison of diagnostic methods in the evaluation of onychomycosis. *J Am Acad Dermatol* 2003;49:193.
4. Padhye A, Weitzman I. The Dermatophytes, in Ajello L, Hay RJ (eds), *Medical Mycology*, 9th ed. London, Arnold, 1998, p 215.
5. Crespo E, Delgado F. *Malassezia* species in skin diseases. *Curr Opin Infect Dis* 2002;15:133.
6. Vander Straten MR, Hossain MA, Ghannoum MA. Cutaneous infections, dermatophytosis, onychomycosis, and tinea versicolor. *Infect Dis Clin North Am* 2003;17:87.
7. Faergemann J. *Pityrosporum* species as a cause of allergy and infection. *Allergy* 1999;54:413.
8. Halder RM, Grimes PE, McLaurin CI, et al. Incidence of common dermatoses in a predominantly black dermatologic practice. *Cutis* 1983;32:388-390.
9. Halder RM, Nootheti PK. Ethnic skin disorders overview. *J Am Acad Dermatol* 2003;48:S143.
10. Child FJ, Fuller LC, Higgins EM, et al. A study of the spectrum of skin disease occurring in a black population in south-east London. *Br J Dermatol* 1999;141:512.
11. Van Hecke E, Bugingo G. Prevalence of skin disease in Rwanda. *Int J Dermatol* 1980;19:526.
12. Gupta AK, Kohli Y, Summerbell RC, et al. Quantitative culture of *Malassezia* species from different body sites of individuals with or without dermatoses. *Med Mycol* 2001;39:243.
13. Nakabayashi A, Sei Y, Guillot J. Identification of *Malassezia* species isolated from patients with seborrhoeic dermatitis, atopic dermatitis, pityriasis versicolor and normal subjects. *Med Mycol* 2000;38:337.
14. Gupta AK, Kohli Y, Summerbell RC, et al. Quantitative culture of *Malassezia* species from different body sites of individuals with or without dermatoses. *Med Mycol* 2001;39:243.
15. Mayser P, Gross A. IgE antibodies to *Malassezia furfur, M. sympodialis* and *Pityrosporum orbiculare* in patients with atopic dermatitis, seborrheic eczema or pityriasis versicolor, and identification of respective allergens. *Acta Dermatol Venereol* 2000;80:357.
16. Gueho E, Boekhout T, Ashbee HR, et al. The role of *Malassezia* species in the ecology of human skin and as pathogens. *Med Mycol* 1998;36:220S.
17. Porro MN, Passi S, Caprilli F, et al. Induction of hyphae in cultures of *Pityrosporum* by cholesterol and cholesterol esters. *J Invest Dermatol* 1977;69:531.
18. King RD, Cunico RL, Maibach HI, et al. The effect of occlusion on carbon dioxide emission from human skin. *Acta Dermatol Venereol* 1978;58:135.
19. Gupta AK, Bluhm R, Summerbell R. Pityriasis versicolor. *J Eur Acad Dermatol Venereol* 2002;16:19.
20. Borgers M, Cauwenbergh G, Van de Ven MA, et al. Pityriasis versicolor and *Pityrosporum ovale:* Morphogenetic and ultrastructural considerations. *Int J Dermatol* 1987;26:586.
21. Gupta AK, Bluhm R, Summerbell R. Pityriasis versicolor. *J Eur Acad Dermatol Venereol* 2002;16:19.
22. Nazzaro-Porro M, Passi S. Identification of tyrosinase inhibitors in cultures of *Pityrosporum*. *J Invest Dermatol* 1978; 71:205.
23. Galadari I, el Komy M, Mousa A, et al. Tinea versicolor: Histologic and ultrastructural investigation of pigmentary changes. *Int J Dermatol* 1992;31:253.
24. Crespo-Erchiga V, Martos AO, Casano AV, et al. Mycology of pityriasis versicolor. *J Mycol Med* 1999;9:143.
25. Savin R. Diagnosis and treatment of tinea versicolor. *J Fam Pract* 1996;43:127.
26. Stern JC, Lucente FE. Otomycosis. *Ear Nose Throat J* 1988;67:804.
27. Stern JC, Shah MK, Lucente FE. In vitro effectiveness of 13 agents in otomycosis and review of the literature. *Laryngoscope* 1988;98:1173.
28. Thrasher RD, Kingdom TT. Fungal infections of the head and neck: An update. *Otolaryngol Clin North Am* 2003;36:577.
29. Knox J, Mullins F, Spiller W. Tinea nigra. *J Invest Dermatol* 1956;27:187.
30. Palmer SR, Bass JW, Mandojana R, et al. Tinea nigra palmaris and plantaris: A black fungus producing black spots on the palms and soles. *Pediatr Infect Dis J* 1989;8:48.
31. Mok WY. Nature and identification of *Exophiala werneckii*. *J Clin Microbiol* 1982; 16:976.
32. McKinlay JR, Barrett TL, Ross EV. Picture of the month: Tinea nigra. *Arch Pediatr Adolesc Med* 1999;153:305.
33. Burke WA. Tinea nigra: Treatment with topical ketoconazole. *Cutis* 1993;52:209.
34. Figueras MJ, Guarro J, Zaror L. New findings in black piedra infection. *Br J Dermatol* 1996;135:157.
35. Smith JD, Murtishaw WA, McBride ME. White piedra (trichosporosis). *Arch Dermatol* 1973;107:439.
36. Guidelines/Outcomes Committee, American Academy of Dermatology. Guidelines of care for superficial mycotic infections of the skin: Piedra. *J Am Acad Dermatol* 1996;34:122.
37. Gupta AK, Chaudhry M, Elewski B. Tinea corporis, tinea cruris, tinea nigra, and piedra. *Dermatol Clin* 2003;21:395.
38. Odom R, James W, Berger T. Diseases resulting from fungi and yeasts, in *Andrew's Diseases of the Skin: Clinical Dermatology*, 9th ed. Toronto, Ontario, Canada, Saunders, 2000, p 358.
39. Drake LA, Dinehart SM, Farmer ER, et al. Guidelines of care for superficial mycotic infections of the skin: Tinea corporis, tinea cruris, tinea faciei, tinea manuum, and tinea pedis. Guidelines/Outcomes Committee, American Academy of Dermatology. *J Am Acad Dermatol* 1996; 34:282.
40. Weinstein A, Berman B. Topical treatment of common superficial tinea infections. *Am Fam Physician* 2002;65:2095.
41. Gupta AK, Einarson TR, Summerbell RC, et al. An overview of topical antifungal therapy in dermatomycoses: A North American perspective. *Drugs* 1998; 55:645.
42. Gupta AK, Chow M, Daniel CR, et al. Treatments of tinea pedis. *Dermatol Clin* 2003;21:431.
43. Perea S, Ramos MJ, Garau M, et al. Prevalence and risk factors of tinea unguium and tinea pedis in the general population in Spain. *J Clin Microbiol* 2000;38:3226.
44. Lupa S, Seneczko F, Jeske J, et al. Epidemiology of dermatomycoses of humans in central Poland: III. Tinea pedis. *Mycoses* 1999;42:563.

45. Ungpakorn R, Lohaprathan S, Reangchainam S. Prevalence of foot diseases in outpatients attending the Institute of Dermatology, Bangkok, Thailand. *Clin Exp Dermatol* 2004;29:87.
46. Cheng S, Chong L. A prospective epidemiological study on tinea pedis and onychomycosis in Hong Kong. *Chin Med J (Engl)* 2002;115:860.
47. Falahati M, Akhlaghi L, Lari AR, et al. Epidemiology of dermatophytoses in an area south of Tehran, Iran. *Mycopathologia* 2003;156:279.
48. Raboobee N, Aboobaker J, Peer AK. Tinea pedis et unguium in the Muslim community of Durban, South Africa. *Int J Dermatol* 1998;37:759.
49. Lopes JO, Alves SH, Mari CR, et al. A ten-year survey of tinea pedis in the central region of the Rio Grande do Sul, Brazil. *Rev Inst Med Trop Sao Paulo* 1999;41:75.
50. Vella ZL, Gatt P, Boffa MJ, et al. Characteristics of superficial mycoses in Malta. *Int J Dermatol* 2003;42:265.
51. Masri-Fridling GD. Dermatophytosis of the feet. *Dermatol Clin* 1996;14:33.
52. Tanuma H. Pathogenesis and treatment of hyperkeratotic tinea pedis in Japan. *Mycoses* 1999;42:21.
53. Pierard G, Wallace R, De Doncker P. Biometrological assessment of the preventive effect of a miconazole spray powder on athlete's foot. *Clin Exp Dermatol* 1996;21:344.
54. Watanabe K, Taniguchi H, Katoh T. Adhesion of dermatophytes to healthy feet and its simple treatment. *Mycoses* 2000; 43:45.
55. Aly R, Fisher G, Katz I, et al. Ciclopirox gel in the treatment of patients with interdigital tinea pedis. *Int J Dermatol* 2003;42:29S.
56. USP DI. *Drug Information for the Health Care Professional*. Greenwood Village, CO, Thompson Micromedex, 2004.
57. Gupta AK, Jain HC, Lynde CW, et al. Prevalence and epidemiology of onychomycosis in patients visiting physicians' offices: A multicenter canadian survey of 15,000 patients. *J Am Acad Dermatol* 2000;43:244.
58. Foster KW, Ghannoum MA, Elewski BE. Epidemiologic surveillance of cutaneous fungal infection in the United States from 1999 to 2002. *J Am Acad Dermatol* 2004;50:748.
59. Ghannoum MA, Hajjeh RA, Scher R, et al. A large-scale North American study of fungal isolates from nails: The frequency of onychomycosis, fungal distribution, and antifungal susceptibility patterns. *J Am Acad Dermatol* 2000;43:641.
60. Tosti A, Piraccini BM, Lorenzi S, et al. Treatment of nondermatophyte mold and *Candida* onychomycosis. *Dermatol Clin* 2003;21:491.
61. Lynde C. Nail disorders that mimic onychomycosis: What to consider. *Cutis* 2001;68:8.
62. Haneke E, Roseeuw D. The scope of onychomycosis: Epidemiology and clinical features. *Int J Dermatol* 1999;38:7S.
63. Gupta AK, Konnikov N, Lynde CW, et al. Onychomycosis: Predisposed populations and some predictors of suboptimal response to oral antifungal agents. *Eur J Dermatol* 1999;9:633.
64. Baran R, Hay RJ, Tosti A, et al. A new classification of onychomycosis. *Br J Dermatol* 1998;139:567.
65. Tosti A, Baran R, Piraccini BM, et al. "Endonyx" onychomycosis: A new modality of nail invasion by dermatophytes. *Acta Dermatol Venereol* 1999; 79:52.
66. Jerasutus S: Histology and histopathology, in Scher RK, Daniel CR III (eds), *Nails: Therapy, Diagnosis, Surgery*, 2nd ed. Philadelphia, Saunders, 1997, pp 55-98.
67. Hull PR, Gupta AK, Summerbell RC. Onychomycosis: An evaluation of three sampling methods. *J Am Acad Dermatol* 1998;39:1015.
68. Hettinger DF, Valinsky MS. Treatment of onychomycosis with nail avulsion and topical ketoconazole. *J Am Podiatr Med Assoc* 1991;81:28.
69. Darmstadt GL, Dinulos JG, Miller Z. Congenital cutaneous candidiasis: Clinical presentation, pathogenesis, and management guidelines. *Pediatrics* 2000; 105:438.
70. Hay RJ. The management of superficial candidiasis. *J Am Acad Dermatol* 1999; 40:35S.
71. Blatchford NR: Treatment of oral candidosis with itraconazole: A review. *J Am Acad Dermatol* 1990;23:565.

CHAPTER 60

Parasitic Infections

Shobita Rajagopalan

Key Points

- Parasitic infestations and infections are encountered commonly in developing countries, where the environment is ideal for them to thrive. International travel to tropical exotic destinations plays an important part in the acquisition of parasitic diseases.
- Factors such as geography, environment, and low socioeconomic status causing overcrowding and pollution, poor hygiene, food and water contamination, malnutrition, delayed access to medical care, and the presence of appropriate vectors play an important role in transmission of parasitic diseases.
- Darker skin differs from light skin in its reactivity and disease presentation. Genetic susceptibility to specific parasites must be recognized; some skin diseases, including those caused by or associated with parasitic infection or infestation, are encountered in darker-skinned race/ethnicities, that is, blacks, Asians, Hispanics/Latinos, and Native Americans.
- Skin manifestations of specific parasitic diseases, although not particularly associated with skin of color, include scabies and cutaneous larva migrans.

Parasitic diseases are common in developing nations but are relatively rare elsewhere. The environment in such countries, that is, overcrowding, malnutrition, pollution, contamination of food and water sources, and the presence of appropriate vectors, enables the efficient transmission of parasitic diseases. From the perspective of industrialized countries, international travel to exotic tropical and subtropical destinations enhances the risk of acquiring parasitic illnesses.

The role of genetic susceptibility to specific parasites, however, also must be recognized. Darker skin differs from light skin in its reactivity and disease presentation. Ethnic differences in skin properties may explain some of the racial disparities seen in dermatologic disorders. These include differences in epidermal melanin content, melanosome dispersion, hair structure, and fibroblast and mast cell size and structure in people of color compared with light-skinned persons.[1–4]

Many skin diseases, including those caused by or associated with parasitic infection or infestation, are common to most people of color, that is, blacks, Asians, Hispanics/Latinos, and Native Americans. Geography, environment, and low socioeconomic status causing overcrowding, malnutrition, and poor or delayed access to medical care in part may explain this health disparity.[3,4]

This chapter will review some common and important parasitic illnesses that are known to cause significant skin disease in humans and focus on possible race-related variation in disease presentation. Skin manifestations of specific parasitic diseases that will be covered include the ectoparasitic infestation *scabies* and the cutaneous migratory endoparasitic phenomenon known as *cutaneous larva migrans* (CLM).

SCABIES

Background

Scabies is a common and highly contagious ectoparasitic infestation of global and public health significance caused by the arthropod *Sarcoptes scabiei* var. *hominis*. Scabies affects all individuals regardless of age, gender, race/ethnicity, or socioeconomic status. Worldwide, an estimated 300 million cases occur annually.[5] Prevalence rates in developing countries are higher than those in developed nations. Overcrowding, poor hygiene, delayed diagnosis and treatment, and lack of public education are among some of the factors that contribute to the prevalence of scabies in both industrial and nonindustrial nations. In developed countries, scabies epidemics occur primarily in institutional settings, such as prisons, long-term care facilities such as nursing homes, and hospitals. Prevalence rates are observed to be higher in children and sexually active individuals than in other persons. The more severe and crusted variant of scabies known as *Norwegian scabies* (so named because its initial description from Norway in the mid-1800s) is common in patients with poor sensory perception owing to entities such as leprosy and persons with immunocompromise owing to post-transplantation, human immunodeficiency virus (HIV) infection, and aging.[6] These populations typically present with clinically atypical lesions and are frequently misdiagnosed, thus delaying treatment and elevating the risk of local epidemics. Although scabies is a readily treatable infestation, it remains relatively common primarily because of diagnostic difficulty, inadequate treatment of patients and their contacts, and improper environmental control measures.

Pathophysiology

The scabies mite is an obligate parasite and completes its entire life cycle on humans.[7] Animal scabies mites may cause mild and transient symptoms in humans that generally do not persist. Prolonged direct contact with infested individuals facilitates transmission. Mites can live up to 3 days away from human skin; thus fomites such as infested bedding or clothing may be an additional rare source of transmission. The life cycle of the scabies mite is approximately 30 days and is spent within the human epidermis. After copulation, the male mite dies, and the female mite burrows into the superficial skin layers and lays a total of 60–90 eggs. The eggs incubate and hatch after 3–8 days. About 90% of the hatched mites die, but those that survive go through various molting stages and reach maturity after approximately 2 weeks. The female adults, who never leave their burrows, die after 1–2 months. In classic scabies, 5–15 mites (range 3–50) may live on the host skin.

During the initial month of scabies infestation, infested individuals remain relatively asymptomatic. However, approximately 4 weeks into and with subsequent infestation, a delayed-type hypersensitivity reaction develops to the mites, eggs, and scybala (packet of feces). With reinfestation, the sensitized individual may develop a rapid reaction (often within hours). The resulting skin eruption and its associated intense pruritus are the hallmark of classic scabies.

In immunocompromised, frail elderly, and physically and/or mentally handicapped persons and in individuals with sensory nerve impairment, the fulminant distinctive and highly contagious hyperinfestation owing to the crusted or Norwegian form of scabies is common. In this variant of scabies, numerous mites infest the host individual. Rare cases have been described in immunocompetent patients. Extensive, widespread crusted lesions appear with thick, hyperkeratotic scales over the elbows, knees, palms, and soles. The number of mites in a patient with crusted scabies can exceed 1 million. In these cases, the mite can survive off the host for up to 7 days, feeding on the sloughed skin in the local environment, such as bedsheets, clothing, and chair covers. Failure to implement environmental control measures in this situation may result in relapse and reinfestation after successful treatment of the host. Serum immunoglobulin E (IgE) and immunoglobulin G (IgG) levels are extremely high in these patients, yet the immune reaction does not seem to be protective. Cell-mediated immune responses in classic scabies demonstrate a predominantly CD4 T-cell infiltrate in the skin, whereas one study suggests CD8 T-cell predominance in crusted scabies. Atypical infestations also can occur in infants and young children.

Clinical Manifestations

The historical aspects of scabies infestations are quite reliable in suggesting the diagnosis.[8] The incubation period prior to onset of symptoms depends on whether the infestation is an initial exposure or a relapse/reinfestation. Previously sensitized individuals can develop symptoms within hours of reexposure. The hypersensitivity reaction is responsible for the intense pruritus that is the clinical hallmark of the disease.

Lesion distribution, intractable pruritus that is worse at night, and similar symptoms in close contacts immediately should raise a high index of suspicion for scabies. Lesion distribution differs in adults and children. Adults manifest lesions primarily on the flexor aspects of the wrists, the interdigital web spaces of the hands, the dorsal feet, axillae, elbows, waist, buttocks, and genitalia.[9] Secondary lesions may occur as a result of rubbing and scratching, and they may be the only clinical manifestation of the disease. Pruritic papules and vesicles on the scrotum and penis in men and the areolae in women are highly characteristic. Infants and small children develop lesions predominantly on the face, scalp, neck, palms, and soles, although any site may be involved. All cutaneous sites are susceptible in immunocompromised and elderly patients, who often have a history of a widespread pruritic eczematous eruptions.

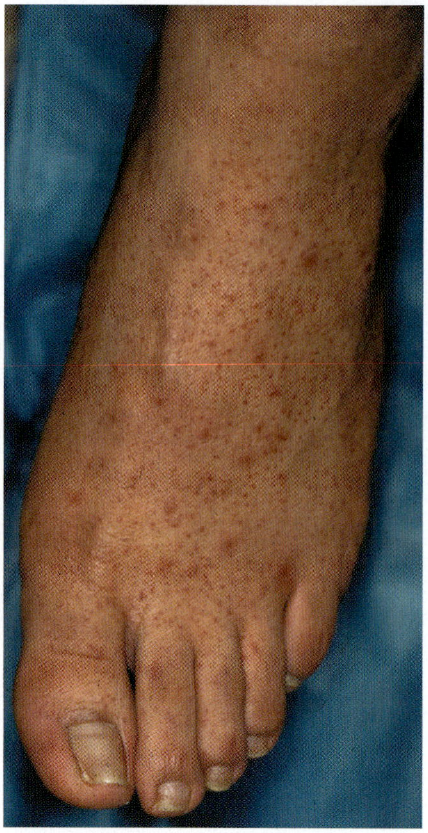

▲ **FIGURE 60-1** Classic scabies eruption showing burrows.

Burrows are a pathognomonic sign of classic scabies and represent the intraepidermal tunnel created by the moving female mite. They appear as inapparent, serpiginous grayish thread-like elevations ranging from 2–10 mm long (Figure 60-1). Common locations for burrows include the webbed spaces of the fingers; the flexor surfaces of the wrists, elbows, and axillae; the belt line; the feet; the scrotum in men; and the areolae in women. In infants, burrows are commonly located on the palms and soles. The actual mites are microscopic and cannot be visualized without microscopy.

Complications of scabies are rare and generally result from vigorous rubbing and scratching. Disruption of the skin barrier puts the patient at risk for secondary bacterial invasion, primarily by *Streptococcus pyogenes* and *Staphylococcus aureus.* Superinfection with *S. pyogenes* can precipitate acute poststreptococcal glomerulonephritis and even rheumatic fever. More common pyodermas include impetigo and cellulitis, which rarely may result in sepsis. Scabies infestations can exacerbate underlying eczema, psoriasis, and other preexisting dermatoses. Even with appropriate treatment, scabies can leave in its wake residual eczematous dermatitis and/or postscabietic pruritus, which can be debilitating and recalcitrant. Crusted or Norwegian scabies can involve the skin extensively and carries an increased mortality rate because of the frequency of secondary bacterial infections resulting in sepsis (Figure 60-2).

Laboratory Diagnosis

LIGHT MICROCOPY The diagnosis is confirmed by light microscopic identification of mites, larvae, ova, or scybala in skin scrapings[10,11] (Figure 60-3). In rare cases, mites are identified in biopsy specimens obtained to rule out other

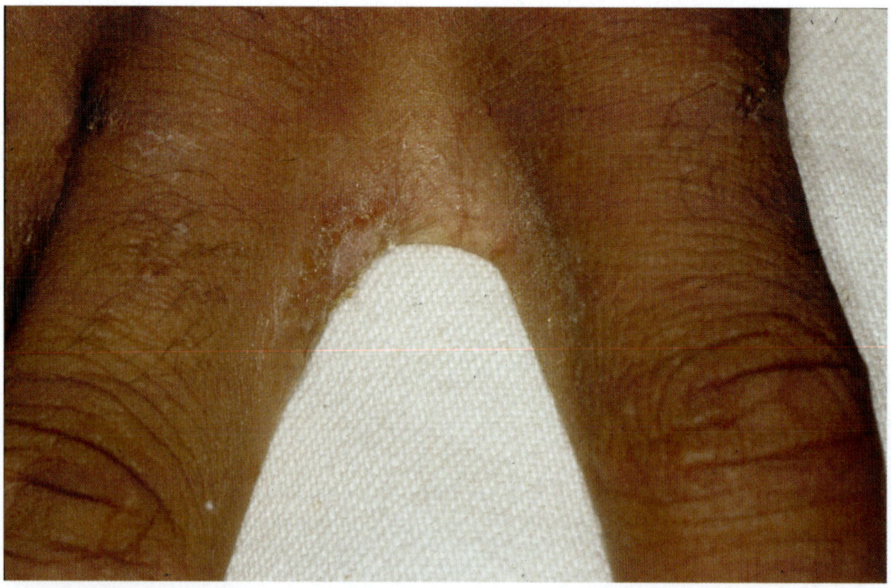

▲ **FIGURE 60-2** Scabies of the finger and web spaces.

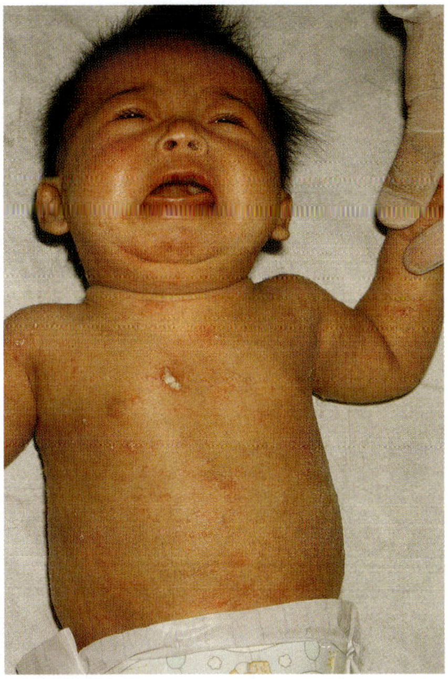

▲ **FIGURE 60-3** A Hispanic infant with generalized scabies.

dermatoses. Characteristic histopathology common to a variety of arthropod reactions in the absence of actual mites also may suggest the diagnosis. Excision of a burrow may reveal mites, larvae, ova, and feces within the stratum corneum. A superficial and deep dermal infiltrate composed of lymphocytes, histiocytes, mast cells, and eosinophils is characteristic. Spongiosis and vesicle formation with exocytosis of eosinophils and occasional neutrophils is present. Biopsy of older lesions may be nondiagnostic and reveal fibrotic and scale crusts. Crusted scabies demonstrates massive hyperkeratosis of the stratum corneum with numerous mites in all stages of development. Psoriasiform hyperplasia of the underlying epidermis with spongiotic foci and occasional epidermal microabscesses is present. The dermis shows a superficial and deep chronic inflammatory infiltrate with interstitial eosinophils. Nodular variants of scabies reveal a dense, mixed, superficial and deep dermal inflammatory cell infiltrate. Lymphoid follicles may be present, and the infiltrate occasionally extends into the subcutaneous fat.

OTHER TESTS Elevated IgE titers and eosinophilia may be found in some patients with scabies. Clinically inapparent infection can be detected by amplification of *Sarcoptes* DNA in epidermal scale by polymerase chain reaction.[12] Immunosuppression, either via medication or disease-related, may be associated with crusted scabies.

Treatment

The mainstay of treatment is the application of topical antiscabietic agents such as permethrin, with repeat application in 7 days.[13] An oral agent, ivermectin, is also available and effective.[14] Ivermectin is a synthetic macrocyclic lactone belonging to the avermectin group of antibiotics. It is active against a number of human and animal endoparasites and ectoparasites. Ivermectin is effective in most cases of typical scabies at a dose of 200–250 μg/kg given at diagnosis and repeated in 7–14 days. Crusted scabies may require three or more doses given at 1- to 2-week intervals. Ivermectin is an ideal agent in patients in whom topical therapy is difficult or impractical, such as in widespread institutional infestations and bedridden patients.[15,16] Ivermectin is contraindicated in patients with allergic sensitization or nervous system disorders and in women who are pregnant or breast-feeding. Children younger than 5 years or weighing less than 15 kg should not be treated with ivermectin.

Patients may experience pruritus for up to 2 weeks after successful treatment. If itching persists beyond this time, the patient must be reevaluated to ensure the correct diagnosis, adequate treatment, and simultaneous treatment of contacts and environment. A second treatment course may be indicated. Rarely, individuals with a history of atopy may require a tapered dose of prednisone for the treatment of severe pruritus. Intranodular injection of dilute corticosteroids may be necessary in patients with nodular scabies. Because of the heavy mite burden, patients with crusted scabies may require repeated applications of topical scabicides or simultaneous treatment with the topical permethrin and oral ivermectin.

Symptomatic treatment may require oral antihistamines and topical antipruritics/anesthetics such as menthol (Sarna) and pramoxine (Prax). More severe symptoms may require a short course of topical or oral steroids. Secondary infections may require antibiotics and should be prescribed based on culture and sensitivity.

Detailed verbal and written instructions are critical for compliance and complete eradication and prevention of spread to contacts and are as follows:

- Family members and close contacts must be evaluated and treated, even if they do not have symptoms. Pets do not require treatment. All carpets and upholstered furniture should be vacuumed and the vacuum bags immediately discarded.
- Patients must be instructed to launder clothing, bed linens, and towels used within the last week in hot water the day after treatment is initiated and again in 1 week. Items that cannot be washed may be professionally dry cleaned or sealed in plastic bags for 1 week.
- Patients with crusted scabies or their caregivers should be instructed to remove excess scale to allow penetration of the topical scabicidal agent and decrease the burden of infestation. This can be achieved with warm-water soaks followed by application of a keratolytic agent such as 5% salicylic acid in petrolatum or Lac-Hydrin cream. (Salicylic acid should be avoided if large body surface areas are involved because of the potential risk of salicylate poisoning.) The scales then are debrided mechanically with a tongue depressor or similar nonsharp device.

Complications

Treatment failures are uncommon if guidelines are followed. Residual pruritus may require antihistamines or a short course of topical or oral corticosteroids. Secondary infection usually as a result of *Streptococcus pyogenes* requires administration of an empirical course of antibiotics; although antibiotic susceptibility is usually predictable, culture and sensitivity data should be followed to appropriately tailor the regimen. Scabietic nodules may require intranodular corticosteroid injection for complete resolution. Flaring or reactivation of preexisting eczema or atopic dermatitis requires the use of standard eczema treatments.

Prognosis

Prognosis is usually excellent with proper diagnosis and treatment in otherwise healthy individuals, as well as in immunocompromised or institutionalized hosts.

CUTANEOUS LARVA MIGRANS (CLM)

Background

CLM is a common dermatologic condition caused by the migratory larvae of animal hookworms characteristically encountered in travelers returning from

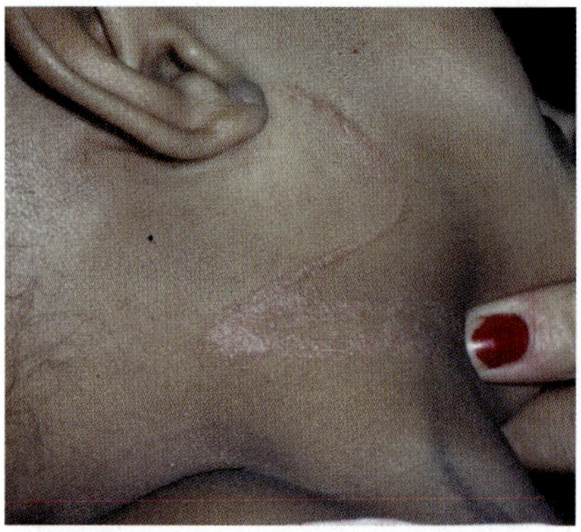

▲ **FIGURE 60-4** Cutaneous larva migrans.

tropical and subtropical destinations.[17] Cases also have been reported from the southwestern United States. CLM is characterized by an erythematous, serpiginous, pruritic cutaneous eruption caused by accidental percutaneous penetration and subsequent migration of larvae of various nematode parasites. The animal hookworm, *Ancylostoma braziliense,* is the species found most frequently in humans.[18,19] These hookworms generally live in the intestines of domestic pets such as dogs and cats and shed their eggs via feces to soil (usually moist soil and sandy areas of beaches or under houses). Humans are incidental hosts and are infected by contact with contaminated soil found in endemic areas of tropical and subtropical regions. The hookworm larvae burrow through intact skin and stay confined to the upper dermis. Migration of larvae through the skin results in an intensely pruritic, linear, or serpiginous track known as a *creeping eruption* (Figure 60-4). Creeping eruptions are not unique to CLM and occur in many other human skin diseases.

In the United States, among helminthic infestations, CLM is rated second to pinworm. The condition is benign and self-limited but can cause a disturbing pruritus. There is neither a specific racial nor gender predilection for CLM, and it largely depends on exposure to animal nematode larvae. In addition, CLM can affect persons of all ages, but it tends to be seen more commonly in children than in adults.

Etiology and Pathogenesis

Common etiologies of CLM include the following:

- *Ancylostoma braziliense* (hookworm of wild and domestic dogs and cats) is the most common cause. It can be found in the central and southern United States, Central America, South America, and the Caribbean.
- *Ancylostoma caninum* (dog hookworm) is found in Australia.
- *Uncinaria stenocephala* (dog hookworm) is found in Europe.
- *Bunostomum phlebotomum* (cattle hookworm).

Rare etiologies include the following:

- *Ancylostoma ceylonicum*
- *Ancylostoma tubaeforme* (cat hookworm)
- *Necator americanus* (human hookworm)
- *Strongyloides papillosus* (parasite of sheep, goats, and cattle)
- *Strongyloides westeri* (parasite of horses)
- *Ancylostoma duodenale*

The life cycle of the parasites begins when eggs are passed from animal feces into warm, moist soil, where the larvae hatch. The larvae initially feed on soil bacteria and molt twice before the infective third stage. By using their proteases, larvae penetrate through follicles, fissures, or intact skin of the new host. After penetrating the stratum corneum, the larvae shed their natural cuticle and begin migration within a few days. In their natural animal hosts, the larvae are able to penetrate into the dermis and are transported via the lymphatic and venous systems to the lungs. They break through into the alveoli and migrate to the trachea, where they are swallowed. In the intestine, they mature sexually, and the cycle begins again as their eggs are excreted. Humans are accidental hosts, and the larvae are believed to lack the collagenase enzymes required to penetrate the basement membrane to invade the dermis. Therefore, the disease remains limited to the skin when humans are infected.

Clinical Features

Patients complain of tingling/prickling at the site of exposure within 30 minutes of penetration of larvae, intense pruritus, erythematous, often linear lesions that advance and are associated with a history of sunbathing, walking barefoot on the beach, or similar activity in a tropical location.[20,21] Predispositions include hobbies and occupations that involve contact with warm, moist sandy soil and tropical/subtropical travel. They include persons who walk barefoot or sunbathe on the beach, children in sandboxes, carpenters, electricians, plumbers, farmers, gardener, and pest exterminators.

Cutaneous signs include pruritic, erythematous, edematous papules and/or vesicles; serpiginous, slightly elevated, erythematous tunnels that are 2- to 3-mm wide and track 3–4 cm from the penetration site; nonspecific dermatitis; vesicles with serous fluid; secondary impetiginization; and tract advancement of 1–2 cm/day. Systemic signs include peripheral eosinophilia (Loeffler syndrome), migratory pulmonary infiltrates, and increased IgE levels but are rarely seen. Lesions typically are distributed on the distal lower extremities, including the dorsal surfaces of the feet and the interdigital spaces of the toes, but also can occur in the anogenital region, the buttocks, the hands, and the knees.

Differential diagnosis includes allergic contact dermatitis, epidermal dermatophytosis, erythema chronicum migrans, migratory myiasis, photoallergic dermatitis, and larva currens caused by *S. stercoralis*.

Laboratory Diagnosis

Diagnosis is based mostly on the classic clinical appearance of the eruption. Some patients may demonstrate peripheral eosinophilia on a complete blood count and increased IgE levels on total serum immunoglobulin determinations.

Skin biopsy samples from the advancing edge of a tract may show a larva (periodic acid–Schiff–positive) in a suprabasalar burrow, basal layer tracts, spongiosis with intraepidermal vesicles, necrotic keratinocytes, and an epidermal and upper dermal chronic inflammatory infiltrate with many eosinophils.

Treatment

Even though the condition is self-limited, the intense pruritus and risk for infection mandate treatment.[22] Topical modalities such as ethyl chloride spray, liquid nitrogen, phenol, carbon dioxide snow, piperazine citrate, electrocautery, and radiation therapy were used unsuccessfully because their effectiveness is limited for multiple lesions and hookworm folliculitis and may need multiple daily applications for several days. Topical application of a 10–15% thiabendazole solution/ointment/cream to the affected area has been shown to be effective.[20,21,23,24]

Systemic treatment with thiabendazole is currently considered the treatment of choice. Other effective alternative treatments include albendazole, mebendazole, and ivermectin. The treatment course results in decreased pruritus within 24–48 hours, and lesions/tracts resolve in 1 week.

THIABENDAZOLE Thiabendazole is the drug with which there has been the most experience in the oral treatment of CLM.[24–27] Thiabendazole is minimally effective when given as a single dose. The 4-weekly-dose regimen with oral thiabendazole at 50 mg/kg per day has been demonstrated to yield the best results. However, thiabendazole is less well tolerated than either albendazole or ivermectin. Reported adverse affects include nausea, vomiting, dizziness, and headache.[28]

ALBENDAZOLE Albendazole is a third-generation heterocyclic antihelminthic drug used in the treatment of intestinal helminthe infection, for example, ascariasis, enterobiasis, ancylostomiasis, trichuriasis, and strongyloidiasis. Albendazole treatment of CLM with single dose of 400 mg, the same dose for 3 and 5 consecutive days, and with an 800-mg daily dose for 3 consecutive days has been shown to yield successful results.[29–32] However, other studies suggest that for tourists with CLM treated with albendazole, the regimen should be 400–800 mg/day for 3–5 days.[33] Albendazole is generally well tolerated when use for the treatment of CLM. However, the rare side effect of gastrointestinal pain and diarrhea after receiving 800 mg albendazole by mouth on three consecutive days has been reported.[34, 35]

IVERMECTIN Ivermectin, briefly described in the section on scabies, is also active against *O. volvulus* and other nematodes, including gastrointestinal helminths. Its mechanism of action is poorly understood.[36,37] A single 12-mg dose of ivermectin resulted in 100% cure rates among patients with CLM.

Complications

Complications such as secondary bacterial infection, usually with *S. pyogenes,* may lead to cellulitis and impetigo and prolonged pruritis, and local or general allergic reactions may occur.

Prognosis

The prognosis of CLM is excellent. This is a self-limiting disease. Humans are accidental, dead-end hosts, with the larva dying and the lesions resolving within 4–8 weeks or as long as a year in rare cases.

Prevention

Persons who travel to tropical regions and pet owners should be made aware of CLM. Because tourists are usually infected by walking or lying on tropical sandy beaches contaminated by dog feces, the best way to prevent CLM is to wear shoes when walking in sandy areas. It also may be prudent to lie on sand washed by the tide or to use a mattress; avoid lying on dry sand, even on a towel.

REFERENCES

1. Bari AU, Khan MB. Pattern of skin diseases in black Africans of Sierra Leone, West Africa. *J Clin Diagn Res* 2007;1: 361-368.
2. Shriver MD. Ethnic variation as a key to the biology of human disease. *Ann Intern Med* 1997;127:401-403.
3. Fitzpatrick TB. The validity and practicality of sun reactive skin type I through VI. *Arch Dermatol* 1988;124:869-871.
4. Maibach HI. Racial (ethnic) differences in skin properties: The objective data. *Am J Clin Dermatol* 2003;4:843-860.
5. Burkhart CG, Burkhart CN, Burkhart KM. An epidemiologic and therapeutic reassessment of scabies. *Cutis* 2000;65: 233-240.
6. Guldbakke KK, Khachemoune A. Crusted scabies: A clinical review. *J Drugs Dermatol* 2006;5:221-227.
7. Burgess I. Sarcoptes scabiei and scabies. *Adv Parasitol* 1994;33:235-292.
8. Elgart ML. Scabies. *Dermatol Clin* 1990;8: 253-263.
9. Fitzpatrick TB, Johnson RA, Wolff K. Inset bites and infestations, in Fitzpatrick TJ, Johnson RA, Wolff K, Polano MK, Suurmond R (eds), *Color Atlas and Synopsis of Clinical Dermatology,* 3rd ed. New York, McGraw-Hill, 1997, pp 836-861.
10. Brodell RT, Helms SE. Bedside testing: The diagnostic cornerstone of dermatology. *Compr Ther* 1997;23:211-217.
11. Johnston G, Sladden M. Scabies: Diagnosis and treatment. *Br Med J* 2005; 331:619-622.
12. Bezold G, Lange M, Schiener R, et al. Hidden scabies: Diagnosis by polymerase chain reaction. *Br J Dermatol* 2001;144:614-618.
13. Karthikeyan K. Treatment of scabies: Newer perspectives. *Postgrad Med J* 2005; 81:7-11.
14. Elgart GW, Meinking TL. Ivermectin. *Dermatol Clin* 2003;21:277-282.
15. Huffam SE, Currie BJ. Ivermectin for *Sarcoptes scabiei* hyperinfestation. *Int J Infect Dis* 1998;2:152-154.
16. Aubin F, Humbert P. Ivermectin for crusted (Norwegian) scabies. *N Engl J Med* 1995;332:612.
17. Caumes E, Carrière J, Guermonprez G, et al. Dermatoses associated with travel to tropical countries: A prospective study of the diagnosis and management of 269 patients presenting to a tropical disease unit. *Clin Infect Dis* 1995;20:542-548.
18. Beaver PC. Larva migrans: A review. *Exp Parasitol* 1956;5:587-621.
19. Chaudhry AZ, Lonworth DL. Cutaneous manifestations of intestinal helminthic infections. *Dermatol Clin* 1989;7:275-290.
20. Davies HD, Sakuls P, Keystone JS. Creeping eruption: A review of clinical presentation and management of 60 cases presenting to a tropical disease unit. *Arch Dermatol* 1993;129:588-591.
21. Jelineck T, Maiwald H, Northdurft HD, Loscher T. Cutaneous larva migrans in travelers: Synopsis of histories, symptoms and treatment of 98 patients. *Clin Infect Dis* 1994;19:1062-1066.
22. Caumes E. Treatment of cutaneous larva migrans. *Clin Infect Dis* 2000;30:811-814.
23. Davis CM, Israel RM. Treatment of creeping eruption with topical thiabendazole. *Arch Dermatol* 1968;97:325-326.
24. Katz R, Hood WR. Topical thiabendazole for creeping eruption. *Arch Dermatol* 1966;94:643-645.
25. Katz R, Ziegler J, Blank H. The natural course of creeping eruption and treatment with thiabendazole. *Arch Dermatol* 1965;91:420-424.
26. Jacksonville Dermatology Society. Creeping eruption treated with thiabendazole. *Arch Dermatol* 1965;91:425-426.
27. Stone OJ, Mullins JF. Thiabendazole effectiveness in creeping eruption. *Arch Dermatol* 1965;91:427-429.
28. Thomas J, Lugagne J, Rosso AM, et al. Traitement de la dermatite vermineuse rampante par le thiabendazole (à propos de 50 cas). *Marseille Med* 1969;9: 718-721.
29. Vakil BJ, Bandisode MS, Gaitonde BB, et al. Clinical trials with a new antihelminthic, thiabendazole. *J Trop Med Hyg* 1955;58:287-295.
30. Coulaud JP, Binet D, Voyer C, et al. Traitement du syndrome de larva migrans cutanée "larbish" par l'albendazole: À propos de 18 observations. *Bull Soc Pathol Exot Filiales* 1982;75:534-537.
31. Wlliams HC, Monk B. Creeping eruption stopped in its tracks by albendazole. *Clin Exp Dermatol* 1989;14:355-356.
32. Orihuela AR, Torres JR. Single dose of albendazole in the treatment of cutaneous larva migrans. *Arch Dermatol* 1990;126:398-399.
33. Jones SK, Reynolds NJ, Oliwiecki S, Harman RRM. Oral albendazole for the treatment of cutaneous larva migrans. *Br J Dermatol* 1990;122:99-101.
34. Sanguigni S, Marangi M, Teggi A, De Rosa F. Albendazole in the therapy of cutaneous larva migrans. *Trans R Soc Trop Med Hyg* 1990;84:831.
35. Pungpak S, Bunnag D, Chindanond D, Radmoyos B. Albendazole in the treatment of strongyloidiasis. *Southeast Asian J Trop Public Health* 1987;18:202-207.
36. Caumes E, Carrière J, Datry A, et al. A randomized trial of ivermectin versus albendazole for the treatment of cutaneous larva migrans. *Am J Trop Med Hyg* 1993;49:641-644.
37. Goa KL, McTavish D, Clissold SD. Ivermectin: A review of its antifilarial activity, pharmacokinetic properties and clinical efficacy in onchocerciasis. *Drugs* 1991;42:640-658.

CHAPTER 61

Onchocerciasis

Edith Nkechi Nnoruka

Key Points

- Onchocerciasis is an age-old disease caused by infestation with a filarial nematode worm, *Onchcerca volvulus*. The bite of the blackfly *Simulum damnosum* transmits the microfilaria worms.
- Onchocerciasis remains a major cause of disabling skin disease, visual impairment, and blindness, with notable geographic variation in clinical expression of the disease.
- An estimated 20–40 million people are afflicted worldwide, with over 99% of cases in sub-Saharan Africa.
- Onchocercoma, a firm, painless nodule in the subcutaneous tissue, is the classic lesion of cutaneous onchocerciasis.
- Onchocercomata are formed predominantly on the head, face, and torso, mainly over bony prominences.
- Unbearable itching and scratching are the most distressing clinical manifestations of cutaneous onchocerciasis.

Onchocerciasis is an age-old disease caused by infestation with a filarial nematode worm. It is associated with severe morbidity that has a significant impact on the quality of life of affected individuals. Onchocerciasis has led to the disintegration and abandonment of families and vast communities. The name *river blindness* reflects the importance of the disease as one of the top five leading preventable causes of visual impairment and blindness in the world, particularly in Africa, Latin America, and Yemen.[1,2] In endemic communities, onchocerciasis is the main public health problem that people face.[3]

An estimated 20–40 million people are afflicted worldwide, and 100 million people are at risk for the disease in 35 endemic countries.[4] Over 99% of the cases of onchocerciasis occur in sub-Saharan African countries stretching between 15°N and 14°S from Senegal in the west to Ethiopia in the east (Figure 61-1). Half the cases in the world are located in Nigeria.[4] In 1875, O'Neill first reported the presence of filaria in "craw-craw," as onchocerciasis is called in West Africa. The term *onchocerca* is derived from the Greek word *ogkos,* meaning "swelling or mass," and *kerkos,* meaning "tail."[5]

Infestation with the filarial nematodal worm *Onchocerciasis volvolus* results in the communicable parasitic disease onchocerciasis. It remains a major cause of disabling skin disease, visual impairment, and blindness in endemic countries. Depending on the degree of host immune response to the parasites, there exists a wide spectrum of clinical manifestations of onchocerciasis—ranging from endemic normal individuals (putatively immune) who are free of the disease and have a good cellular immune response to the parasite to individuals with depressed cellular immunity (with or without generalized onchodermatitis) and remarkable immune tolerance to millions of microfilariae, tissue damage accruing only gradually over many years. At the other extreme are those with a vigorous antibody response and hyperreactive onchodermatitis to human immunodeficiency virus (HIV)–positive patients with an impaired antibody response.

The major physical, emotional, psychosocial, and economic burden posed by cutaneous onchocerciasis, particularly from rain forest ecologic areas, has been reported extensively.[6,7] Most of the burden of onchocercal skin disease is due to the severe unbearable pruritus. This chapter reviews the cutaneous manifestations of onchocerciasis.

EPIDEMIOLOGY

Several factors determine the epidemiology of onchocerciasis, which includes the host response, the parasite and vector competence, the geographic environment, and social and demographic influences. Within the same geographic area, onchocerciasis has markedly variable endemic rates. The flight range of the vector, the blackfly (*Simulium damnosum* complex for Africa) and breeding sites determine the focal and rural distribution of the disease. Differences between West Africa and Central/South America with respect to features of onchocerciasis, parasite strain, and vector species complexes probably reflect long-term evolutionary divergence. Variation exists in the blindness rate in different geographic areas possibly because of distinct strains or biologic variants. Onchocerciasis is more likely to lead to blindness in Africa than in Latin America, and it is several times less frequently blinding in the rain forest areas than in the savannah (nonforested) areas. The focal microfilarial prevalence and load in onchocerciasis increase with age and are higher in males than in females. Lymphatic involvement and skin manifestations (e.g., pruritus, chronic papular dermatitis, nodules, and depigmentation) are more common in the rain forest than in the savannah.

ETIOLOGY AND PATHOGENESIS

O. volvulus, a member of the family Filarioidae, is a parasitic filarial nematode worm. *Homo sapiens* are the only natural vertebrate host, although infection of nonhuman primates such as the chimpanzee is possible. Blackflies of the genus *Simulium,* which are tiny ferocious biters, are the only vectors of *O. volvulus*. At least 15 different species of blackflies can transmit onchocerciasis, and they vary by terrain and continent (e.g., *S. damnosum* in Africa). Their eggs require fast-running rivers for breeding grounds. As a result, the numbers of flies produced fluctuate with the season. They have a life span of 4 weeks. The life cycle of *O. volvulus* is depicted in Figure 61-2.

Infected *O. volvulus* larvae are inoculated into the human host by the *Simulium* fly. The infected larvae molt to the L_4 and juvenile adult stages within 1–2 months, whereas mature adult worms capable of producing microfilariae develop within 10–15 months of infection. Development to the adult stage occurs in humans. The adult worms pair and mate in the human host, and unlike most nematodes that produce eggs, the female *Onchocerca* gives birth daily to thousands of microscopic larvae known as *microfilariae.* These larvae mature into adult worms in about 1 year. The life span of microfilariae is 6–30 months. The adult worms that complete their life circle may survive a decade, during which time they release millions of microfilariae.

The classic lesion of onchocerciasis is the *onchocercoma,* a firm, painless nod-

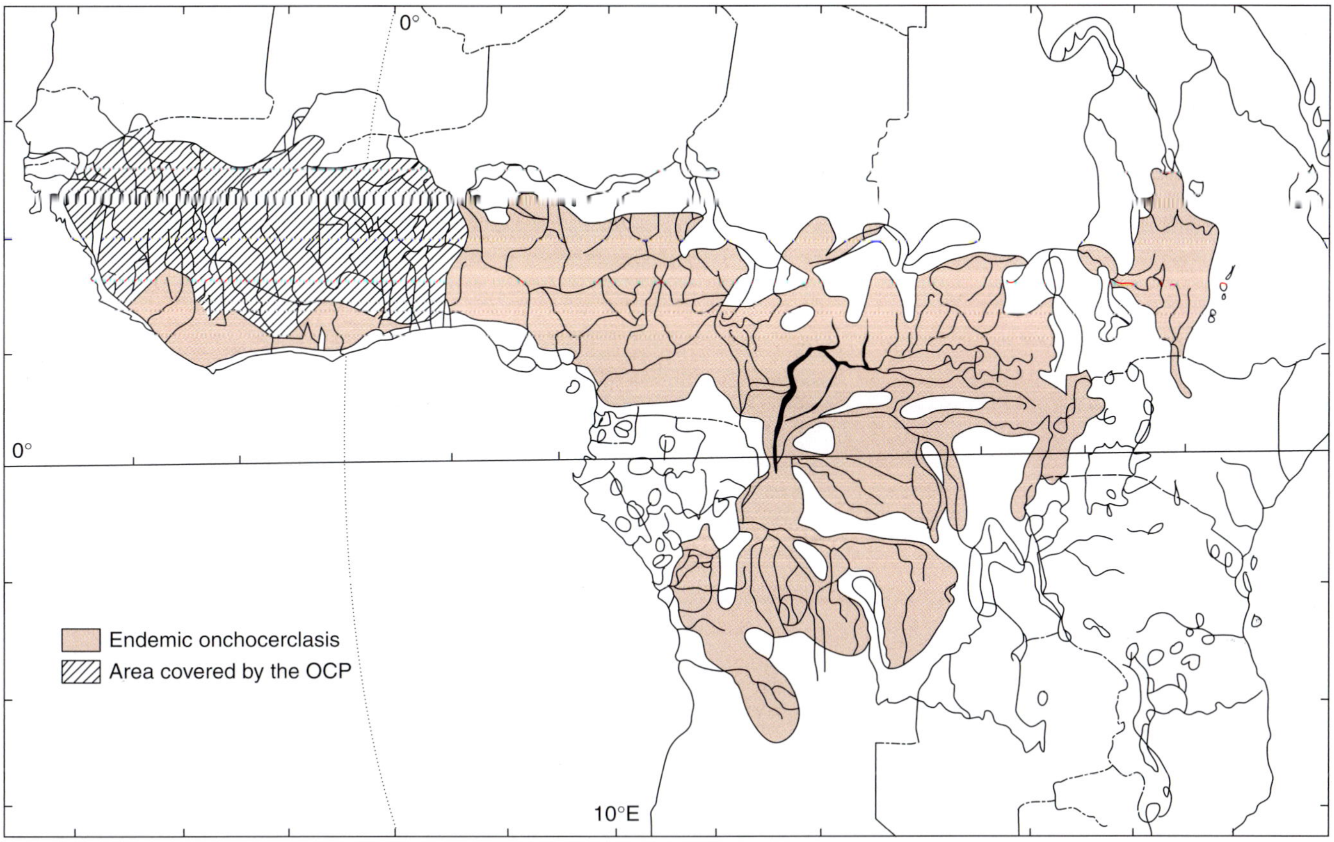

▲ **FIGURE 61-1** Map of the geographic distribution of onchocerciasis in Africa and Arabian Peninsula reflecting endemic onchcerciasis and areas of OCP and APOC. (WHO/APOC).

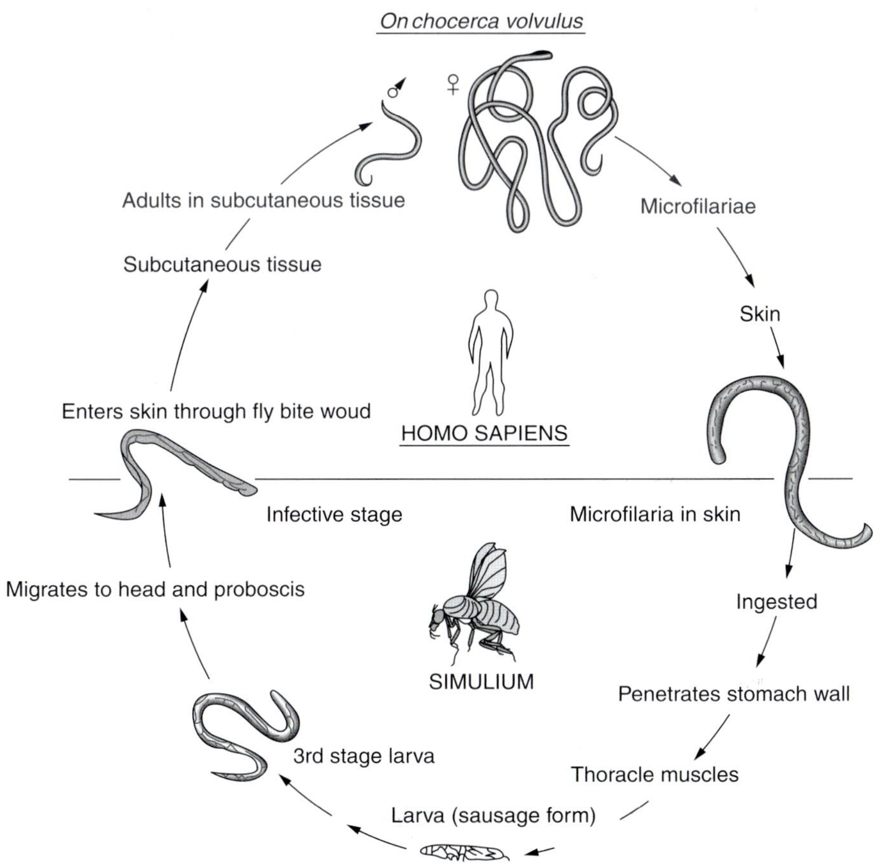

▲ **FIGURE 61-2** Life cycle of *Onchocerca volvulus.* (WHO/APOC).

ule in the subcutaneous tissue (Figure 61-3). Onchocercomata are formed predominantly on the head, face, and torso, but they may be found on the pelvic girdle and lower extremities deep-seated against the bones or near the joints. Nodules may vary in size from as small as 0.2 cm in diameter to as large as 6.0 cm and occasionally even larger. The nodule usually is composed of two or three females and daughter microfilariae encapsulated in a fibrous coat. Dead worms may calcify within the nodules. Various factors may account for nodule location. These may be mechanical restrictions to worm migration such as bony prominences and the biting proclivities of the local vector.

The ocular tissues are involved via migration of the microfilariae from the neighboring tissues, through the bloodstream, or along the nerves. Intraocular organisms are evident early in the disease by direct invasion from the conjunctiva, through the sclera, or through the cornea.

Most microfilariae die as immature worms in the host. Their death triggers an intense inflammatory reaction that is responsible for most of the morbidity of onchocerciasis. Antigens of the infec-

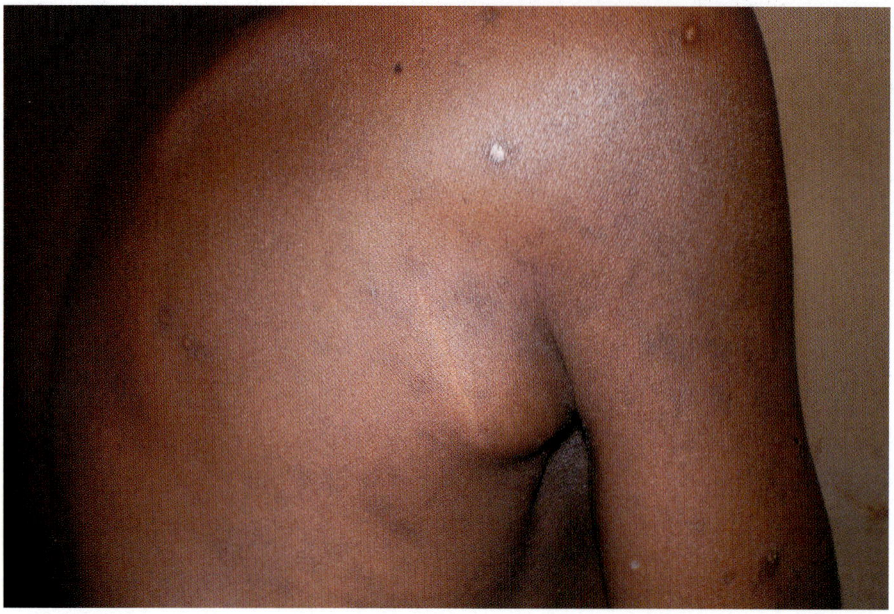

▲ **FIGURE 61-3** Onchocercoma—subcutaneous nodule (3 × 5 mm) over the lower lateral edge of the right shoulder.

1. A simple classification that subdivides onchocercal skin diseases into early and late skin lesions.[9] Early skin lesions include alterations in pigmentation and inflammatory skin diseases.
2. Mackenzie and colleagues[10] referred to these as *reactive* and *long-term disorders*.
3. The classification of Mudorch and colleagues[6] describes five main categories of onchocercal skin diseases: (a) acute papular onchodermatitis (APOD), (b) chronic papular onchodermatitis (CPOD; Figure 61-4), (c) lichenified onchodermatitis (LOD)/sowda, (d) atrophy, and (e) depigmentation (DPM; Figure 61-5)—with activity, severity (presence of itching or excoriation), and distribution grading as appropriate. Four of the associated

tive larvae seem to induce cell-mediated and humoral responses. Circulating immune complexes have been identified and implicated in the inflammatory response to infection. Perivascular deposits of immune complexes have been shown in various tissues. Immunoglobulin E (IgE) levels are also very high, thus implicating all the known mechanisms of pathologic immune destruction. The lymph nodes that drain infected areas show granulomatous inflammation, fibrosis, and atrophy on histologic examination.

CINICAL FINDINGS

Onchocerciasis, or river blindness, is characterized by dermal, lymphatic, and ocular manifestations with notable geographic variation in the clinical expression of the disease. These variations arise from variability of host response, parasite strain, and biting habits of different *Simulium* vector species. Cutaneous manifestations of onchocerciasis may be broadly divided into early and late skin lesions (Table 61-1).

Classification of Cutaneous Onchocerciasis

Various classifications are in existence for onchocerciasis. However, a classification scheme for standardization and comparison of surveys conducted from different parts of the world has been proposed by Mudorch and colleagues.[6]

TABLE 61-1
Clinical Features of Cutaneous Onchocerciasis

Symptoms

Pruritus
- Severe pruritus is the most distressing clinical manifestation of cutaneous onchocerciasis, interfering with the ability to sleep, work, farm, or interact socially.

Scratching
- The itching may be so severe that victims resort to scratching with twigs, stones, and knives, resulting in bleeding wounds, sores, and pain.[7]

Emotional disturbance
- Agitation, emotional disturbances, and stigmatization may drive the victim to suicide.[8]

Signs
- Itching may be mild and intermittent or severe and continuous, leading to superficial excoriation, crusts, secondary infection, and ulceration.
- Early skin lesions include alterations in pigmentation and inflammatory skin diseases (onchodermatitis). Features of onchodermatitis thus include
  - Urticaria
  - Macules
  - Papules
  - Subcutaneous edema (swelling of limbs or groin area)
  - Pustules
  - Scaling
  - Lichenification
  - Lymphadenopathy (particularly in the inguinal and femoral region)
  - Cellulitis, lympangitis, and lymphadenitis
  - Excoriations
  - Nodules (onchocercomata) found over bony prominences
  - Sowda (seen in chronic hypereactive onchodermatitis and characterized by intensely itchy localized papules, pustules, pachydermia, and darkening of the skin)
- Late skin lesions develop after years of chronic infestation and manifest as the following:
  - Atropy (resulting in the shiny, fragile skin described as "lizard skin")
  - Dermal scaring and loss of elasticity
  - Loose and hanging skin (face—leonine facies; axilla and groin—hanging groin)
  - Spotty depigmentation over the shin (leopard skin; see Figure 61-5)
  - Genital elephantiasis
  - Elephantiasis of the limbs also may occur with sowda.

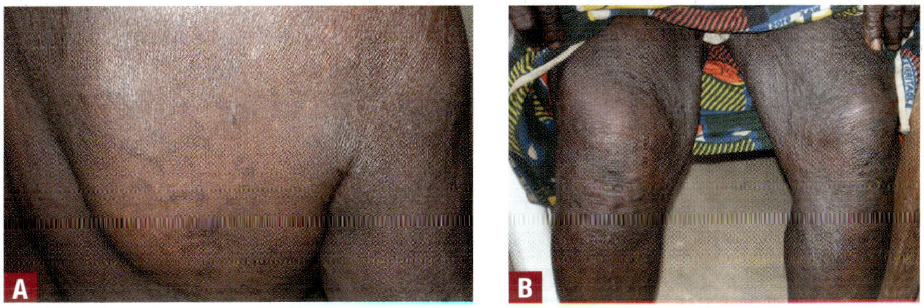

▲ **FIGURE 61-4** *A,B.* Chronic papular onchodermatitis with severe atrophy over the entire body (upper back and limbs).

features also may be recorded, namely, palpable onchocercal nodules, lymphyadenopathy, hanging groin, and lymphoedema—each with a corresponding grading scheme.

DIFFERENTIAL DIAGNOSIS

The differential diagnosis of cutaneous onchocerciasis depends on the various clinical manifestiations of the disease. Table 61-2 outlines the possible differential diagnoses.

TABLE 61-2
Differential Diagnosis of Cutaneous Onchocerciasis

Most Likely

Localized nodules/rash
- Epidermoid cyst
- Juxtaarticular nodules
- Fibroma
- Lymphoedema
- Urticaria

Generalized/eruptive rash
- Pyoderma
- Dermatitis herpertiformis
- Pityriasis lichenoides chronica
- Lichen planus

Consider

Localized rash
- Lichen simplex chronicus
- Podoconiosis

Generalized/eruptive
- Tinea incognito
- Drug eruption
- Chronic idiopathic urticaria

Always Rule Out

Localized nodules/lesions
- Lipoma
- Epidermoid cysts

Generalized
- Papular urticaria
- HIV infection

Eruptive
- Scabies
- Secondary syphilis

COMPLICATIONS

Complications include secondary bacterial infection, cellulitis, lymphangitis or recurrent lymphangitis, and blindness in the eruptive phase. The impaired social activity, low morale, stigmatization, and socioeconomic impact of the disease must be emphasized. The manifestations of the disease have resulted in abandonment of vast areas of fertile land and a poor attitude with regard to work.

TREATMENT

Clinical features of cutaneous onchocerciasis, together with recent observations that the disease can have major adverse psychosocial and socioeconomic effects, justified the inclusion of regions in Africa in control programs for ivermectin distribution. The World Health Organization (WHO) launched a control program for onchocerciasis, the African Programme for Onchocerciasis Control (APOC), which currently covers 19 endemic countries in Africa. Treatment of cnchocerciasis is outlined in Table 61-3.

Other Therapeutic Measures

Nodulectomy ± ivermectin or diethlcarbamazine. (Nodulectomy may be undertaken for cosmetic purposes.)

CONTROL/PREVENTION

Great progress has been made in the last 30 years in the control of onchocerciasis both in Africa and in the Americas, and this progress has been due largely to international public-private partnerships, sustained funding of regional programs, and new tools and technology. Until the advent of ivermectin, larvicidal campaigns against the insect vector were the only practical approach to onchocerciasis control. The insecticides used were effective against the vectors but safe for the remainder of the environment because they were biodegradable. They included the organophospate temephos, chlorphoxin, and pyracolos. Although dichlorodiphenyltrichloroethane (DDT) was relatively cheap, it later fell out of favor because of its persistence in the environment and fears of toxicity. Newer larvicides in use include biocides such as *Bacillus thuringenesis* sp. *isrealensis*[11] (serotype BT H14). This bacterium infects and kills mosquitos and blackfly larvae.

Vector reinvasion was a problem. This reinvasion phenomenon was handled by larviciding into expansion zones, supplemented by mass ivermectin chemotherapy. With the phasing out of the Onchocercal Control Programme (OCP) and the mass distribution of ivermectin, the Mectizan Expert Committee and the Mectizan Donation Program were able to organize and promote distribution of the drug.

TABLE 61-3
Treatments for Cutaneous Onchocerciasis

Systemic (microfilaricidal)	
Ivermectin (Mectizen)	150–100 μg/kg (repeat dose at 3 months, 6 months, or yearly. depending on symptoms until the worm dies (i.e., about 10–15 years)
Banocide (Hetrazan)*	25–50 mg tds increased weekly by 25 mg up to 100 mg. Treatment was continued until microfilarial negative in skin snips. Was the most effective microfilaricidal drug before the advent of ivermectin.
Suramin (macrofilaricidal drug with a narrow therapeutic margin/toxicity)	4 g over 6 weeks for adults over 60 kg, starting with a test dose of 0.2 g
Prospective macrofilaricidals	
Amorcazine	3 mg/kg twice daily
Moxidectin	Showing promising results in animal screens

*Associated with a significant Mazotti reaction

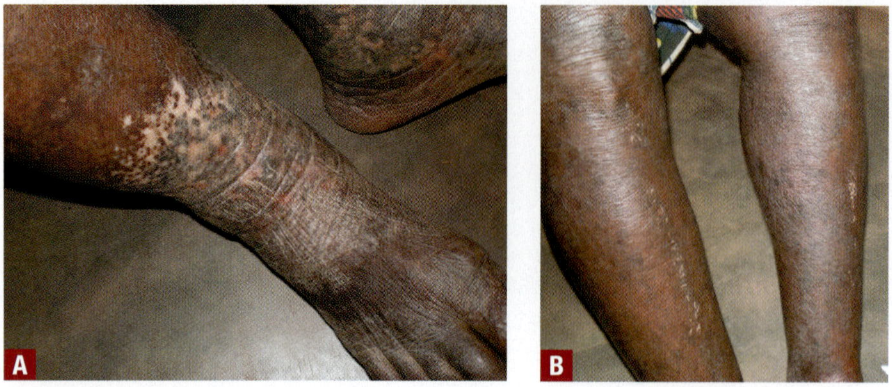

▲ **FIGURE 61-5** **A, B.** Depigmentation over the shin of the lower limbs (leopard skin).

A unique global partnership was launched in 1995 by the APOC (among 19 endemic African countries), WHO, the World Bank, and afflicted communities with the objective "To establish, within a period of 12 years, effective and self-sustainable, community-directed treatment with ivermectin throughout the remaining endemic areas in Africa and to eliminate the disease by vector control in selected foci.[12,13]

Over the years, constraints to the sustainability of ivermectin distribution[14] has been identified as a threat to the gains achieved in the prevention and treatment, coupled with the decreased prevalence of this disease in localized areas of Africa and Latin America.

REFERENCES

1. World Health Organization. *Report on Infectious Diseases: Removing Obstacles to Healthy Development.* Document WHO/CDS/99.1. Geneva: WHO, 1999; *www.who.int/infectious-disease-eport/index.html.*
2. Ahmad K. Global onchocerciasis programme under threat. *Lancet* 1999;356:1523.
3. World Health Organization. *Prevention and Control of Intestinal Parasitic Infections: Report of a WHO Expert Committee.* Geneva: WHO, 1987.
4. World Health Organization. *Onchocerciasis and Its Control: Report of a WHO Expert Committee on Onchocerciasis Control.* Technical Repot Series no 852. Geneva: WHO, 1995.
5. Brown L, Huges AM, Sykes J, et al (eds). *The New Shorter Oxford English Dictionary on Historical Principles.* Oxford, England, Oxford University Press, 1993.
6. Mudorch ME, Hay RJ, Mackenzie CD, et al. A clinical classification and grading system of the cutaneous changesin onchocerciasis. *Br J Dermatol* 1993;129:260-269.
7. World Health Organization. *The Importance of Onchocercal Skin Diseases: Report of a Multicountry Study by the Pan-African Study Group on Onchocercal Skin Diseases.* Document TDR/AFR/RP/95.1. Geneva: WHO, 1995.
8. Nwokolo C. Studies in onchocerciasis: A review of 100 cases from Enugu District of Eastern Nigeria. *Trans R Soc Trop Med Hyg* 1950;43:493-501.
9. World Health Organization. *Expert Committee on Onchocerciasis: Third Report.* Technical Report Series No 752. Geneva: WHO, 1987.
10. Mackenzie CD, Williams JF, Sisely BM, et al. Variations in host responses and the pathogenesis of human onchocerciasis. *Rev Infect Dis* 1985;7:802-808.
11. Hougard JM, Back C. Perspectives on the bacterial control of vectors in the tropics. *Paristol Today* 1992;8:364-368.
12. APOC/WHO Web site; updated December 3, 1997; *www.who.int/ocp/apoc.*
13. Seketeli A, Adeoye G, Eyamba A, et al. The achievements and challenges of the African Programme for Onchocerciasis Control (APOC). *Ann Trop Med Parasitol* 2002;96:S15-28.
14. Abiose A, Homeida M, Lisse B, et al. Onchocerciasis control strategies. *Lancet* 2000;356:1523.

CHAPTER 62

Leprosy

Yemane-Berhan Tebebe
Shobita Rajagopalan

Key Points

- Leprosy is a chronic bacterial infection caused by *Mycobacterium leprae.*
- The variety of clinical manifestations of the disease is determined by the host immune response.
- Leprosy primarily affects the skin, the peripheral nerves, the upper respiratory tract, and the eyes. Peripheral nerve involvement results in neuropathy, a cardinal manifestation of the disease.
- Early detection of leprosy and treatment with multiple drugs are the most important steps in preventing long-term deformity and disability.
- The World Health Organization recommends a protocol of multidrug therapy that effectively controls the disease and contributes to global elimination of leprosy.

Leprosy is a chronic bacterial infection caused by the intracellular microorganism *Mycobacterium leprae*. The disease triggers a broad range of immune responses that eventually determine the clinical spectrum of the disease.[1] Leprosy is characterized by a wide variety of clinical disease manifestations that are determined by an interplay between the disease burden and host immune responses (Table 62-1). The bacteria have an affinity for the peripheral nerves, resulting in neuropathy, which is a cardinal manifestation of the disease.[2] Skin lesions are common and the primary external symptom (Table 62-2). The clinical features of the disease depend primarily on the balance between bacillary multiplication and the host cells that mediate immune response. The progressive nature of this chronic infectious disease causes long-term damage to facial skin, limbs, nerves, and eyes (Figures 62-1 and 62-2). Leprosy has been determined to also affect animals and is now also considered a zoonotic disease[3] (Table 62-3).

TABLE 62-1
Neuropathology of Leprosy

- Congenital sensory neuropathy
- Primary amylodosis of nerves
- Nerve tumors
- Polyneuropathy
- Facial nerve paralysis
- Entrapment neuropathy
- Acute idiopathic polyneuropathy
- Neurogenic muscular atrophy (Tooth-Charcot-Hoffmann syndrome)
- Hereditary sensory neuropathy (Thevenard syndrome)
- Dejerine-Sottas syndrome
- Syringomyelia

Leprosy is seen most commonly in people with skin of color. Today, leprosy is found predominantly in developing countries in subtropical and tropical regions. Socioeconomic factors (e.g., lack of resources, overcrowding, and poor sanitation) and environmental factors (e.g., warm and moist climates that provide an ideal environment for microorganisms to thrive) are likely to play a significant role in the increased disease prevalence in these regions.

TABLE 62-2
Leprosy: Skin Lesions

Annular Lesions
- Tinea corporis
- Granuloma annulare
- Necorobiosis lipoidica
- Granuloma disciformis (Miecher)
- Granuloma Multiforme (Leiker)
- Erythema annulare centrifugum
- Erythema multiforme

Nodular Lesions
- Neurofibromatosis (von Recklinghausen disease)
- Sarcoma idiopathicum haemorchagicium (Kaposi sarcoma)
- Dermal leishmaniasis
- Postkalaazar dermal leishmaniasis
- Mollusca contagiosum

Infiltrated Patches
- Psoriasis
- Seborrhaic dermatitis
- Pityriasis rosea (Gilbert)
- Scleroderma
- Lichen planus
- Lichen nitidus
- Sarcoidosis (Boeck)
- Tuberculosis
- Lupus vulgaris
- Lupus erythematosus
- Mycosis

Disseminated Diffuse Infiltrates
- Diffuse cutaneous lesishmaniasis
- Mycosis fungoides
- Reticulosis
- Syphilis

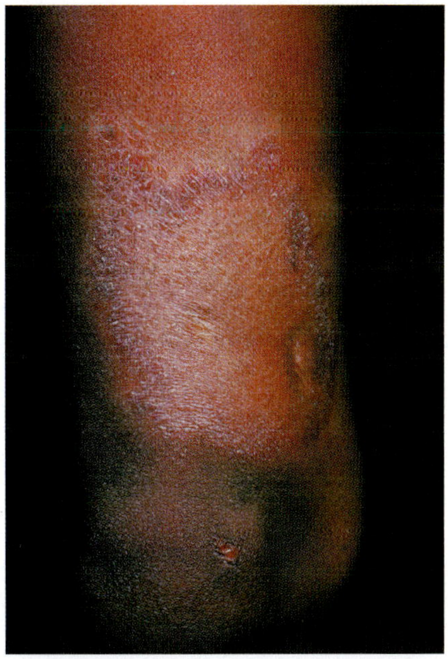

▲ **FIGURE 62-1** Tuberculoid leprosy (TT). Single anesthetic plaque on the leg. Courtesy of Barbara Leppard, M.D.

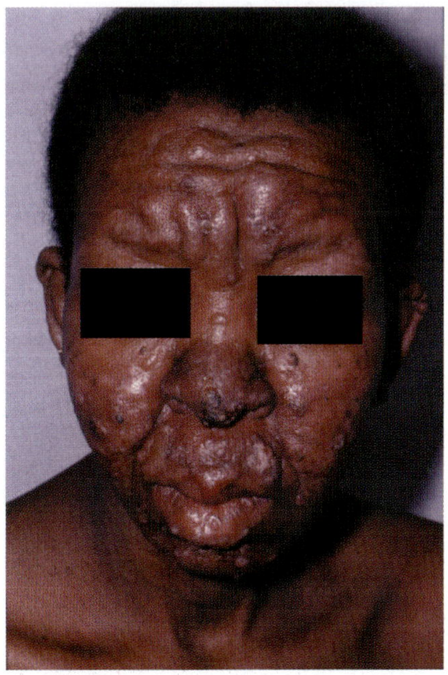

▲ **FIGURE 62-2** Lepromatous leprosy (LL). Extensive papules, nodules, and plaques. Note loss of eyebrows and leonine facies. Courtesy of Barbara Leppard, M.D.

TABLE 62-3
A Zoonotic Disease: Animals that can be Infected with Leprosy

- Humans
- Armadillo
- Chimpanzee
- Mangabey monkey

EPIDEMIOLOGY

Leprosy is found largely in developing countries around the tropics and subtropics. Sporadic cases encountered in developed nations occur among immigrants from countries where the disease is endemic.

ETIOLOGY AND PATHOGENESIS

M. leprae, or the lepra bacillus, an acid-fast organism, was first discovered by Armauer Hansen in the year 1874. The organism is about 0.2 μm thick and 8 μm long. Although the organism is not cultured in any laboratory media, limited multiplication can be obtained in the foot pads of mice. Lepra bacilli have been found in many different types of cells, as shown in Table 62-4.

The incubation period (IP) of leprosy typically ranges from 1–5 years, thus increasing the likelihood of spread of infection to children and family members. The IP can vary from several months to 30 years, with an average of 4–10 years.[4]

The mode of transmission is not yet known, but three potential portals of entry have been considered: the skin, the gastrointestinal tract, and the respiratory tract. Until recently, lepra bacilli have not been known to cross the placenta; current literature suggests rare transplacental transmission of *M. leprae.*[5]

The causative organism evokes three possible responses in a given host. One type of host is able to completely destroy the organism owing to natural or acquired immunity. The second type of host has partial resistance and develops a localized disease. The third type of host has a near-complete absence of immunity to *M. leprae* and develops a generalized disease. Regardless of the route of entry into the human body, only a small proportion of infected persons develops overt symptoms and signs of the disease after the usual incubation period; the vast majority of infected individuals develop only a subclinical infection.[6]

TABLE 62-4
Cells Where Lepra Bacilli are Found

- Macrophages
- Schwann's cells of nerves
- Muscle cells
- Endothelial cells of blood vessels
- Skin melanocytes
- Chondrocytes of cartilage

IMMUNOLOGY

Leprosy triggers a very complex mix of humoral and cell-mediated immune responses The circulating antibodies produced in leprosy have no protective function and potentially may aggravate the disease process.

The total absence of immune response to *M. leprae* in certain patients is specific to this particular organsm, and it may be genetically determined. The recent response to *M. leprae* can be observed in several lepromatous leprosy patients after the addition of interleukin 2 (IL-2). Also, the type of response seems to correlate with specific human leukocyte antigen (HLA) types: Patients with HLA-DR2 and HLA-DR3 are more likely to develop tuberculoid-type leprosy (TT), whereas those with HLA-DQ1 are more likely to develop lepromatus leprosy (LL).[3,4]

In TT, effective cell-mediated immunity (CMI) to *M. leprae* results in phagocytosis and digestion of the lepra bacilli by macrophages, which, in turn, mature into epitheloid cells. Circulating antibodies to antigens of *M. leprae* are not demonstrable. In LL, a predominantly Th1 CD4 and Th2 response is seen.[5] In borderline-tuberculoid leprosy (BT), depending on its place in the immunologic spectrum, there are varying degrees of CMI response; significant CMI responses are seen toward the tuberculoid end of the spectrum and minimal to none toward the lepromatous end.

CLINICAL ASPECTS OF LEPROSY

A proper classification of the disease should be based on clinical appearance, histopathologic changes, bacteriologic load, and immunologic status of the patient. Depending on the susceptibility of a patient, infection with *M. leprae* may produce (1) a localized disease in a highly resistant patient, namely, the tuberculoid type, (2) a disseminated generalized disease in a highly susceptible patient with no immunity at all, namely, the lepromatous type, (3) a disease spectrum between the two polar varieties, manifesting in different degrees the characteristics of the polar varieties and referred to as the *borderline type,* (4) an *indeterminate* group, which consists of the development of an early lesion before the disease becomes active, and (5) a purely *neural* variety in which a small number of patients present with disease that solely involves the nerves.

CLASSIFICATION OF LEPROSY

In 1996, Ridley and Jopling[7] defined TT, BT, BB (mid-borderline), BL (borderline lepromatous leprosy), and LL groups on the basis of all the findings (i.e., clinical, bacteriologic, histologic, and immunologic). The pure neural and indeterminate dermal patients did not fall within this spectrum. Two principal manifestations of LL deserve mention: First, *histioid leproma,* the term introduced by Haregewoin and colleagues,[8] was applied to the firm, erythematous, round or oval, shiny, glistering nodules that appear on the skin of patients whose disease is relapsing either because they have stopped treatment or because *M. leprae* has become drug resistant.[2] Second, *lucio leprosy* is the term applied to the diffuse nonnodular type of leprosy that presents as shiny thickened skin, loss of body hair (including eyebrows and eyelashes), puffy hands, and widespread sensory loss owing to involvement of dermal nerves because the nodules and other types of skin lesions are absent. The different types of leprosy are listed in Table 62-5.

Indications of Leprosy

Enlarged peripheral nerves are found very rarely in any other disease and can be considered pathognomonic of leprosy. Comparison of enlarged nerves on contiguous sides must be evaluated. Leprosy is also the only disease in which there can be a massive invasion of the dermis or nasal mucosa with acid-fast bacilli.[9]

The signs and symptoms of leprosy are related to three processes: (1) the multiplication and dissemination of *M. leprae,* (2) the patients immune response to *M. leprae* and its antigens, and (3) complications resulting from peripheral nerve damage that occurs owing to the first two processes.

When the disease has moved into the spectrum, eight characteristics are especially useful in determining where on the spectrum the disease may be:

TABLE 62-5
Classifications of Leprosy

LL = lepromatous leprosy
TT = tuberculoid leprosy
BL = borderline lepromotous leprosy
BT = borderline teberculoid leprosy
BB = mid-borderline leprosy
IL = indeterminate leprosy

1. The number of skin lesions
2. The distribution and symmetry of skin lesions
3. Definition and clarity of skin lesions
4. Anesthesia
5. Loss of sweating and reduced hair growth
6. The distribution, extent, and nature of peripheral nerve involvement
7. Mucosal and systemic involvement
8. The number of *M. leprae*

The type of leprosy that develops is determined by the way in which the defensive cells respond to the challenge once they have "recognized" the infection. The different types of leprosy are listed in Table 62-5. Once lepra bacilli gain entry into the host, they have an affinity for neural tissue; Schwann cells within the neural tissue engulf the lepra bacilli.[10] The subsequent fate and type of leprosy that ensues depend on host immune responses. Resistance is highest in TT, diminishes through the borderline spectrum, and is lowest in LL.

Not only do leprosy bacilli have a predilection for nerves, but they also are the only bacteria to have the capacity to enter nerves. Nerves invaded by leprosy bacilli are either dermal nerves or trunk nerves.

Tuberculoid Leprosy (TT)

TT affects skin and peripheral nerves (see Figure 62-1). Skin lesions are single with sharp borders. They may be macules or plaques. The lesions are hyperesthetic or definitely anesthetic, except when on the face, where the skin sensory innervation compensates for the damage. Autonomic nerve damage within the lesions is often severe; the skin texture is rough and dry. By usual methods of examination, no *M. leprae* can be found in TT. The lepromine test generally is positive.

Lepromatous Leprosy (LL)

The early lesions of LL usually are macules that are widely and symmetrically distributed (see Figure 62-2). They are usually ill-defined, slightly hypopigmented, and mildly erythematous. The surface may be shiny and moist, so they are seen with difficulty except with very good illumination. Sensation to touch and a pin prick is usually unimpaired in early lepromatous macules, but sweating may be diminished. Hair is lost in all skin lesions, especially on the face. Loss of eyelashes and eyebrows, a condition known as *madarosis,* is characteristic. Bacillary destruction of the bony nasal spine leads to collapse of the nose. Other facial bones may be eroded too. The continuous bacillemia in LL, estimated to be 10 organism per milliliter of blood, ensures the constant bombardment of internal organs by *M. leprae.*[11,12]

Borderline Tuberculoid Leprosy (BT)

Borderline tuberculoid leprosy skin lesions resemble those of TT in that they tend to be well defined and hypopigmented, but there are clear differences (Figure 62-3). Marginal definitions of the lesion are less pronounced and infiltrate less on the margins. They stream off gradually into the normal skin, but satellite lesions lie near the edges. The margins may be raised and well defined or flat and vague. The number of lesions is up to 8–10 or more. One of the important features of BT is the frequency with which nerves are damaged; it is not uncommon for a prolonged polyneuritic phase to precede the appearance of the skin lesion, and several nerves are likely to be involved asymmetrically. Bacilli are scanty or absent from skin smears.[9]

Mid-Borderline Leprosy (BB)

BB is the most unstable form of leprosy. It has dimorphic features that can readily downgrade or revert to normal. BB lesions tend to be numerous and symmetric. BB lesions are mostly macules, plaques, and/or papules with a punched-out appearance. The edges of the punched-out portions of the lesions are distinctly palpable, with some degree of anesthesia. Lepra bacilli are found readily in skin smears obtained from affected areas. Large nerve involvement is common, with variable and asymmetric enlargement.

Indeterminate Leprosy (IL)

IL is an early and transitory stage of leprosy found in patients (usually children) whose immunologic status has yet to be determined. There is scattered nonspecific histiocytic and lymphocytic infiltration, histopathologically resembling leprosy. In some cases, cellular reaction within dermal nerves or the presence of one or more lepra bacilli in dermal nerves, the subepidermal zone, or the arrectores pilorum muscles may be found.

Pure Neural Leprosy

In the purely neural form of leprosy, there may be involvement and enlargement of

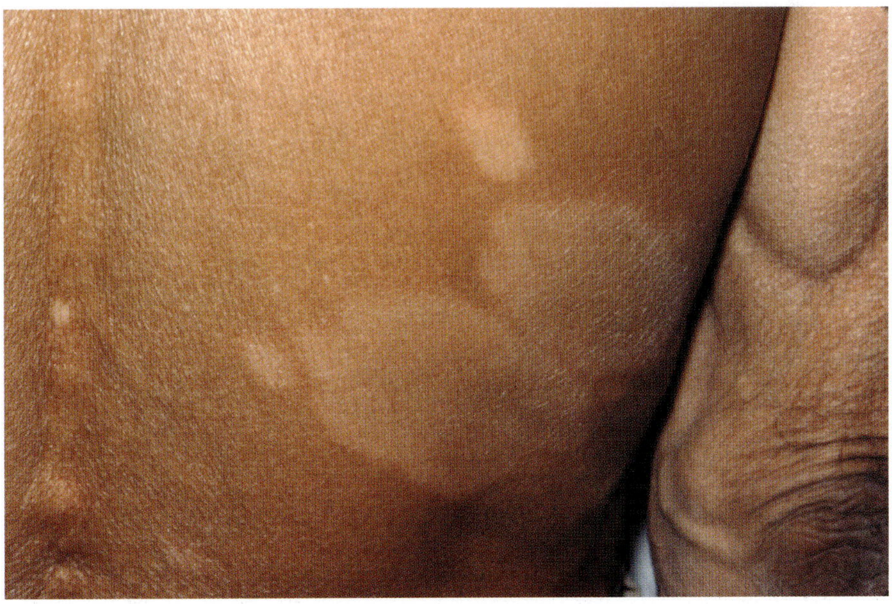

▲ **FIGURE 62-3** Borderline tuberculoid leprosy (BT). Few hypopigmented, anesthetic plaques localized to one area of the body. Courtesy of Barbara Leppard, M.D.

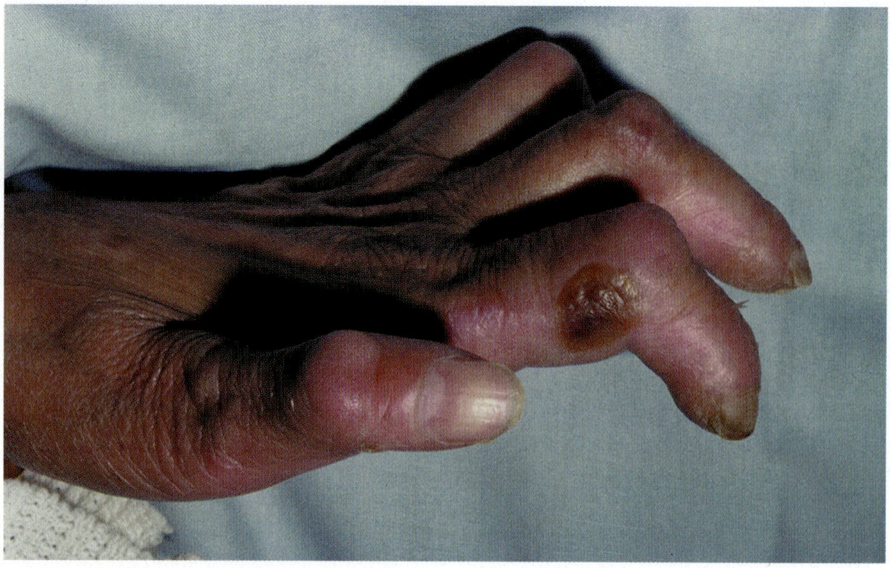

▲ **FIGURE 62-4** Claw hand owing to ulnar and median nerve palsy. Courtesy of Barbara Leppard, M.D.

one or more peripheral nerves without skin involvement (Figure 62-4). This form usually presents with signs and symptoms of nerve deficit, such as gradual weakness in a hand or a sudden foot drop or anesthesia in an extremity. The diagnosis usually can be made based on the presence of definite nerve enlargement.

COMPLICATIONS

There are two main types of complications: (1) those owing to massive invasion of tissue by *M. leprae* and (2) those owing to reactions. Reactions represent episodes of acute hypersensitivity to antigens of *M. leprae* brought about by a disturbance in the preexisting immunologic balance. Three types of reactions are recognized. Type I reaction is associated with cell-mediated hypersensitivity. Type II reaction is associated with immune complexes. The Luci phenomenon occurs because of necrosis of the endothelium of arterioles that are massively invaded by *M. leprae.*[13]

DIAGNOSIS

There are three cardinal signs of leprosy: (1) loss or impairment of sensations (2) thickening of the above-mentioned nerves and (3) the presence of M. leprosy bacilli in smears from skin and/or nasal mucosa. The presence of one of the three signs is sufficient to establish a diagnosis. A full physical examination, however, is needed to determine the extent of disease and its likely complications.

Clinical diagnosis is confirmed by obtaining skin smears from affected areas of the body. Lepra bacilli grow best at a temperature around 35°C; thus they thrive in cooler areas of the body, such as the earlobes, testicles, nose, and areas where the peripheral nerves are close to the skin. Skin smears are the most important laboratory test used in the diagnosis and prognosis of leprosy. The epidermis is slit open to a depth of 2–3 mm using a very sharp sterile scalpel. Care should be taken not to go deep and draw blood. The smear can be stained for acid-fast bacilli.[14,15]

Bacteriologic Index

The evaluation of smears from each site is made according to grades 1–6. The average grade arrived at after examining the smears from the four sites is calculated to find the bacteriologic index (BI). The BI continues to be a valuable test to diagnose and assess a patient's progress.

Morphologic Index (MI)

This is a very sensitive index used to evaluate the efficacy of antileprosy drugs in a given patient. Each bacillus should be examined separately and carefully.[16]

TREATMENT

Chemotherapy

A common regimen for the treatment of both paucibacillary (PB) and multibacillary (MB) leprosy is desirable. The World Health Organization (WHO) Technical Advisory Group recommends that all leprosy patients, both PB and MB, should be treated with a multiple-drug therapy (MDT) regimen for a period of 6–12 months. The rationale for these recommendations is as follows:

- MDT has been proven to be robust in terms of treatment efficiency and safety.
- Relapse rates are less than 1%.
- Resistance to MDT has been virtually nonexistent.

MDT treatment may vary based on the age of the patient and the type leprosy of and is determined by bacilloscopy for number of lesions.[17] Table 62-6 outlines

TABLE 62-6
Treatment of Leprosy with Multidrug Therapy

Multidrug Therapy for Multibacillary Leprosy

	Rifampicin	Dapsone	Clofazimine
Adult, 50–70 kg	600 mg/month*	100 mg/day	50 mg/day and 300 mg/month*
Child, 10–14 years	450 mg/month*	50 mg/day	50 mg/day and 150 mg/month*
Younger than 10	300 mg/month*	25 mg/day	50 mg twice/week and 100 mg/month*

Multidrug Therapy for Paucibacillary Leprosy

	Rifmpicin	Dapsone
Adult, 50–70 kg	600 mg/month*	100 mg/day
Child 10–14 years	450 mg/month*	50 mg/day
Younger than 10	300 mg/month*	25 mg/day

*Monthly doses are administered via direct observation.
Source: Modified from Ref 2.

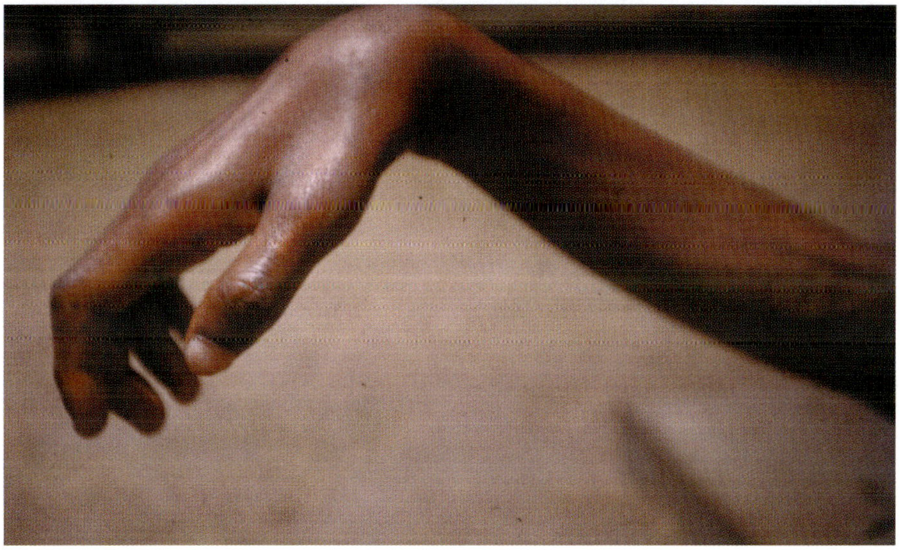

▲ **FIGURE 62-5** Type 1 leprosy reaction: wrist drop. Courtesy of Barbara Leppard, M.D.

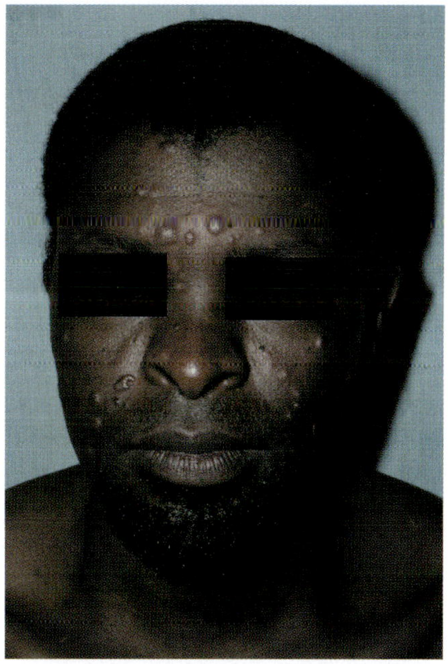

▲ **FIGURE 62-6** Type 1 leprosy reaction: swelling of old lesions. Courtesy of Barbara Leppard, M.D.

treatment for PB and MD leprosy recommended by the WHO. Ishii[2] provides a concise update on MDT regimens, mode of action, side-effect profile, and laboratory monitoring.

PREVENTION AND CONTROL

Early case detection and timely and appropriate initiation of MDT are appropriate critical to minimize leprosy-related impairment. Rehabilitation also needs to be addressed. BT, BB, and BL patients tend to develop a type 1 reversal reaction (Figures 62-5 through 62-7).

Multibacillory Patients

LL patients tend to develop an erythema nodosum leprosum (Figures 62-8 and 62-9) type 2 reaction, which usually responds satisfactorily to anti-inflammatory treatment (e.g., predonisolone and thalidomide).

CONCLUSION

Early diagnosis of leprosy is vitally important to reduce peripheral nerve damage, such as loss of sensory, motor, and autonomic nerve function, with subsequent deformity resulting from repeated trauma of the skin. Recognition and management of leprosy reactions always lead to reduced consequences of nerve damage and have an impact on the quality of life for those affected by the disease and the stigma it generates. Prevention of nerve damage and management of impairment are important

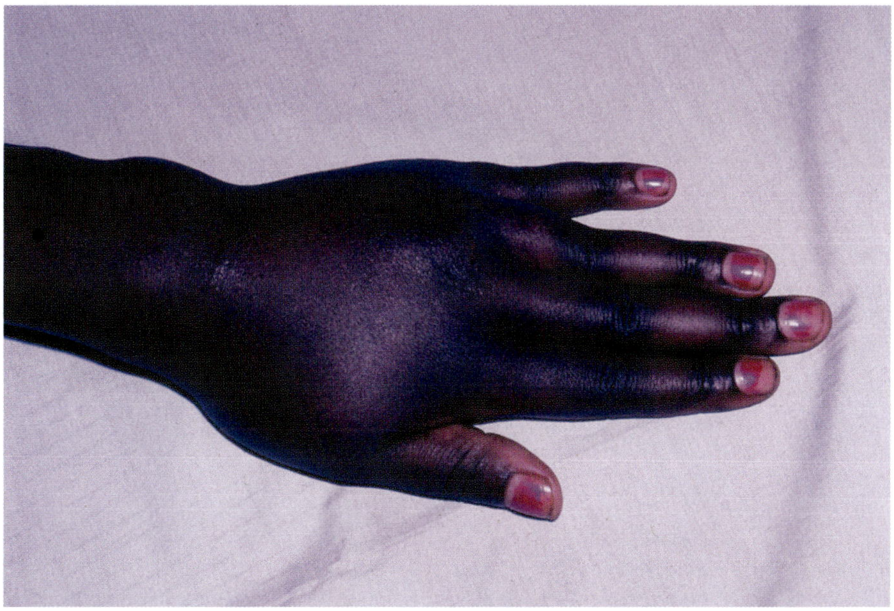

▲ **FIGURE 62-7** Type 1 leprosy reaction: swelling of hand. Courtesy of Barbara Leppard, M.D.

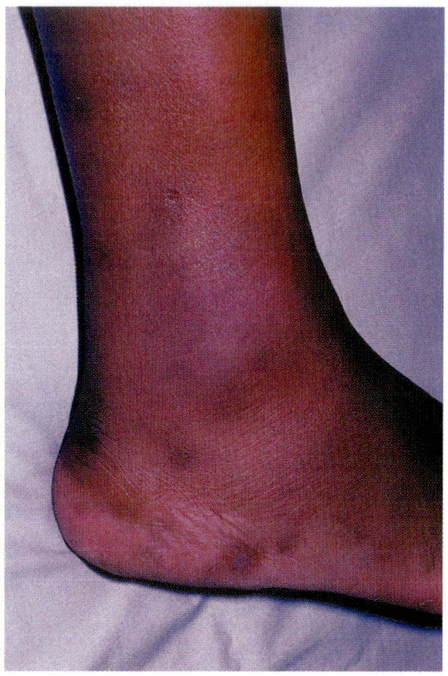

▲ **FIGURE 62-8** Type 2 leprosy reaction: erythema nodosum leprosum. Courtesy of Barbara Leppard, M.D.

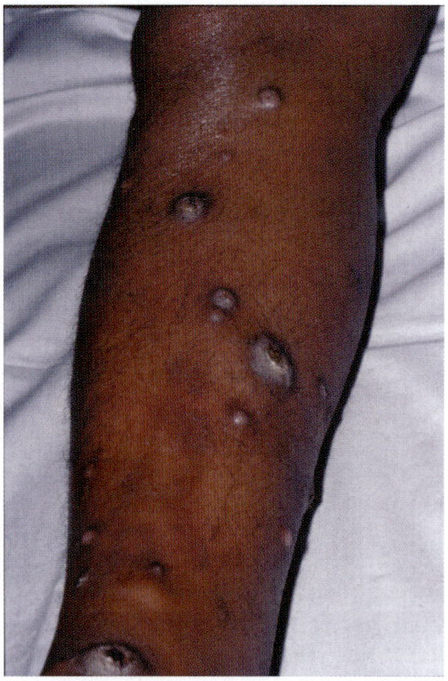

▲ **FIGURE 62-9** Type 2 leprosy reaction: erythema nodosum leprosum. Courtesy of Barbara Leppard, M.D.

components of a leprosy program. Since leprosy leaves a great number of patients with permanent disabilities, a well-thought-out plan of integration of the disabled person into the larger society should be a goal in a successful leprosy control program.

REFERENCES

1. Sasaki S, Takeshita F, Okuda K, Ishii N. *Mycobacterium leprae* and leprosy: A compendium. *Micribiol Immunol* 2001;45:729-736.
2. Ishii N. Recent advances in the treatment of leprosy, *Dermatol Online J* 2003;9:2.
3. Rojas-Espinoza O, Lovik M. *Mycobacterium leprae* and *Mycobacterium lepraemurium* infections in domestic and wild animals. *Rev Off Int Epizoot* 2001;20:219-251.
4. Nsibambi J, Berhan TY, Warndorff Van Diepen T. Multibacillary leprosy in an 18-month-old child: A case report. 1984.
5. Ryan KJ (ed). *Sherris Medical Microbiology*, 4th ed. New York, McGraw-Hill, 2004, pp 451-453.
6. Britton W. Leprosy, in Armstrong D, Cohen J (eds), *Infectious Diseases*. London, Mosby, 1991, pp 16.1-16.6.
7. Ridley DS, Jopling WH. Classification of leprosy according to immunity. *Int J Leprosy* 1996;34:255-273.
8. Haregewoin T, Godal AS, Mustafa A, et al. T-cell conditioned media reverse, T-cell unresponsiveness in lepromatous leprosy. *Nat Int Wkly J Sci* 1983;303:342-344.
9. Jopling WH. Borderline (dimorphous) leprosy maintaining a poluneuritic form for eight years: A case report. *Trans R Soc Trop Med Hyg* 1956;50:478-480.
10. Rea TH, Ridley DS. Lucio's phenomenon: A comparative histological study. *Int J Leprosy* 1979;47:161-166.
11. Drutz DJ, Chen TSN, Lu W-H. The continuous bacteraemia of lepromatous leprosy. *N Engl J Med* 1972;287:159-164.
12. Wade HW. The histoid variety of lepromatous leprosy. *Int J Leprosy* 1963;31:129-142.
13. Reich CV. Leprosy: Cause, transmit ion, and a new theory of pathogenesis. *Rev Infect Dis* 1987;9:590-594.
14. Alcais A, Mira M, Casanova JL, et al. Genetic dissection of immunity in leprosy. *Curr Opin Immunol* 2005;17: 44-48.
15. Chehl S, Job C, Hastings R. Transmission of leprosy in nude mice. *Am J Trop Med Hyg* 1985;34:1161-1166.
16. World Health Organization. *Epidemiology of Leprosy in Relation to Control: Report of a WHO Study Group*. WHO Technical Report Series 716. Geneva, WHO, 1985, pp 1-60.
17. World Health Organization. Report on the Third Meeting of the WHO Technical Advisory Group on the Elimination of Leprosy, Brasilia, February 1-2, 2002.

CHAPTER 63

Leishmaniasis

Yemane-Berhan Tebebe
Edith Nkechi Nnoruka

Key Points

- Leishmaniasis is caused by unicellular fagellate protozoa of the genus *Leishmania.*
- The disease is endemic in warm regions such as the the Mediterranean, North and East Africa, the Middle East, India, China, and South and Central America.
- Vectors include female sandflies of the genus *Phlebotomus* (old world), *Lutzomyia,* and *Psychodopygus* (new world).
- Other modes of transmission (e.g., parenteral, congenital, sexual, occupational, and person to person) may be more relevant in human immune deficiency virus (HIV)–positive patients.
- Leishmaniasis manifests clinically as four major syndromes: cutaneous leshmaniasis (CL), mucocutaneous leshmaniasis (ML), diffuse cutaneous leshmaniasis, and visceral leshmaniasis (VL).
- CL is characterized by single or multiple cutaneous papules at the site of a sandfly bite, often evolving into nodules and ulcers.

Leishmaniasis is a parasitic disease caused by unicellular flagellate intracellular protozoa of the genus *Leishmania,* which are members of the order Kinetoplastida. Parasties of the genus *Leishmania* infect macrophages of mammals, including humans.[1] There are many species and serologic strains, giving rise to a variety of clinical types of the disease (Table 63-1)

TABLE 63-1
Synonyms and Types Of Leishmaniasis

- Old world cutaneous leishmaniasis
  - Oriental sore
  - Baghdad boil
- New world cutaneous and mucocutaneous leishmaniasis
  - Leishmaniasis Americana
  - Uta
  - Espundia
  - Chirleru ulcer
- Visceral leishmaniasis
  - Kala-azar
  - Dum-dum fever
- Leishamania infantum
- Leishmania clonovani
- Leishmania cha chagasi

WORLDWIDE GEOGRAPHIC DISTRIBUTION

Leishmaniasis is endemic to 82 countries (10 developed and 72 developing, including 13 of the least developed countries[2]). The World Health Organization (WHO) estimates an incidence of 12 million cases among 350 million at risk and an annual incidence of 600,000 cases. Despite its wide geographic distribution, human leishmaniasis is often very focal within an endemic area, leading to outbreaks of the disease. The disease is endemic to warm regions such as the Mediterranean, North and East Africa, the Middle East, India, China, and South and Central America.

LIFE CYCLE

The protozoan parasites *Leishmania,* which resides in a hydrolytic environment, have two developmental stages in their life cycle.

Promastigote

This is a slender elongation of the parasites with the flagellum located interiorly. This stage of the parasite is formed in the gut of the sandfly vector and is the form maculated into the body of the vertebrate host. Transmission of the *Leishmania* parasite from the sandfly vector of the mammalian host.

Amastigote

This is an oval-shaped form of the organism found in the macrophage of the vertebrate host. Although the general configuration of all amastigotes is smaller than promastigotes, electron microscopy reveals the presence of a flagellum protruding from the reservoirs of amastigotes.

RESERVOIR HOSTS

Domestic dogs, wild animal canidae (e.g., foxes, jackals, wolves), raccoons, hyraxes, and rodents are the principal reservoirs. However, not all species of *Leishmania* are thought to have an animal reservoir, as evidenced by *L. donovani* in India.

THE VECTOR

Sandflies responsible for transmission of leishmaniasis are divided in two groups: *Phlebotomus* in the old world and *Lutzomyia* in new world.[3] *Psychodopygus* also has been described.[4] Other modes of transmission (i.e., parenteral, congenital, sexual, occupational, and person to person) may be becoming more relevant in HIV-positive patients.

THE DISEASE OF LEISHMANIASIS

Worldwide, leishmaniasis still can be considered to be a childhood disease, even though a changing clinical picture has been emerging. There are basically three broad clinical manifesatations—cutaneous leishmanisis (CL), mucocutaneous leishmanisis (ML), and visceral leishmaniasis (VL). Both CL and VL can be seen in all age groups.[5–7]

Human leishmaniasis is caused by at least 14 different species or subspecies of *Leishmania.* Leishmaniasis presents as a large variety of disease manifestations, differing markedly in their severity and health impact.[2] Outcome of infection and clinical patterns of the disease vary according to parasite strain, size of inoculum, site of inoculum, host genetics (i.e., immunologic competence of the host), acquired immunity, and nutritional state of the host.[8] The spectrum of clinical manifestations of the disease is grouped into four major clinical forms (Tables 63-2 and 63-3)

1. *Cutaneous leishmaniasis* is normally caused by *L. tropica, L. aethiopica,* and *L. major* in the old world.[9] The clinical characteristics of cutaneous leishmaniasis tend to vary from region to region depending on parasite, host, and zoonotic cycles involved. The classic disease is characterized by one or more nodular lesions at the site of inoculation. The lesions may heal spontaneously, leaving a scar. Nonhealing forms are also known. The nodule appears 3–7 weeks after incubation. After 2–4 months, the nodule

TABLE 63-2
Major *Leishmania* Species Causing Human Disease

Type of Disease	Leishmania Species	Primary Locations
Cutaneous leishmaniasis (CL)	*L. mexicana*	Central America
	L. amazonensis	Brazil
	L. venezuelensis	Venezuela
	L. pifanoi	Venezuela
	L. tropica	Mediterranean countries
	L. major	Asia, Far East, Africa
	L. aethiopica	Ethiopia
	L. guyanensis	Brazil
	L. peruviana	Peru, Argentina, Panama, Costa Rica,
	L. panamanesis	Colombia
Diffused cutaneous leishmaniasis (DCL)	*L. aethiopica*	Ethiopia
	L. amazonesis	Brazil
	L. pifanoi	Venezuela
Mucocutaneous leishmaniasis (MCL)	*L. braziliensis*	Brazil
	L. aethiopica	Ethiopia
Visceral leishmaniasis (VL)	*L. donovani, L. infantum*	India, Ethiopia
	L. chagasi	Mediterranean countries
	L. archibaldi	South and Central America
		Sub-Sahara Africa

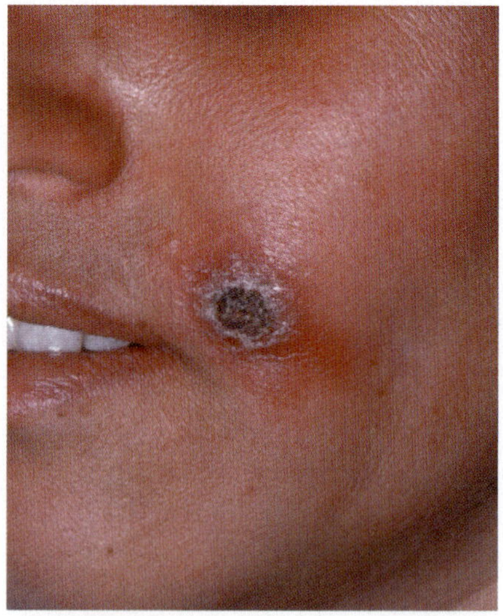

▲ **FIGURE 63-2** Cutaneous leishmaniasis. The same female patient as in Figure 63-1 two months later.

ulcerates and becomes crusted (Figures 63-1 through 63-6). Self-healing gradually takes place within 6–10 months or so, leaving a characteristic scar. If cutaneous leishmaniasis

TABLE 63-3
Clinical Forms of Leishmaniasis

- Cutaneous leishmaniasis (CL), where infection is restricted to the skin
- Diffused cutaneous leishmaniasis (DCL), where infection is restricted to the skin in diffuse form
- Mucocutaneous leishmaniasis (MCL), where infection is restricted to the mucous membranes
- Visceral leishmaniasis (VL), where infection is predominantly visceral
- HIV-visceral leshmaniasis coinfection

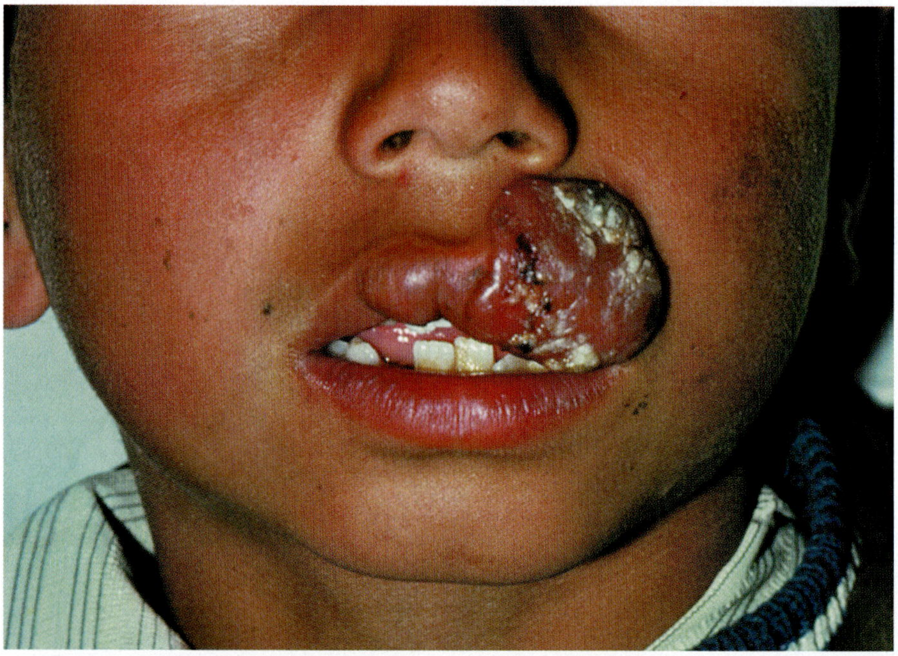

▲ **FIGURE 63-3** Cutaneous leishmaniasis on the lip of an 8-year-old boy.

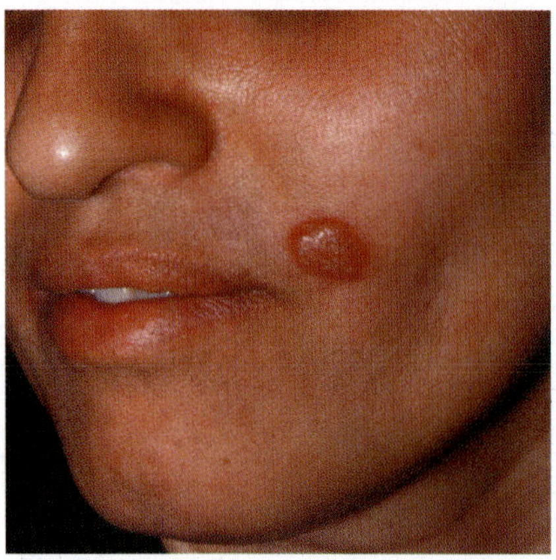

▲ **FIGURE 63-1** Cutaneous leishmaniasis. Early lesion with a red papule on the cheek.

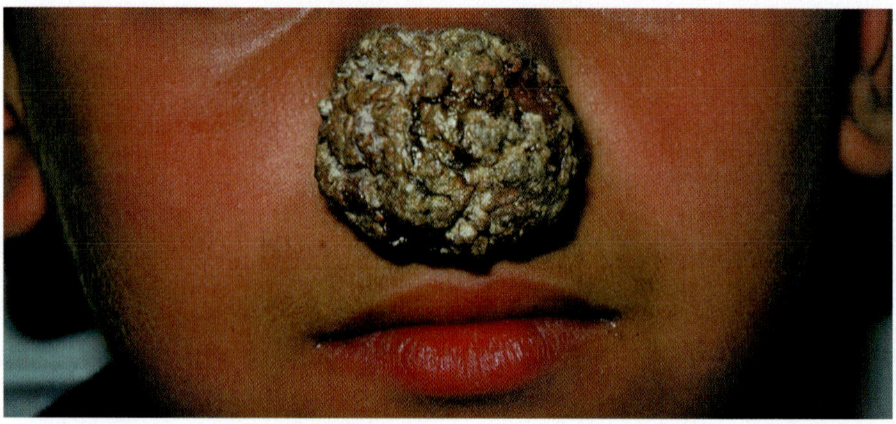

▲ **FIGURE 63-4** Cutaneous leishmaniasis with crusting lesions destroying the nose tip of the child.

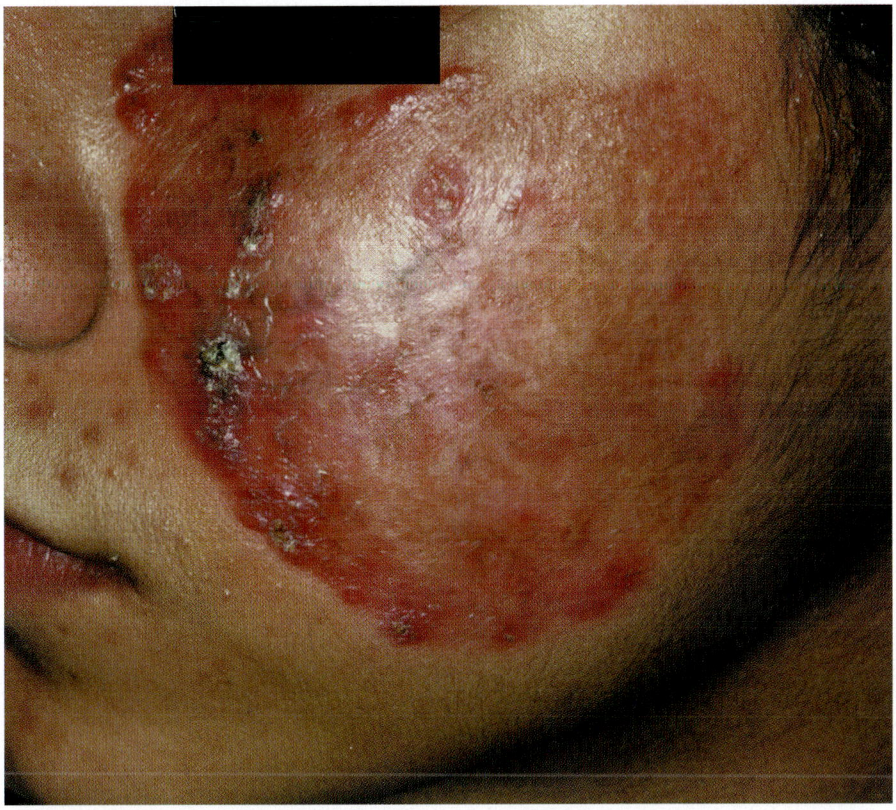

▲ **FIGURE 63-5** Leishmaniasis on the cheek of a 12-year-old girl showing an extensive area with resolving papules and active edematous papules at the periphery.

heals on its own, permanent immunity to reinfection ensues. This is accompanied by a strong delayed cutaneous hypersensitivity to leishmanial antigens.

2. *Mucocutaneous leishmaniasis* is caused by *L. braziliensis* complex in the new world, and *L. aethopica* may give rise to oronasal, mucosal leishmaniasis. Mucocutaneous leishmaniasis affects the mouth, nose, and throat, causing severe destruction and permanent disfiguration. The disease never heals spontaneously.[2]

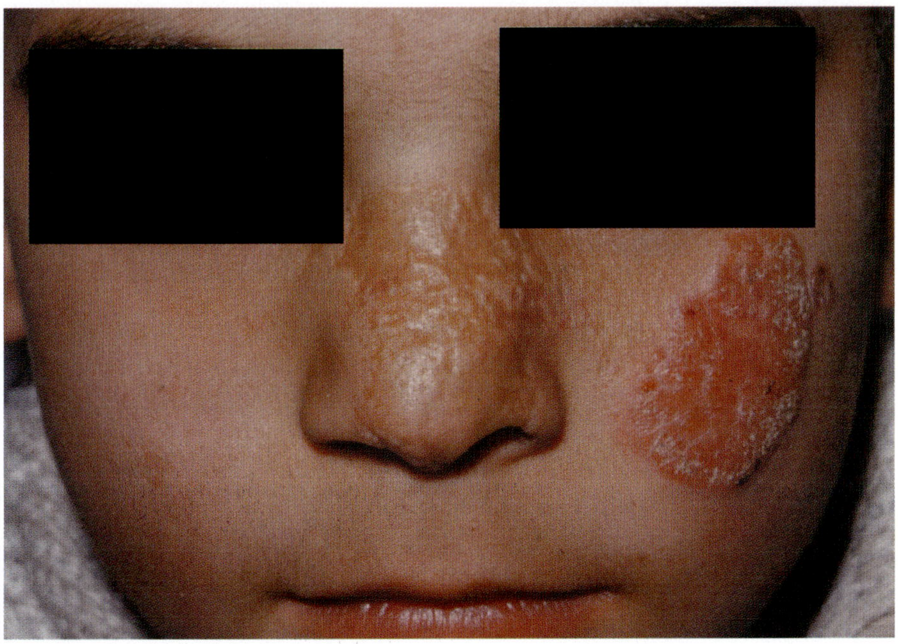

▲ **FIGURE 63-6** Lupoid leishmaniasis in an 8-year-old boy on the edge of a previous leishmaniasis scar with healed lesions over the nose and active plaques occurring laterally.

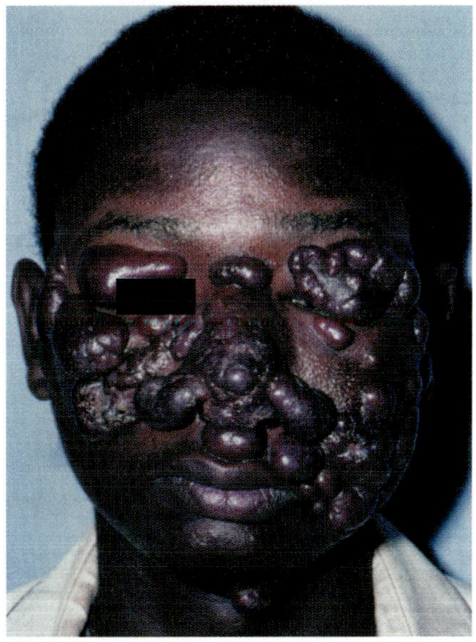

▲ **FIGURE 63-7** Mucocutaneous leishmaniasis in a 25-year-old man with multiple nodules clustered on his face, destroying the nasal cartilage.

Acquisition of resistance to mucocutaneous leishmaniasis has not been explained with certainty. Both cellular and humeral responses have been shown to be strong in the majority of mucocutaneous leishmaniasis patients (Figure 63-7).

3. *Diffuse cutaneous leishmaniansis.* It is not known whether diffuse cutaneous leishmaniasis starts as a single lesion owing to a single bite or as multiple lesions from multiple bites. Usually the patient's skin test is unresponsive to leshmanial antigens. In diffuse cutaneous leishmaniasis patients, the lesions are full of parasites inside macrophages, with very few lymphocytes but with a considerable number of plasma cells. There is no self-cure in diffuse leishmaniasis.[10]

4. *Visceral leishmaniasis* is caused by *L. donovani* complex (*L. donovani, L. chagasi, L. infantum*). Human infections with *L. donovani* can take one of two courses. While it is often severe, in some individuals, it remains a subclinical infection with no or a few, mild symptoms, detectable only by development of specific immune responses to leishmanial antigens.[11] A late event that may occur in course of kala-azar is *post-kala-azar dermal leishmaniasis* (PKDL). Parasites are quite numerous in the body but are apparently restricted to the skin. The disease responds poorly to chemotherapy. The infections often return following apparent cure. HIV-induced immunosuppression increases the risk of contracting visceral leishmaniasis.

TABLE 63-4
Differential Diagnosis of Leishmaniasis

Nodular Form
- Furuncle
- Carbuncle
- Basal cell carcinoma
- Keratoaconthoma
- Lupus erythematosus
- Sarcoidosis
- Pseudolymphoma

Ulcerous Form
- Ecthyma
- Tropical ulcer
- Yaws
- Malignant tumors
- Syphilitic chancre
- Inoculation tuberculosis

Recidivans Form
- Lupus vulgaris
- Tuberoserpiginous syphilid
- Sarcoidosis
- Tuberculoid leprosy
- Sporotrichosis
- Atypical mycobacterial infection (*M. marinum, M. ulcerous*)

Atypical clinical presentations of visceral leishmaniasis in patients coinfected with HIV poses a diagnostic challenge.[12]

DIAGNOSIS

The diagnosis of leishmaniasis depends on clinical, parasitologic, and serologic grounds (Table 63-4). The following are general diagnostic methods for leishmaniasis:

1. *Demonstration of parasites.* Parasites may be detected by direct-smear culture or animal inoculation.
2. *Skin test.* The type of test applied for the diagnosis of previous leishmaniasis infection is the leishmaniasis antigen test also known as Montenegro test.
3. *Serologic methods.* For serologic tests, antigens prepared from sonicated promastigotes (or alternatively amastigotes) of any species of *Leishmania* have provided satisfactory results. Enzyme linked immunosorbant assay (ELISA) and the direct agglutination test (DAT) have been evaluated.

TREATMENT

Among all antileishmanial drugs, pentavalent antimony is the drug of choice for all forms of leishmaniasis. Two pentavalent antimonials are available: meglumine antimonate and sodium stiboglucunate. Other drugs are amphotercin B (conventional or lipid formulations such as Abelcet or AmBisome), miltefosine, and paramomycin, as well as lowidine and oxiconazole (Table 63-5).

TABLE 63-5
Treatment of Leishmaniasis

- Pentostam (sodium stibogluconate)
- Crystalline glucocorticosteroid
- Physical treatment
  - Cryotherapy
    - Carbon dioxide/acetate
    - Liquid nitrogen
  - Electrocoagulation 39–42°C
- Antimalarial agents
  - Antimony
  - Ketoconazole

Treatment of Cutaneous Leshmaniasis

Treatment should be individualized on the basis of the causative organism, severity of the lesions, availability of drugs, tolerance of the patient for toxicity, and local resistance partterns:

1. Small lesions may be treated by freezing with liquid nitrogen or curettage.
2. Topical application of paramomycin 15% plus methlbenzethonium chloride 12% is beneficial for both old and new world cutaneous leshmaniasis.
3. When lesions are multiple or in a disfiguring site, it is better to treat with parenteral sodium stilbogluconate (Pentostam), 20 mg/kg intramuscularly daily for 20 days. Intralesional sodium stilbogluconate also may be used.
4. Intralesional antimony (0.2–0.8 mL per lesion up to 2 g) is safe in patients with cardiac, liver, or renal disease.
5. Two to four doses (2–4 mg/kg) of alternate-day pentamidine is effective in new world cutaneous leshmaniasis.
6. Ketoconazole, 600 mg daily for 4 weeks, has shown some potential against *L. mexicana*, whereas in India, itraconazole, 200 mg daily for 6 weeks, has been effective for cutaneous leshmaniasis.
7. For refractory cutaneous leshmaniasis or mucocutaneous leishmaniasis, conventional or liposomal amphotericin B has been effective.

Treatment for Visceral Leismaniasis

1. Sodium stilbogluconate (Pentostam), 20 mg/kg intramuscularly or intravenously daily for 20 days
2. Ampotericin B

Treatment for Post-Kala-Azar Dermal Leshimaniasis

1. Sodium stilbogluconate (Pentostam)
2. Pentamidine
3. Allopurinol

CONTROL AND TRANSMISSION

The control of leishmaniasis is determined by the ecology of the diseases.

Anthroponotic Leishmaniasis

Humans are the main reservoir, and the source of infection and vector are represented by synanthropic sandflies.

Zoonotic Leishmaniasis

Wild animals are the source of infection, and wild sandflies are the vector. Four groups of measures should be considered for effective control of leishmaniasis:

- Control of vectors
  - Chemical methods
  - Biologic methods
  - Genetic methods
  - Ecological methods
- Control of the parasites
- Control of reservoirs
- Zonal control
  - Total control
  - Protection of people from infection

VACCINATION

Lastly, vaccination is considered to be the simplest, most convenient, and reliable way to protect humans from infection, but there is not yet a safe and broad-spectrum vaccine. While some vaccines have been tried in different parts of the world, they have some negative side effects.

REFERENCES

1. Bernier R, Turco SJ, Olivier M, et al. Activation of human immunodeficiency virus type 1 in monocytoid cells by the protozoan parasite *Leishmania donovani*. *J Virol* 1995;69:7282-7285.

2. World Health Organization. Global health situation: IV. Selected infectious and parasitic diseases due to identified organisms. *Week Epidemiol Rec* 1993;6:41-48.
3. Killick-Kendrik R. Phleobotine vectors of the leishmaniasis: A review. *Med Vet Entomol* 1990;4:1.
4. World Health Organization Expert Committee. *Control of the Leishmaniases.* WHO Technical Report Series 793. Geneva, WHO, 1990, p 1.
5. Evans T, Teixira M, McAuliffe I, et al. Epidemiology of visceral leishmaniasis in northeast Brazil. *J Infect Dis* 1992;166:1124.
6. Belazzoug S. Leishmaniasis in Mediterranean countries. *Vet Pathol* 1992; 44:15.
7. Aggarwal P, Prakash-Wali J. Profile of kala-azar in North India. *Asia-Pacific J Public Health* 1991;5:90.
8. Molyneux DH, Ashford RW. *The Biology of Trypanosoma and Leishmania, Parasites of Man and Domestic Animals.* London, Taylor and Francis, 1983, p 294.
9. Bray RS, Bryceson ADM. The identity of strains of *Leishmania* from Ethiopian diffuse cutaneous leishmaniasis. *Trans R Soc Trop Med Hyg* 1969;63:523.
10. Turk JK, Bryceson ADM. Immunological phenomenon in leprosy and related diseases. *Adv Immunol* 1971;13:209.
11. Badarù R, Carvalho EM, Rocha H, et al. *Leishmania donovani:* An opportunistic microbe associated with progressive disease in three immunocompromised patients. *Lancet* 1986;1:647-648.
12. Fernández-Guerrero ML, Aguado JM, Buzùn L, et al. Visceral leishmaniasis in immune-compromised hosts. *Am J Med* 1987;83:1098-1102.

CHAPTER 64

Cutaneous Manifestations of HIV

Wilbert C. Jordan

Key Points

- A cutaneous presentation may be the first sign or symptom of human immunodeficiency virus (HIV) infection.
- Because AIDS is the end result of many years of HIV infection, the HIV-infected person may be truly asymptomatic or mildly symptomatic with vague infections not necessarily pointing to HIV.
- Cutaenous presentations of HIV disease may be more invasive and rapid as the CD4 count declines.
- The same isolation techniques apply for cutaneous presentations in HIV-positive persons as in HIV-negative persons.
- Some of the principal cutaneous manifestations of HIV disease in skin of color are Karposi sarcoma, psoriasis, scabies, secondary syphilis, tinea versicola, rash on early HIV viremia, HIV drug eruptions, HIV abscesses, herpes simplex, herpes zoster, candidiasis, and veneral warts.

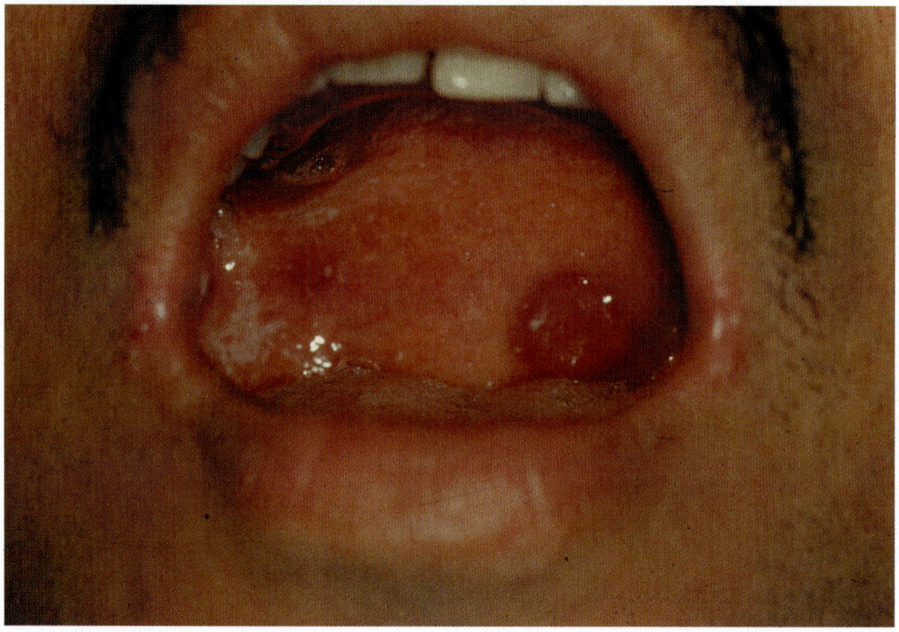

▲ **FIGURE 64-1** Karposi sarcoma.

BRIEF OVERVIEW OF HIV

The human immunodeficiency virus (HIV) has been identified as the causative agent for acquired immune deficiency syndrome (AIDS).[1,2] Since the first cases were reported in 1979, the number of cases has increased steadily in the United States and worldwide.[3] How HIV infects the host is now well documented.[4,5] This is a complex process; AIDS is the end result of many years of infection with HIV, and throughout the years of infection, the HIV-infected person may be truly asymptomatic or mildly symptomatic with vague infections not necessarily pointing to HIV. Sometimes the infection may suggest HIV, although the health care provider may not be aware of the relationship. Later in the infection, symptoms occur that are more suggestive of HIV infection.[6–8]

Over time, viral replication continues, and ongoing depletion of CD4 cells occurs. The production of CD4 cells occurs continuously, with an average life span of 4 days. As more and more cells and CD4 cells are infected, there is a depletion of CD4 cells. As this occurs, the body is more susceptible to T-cell-mediated infections.

KAPOSI SARCOMA

Kaposi sarcoma (KS) was one of the first diseases reported in association with what later became known as AIDS. It remains the malignancy most widely associated with HIV. KS commonly presents as a lesion(s) of the skin in various forms (Figure 64-1). The lesions are usually painless, easily visible and palpable, and highly vascular. KS can present internally, especially in the gastrointestinal tract and lungs. KS usually occurs as the CD4 count falls, but it can occur in HIV-positive persons with CD4 counts as high as 700. KS is a vascular lesion. In darker-skinned persons, the lesions appear purplish to red, whereas in lighter-skinned persons, the lesions appear to be some shade of red.

Diagnosis is made by biopsy. A biopsy can bleed excessively, so it is important to observe the patient after the procedure. It also is important to involve what appears to be normal tissue as well as affected tissue in the biopsy. That is, it is not wise to biopsy in the center of a lesion because it is so vascular that it may hemorrhage. It is safer to take tissue from an area bordering and including normal-appearing tissue. In darker-skinned persons, KS lesions often can appear similar to psoriatic lesions. Any patient found to have KS without a prior HIV test should be tested for HIV.

Treatments vary depending on the extent of the lesions. In patients with few lesions, topical treatment may suffice. Patients with more extensive lesions may require chemotherapy, radiation, interferon, and investigation studies or a combination of these.

In darker-skinned patients, lesions of psoriasis and chronic dermatitis can be mistaken for KS. Biopsy determines whether the lesion is KS, and treatment should not commence without biopsy confirmation.

Recent reports have indicated that protease inhibitors are potent antiangiogenic molecules that promote regression of KS. KS is associated with the KS-associated herpes virus (KSHV), a gamma herpesvirus that is widely prevalent in immunosuppressed populations. Immune reconstitution by highly active antiretroviral therapy (HAART) has been reported to cause KS regression.

PSORIASIS

In HIV-positive blacks, psoriasis can be mistaken for secondary syphilis.

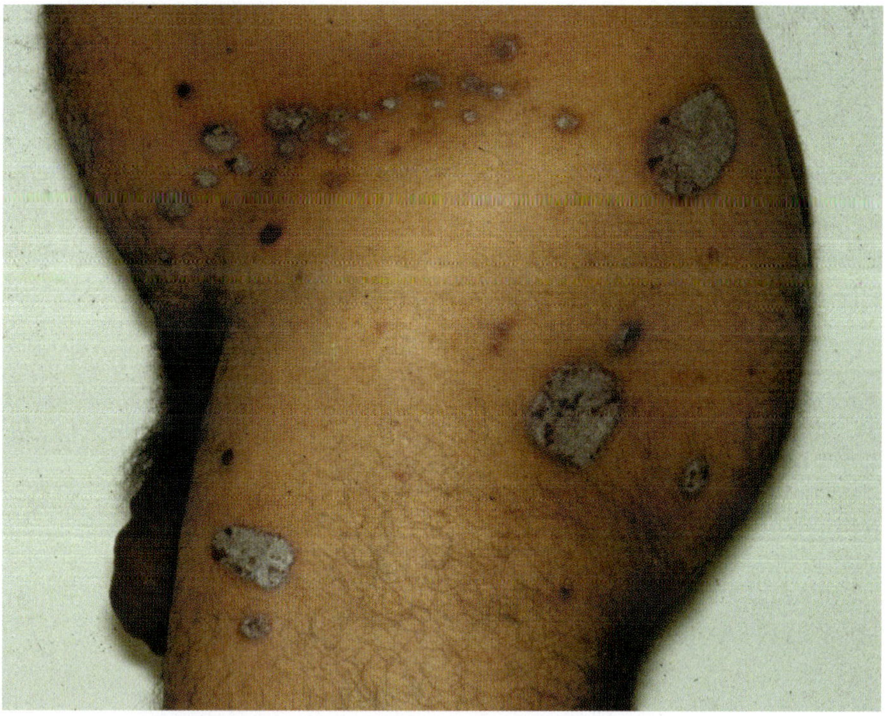

▲ **FIGURE 64-2** Psoriasis.

Psoriasis can present like a chronic fungal infection, often under the breasts in women and around the elbows in men (Figure 64-2). There may or may not be symptoms of arthritis, pruritus, or joint pain. A detailed sexual history may disclose early that the rash is psoriasis and not syphilis. Patients with a family history of psoriasis or eczema may present with skins lesions that look like psoriasis.

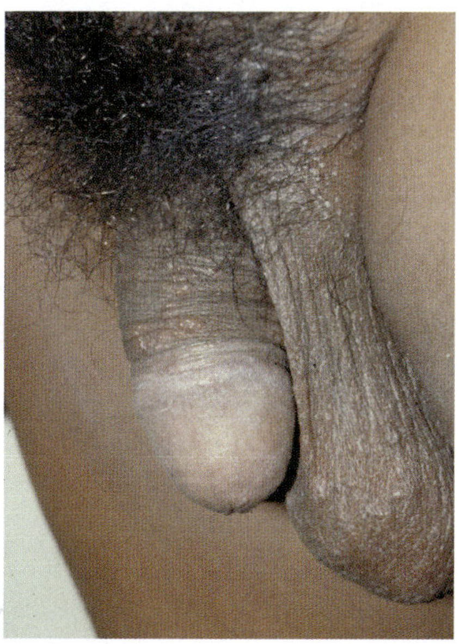

▲ **FIGURE 64-3** Scabies.

SCABIES

Scabies (Figure 64-3) is often overlooked. In HIV-positive patients, the area of involvement may be larger, and the spread faster, especially in persons with low CD4 counts. Men who have sex with men often present with a facial eruption that resembles lupus, except for the itching. A thorough history will reveal the appropriate facial contact. Treatment is the same as for uninfected patients, although often it is necessary to apply the medication for twice as long.

SECONDARY SYPHILIS

The varied rashes of secondary syphilis are the same in HIV-positive patients (Figure 64-4). Someone treated late for secondary syphilis who then gets reinfected may have a primary or secondary lesion. And someone treated late for primary syphilis who gets reinfected may bypass the presentation of primary syphilis and present with lesions of secondary syphilis. Taking a sexual history routinely with each visit of the sexually active patient is necessary to alert the physician to possible reexposure. In these situations, the titers of the Venereal Disease Research Laboratory (VDRL) test can be helpful and diagnostic. Treatment for primary and secondary syphilis in the HIV-positive patient is recommended as two injections of bacillim 2.4 million units given 1 week apart.

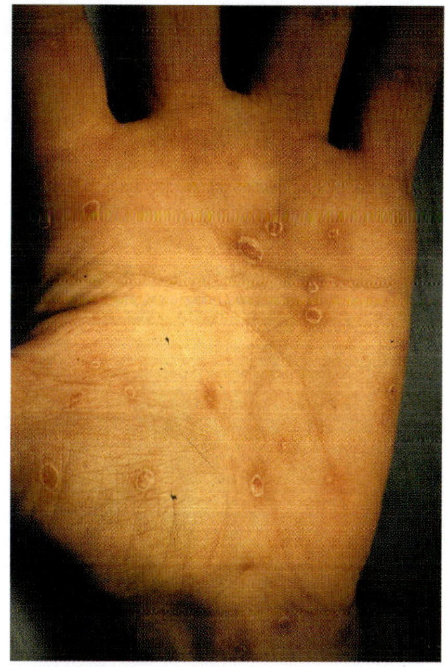

▲ **FIGURE 64-4** Secondary syphilis.

TINEA VERSICOLOR

As the CD4 count falls below 350, eruptions of tinea vericolor are more likely to occur (Figure 64-5). These may be in one area or several, and they spread rapidly over time compared with lesions in HIV-negative persons.

RASH OF EARLY HIV VIREMIA

This is a typical rash of viremia and not distinct for HIV. Diagnosis comes from a detailed history that associates recent intravenous drug use or at-risk sexual behavior. This rash is illustrated in Figure 64-6.

DRUG ERUPTIONS

There are several forms of drug eruptions (Figure 64-7). The most dangerous are the hemorrhagic eruptions. These are seen often in those who use nonconventional drugs. Hemorrhagic drug eruptions probably were seen more in the early 1980s, when it was common for patients to undergo a variety of nontested regimens. Platelet dysfunction may be associated with this. Patients may give a history of easy bruising.

ABSCESSES

Abscesses (Figure 64-8) have always been a part of the differential diagnosis of body masses; they are usually distinguished by

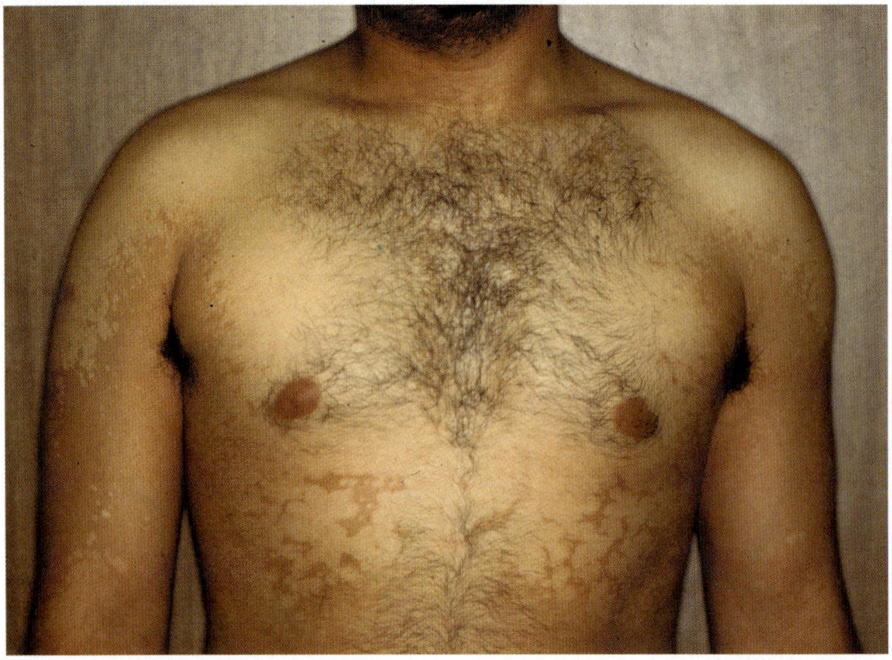

▲ **FIGURE 64-5** Tinea Versicola.

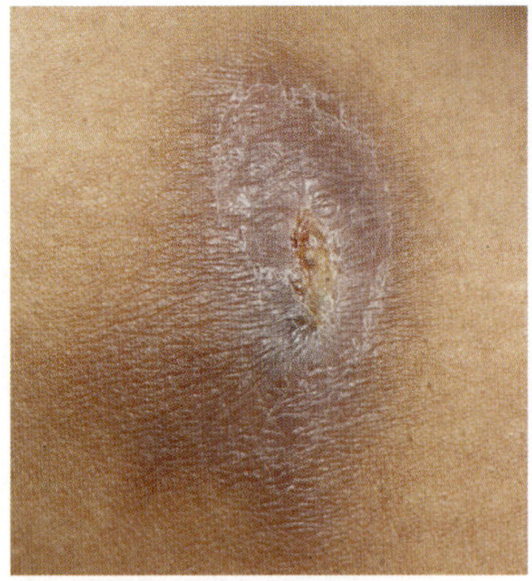

▲ **FIGURE 64-7** HIV drug eruptions.

increased warmth, tenderness, and redness. They are caused primarily by *Staphylococcus aureus* and often methicillin-resistant *S. aureus* (MRSA). In some communities, there are clusters of MRSA skin infections associated with jails, piercings, and instrumentation. These tend to be seen more often in people with CD4 counts above 200 because such people are less likely to be on prophylactic antiopportunistic infection therapies. Treatment is usually intravenous vancomycin, intravenous or oral bactrim, or oral rifampin.

HERPES SIMPLEX

Herpes simplex viruses (HSV-1 and HSV-2) cause a variety of infections involving the central nervous system, mucocutaneous surfaces, and occasionally, internal organs. HSV is a double-stranded DNA virus that can be isolated from nearly all visceral and mucocutaneous surfaces. Both types can cause genital and orofacial infections, and they are indistinguishable clinically (Figure 64-9). In HIV-positive patients, these infections tend to be chronic and more necrotizing and ulcerating. The pain is more widespread, and the open lesions are infectious.

HERPES ZOSTER

Concomitant with the fall in CD4 count, the occurrence of shingles (Figure 64-10) can increase. In the HIV-positive patient, shingles may be more severe and last longer, usually requiring intravenous therapy instead of oral antiherpes therapy. Prophylactic antiherpes treatment with acyclovir, 200 mg tid or 800 mg bid, or famciclovir, 500 mg bid, should be considered if there have been recurrences, especially when the outbreaks tend to travel up the spinal cord (i.e., the last outbreak involving a dermatome at a higher spinal level than the prior). A subsequent outbreak may involve the central nervous system and not be cutaneous.

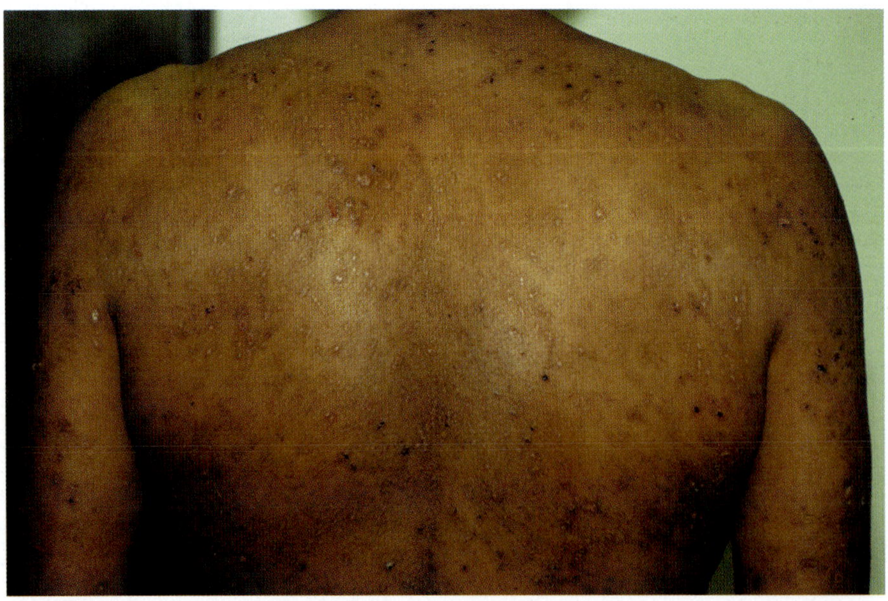

▲ **FIGURE 64-6** Rash on early HIV viremia.

CANDIDIASIS

One of the most common presentations of early HIV is oral candidiasis (Figure 64-11). Unexplained thrush should raise the suspicion for HIV infection, and the clinician should test the patient. Thrush also can be seen in someone on steroids or with signs of early diabetes. Therefore, clinical judgment is important. Treatments are available with oral antifungals such as Nilstat oral suspension used thrice daily or more or Mycelex troches 10 mg three to four times daily. In more demanding situations, treatment may require oral sysgtemic medication. Diflucan, 100 mg daily, is the drug of choice; itraconizole, 100 mg daily, is the second drug of choice. In patients with CD4 counts below 200, diflucan is given prophylactically and definitely when the CD4 count falls below 100.

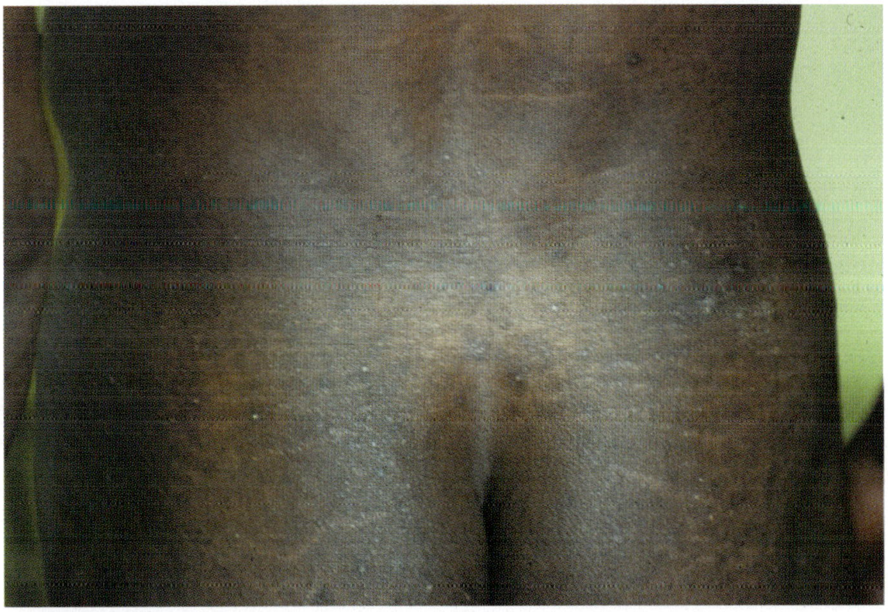

▲ **FIGURE 64-8** HIV abscesses.

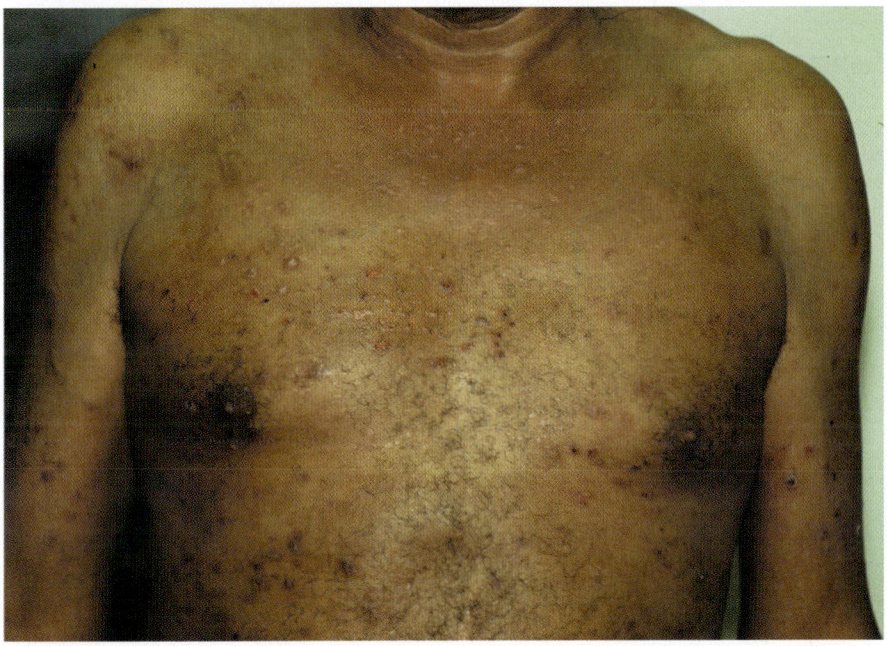

▲ **FIGURE 64-9** Herpes simplex.

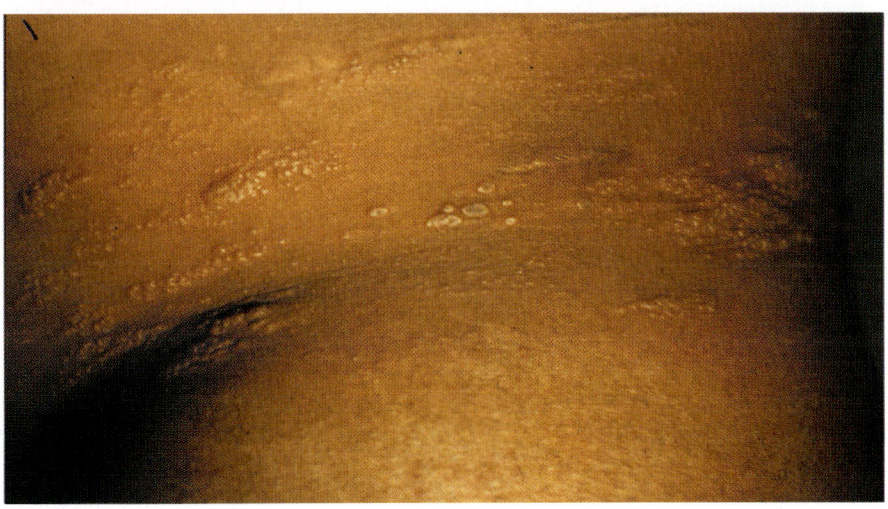

▲ **FIGURE 64-10** Herpes zoster.

VENEREAL WARTS

In many areas of the country, venereal warts, or condyloma accuminata, are the fastest rising venereal disease among young people. Caused by the papillomavirus, venereal warts produce an increase in tissue. Usually, they are painless, but they can be painful when obstruction and pressure caused by rubbing or friction, seed of the infected tissue into a second tissue. A simple touch does not cause infection. The most difficult infection, oral warts, has had a marked increase in reported cases Figure 64-12. Venereal warts can be seen in Figure 64-13.

CONCLUSION

It is important to note that the presentation of skin disease is the same in an HIV-positive person as in an HIV-negative person. What is different is not the color of the lesion but the rapidity and invasiveness. As the HIV-positive person's CD4 count declines, they may present more rapidly and appear more invasive.

Many persons of color do not consider themselves to be at risk for HIV infection and will not associate a cutaneous process as indicative of HIV infection. When in doubt, the health care provider should test for HIV.

In all the preceding cutaneous presentations of HIV, except primary and secondary syphilis, the HIV antibody titer is already present. The health care provider is encouraged to order an HIV antibody test to rule out HIV infection. In terms of primary and secondary syphilis, an HIV antibody titer is suggested because the person has obviously engaged in unprotected sex. However, to rule out HIV as also occurring, the patient should be retested in 3–6 months. A negative HIV test then will ensure that HIV is not a comorbidity.

Treatment for HIV is constantly changing. There are treatment guidelines from several sources. To determine if treatment is necessary, one of the following three sources can be reviewed:

- Department of Health and Human Services (DHHS) Adult and Adolescent Antiretroviral Treatment Guidelines: *AIDSinfo.nih.gov*
- National Medical Association Guidelines: *NMAnet.org*
- International AIDS Society Guidelines: *www.IAS-USA.org*

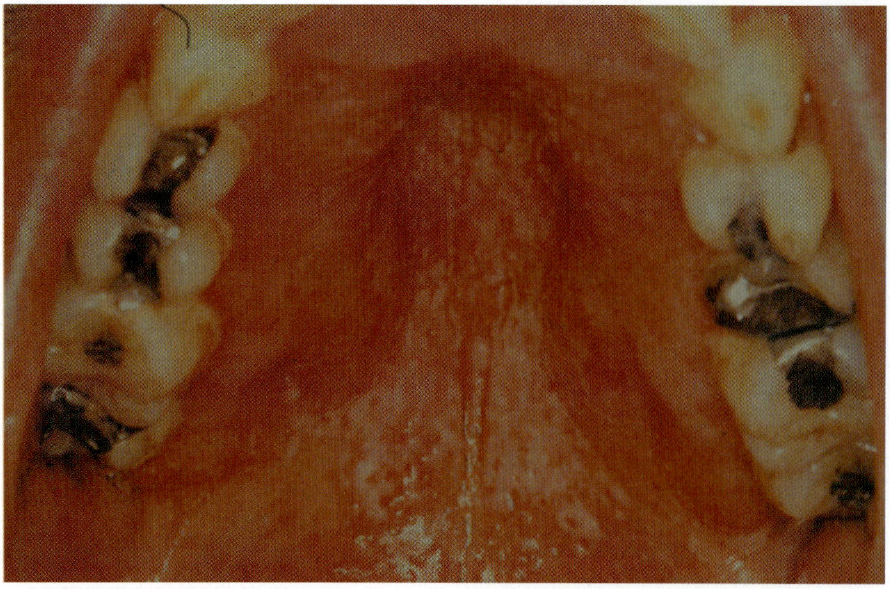

▲ **FIGURE 64-11** Candidiasis.

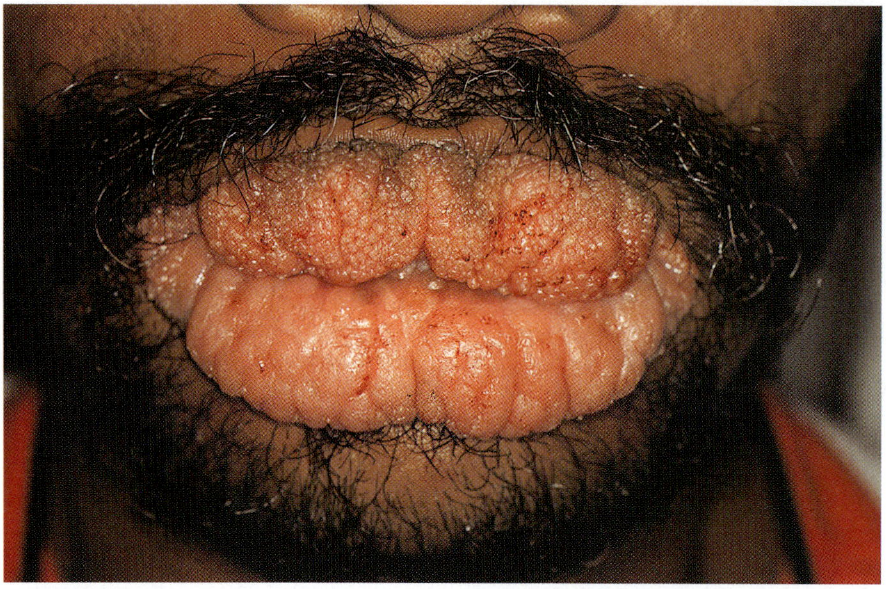

▲ **FIGURE 64-12** Condyloma acuminatum on the lips of an African-American man.

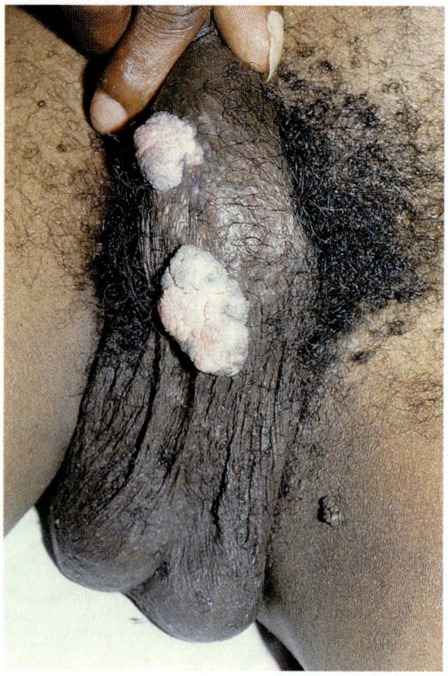

▲ **FIGURE 64-13** Venereal warts.

REFERENCES

1. Ansary MA, Hira SK, Bayle AC, et al. *Color Atlas of AIDS in the Tropics.* Ipswich, England, Wolfe Medical Publications Ltd, 1989, slides 19, 20, 27, 38, 40, 46, 56, 192, 266, 306, 309, 339.
2. Farthing C, Staughton R, Brown S, et al. *Color Atlas of AIDS and HIV Disease,* 2nd ed. London, England Ortho Pharmaceutical Corporation, 1988, slides 51, 53, 61, 67, 104, 109, 175, 176, 246.
3. Republic of Namibia, Ministry of Health and Social Services. *Guidelines for Clinical Management of HIV/AIDS.* Windhoek 2006.
4. Centers for Disease Control and Prevention. *Statistics from the Division of HIV/AIDS.* Atlanta, CDC, 2008.
5. Jordan WC. Slides from OASIS Clinic clients, 1984-2004.
6. US Department of Health and Human Services. *The Adult Guidelines for the Treatment of HIV/AIDS.* Washington, US Government Printing Office, 2008.
7. International AIDS Society, USA. *Adult Guidelines for the Treatment of HIV/AIDS.* New York, NY, 2007.
8. National Medical Association. *Guidelines for the Treatment of HIV/AIDS in Adults.,* Washington, DC 2008.

SECTION 10

Effects of Ultraviolet Radiation and Topical Agents

CHAPTER 65

Acute and Chronic Effects of Ultraviolet Radiation, Including Photocarcinogenesis

Dakara Rucker Wright
Lawrence S. W. Khoo
Henry W. Lim

TABLE 65-1
Electromagnetic Radiation

Radiation	Wavelength (nm)	Biologic Effects
UVC	200–290	Erythema; use as germicidal lamp
UVB	290–320	Erythema; delayed tanning
UVA_2	320–340	Erythema; immediate pigment darkening; persistent pigment darkening; delayed tanning
UVA_1	340–400	
Visible	400–760	General illumination; vision

Key Points

- Owing to the effect of melanin, individuals with skin of color are less prone to develop ultraviolet (UV)–associated skin cancers compared with fair-skinned individuals. However, they are more likely to have a low serum vitamin D level.
- Pigment darkening is divided into three types: immediate pigment darkening (IPD), persistent pigment darkening (PPD), and delayed pigment darkening (DPD), or tanning.
- Acute effects of UV light include erythema, pigment darkening, epidermal hyperplasia, vitamin D synthesis, and photoimmunosuppression.
- New melanin synthesis occurs only during delayed pigment darkening.
- UV radiation is divided into UVC (200–290 nm), UVB (290–320 nm), UVA_2 (320–340 nm), and UVA_1 (340–400 nm).
- Chronic effects of UV include photoaging and photocarcinogenesis, or skin cancer.
- There are three primary types of skin cancer associated with UV light: basal cell carcinoma, squamous cell carcinoma, and melanoma.
- Sunscreens provide some protection against UV light and can be divided into organic (chemical) and inorganic (physical/nonchemical) UV filters.

DEFINITION OF ULTRAVIOLET RADIATION

Ultraviolet (UV) radiation is a component of the electromagnetic radiation emitted by the sun. Unlike the earth, which is solid, the sun consists entirely of gas: 70% hydrogen, 28% helium, and 2% heavy elements.[1] The sun, which has been in existence for 4.6 billion years, emits an extremely wide range of electromagnetic radiation, from 0.1 to more than than 10^6 nm. The earth's atmosphere filters out most of the radiation, and only radiation with wavelengths from 290–4000 nm reaches the earth's surface. The radiation that reaches the earth's surface is subdivided by convention into UV radiation (290–400 mn), visible light (400–760 nm), and infrared radiation (IR; >760 nm).

The radiation that has the most photodermatologic and photobiologic significance is UV radiation. In the Second International Congress on Light held in Copenhagen in August 1932, it was recommended that UV radiation be divided into UVC (100–280 nm), UVB (280–315 nm), and UVA (315–400 nm).[2] However, in photodermatology, the following subdivisions are now commonly used: UVC: 200–290 nm; UVB: 290–320 nm; UVA_2: 320–340 nm; and UVA_1: 340–400 nm (Table 65-1). Visible light is the only spectrum of radiation that results in a sensation of vision and is used for general illumination purposes. Infrared radiation (IR) is imperceptible to the human eyes. It is used in various remote-control devices (e.g., televisions, computers, etc.) and is responsible for the heat coming from sunlight.

It should be noted that because of the presence of atmosphere, UVC from sunlight does not reach the earth's surface, and therefore, it has no biologic significance. Exposure to UVC occurs only through exposure to artificial light sources, for example, germicidal lamps used in research and clinical laboratories. Ninety-five percent of the UV radiation reaching the earth's surface is UVA, and 5% is UVB.[3] UVB can be blocked by glass, but UVA can penetrate through glass.[4] Since UVB has the shorter wavelengths, it is mostly absorbed in the epidermis, with a small proportion reaching the upper dermis, whereas UVA penetrates deeper into the dermis. Subdivision of UVA into UVA_1 and UVA_2 is done because UVA_2, being of a shorter wavelength range, has biologic effects closer to those of UVB. Because of its longer wavelength and hence deeper penetration, UVA has an intensity that does not vary as much as UVB with the seasons or the time of day.[3]

The main cellular chromophores for UV are DNA, RNA, and reactive oxygen species (ROS) generating chromophores.[3] The normal effects of UV radiation can be broken into its *acute effects,* namely, erythema, sunburn, pigment darkening, tanning, epidermal hyperplasia, vitamin D synthesis, and immunosuppression, and its *chronic effects,* namely, photoaging and carcinogenesis (Table 65-2). Photodermatoses, including photosensitivity and photoaggravated disorders, are "abnormal" responses to UV radiation owing to various immune abnormalities, biochemical disorders, or DNA repair deficiencies; they will not be discussed in this chapter.

ACUTE EFFECTS OF UV RADIATION

Erythema

UVB is the predominant spectrum in UV radiation responsible for cutaneous erythema owing to underlying vasodilation caused by vasoactive mediators such as

TABLE 65-2
Cutaneous Effects of UV Radiation

Acute Effects
Erythema
Pigment darkening (immediate and persistent)
Delayed tanning
Epidermal hyperplasia
Vitamin D synthesis
Immunosuppression
Chronic Effects
Photoaging
Photocarcinogensis

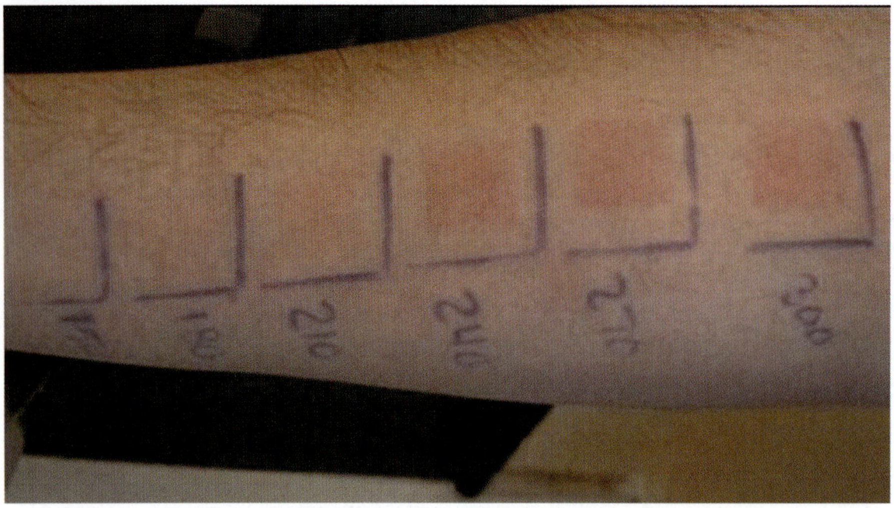

▲ **FIGURE 65-1** Minimal erythema dose (MED) testing on arm of an East Asian man (skin phototype IV) using targeted UVB source. Courtesy of Ilefat Hamzavi, M.D.

prostaglandin (PG) E_2 at higher UVB doses and nitric oxide (NO) at lower doses around the minimal erythema dose (MED).[5] MED is the lowest UV dose that causes skin redness after 24 hours (Figure 65-1); it is induced by UVB and, less efficiently, by UVA. It is used as an indicator of UV sensitivity but does not necessarily correlate with skin color or ethnicity, although it may predict levels of DNA damage.[6] Generally speaking, the lowest MED doses are found among fair-skinned Caucasians and the highest among dark-skinned blacks, although there are considerable interracial/ethnic overlaps. For example, for individuals with skin phototype I, MED to UVB (MED-B) is in the range of 20–40 mJ/cm^2, whereas for those with skin phototype VI, the MED-B could be greater than 108 mJ/cm^2. UVB-induced erythema is visible 3–6 hours after exposure and peaks around 24 hours. Erythema fades over a day or longer (especially in fair skin) and is followed by desquamation and tanning. Sunburn is an acute inflammatory response of the skin above a threshold dose of UVB, the MED-B. The mediators of the sunburn response include ROS; transcription factors, that is, NFκB and AP-1; vasoactive mediators, that is, PGE_2 and nitric oxide (NO); proinflammatory cytokines, that is, tumor necrosis factor α (TNF-α), interleukin 1 (IL-1), IL-6, IL-8, and IL-12; and adhesion molecules, that is, ICAM-1 and E-selectin.[3]

Signs and symptoms of UVB exposure include erythema, burning, pain, heat, edema, and if severe, blistering. Systemic symptoms may occur in cases of severe generalized sunburn in some people. The risk of sunburn owing to sun exposure is greater during peak hours (typically between 10 a.m. and 4 p.m. in summer months), in areas closer to the equator, and in persons with Fitzpatrick skin phototypes I and II. Although the risk of sunburn is less in individuals of skin of color (typically phototypes IV–VI), they do indeed burn. Of note, there is not a strong correlation between a person's self-reported Fitzpatrick skin type, the actual sensitivity to UV radiation, and skin color.[7,8] Moreover, erythema can be difficult to evaluate by the naked eye in darker-pigmented persons. Histologically, "sunburn cells," which are damaged keratinocytes undergoing apoptosis with shrunken chromatin and eosinophillic cytoplasm, may be seen within 30 minutes following UVB exposure. Sunburn cell formation is a protective mechanism to eliminate DNA-damaged cells, and it can occur in the absence of inflammation. Dermal endothelial swelling is also evident within 30 minutes of UVB exposure. Other changes seen histologically include epidermal spongiosis, morphologic changes and decreased numbers of Langerhans cells, and a perivascular infiltrate of neutrophils early on and mononuclear cells later.[9,10]

UVA also can cause skin erythema, but at 1000-fold higher doses than UVB. UVA erythema is more immediate, peaks at 1–6 hours after exposure, and resolves gradually in 48–72 hours.[11]

Pigment Darkening

UV radiation–induced skin pigmentation occurs in three distinct phases: (1) immediate pigment darkening, (2) persistent pigment darkening, and (3) delayed tanning. Minimal pigmentation dose (MPD) is the lowest UV dose that causes increased skin pigmentation; depending on the skin phototype and the spectrum of the radiation source, pigment darkening may require doses higher, lower, or the same as those causing erythema. Generally, individuals with lower MEDs need higher doses of UV MEDs to produce new pigmentation than do subjects with higher MEDs; in other words, fair-skinned individuals do not tan as readily as those with dark skin.

Immediate pigment darkening (IPD) is primarily due to low-dose UVA (1–5 J/cm^2). It occurs right after exposure and usually fades within 10–20 minutes; at UVA doses of more than 10 J/cm^2, IPD may persist longer and will fade in 2 hours. IPD results from oxidation and redistribution of preexisting melanin, not new melanin synthesis. Clinically, it manifests as a grayish blue color; it is more apparent in individuals with skin of color. The biologic significance of IPD is not completely understood.

Persistent pigment darkening (PPD) follows IPD and persists from 2–24 hours.[11] It is induced by higher UVA doses (>10 J/cm^2 in fair skin and >60 J/cm^2 in darker skin).[3] PPD, like IPD, is due to oxidation and redistribution of preexisting melanin from the lower to middle layer of the skin; this process is more dramatic in darker skin.[12] No new melanin is synthesized. Clinically, it appears as a brownish color.

Delayed pigment darkening, also known as *tanning*, is a delayed effect of UV radiation, becomes visible after about 3 days, and is associated with the synthesis of new melanin. The term *tanned* does not seem to apply to skin of color, which is inherently tan or of varying shades of brown. It should be emphasized that pigment darkening (IPD, PPD, and delayed tanning) does occur in all skin types, including skin of color.

Tanning became popular in the West during the 1920s. Famous fashion designer Coco Chanel is thought to have glamorized the bronzed look after she traveled the French Riviera and was suntanned. Before then, fair skin was considered a sign of wealth and beauty, corresponding to a higher socioeconomic status that did not have to work in the sun doing manual labor. After World War II, this trend reversed, and suntanned skin signified wealth because of the ability to travel to warmer climates and enjoy leisurely outdoor activities. Moreover, tanned skin became associated with health and strength as bodybuilders and the fitness industry use tanned skin to highlight muscle definition and tone. Ironically, in postcolonial Africa and in many parts of Asia, dark skin is sometimes perceived to be associated with lower social class, and for some, lighter skin may be more socially desirable.[13]

Both UVB and UVA can induce tanning, but in the case of UVB, erythema always precedes tanning, especially in fair skin, whereas UVA can induce tanning without noticeable erythema. Interestingly, in a recent study of human subjects (skin types II–VI) exposed to UVA, inhibition of UVA-induced accelerated blood flow with epinephrine resulted in partial or complete inhibition of IPD and delayed tanning, leading the authors to conclude that vascular change is an important process in IPD and delayed tanning.[14] Tanning is an inherent protective mechanism of the skin against DNA damage. Fitzpatrick skin types III and higher have a greater ability to tan, whereas skin types I and II have a poor ability to tan and thus have minimal protection against UV radiation–induced DNA damage.[15] Delayed tanning fades rapidly if it is the result of UVB exposure. However, if tanning is induced by UVA, it can last for months. In darker-skinned individuals, the UVA-induced delayed tanning tends to last even longer.[11] Recent studies using pure visible light spectrum (400-700 nm) is capable of inducing immediate, persistent and delayed pigment darkening as well (personal communication, Oct 15, 2008 Mahmoud, B).

In a study of erythema and melanogenic responses in a group of European Americans, Hispanics, and East Asians, it was found that there was a significant difference in the melanogenic responses of the Hispanics and East Asians, although there was no significant difference between the constituitive pigmentation (background skin color) as determined by an optical instrument. The melanogenic response was two times higher in East Asians than in Hispanics.[16,17] The histology of solar-induced pigment darkening is the same in all ethnic groups in that there is an increase in the number of melanocytes and melanocytic activity characterized by an increase in tyrosinase activity, elongation of dendrites, and increased transfer of melanosomes to keratinocytes.[18]

Keratinocytes release substances such as α-melanocyte-stimulating hormone (α-MSH), which stimulates melanocytic production of melanin through activation of the melanocortin 1 receptor (MC1R) on melanocytes. Adrenocorticotropic hormone (ACTH) is another even more potent agonist of the MC1R.[19] MC1R regulates the types of melanin formed—eumelanin, the black to brown melanin pigment, and pheomelanin, the reddish brown variant. Eumelanin acts more as a free-radical scavenger, offering protection against UV cell damage, whereas pheomelanin increases oxidative stress.[3] The morphology of the melanin granules and transitional elemental binding properties may add to melanin's photoprotective function.[20] Melanocytic dendritic processes distribute melanin contained within the melanosomes; melanin serves to absorb and scatter UV radiation, thus protecting other epidermal cells from UV-induced DNA damage. Melanin forms supranuclear caps over the nuclei of basal keratinocytes, even in unirradiated skin.[21] Days after sun exposure, as epidermal cells migrate upward, melanin eventually reaches the stratum corneum; as skin sheds, the tan or pigmentation fades. UVA-induced melanization tends to occur in the deeper part of the epidermis compared with that induced by UVB. This is the reason that UVA-induced DPD lasts longer than that induced by UVB.

Some melanocytes are not responsive to α-MSH; in skin phototypes I and II, these are associated with MC1R variants. Therefore, little eumelanin is produced; clinically, these persons show weak or no tanning response. In black skin with more melanin production, the sun protection factor (SPF) is 13.4 compared with 3.4 in whiter skin following exposure to UVB.[22] Approximately 7% of UVB and 18% of UVA is transmitted to the dermis of black skin. On the contrary, 30% of UVB and more than 55% of UVA can penetrate the dermis of white skin. The UV radiation that is filtered in black skin occurs mainly in the malpighian layer, whereas in white skin the major area of filtration is in the stratum corneum.[22] In a study on Asian, white, and black skin, it was observed that the density of melanocytes was similar in all three groups, and blacks have the highest melanin content. One week after exposure to 1 MED of UVB/UVA, total melanin content is only slightly increased by 5–10% in all three groups. However, the change in the distribution of melanin from the lower to the middle layer of the skin was most dramatic in darker skin, which accounted for the increase in skin pigmentation several days after exposure.[18]

Mediators of melanogenesis include DNA excision repair fragments, which initiate DNA excision repair enzymes, α-MSH, NO, and histamine.[23,24] T_4 endocnuclease V, a DNA repair enzyme that catalyzes the initial and rate-limiting steps in excision of cyclopyrimidine dimers (CPDs), has been shown to result in greater melanogenesis in vitro.[24] Increased expression of nitric oxide synthase (NOS) has been noted in skin after exposure to UV radiation, and topical application of the NOS inhibitor *N*-nitro-L-arginine methylester hydrochloride (L-NAME) was shown to reduce the melanin content of melanocytes in animal studies.[3]

Epidermal Hyperplasia

In addition to erythema and pigmentation, UVB exposure causes epidermal hyperproliferation, especially of the stratum corneum, which appears clinically as a several-fold increase in thickness. Dermal thickening also may occur. This is evident histologically within days and persists for weeks. The epidermal hyperplasia, along with melanogenesis, is responsible for further protection against UV radiation damage, but the exact contribution of either process is unclear. Repeated UVA exposures may cause some epidermal thickening, but not to the degree of UVB radiation; hence a UVA-induced tan, such as from sunbed use, only provides a protection factor of 1.3 against sunburn from subsequent UV exposure, whereas a UVB-induced tan gives a protection factor of 3.[23,25]

Vitamin D Synthesis

Synthesis of vitamin D_3 is a major beneficial acute effect of UV radiation, specifically UVB (300 ± 5 nm). Vitamin D_3 is synthesized in the epidermis from pre-vitamin D_3 (cholecalciferol), which is rapidly converted by UVB from 7-dehydrocholesterol. An equilibrium exists between pre-vitamin D_3 and vitamin D_3 in which further UVB exposure does not result in increased production.[25,26] Other sources of vitamin D_3, although in low quantity at around 10%, are foods such as salmon, sardines, liver, and egg yolk. Vitamin D_2 is present in plants and fortified milk, butter, and cereals. Most vitamin supplements contain vitamin D_2, but vitamin D_3 supplement is also widely available.

Vitamin D formed from the skin or from dietary intake is biologically inactive and must undergo two hydroxylation steps in the liver to 25-hydroxyvitamin D [25(OH)-D, which is measured in serum] and then to 1,25-dihydroxyvitamin D [1,25$(OH)_2$-D] in the kidney under tight metabolic control. The biologically active form of vitamin D [1,25(OH)$_2$-D] promotes intestinal absorption of calcium and bone mineralization.[3] People with darker skin, the elderly, and those who are not exposed to any natural sunlight are at risk for vitamin D insufficiency. Severely low serum levels (<20 nmol/L) can manifest as rickets or osteomalacia. Levels between 20 and 80 nmol/L may manifest as secondary hyperparathyroidism, which results in bone loss and osteoporotic fractures. Optimal circulating vitamin D levels are suggested to be around 80 nmol/L, or 32 μg/L,[27] which is adequate for bone health and perhaps has other potential health benefits. While an adequate vitamin D level can be achieved by incidental sun exposure in many individuals, for those at risk for vitamin D insufficiency (e.g., those with darker skin, the elderly, institutionalized persons, and those whose cultural or religious practice require them to cover exposed skin with a dark fabric), 800–1000 IU (20–25 μg) of daily vitamin D_3 or 50,000 IU of monthly vitamin D_3 is recommended.[3,28]

Photoimmunosuppression

UV radiation suppresses the skin's immune system in a localized (direct) and systemic manner (at a distant unirradiated site).[29] Clinical examples of UV immunosuppression are the reactivation of herpes simplex infections after solar exposure[30] and the increased risk of certain skin cancers in chronically immunosuppressed solid-organ transplant patients. Previously, it was thought that mainly UVB induces immunosuppression, but UVA radiation also may play a role by inducing oxidative damage.[3,25] The mechanism of UV radiation–induced immunosuppresion is complex and not completely understood. It depends on wavelength, dose (suberythemal or erythemal, single or multiple), type of antigen, and type of immune response involved.[29,31] The role of pigmentation and susceptibility to UV immunosuppression is not clear because the data are conflicting. The following is a brief discussion of the some of the mechanisms.

The chromophore in the epidermis responsible for initiating the skin's immune modulation and downstream signaling in response to UV radiation is unknown but is presumed to be DNA and urocanic acid (UCA). In addition, membrane damage and activation of transcription factors probably also play critical roles.[31] UCA, produced from histidine by the enzyme histidase, is found in the stratum corneum and is converted from *trans*-UCA to *cis*-UCA by UV radiation.[31] DNA also absorbs UV radiation and forms various dimers such as cyclobutane-pyrimidine (CPD), which has been associated with UV radiation–induced immunosuppression. In studies that delivered liposomal DNA excision repair enzyme T_4 endonuclease V, UV radiation–induced suppression of contact hypersensitivity (CHS) and delayed hypersensitivity (DHT) were reversed.[32]

UV radiation increases a variety of pro- and anti-inflammatory mediators such as TNF-α; IL-1α and IL-1β; IL-6, IL-8, IL-10, and IL-12; PGE_2, and histamine production from a variety of cells in the skin, such as keratinocytes, Langerhans cells (the major antigen-presenting cells of the epidermis), mast cells, antigen-presenting dermal macrophages, dendritic cells, dermal fibroblasts, and/or melanocytes. In addition, a range of neuropeptides and neurohormones is involved in skin immunity, such as calcitonin gene–related peptide (CGRP), which is released from cutaneous sensory C fibers near epidermal Langerhan cells. CGRP alters antigen presentation cell function and adhesion molecule expression and has vasodilatory properties, thus contributing to UV-induced erythema and edema.[33] TNF-α is a major cytokine involved in immunosuppression of the skin. TNF-α, IL-1β, and the eicosanoid PGE_2 may be involved in stimulating the migration of Langerhan cells out of the epidermis, resulting in diminished antigen presentation function and reduced immunosurveillance. UV radiation also can stimulate T-suppression cells or T-regulatory cells and inhibit the activity of natural killer cells involved in innate immunity and tumor suppression.[3]

UV radiation also alters the Th1/Th2 cytokine profile in favor of Th2 cytokines IL-10 and IL-4 and reduces secretion of IL-12 and interferon-γ (IFN-γ) which mediates the CHS and DTH responses.[33] IL-10 induction after UV radiation was shown to be due to UV-induced skin infiltrating CD11+ macrophages that are potent sources of IL-10. IL-12 can reverse IL-10 UV radiation–induced immunosuppression and establish tolerance (unresponsiveness to a sensitizing hapten).[34]

UV radiation exposure of human skin causes a downregulation of DTH reseponse to intradermally and subcutaneously injected antigens and CHS response to applied haptens via overall reduction of T-cell function. This concept has implications for suppressing allergic contact dermatitis with phototherapy.

CHRONIC EFFECTS OF UV RADIATION

Photoaging and epidermal carcinogenesis are the primary long-term effects of chronic UV radiation to skin.

Photoaging

Photoaging is distinct from intrinsic aging because intrinsic skin aging is owing to the passage of time, whereas photoaging results from damage to the skin from UV radiation superimposed on intrinsically aged skin. Intrinsically aged skin appears finely wrinkled, lax, dry, and pale with benign neoplasms. Photoaged skin is coarser, rougher, deeply wrinkled, leathery, inelastic, and telangiectatic, with persistent constitutive hyperpigmentation, irregular hyperpigmentation, reticular hyperpigmentation (poikiloderma of Civatte), gutate hypomelanosis, freckling, and/or solar lentigines. Open comedones (Favre-Racouchot), sebaceous hyperplasia, erosive pustulosis also may be present in photodamaged skin. The development of irregular hyperpigmented macules ("sunburn freckles") can be seen just several months after a sunburn. Repeated suberythemogenic UVB doses can change the morphology of acquired melanocytic nevi by increasing their size, darkening their color, and changing their dermoscopic pattern to potentially simulating melanoma in situ.[24] The skin loses resilience and elasticity and has increased fragility and decreased capacity for wound healing. Darker-skinned individuals are less severely affected by photoaging, but the same changes do occur. However, in Asians, a greater number and larger size of pigmented seborrheic keratoses (Figure 65-2) were found in chronically sun-exposed skin than in occasionally sun-exposed or protected skin.[35] Thus aging and sunlight exposure are independent contributory factors to the development of seborrheic keratosis in Asians.[35] Fair-skinned Hispanics display clinical photoaging signs similar to those of darker-skinned Caucasians, and darker-skinned Hispanics show photoaging signs similar to those of Asians, with fine wrinkling and mottled pigmentation occurring in the late fourth through sixth decades.[36] Histologically, there can be acanthosis or atrophy, loss of polarity, cellular atypia in the epidermis, and increased melanin in keratinocytes, especially in skin of color. In the dermis, reduced anchoring fibrils, loss of mature collagen, basophilic collagen degeneration, elastosis, increased ground sub-

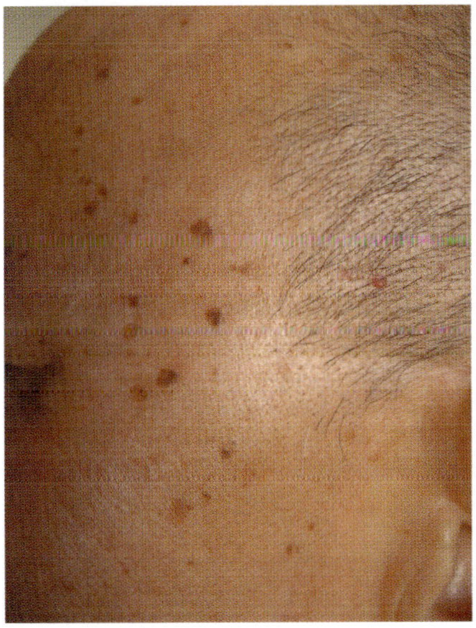

▲ **FIGURE 65-2** Photoaging in an Asian man. Note numerous pigmented seborrheic keratoses on the temple and cheek.

stance, and in skin of color, increased numbers of large, densely melanin-packed melanophages are seen.[36] There is also increased numbers of mast cells, histiocytes, fibroblasts, and mononuclear cells, although in the epidermis there is decreased numbers of Langerhan cells.[37] There is less elastotic tissue, reducing the dermal volume, and greater presence of fiber fragments, hypertrophied multinucleated fibroblasts, and macrophages in older black skin, which may represent active biosynthesis, degradation, and turnover, accounting for the clinical appearance of less wrinkling in black skin.[36]

The action spectrum for photoaging has not been completely elucidated. UVA is thought to play more of a role in photoaging than UVB because of its greater average depth of penetration into the dermis, more abundance in terrestrial sunlight, and persistent irradiance day long and year round. Studies also have shown that human skin exposed daily for only 1 month to suberythemogenic doses of UVA alone demonstrates stratum corneum thickening, Langerhans cell depletion, and dermal inflammatory infiltrates with deposition of lysozyme on the elastic fibers, suggesting that frequent casual exposure to sunlight containing primarily UVA eventually may result in dermal collagen and elastin damage, contributing to photoaging. UVA increased the cross-linking of collagen fibers, rendering dermal collagen more resistant to degradation, whereas UVB renders collagen more susceptible to enzymatic degradation. Studies using reconstructed skin in vitro containing live fibroblasts in a dermal matrix and differentiated epidermis showed that UVA induced fibroblast apoptosis in the upper dermis and secretion of matrix metalloproteinases (MMPs), whereas UVB affected epidermal cells, giving rise to CPDs and sunburn cells (apoptotic keratinocytes).[38] Interestingly, IR (760 nm–1 mm) contributes independently to the physiologic changes of photoaging, as well as in conjunction with the changes induced by UV radiation.[39]

The hallmark of aged nondividing cells is lipofuscin, a yellow-brown granular pigment that is the result of an accumulation of oxidized, cross-linked proteins that were not degraded by the proteasome; the latter is known to have diminished activity in aging human keratinocytes and fibroblasts.[24]

On a molecular level, UV irradiation directly activates cell surface receptors partly through ROS, which, in turn, initiate intracellular signaling. This results in activation of the nuclear transcription complex AP-1, which is composed of proteins c-Jun and c-Fos. Increased AP-1 blocks the effect of the cytokine transforming growth factor β (TGF-β) and its receptors, thus inhibiting collagen transcription. Other effects of increased AP-1 activity include increasing the levels of several MMPs that degrade collagen. MMP-8 (collagenase) from UV-induced neutrophillic infiltration further exacerbates matrix degradation. Tissue inhibitors of metalloproteinases (TIMPs), although are also upregulated, are not sufficient to completely block cumulative dermal collagen damage. Collagen degradation products not only reduce the integrity of the skin but also prevent new collagen synthesis.[38]

Not only does UV radiation–induced generation of ROS damage the dermal matrix, but ROS also damage mitochondrial DNA (mtDNA). Photoaged skin has more mtDNA mutations than sun-protected skin, which leads to poor mitochondrial function and further accumulation of ROS through a dysfunctional respiratory chain system.[38]

Telomeres also may play a role in photoaging of the skin. Telomeres protect the chromosome from degradation or fusion; they also serve as a biologic clock. Older epidermal cells and dermal fibroblasts have shorter terminal sequences or telomeres because DNA polymerase cannot replicate the final base pairs of each chromosome. Therefore, these older cells are less protected from the damage caused by repeated UV radiation exposure or prolonged exposure to ROS, resulting in accelerated cellular senescence.[38]

Photocarcinogenesis

UV exposure has been associated with the development of actinic keratoses, squamous cell carcinomas, basal cell carcinomas, and possibly melanomas (Figures 65-3–65-8). Both UVB and UVA are capable are inducing DNA damage, although through different mechanisms.

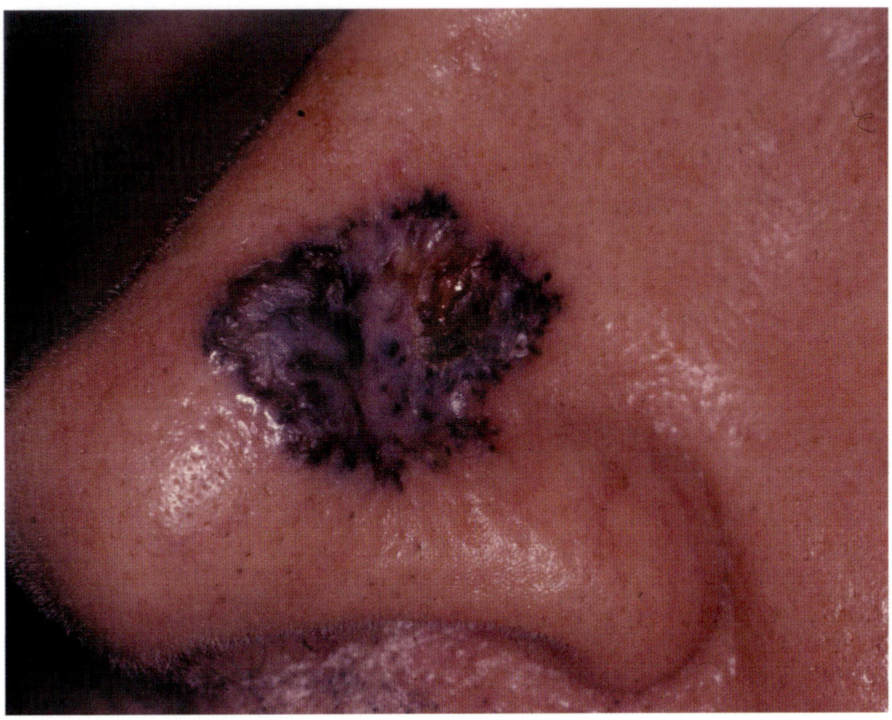

▲ **FIGURE 65-3** A Hispanic man with pigmented basal cell carcinoma on the left side of his nose.

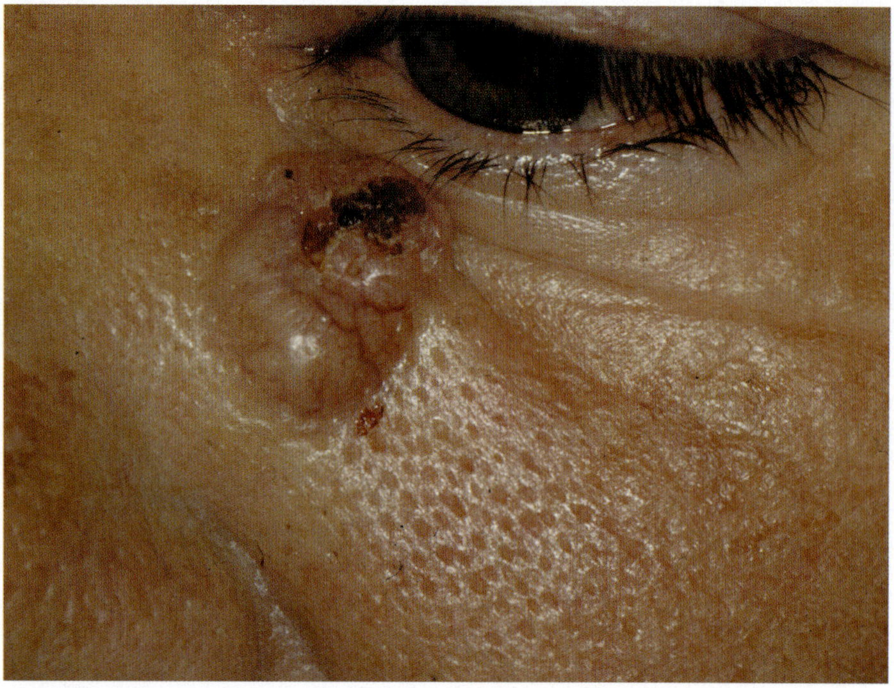

▲ **FIGURE 65-4** An Asian man with classical basal cell carcinoma below left medial eye.

UVB is most efficient in inducing DNA damage through the formation of CPDs and pyrimidine-pyrimidone (6-4) photoproducts, with the latter occurring at a lower frequency than the former. The most common dimers induced by UVB, in decreasing frequency, are thymine-thymine (T-T) dimers, cytosine-thymine (C-T) dimers, thymine-cytosine (T-C) dimers, and cytosine-cytosine (C-C) dimers. The (6-4) photoproduct formation is also most efficiently induced by UVB, with thymine-cytosine (6-4) dimers as the most common product.[40] Cytosine-cytosine (6-4) dimers and thymine-thymine (6-4) dimers are also observed. It should be noted that the in vitro action spectra for the formation of CPDs and (6-4) photoproducts are very similar, correlating well with the absorption spectrum of DNA.[41] The (6-4) photoproducts could be converted to their corresponding Dewar photoproducts by a photoisomerization process following exposure to 280–360 nm of UV radiation.[42]

In contrast to UVB, which produces DNA damage through direct effect, as described earlier, UVA radiation produces DNA damage mainly through indirect mechanisms. UVA induces the generation of single-oxygen, hydrogen peroxide, and superoxide radicals. ROS react predominately with guanine, resulting in the generation of 8-hydroxy-2'-deoxyguanosine.[43,44] However, it should be noted the action spectra in inducing DNA damage in mammalian cells by UVB and UVA are not mutually exclusive.[44] While UVA predominately induces DNA damage through generation of ROS, in vivo, UVA has been shown to also induce CPD formation in human skin.[15] UVB is also known to induce oxidative damage on the DNA (Table 65-3).

The in vivo relevance of these findings was demonstrated in a photocarcinogenesis study using an albino mouse model. It was shown that the maximum efficacy for skin cancer induction was 293 nm.[45] This corresponds to the action spectrum of CPD formation.

Pyrimidine dimers as well as DNA oxidative photoproducts are mutagenic. CPDs and pyrimidine-pyrimidone (6-4) photoproducts are formed by covalent linkage of two adjacent bases on the DNA, resulting in structurally "bulky" products. These are repaired by the nucleotide excision repair pathway. This pathway involves incision of the DNA strand containing the photoproduct, followed by DNA synthesis and gap closure by DNA ligase to replace the excised oligonucleotide (24–34 residues usually).[46]

Oxidative DNA photoproducts, formed predominately by UVA, consist of incorporation of an oxygen atom into a base. These "nonbulky" lesions are repaired by the base excision repair pathway.[47] DNA glycosylase is the enzyme responsible for base exision repair; this enzyme has substrate specificity for the type of DNA base damage. Base excision repair results in a single-nucleotide replacement. A less common base repair mechanism exists where the damaged nucleotide, together with several surrounding nucleotides, is replaced.

Darker skin following UV exposure shows less DNA damage and a higher rate of apoptotic cell formation and may be more efficient than lighter skin at removing damaged cells, which could be a factor resulting in the reduced risk of photocarcinogenesis.[6,8] In addition,

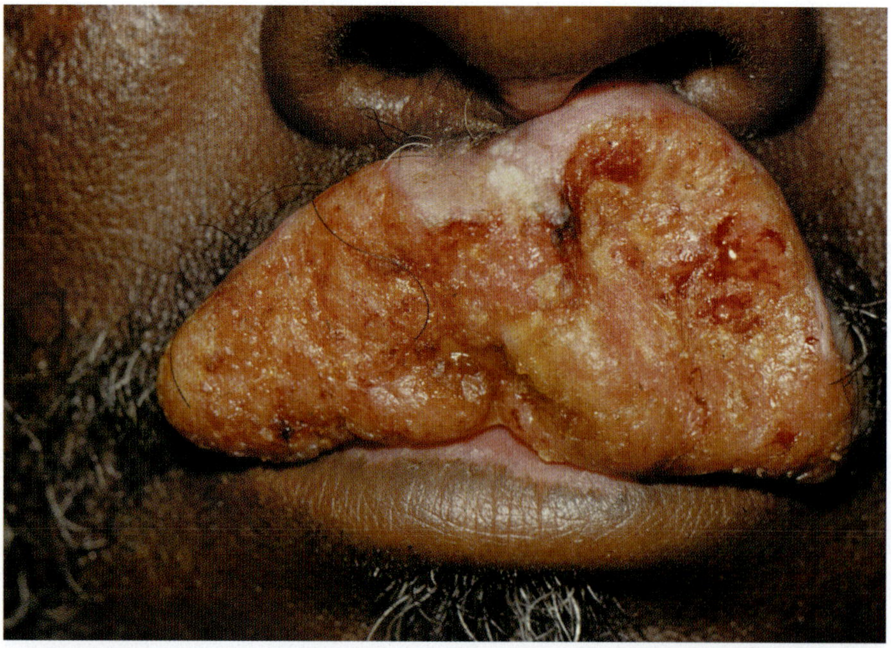

▲ **FIGURE 65-5** An African-American man with a large squamous cell carcinoma involving the upper lip of a patient with discoid lupus erythematosus.

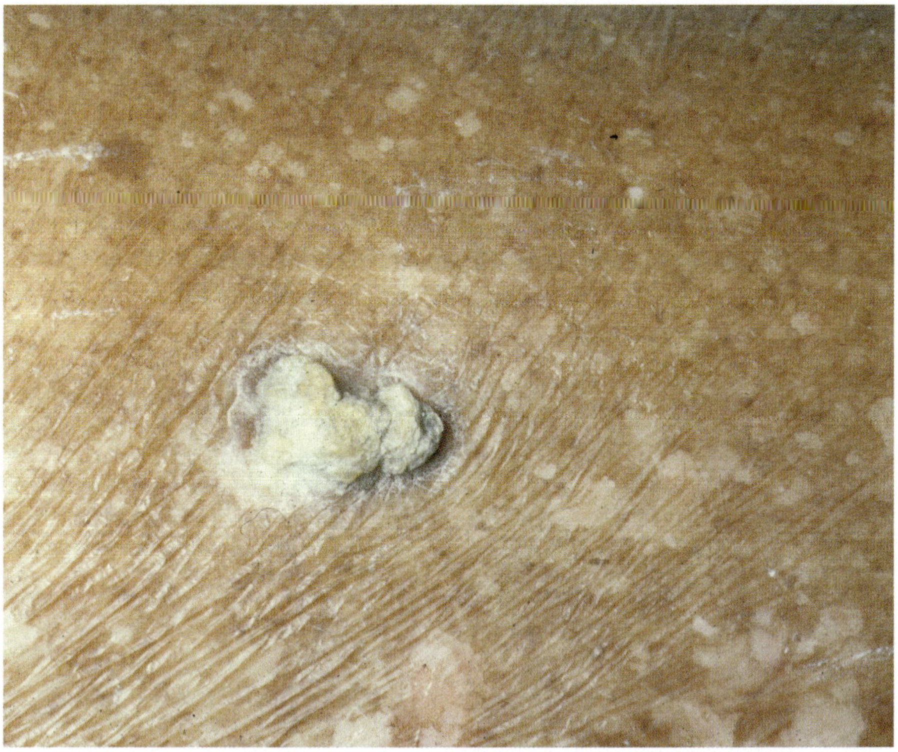

▲ **FIGURE 65-6** Bowen's disease (squamous cell carcinoma in situ) and actinic keratoses on the forearm of a skin of color patient.

because melanin acts as a natural UV filter, there is less damage of keratinocyte stem cells and basal melanocytes.[48]

Gene Mutations and Skin Cancers (Table 65-4)

The p53 protein is the product of the *p53* tumor suppressor gene. The p53 protein has been regarded as the "guardian of the genome."[49] It regulates cell cycle progression, DNA repair, and apoptotic cell death. Mutations of the *p53* gene had been detected in lesions of actinic keratoses, squamous cell carcinomas, and basal cell carcinomas, as well as in surrounding normal skin. The mutations found in these lesions are predominately C→T mutations or, much less commonly, tandem CC→TT mutations. Because these types of mutation are rarely seen in *p53* mutation in internal malignancies, they have been called *UV signature mutations.*

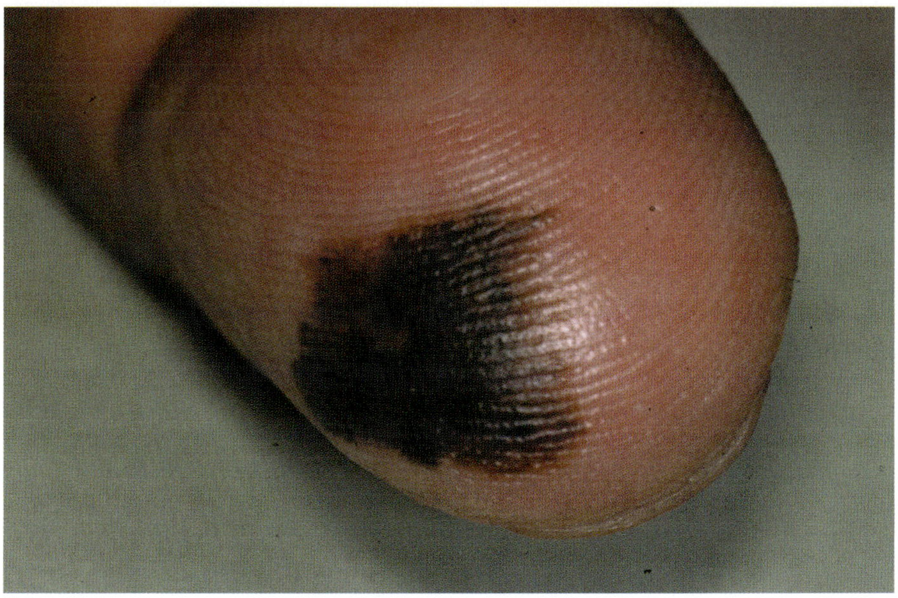

▲ **FIGURE 65-7** Acral lentiginous melanoma of the right index finger of a Hispanic man

The Hedgehog-Patched signaling pathway has been shown to be important in the development of basal cell carcinomas. The human *PTCH* gene was identified in 1996. The product of this gene, Patched, is the Hedgehog membrane receptor protein. Patched protein normally binds to another membrane receptor protein called *Smoothened.* Binding of the Patched protein to Smoothened protein results in suppression of the latter. Mutations of the *PTCH* gene result in the inability of the Patched protein to suppress the activity of Smoothened. Alternatively, mutations in the *Smoothened* gene also could result in the release of suppression on the Smoothened protein. Either of these events results in cell proliferation and lack of suppression of apoptosis.[50,51] The effect of UV radiation on the Hedgehog-Patched signaling pathway has not been completed elucidated.

The development of melanoma is associated with mutations of the *CDKN2A* gene (also known as the *INK4a/ARF* gene), located on chromosome 9p21. This gene encodes two products, p16 protein and p14ARF (alternative reading frame) protein. p16 is essential for cycle arrest; gene mutations resulting in the loss of p16 functions lead to an increased probability of a lack of repair of DNA mutations before cell division. Germ-line mutations in the *p16* gene are found in 38% of melanoma-prone families.[52] Mutations of the *CDKN2A* gene also can result in the loss of p14ARF functions, which leads to accelerated destruction of p53 protein, resulting in uncontrolled proliferation of cells.[52,53] It should be noted that UV signature mutations (C→T and CC→TT) are only infrequently detected in the *CDKN2A* gene.[54]

Epidemiology of Skin Cancers

Differences in the incidence and trend of skin cancers vary among populations of different skin types and geographic locations, occupational exposure, behavior in terms of sun exposure and skin protection, and differences in disease awareness and surveillance. Among white populations, since 1960s, the incidences of basal cell carcinoma (BCC), squamous cell carcinoma (SCC), and melanoma have increased at a rate of between 3% and 8% annually.

Basal Cell Carcinoma

There is great variation in incidence of BCC at different geographic locations.

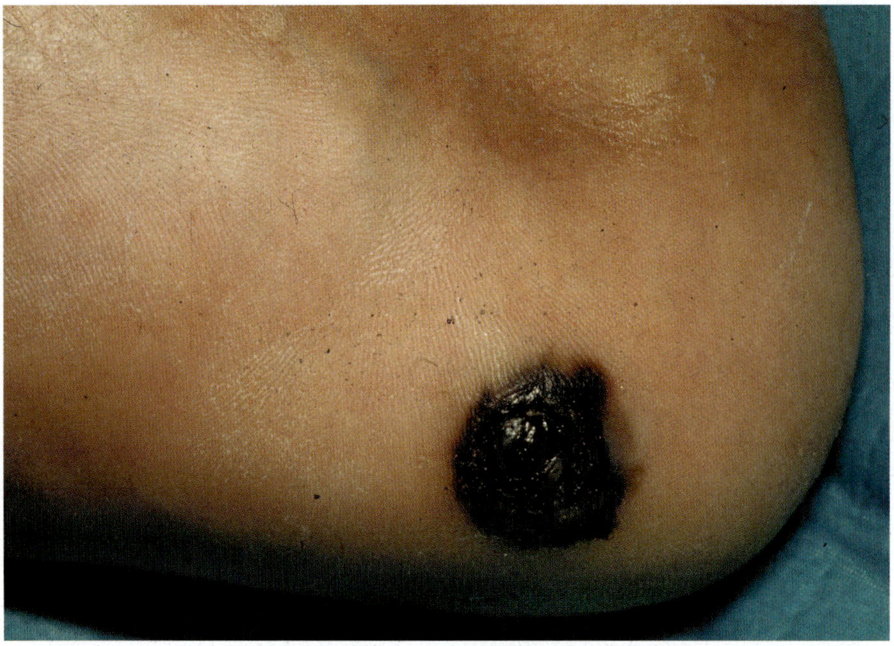

▲ **FIGURE 65-8** Acral lentiginous melanoma of the heel of a skin of color patient.

The incidence of BCC is 10 per 100,000 per annum in Iceland, 191 per 100,000 in white Americans, and 692 per 100,000 per annum in Hawaii.[55] This geographic variation in incidence corresponds with variation in latitude; it correlates well with the latitudinal variation in UV radiation exposure, supporting the proposal that sun exposure is an important etiologic factor in the causation of BCC. However, despite locations at lower latitudes, the relatively lower incidence rates of 5.5 per 100,000 person-years in Singapore[56] and 30 per 100,000 person-years among Japanese in Hawaii[57] suggest that variation in race and skin type are an important factor too. The difference in incidence rates between Singaporean Chinese (4.8 per 100,000 person years) and Japanese Hawaiians (30 per 100,000 person years) suggests ethnic variation in the incidence of BCC.[56] Ethnicity encompasses both skin type and sociocultural differences. Both inherent genetic differences and varying environmental exposure to UV radiation can account for ethnic differences.

There is a male predominance in the incidence of BCC in white population, with a male-to-female ratio of 2:1[58]; however, there is no difference in incidence rates of BCC between males and females among the different ethnic groups in an Asian population.[56] There is an increased incidence of BCC with age, with 80% of patients over 50 years of age and 30% older than 70 years of age.[59] In addition, there is an increasing trend in incidence of BCC over the years, especially among the fair-skinned populations. For example, the incidence of BCC in Tasmania increased by 8% per year,[60] the incidence of BCC increased by 60.6% in males and 48.4% in females in British Columbia, Canada, over a 12-year period,[61] and the incidence of BCC increased 2.4 times in Finland over a 25-year period.[62] In comparison, the incidence of BCC in Singapore, which has a darker-skinned population, increased only 3% annually over almost three decades.[56]

Although sun exposure is a definite risk factor for development of BCC, it has been postulated that intermittent sun exposure may play a greater role than cumulative sun exposure, especially among poor tanners.[63] It was postulated that good tanners may have protective effects such as increased melanization, which may provide some protection from the sun, even with intermittent sun exposure, in comparison with the poor tanners. BCCs in good tanners tend to be more pigmented too.

The development of various BCC subtypes also may differ with regard to the role of sun exposure.[64] Superficial BCCs were found more commonly in younger subjects and were seen most commonly on the trunk in males and lower extremities in females. Nodular BCCs were found more commonly in the head and neck areas in older subjects. It was postulated that since superficial BCCs were found more commonly on areas not subjected to constant UV radiation, intermittent sun exposure may be more important for this subtype of BCC. In contrast, because nodular BCCs were found more commonly on chronically sun-exposed areas, chronic sun exposure may be a more important etiologic factor for this subtype.

BCCs are also seen commonly adjacent to the inner canthus and in the nasolabial fold. When BCC spreads, there is a tendency to do so by direct invasion, very often along embryologic fusion planes. It thus was postulated that a relationship between development of BCC and embryologic closure lines may exist.[65]

Some of the less common etiologic factors for development of BCC include psoralen with UVA (PUVA) photochemotherapy,[66] genetic disorders (such as Gorlin syndrome, Basex syndrome, and xeroderma pigmentosa), preexisting sebaceous nevi,[67] arsenic ingestion,[68] immunosuppression (especially among transplant recipients),[69–71] after radiation therapy,[72] and in areas of chronic trauma.[73,74]

Squamous Cell Carcinoma

SCC is the less common form of nonmelanoma skin cancer compared with

TABLE 65-3
UV-Induced DNA Damage

Predominant Effects of UVB

Cyclobutane-pyrimidine dimers:
- Thymine-thymine
- Cytosine-thymine
- Thymine-cytosine
- Cytosine-cytosine

Pyrimidine-pyrimidone (6-4) photoproducts:
- Thymine-cytosine (6-4) dimers
- Cytosine-cytosine (6-4) dimers
- Thymine-thymine (6-4) dimers

Predominant Effects of UVA

Generation of reactive oxygen species
8-Hydroxy-2′-deoxyguanosine

TABLE 65-4
Gene Mutations and Skin Cancers

Condition	Gene Mutations
Actinic keratosis	
Squamous cell carcinoma	*p53*
Basal cell carcinoma	
Basal cell carcinoma	*PTCH* *Smoothened*
Melanoma	*CDKN2A* (or *INK4a/ARF*)

BCC, with a BCC:SCC ratio of 4:1. There is a more direct dose-response relationship between exposure to UV radiation and the development of SCC compared with that of BCC. Rates of SCC rise more rapidly than those of BCC with increasing UVB exposure.[75] Among the fair-skinned populations, the incidence of SCC corresponds with the latitudinal locations relative to the equator. The age-standardized rates of SCC per 100,000 person-years for males and females were reported to be 7.2 and 4.2, respectively, for Finland,[62] 64 and 20, respectively, for Tasmania,[60] and 270 and 112, respectively, for Arizona.[76] Besides sun exposure, skin types and thus ability to tan are also important determinants for development of SCC. Singapore, which is located very near to the equator, but with a predominant Asian population, has an age-standardized rate of only 2.2 per 100,000 person-years.[56]

In addition to sun exposure, there are numerous other predisposing factors for SCC. These include various environmental carcinogens, chronic immunosuppression, chronic infections, chronic scarring, inflammatory processes, and a number of heritable diseases. The environmental carcinogens include ionizing radiation, aromatic hydrocarbons, and arsenic toxicity. An 18-fold increase in SCC has been reported in renal transplant patients.[77] The skin cancers tend to appear 3–7 years after the onset of prolonged immunosuppressive therapies, especially with azathioprine, corticosteroids, and cyclosporine.[78] Chronic infections such as osteomyelitis,[79] lupus vulgaris,[80] and leprosy[81] have been reported to be associated with development of SCC. Chronic scarring inflammatory processes such as discoid lupus erythematosus,[82] chronic venous ulcer,[83] and lichen planus[84] also have been reported to be associated with SCC. Periungual SCC[85] has been associated with human papillomavirus (HPV) type 16, whereas one-third of patients with epidermodysplasia verruciformis (who are commonly infected with HPV-5) developed SCC.[86,87] The heritable diseases that are associated with increased risks of SCC include oculocutaneous albinism and xeroderma pigmentosum.

Melanoma

Melanoma is an important skin cancer predominantly among the fair-skinned population. The incidence rates ranges from 0.5 per 100,000 person-years in Singaporean Chinese, to 0.2 per 100,000 person-years in Singaporean Indians,[56] to 2.8 and 3 per 100,000 person-years among Hispanics in California,[88] to 55.8 and 42.9 per 100,000 person-years among Australians.[89] Among fair-skinned populations, there is a correlation between the latitudinal location of a region and the incidence of melanoma; the nearer a region is to the equator, the higher is the incidence of melanoma. In comparison with the data from Australia, the incidences of melanoma were 6.4 and 5.3 per 100,000 person-years among males and females in Finland[90] and 4.8 per 100,000 person-years for both males and females in Germany.[91] An earlier report from Australia also noted that the lower the latitude, the higher is the mortality from melanoma.[91] However, in a multicentered study, no significant association existed between the UV index and latitude and the incidence of melanoma among Hispanic or black populations compared with whites.[92]

However, the relationship between UV radiation and melanoma is complex and does not follow a simple linear correlation. For example, the sites affected most frequently generally are not the areas that receive the highest cumulative sun exposure; melanoma has a relative peak incidence in midlife instead of in an older age group, who would have higher cumulative effects of sun exposure; and melanoma occurs more frequently in indoor versus outdoor workers.[58] Despite these observations, there is still significant epidemiologic evidence linking UV irradiation and melanoma. Migration studies have documented an increased incidence of melanoma in people migrating to regions with higher levels of solar radiation compared with individuals in their native land.[93,94]

Lack of pigmentation has been shown to be a risk factor for melanoma, as evidenced by the wide differences in incidence of melanoma among populations with different predominant skin types. Within the Caucasian population, those with fair skin, blue eyes, and blond or red hair are especially at risk. The relative risk for individuals with blond hair ranges from 1.4–7.1, and for those with red hair, from 2.9–4.7.[95] Others have found sun sensitivity to be more closely associated with an increased risk rather than individual pigmentary characteristics.[96] A history of sunburns, especially in childhood, has been associated with an increased risk of melanoma.[96–99] However, the tendency to sunburn, rather than the total number of sunburns, is a more important factor for development of melanoma.[100] It has been postulated that the risk of melanoma is related to episodes of intermittent, intense sun exposure of normally unexposed skin.[95] This may account for the fact that melanomas are found most frequently on the trunk in men and the lower extremities in women, instead of areas that are more exposed to the sun, such as the head and neck areas.[95] This also may account for the observation that melanoma is more common in individuals from high socioeconomic classes and in indoor workers.[101] This hypothesis has been supported further by observations that the risk of melanoma is apparently not increased by total or occupational exposure but is increased with increasing recreational exposure of untanned skin to intense sunlight.[100]

The different histologic subtypes of melanoma appear to differ with respect to location and pattern of sun exposure. Superficial spreading melanoma (SSM) has been associated with recreational patterns of sun exposure; it is found mainly on the trunk and extremities. Lentigo maligna melanoma (LMM) occurs most commonly on the head and neck, areas of skin chronically exposed to the sun. In addition, the incidence of LMM has been shown to increase progressively with age. Acral lentiginous melanoma (ALM) is the most common subtype among patients with darker skin types; it commonly occurs on the palms and soles, which are shielded from the sun. This suggests that ALM subtype may be associated with other etiologic factors rather than UV exposure.[95,102]

It is clear that there are differences in the effects of UV radiation and in the incident of skin cancers between various racial and ethnic groups. In addition to skin type, other important variables include geographic location, sun exposure and protection, and occupational exposure. Individuals with all skin types must be made aware of the importance of sun protection.

SUNSCREEN

Sunscreens can be divided into organic (chemical) and inorganic (physical/nonchemical) UV filters. The organic sunscreens can be further divided into primarily UVB and UVA filters. *Sun protection factor* (SPF) is the dose of UV radiation required to produce 1 MED on protected skin after the application of 2 mg/ cm^2 of sunscreen product divided by the dose of UV radiation to produce

1 MED on unprotected skin. The endpoint of evaluation is cutaneous erythema; therefore, SPF is a reflection of predominantly protection against the effect of UVB, the main erythemogenic spectrum of UV radiation. A product with an SPF of 30 is able to filter 97% of UVB radiation. In August 2007, the Food and Drug Administration (FDA) has released a proposed revision to the 1999 FDA sunscreen monograph; among the proposed revisions is a rating system for the UVA protection of sunscreens.[25] The acute and chronic effects of UV radiation that are summarized in this chapter affect skin of color to a lesser degree than white skin primarily because of some of the protective properties of melanin. However, photoprotective measures, which include seeking shade during the peak UV hours of 10 a.m. to 4 p.m., the use of photoprotective clothing and wide-brimmed hats, and the use of sunscreens and sunglasses, should be taken by individuals with skin of color to avoid the deleterious effects of the sun. These should be balanced with appropriate dietary intake of vitamin D–containing food (e.g., saltwater fish and vitamin D–fortified foods) and vitamin D_3 supplements.

CONCLUSION

This chapter has summarized the cutaneous acute and chronic effects of UV radiation in general and how it affects skin of color in particular. Owing to the effect of melanin, individuals with skin of color are less prone to develop UV-associated skin cancers than fair-skinned individuals. The acute effects are erythema, pigment darkening, epidermal hyperplasia, vitamin D synthesis, and photoimmunosuppression. The chronic effects are photoaging and photocarcinogenesis. The types of skin cancers associated with UV radiation are BCC, SCC, and melanoma. However, people with skin of color are more susceptible to having low serum vitamin D levels. The use of sunscreen, in addition to sun avoidance during peak hours and photoprotective clothing, can help to reduce the effects from the sun.

REFERENCES

1. Suplee C. The sun: Living with a stormy star. *National Geographic* 2004;206:2-33.
2. Diffey BL. What is light? *Photodermatol Photoimmunol Photomed* 2002;18:68-74.
3. Rhodes L, Lim H. Acute effects of ultraviolet radiation on the skin, in Lim H, Honigsmann H, Hawk J (eds), *Photodermatology*. New York, Informa Healthcare USA, 2007, pp 76-89.
4. Tuchinda C, Srivannaboon S, Lim H. Photoprotection by window glass, automobile glass and sunglasses. *J Am Acad Dermatol* 2006;54:845-854.
5. Rhodes L, Belgi G, Parslew R, et al. Ultraviolet-B-induced erythema is mediated by nitric oxide and prostaglandin E_2 in combination. *J Invest Dermatol* 2001; 117:880-885.
6. Tadokoro T, Kobayashi N, Zmudzka B, et al. UV-induced DNA damage and melanin content in human skin differing in racial/ethnic origin. *FASEB J* 2003;17: 1177-1179.
7. Park S, Suh D, Youn J. Realiability of self-assessment in determining skin phototype for Korean brown skin. *Photodermatol Photoimmuol Photomed.* 1998;14:5-6.
8. Beer J, Hearing V. Skin color, melanin, race/ethnicity and UV-induced DNA damage, in Giacomoni PU (ed), *Biophysical and Physiological Effects of Solar Radiation on Human Skin,* Vol 10. Melville, SC, RSC Publishing, 2007, pp 99-125.
9. Rosario R, Mark G, Parrih J. Histological changes produced in skin by equally erythemogenic doses of UVA, UVB, UVC and UVA with psoralens. *Br J Dermatol* 1979;120:767-777.
10. Hawk J, Murphy G, Holden C. The presence of neutrophils in human cutaneous ultraviolet-B-induced inflammation. *Br J Dermatol* 1988;118:27-30.
11. Moyal D, Fourtanier A. Acute and chronic effects of UV on skin: What are they and how to study them? in Rigel D, Weiss R, Lim H, Dover J (eds), *Photoaging*. New York, Marcel Dekker, 2004, pp 15-32.
12. Taketsugu T, Yamaguchi Y, Batzer J, et al. Mechaisms of skin tanning in different racial/ethnic groups in response to ultraviolet radiation. *J Invest Dermatol* 2005;124: 1326-1332.
13. Wikimedia Foundation, Inc. Sun Tanning *Wikipedia: The Free Encyclopedia* (Internet),. February 3, 2008; available at *http://en.wikipedia.org/w/index.php?titleSun_tanning & oldid=188765591. Accessed Jan 27, 2008.*
14. Yamashita T, Akita H, Astner S, et al. In vivo assessment of pigmentary and vascular compartments changes in UVA exposed skin by reflectance-mode confocal microscopy. *Exp Dermatol* 2007;16: 905-911.
15. Young AR, Potten CS, Nikaido O, et al. Human melanocytes and keratinocytes exposed to UVB or UVA in vivo show comparable levels of thymine dimers. *J Invest Dermatol* 1998;111:936-940.
16. Wagner J, Jovel C, Norton H, et al. Comparing quantitative measures of erythema, pigmentation and skin responses using reflectometry. *Pigment Cell Res* 2002;15:379-384.
17. Wagner J, Parra E, Norton L, et al. Skin responses to ultraviolet radiation:effects of consitutive pigmentation, sex, and ancestry. *Pigment Cell Res* 2002;15:385-390.
18. Tadokoro T, Yamaguchi Y, Batzer J, et al. Mechanisms of skin tanning in different racial/ethnic groups in response to ultraviolet radiation. *J Invest Dermatol* 2005; 124:1326-1332.
19. Thody A. α-MSH and the regulation of melanocyte function. *Ann NY Acad Sci* 1999;885:217-229.
20. Cheng J, Moss S, Eisner M. X-ray characterization of melanins, parts I and II. *Pigment Cell Res* 1994;7:255-273.
21. Kobayashi N, Nakagawa A, Muramatsu T, et al. Supranuclear melanin caps reduce ultraviolet induced DNA photoproducts in human epidermis. *J Invest Dermatol* 1998;110:806-810.
22. Kaidbey K, Agin P, Sayre R, Kligman A. Photoprotection by melanin: A comparison of black and Caucasian skin. *J Am Acad Dermatol* 1979;1:249-260.
23. Hönigsmann H. Erythema and pigmentation. *Photodermatol Photoimmunol Photomed* 2002;18:75-81.
24. Calzavara-Pinton P, Ortel B. Pigmentation after solar radiation, in Giacomoni PU (ed), *Biophysical and Physiological Effects of Solar Radiation on Human Skin,* Vol 10. Melville, SC, RSC Publishing, 2007, pp 65-97.
25. Kullavanijaya P, Lim H. Photoprotection. *J Am Acad Dermatol* 2005;52:937-958.
26. Wolpowitz D, Gilchrest B. The vitamin D questions: How much do you need and how should you get it? *J Am Acad Dermatol* 2006;54:301-317.
27. Hollis B. Symposium—Vitamin D insufficiency: A significant risk factor in chronic disease and potential disease-specific biomarkers of vitamin D sufficiency. *J Nutr* 2005;135:317-322.
28. Lehmann B. The vitamin D_3 pathway in human skin and its role for regulation of biological processes. *Photochem Photobiol* 2005;81:1246-1251.
29. Schwartz T. Photoimmunosuppression. *Photodermatol Photoimmunol Photomed* 2002; 18:141-145.
30. Perna J, Mannix M, Rooney J, et al. Reactivation of latent herpes simplex virus infection by ultraviolet light: A human model. *J Am Acad Dermatol* 1987; 17:473-478.
31. Norval M. The impact of ultraviolet radiation on immune responses. *Radiat Prot Dosimetr.* 2000;91:51-56.
32. Applegate L, Levy R, Alcalay J. Identification of the molecular target for the suppression of contact hypersensitivity by UV radiation. *J Exp Med* 1989;170: 1117-1131.
33. Norval M. Effects of solar radiation on the human immune system, in Giacomoni PU (ed), *Sun Protection in Man.* New York, Elsevier, 2001.
34. Kang K, Hammerberg C, Meuier L, Cooper K. CD11b+ macrophages that infiltrate human epidermis after in vivo ultraviolet exposure potently produce IL-10 and represent the major secretory source of epidermal IL-10 protein. *J Immunol* 1994;153:5256-5264.
35. Kwon O, Hwang E, Bae J, et al. Seborrheic keratosis in the Korean males: Causative role of sunlight. *Photodermatol Photoimmunol Photomed* 2003;19:73-80.
36. Halder R, Richards G. Photoaging in patients of skin of color, in Rigel D, Weiss R, Lim H, Dover J (eds), *Photoaging*. New York, Marcell Dekker, 2004, pp 55-63.
37. Wlaschek M, Tantcheva-Poor I, Naderi L. Solar UV irradiation and dermal photoaging. *J Photochem Photobiol B* 2001;63:41-51.
38. Yaar M. The chronic effects of ultraviolet radiation on the skin: Photoaging, in Lim H, Honigsmann H, Hawk J (eds), *Photodermatology*. New York, Informa Healthcare USA, 2007, pp 92-106.

39. Schieke S, Schroeder P, Krutmann J. Cutaneous effects of infrared radiation: From clinical observations to molecular response mechanisms. *Photodermatol Photoimmunol Photomed* 2003;19:228-234.
40. Bykov VJ, Hemminki K. Assay of different photoproducts after UVA, B, and C irradiation of DNA and human skin explants. *Carcinogenesis* 1996;17:1949-1955.
41. Matsunaga T, Hieda K, Nikaido O. Wavelength dependent formation of thymine dimers and (6-4) photoproducts in DNA by monochromatic ultraviolet light ranging from 150 to 365 nm. *Photochem Photobiol* 1991;54:403-410.
42. Matsunaga T, Hatakeyama Y, Ohta M, et al. Establishment and characterization of a monoclonal antibody recognizing the Dewar isomers of (6-4) photoproducts. *Photochem Photobiol* 1993;57: 934-940.
43. Hattori Y, Nishigori C, Tanaka T, et al. 8-Hydroxy-2′-deoxyguanosine is increased in epidermal cells of hairless mice after chronic ultraviolet B exposure. *J Invest Dermatol* 1996;107:733-737.
44. Kielbassa C, Roza L, Epe B. Wavelength dependence of oxidative DNA damage induced by UV and visible light. *Carcinogenesis* 1997;18:811-816.
45. de Gruijl FR, Sterenborg HJ, Forbes PD, et al. Wavelength dependence of skin cancer induction by ultraviolet irradiation of albino hairless mice. *Cancer Res* 1993;53: 53-60.
46. Lindahl T, Wood RD. Quality control by DNA repair. *Science* 1999;286:1897-1905.
47. Demple B, Harrison L. Repair of oxidative damage to DNA: Enzymology and biology. *Ann Rev Biochem* 1994;63: 915-948.
48. Yamaguchi Y, Takahashi K, Zmudzka B, et al. Human skin responses to UV radiation: Pigment in the upper epidermis protects against DBA damage in the lower epidermis and facilitates apoptosis. *FASEB J* 2006;20:1486-1488.
49. Lane DP. Cancer: p53, guardian of the genome. *Nature* 1992;358:15-16.
50. Hahn H, Wicking C, Zaphiropoulous PG, et al. Mutations of the human homolog of *Drosophila patched* in the nevoid basal cell carcinoma syndrome. *Cell* 1996;85: 841-851.
51. Johnson RL, Rothman AL, Xie J, et al. Human homolog of *patched,* a candidate gene for the basal cell nevus syndrome. *Science* 1996;272:1668-1671.
52. Piepkorn M. Melanoma genetics: An update with focus on the *CDKN2A (p16)/ARF* tumor suppressors. *J Am Acad Dermatol* 2000;42:705-722.
53. Tsao H. Update on familial cancer syndromes and the skin. *J Am Acad Dermatol* 2000;42:939-969.
54. Peris K, Chimenti S, Fargnoli MC, et al. UV fingerprint *CDKN2a* but no *p14ARF* mutations in sporadic melanomas. *J Invest Dermatol* 1999;112:825-826.
55. Gloster HM Jr, Brodland DG. The epidemiology of skin cancer. *Dermatol Surg* 1996;22:217-226.
56. Koh D, Wang H, Lee J, et al. Basal cell carcinoma, squamous cell carcinoma and melanoma of the skin: Analysis of the Singapore Cancer Registry data 1968-1997. *Br J Dermatol* 2003;148: 1161-1166.
57. Chuang TY, Reizner GT, Elpern DJ, et al. Nonmelanoma skin cancer in Japanese ethnic Hawaiians in Kauai, Hawaii: An incidence report. *J Am Acad Dermatol* 1995; 33:422-426.
58. Armstrong BK, Kricker A. Skin cancer. *Dermatol Clin* 1995;13:583-594.
59. Healy E, Collins P, Barnes L. Nonmelanoma skin cancer in an Irish population: An appraisal of risk factors. *Ir Med J* 1995;88:58-59.
60. Kaldor J, Shugg D, Young B, et al. Nonmelanoma skin cancer: Ten years of cancer-registry-based surveillance. *Int J Cancer* 1993;53:886-891.
61. Gallagher RP, Ma B, McLean DI, et al. Trends in basal cell carcinoma, squamous cell carcinoma, and melanoma of the skin from 1973 through 1987. *J Am Acad Dermatol* 1990;23:413-421.
62. Hannuksela-Svahn A, Pukkala E, Karvonen J. Basal cell skin carcinoma and other nonmelanoma skin cancers in Finland from 1956 through 1995. *Arch Dermatol* 1999;135:781-786.
63. Kricker A, Armstrong BK, English DR, Heenan PJ. Does intermittent sun exposure cause basal cell carcinoma? A case-control study in western Australia. *Int J Cancer* 1995;60:489-494.
64. Bastiaens MT, Hoefnagel JJ, Bruijn JA, et al. Differences in age, site distribution, and sex between nodular and superficial basal cell carcinoma indicate different types of tumors. *J Invest Dermatol* 1998; 110:880-884.
65. Panje WR, Ceilley RI. The influence of embryology of the mid-face on the spread of epithelial malignancies. *Laryngoscope* 1979;89:1914-1920.
66. Stern RS, Laird N. The carcinogenic risk of treatments for severe psoriasis. Photochemotherapy follow-up study. *Cancer* 1994;73:2759-2764.
67. Helwig EB, Hackney VC. Syringadenoma papilliferum: Lesions with and without naevus sebaceous and basal cell carcinoma. *Arch Dermatol* 1955;71:361-372.
68. Alain G, Tousignant J, Rozenfarb E. Chronic arsenic toxicity. *Int J Dermatol* 1993;32:899-901.
69. Glover MT, Niranjan N, Kwan JT, Leigh IM. Non-melanoma skin cancer in renal transplant recipients: The extent of the problem and a strategy for management. *Br J Plast Surg* 1994;47:86-89.
70. Hardie IR, Strong RW, Hartley LC, et al. Skin cancer in Caucasian renal allograft recipients living in a subtropical climate. *Surgery* 1980;87:177-183.
71. McGregor JM, Morris R, Smith CH, MacDonald DM. Skin cancer morbidity amongst renal allograft recipients: A 25-year retrospective follow-up study. *Br J Dermatol* 1995;133:40.
72. Landthaler M, Hagspiel HJ, Braun-Falco O. Late irradiation damage to the skin caused by soft x-ray radiation therapy of cutaneous tumors. *Arch Dermatol* 1995; 131: 182-186.
73. Ewing MR. The significance of a single injury in the causation of basal-cell carcinoma of the skin. *Aust NZ J Surg* 1971; 41:140-147.
74. Rustin MH, Chambers TJ, Munro DD. Post-traumatic basal cell carcinomas. *Clin Exp Dermatol* 1984;9:379-383.
75. Vitaliano PP, Urbach F. The relative importance of risk factors in nonmelanoma skin cancer. *Arch Dermatol* 1980;116:454-456.
76. Harris RB, Griffith K, Moon TE. Trends in the incidence of nonmelanoma skin cancers in southeastern Arizona, 1985-1996. *J Am Acad Dermatol* 2001;45: 528-536.
77. Gupta AK, Cardella CJ, Haberman HF. Cutaneous malignant neoplasms in patients with renal transplants. *Arch Dermatol* 1986;122:1288-1293.
78. Penn I. Immunosuppression and skin cancer. *Clin Plast Surg* 1980;7:361-368.
79. Hejna WF. Squamous-cell carcinoma developing in the chronic draining sinuses of osteomyelitis. *Cancer* 1965;18: 128-132.
80. Forstrom L. Carcinomatous changes in lupus vulgaris. *Ann Clin Res* 1969;1:213-219.
81. Majoroh TO, Imongan WI. Carcinoma in plantar ulcers of leprosy patients. *Trop Geogr Med* 1988;40:365-368.
82. Goh CL, Ang LC, Ho J. Squamous cell carcinoma complicating discoid lupus erythematosus. *Int J Dermatol* 1987;26: 110-111.
83. Halliday JP. Squamous carcinoma in a venous ulcer. *Med J Aust* 1968;1:449-451.
84. Gawkrodger DJ, Stephenson TJ, Thomas SE. Squamous cell carcinoma complicating lichen planus: A clinico-pathological study of three cases. *Dermatology* 1994;188:36-39.
85. Moy RL, Eliezri YD, Nuovo GJ, et al. Human papillomavirus type 16 DNA in periungual squamous cell carcinomas. *JAMA* 1989;261:2669-2673.
86. Jablonska S, Orth G. Epidermodysplasia verruciformis. *Clin Dermatol* 1985;3: 83-96.
87. Ostrow RS, Bender M, Niimura M, et al. Human papillomavirus DNA in cutaneous primary and metastasized squamous cell carcinomas from patients with epidermodysplasia verruciformis. *Proc Natl Acad Sci USA* 1982;79:1634-1638.
88. Cress RD, Holly EA. Incidence of cutaneous melanoma among non-Hispanic whites, Hispanics, Asians, and blacks: An analysis of California cancer registry data, 1988-1993. *Cancer Causes Control* 1997;8:246-252.
89. Garbe C, McLeod GR, Buettner PG. Time trends of cutaneous melanoma in Queensland, Australia and Central Europe. *Cancer* 2000;89:1269-1278.
90. Magnus K. The Nordic profile of skin cancer incidence: A comparative epidemiological study of the three main types of skin cancer. *Int J Cancer* 1991; 47:12-19.
91. Lancaster HO. Some geographical aspects of the mortality from melanoma in Europeans. *Med J Aust* 1956;43: 1082-1087.
92. Eide M, Weinstock M. Association of UV index, latitude, and melanoma incidence in nonwhite populations. US Surveillance, Epidemiology, and End Results (SEER) Program, 1992-2001. *Arch Dermatol* 2005; 141:477-481.
93. Holman CD, Armstrong BK. Cutaneous malignant melanoma and indicators of total accumulated exposure to the sun: An analysis separating histogenetic types. *J Natl Cancer Inst* 1984;73:75-82.
94. Langley RG, Sober AJ. A clinical review of the evidence for the role of ultraviolet

radiation in the etiology of cutaneous melanoma. *Cancer Invest* 1997;15:561-567.
95. Katsambas A, Nicolaidou E. Cutaneous malignant melanoma and sun exposure: Recent developments in epidemiology. *Arch Dermatol* 1996;132:444-450.
96. Weinstock MA, Colditz GA, Willett WC, et al. Melanoma and the sun: The effect of swimsuits and a "healthy" tan on the risk of nonfamilial malignant melanoma in women. *Am J Epidemiol* 1991;134:462-470.
97. Elder DE. Human melanocytic neoplasms and their etiologic relationship with sunlight. *J Invest Dermatol* 1989;92: 297-303S.
98. Elwood JM, Whitehead SM, Davison J, et al. Malignant melanoma in England: Risks associated with naevi, freckles, social class, hair colour, and sunburn. *Int J Epidemiol* 1990;19:801-810.
99. Green A, Siskind V, Bain C, Alexander J. Sunburn and malignant melanoma. *Br J Cancer* 1985;51:393-397.
100. Elwood JM, Gallagher RP, Davison J, Hill GB. Sunburn, suntan and the risk of cutaneous malignant melanoma: The Western Canada Melanoma Study. *Br J Cancer* 1985;51:543-549.
101. Gallagher RP, Elwood JM, Yang CP. Is chronic sunlight exposure important in accounting for increases in melanoma incidence? *Int J Cancer* 1989;44:813-815.
102. Elder DE. Skin cancer: Melanoma and other specific nonmelanoma skin cancers. *Cancer* 1995;75:245-256.

CHAPTER 66

Topical Steroids

Ncoza Dlova
Nilesh Morar

Key Points

- Hydrocortisone was the first topically effective synthetic glucorcoticoid to be introduced (56 years ago).
- The potency of topical steroids depends on their vasoconstrictor effect.
- Clinical use is based on their ability to cause vasoconstriction, immunosuppression, and anti-inflammatory and antiproliferative effects.
- Indications include dermatoses that are highly responsive, moderately responsive, and least responsive.
- Abuse of topical steroids has been widespread, particularly in Africa.

The illicit availability of topical corticosteroids in Africa has led to widespread abuse of these creams. In South Africa there is a misconception that topical corticosteroids will improve the complexion. This is particularly rife among the low-income and illiterate black women. Potent steroids are often applied on the face without medical advice and are intended by the user to clear postinflammatory hyperpigmentation, melasma, and sometimes acne. The long latency of topical corticosteroid side effects usually inspires some confidence in the treatment by users, with the skin looking smooth and brighter for a period of time.

HISTORY

Hydrocortisone was the first effective topical synthetic glucocorticoid to be developed. When introduced by Sulzberger and Witten in 1952, it revolutionalized therapeutic modalities in dermatology. Topical steroids are the leading prescribed drug in dermatology.[1]

Inactive cortisone is reduced to 11-hydroxyl hydrocortisone, which then becomes more active. This reaction does not occur effectively in the skin.[2] Variations in vehicles, concentrations, and modifications of the original hydrocortisone molecule have led to the availability of numerous topical steroids with different potencies and the development of a new market in the pharmaceutical industry.

PHARMACOLOGY

Topical corticosteroid preparations are available as fluorinated and nonfluorinated compounds. Fluorination or chlorination of a compound increases its potency and anti-inflammatory effects, but it also increases its side effects when compared with the nonfluorinated steroids.

Halogenation at the 9α position increases the strength of a steroid and decreases breakdown into inactive metabolites.[3] These corticosteroids have increased mineralocorticoid effects and are often considered to cause more adverse effects than the nonhalogenated preparations with similar clinical efficacy.

The vasoconstriction assay, which is the most commonly used test to estimate clinical effect, has been shown to be of great value. It is based on the property of glucocorticosteroids to produce transient vasoconstriction, and it usually correlates well with clinical efficacy and is also reproducible.[2]

PHARMACOKINETICS

The clinical potency of a topical corticosteroid depends on three interrelated factors—the structure of the corticosteroid molecule, the vehicle, and the skin onto which it is applied.[2] The basic configuration of most topical corticosteroids is represented in Figure 66-1. Further addition or change of functional groups (e.g., hydroxy, hydrocarbon, ester, fluoro, chloro, acetonide, and ketone) at certain positions can have a great impact on the pharmacokinetic characteristics of a particular molecule. Changing the vehicle of a topical corticosteroid may affect the amount of steroid that is released and its penetration into the epidermis. Using an ointment rather than a cream potentiates topical corticosteroid efficacy, as does a propylene glycol vehicle. This explains why a topical corticosteroid in an ointment vehicle is more potent than the cream or lotion equivalent. Use of keratolytics, α-hydroxy acids, tape stripping, wetting of the skin, and occlusive dressings also has been shown to increase the absorption of hydrocortisone.

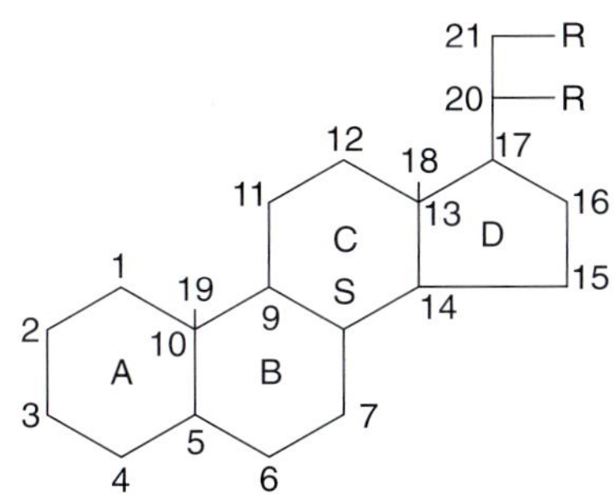

The configuration of the basic corticosteroid structure

▲ **FIGURE 66-1** Basic corticosteroid structure.

MECHANISM OF ACTION

Percutaneous absorption follows the application of a topical corticosteroid to the skin's surface. The steroid first diffuses into the stratum corneum. Hydrophilic steroids have a greater rate of penetration through the stratum corneum than hydrophobic topical corticosteroids, whereas penetration into the keratinocytes is more rapid with lipophilic steroids. This helps to explain the wide range of clinical efficacy among different topical corticosteroids. The corticosteroid then diffuses into the keratinocyte and binds to the glucorcorticoid receptor in the cytoplasm.[4] This is followed by a cascade of reactions with resulting modulation of messenger RNA production. Receptor binding by the cytoplasm is also greater with increasing lipid solubility of the topical corticosteroid. Receptor-binding affinity also determines the clinical potency of a particular steroid.

Most cells in the body possess glucorcoticoid receptors, and this may explain the numerous glucocorticoid receptor–mediated effects. Topical steroids affect all the cells that are involved with inflammation, such as Langerhans cells, antigen-presenting cells, and polymophonuclear leukocytes (reducing their phagocytic and antibacterial capabilities).[2] Synthesis and secretion of cytokines and inflammatory proteins necessary to initiate and sustain immune response are also reduced by the application of topical corticosteroids.

CLINICAL USES

Use of topical steroids in dermatology is based on their ability to cause

TABLE 66-1
List of Steroid Responsive Dermatosis

Highly Responsive to Steroids
- Atopic dermatitis
- Seborrhoeic dermatitis
- Psoriasis (flexural)
- Napkin dermatitis
- Intertrigo

Moderately Responsive
- Psoriasis
- Lichen simplex chronicus
- Irritant dermatitis
- Pityriasis rosea
- Discoid eczema
- Vitiligo

Least Responsive
- Palmoplantar psoriasis and nail psoriasis
- Dyshidrotic eczema
- Lupus erythematosus
- Lichen planus
- Pemphigus
- Granuloma annulare
- Necrobiosis lipoidica diabeticorium
- Sarcoidosis
- Acne keloidalis nuchae
- Morphea
- Chondrodermatitis nodularis

vasoconstriction, immunosuppression, and anti-inflammatory and antiproliferative effects. Table 66-1 lists dermatologic conditions and their responsiveness to topical steroids.

TABLE 66-2
Potency Ranking of Some Commonly Used Topical Steroids

Very Potent	
• Fluocinolone acetonide	0.2%
• Clobetasol propionate	0.05%
• Bethamethasone dipropionate	0.05%
• Diflucortolone valerate	0.3%
• Halcinonide	0.1%
Potent	
• Budesonide	0.025%
• Bethamethasone valerate	0.1%
• Fluocinolone acetonide	0.025%
• Diflucortolone valerate	
• Hydrocortisone butyrate	0.1%
• Beclometasone dipropionate	0.1%
• Betametosone dipropionate	0.025%
• Mometasone furoate	0.05%
• Fluticasone propionate	
• Methylprednisolone	0.1%
• Fluclorolone acetonide	0.025%
• Triamcinolone acetonide	0.1%
Moderately Potent	
• Clobetasone butyrate	0.05%
• Alclometasone dipropionate	0.05%
• Betamethasone valerate	0.05%
Hydrocortisone17-butyrate 1 mg/g	
• Hydrocortisone 1% with urea	
• Fluocortolone hexanoate	0.25%
• Flurandrenolone	0.05%
Lowest Potency	
• Hydrocortisone	1%
• Hydrocortisone	0.05%
• Aclometasone dipropionate	0.05%
• Fluocinolone acetonide	0.0025%

ADVERSE EFFECTS

With the introduction of super-high-potency topical corticosteroids, the potential for both local and systematic side effects has increased (Table 66-2). The side effects of topical corticosteroids can be either local or systemic. Increased percutaneous penetration of superpotent topical steroids leads to adverse systemic effects such as suppression of the hyphothalamic-pituitary-adrenal (HPA) axis.[5] Cushing syndrome as a result of superpotent topical corticosteroid use has been reported.[6] Local side effects of topical corticosteroids are listed in Table 66-3.

TABLE 66-3
Side Effects of Topical Steroid Use

Epidermal atrophy
Hypertrichosis lanuginosa
Striae distensae
Steroid purpura
Telangectasia
Miliaria
Steroid dermatitis
Steroid induced acne.
Steroid induced rosacea
Perioral dermatitis
Hyper- and hypopigmentation
Granuloma gluteale infantum
Folliculitis
Tinea incognito
Opportunistic skin infections
Delayed wound healing
Tachyphylaxis

ABUSE OF TOPICAL STEROIDS

Improper use of steroids can induce a variety of iatrogenic cutaneous conditions. In Africa, there is widespread abuse of topical steroids as skin lighting creams with or without hydroquinone (Figure 66-2).

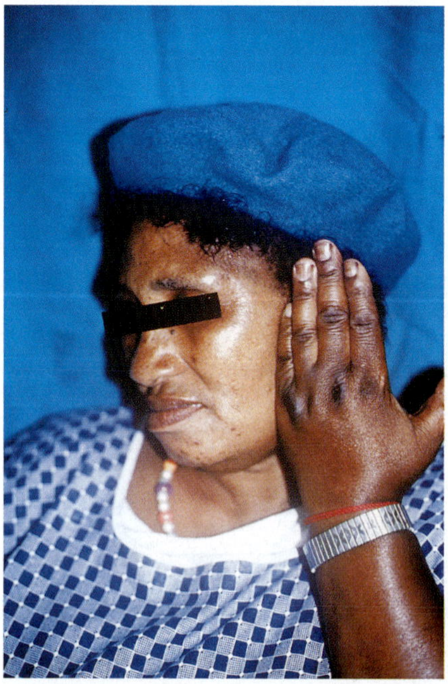

▲ **FIGURE 66-2** Skin lightening owing topical steroids. Note that the face is lighter than the hand.

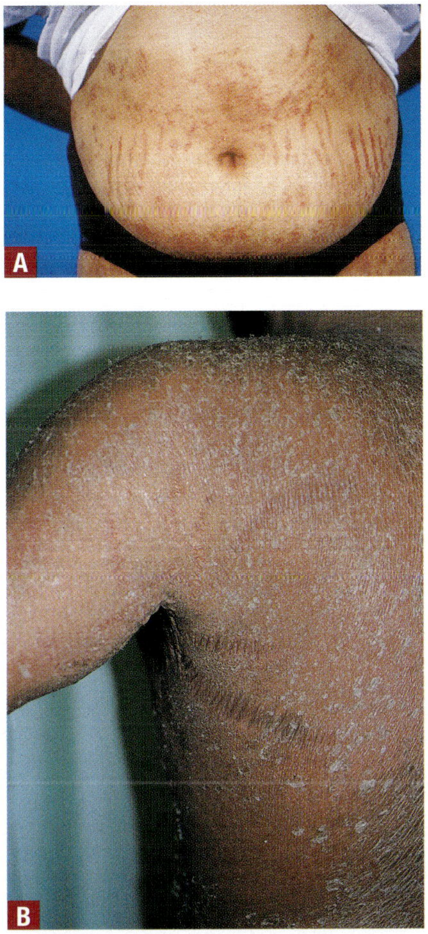

▲ **FIGURE 66-3** *A.* Steroid-induced striae on the abdomen. Courtesy of King Edward Hospital. *B.* Steroid- induced striae on the axilla.

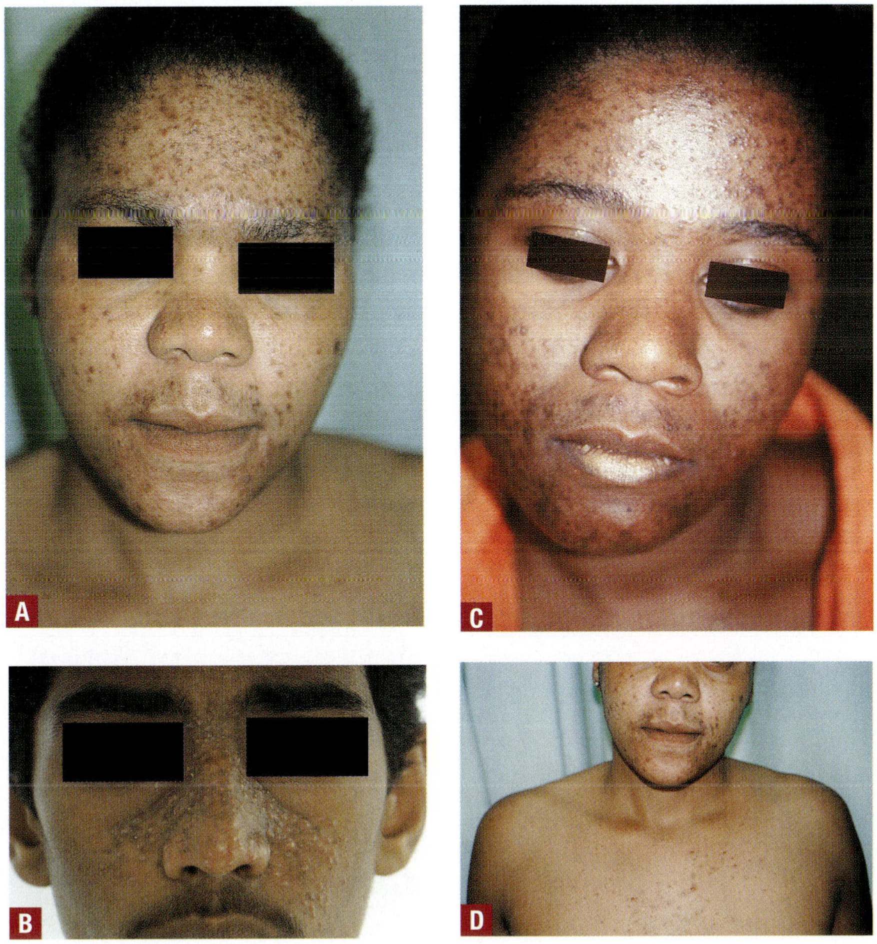

▲ **FIGURE 66-4** Steroid-induced acne. *A, B, C.* Face. *D.* Anterior chest.

Striae and atrophy commonly occur on the groin and axilla and unfortunately are irreversible (Figure 66-3). Steroid acne usually occurs in early adulthood, in elderly patients, and rarely in adolescents (Figure 66-4). It is characterized by monomorphic crops of dense, inflamed pustules and papules. The ability of topical steroids to induce acne is directly related to the potency class of the steroid. Response of steroid-induced acne to antiacne therapy, however, may take longer than that of acne vulgaris. Perioral dermatitis induced by steroids usually improves with cessation of the steroid. Steroid rosacea also may complicate abuse of steroids, particularly in patients who have a predisposition to rosacea and blush easily (Figure 66-5). An eruption of acneiform lesions causes anxiety for the patient, which results in the overenthusiastic application of topical steroids to try to control the acne. An attempt to withdraw the topical steroids at this stage provokes a full-blown rebound eruption, which results in a vicious cycle.

Steroid dermatitis is another common manifestation of steroid abuse that is seen in South Africa (Figure 66-6). Usually one finds intermingled elements such as epidermal atrophy, telangectasias, burning,

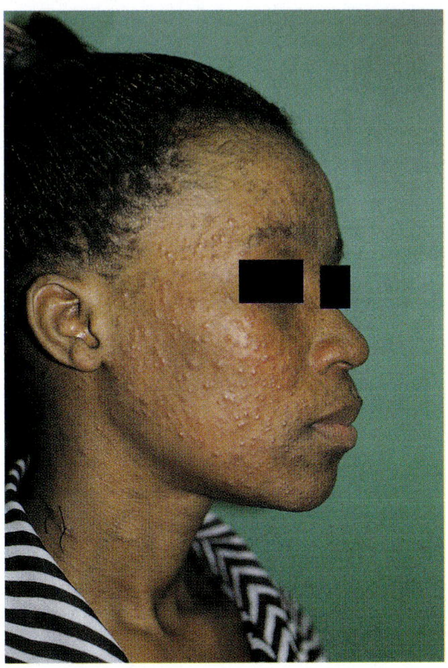

▲ **FIGURE 66-5** Steroid-induced rosacea.

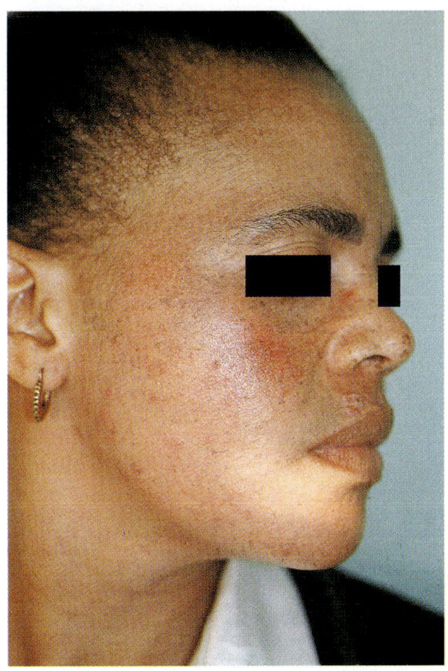

▲ **FIGURE 66-6** Steroid-induced dermatitis.

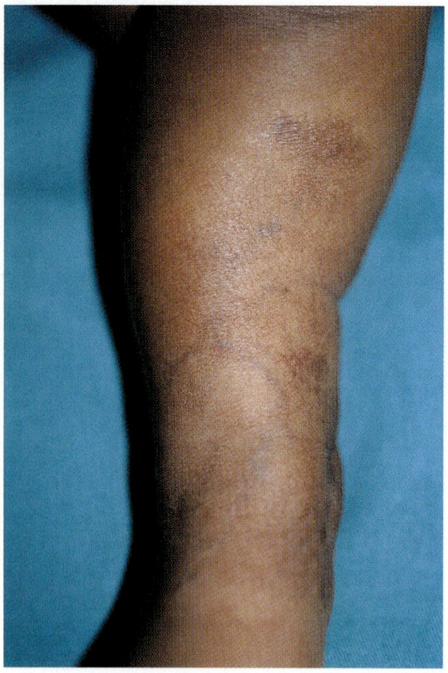

▲ **FIGURE 66-7** Steroid-induced talengiectasia and atrophy.

and stinging with occasional folliculitis and papulopustules without a background of acne or rosacea. Fixed vasodilatation and atrophy sometimes are observed as well (Figure 66-7).

Allergic contact dermatitis has been reported in the literature.[8] This reaction is suspected when there is failure of a steroid-sensitive dermatitis to respond to topical steroid therapy.

DRUG INTERACTIONS

Topical steroids have few, if any, known drug interactions.

PRECAUTIONS

Therapy with topical corticosteroids should be supervised in order to avoid adverse side effects and maximize the therapeutic effects. Proper follow-up and patient education, accompanied by simplified handouts, have been found to be beneficial. Manufacturers of clobetasol propionate do not recommend use of more than 50 g/week in an adult.[9] Systemic side effects with clobetasol are likely to be seen in infants because of their large surface area to body weight ratio compared with adults.[9]

REFERENCES

1. Sulzberger MD, Witten VH. The effect of topically applied compounds in selected dermatoses. *J Invest Dermatol* 1952;19:101.
2. Warner M, Canisa C. Topical corticosteroids, in Wolverton SE (ed), *Comprehensive Dermatologic Drug Therapy*. Philadelphia, Saunders, 2001.
3. Brattsand R. Influence of 16 α,17α acetyl substitution and steroid nucleus fluorination on the topical to systematic activity ratio of corticosteroids. *J Steroid Biochem* 1982;16:779.
4. Catt KJ, Dufau ML. Hormone action: Control of target cell function by peptide, thyroid and steroid hormones, in Felig P, Baxter JD, Broadus AE, et al (eds), *Endocrinology and Metabolism*. New York, McGraw-Hill, 1981, pp 61-105.
5. Walsh P, Aeling JL, Huff L, et al. Hypothalumus-pituitary-adrenalin axis suppression by super potent topical steroids. *J Am Acad Dermatol* 1993;29: 501-503.
6. Gilbertson EO, Spellman MC, Piacquadio DJ, et al. Super potent topical corticosteroid use associated with adrenal suppression: Clinical considerations. *J Am Acad Dermatol* 1998;38: 318-321.
7. Pascal del Giudice, Pinier Yves. The widespread use of skin lightening creams in Senegal: A persistent public health problem in West Africa. *Int J Dermatol* 2002;41:69-72.
8. Lauerna A. Contact hypersensitivity to glucocorticosteroids. *Am J Contact Dermatitis* 1992;3:112-132.
9. Harris DW, Hunter JA. The use and abuse of 0.05% clobetasol propionate in dermatology. *Dermatol Clin* 1988;6: 643-647.

CHAPTER 67

Topical Hydroquinones

Nilesh Morar
Ncoza Dlova

Key Points

- Exogenous ochronosis is a cosmetically induced pigmentation of the skin owing to the deposition of polymerized homogentisic acid in collagen.
- It can occur as a result of prolonged use and application of hydroquinone-containing skin-lightening creams.
- The skin lesions, characterised by coarsening and darkening, are in areas where the cream has been rubbed in effectively and at sites of greatest sun exposure.
- Hydroquinone concentrations above 5% increase the incidence of side effects without improving the efficacy of bleaching.
- Once pigmentation has occurred, there is no effective treatment.

Hydroquinone (HQ) is still a widely used hypopigmenting agent in dermatology. In South Africa, HQ-containing products were widely abused, which resulted in several adverse reactions. Most notably, the use of HQ at concentrations of 3.5–7.5% for many years resulted in an epidemic of exogenous ochronosis in South Africa. The skin lesions developed over a 6-month to 3-year period. Fortunately, the epidemic is now over, and few new cases are seen, which is attributed to legislation prohibiting over-the-counter (OTC) sale of cosmetics containing more than a 2% concentration of HQ. However, the safety of 2% HQ preparations is being questioned because patients have acquired ochronosis despite using OTC HQ preparations. Safety can be determined not only by the concentration on the label but also by the amount, frequency, and vigor of application.

In the United States, the Food and Drug Administration (FDA) approved the OTC HQ up to 2% concentration and 3–4% HQ concentrations under a doctor's supervision. This decision was based on Findlay's documentation in 1975, which highlighted that 3.5–7.5% concentrations of HQ caused exogenous ochronosis.[1] In 2007, the FDA proposed a ban on OTC HQ-containing products and a requirement for an approved drug application for all prescription-strength HQ preparations. The proposed ban was based on possible safety concerns. A ban of this type would severely limit the availability of HQ in the United States.

BACKGROUND

Ochronosis is a descriptive term initially coined by Virchow in 1866 in describing pigmentation in the knee and hip joints in a 67-year-old man that was blue-black on macroscopic examination but ochre-colored histologically. Exogenous ochronosis is a cosmetically induced pigmentation of the skin from the abuse of mainly HQ-containing creams owing to the deposition of polymerized homogentisic acid in collagen. It also occurs following use of antimalarials and products containing phenol, mercury, picric acid, and resorcinol. Exogenous ochronosis was first reported in 1906 from the prolonged use and absorption of phenol. Endogenous ochronosis owing to alkaptonuria is a different entity, owing to the lack of homogentisic acid oxidase, where homogentisic acid accumulates in various organs, including the sclera, skin, cartilage, tendons, and heart valves.

EPIDEMIOLOGY

Exogenous ochronosis occurring as a consequence of topical application of HQ-containing skin-lightening creams was described for the first time in South Africa by Findlay in 35 black women.[1] The largest number of cases were seen in South Africa, where epidemic proportions were reached owing to lack of regulation and indiscriminate use of HQ. There are several published papers[1–7] on this entity from South Africa, the largest being that by Phillips and colleagues,[4] in which, over a period of 1 year, 395 patients with ochronosis were seen in Johannesburg. In Findlay's series,[1] all patients presenting to dermatology clinics were black women between 30 and 39 years of age (this higher age is due to slow emergence of the disorder) who had used these preparations for prolonged periods of up to 8 years. The concentrations used ranged from 3.5–7.5%, and the skin lesions developed over a period of 6 months to 3 years.

In South Africa, the epidemic is now over, and few new cases are seen. This could be attributed to legislation prohibiting OTC sale of cosmetics containing more than 2% HQ.

Exogenous ochronosis was first described in blacks in the United States in 1983.[8] Here, the condition is reported to be rare, with only eight cases being described to date.[8–13] The mean age of patients in these reports was 49.5 years, with all patients being women, and the majority of the Negroid race. It also has been reported to occur in Hispanics and Caucasians.[11,14] Bleaching creams in concentration of 1–4% were used for 3 months to 3 years prior to the onset of the lesions. This differed from the South African patients, in whom higher concentrations of HQ of up to 7.5% were used in some reports.[4]

The reason why exogenous ochronosis is relatively uncommon in the United States is unclear. It could be the result of skin care products containing resorcinol in combination with HQ or the use of HQ in a hydroalcohol lotion in Africa.[14]

PATHOGENESIS

Individuals use HQ-containing creams to brighten or lighten their complexions. HQ creams are also used to treat postinflammatory hyperpigmenation, melasma, lentigines, and freckles. Although these creams are called *bleaching creams,* they do not significantly bleach pigment but instead inhibit melanin formation, blocking the conversion of tyrosine to melanin. HQ inhibits melanogenesis in vitro and in vivo. Lightening effects can be seen in concentrations as low as 1.5%. Using patch-test trials over a 6-year period, it was proposed that 3% was the optimal HQ concentration for use in lightening creams.[5] Concentrations above 5% increase the incidence of side effects without improving efficacy. The success of these preparations is confined to pigmentary changes in the epidermis. The preparations oxidize easily at pH > 6 and lose potency after about 2 months.

The exact pathogenesis of exogenous ochronosis is unclear, although several theories exist. Findlay and colleagues suggested that prolonged applications of HQ, together with sun stimulation, causes melanocytes to overcome the damaging effects of HQ and become overactive.[1] HQ enters the papillary dermis and is taken up by fibroblasts, resulting in abnormal fiber production.

It has been suggested that melanin-HQ complexes form ochronotic pigment and that the melanocyte is the essential cell for developing ochronosis. This may explain why patients with lighter skin pigmentation may not readily develop clinical lesions because of subthreshold quantities of melanin-HQ complexes being formed. Penneys proposed a different pathogenetic theory for exogenous ochronosis similar to that in alkaptonuria—that HQ applied topically could inhibit cutaneous homogentisic acid oxidase activity, resulting in localized accumulation and polymerization of homogentisic acid and hence ochronotic pigment.[15]

There also may be genetic factors that predispose blacks to developing this condition. This may explain why Caucasians with this entity have not been reported, despite the widespread use of HQ bleaching creams for the treatment of melasma, lentigines, and ephelides.

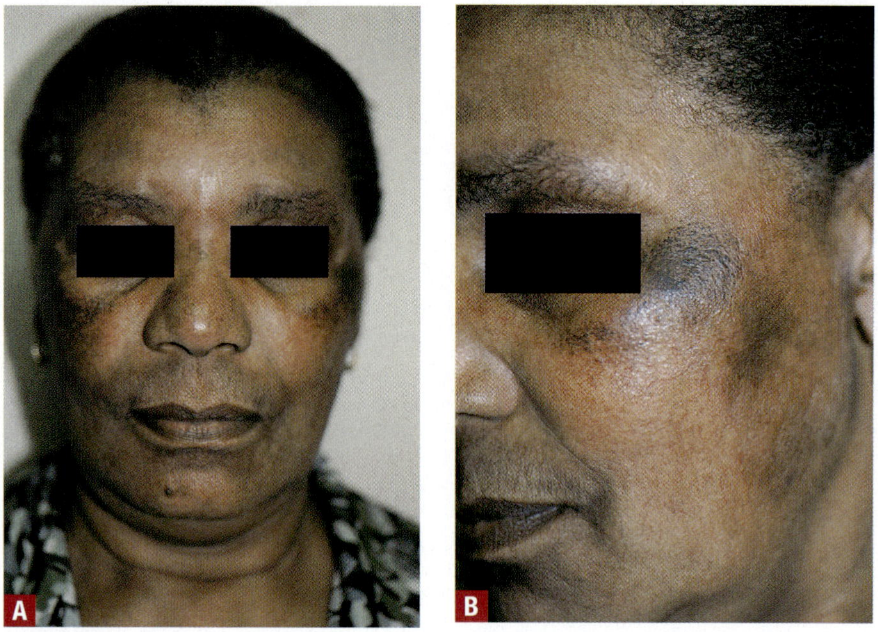

▲ **FIGURE 67-1** Sooty pigmentation with areas of erythema and mild hyperpigmentation.

PREPARATIONS

In 1975, Kligman reported a formula containing 5% HQ, 0.1% dexamethasone, and 0.1% tretinoin that was effective for the treatment of melasma, ephelides, and postinflammatory hyperpigmentation. This preparation tended to darken owing to oxidation when stored for more than 1 month.

Several other variants formed by the addition of tretinoin, salicylic acid, and corticosteroids also may be used, for exaqmple, 0.05% tretinoin cream, 0.1% betamethasone valerate, and 2% HQ daily or 2% salicylic acid, 5% HQ, and 0.05% desonide cream. With all these formulations, strict sun protection is advised.

CLINICAL FEATURES

There are three clinical stages of exogenous ochronosis, each of which may coexist in individual patients. Phillips and colleagues described mild ochronotic changes of coarsening and darkening of the skin with minute black papules, moderate ochronosis with large black papules, and severe ochronosis composed of intensely black caviar-like larger coalescent papules.[3] According to Dogliotti, there are three stages, with stage 1 being characterized by erythema and mild reticulate, ripple-like sooty pigmentation with paler normal skin in between[16] (Figure 67-1). Stage 2 is characterized by black colloid milium-like or caviar-like papules that are darker than normal skin and which range from gray to black with mild atrophy (Figure 67-2). Stage 3 lesions are papulonodular

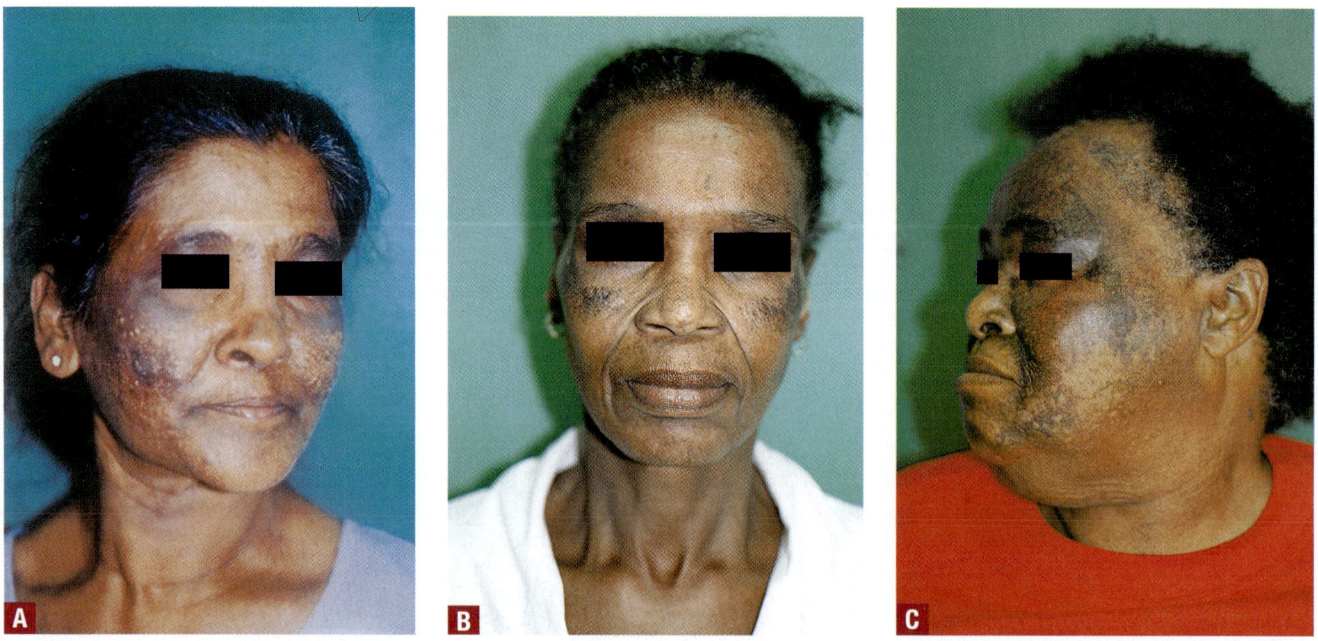

▲ **FIGURE 67-2** Black colloid milium–like papules.

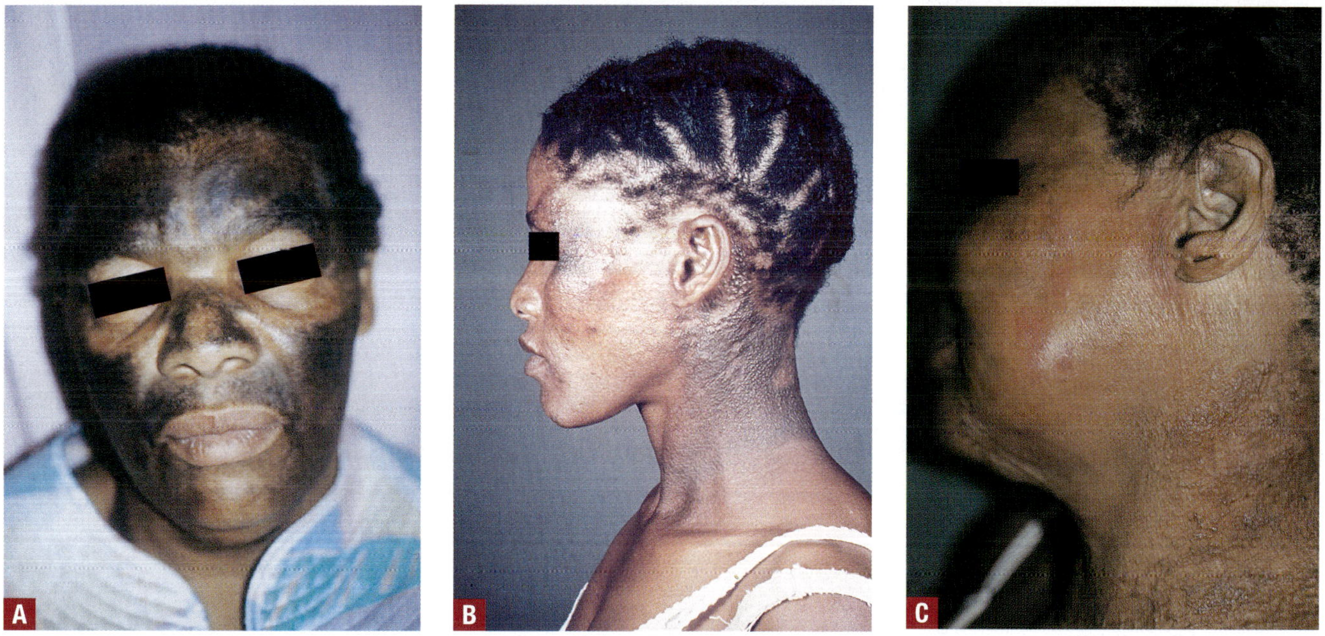

▲ **FIGURE 67-3** Papulonodular lesions on the face and neck where cream has been rubbed.

(Figure 67-3). The lesions classically occur in areas where the cream has been applied and that have received the greatest sun exposure. On the face, these are typically over the bony prominences—forehead, temples, nose, malar area, lower cheeks, and lower jaws. The lateral aspects of the neck are also affected. The lesions also can be accentuated where the cream remains "trapped," for example, the eyebrows, creases around eyes, and the cavity of the pinna. HQ also may cause brown pigmentation of the nails owing to deposition in the nails during application of the cream.

Allergic sensitisation to HQ also can occur, and this can be tested using freshly prepared 1% HQ in petrolatum and a standard closed patch test. Most reactions, though, are irritant, and this is more common with the higher concentrations used.

HISTOLOGY

The histologic features of exogenous ochronosis are mainly confined to the papillary dermis.[1,3] Melanophages are observed in the upper dermis. The changes in exogenous ochronosis arise from the breakdown of normal collagen. Collagen fibers become basophilic and then yellow or ochronotic, forming amorphous eosinophilic material (ochronotic colloid milium); the fibers are curved and banana-shaped and may have transverse fracturing. A variable cellular infiltrate is seen consisting of fibroblasts, macrophages, lymphocytes, and epitheliod or giant cells. Although the initial basophilic fibers are similar to solar elastoses, they are morphologically different because in solar elastosis the fibers are short, curved, and irregularly oriented. The yellow ochronotic fibres do not stain as elastic fibres. The colloid milia seen in ochronosis from HQ bear no resemblance to colloid milia owing to sun damage, which appear more filamentous and have elastic fibers as their precursors.

Other histologic types show a granulomatous infiltrate of the foreign-body type reaction, imitating sarcoidosis owing to a reaction to the ochronotic particles and transepidermal elimination of ochronotic material.[6,16] Clinical stages 1 and 2, described by Dogliotti, correspond to the histologic features of hyperkeratosis, epidermal thinning, melanocyte depletion, pigmentary incontinence, and ochronotic material in the dermis.[16] Stage 3 demonstrated sarcoid-like granulomas attached to ochronotic material (Figure 67-4).

ELECTRON MICROSCOPY

In exogenous ochronosis, the collagen bundles lose their normal banding pattern and become variable in diameter.[3] The fibrils are electron dense, which corresponds to the yellow ochronotic fibers seen on light microscopy. Breakdown of the electron-dense material near the periphery of the collagen fibers form electron-dense material corresponding to the eosinophilic miliary material.

TREATMENT

Treatment is difficult and is mainly aimed at avoiding the offending agent. A number of techniques such as dermabrasion and the use of the carbon dioxide or Q-switched alexandrite lasers have been tried, but controlled studies are required to determine the true efficacy of these treatments.

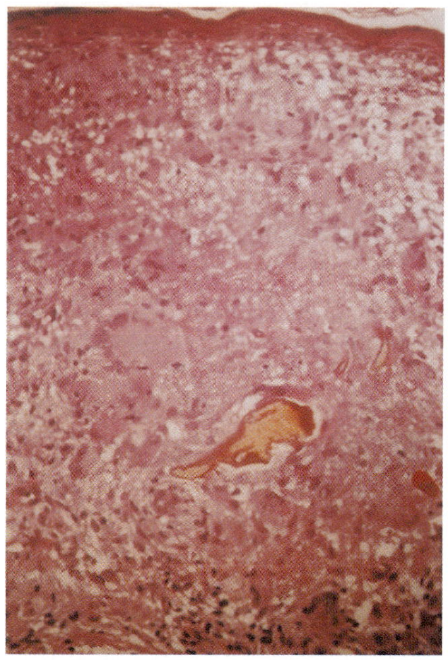

FIGURE 67-4 Ochronotic material in the dermis with sarcoid-like granulomas attached to ochronotic material.

CONCLUSION

HQ products are widely used in skin of color populations throughout the world. They are used commonly in South Africa as well as in the United States as a hypopigmenting agent. It is thought that frequency of use, concentration of the active ingredient, intensity of sun exposure, and possibly genetics may account for the differences in occurrence of exogenous ochronosis in these two countries.

REFERENCES

1. Findlay GH, Morrison JGL, Simonson IW. Exogenous ochronosis and pigmented colloid milium from hydroquinone bleaching creams. *Br J Dermatol* 1975;93:613-622.
2. Findlay GH. Ochronosis following skin bleaching with hydroquinone. *J Am Acad Dermatol* 1982;6:1092-1093.
3. Phillips JI, Isaacson C, Carmen H. Ochronosis in black South Africans who use skin lighteners. *Am J Dermatopathol* 1986;8:14-21.
4. Findlay GH, De Beers HA. Chronic hydroquinone poisoning of the skin from skin-lightening cosmetics. *S Afr Med J* 1980;57:(6)187-190.
5. Bentley- Phillips B, Bayles MH. Cutaneous reactions to topical applications of hydroquinone. *S Afr Med J* 1975; 49: 1391-1395.
6. Jordaan HF, Van Niekerk DJT. Transepidermal elimination in exogenous ochronosis. *Am J Dermatopathol* 1991; 13:418-424.
7. Jacyk W. Annular granulomatous lesions in exogenous ochronosis are manifestations of sarcoidosis. *Am J Dermatopathol* 1995;17:18-22.
8. Cullison D, Abele DC, O'Quinn JL. Localized exogenous ochronosis: A report of a case and review of the literature. *J Am Acad Dermatol* 1983;8:882-889.
9. Hoshaw RA, Zimmerman KG, Menter A. Ochronosis like pigmentation from hydroquinone bleaching creams in American blacks. *Arch Dermatol* 1985;121: 105-108.
10. Connor T, Braunstein B. Hyperpigmentation following use of bleaching creams. *Arch Dermatol* 1987; 123:105.
11. Howard KL, Furner BB. Exogenous ochronosis in a Mexican-American woman. *Cutis* 1990;45:180-182.
12. Lawrence N, Bligard CA, Reed R, et al. Exogenous ochronosis in the United States. *J Am Acad Dermatol* 1988;18: 1207-1211.
13. Fisher AA. Tetracycline treatment for sarcoid-like ochronosis due to hydroquinone. *Cutis* 1988;18 1207-1211.
14. Levin CY, Maibach H. Exogenous ochronosis: An update on clinical features,causative agents and treatment options. *Am J Dermatol* 2001;2:213-217.
15. Penneys NS. Ochronosis-like pigmentation from hydroquinone bleaching creams. *Arch Dermatol* 1985;121: 1219-1240.
16. Dogliotti M, Leibowitz M. Granulomatous ochronosis: A cosmetic-induced skin disorder in blacks. *S Afr Med J* 1979;56: 757-760.

SECTION 11

Cutaneous Manifestations of Systemic Diseases

CHAPTER 68

Cutaneous Manifestations of Systemic Diseases

Lynn McKinley-Grant
Meredith Warnick
Saurabh Singh

Key Points

- The importance of early recognition of the cutaneous signs of systemic diseases that have a high morbidity and mortality in people of color will be discussed in this chapter.
- Each section describes the disease and discusses the epidemiology and genetics, clinical findings, and treatment.
- Clinicians can use the clinical findings and clinical photographs to increase their diagnostic acumen of systemic diseases in patients of color.

Cutaneous manifestations of systemic diseases are seen daily in the practice of all medical specialties. The U.S. Census Bureau projects that by the year 2050, the U.S. population will shift from 75–50.1% white, the Latino/Hispanic population will increase to 24.4%, the African-American population to 14.6%, and the Asian-American population to 8%.[1] The patient population seen by health care providers will change. All the systemic diseases discussed in this chapter can be detected by a physician who is aware of the clinical manifestations of systemic diseases in skin of color.

Many systemic diseases associated with skin manifestations are also associated with higher morbidity and mortality rates in people of color. For example, the incidence of type 2 diabetes, renal disease, sarcoidosis, lupus, hepatitis C, and sickle cell anemia are higher in African-Americans than in Caucasians. The incidence of diabetes, systemic lupus, chronic liver disease, and thyroid disease are higher in Latinos than in Caucasians. Thyroid cancer occurs more often in the Asian population than in Caucasians, and East Asians have demonstrated more cases of systemic lupus erythematosus (SLE) than Caucasians in Hawaii and Asia. Unfortunately, people of color tend to be diagnosed with many systemic diseases at a later stage than Caucasians, when the disease is less treatable because of the advanced stage, partly because of socioeconomic factors and lack of access to health care.

Discussed in this chapter are the systemic diseases that have a high morbidity and mortality in people of color and present with early and late dermatologic findings. This chapter also includes systemic diseases that have different and distinct skin findings based on skin color and race

DIABETES MELLITUS

An estimated 19–20 million Americans have type 2 diabetes, and approximately one-third are unaware of their condition.[3] Diabetes is classified by type: Type 1 diabetes is a disease characterized by complete lack of insulin secretion. Type 2 diabetes is a disease in which there is impaired insulin secretion and/or insulin resistance, which often occur simultaneously. The primary contributing factor to the increase in type 2 diabetes is obesity.

Epidemiology

- Type 2 diabetes is the most common form of diabetes, accounting for up to 95% of cases, and almost always occurs in overweight or obese individuals.[2]
- While type 2 diabetes occurs most commonly in adulthood, pediatric type 2 diabetes is becoming increasingly common as obesity becomes a growing problem in children and adolescents.
- African-Americans have a higher prevalence of type 2 diabetes than other racial groups. In 2005, the age-adjusted prevalence in the African-American population was 8.2 per 100 persons compared with 7.3 per 100 in Hispanic Americans and 5 per 100 in Caucasian Americans.[5]
- From 30% to greater than 80% of patients with diabetes mellitus report some sort of dermatologic symptom.[2,6]

Etiology/Genetics

- Type 1 diabetes is caused by autoimmune destruction of the insulin-producing beta cells and a total lack of insulin.
- Type 2 diabetes is caused by a range of abnormalities, some of which are genetic in nature.[7]

Clinical Findings

Infections of the skin can be the earliest presenting sign of diabetes mellitus. They include:

- *Candida albicans*—intertrigo, vaginitis, and balanitis (Figure 68-1)
- Corynebacterium minutissimum—Erythrasma

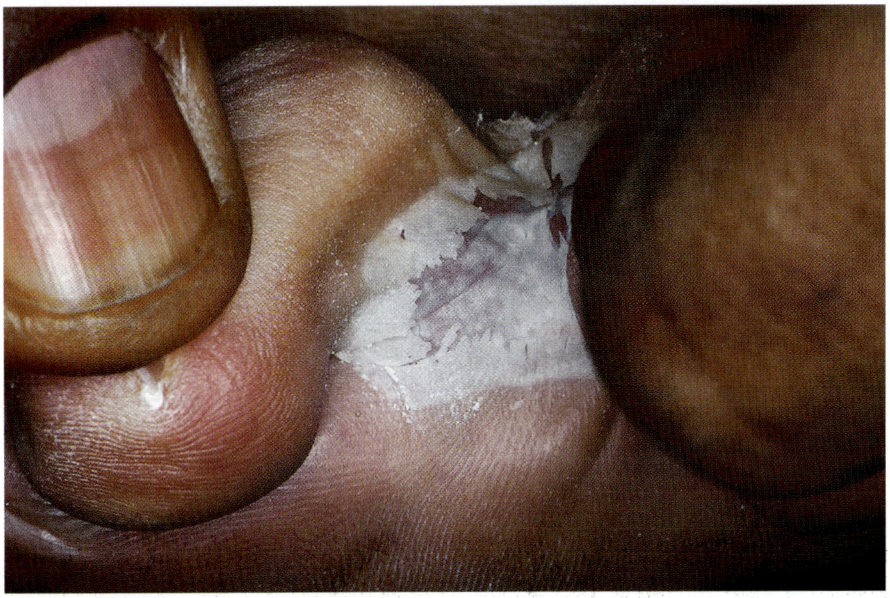

▲ **FIGURE 68-1** Intertrigo. Courtesy of Department of Dermatology, Washington Hospital Center, Washington DC.

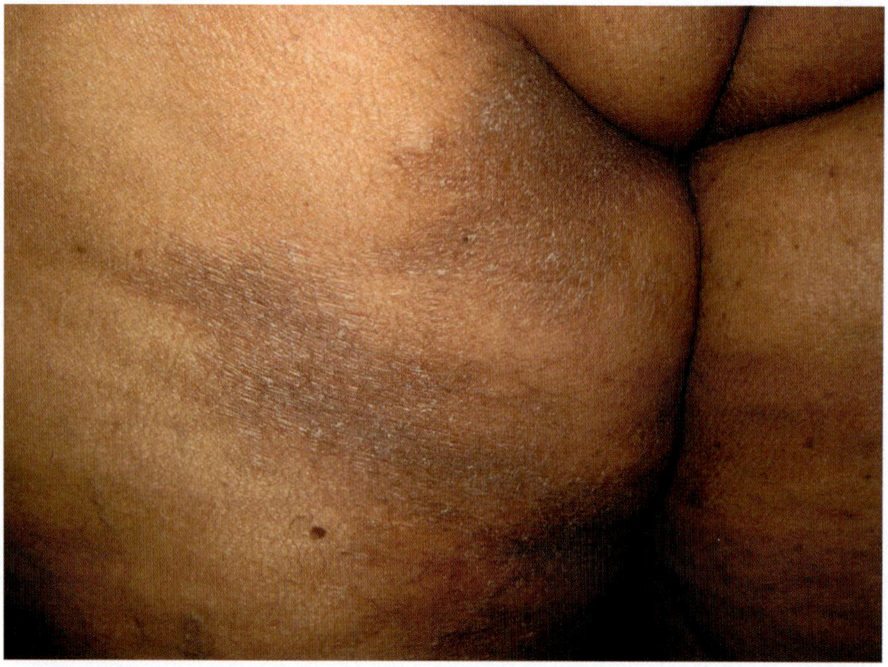

▲ **FIGURE 68-2** Tinea corporis. Courtesy of Department of Dermatology, Washington Hospital Center, Washington DC.

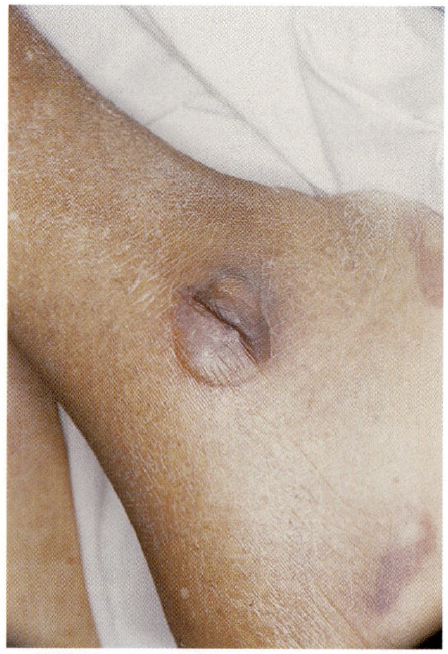

▲ **FIGURE 68-5** Diabetic bulla.

- Tinea corporis with *Trichophyton rubra* (Figure 68-2)
- *Streptococcus, Staphylococcus,* and methicillin-resistant *Staphylococcus aureus* (MRSA) cellulitis and folliculitis
- Necrotizing fasciitis (Figure 68-3)
- Malignant external otitis
- Rare rhinocerebral mucormycosis—elderly present with facial cellulitis, periorbital edema, and fever (fatal)

GRANULOMA ANNULARE (Figure 68-4)

- Very common dermatosis in children
- Controversial association with diabetes

DIABETIC BULLA (Figure 68-5)

- While bullae are seen most often in patients with long-standing diabetes, they are sometimes present when diabetes is diagnosed.
- Bullae occur equally in men and women. The cause is unknown, and onset is often sudden.[2]
- Bullae appear on a pigmented base as round pale-yellow blisters with clear fluid. If the bullae have ruptured, there will be a gray or yellowish flaccid piece of skin overlying a pink base and surrounded by normal brown skin with no inflammation.
- Spontaneous tense serous bullae occur primarily on the lower extremities.
- Bullae are painless and heal without scarring.
- Histology shows that bullae are subepidermal.

DIFFERENTIAL DIAGNOSIS

- Fixed drug eruption
- Porphyria cutanea tarda
- Bullous pemphigoid
- Other autoimmune bullous diseases

LEG AND FOOT ULCERS (Figure 68-6)

- Leg and foot ulcers result from large- and small-vessel disease and inadequate perfusion. They are associated with sensory neuropathy.
- While the cause is often undetermined, ulcers are associated with altered foot biomechanics and limited joint mobility.
- Diabetic skin ulcers have the greatest impact on general health of any cutaneous disease and can lead to gangrene and amputation.
- Leg and foot ulcers are seen in approximately 15% of people with diabetes and are a leading cause of hospitalization in this population.[8]
- The ulcers are non-painful and seen most commonly on the foot.

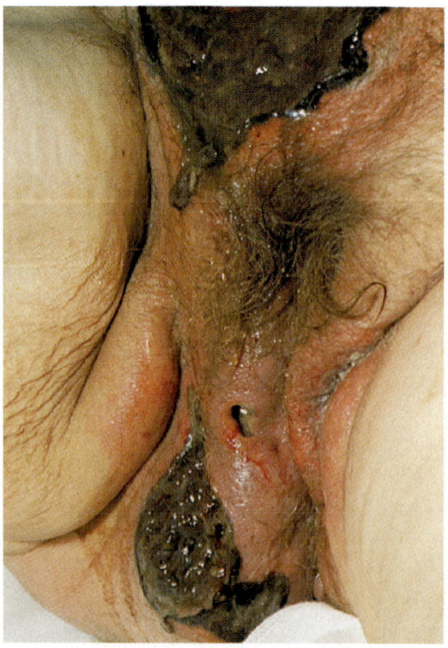

▲ **FIGURE 68-3** Necrotizing fasciitis with MRSA.

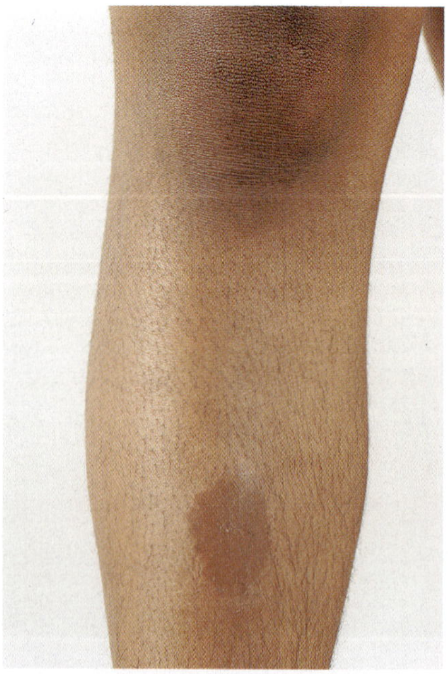

▲ **FIGURE 68-4** Granuloma annulare.

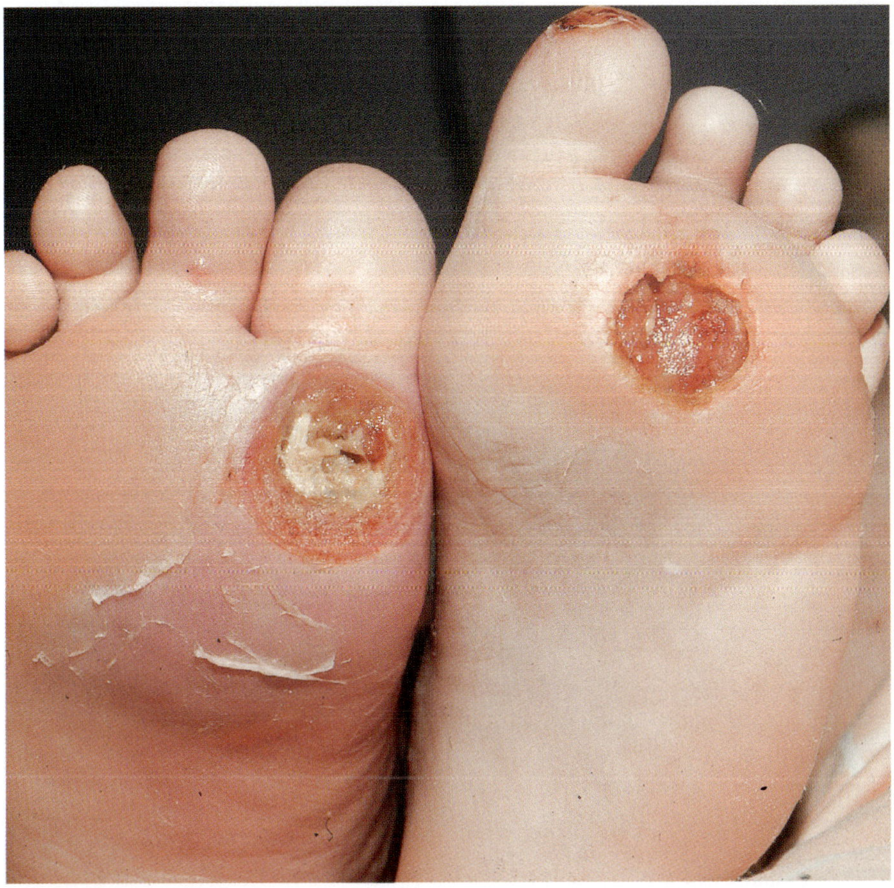

▲ **FIGURE 68-6** Diabatic ulcers.

ACANTHOSIS NIGRICANS (Figure 68-7)

- Acanthosis nigricans (AN) is associated with insulin resistance, obesity, lipodystrophy, and polycystic ovary disease. It can be seen in other hormonal disorders such as acromegaly, Cushing syndrome, and leprechaunism (all insulin resistant). Also seen in internal malignancy.
- The prevalence of AN in children with type 1 diabetes but no evidence of microvascular disease suggests that the condition is not related to microangiopathy.[8]

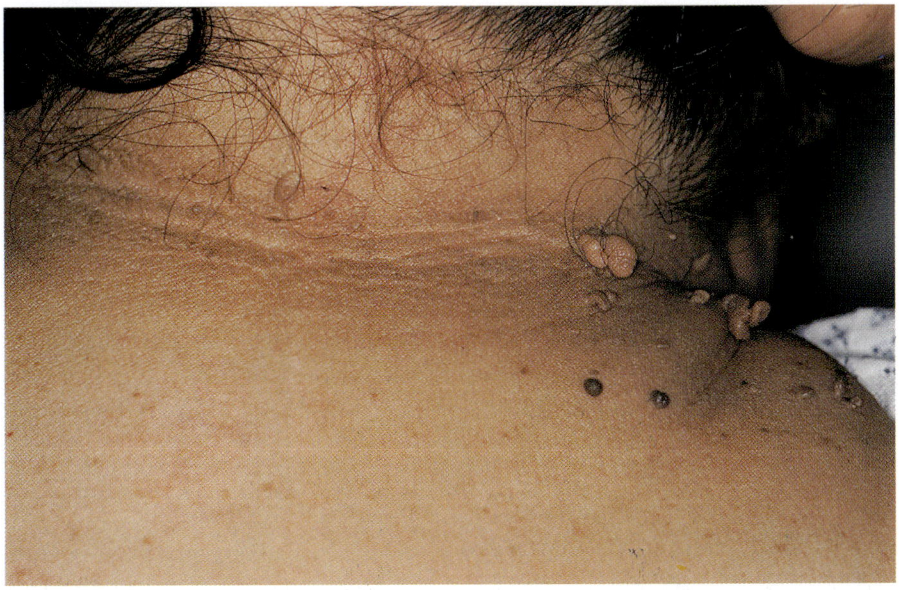

▲ **FIGURE 68-7** Acanthosis nigricans. Courtesy of Department of Dermatology, Washington Hospital Center, Washington DC.

- In adults with type 2 diabetes, the prevalence increases with obesity.[9]
- AN consists of thick velvety hyperpigmented plaques, most commonly in the neck and axillae. It is seen more commonly in skin of color. In African-American skin, the plaques are dark brown to black; in Asian or Hispanic skin, they are light brown to dark brown.
- Histology shows papillomatosis, hyperkeratosis, and acanthosis.

SCLEREDEMA (SCLEREDEMA ADULTUORUM OF BUSCHKE) (Figure 68-8)

- Scleredema is thought to be secondary to glycosaminoglycan and collagen deposition. It is usually seen in obese patients with poor glycemic control and is 10 times more common in men than in women.[8]
- Scleredema is characterized by hard, thickened erythematous skin of the upper back, shoulders, and neck. It is slowly progressive, and as it progresses, it can lead to restricted range of motion.[10]
- Histologic examination reveals thickened dermis with subcutaneous fat replaced by connective tissue and increased collagen and glycosaminoglycans.[2]

DIFFERENTIAL DIAGNOSIS

- Scleroderma
- Dermatomyositis

DIABETIC DERMOPATHY (Figure 68-9)

- Diabetic dermopathy is possibly precipitated by trauma, and its frequency increases with age and duration of disease.
- This is seen more commonly in people with type 1 diabetes and elderly patients and in males. It is common and documented in as many as 40% of people with diabetes.[2]
- Diabetic dermopathy presents with hyper- and hypopigmented macules and patches, some with atrophic and hypertrophic scars. It typically occurs on the lower extremities.
- Histology shows thickening of the basement membrane, thickened capillaries in the dermis, and edema of the epidermis and papillary dermis.

NECROBIOSIS LIPOIDICA DIABETICORUM (Figure 68-10)

- Necrobiosis lipoidica diabeticorum (NLD) is a rare condition, seen in

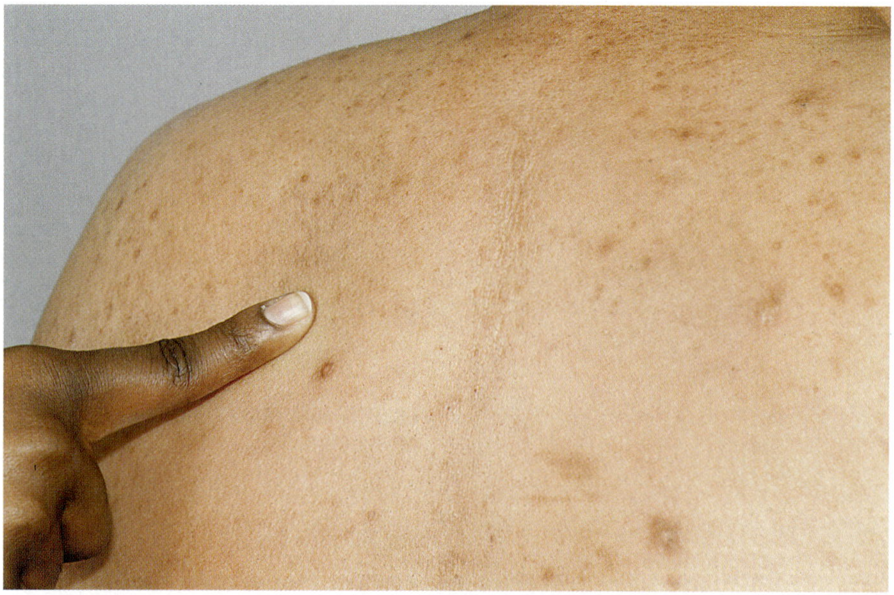

▲ **FIGUTE 68-8** Scleredema.

fewer than 0.5% of people with diabetes, most of them women. It is also seen in people without diabetes.

- NLD typically develops in people in their thirties and may predate the onset of diabetes.[2] Both immune and antibody mediation has been suggested.[8]
- Lesions are seen most often on the anterior tibial surfaces of both lower legs. In pigmented skin, they begin as small yellow to brown to bluish purple patches (depending on the background pigment), with a reddish border and yellowish brown center. As lesions grow, the central area will atrophy and turn waxy, with the outer border darkening. In about one-third of cases, ulceration will occur.[2]
- Lesions subject to trauma are likely to progress to ulceration.[8]
- Histologically, lesions are marked by collagen degeneration as well as granulomatous inflammation of subcutaneous tissues. Inflammation of blood vessels, capillary basement membrane thickening, and obliteration of vessel lumina are also observed.[2]

DIFFERENTIAL DIAGNOSIS

- Pretibial myxedema
- Stasis dermatitis

Treatment

DIABETIC BULLA

- Large bullae may be aspirated if they cause discomfort to the patient.
- Otherwise, treatment is focused on preventing complications, that is, infection.

LEG AND FOOT ULCERS

- Preventive foot care with regular visits to a podiatrist
- Antibiotics
- Surgical grafting
- Hyperbaric oxygen therapy

ACANTHOSIS NIGRICANS

- Primary treatment is tight glycemic control and weight loss. Patients with AN are likely to require much higher insulin doses than are usually given to achieve good control.[9]
- Retinoic acid, α-hydroxy acids, hydroquinones, Nd:YAG laser, cream, and accutane also have been used for treatment.

SCLEREDEMA

- Scleredema in people with diabetes has been found to respond poorly to treatment. Tight diabetic control is currently the best treatment.
- Treatments include intralesional and topical steroids, extracorporeal photopheresis, and psoralen plus ultraviolet A (PUVA) therapy.[2]

DIABETIC DERMOPATHY

- Therapy is focused on prevention of complications, particularly infection.

NECROBIOSIS LIPOIDICA DIABETICORUM (NLD)

- There are reports of successful treatment of NLD with hyperbaric oxygen therapy.[8]
- Intralesional and topical steroids.

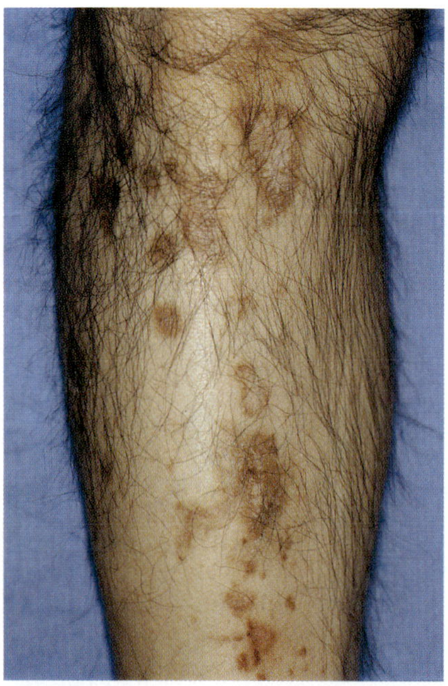

▲ **FIGURE 68-9** Diabetic dermopathy.

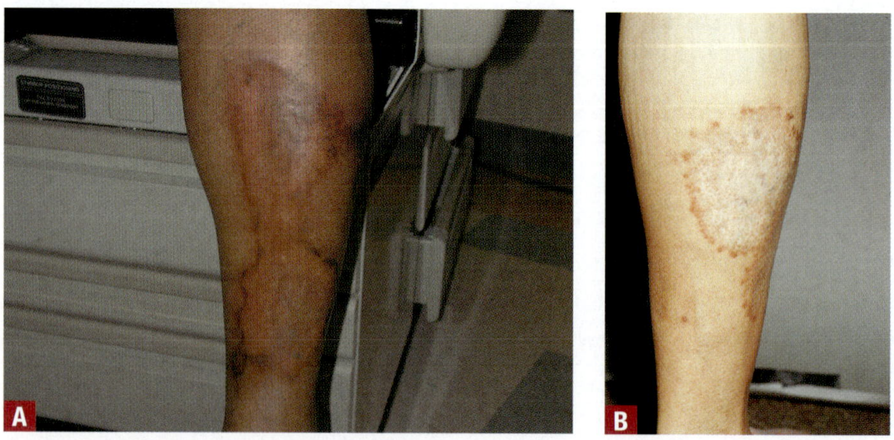

▲ **FIGURE 68-10** **A.** Necrobiosis lipoidica diabeticorum on an anterior tibia. **B.** Red-brown yellowish shiny plaque with dark brown red serpeiginous border with few punctuates lesions with scale and loss of hair follicles. Courtesy of Department of Dermatology, Washington Hospital Center, Washington DC.

THYROID DISEASE

The dermatologist is the first to see patients with hypo- and hyperthyroid disease with common dermatoses such as xerosis, hair loss, hyperhydrosis, brittle nails, and loss of eyebrows. There are several medications that will cause hypothyroidism, and a careful drug history should be taken. Thyroid cancer is seen most commonly in women ages 15–30 and then over 60. It is rarely fatal if detected early. There are several rare syndromes that have cutaneous manifestations and are associated with thyroid cancer.

Definitions

HYPERTHYROIDISM

- Hyperthyroidism is a condition of the thyroid gland in which there is overproduction of thyroid hormone.
- Graves disease is the thyroid disorder most commonly associated with dermatologic manifestations. Graves disease is an autoimmune disorder in which B-lymphocytes produce thyroid-stimulating immunoglobulins that activate the thyroid gland's thyroid-stimulating hormone (TSH) receptor to cause increased thyroid hormone production.[11,12]

HYPOTHYROIDISM

- Hypothyroidism is a condition of the thyroid gland in which there is impaired production of thyroid hormones T_3 (triiodothyronine) and T_4 (thyroxine).[11]
- Most commonly caused by Hashimoto thyroiditis, an autoimmune disorder. Patients with Hashimoto thyroiditis develop antibodies against the thyroglobulin protein and/or the peroxidase enzyme in the thyroid gland.[11]
- Can be primary (e.g., disease of the thyroid gland, previous external radiation to the head or neck, or a partial or total thyroidectomy) or secondary (e.g., disease of the pituitary gland or hypothalamus).[11]
- Autoimmune primary hypothyroidism is the most common type of hypothyroidism.

THYROID CANCER

- Medullary carcinoma
- Papillary carcinoma
- Anaplastic carcinoma
- Lymphoma

Epidemiology

HYPERTHYROIDISM

- Several studies have found a lower prevalence of thyroid disease in the African-American population.[13,14]
- Autoimmune thyroid disease is associated with other autoimmune diseases, including vitiligo, alopecia, and diabetes mellitus.[15–17]

THYROID CANCER

- Incidence of thyroid cancer is increasing more rapidly in women than any other cancer, and it is the third most rapidly rising cancer in men.[11]
- Low mortality.
- There is a lower rate of thyroid cancer in African-Americans than in Caucasians.[23]
- Ages 14–45 white non-Hispanics and Asians/Pacific Islanders are at highest risk.[24]

Etiology/Genetics

HYPERTHYROIDISM

- Multinodular goiter, Graves disease, solitary nodule, and thyroiditis

HYPOTHYROIDISM[25]

- Drug-induced—lithium, targretin, interferon-alfa, interleukin 2
- Autoimmune Hashimoto thyroiditis
- Thyroidectomy
- Radiation exposure (external and internal)
- Sarcoidosis

THYROID CANCER

- Radiation exposure (Chernobyl and atomic bombs)

Clinical Findings

HYPERTHYROIDISM

Infiltrative Dermopathy

- Occurs almost exclusively in Graves hyperthyroidism.[11]
- Occurs in only 4% of patients.[18]
- Secondary to glycosaminoglycan deposition in the dermis.[12,19]
- Most commonly occurs on the lower extremities (pretibial myxedema; Figure 68-11).
- Presents as hyperpigmented or violaceous papules and plaques, nonpitting edema, and induration, frequently referred to as a *peau d'orange* appearance.[20]

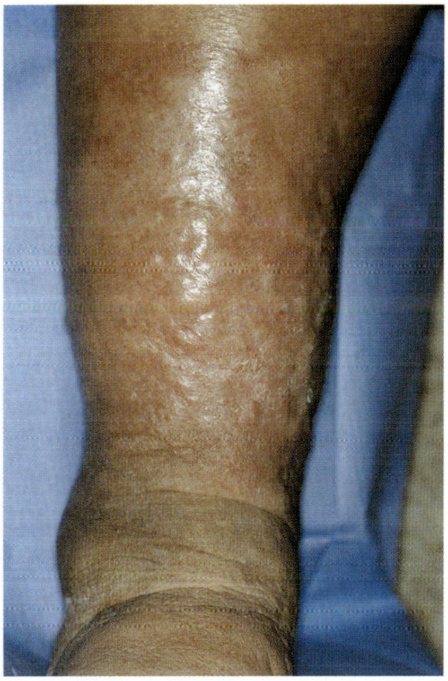

▲ **FIGURE 68-11** Pretibial myxedema. Courtesy of Department of Dermatology, Washington Hospital Center, Washington DC.

- Typically asymptomatic but can cause pruritus and rarely pain.[18]
- Treatment is directed at both pruritus and cosmesis with topical steroids under occlusion.[20,21]

THYROID ACROPACHY

- Occurs in fewer than 1% of patients with Graves disease.[20,22]
- Usually occurs in conjunction with infiltrative dermopathy and ophthalmopathy.[20,22]
- Presents as clubbing and edema of the digits.[20,22]
- Patients also may have a periosteal reaction and pain at the distal bones.[20,22]
- Therapy is limited to treatment of Graves disease and symptomatic treatment if needed.[22]

HYPOTHYROIDISM

Hair/Nails/Skin[12]

- Dry, coarse, brittle
- Skin is also cool to touch
- Hair loss in lateral eyebrows
- Diffuse pattern of nonscarring alopecia

THYROID CANCER Rare syndromes associated with thyroid cancer:

- Multiple endocrine neoplasia (MEN) type 2 is a rare familial disorder caused by mutations in the *RET* protooncogene. MEN 2A is associated with medullary thyroid cancer, whereas MEN 2B is associated with medullary thyroid cancer. MEN 2A and MEN 2B are autosomal dominant and have very high, if not complete, penetrance.[11]

- Carney complex (a very rare autosomal dominant disease), LAMB syndrome (mucocutaneous lentigines, cardiomucocutaneous myxomas, and multiple blue nevi).
- NAME syndrome (nevi, atrial myxoma, mucinosis of the skin, and endocrine overactivity).
- Cowden syndrome (caused by a mutation in the *PTEN* suppressor gene) might be associated with thyroid cancer.
- Gardner syndrome (familial adenomatous polyposis).[11]

Treatment

HYPERTHYROIDISM

- Radioactive iodine
- Antithyroid medications (propylthiouracil/methimazole)
- Partial thyroidectomy

HYPOTHYROIDISM

- Thyroid hormone replacement (levothyroxine)
- Removal of offending medication or toxin

THYROID CANCER

- Early detection of thyroid cancer using physical examination of the neck and other signs of thyroid disease
- Genetic testing if indicated

RENAL DISEASE

All adults and children with renal disease will develop cutaneous manifestations from either the uremic state, the medical treatment, dialysis, or kidney transplant.[26] Many systemic diseases that affect people of color are diseases that have end-organ involvement of the kidney.

Diabetes and hypertension are numbers one and two in the etiology of renal disease in people of color. Other diseases linked to renal problems include connective tissue diseases, SLE, scleroderma, gout, and sickle cell anemia. Medical science has increased the lifespan of people with renal diseases, but with treatment—which can include medications, dialysis, and kidney transplants—dermatologic conditions will develop.

Definitions

ACUTE RENAL FAILURE

- Acute renal failure is a rapid fall in renal function occurring over a period of hours to days.
- It can be a result of prerenal, intrarenal, or postrenal obstruction and is frequently reversible with early intervention.[27]

CHRONIC RENAL FAILURE

- Chronic renal failure is a slowly progressive decrease in renal function.
- It is generally irreversible and, without intervention, progresses to end-stage renal disease (ESRD).[28]

Epidemiology

- Incidence of renal failure in African-Americans in 2004—968 per 1 million population, compared with Caucasian American—263 per 1 million population[29]
- Mean age at therapy initiation for renal failure in African-Americans in 2006—56.4 years, compared with Caucasian Americans—59.6 years[29]
- Diabetes mellitus is the number one cause of renal failure in African-Americans.[29]

Etiology

- Uremia
- Medical treatment for kidney disease
- Hemodialysis and peritoneal dialysis
- Medical treatment for kidney transplantation

Clinical Findings

CUTANEOUS MANIFESTATIONS OF UREMIA[33]

- Generalized xerosis, acquired ichthyosis, and decreased skin turgor
- Pruritus with and without excoriation and lichen simplex chronicus (58–90% undergoing dialysis) (Figure 68-12)
- Pallor from anemia of chronic disease
- Ecchymoses—secondary to decreased platelet function
- Uremic frost—in skin of color, a gray hue to the skin with underlying hyperpigmentation, pallor, and fine scale

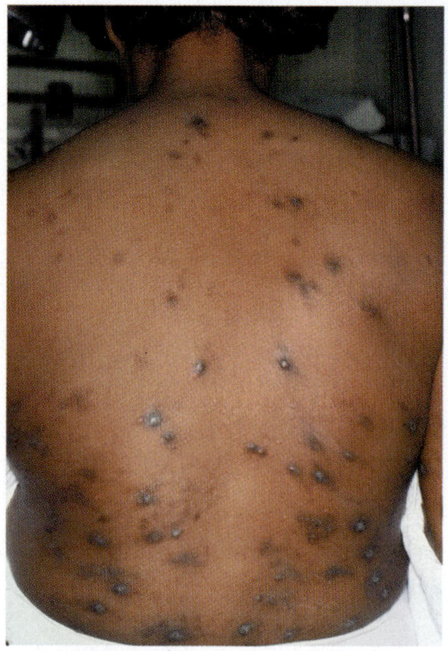

▲ **FIGURE 68-12** Prurigo nodularis. Courtesy of Department of Dermatology, Washington Center, Washington DC.

- Half-and-half nails
- Skin infections—fungal, viral, and bacterial
- Drug eruptions—most commonly penicillin, sulfa drugs, and cephalosporins

CUTANEOUS MANIFESTATIONS OF DIALYSIS

- Graft site complications
- Generalized hyperpigmentation
- Pruritus
- Onychoschizia
- Calcinosis cutis and calciphylaxis (deposition of calcium and phosphate salts in the skin, extruded via transepidermal elimination[31,32]) (Figure 68-13)
  - Lesions are firm papules, plaques, or nodules.[31–33]
  - When extrusion occurs, it appears as white material.[31–33]
  - Occurs primarily in patients with end-stage renal disease.[31,34]
  - Caused by hyperphosphatemia (impaired phosphate clearance) and hyperparathyroidism (hypocalcemia owing to impaired 1,25-dihydroxyvitamin D_3 production).[31–33]

Acquired Perforating Dermatosis (Kyrle's disease) (Figure 68-14)

- Most often found in African-Americans with renal failure.
- Most often associated with diabetes, and usually seen in patients on dialysis.[35]

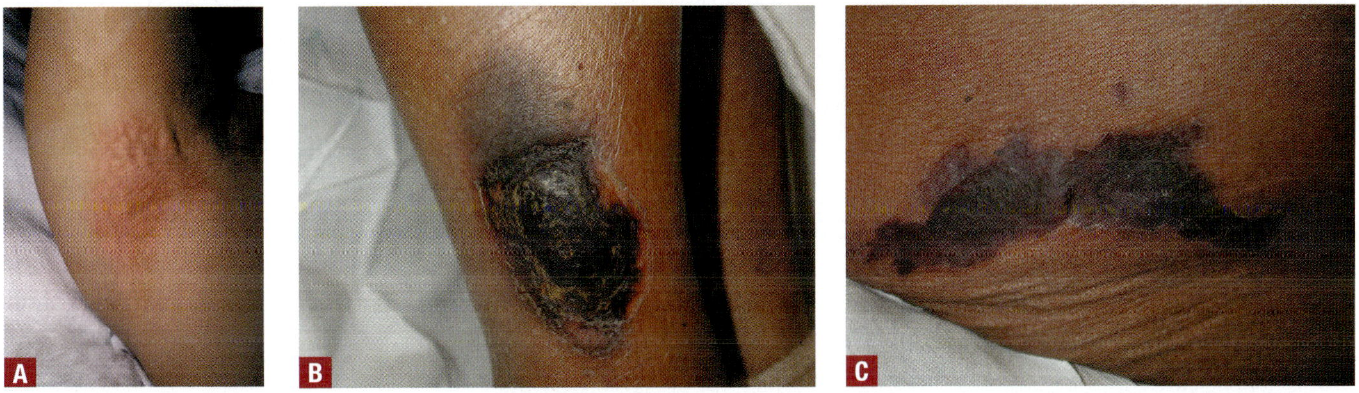

▲ **FIGURE 68-13** **A.** Calcinosis cutis axilla in a Hispanic female. **B.** Calciphylaxis on lower extremity. This is a dermatologic emergency with high mortality in an African-American patient on dialysis with necrotic plaque on edematous erythematous base. **C.** Calciphylaxis on proximal lower extremity. Painful burgundy, necrotic, depressed plaque with acute onset in patient on dialysis. Courtesy of Department of Dermatology, Washington Center, Washington DC.

- Pathogenesis is unknown.[36,37]
- Patients present with pruritic hyperkeratotic papules most commonly on the lower extremities.[37–39]
- Frequently present as hyperpigmented papules.[33]
- Histology shows the epidermis surrounding a plug of necrotic material made up of collagen, elastin, nuclear debris, and leukocytes that is extruded though the epithelium.[37,38]

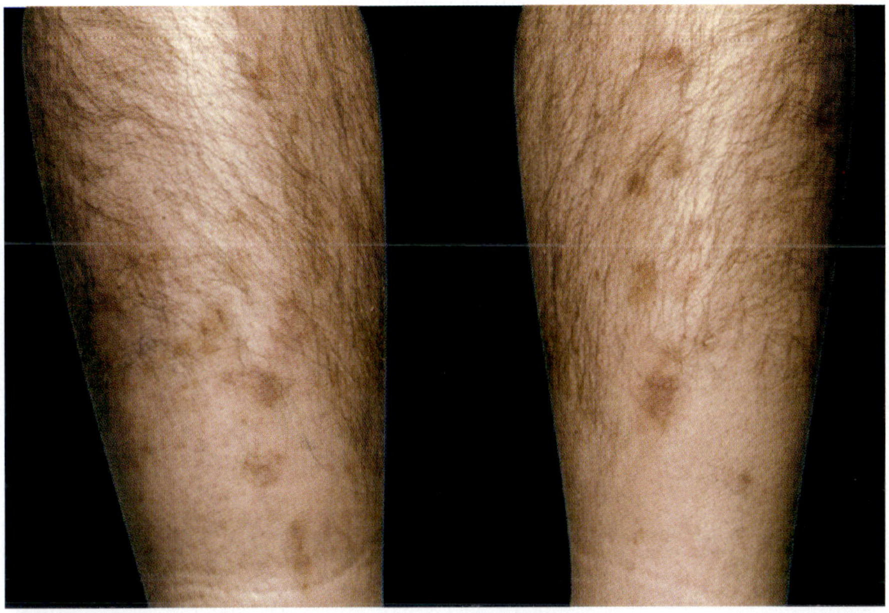

▲ **FIGURE 68-14** Kyrle's disease.

Porphyria Cutanea Tarda (Figure 68-15)

- Uroporphyrinogen decarboxylase deficiency.[33,40,41]
- Occurs in patients with ESRD on dialysis.[33]
- Patients present with noninflammatory vesicles and bullae in a photodistribution.[40,41]
- Vesicles and bullae are subepidermal.[33,41]
- Crusts and erosions are often present, and lesions heal with milia and scars.[33,41]

CUTANEOUS MANIFESTATIONS OF ORGAN TRANSPLANTATION

- More common in Hispanic and African-American children and adults.[26]
- Steroid acne.
- Cushingoid facies and habitus (Figure 68-16)
- Hypertrichosis and gingival hypertrophy secondary to cyclosporine and minoxidil (more common in African-Americans and Hispanics than in Caucasians).
- Palmar warts—secondary to immunosuppression (human papillomavirus [HPV])

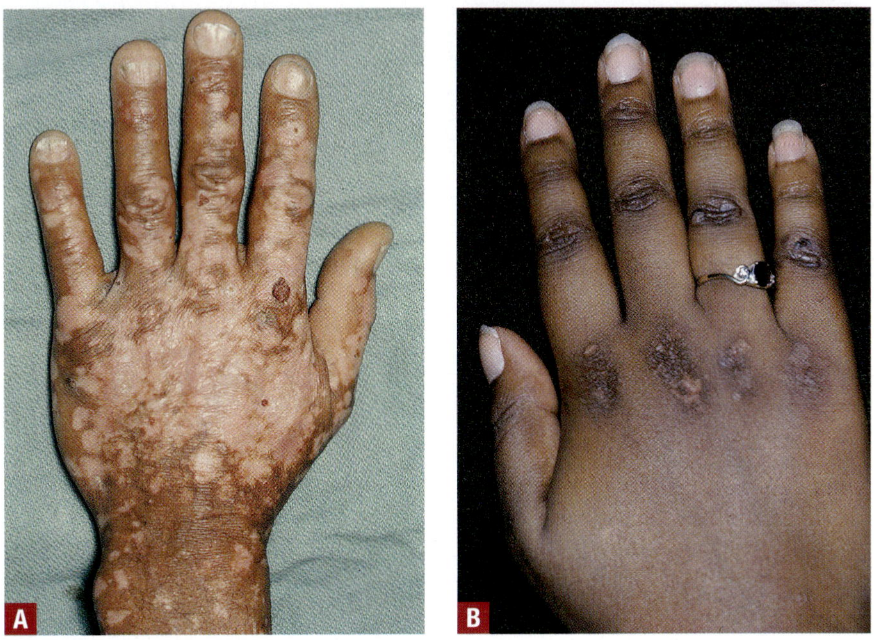

▲ **FIGURE 68-15** **A.** and **B.** Porphyria cutanea tarda.

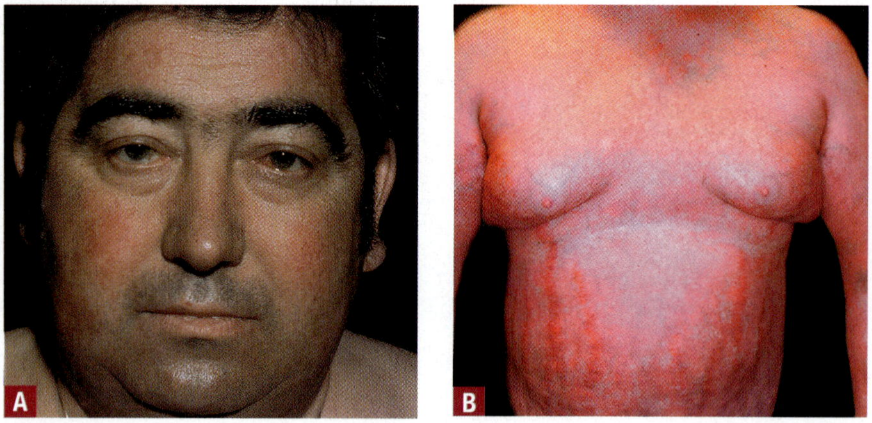

FIGURE 68-16 A. Cushingoid face. B. Stria Hyperplasia.

- Increased number of acral nevi (secondary to immunosuppression).
- Half-and-half nails (Lindsey nails)—distal darkening of the nail bed and proximal white nail.
- Lingual fungiform papillae hypertrophy—secondary to cyclosporine use. Also associated with increased risk of rejection. Resolved with discontinuing cyclosporine.

Diagnosis

- Skin biopsy and/or 24-hour urine or blood for porphyrins or viral or bacterial culture where clinically indicated.

Treatment

PRURITUS AND ACQUIRED PERFORATING DERMATOSIS (KYRLE'S DISEASE)

- No single treatment has proved to be uniformly effective.[33]
- Treatment is difficult and focused on relief of pruritus, including antihistamines, phototherapy, steroids, and retinoids.[33,37]

CALCINOSIS CUTIS/CALCIPHYLAXIS

- Smaller deposits are generally asymptomatic and resolve after correction of phosphate and calcium levels.[33]
- Does not require treatment unless deposits are unusually large.[33]
- A low-phosphate diet is frequently recommended.[31,33]
- Calciphylaxis is a medical emergency and can result in death.

PORPHYRIA CUTANEA TARDA (PCT)

- Patients are photosensitive and should avoid UV light.[33,41]
- Standard treatment for acquired PCT is phlebotomy, which reduces hepatic iron and therefore decreases iron's inhibition of uroporphyrinogen decarboxylase (UROD) oxidation.[40,42]
- Treatment for PCT must be altered in patients with ESRD to smaller volumes for longer periods of time.[33]
- Erythropoietin alone or in addition to small-volume phlebotomy is often recommended for PCT in ESRD patients.[40,44]

NEPHROGENIC SYSTEMIC FIBROSIS

First described in 1997, nephrogenic systemic fibrosis (NSF) is a cutaneous thickening and multiorgan fibrosis in patients with renal failure or renal insufficiency.[45,46] The pathogenesis of NSF is still not known entirely. Gadolinium exposure has been proposed as a precipitating factor, although erythropoietin also has been implicated.[47]

Epidemiology

- First described as a scleromyxedema-like disease in Caucasians and renal dialysis patients from Asia, India, the Middle East, Latin America, and Africa.[52]
- No cases reported before 1997.[46]
- In one study, six of eight patients had previous thrombotic event.[46]
- As of the date of this publication, data not obtained on the ethnicity of patients with NSF. However, we know that there is a higher percentage of people of color on hemodialysis than Caucasians on dialysis. In our clinical experience, 9 of 10 patients diagnosed and/or treated between 2005 and 2008 with extracorporeal photopheresis have been African-American

Etiology/Genetics

- The pathogenesis of NSF is still not known entirely.
- Possible mechanism: Free gadolinium (Gd) dissociates from its chelate in an acidodic environment and interacts with phosphates and other ions, forming a precipitate.[50] It is reported to occur anywhere from 2 days to 18 months after exposure to gadolinium.[51]
- Other mechanisms that have been implicated include bone marrow–derived fibrocytes and transforming growth factor β1 (TGF-β1).[57,58]
- It is also thought that the increased amount of contrast material used in vascular magnetic resonance imaging (MRI) compared to the traditional MRI has contributed to the development of this condition.[50,56]

Clinical Findings

- NSF presents as dark brown to purple indurated papules and plaques that coalesce to cause a diffuse hardening of the skin, woodlike texture, *peau d'orange* plaques, and subcutaneous nodules typically beginning in the lower extremities and moving upward and proximally to involve the trunk and upper extremities[48,57,59] (Figure 68-17).
- NSF can progress to joint contractures and sclerodactyly.[45,60]
- Patients often report pain, burning, and pruritus in affected areas.[45,59]
- Systemic involvement of various organ systems has been reported to include the heart and lungs, kidneys, and muscle.[48–50]
- Gadolinium has been found in the tissues on histology.[65]

Diagnosis

- Clinical history
- Skin biopsy
- Thickening of the reticular dermis and dermal fibrosis with CD34-positive fibrocytes, increased dermal mucin, and thick collagen bundles with surrounding clefts.[45,49,50]
- There is not a sizable lymphocytic infiltrate.[45,49]

Treatment

- Symptoms can persist even with natural improvement in renal failure or

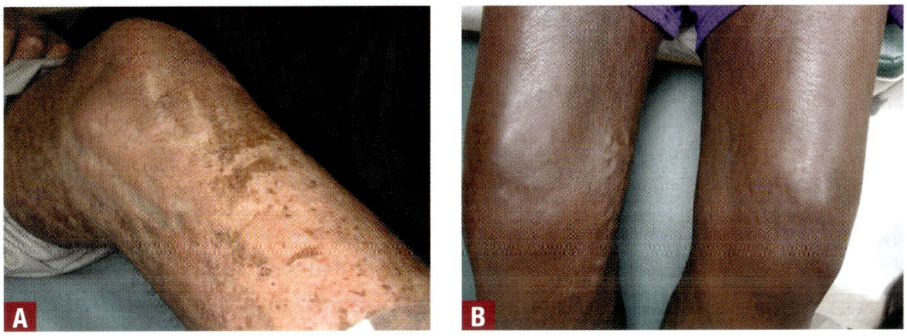

▲ **FIGURE 68-17** **A.** Nephrogenic systemic fibrosis after anasarca in a 23-year-old African-American man with kidney transplant rejection requiring hemodialysis. Clinical findings include a sclerotic band on the medial aspects of the legs and thighs. **B.** Nephrogenic systemic fibrosis of bilateral knees after an MRI in an African-American man on hemodialysis. Note the smooth shiny sclerotic skin with the knees in a fixed position. Courtesy of Department of Dermatology, Washington Center, Washington DC.

with dialysis or renal transplantation.[50,62]

- Extracorporeal photopheresis (ECP) is the most successful treatment in early disease.[46,50,63,65,66]
- Physical therapy.
- ECP and acetretin.
- PUVA.
- Plasmapheresis.
- Methotrexate.
- Thalidomide.
- Imatinib mesylate to reduce fibrosis in mice.[64]

SARCOIDOSIS

Sarcoidosis is a systemic inflammatory, immune-modulated disease involving multiple organs. The disease's etiology is unknown, but evidence suggests that an unknown antigen (e.g., bacterial, viral, or environmental) and a genetic susceptibility interact to initiate the immunologic cascade to produce the noncaseating granulomas most commonly found in the lung, skin, heart, and liver (Figure 68-18).

William Osler published a case in 1884 of a well-nourished 11-year-old black girl with parotid gland swelling and no evidence of tuberculosis (TB) at the time. TB rarely involved the partotid.[7]

Sarcoid skin lesions are classified as specific and nonspecific. Specific lesions reveal noncaseating granulomas on histology. Nonspecific cutaneous eruptions are reactive processes that do not demonstrate granulomas on histology.

Epidemiology

- Sarcoidosis affects all races and ethnicities and occurs on all continents of the world.[67]
- Northern Europe has the highest incidence; Japan, the lowest. High incidence among women across all ethic and racial groups.[67]
- In the United States, sarcoidosis tends to occur in African-Americans in their forties.[67]
- More common in African-Americans (35 cases per 100,000) than whites (10.9 per 100,000) in the United States.[67]

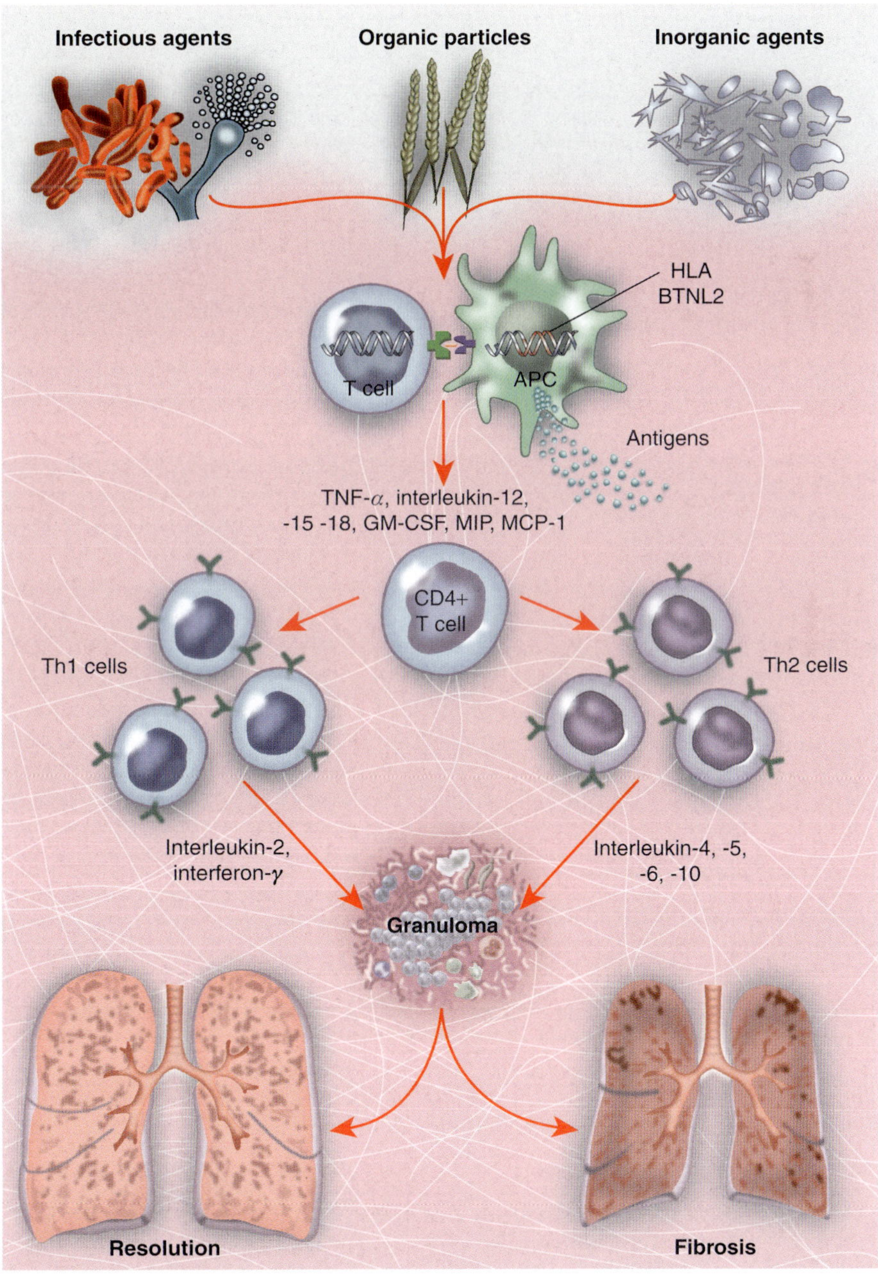

▲ **FIGURE 68-18** Molecular cascade suspected in sarcoidosis.

- Morbidity and mortality are higher in African-Americans than in whites.[67]
- African-Americans are more likely to have skin sarcoidosis (other than nodosum) and eye, liver, bone, and lymph node involvement.[82]
- A study of 165 African-Americans with sarcoidosis in Georgia found that 90% had comorbid illnesses.[68] The most frequent chronic comorbid illnesses were.
  - Hypertension
  - Diabetes mellitus
  - Anemia
  - Asthma
  - Gastroesophageal reflux disease (GERD)
  - Depression
  - Heart failure[75]
- The Georgia study found that females had increased frequency and clustering of chronic illnesses.[75]
- Lower prevalence of sarcoidosis in smokers than in nonsmokers.[68]

Prognosis[70]

- Sixty percent of patients experience spontaneous resolution.
- Between 10% and 20% of cases resolve with steroid use.
- More than 80% of patients with erythema nodosum (EN) and acute inflammatory manifestations of sarcoidosis have spontaneous remissions.
- Between 10% and 20% have a chronic and progressive disease.
- Up to 10% with cardiac and neurologic disease die from this illness.
- Death from sarcoidosis is mostly due to failure of vital organs such as heart and lungs.

Mortality Rates[70]

- 2.1 per 1 million in 1991
- Mortality higher for females and for African-Americans.
- Higher mortality rates in black patients noted in the Middle Atlantic and northern Midwestern states.
- Between 1% and 5% of patients eventually die of the disease.

Etiology/Genetics

- The etiology of sarcoidosis is unknown, but some evidence indicates that an unidentified bacterial, viral, or environmental antigen interacts with a genetic susceptibility to initiate a cascade that produces noncaseating granulomas in the body's major organs, usually the lung, skin, heart, and liver.[70]
- A study of 68 patients with chronic hepatitis C infection found that 66% developed sarcoidosis within 6 months of starting therapy.[69]
- Reported case of an acquired immune deficiency syndrome (AIDS) patient after highly active antiretroviral therapy (HAART) developing sarcoidosis as a manifestation of immune reconstitution inflammatory syndrome.[79,80]
- Environmental and occupational exposures:
  - Farming, raising birds, and teaching middle or high school
  - Exposures to insecticides, pesticides, and damp environments[81]
  - Increased incidence in New York City fire and rescue workers at World Trade Center 2001[67]
- Infectious etiologies reported: *Propionibacterium* and *Mycobacterium* used in animal models to induce granulomas.[71]
- Findings from the A Case Control Etiologic Sarcoidosis Study (ACCESS), sponsored by the National Heart and Lung and Blood Institute (NHLBI) and 10 clinical centers:
  - Although sarcoidosis can be transferred from organ donors and is found in families and people living in close proximity, the ACCESS study shows that sarcoidosis is not an infection (does not follow Koch's postulates).[71]
  - African-Americans, in particular, those with lung-only sarcoidosis, were more likely to have been exposed to burning wood, whereas Caucasians were more likely to have a history of agricultural dust exposure.[72]
  - People with sarcoidosis were more likely than controls to have been educators and to have worked in a school and less likely to have worked in a child-care center.[72]
  - Family clusters of sarcoidosis and differences in incidence by race have been identified.[73]
  - Siblings of patients with sarcoidosis have a risk of sarcoidosis that is about five times higher than that of the general population.[73]
  - Linkage to chromosome 5 in African-American families and to chromosome 6 in German families.[73]
- Based on the ACCESS trial results, an NHLBI working group recommended:
  - Development of a tissue bank
  - Use of new methods to identify genetic factors
  - More research on the disease's development in human and animal models
  - Studies testing new approaches for diagnosing and managing the disease
  - Randomized, controlled trials to assess new therapies[74]
- A study of 225 families in Detroit, Michigan, demonstrated that the angiotensin-converting enzyme, vitamin D receptor, and tumor necrosis factor α genes are not associated with an increased risk of sarcoidosis in African-Americans.[75]
- Genetic susceptibility to sarcoidosis was identified on the *BTNL2* gene.[80]
- A follow-up to the Sarcoid Genetic Analysis study found that in African-American nuclear families that included two or more siblings with sarcoidosis, the strongest signal was at marker D5S407 ($P = 0.005$) on 5q11.2-based full- and half-sibling pairs. The results suggest a sarcoidosis-susceptibility gene in African-Americans on chromosome 5q11.2 and a gene that protects this population from sarcoidosis on 5p15.2.[76]
- In African-Americans, genetic susceptibility is found on the HLA-DQB1 locus and an environmental association is exposure to damp environments.[67]

Clinical Findings

- One-quarter of patients with systemic sarcoidosis also have cutaneous involvement. A recent review of cutaneous sarcoidosis found that 73% of the patients have specific lesions at the beginning of their disease, 70% of these patients have systemic manifestations concomitantly, and the remaining 30% develop systemic disease 6 months to 3 years later.[82]
- In many cases, skin involvement is an early finding, and 25–35% of patients with sarcoidosis have cutaneous lesions. Skin findings in African-Americans often include scars, pits, and depigmented areas.[67]
- Cutaneous sarcoidosis has many different morphologies, including

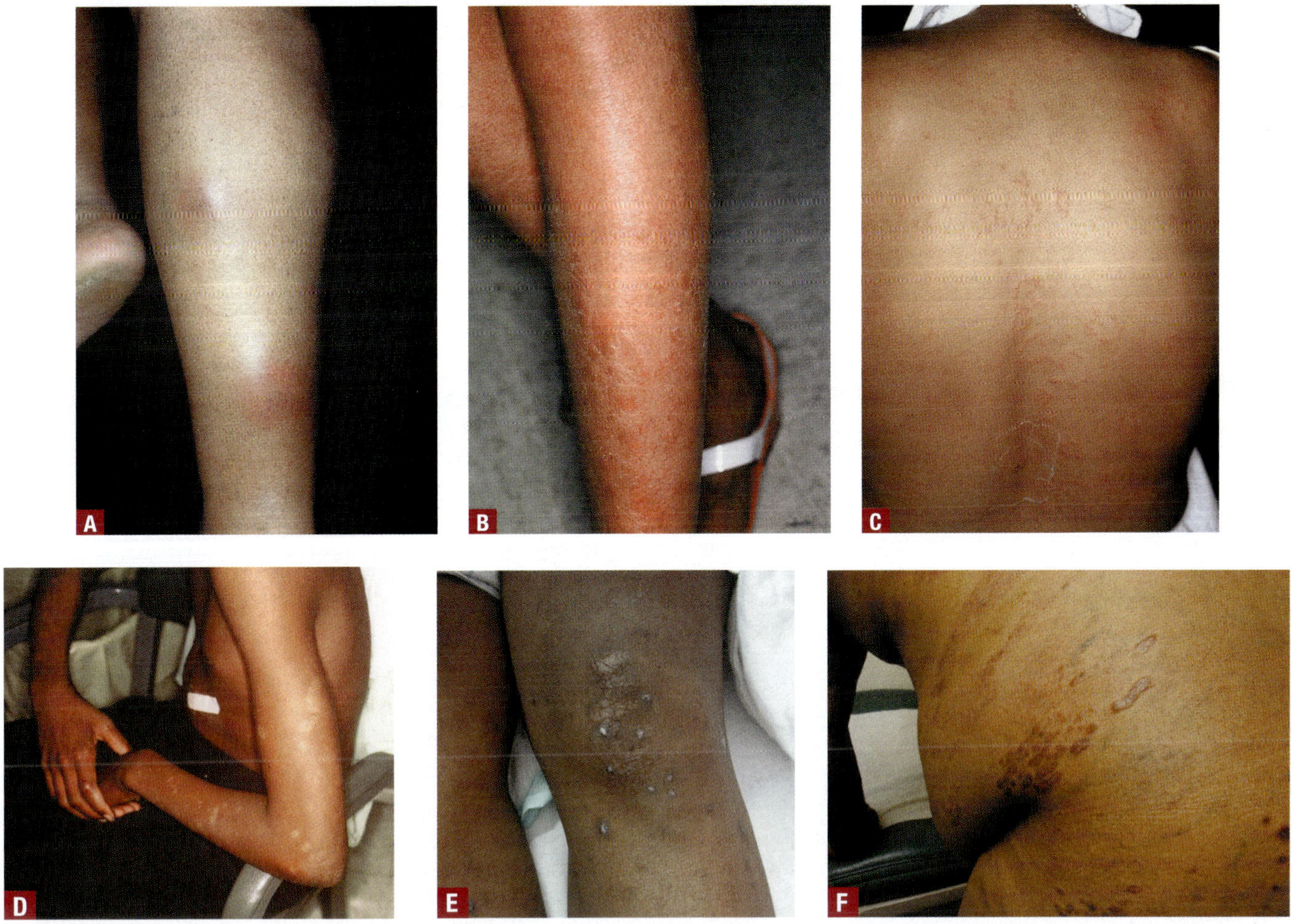

▲ **FIGURE 68-19** **A.** Erythema nodosum in an African-American woman with multiple tender red nodules on the posterior tibia. **B.** Sarcoidosis ichthyosis in an African-American woman with ichthyotic red-brown scale on the lower extremities. **C.** Sarcoidosis in an African-American with discrete brown granulomatous annular papules and plaques on the back. **D.** Sarcoidosis in an African-American woman with hypopigmented macules and patches that on palpation have some induration. **E.** Sarcoidosis in an African-American woman with multiple scars on the knee specked with purple-brown hyperkeratotic papules in the scars and surrounding area. **F.** Sarcoidosis in an obese African-American man with brown granulomatous linear plaques, some ulcerated, on the abdomen. Courtesy of Department of Dermatology, Washington Hospital Center, Washington DC.

indurated, violaceous plaques and nodules on the face (lupus pernio); firm red to brown papules on the face and neck that have an "apple jelly" appearance on diascopy; and nonspecific lesions of septal panniculitis (known as *erythema nodosum;* Figure 68-19*A*).[67]

- Other clinical findings can include pulmonary, liver, spleen, neurologic, ophthalmologic, cardiac, renal, and musculoskeletal involvement.[67]

PAPULES (see Figure 68-19*C*)

- Localized or generalized, typically firm, red-brown to violaceous in color, less than 1 cm in size[82]
- Commonly involve the face, particularly the eyelids and around the orbits, and the nasolabial folds; other areas include the neck, trunk, extremities, and rarely, mucous membranes.
- Diascopy can demonstrate an "apple jelly" color. Maculopapular lesions are commonly associated with acute forms of sarcoidosis, such as hilar lymphadenopathy, acute uveitis, peripheral lymphadenopathy, and parotid enlargement.
- Scarring alopecia of the scalp has been reported.
- Annular plaques involve the forehead.

ANGIOLUPOID PLAQUES

- Large telangiectasias are present within the plaques and are associated with chronic and systemic sarcoidosis[82] (Figure 68-20).

SUBCUTANEOUS NODULES OF DARIER-ROUSSY SARCOIDOSIS (Figure 68-21)

- Painless, firm, mobile nodules measuring 0.5–2 cm without epidermal involvement and potentially numerous

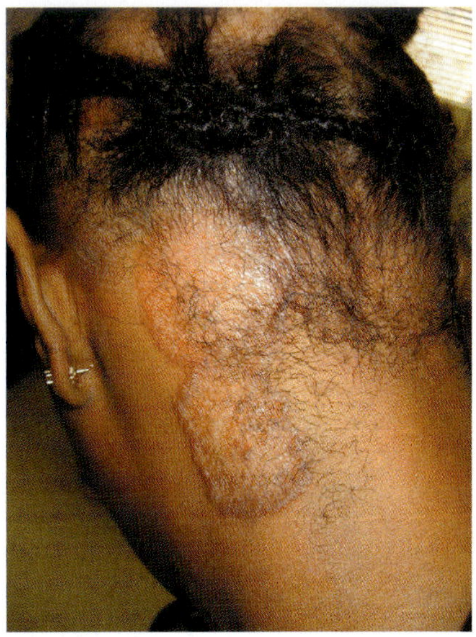

▲ **FIGURE 68-20** Systemic sarcoidosis in an African-American woman after liver transplant with annular plaque on posterior neck and scalp. Courtesy of Department of Dermatology, Washington Hospital Center, Washington DC.

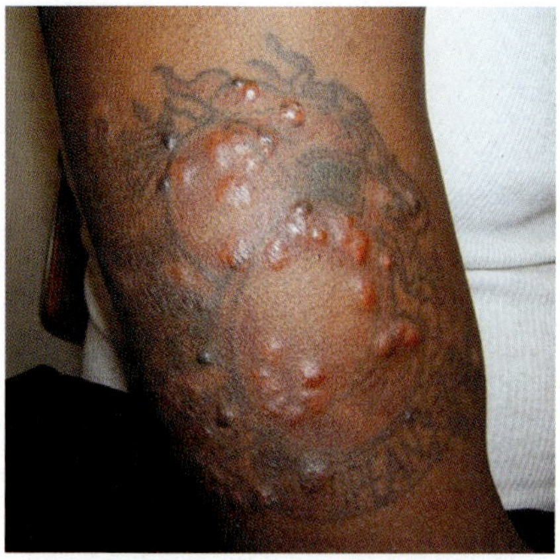

▲ **FIGURE 68-21** Darier-Roussy sarcoidosis. Multiple red nodules and papules in the markings of a tattoo on the upper extremity, sparing areas with no ink. Courtesy of Department of Dermatology, Washington Hospital Center, Washington DC.

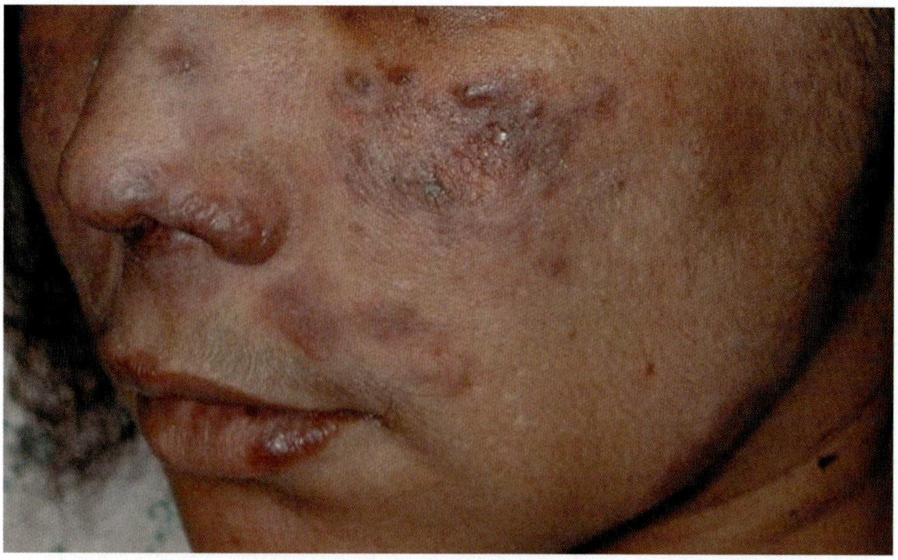

▲ **FIGURE 68-22** Lupus pernio sarcoidosis in an African-American woman with multiple dark brown and burgundy papules on the cheek, rim of the nares, and lip. Courtesy of Department of Dermatology, Washington Hospital Center, Washington DC.

- Commonly associated with liver, lung, and spleen sarcoidosis
- Usually involve the trunk and extremities
- Form of panniculitis that exclusively involves the subcutaneous tissue and does not extend into the dermis

INACTIVE SCARS[82] (see Figure 68-19*E*)

- Can become infiltrated with sarcoidosis and develop a red or purple hue with induration
- May appear early in the disease process before the onset of pulmonary disease or parallel chronic systemic findings

LUPUS PERNIO[67,82] (Figure 68-22)

- Common in African-American women.
- Hallmark of fibrotic disease.
- Consists of indolent, indurated, red-brown to purple, swollen, shiny skin changes on the nose, lips, cheeks, and ears.
- When the nose is involved, frequently associated with a granulomatous infiltration of the nasal mucosa and bone.
- Ulceration and septal perforation can occur (see Figure 68-19*F*).
- Can be quite disfiguring.
- Coexists with chronic fibrotic sarcoidosis of the upper respiratory tract with nasal, pharyngeal, and laryngeal involvement; pulmonary fibrosis; chronic uveitis; and bone cysts.
- Atypical specific presentations: ichthyosiform, ulcerative, morpheaform, vulvar, penile, psoriasiform, hypopigmented (see Figure 68-19*D*), faint erythema, verrucous, folliculitis, lichenoid, eruptive, erythrodermic, cicatricial alopecia, scalp nodules, mutilating lesions, erythematous plaques of the palms and soles, unilateral lower extremity edema, nodular fingertip lesions, granulomatous chelitis, erythema annular centrifugum, annular elastolytic, palmar erythema, rosacea-like syndrome, light-exposed papules, angiolupoid, perforating, lupus erythematosus–like, umbilicated, and nail changes.

ICHTHYOSIFORM SARCOIDOSIS (APPEARS AS AN ACQUIRED ICHTHYOSIS) (see Figure 68-19*B*)

- Has been reported; appears as large rhomboidal hyperpigmented scaling plaques that are usually asymptomatic and usually involve the lower portion of the legs.
- Histology reveals compact orthokeratosis with diminished or absent granular layer and multiple noncaseating granulomas within the dermis.[85]

MORPHEAFORM SARCOIDOSIS

- Mimics morphea and is usually symmetric on lower extremities.
- On histology, see epithelioid granulomas and dermal sclerosis.
- Hydroxychloroquine may be helpful.[68]

SARCOIDOSIS OF THE VULVA

- Three reported cases and one reported case of sarcoid involving the fallopian tubes, ovaries, and uterus[87]

ULCERATIVE SARCOIDOSIS

- Thirty-five reported cases and most commonly affects women and blacks in young adulthood.
- Lower extremities are involved most commonly, but the disease also can be generalized.
- Treatment includes corticosteroids and methotrexate for refractory cases.
- Tends to heal with scarring.[88]

SARCOIDOSIS OF THE SCALP

- Twenty-eight reported cases, most commonly affecting black women
- Usually presents as scarring alopecia that can be localized or present as total alopecia
- Most commonly associated with systemic sarcoidosis and resistant to therapy[90]

NONSPECIFIC/REACTIVE CUTANEOUS ERUPTIONS

Erythema Nodosum (EN)

- Hallmark of acute and benign sarcoidosis
  - Associated with a good prognosis and spontaneous resolution of the disease
  - Eighty-three percent of patients with EN have resolution of their sarcoid within 2 years.
  - Panniculitis with widened and edematous septa with lymphocytic and neutrophilic infiltrate on histology

Löfgren Syndrome

- EN associated with bilateral hilar adenopathy with or without pulmonary infiltrates, symmetric arthralgias or arthritis, fever, and anterior uveitis
- Usually affects young women with tender subcutaneous nodules most commonly located on the anterior tibial area
- Variant—swelling of both ankles with acute inflammation, preserved articular motion, bilateral hilar adenopathy, with or without EN
  - Calcifications
  - Prurigo
  - Pruritus
  - Erythema multiforme
  - Leonine facies
  - Nail changes—clubbing, dystrophy with and without underlying bone cysts, subungual hyperkeratosis, and onycholysis

Diagnosis

- Clinicians should remember that sarcoidosis is a great mimicker of many diseases.
- Clinicians should screen patients with sarcoidosis for comorbid illnesses.[68]
- The clinician should take a very thorough occupational and environmental history at the initial evaluation, including a drug history (e.g., for methotrexate pneumonitis).
  - A skin biopsy can give a definitive diagnosis and is easy; without a skin biopsy, a diagnosis of sarcoidosis becomes a diagnosis of exclusion.
  - A wedge, incisional or excisional, full-thickness biopsy involving subcutaneous fat should be taken to confirm the diagnosis.
- The differential diagnosis of sarcoidosis involves all granulomatous infectious and inflammatory diseases.
- Angiotension-converting enzyme is used to follow disease activity.

Treatment

CUTANEOUS SYSTEMIC SARCOIDOSIS, LUPUS PERNIO, AND SARCOIDAL PLAQUES AND NODULES

- Prednisone 20–40 mg/day
- Methotrexate 10–15 mg/week
- Hydroxychloroquine 400 mg/day
- Thalidomide 100–150 mg/ day
- Infliximab to treat lupus pernio[83]

CUTANEOUS LUPUS ERYTHEMATOSUS

Systemic lupus erythematosus (SLE) is a chronic, multisystem, heterogeneous autoimmune disorder in terms of presentation, course, and outcome.[91] In over 80% of patients, skin and mucous membranes are involved.[92–94] Diagnosis is based on the American College of Rheumatology (ACR) 1982 Revised Criteria for Classification of SLE, in which any 4 of the 11 criteria must be present; of note, the ACR updated its criteria by adding "positive finding of antiphospholipid antibodies" to the immunologic disorder category in 1997.[95]

Epidemiology

- SLE is a complex disorder with many clinical presentations, and the extent and degree of disease activity vary greatly among different ethnic groups.[96–98]
- SLE prevalence has been reported to be 40–150 cases per 100,000.[99,100]
- This autoimmune disorder is found throughout the world, but certain ethnic groups within particular countries are more likely to develop the disease.[101]
  - Estimated incidence rates in North America, South America, and Europe vary from 1–32 cases per 100,000 per year,[102] with the prevalence higher among Asians, African-Americans, African Caribbeans, Hispanic Americans, and Asian Indians.[99]
  - Conversely, SLE occurs less frequency in Africans.[103]
  - The incidence rates among Native Americans are also higher than for the rest of the North American population,[104] and East Asians have demonstrated more cases of SLE than Caucasians in Hawaii and Asia.[105,106]
  - Aborigines have even been found to have a higher prevalence of disease than whites in central Australia.[107]
- Lupus affects close to 2 million people in the United States, with an estimated 16,000 people developing the disease annually. Women comprise more than 90% of patients diagnosed with SLE.[108]
- SLE is three to four times more prevalent in African-American women than Caucasian women,[101] and this disorder afflicts 1 in every 250 black women.[109]
- African-Americans and Hispanics tend to develop SLE at an earlier age and carry a poorer prognosis than Caucarians.[101]
- African-Americans are more likely to have active disease with more serious organ-system involvement. Specifically, African-Americans have a higher likelihood of developing lupus-related kidney failure and skin damage.[109] In addition, blacks are more likely to demonstrate proteinuria, psychosis, and serositis.[110,111]
- Arthritis and renal, hematologic, and immunologic involvement are more common in Texas Hispanics and African-Americans than in other groups.[91]
- Lupus nephritis is also more common in Hispanic Americans, Chinese, and other Asians.[101]
- Occurrence of specific autoantibodies also varies according to ethnicity. Southern Chinese and North African patients are more likely to have anti-Ro antibodies, whereas anti-Sm antibodies have a higher prevalence in North and South Africans, African-Americans, Saudis, and Vietnamese. Antiphospholipid antibodies are less likely to occur in Chinese and African-Americans, whereas antiribosomal P protein antibodies are observed more commonly in Japanese and Malaysian Chinese.[101]
- Prognosis is poorer in patients with less education,[122] which could reflect poor compliance.[113] It is also worse in individuals with a lower socioeconomic status or with inadequate access to medical care.[96]
- The mortality rates for SLE among African-Americans and Asians have been demonstrated to be greater than among Caucasian whites.[101]

Etiology/Genetics

- SLE is a multifactorial disease with genetic, hormonal, immunologic, and environmental factors all thought to play a role.
- While the pathogenesis of lupus remains unclear, many of the clinical findings of SLE are directly or indirectly involved with the creation of autoantibodies and the formation of

immune complexes.[114,115] These vary among different ethnic groups[91]:

- HLA-DRB1*1503 and HLA-DQB1*0602 have been found to be more frequent in African-American patients with SLE.[116]
- HLA-DRB1*08 has been linked to Hispanic-American patients with SLE.[117]
- HLA-DRB1*0301 has been connected to SLE in Caucasians and Texas Hispanics.[91]

Clinical Findings

- Several variants of cutaneous lupus exist and are classified according to the chronicity of skin lesions (i.e., acute, subacute, chronic) or the histologic location of the inflammatory infiltrate.
- Acute cutaneous lupus (ACLE) is classically illustrated by the malar butterfly rash (Figure 68-23*A*), which develops in approximately half of patients, usually after UV exposure.
- Subacute cutaneous lupus (SCLE; see Figure 68-23*B*) lesions begin as small, erythematous, slightly scaly papules that evolve into either an annular or a papulosquamous form, most commonly seen on the shoulders, forearms, neck, and upper torso.
- Chronic discoid lesions are found in up to 25% of SLE patients and are located most commonly on the face, neck, scalp, and ears but can be present in a widespread distribution (Figure 68-24).
- Discoid lesions are characterized by discrete, erythematous, slightly infiltrating plaques covered by an adherent scale, and they have the potential for scarring. Discoid lupus rash is more common in African-Americans than in other groups.
- Follicular plugging and scarring alopecia are often observed in patients with chronic cutaneous lupus erythematosus.
- Lupus panniculitis lesions are characterized by indurated plaques secondary to intense inflammation in the fat and can develop into disfiguring depressed areas.

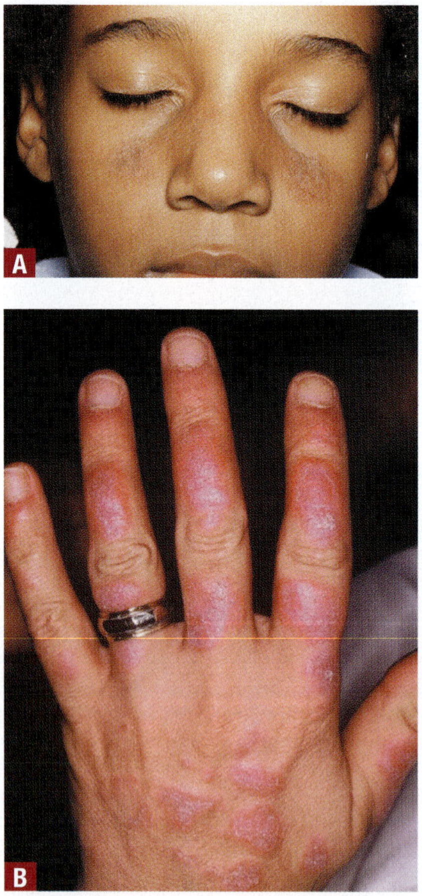

▲ **FIGURE 68-23** **A.** Malar rash. **B.** Subacute cutaneous lupus erythematosus in a Hispanic man with pink-red plaques on the dorsum of his hand, sparing the proximal and distal interphylangeal joints. Courtesy of Department of Dermatology, Washington Hospital Center, Washington DC.

Diagnosis

- The top four ACR criteria for SLE are
  - Arthritis
  - Photosensitivity
  - Malar rash
  - Antinuclear antibody (ANA) positivity
- The most common combination of two presenting criteria are arthritis and ANA positivity, followed by malar rash and photosensitivity.[91]

Pathology

- Histology differs according to the variant of cutaneous lupus.
- ACLE and SCLE involve the epidermis and upper dermis.
- Lupus panniculitis involves the subcutaneous tissue.
- Discoid lesions of lupus involve the epidermis, upper and lower dermis, and adnexal structures.
- In direct immunofluorescence, the most characteristic finding in cutaneous lupus is antibody deposition at the dermal-epidermal junction and around hair follicles. These deposits are typically granular and are composed primarily of IgG and/or IgM. Deposits of complement proteins also can be found.

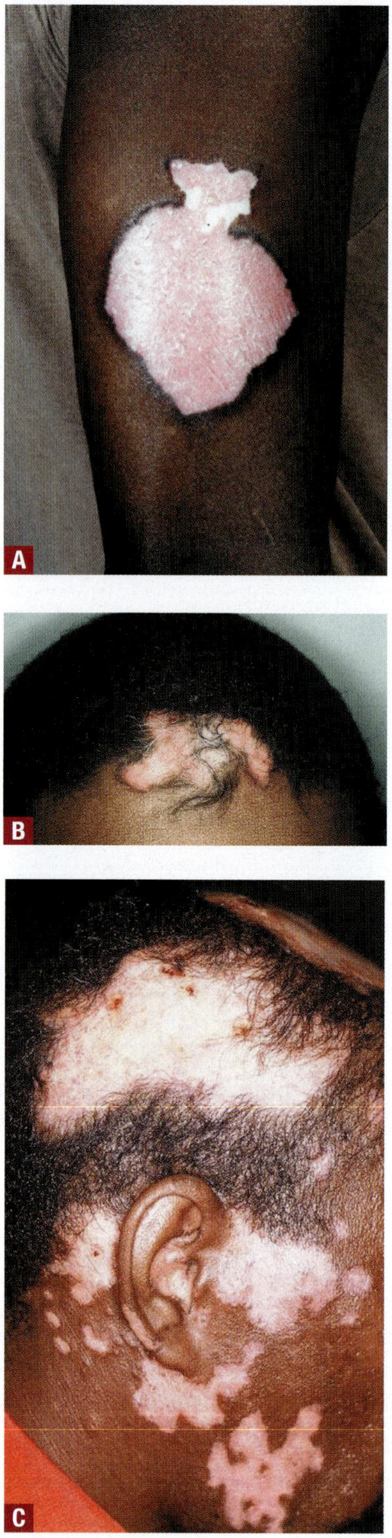

▲ **FIGURE 68-24** **A.** Discoid lupus. Pink-white scarred atrophic plaque on lower extremity with dark brown well-demarcated border in an emblem-shaped erythematosus. **B.** Discoid lupus in an African-American man with pink, scarred with brown serpiginous border, well-defined plaque with white hairs in an erythematosus scalp. **C.** Discoid lupus erythematosus in an African-American man with multiple hypopigmented and depigmented white plaques with hyperpigmented borders. Courtesy of Department of Dermatology, Washington Hospital Center, Washington DC.

Differential Diagnosis

- Polymorphous light eruption
- Drug-induced photosensitivity
- Porphyria cutanea tarda
- Pseudoporphyria
- Rosacea
- Eczema
- Dermatomyositis
- Granuloma annulare
- Erythema annulare centrifugum
- Lymphoma cutis
- Granuloma faciale
- Jessner lymphocytic infiltrate
- Sarcoidosis

Treatment

- Preventive measures such as avoidance of sun will preclude the development of skin lesions in most patients.
- Photosensitive patients should use sunscreen on a daily basis.
- Cessation of smoking[118] also must be emphasized.
- An effective therapeutic regimen takes both disease activity and severity into account.
- Nonsteroidal anti-inflammatory drugs, antimalarial agents, and immunosuppressive agents are all used in the treatment of SLE.

SCLERODERMA

Scleroderma—also known as *systemic sclerosis* (SSc)[119]—is a multisystem autoimmune connective tissue disease that presents clinically with thickening of the skin and organs, vascular injury, and a widespread immune fibrotic process.[120] The subtypes of the disease are diffuse cutaneous systemic sclerosis (dcSSc) and limited (acral) cutaneous systemic sclerosis (lcSSc).[119] The prognosis for patients with diffuse SSc is much poorer than for patients with limited SSc.[119]

Epidemiology

- Some studies have found significant differences in the clinical characteristics and course of SSc in different races and ethnic groups. However, many of these studies had small sample sizes or did not account for variations in disease duration or differences in the proportion of patients with limited versus diffuse cutaneous disease.[119]
- The incidence of SSc in the United States rose from 1947–1973; since 1973, the rate has been relatively stable.[121]
- The average length of survival from diagnosis is 13 years.[121]
- Scleroderma occurs much more frequently in women than in men.[121]
- Some studies have found that SSc is more common in the United States than in other countries.[121]
- About 240 per 1 million adults in the United States have SSc.[121]
- Several studies in the United States have shown that blacks appear to have a higher age-specific incidence rate than whites, and the disease is more severe in blacks. For example, peak age-specific incidence (20/million/year) of diffuse SSc is higher and occurs at a younger age in black women age 35–44 than in white women (8/million/year). In addition, approximately 70% of cases of SSc in blacks are diffuse disease compared with 30–40% of cases in whites. Research also shows that age of onset in black men is earlier than in white men.[121]

Etiology/Genetics

- The etiology of scleroderma is unknown. SSc can begin with endothelial inflammation and edema that leads to vasculopathy and recurrent vasoconstriction and reperfusion episodes. The vasoconstriction and reperfusion progress to episodic and sustained tissue ischemia and a diminished immunologic ability to respond to and repair injuries.[120]
- African-Americans have more severe symptoms than whites, including more extensive lung involvement and renal involvement and higher mortality rates. It is not clear whether these racial differences are genetic, environmental, or a combination.[119]
- Antibodies to topoisomerase I (Scl-70) are associated with an increased risk of interstitial lung disease in patients with SSc. Research has shown that blacks with SSc are more likely than whites to test positive for antibodies to topoisomerase I (Scl-70) and less likely to test positive for anticentromere autoantibodies.[119]
- Anti–RNA polymerase I or II reactivity, but not anti–toposiomerase I (Scl-70), is an independent risk factor for renal crisis associated with SSc. In addition, pulmonary hypotension, which is common in patients with SSc, is associated with anticentromere antibody and antifibrillarin reactivity.[122]
- In one study, anti-U3RNP (fibrillarin) was detected in nearly half of black SSc patients but in fewer than 5% of white and Japanese patients.[122]
- SSc-associated death is caused primarily by pulmonary complications. Pulmonary interstitial fibrosis is the primary cause of morbidity and mortality in patients with SSc, and it has a major impact on survival in patients who have had SSc for 8–9 years.[122]
- Evidence supports the existence of genetic susceptibility to familial SSc, and some cluster studies have shown a high incidence of the disease. For example, the Choctaw Native Americans in southeastern Oklahoma have a high prevalence (610/million) of SSc; a single-nucleotided polymorphism in the 5′ untranslated region of *FBN1* is strongly associated with SSc in this population.[121]

Clinical Findings

- Patients present to the dermatologist with tightening of the skin in the upper extremities, a feeling of hands turning cold, or actual Raynaud phenomenon[123] (Figure 68-25).
- They will have tightening of facial skin and then symptoms of shortness of breath on exertion.[123]
- The many cutaneous findings in patients with SSc include diffuse hyperpigmentation, particularly in areas of pressure; localized areas of depigmentation, with sparing of perifollicular skin (salt-and-pepper; Figures 68-26 and 68-27); edema of the fingers; telangiectasias; capillary abnormalities of the proximal nail fold; calcinosis cutis; cutaneous ulcers, especially on the digits; pitting at the fingertips; and sclerodactyly.[123,124]
- Blacks have a higher rate of digital ulcer, digital tip pitting, and digital gangrene and more diffuse and severe skin involvement.[119]
- Patients with limited cutaneous SSc typically have skin findings on the hands and, to a lesser extent, on the face and neck. A distinct subset of patients with lcSSc have CREST syndrome (calcinosis cutis, Raynaud

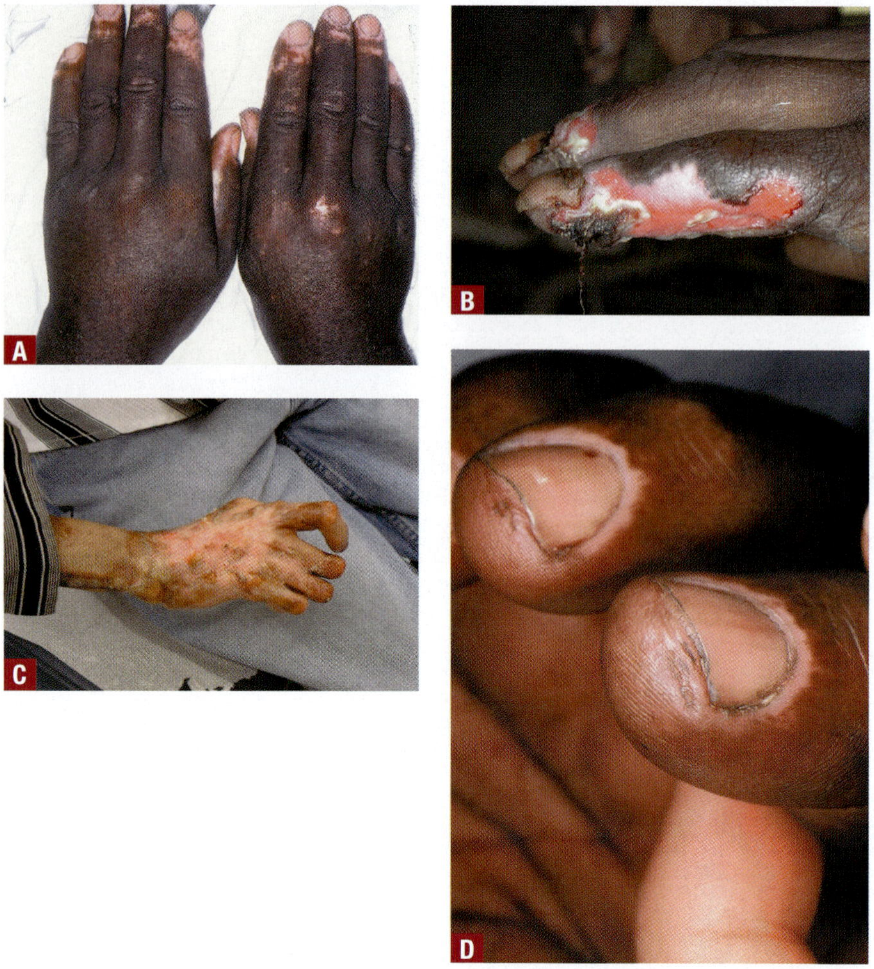

▲ **FIGURE 68-25** **A.** Scleroderma in an African-American man with distal hypopigmentation and depigmentation on bound down skin on 10 tapering fingers. **B.** Scleroderma in an African-American man with marked clubbing o fingernails, hyperpigmentation of the skin, tapering of fingers, and ulceration of the fifth digit with a serpigimou border around granulation tissue and an area of eschar. **C.** Scleroderma in an African-American woman with widespread atrophic, scarred, hypopigmenterd plaques with brown borders and some scale on the right hand with contractures. Courtesy of Atlantic Dermatology Conference, 2006. **D.** Scleroderma. Periungal hypopigmentation and digital pitting at the tips of the fingers in an African-American man. Courtesy of Department of Dermatology, Washington Hospital Center, Washington DC.

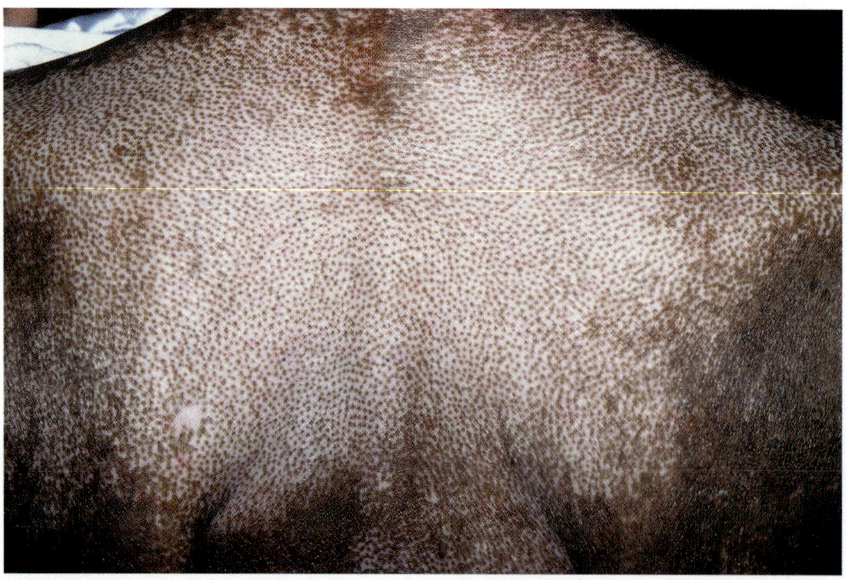

▲ **FIGURE 68-26** Scleroderma in an African-American woman with salt and pepper pattern of depigmentation with perifollicular hyperpigmentation. Courtesy of Department of Dermatology, Washington Hospital Center, Washington DC.

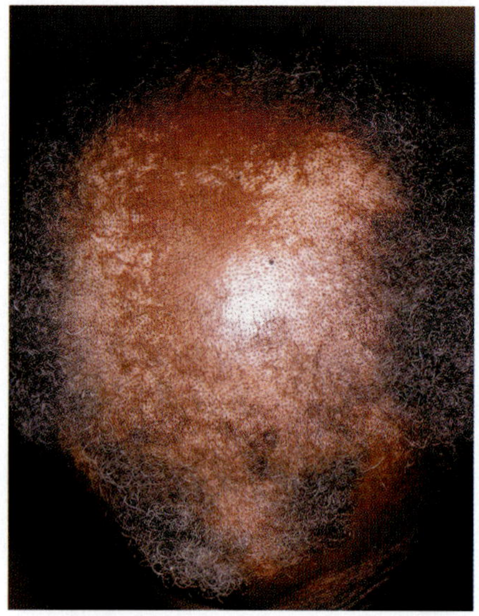

▲ **FIGURE 68-27** Scleroderma in an elderly African-American man with salt and pepper perifollicular hypo- and hyperpigmentation with scarring in an androgenic distribution on the scalp. Courtesy of Department of Dermatology, Washington Hospital Center, Washington DC.

phenomenon, esophageal involvement, sclerodactyly, and telangiectasia).[125,126]

- Patients with diffuse cutaneous SSc have skin findings that extend to the chest, abdomen, or upper arms and shoulders. These patients are more likely to have or develop internal organ injury secondary to ischemia or fibrosis.[125,126]
- Patients who have had diffuse SSc for several years often present with SSc renal crisis, including malignant hypertension, renal insufficiency, and microangiopathic hemolytic anemia.[122]
- Up to 90% of patients with both diffuse and limited SSc present with upper and/or lower gastrointestinal involvement. Symptoms can range from subclinical to severe paresis and can occur in any area of the tract between the mouth and and the anus. The most common gastrointestinal manifestations in patients with SSc are gastroesophageal reflux disease and esophageal dysmotility.[122]

Diagnosis

- Serologic markers in blacks include anti–topoisomerase Scl-70, anti-RNP, and anti-Ro antibodies.[122]
- Blacks are more likely to have more than one antibody, and they have a lower rate of speckled-pattern ANAs and higher rate of nucleolar-pattern ANAs than whites.[122]

- Clinicians should conduct follow-up studies annually or earlier if patients develop new dyspnea symptoms.[122]
- Clinicians also should screen for arterial pulmonary hypertension with pulmonary function testing, diffusion capacity of the lung, high-resolution computed tomography (HRCT), and echocardiography.[122]
- Interstitial fibrosis can be assessed by HRCT or bronchoalveolar lavage.[122]
- All patients with SSc should be referred for baseline pulmonary testing after their initial diagnosis.[127]
- The diagnosis of SSc is multifactorial and includes patient history, family history, physical examination, serologic testing, and a skin biopsy in an area that will heal easily.[128] The differential diagnosis includes
  - Scleredema
  - Scleromyxedema
  - Diabetic sclerodactyly
  - Myxedema
  - Nephrogenic systemic fibrosis
  - Amyloidosis
  - Eosinophilic fasciitis
  - Chronic graft-versus-host disease
  - Drug-induced scleroderma
  - Generalized morphea
  - Environmental exposures

Treatment

- The most successful treatments for SSc to date have been strategies aimed at treating the disease's vascular complications (especially with the use of angiotensin-converting inhibitor drugs), especially for managing renal crisis and pulmonary arterial hypertension. These can increase quality of life and survival. Cyclophosphamide is also effective.[128]
- PUVA, narrow-band UVB, and extracorporeal photopheresis have been used to improve and increase the mobility of the skin.[128]
- Currently available strategies to reduce or control fibrosis directly have not shown effectiveness, although new approaches are in development.[128]

HEPATITIS C VIRUS INFECTION AND HEPATIC FAILURE

The epidemiology of liver disease shows a prevalence in people of color, and the skin will give the first clues to the signs and symptoms of liver disease. Chronic liver disease and cirrhosis were the fifth most common cause of death in 2001 among Native Americans and Alaska Natives according to the Centers for Disease Control and Prevention (CDC).[129] In Hispanic/Latino populations, it was the seventh most common cause of death.

Viral hepatitis A and B have been well described in the literature, and a vaccine is now available for hepatitis B. However, acute hepatitis C can be symptomatic, and chronic hepatitis C is associated with autoimmune thyroid disease, sialadenitis autoimmune thrombocytopenic purpura, lymphoma, and hepatic carcinoma.[130]

The epidemiology of the disease shows a prevalence in people of color. The skin will give the first clue to the cutaneous signs and symptoms of liver disease.

- The hepatitis C virus (HCV) is an RNA virus of the flaviviridae family.
- It affects the liver, with both acute and chronic courses of infection.
- Acute HCV infection is frequently asymptomatic and can be self-limiting or fulminant (hepatic encephalopathy), but most (60–80%) patients progress to a chronic infection.[131,132]
- Chronic HCV infection is a state of chronic inflammatory damage to the liver for 6 months or more and can lead to cirrhosis and hepatocellular carcinoma.
- The African-American population has a weaker HCV-specific immunity.[133]

Epidemiology

- HCV is most prevalent among blood transfusion and organ recipient patients prior to 1992, intravenous drug users, dialysis patients, health care workers, and people who engage in high-risk sexual behaviors.[140,130]
- The prevalence of HCV antibodies in African-Americans is double that in Caucasian Americans.[134]
- Viral persistence is higher in the African-American population.[135]
- There is a higher incidence of hepatocellular carcinoma secondary to chronic HCV infection in the African-American population.[136]
- African-American patients with HCV have a poorer response to interferon therapy than the Caucasian-American population.[137–139]
- A 2004 study found that Latino patients showed statistically significant higher serum alanine transaminase, aspartate transaminase, and bilirubin levels and lower serum albumin levels than Caucasian, Asian, and African-American populations.[141]

Systemic Signs and Symptoms

- Pruritis
- Fatigue
- Nausea
- Anorexia
- Right upper quadrant pain and tenderness to palpation
- Hepatosplenomegaly
- Jaundice
- Muscle weakness
- Dark urine

Clinical Findings

HEPATIC FAILURE

- Spider angiomata—seen in lighter browns on the chest
- Alopecia—usually with seborrheic dermatitis or a scaly, pruritic scalp with lichenification and hair breakage
- Livedo reticularis—difficult to detect in darkly pigmented skin; brown skin will have hyperpigmented reticulated pattern.
- Palmar erythema—can present as hyperpigmented palms

LICHEN PLANUS (Figure 68-28)

- Violaceous shiny polygonal papules and plaques with overlying delicate white lines (Wickhams's striae)[142]

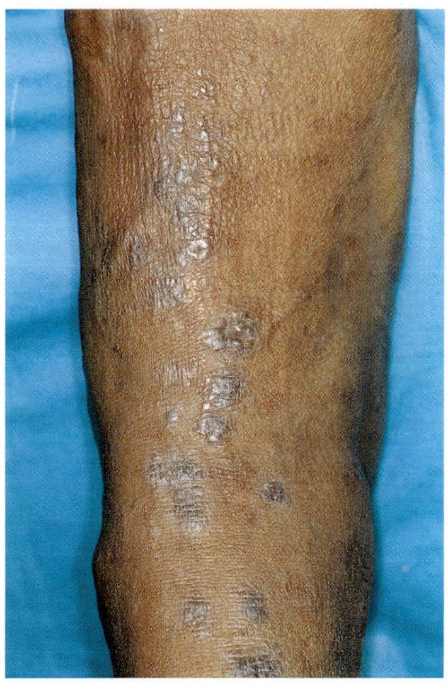

▲ **FIGURE 68-28** Lichen planus.

- Occurs on skin (especially flexor surfaces), nails, and mucosa (oral and genital lesions)[143]
- Lesions are typically extremely pruritic.[142]
- Oral mucosa commonly involved when associated with hepatitis C[144,145]
- Treatment of oral lesions includes topical corticosteroids, superpotent topical steroids, topical retinoids, topical calcineurin inhibitors, and intralesional corticosteroids, among others.[142,146,147]
- Skin lesions are treated initially with topical steroids and superpotent topical steroids.[142]
- Topical calcineurin inhibitors, intralesional corticosteroids, systemic corticosteroids, retinoids, narrow-band UVB, and PUVA also can be used when topical steroids fail.[142,148]

MIXED CRYOGLOBULINEMIA (Figure 68-29)

- Precipitation of polyclonal IgG and monoclonal IgM in small- to medium-sized blood arteries[142,144]
- Anti-HCV antibody and HCV RNA can be found in plasma and cryoprecipitate.[144,149]
- Clinical presentation includes palpable purpura, arthralgias, lymphadenopathy, hepatosplenomegaly, and weakness.[142,144]
- The mainstay of treatment includes treatment of HCV with interferon.[150,151]
- Therapies under investigation for disease recalcitrant to interferon include rituximab.[152]

NECROLYTIC ACRAL ERYTHEMA

- Rare, pruritic, acrally located psoriasis-like manifestation of HCV[153–155]
- Lesions are erythematous to violaceous and hyperpigmented papules and plaques with sharp borders; scales and erosion are also seen.[153–155]
- Lesions typically occur on the lower extremities.[153–155]
- Histologic examination shows psoriasiform changes with epidermal necrosis.[153–155]
- Treatment includes treatment of HCV, topical and systemic corticosteroid therapy, and oral zinc.[153–155]

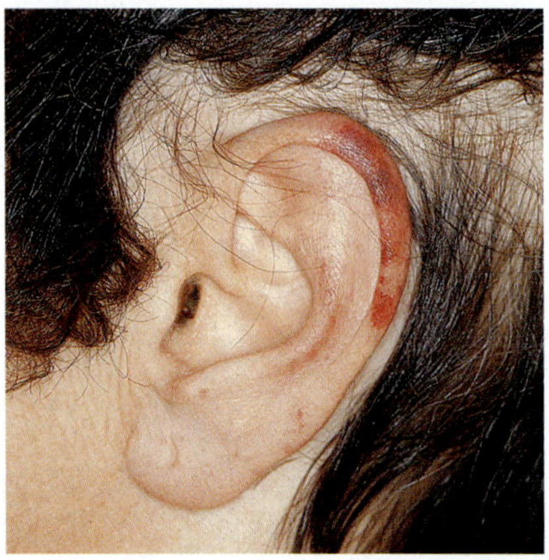

▲ **FIGURE 68-29** Cryoglobulinemia.

PORPHYRIA CUTANEA TARDA (PCT)

- Decreased activity of UROD in the liver only.[156]
- Patients present with noninflammatory vesicles and bullae in a photodistribution.[156]
- Vesicles and bullae are subepidermal.[156,157]
- Crusts and erosions are often present, and lesions heal with milia and scars.[156.157]
- Patients are photosensitive and should avoid UV light.[156]
- Standard treatment for acquired PCT is phlebotomy, which reduces hepatic iron and therefore decreases iron's inhibition of UROD oxidation.[158]

TOXIC EPIDERMAL NECROLYSIS

Toxic epidermal necrolysis (TEN) is a life-threatening drug reaction involving an immune mechanism that causes the separation of the epidermis from the dermis, resulting in necrolysis of the skin surface and mucous membranes. Separation of the skin occurs at the dermal-epidermal junction.[159]

Many of the drugs used to treat the diseases that have higher prevalence and incidence in people of color (e.g., HIV/AIDS, gout, hypertension, and connective tissue diseases) can cause drug reactions. People of color may be at more risk because they are taking more of the medications that may cause TEN. Early detection in skin of color requires recognition of red in all shades of brown skin. Early treatment and withdrawal of the drug will decrease morbidity and mortality.

Diagnosis

- Acute HCV diagnosis is usually made by finding HCV RNA in the serum of a patient with a clinical picture consistent with acute HCV infection.
- Chronic HCV diagnosis can be made by finding HCV RNA in the serum of a patient with a clinical and laboratory picture consistent with inflammatory liver damage for 6 months or more (elevated transaminases, as well as alkaline phosphatase, albumin, prothrombin time, direct bilirubin, and γ-glutamyltranspeptidase in severe disease).

Treatment of Hepatitis C Virus Infection

ACUTE VIRAL HEPATITIS

- Interferon or peg interferon 2–4 months after onset for viral clearance and prevention of chronic HCV[140]

CHRONIC VIRAL HEPATITIS

- Standard treatment is peg interferon plus ribavirin.[140]
- Treatment can be individualized depending on the specific viral genotype, comorbid conditions, age of the patient, severity of disease, and laboratory values.[140]

Epidemiology

- TEN incidence varies between 0.4 and 1.2 cases per 1 million per year,[161] and it affects women more than men at a ratio of 1.5:1, with the incidence increasing with age.[162]
- Mortality rate of 25–40%, highest in elderly and HIV-infected patients[160,166]
- HIV-positive patients have a thousand-fold greater risk of developing TEN than the general population.[163]
- No racial predilection has been noted in the literature.
- Genetic link to carbamazepine-induced TEN among HLA-B502-positive Han Chinese patients[168]
- In Asian populations, phenytoin and allopurinol are observed.[169] (100% of Han Chinese had HLA-B*5801)

Etiology/Pathogenesis

- The medications most often involved in TEN include antibiotics (especially sulfonamide, trimethoprim-sulfamethoxazole), oxicam, nonsteroidal anti-inflammatory drugs, anticonvulsants (e.g., Dilantin, phenobarbital, and carbamazepine), and allopurinol, furosemide, captopril, thiazide diuretics, antibiotics, COX-2 inhibitors, and antiretroviral medication.[161,164]
- TEN has occurred with mupirocin, natural topical medications, Chinese herbal medicines, and cold remedies with pseudoephedrine.[169]
- Five percent etiology associated with *Mycoplasma pneumoniae,* herpes virus,

immunizations, and bone marrow or solid-organ transplantation.[169]

Clinical Findings

- A prodrome of fever, sore throat, and burning eyes.
- Mucosal lesions also can precede skin lesions. Mucosal involvement includes the conjunctiva, mouth, trachea, bronchi, genitourinary tract, and gastrointestinal tract.[160,165]
- Burning and itching and pain in the skin involving more than 10–30% of body surface area.[169]
- Skin lesions dusky, violaceous, erythematous macules, patches, and plaques that coalesce and form bullae (Figure 68-30)
- Positive Nikolsky sign
- Flacid bullae with few intact bullae
- Widespread red-pink, moist erosions surrounded by gray-brown sheets of epidermis representing the roofs of coalesced flaccid bullae
- Postinflammatory hyper- and hypopigmentation and some scarring after resolution of condition[159]

Diagnosis

- History and very careful drug history to include 60 days before onset of symptoms (our recommendation)
- Family history of first-degree relative having a drug reaction to a medicine[169]

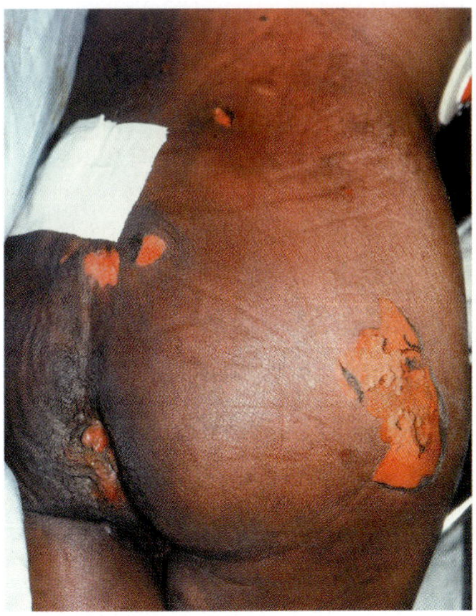

▲ **FIGURE 68-30** Toxic epidermal necrolysis (TEN) in an HIV-positive African-American woman with complaints of painful skin. There is generalized erythema with gray-roofed denuded bullae with bright red-orange bases. Courtesy of Department of Dermatology, Washington Hospital Center, Washington DC.

- Complete skin examination
- Skin biopsy—frozen section and hematoxylin and eosine
- Histology—necrotic keratinocytes and confluent epidermal necrosis with vacuolar changes of the dermal-epidermal junction and subepidermal blistering[167]
- Workup for sepsis

Treatment

- Early diagnosis, removal of the causative drug, supportive care, and supervision in a burn center or intensive care unit for optimal treatment of TEN.[160,165]
- Supportive care includes strict fluid management, ocular care, environmental support, and burn management for skin care.[165,166]
- IV immunoglobulin is advocated by several published studies.[160,165]
- Steroid use is still controversial and in most cases not indicated.
- Plasmapheresis.[165]

MENINGOCOCCEMIA

Meningococcemia is a bacteremia caused by *Neisseria meningitidis,* a gram-negative aerobic diplococcus.[170,171] It can occur with or without clinically apparent meningitis.[171,172]

Epidemiology

- In the United States, meningococcal infection is endemic.
- In the 1990s, one study estimated that the annual incidence of meningococcemia was 1.1 per 100,000 population in the United States.[173]
- The same study found that serotype Y was more common in African-Americans (50%) than in other populations (23%), and conversely, patients with serotype Y were more likely to be African-American than Caucasian American.[173]
- Another study from the 1990s found that rates of meningitis to *S. pneumoniae, N. meningitidis,* and group B *Streptococcus* were all higher in African-Americans.[174]
- College students living in college dormitories have a higher rate of meningococcal infection than their off-campus counterparts.[175]
- Up to 2% of the worldwide incidence of meningococcal disease occurs in epidemics in Africa.[176]
- Worldwide, the incidence of endemic disease is 0.5–5 cases per 100,000 population per year.[176]
- Epidemics in Africa occur in the "meningitis belt," which includes parts of Benin, Burkina Faso, Cameroon, Central African Republic, Chad, Côte d'Ivoire, Eritrea, Ethiopia, Ghana, Kenya, Mali, Niger, Nigeria, Senegal, Sudan, Togo, and Uganda.[177]
- Meningococcal disease is endemic in Delhi, India.[172]
- As recently as 2005, a new serotype of *N. meningitides,* serogroup C, caused outbreaks in China.[178]

Diagnosis

- Gram stain and culture of cerebrospinal fluid or blood for isolation of organism and antibiotic susceptibility testing[171,172]
- Cerebrospinal fluid analysis for high white blood cell count (100–10,000), high protein (>40 mg/dL), and low glucose (<40 mg/dL or <50% blood glucose)[171]
- Clinical picture consistent with *N. meningitidis* infection (see systemic and cutaneous manifestations below).

Clinical Findings

SYSTEMIC MANIFESTATIONS

- Fever, nausea, vomiting, headache, stiff neck, myalgia, photophobia, altered mental status[170]
- Hypotension, tachycardia, diaphoresis, positive Kernig and Brudzinski signs[170]
- Diffuse intravascular coagulation[179]
- Myocardial dysfunction and heart failure[179]

CUTANEOUS MANIFESTATIONS

Petechiae, Purpura, and Ecchymoses (Figure 68-31)

- Petechiae are a hallmark of meningococcemia and occur on the skin and mucous membranes (soft palate and conjunctivae).[170,171,179]
- Splinter hemorrhages are petechiae under the nail.
- Over 50% of patients have petechiae on presentation.[180,181]
- Petechiae can progress to purpura and ecchymoses.[179]
- These findings can be subtle initially, and therefore, these important diagnostic clues may not been noticed in patients with skin of color.[171]
- Less often, an eruption described as a pink maculopapular or morbilliform

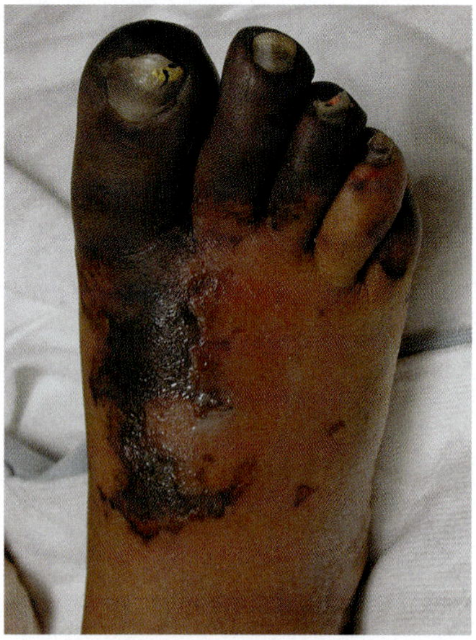

▲ **FIGURE 68-31** Meningococcemia purpura fulminans in a 32-year-old African-American woman presents with fever, vomiting, and arthralgias. She presented with generalized petechiae and hemorrhagic pustules and retiform purpuric plaques on both extremities. Note the edema and hemorrhagic black necrotic toes and dorsum of the foot. With antibiotics and nitropaste, she regained perfusion to this foot. Courtesy of Department of Dermatology, Washington Hospital Center, Washington DC.

also occurs in patients with meningococcal infection.[182,183]

PURPURA FULMINANS

- Purpura fulminans is a common cause of complications and death in people with meningococcal infection, particularly children and young adults.[184]
- Purpura fulminans occurs in 15–25% of meningococcemia patients.[185,186]
- Initially presenting as petechiae and ecchymoses, inflammatory and coagulation factors lead to the development of disseminated intravascular coagulation and vascular thrombosis, which, in turn, cause cutaneous gangrenous necrosis and organ failure.[170,172,184]
- Less often this necrosis can spread to the subcutis, muscle, and bone.[187]

Treatment and Prevention

- Owing to the severe complications and sequelae of meningitis and meningococcemia, a confirmed diagnosis via analysis of cerebrospinal fluid should never delay antibiotic administration.[170,172,179]
- Antibiotics currently used include penicillin and cephalosporins, particularly third-generation cephalosporins such as ceftriaxone, cefotaxime, ceftizoxime, and ceftazidime.[191–193]
- Activated protein C also has shown to improve survival and decrease the need for amputation.[188,189]
- In severe cases, surgical interventions ranging from debridement to skin grafts to amputation may be required.[190]
- In the United States, two vaccines have been approved to help prevent meningococcal infection:
  - The polysaccharide vaccine, also known as *MPSV4* and *Menomune,* was first used in 1981 and is recommended for children ages 2–10 years and adults over age 55.[194]
  - The conjugate vaccine, also known as *MCV4* or *Menactra,* was approved in 2005 and is recommended for people who are susceptible to encapsulated organisms (e.g., those with poor spleen function or asplenic), all children age 11–12 years , all those entering college or the military who will be living in dormitories, and anyone at risk of meningococcal infection between the ages of 11 and 55 years.[194]
- Both the polysaccharide and conjugate vaccine prevent four serotypes of *N. meningitides* (A, C, Y, and W-135).[194]

TUBEROUS SCLEROSIS

Tuberous sclerosis complex (TSC) is a neurocutaneous syndrome that affects multiple organ systems, including the brain, kidney, skin, retina, heart, and lung.[195] This autosomal dominant disorder has a wide range of clinical presentations, and the classic triad of seizures, mental retardation, and facial angiofibromas (Vogt triad) is seen in only 29% of cases;[196] 96% of affected individuals will have skin findings at varying ages. Early diagnosis is important because of the neurologic findings.

Epidemiology

- TSC has an incidence of approximately 1 in 5,000–10,000 live births.
- Its true incidence is likely underreported because many asymptomatic or mildly affected patients are never diagnosed.[195]
- Two-thirds of patients are nonfamilial cases, which are due to spontaneous mutations or mosaicism.[197–199]
- No racial predilection has been noted in the literature.

Etiology/Genetics

- Mutations of two separate gene products are responsible for TSC.
- *TSC1* encodes the protein hamartin and maps to chromosome 9q34,[200] and *TSC2* encodes the protein tuberin and maps to chromosome 16p13.3.[201]
- *TSC1* and *TSC2* are believed to play a role in controlling cellular growth and proliferation.[195]

Clinical Findings

- Onset of skin findings varies by age. Hypomelanotic macules, forehead plaques, and shagreen patches occur early; periungal fibromas and facial angiofibromas occur later (Figures 68-32 and 68-33).
- The color of the skin lesions is affected by the background color of the skin. Lesions that are hypopigmented are light brown compared with the background skin, and papules and plaques will be red brown to dark brown instead of pink.
- In 1998, the Tuberous Sclerosis Alliance held a consensus conference to revise the diagnostic criteria for TSC. Major and minor criteria were established, and either two major features or one major feature plus two minor features were required for a definite diagnosis of TSC. Of the 11 major clinical features, the following are found in the skin:
  - Facial angiofibromas or forehead plaque
  - Nontraumatic ungual or periungual fibroma (Koenen tumor; Figure 68-34)
  - Three or more hypomelanotic macules (ash leaf spots or Fitzpatrick patches; Figure 68-35*A*)
  - Shagreen patch (connective tissue nevus; Figure 68-35*B*)
- The nine minor clinical features include:
  - Multiple, randomly distributed pits in dental enamel.
  - Hamartomatous rectal polyps.

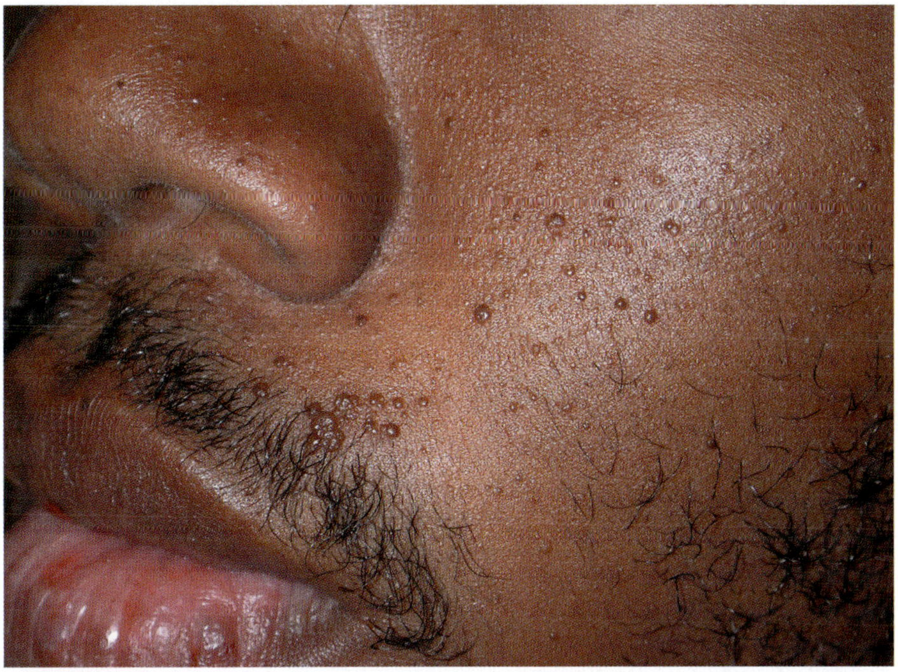

▲ **FIGURE 68-32** Tuberous sclerosis angiofibromas in an African-American adolescent with dome-shaped, close-to-skin-colored, shiny papules, some in a cluster in the midface. Courtesy of Department of Dermatology, Washington Hospital Center, Washington DC.

- Bone cysts
- Cerebral white matter radial migration lines
- Gingival fibromas
- Nonrenal hamartomas
- Retinal achromic patch
- Confetti skin lesions
- Multiple renal cysts[202]

- Facial angiofibromas are dark brown to purple papules that usually involve the malar areas of the face and spare the upper lips.
- Fitzpatrick patches are polygonal hypopigmented to white areas seen most commonly on the trunk and buttocks and are the earliest cutaneous findings in TSC.

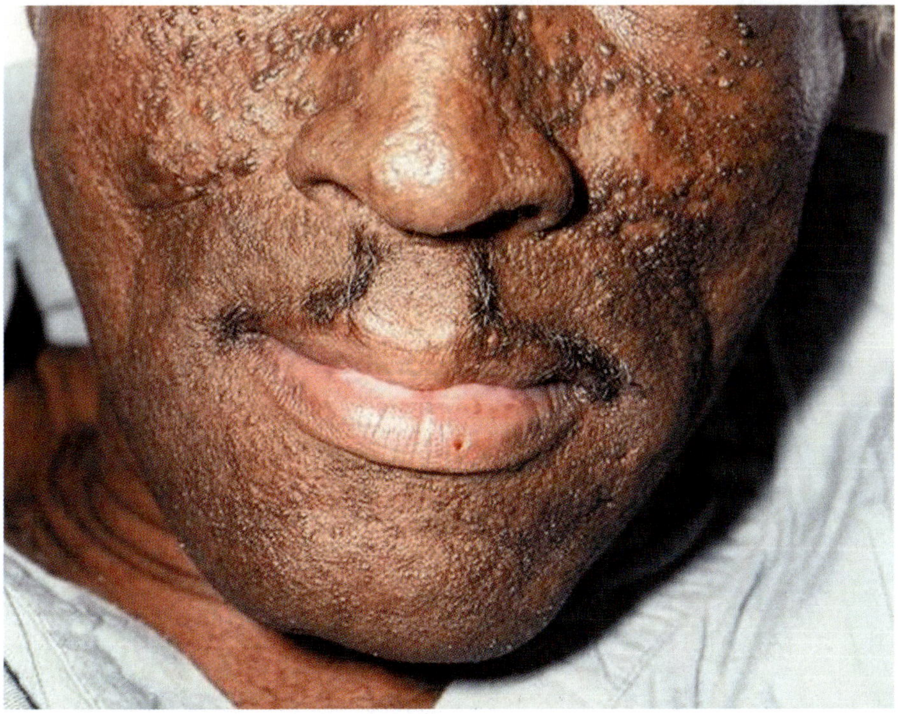

FIGURE 68-33 Tuberous sclerosis angiofibromas in an older African-American man with known seizure disorder showing hyperpigmented, clustered, dome-shaped shiny papules in the midface. Courtesy of Department of Dermatology, Washington Hospital Center, Washington DC.

- A shagreen patch can be slightly elevated, and its rough surface on palpation is reminiscent of an orange peel.
- Confetti skin lesions are multiple small white macules found on the extremities.[195]

Treatment

- Treatment of TSC is largely symptomatic.
- CO_2 laser, argon laser, pulsed-dye laser, dermabrasion, curettage, cryosurgery, chemical peel, limited excision, shave excision, 13-*cis*-retinoic acid, and combinations of any of the aforementioned therapeutic modalities all have been used to varying degrees of success in the treatment of facial angiofibromas.[203,204]
- Rapamycin (Sirolimus) is currently being researched as a nonsurgical therapy for TSC.[195]

SICKLE CELL DISEASE

Sickle cell anemia is an inherited autosomal recessive disorder that causes the bone marrow to produce red blood cells with hemoglobin S.[205] During times of stress or poor oxygenation, this substitution causes red blood cells to sickle, after which they then become caught in capillaries within and outside organs.[205]

Epidemiology

- Affects people around the world, particularly in sub-Saharan Africa, South America, Cuba, Central America, Saudi Arabia, India, and Mediterranean countries.
- The sickle cell gene occurs where malaria is or was prevalent. This is due to the protection that the heterozygous condition provides against malaria.[206]
- In West and Central Africa, 25% of the population has sickle cell trait, and 1–2% of babies are born with the disease.[206]
- In Nigeria, 45,000–90,000 babies are born each year with sickle cell disease.[206]
- In the United States
  - 1 in 500 African-Americans has sickle cell disease.
  - 1 in 12 African-Americans has sickle cell trait.
  - 1 in 1,000–1,400 Hispanic Americans has sickle cell disease.

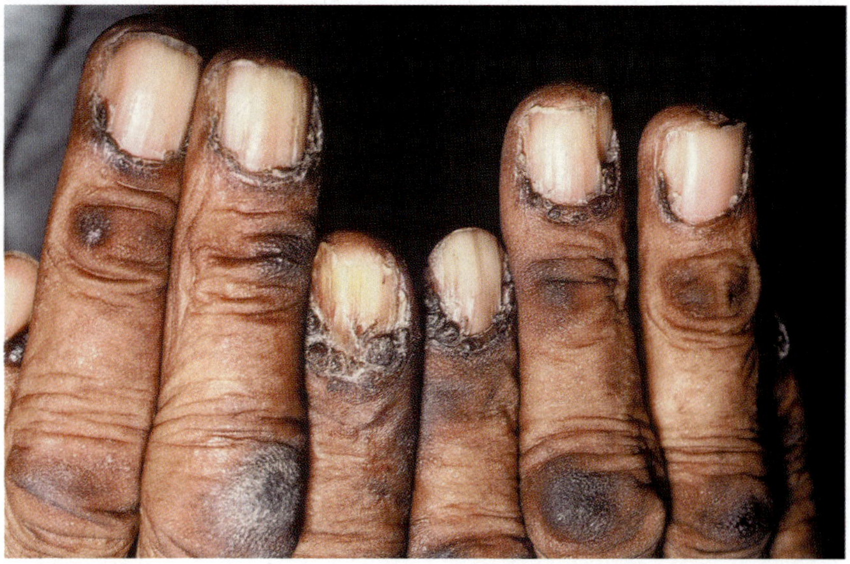

▲ **FIGURE 68-34** Tuberous sclerosis periungal fibromas (Koenens tumors) in the same patient as in Figure 68-33 with periungal dark brown fibrotic plaques and dystrophic nails. Courtesy of Department of Dermatology, Washington Hospital Center, Washington DC.

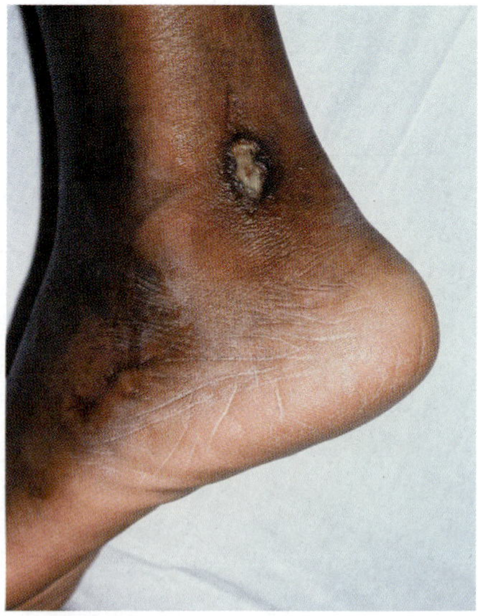

▲ **FIGURE 68-36** Sickle cell disease in an African-American man with a persistent ulcer after a sickle cell crisis.

- 2 million people have sickle cell trait.
- 1,000 babies are born with sickle cell disease.[206]

Cutaneous Epidemiology

- The incidence of leg ulcers in people with sickle cell disease is 25.7–75%.
- Risk factors for leg ulcers:[236]
  - 20 years of age and over
  - Male
  - Low level of fetal hemoglobin and hemoglobin level less than 6 g/dL[221,223,224]
  - Antithrombin III deficiency
  - HLA types B35 and CW4
  - Geographic region, that is, Jamaica (75%) and Saudi Arabia (0%)
  - High risk if previous ulcer

Etiology/Genetics

- In the gene encoding the human β-globin subunit, there is replacement glutamic acid at position 6 by valine on the β chain of hemoglobin.[205]

Diagnosis

- Hemoglobin SS on hemoglobin electrophoresis
- Sickled red blood cells on peripheral blood smear
- DNA polymerase chain reaction (PCR)[207,208]
- Clinical examination and skin biopsy if necessary for cutaneous manifestations

Clinical Presentation of Cutaneous Manifestations

- Most sickle cell patients will have cutaneous manifestations in the form of skin color and leg ulcer (Figure 68-36).
- Other cutaneous manifestations of sickle cell anemia are pseudoxanthoma elasticum (PXE; Figure 68-37), and dactylitis.[221]

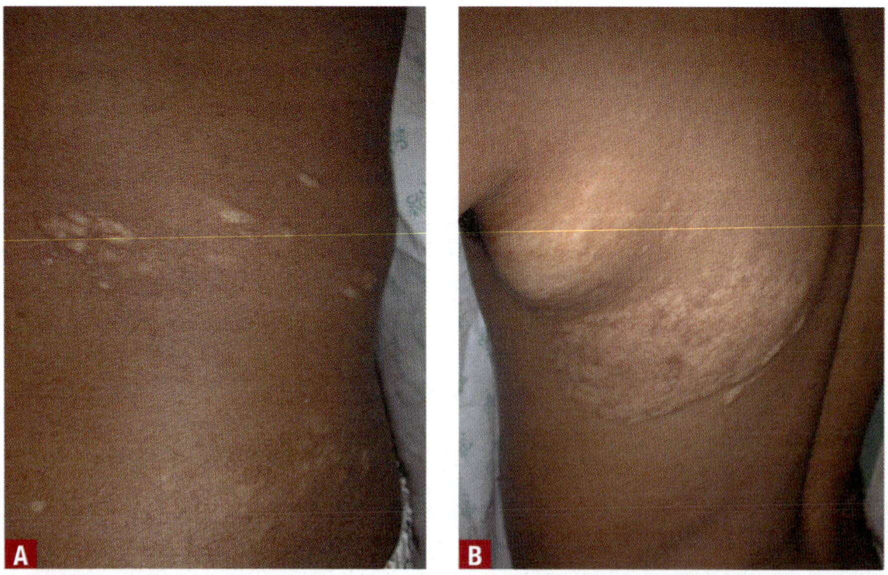

▲ **FIGURE 68-35** **A.** Tuberous sclerosis. Hypopigmented macules and papules on the trunk. **B.** Tuberous sclerosis shagreen patch in an African-American woman with hypopigmented plaques on the upper trunk with lumpy surfaces and a leathery appearance. Courtesy of Department of Dermatology, Washington Hospital Center, Washington DC.

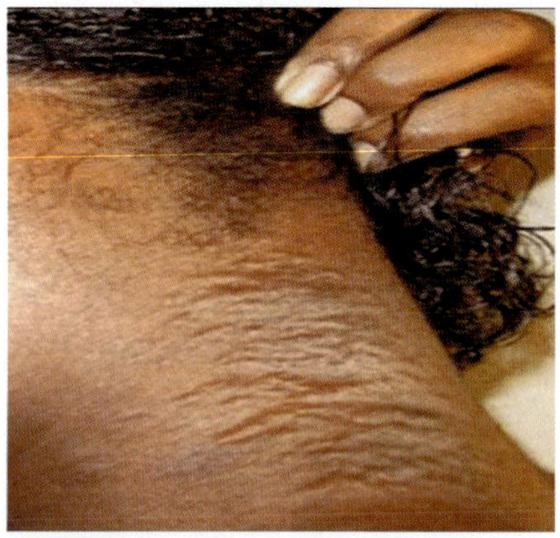

▲ **FIGURE 68-37** Sickle cell disease in an African-American woman with pseudoxanthoma elasticum on the neck that waxes and wanes with reduction in hydroyurea dosing. Courtesy of Department of Dermatology, Washington Hospital Center, Washington DC.

- Cutaneous manifestations typically occur in patients over 10 and under 30 years of age.[221,222]

LEG ULCERS

- Start as round and punched-out ulcerations with a raised border and a deep necrotic base and very tender.
- Dark hyperpigmentation and hardening of the skin surrounding the ulcer.
- Postinflammatory hyperpigmentation in areas of previous ulcers.
- Ulcers occur in areas of less subcutaneous fat and decreased blood flow. The skin overlying the medial and lateral malleoli is the most frequent site of ulcers, but ulcers also are found on the dorsum of the foot and Achilles tendon area.[221,223]
- Often appear in areas of trauma.[221]
- Ulcers are slow to heal, resistant to treatment, and often recurrent.[221,225,226]

SKIN COLOR

- Pale yellowish hue
- Jaundiced sclera
- Pallor and jaundice increase during crises.

PSEUDOXANTHOMA ELASTICUM

- A known but relatively rare association with sickle cell anemia, PXE is a disorder of fragmented elastic fibers and calcium deposition in the mid-dermis.[233–236]
- The relationship between the two disorders is not completely understood.[233]
- There is great variation in clinical phenotype.[234]
- In patients with sickle cell anemia, PXE usually occurs after age 20.[235]
- Often it is reported to be milder than the hereditary form of PXE.[233,235]
- Most commonly involves the skin, eyes, and cardiovascular system.[233–235]
- Lesions are typically described as 1- to 5-mm yellow papules and plaques called *pseudoxanthomas.*[234,235]
- In pigmented skin, lesions are oval-shaped, hyperpigmented plaques along the skin line and mildly pruritic.
- Lesions tend to occur in flexural areas such as the neck and axillae.[234]
- PXE can lead to both lax and redundant skin.[234]
- Treatment of PXE is focused on ophthalmologic and cardiovascular aspects of the disease.

DACTYLITIS

- Swelling of hands and feet during first 3 years of life

Clinical Presentation of Systemic Manifestations

- Chronic hemolytic anemia
- Aplastic crises
- Pain crises
- End-organ damage
- Recurrent infection

Treatment

- Prevention of infection via vaccination, especially for encapsulated organisms.[209,210]
- Prophylactic penicillin in children.[211,212]
- Transfusion.[213,214]
- Pain management.[215]
- Folic acid to help with production of red blood cells.[216]
- Hydroxyurea to increase fetal hemoglobin.[217–220]
- Treatment includes wound debridement, wet-to-dry dressings, and hydrocolloid dressings.[221,227,228]
- Oral zinc also has been shown to hasten ulcer healing.[225]
- Larger ulcers may require surgical intervention, including grafts and flaps.[229–232]

NEUROFIBROMATOSIS TYPE I

Neurofibromatosis type I (NF1), also known as *von Recklinghausen disease,* is an autosomal dominant neurocutaneous disorder.[237,238] Neurofibromatosis type II (NF2) is rare. NF1 affects the skin and nervous and musculoskeletal systems.[237–239]

Etiology/Pathogenesis

- Mutations in the *NF1* gene (chromosome 17q11).
- Protein product is neurofibromin, which has tumor-suppressor activity.[240,241]
- Both familial and sporadic cases occur.[237,238]
- There is complete penetrance but variable expression.[242]

Epidemiology

- Occurs in approximately 1 in 3,000 people.[243]
- NF1 shows no racial predilection.[244]
- Increased risk for malignancy. Most common are neurofibrosarcomas, optic pathway tumors, astrocytomas, ependymomas, medulloblastomas, and myeloid leukemias. There is a 200-fold increased risk for chronic myelomonocytic leukemia (CML).[245,246]

Diagnosis

- Two or more of the following must be present, as determined by the NIH consensus conference:[239]
  - Six or more café-au-lait spots greater than 5 mm in diameter in children and greater than 15 mm in diameter in adults
  - Two or more neurofibromas of any type or one plexiform
  - Axillary or inguinal freckling
  - Optic glioma
  - Two or more Lisch nodules
  - Sphenoid bone dysplasia
  - A first-degree relative with NF1

Clinical Findings

- Café-au-lait spots. (Figure 68-38)
  - Tan to brown macules and patches with homogeneous pigmentation; may appear hypopigmented in darker skin types.
  - Must be distinguished from Mongolian spots, which are blue to black macules and patches.
- Peripheral neurofibromas: cutaneous (skin-colored, tan to dark brown soft papules and nodules), subcutaneous (soft dermal nodules), and plexiform (thought to be congenital but not clinically apparent for 4–5 years and preceded by overlying hyperpigmentation and/or hypertrichosis).[247]
- Axillary and inguinal freckling.
- Giant pigmented nevi.
- Several reports of cutis vertices gyrata (furrows and cerebriform folds of the scalp); on biopsy, neurofibromas are present.[248]

Systemic Manifestations

- Pseudoarthoses
- Learning disabilities
- Macrocephaly
- Peripheral neuropathy

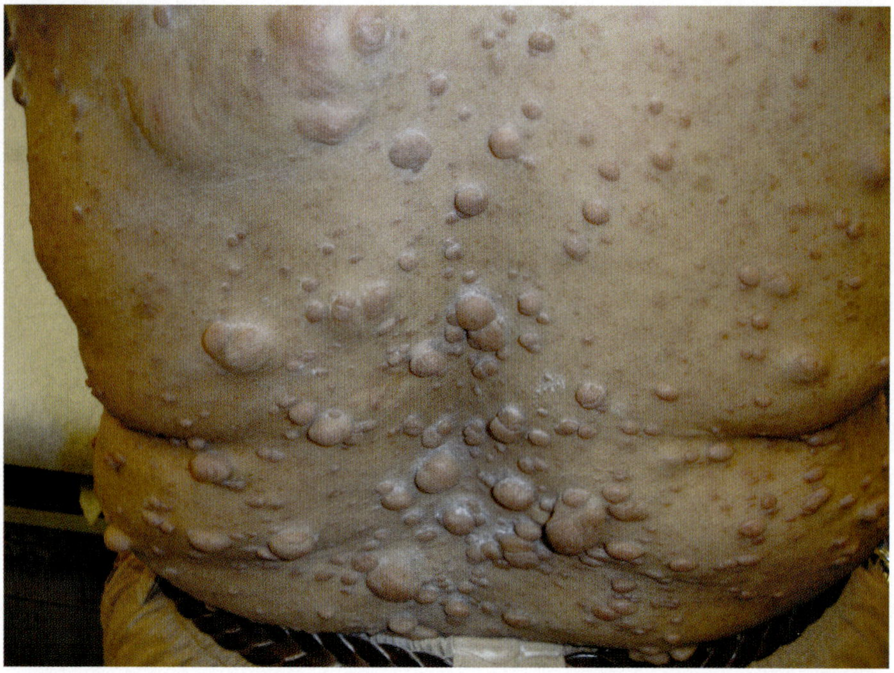

▲ **FIGURE 68-38** Neurofibromatosis. Multiple soft brown-pink papules and nodules. Note on upper back a small plexiform neurofibroma with hyper- and hypopigmentation. Patient has a seizure disorder and a history of resection of multiple brain tumors. Courtesy of Atlantic Dermatology, 2006.

- Short stature
- Hypertension
- Epilepsy
- Mental retardation
- Scoliosis
- Renal artery stenosis
- Bone lesions (e.g., sphenoid bone dysplasia, vertebral defects, and long bone thinning)
- Benign and malignant tumors (e.g., pheochromocytoma, optic gliomas, astrocytomas, brain stem gliomas, soft tissue sarcomas, and others)

Treatment

- Excision of painful or disfiguring neurofibromas[237]
- Surgical removal of tumors involving the spine and brain[249]
- Radiation therapy for optic nerve gliomas[250]
- Genetic counseling/testing
- Prenatal testing
- At least yearly physical examinstion and ophthalmologic examination

INTERNAL MALIGNANCY

Metastatic cancer with lymphoproliferative disease to the skin is usually a very late sign of disease; however, it may be the only sign that brings the patient to the dermatologist. As discussed in this chapter, people of color present later to the health care system in the course of the disease and therefore have a poorer prognosis. The health care provider initially must make an assessment of the patient's health status, perform a complete skin examination, biopsy any growths, and refer the patient to his or her internist for a complete metastatic workup.

Epidemiology[251]

AFRICAN-AMERICANS

For the majority of cancers, African-Americans have the highest death rates and the shortest survivals. These health disparities have been attributed to socioeconomic inequalities. In 2003, the death rate for all cancers combined was 35% higher among African-American men and 18% higher among African-American women than among their Caucasian counterparts.

The most common types of cancer among African-American women are breast (27%), lung (13%), and colorectal (12%) cancers. The most common types of cancer among African-American men are prostate (37%), lung (15%), and colorectal (9%) cancers.

Cancer deaths among African-Americans are primarily due to lung cancer, followed by prostate and colorectal cancers in men and breast and colorectal cancers in women. Racial discrepancies in cancer death rates are mainly due to breast and colorectal cancers in women and prostate, lung, and colorectal cancers in men. This is because of higher incidence rates among African-Americans and poorer survival secondary to later stage of diagnosis and decreased access to treatment.

HISPANICS/LATINOS

In the Hispanic/Latino population, the incidence and death rates for all cancers combined and the most common malignancies are lower than for non-Hispanic whites. Malignancies that have higher rates in this population include stomach, liver, cervix, and gallbladder cancers and acute lymphocytic leukemia.

The most common malignancies among Hispanic men are prostate (30%), colorectal (11%), and lung (8%) cancers, with lung cancer causing most cancer deaths, followed by colorectal and prostate cancers. Among Hispanic women, the most common malignancies are breast (34%), colorectal (9%), and lung (6%) cancers, with breast cancer accounting for the most cancer deaths, followed by lung and colorectal cancers.

Although Hispanics/Latinos have lower incidence and death rates, they are more likely to present with a higher stage of disease than non-Hispanic whites.

ASIAN AMERICANS AND PACIFIC ISLANDERS

Asian Americans and Pacific Islanders have a lower incidence rate than the non-Hispanic white population for most common cancers. This population also has a higher incidence of cancers associated with infection, including hepatocellular and stomach cancers.

NATIVE AMERICANS AND ALASKAN NATIVES

Data for Native Americans and Alaskan Natives are limited, but the Cancer Registry and Indian Health Service are currently working together to resolve this problem. It is known that this population has a higher incidence of renal carcinoma than any other racial or ethnic population.

TREND IN INCIDENCE

Data from 1999–2003 show the following trend in incidence of cancer for all sites:

- *Men:* African-American > Caucasian American > Hispanic/Latino > Asian American/Pacific Islander > Native American/Alaskan Native

- *Women:* Caucasian American > African-American > Hispanic/Latino > Native American/Alaska Native > Asian American/Pacific Islander

Breast Cancer (Figure 68-39*A*)

Among African-American women, breast cancer is the most common malignancy and second most common cause of cancer death. The incidence rate is approximately 12% lower among American women overall. Among women under age 40, the incidence rate is higher than for Caucasian women.[251]

Breast cancer survival rates are lower among African-American women than Caucasian women for two reasons: later stage of detection and worse stage-specific survival. Caucasian women are more likely to be diagnosed with breast cancer at a local stage and tend to participate more in early detection and treatment strategies.[251] There is some evidence that the biologic behavior of breast cancer may be more aggressive in African-Americans than in Caucasians.[252]

Breast cancer is the most common malignancy and the primary cause of cancer death among Hispanic women. Breast cancer incidence is roughly 40% lower among Hispanic women than among non-Hispanic white women. This may be due in part to a reduced use of hormone-replacement therapy among Hispanic women, protective reproductive patterns such as lower age of first birth and larger number of children, and to underdiagnosis secondary to fewer Hispanic women using mammography.[251]

Hispanic women are approximately 20% more likely to die from breast cancer than Caucasian women at a similar age and stage of diagnosis.[254] Caucasian women are more likely to be diagnosed with breast cancer at an earlier stage and with a smaller-sized tumor.[253]

Colorectal Cancer

Colorectal cancer is the third most common malignancy and third most common cause of cancer death among African-American men and women.[251] Incidence rates are higher and survival rates are lower among African-Americans than among Caucasians.[251] A reason for the former has not been elucidated, whereas the latter is secondary to decreased access to care, reduced delivery of treatment, and a possible difference in tumor biology.[255]

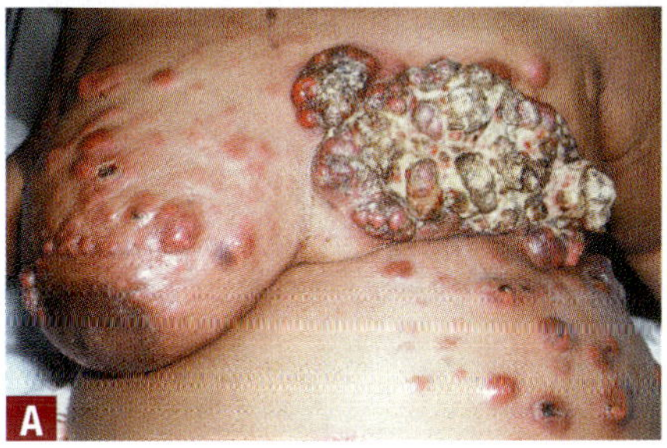

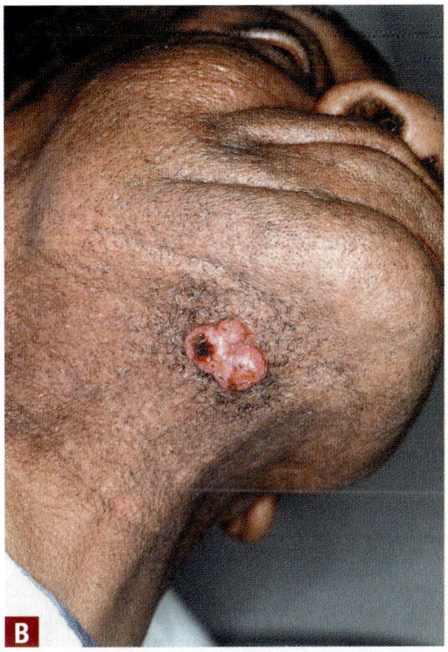

▲ **FIGURE 68-39** **A.** Metastatic breast disease in an African-American woman after a mastectomy with multiple dome-shaped nodules in both breasts and the skin of the chest and abdomen. Both nodules and plaques have necrosis. **B.** Metastatic lung disease in an elderly African-American man with multilobule nodule on chin with unshaven surrounding area. Courtesy of Department of Dermatology, Washington Hospital Center, Washington DC.

Among Hispanics/Latinos, colorectal cancer is the second most common malignancy, and incidence rates are 20–30% lower than in non-Hispanic whites.[251] Hispanics are more likely to be diagnosed at an advanced stage and are less likely to survive after diagnosis.[254] Malignancies of the colon and rectum are the second most common cause of cancer death among Hispanic men and the third most common cause of cancer death among Hispanic women.[251]

Lung Cancer (see Figure 68-39*B*)

Malignancies of the lung and bronchus are the second most common type of cancer and the number one cause of cancer death among African-Americans.[251] Incidence rates are about the same between African-American women and Caucasian women but are almost 40% higher among African-American men than among Caucasian men.[251] Survival rates are slightly lower among African-Americans.[251] One study demonstrated that African-Americans diagnosed with early-stage lung cancer were less likely to receive surgical intervention, which is the only treatment that results in a cure.[256]

Lung cancer is the third most common malignancy among Hispanics/Latinos.[251] Incidence rates are approximately 50% lower in the Hispanic/Latino population than in the non-Hispanic white population.[251] This can be attributed to lower rates of cigarette use among Hispanics/Latinos.[251] Lung cancer accounts for the most cancer-related deaths among Hispanic men, but this malignancy is second to breast cancer for number of deaths among Hispanic women.[251]

Prostate Cancer

Among African-American and Hispanic men, prostate cancer is the most common malignancy.[251] Prostate cancer is the second most common cause of cancer death in African-American men.[251] Prostate cancer is the third most common cause of cancer death in Hispanic men.[251]

The annual incidence rate is approximately 60% higher among African-American men than among Caucasian men, the reason for which is not well understood.[251] Among Hispanic men, prostate cancer rates are about 20% lower than in non-Hispanic whites.[251] The death rate is 2.4 times higher among African-American men, and prostate cancer is more likely to be diagnosed at an earlier stage in Caucasian men.[251]

ACKNOWLEDGMENT

We would like to thank Katina Byrd-Miles, M.D., of the Washington Hospital Center, for the research on sarcoidosis.

REFERENCES

1. US Census Bureau, *www.census.gov/Press-Release/www/releases/archives/population/001720.html.*

Diabetes Mellitus

2. Ahmed I, Goldstein B. Diabetes mellitus. *Clin Dermatol* 2006;24:237-246.
3. National Institutes of Health. Fact Sheet: Type 2 Diabetes, 2007, *www.nih.gov/about/researchresultsforthepublic/Type2Diabetes.pdf.*

4. Pinhas-Hamiel O, Zeitler P. The global spread of type 2 diabetes mellitus in children and adolescents. *J Pediatr* 2005;146:693-700.
5. Centers for Disease Control and Prevention. Prevalence of Diabetes, 2007, *www.cdc.gov/diabetes/statistics/prev/national/menuraceethsexage.htm.*
6. Wahid Z, Kanjee A. Cutaneous manifestations of diabetes mellitus. *J Pak Med Assoc* 1998;48:304-305.
7. American Diabetes Association. Diagnosis and classification of diabetes mellitus. *Diabetes Care* 2007;30: 1(Suppl 1):S42-7.
8. Ngo BT, Hayes KD, DiMiao DJ, et al. Manifestations of cutaneous diabetic microangiopathy. *Am J Clin Dermatol* 2005;6:225-237.
9. Litonjua P, Piñero-Piloña A, Aviles-Santa L, Raskin P. Prevalence of acanthosis nigricans in newly diagnosed type 2 diabetes. *Endocr Pract* 2004;10:101-106.
10. Schmults CA. Scleredema. *Dermatol Online J* 2002;9:11, *http://dermatology.cdlib.org/94/NYU/Jan2002/6.html.*

Thyroid Disease

11. Burman KD, McKinley-Grant L. Dermatologic aspects of thyroid disease. *Clin Dermatol* 2006;24:247-255.
12. Ai J, Leonhardt JM, Heymann WR. Autoimmune thyroid diseases: Etiology, pathogenesis, and dermatologic manifestations. *J Am Acad Dermatol* 2003;48:641-659.
13. Kanaya AM, Harris F, Volpato S, et al. Association between thyroid dysfunction and total cholesterol level in an older biracial population. The Health, Aging and Body Composition Study. *Arch Intern Med* 2002;162:773-779.
14. Sichieri R, Baima J, Marante T, et al. Low prevalence of hypothyroidism among black and mulatto people in a population-based study of Brazilian women. *Clin Endocrinol* 2007;66:803-807.
15. Daneshpazhooh M, Mostofizadeh G M, Behjati J, Akhyani M, Robati RM. Anti-thyroid peroxidase antibody and vitiligo: A controlled study. *BMC Dermatol* 2006;6:3.
16. González GC, Capel I, Rodríguez-Espinosa J, et al. Thyroid autoimmunity at onset of type 1 diabetes as a predictor of thyroid dysfunction. *Diabetes Care* 2007;30:1611-1612.
17. Seyrafi H, Akhiani M, Abbasi H, Mirpour S, Gholamrezanezhad A. Evaluation of the profile of alopecia areata and the prevalence of thyroid function test abnormalities and serum autoantibodies in Iranian patients. *BMC Dermatol* 2005;5:11.
18. Fatourechi V, Pajouhi M, Fransway AF. Dermopathy of Graves' disease (pretibial myxedema): Review of 150 cases. *Medicine (Baltimore)* 1994;73:1-7.
19. Fatourechi V. Pretibial myxedema: Pathophysiology and treatment options. *Am J Clin Dermatol* 2005;6: 295-309.
20. Anderson CK. Triad of exophthalmos, pretibial myxedema, and acropachy in a patient with Graves' disease. *J Am Acad Dermatol* 2003;48:970-972.
21. Georgala S, Katoulis AC, Georgala C, et al. Pretibial myxedema as the initial manifestation of Graves' disease. *J Eur Acad Dermatol Venereol* 2002;16:380-383.
22. Fatourechi V. Thyroid acropachy: Report of 40 patients treated at a single institution in a 26-year period. *J Clin Endocrinol Metab* 2002;87:5435-5441.
23. Luc GT, Andrew GS, David JM, Mark D. Racial patterns of thyroid cancer incidence in the U.S. Presented at American Academy of Otolaryngology Head and Neck Surgery (AAOHNS) Meeting, September 17, 2007, *www.entnet.org.*
24. Waguespack S, Wells S, Ross J, Bleyer A. Thyroid Cancer. In: Bleyer A, O'Leary M, Barr R, Ries LAG (eds): *Cancer Epidemiology in Older Adolescents and Young Adults 15 to 29 Years of Age, Including SEER Incidence and Survival: 1975-2000.* National Cancer Institute, NIH Pub. No. 06-5767. Bethesda, MD 2006.
25. Ross D. Disorders that cause hypothyroidism. *Up To Date* (online journal), 2008, *www.uptodate.com.*

Renal Disease

26. Silverberg NB, Singh A, Laude TA. Cutaneous manifestations of chronic renal failure in children of color. *Pediatr Dermatol* 2001;18:199-204.
27. Mitch WE. Acute renal failure, in Goldman L, Ausiello D (eds), *Cecil Textbook of Medicine* 22nd ed. Philadelphia, Saunders, 2004, pp 703-708.
28. Luke RG. Chronic renal failure, in Goldman L, Ausiello D (eds), *Cecil Textbook of Medicine* 22nd ed. Philadelphia, Saunders, 2004, pp 708-716.
29. National Kidney Foundation. Ten Facts About African-Americans and Kidney Disease, 2008, *www.kidney.org/news/newsroom/fsitem.cfm?id=2.*
30. Centers for Disease Control and Prevention. Prevalence of Diabetes, 2007, *www.cdc.gov/diabetes/statistics/prev/national/menuraceethsexage.htm.*
31. Enelow TJ, Huang W, Williams CM. Perforating papules in chronic renal failure: Metastatic calcinosis cutis with transepidermal elimination. *Arch Dermatol* 1998;134:98-99, 101-102.
32. Tan O, Atik B, Kizilkaya A, Ozer E, Kavukcu S. Extensive skin calcifications in an infant with chronic renal failure: Metastatic calcinosis cutis. *Pediatr Dermatol* 2006;23:235-238.
33. Robinson-Bostom L, DiGiovanna JJ. Cutaneous manifestations of end-stage renal disease. *J Am Acad Dermatol* 2000;43:975-986.
34. Rivet J, Lebbé C, Urena P, et al. Cutaneous calcification in patients with end-stage renal disease: A regulated process associated with in situ osteopontin expression. *Arch Dermatol* 2006;142:900-906.
35. Callen JP. Dermatologic manifestations in patients with systemic disease, in Bolognia JL, Jorizzo JL, Rapini RP (eds), *Dermatology,* 2nd ed. New York, Elsevier, 2008, pp 675-692.
36. Headley CM, Wall B. ESRD-associated cutaneous manifestations in a hemodialysis population. *Nephrol Nurs J* 2002;29: 525-527, 531-539.
37. Rapini RP. Perforating diseases, in Bolognia JL, Jorizzo JL, Rapini RP (eds), *Dermatology,* 2nd ed. New York, Elsevier, 2008, pp 1461-1467.
38. Saray Y, Seçkin D, Bilezikçi B. Acquired perforating dermatosis: Clinicopathological features in twenty-two cases. *J Eur Acad Dermatol Venereol* 2006;20:679-688.
39. Udayakumar P, Balasubramanian S, Ramalingam KS, et al. Cutaneous manifestations in patients with chronic renal failure on hemodialysis. *Indian J Dermatol Venereol Leprol* 2006;72:119-125.
40. Anderson KE. The porphyrias, in Goldman L, Ausiello D (eds), *Cecil Textbook of Medicine,* 22nd ed. Philadelphia, Saunders, 2004, pp 1292-1300.
41. Frank J, et al. Porphyria, in Bolognia JL, Jorizzo JL, Rapini RP (eds), *Dermatology,* 2nd ed. New York, Elsevier, 2008, pp 641-652.
42. Ramsay CA, Magnus IA, Turnbull A, Baker H. The treatment of porphyria cutanea tarda by venesection. *Q J Med* 1974;43:1.
43. Anderson KE, Goeger DE, Carson RW, Lee SM, Stead RB. Erythropoietin for the treatment of porphyria cutanea tarda in a patient on long-term hemodialysis. *N Engl J Med* 1990;322: 315-317.
44. Peces R, Salamanca R, Fontanellas A, et al. Successful treatment of haemodialysis-related porphyria cutanea tarda with erythropoietin. *Nephrol Dial Transplant* 1994;9:433.

Nephrogenic Systemic Fibrosis

45. Introcaso CE, Hivnor C, Cowper S, Werth VP. Nephrogenic fibrosing dermopathy/nephrogenic systemic fibrosis: A case series of nine patients and review of the literature. *Int J Dermatol* 2007;46:447-452.
46. Richmond H, Zwerner J, Kim Y, Fiorentino D. Nephrogenic systemic fibrosis: Relationship to gadolinium and response to photopheresis. *Arch Dermatol* 2007;143:1025-1030.
47. Swaminathan S, Ahmed I, McCarthy JT, et al. Nephrogenic fibrosing dermopathy and high-dose erythropoietin therapy. *Ann Intern Med* 2006;145:234-235.
48. Daram SR, Cortese CM, Bastani B. Nephrogenic fibrosing dermopathy/nephrogenic systemic fibrosis: Report of a new case with literature review. *Am J Kidney Dis* 2005;46:754-759.
49. Piera-Velázquez S, Sandorfi N, Jiménez SA. Nephrogenic systemic fibrosis/nephrogenic fibrosing dermopathy: clinical aspects. *Skinmed* 2007;6:24-27.
50. Todd DJ. Nephrogenic systemic fibrosis: What nephrologists need to know. *Nephrol Rounds* 2007;5:1-6.
51. Update on Magnetic Resonance Imaging (MRI) Contrast Agents Containing Gadolinium and Nephrogenic Fibrosing Dermopathy, 2006, *www.fda.gov/cder/drug/advisory/gadolinium_agents_20061222.htm.*
52. Cowper SE, Robin HS, Steinberg SM, et al. Scleromyxoedemalike cutaneous diseases in renal-dialysis patients. *Lancet* 2000;356:1000-1001.

53. Cowper SE. Nephrogenic fibrosing dermopathy: The first 6 years. *Curr Opin Rheumatol* 2003;15:785-790.
54. Cowper SE, Bucala R, LeBoit PE. Case 35-2004: Nephrogenic fibrosing dermopathy. *N Engl J Med* 2005;352:1723-1724.
55. National Kidney Foundation. Ten Facts About African-Americans and Kidney Disease, 2008, *www.kidney.org/news/newsroom/fsitem.cfm?id=2.*
56. Peak AS, Sheller A. Risk factors for developing gadolinium-induced nephrogenic systemic fibrosis. *Ann Pharmacother* 2007;41:1481-1485.
57. Mendoza FA, Artlett CM, Sandorfi N, et al. Description of 12 cases of nephrogenic fibrosing dermopathy and review of the literature. *Semin Arthritis Rheum* 2006;35:238-249.
58. Cowper SE, Su LD, Bhawan J, Robin HS, LeBoit PE. Nephrogenic fibrosing dermopathy. *Am J Dermatopathol* 2001; 23:383-393.
59. Galan A, Cowper SE, Bucala R. Nephrogenic systemic fibrosis (nephrogenic fibrosing dermopathy). *Curr Opin Rheumatol* 2006;18:614-617.
60. Yerram P, Saab G, Karuparthi PR, Hayden MR, Khanna R. Nephrogenic systemic fibrosis: A mysterious disease in patients with renal failure—Role of gadolinium-based contrast media in causation and the beneficial effect of intravenous sodium thiosulfate. *Clin J Am Soc Nephrol* 2007;2:258-263.
61. Cheung PP, Dorai Raj AK. Nephrogenic fibrosing dermopathy: A new clinical entity mimicking scleroderma. *Intern Med J* 2007;37:139-141.
62. Hamilton-Persaud K, Ezell LD, Macklin JG. Nephrogenic fibrosing dermopathy/nephrogenic systemic fibrosis. *Nephrol Nurs J* 2007;34:283-287.
63. Gilliet M, Cozzio A, Burg G, Nestle FO. Successful treatment of three cases of nephrogenic fibrosing dermpathy with extracorporeal photopheresis. *Br J Dermatol* 2005;152:531-536.
64. Distler JH, Jüngel A, Huber LC, et al. Imatinib mesylate reduces production of extracellular matrix and prevents development of experimental dermal fibrosis. *Arthritis Rheum* 2007;56:311-322.
65. Boyd AS. Gadolinium deposition in nephrogenic fibrosing dermopathy. *J Am Acad Dermatol* 2007;56:27-30.
66. Auron A. Nephrogenic fibrosing dermopathy in children. *Pediatr Nephrol* 2006;21:1307-1311.

Sarcoidosis

67. Iannuzzi MC, Rybicki BA, Teirstein AS. Sarcoidosis. *N Engl J Med* 2007;357: 2153-2165.
68. Westney GE, Habib S, Quarshie A. Comorbid illnesses and chest radiographic severity in African-American sarcoidosis patients. *Lung* 2007;185(3): 131-137.
69. Ramos-Casals M, Mañá J, Nardi N, et al. HISPAMEC Study Group. Sarcoidosis in patients with chronic hepatitis C virus infection: analysis of 68 cases. *Medicine (Baltimore)* 2005;84:69-80.
70. English JC 3rd, Patel PJ, Greer KE. Sarcoidosis. *J Am Acad Dermatol* 2001; 44:725-743.
71. Ezzie ME, Crouser ED. Considering an infectious etiology of sarcoidosis. *Clin Dermatol* 2007;25:259-266.
72. Kreider ME, Christie JD, Thompson B, et al. Relationship of environmental exposures to the clinical phenotype of sarcoidosis. *Chest* 2005;128:207-215.
73. Gray-McGuire C, Sinha R, Iyengar S, et al. SAGA Study Consortium. Genetic characterization and fine mapping of susceptibility loci for sarcoidosis in African Americans on chromosome 5. *Hum Genet* 2006; 120(3):420-430.
74. NHLBI Working Group. Future directions in sarcoidosis research. *Am J Respir Crit Care Med* 2004;170:567-571.
75. Rybicki BA, Maliarik MJ, Poisson LM, Iannuzzi MC. Sarcoidosis and granuloma genes: A family-based study in African-Americans. *Eur Respir J* 2004;24: 251-257.
76. Iannuzzi MC. Genetics of sarcoidosis. *Semin Respir Crit Care Med* 2007;28: 15-21.
77. Sharma OP, James DG. Did Osler's patient, Hannah W, have sarcoidosis? An historical footnote. *Chest* 1984;86: 263-264.
78. Sharma OP. Sarcoidosis: In a historical perspective. *Clin Dermatol* 2007;25: 232-241.
79. Mirmirani P, Maurer TA, Herndier B, et al. Sarcoidosis in a patient with AIDS: A manifestation of immune restoration syndrome. *J Am Acad Dermatol* 1999; 41:285-286.
80. Noor A, Kox KS. Immunopathogenesis of sarcoidosis. *Clin Dermatol* 2007;25: 250-258.
81. Newman L. A case control etiologic study of sarcoidosis: Environmental and occupational risk factors. *Am J Respir Crit Care Med* 2004;170:1324-1330.
82. Mana J, Marcova J. Cutaneous involvement in sarcoidosis: Relationship to systemic disease. *Arch Dermatol* 1997;133: 882-888.
83. Baughman RP, Lower EE. Infliximab for refractory sarcoidosis. *Sarcoidosis Vasculitis Diffuse Lung Dis* 2001;18: 70-74.
84. Giuffrida TJ, Kerdel FA. Sarcoidosis. *Dermatol Clin* 2002;20:435-447.
85. Cather JC, Cohen PR. Ichthyosiform sarcoidosis. *J Am Acad Dermatol* 1999;40: 862-865.
86. Burov EA, Kantor GR, Isaac M. Morpheaform sarcoidosis: Report of three cases. *J Am Acad Dermatol* 1998;39: 345-348.
87. Klein PA, Appel J, Callen JP. Sarcoidosis of the vulva: A rare cutaneous manifestation. *J Am Acad of Dermatol* 1998;39: 281-283.
88. Albertini J, Tyler W, Miller OF. Ulcerative sarcoidosis: Case report and review of the literature. *Arch Dermatol* 1997;133:215-219.
89. Barnard J, Newman LS. Sarcoidosis: Immunology, rheumatic involvement, and therapeutics. *Curr Opin Rheumatol* 2001;13:84-91.
90. Katta R, Nelson B, Chen D, Roenigk H. Sarcoidosis of the scalp: A case series and review of the literature. *J Am Acad of Dermatol* 2000;42:690-692.

Cutaneous Lupus Erythematosus

91. Alarcón GS, McGwin G Jr, Roseman JM, et al. Systemic lupus erythematosus in three ethnic groups: XIX. Natural history of the accrual of the American College of Rheumatology Criteria prior to the occurrence of criteria diagnosis. *Arthritis Rheum* 2004;51:609-615.
92. Patel P, Werth V. Cutaneous lupus erythematosus: A review. *Dermatol Clin* 2002;20:373.
93. Gilliam JN, Sontheimer RD. Skin manifestations of SLE. *Clin Rheum Dis* 1982;8:207.
94. Callen JP. Update on the management of cutaneous lupus erythematosus. *Br J Dermatol* 2004;151:731.
95. Hochbeg MC. Updating the American College of Rheumatology revised criteria for the classification of systemic lupus erythematosus. *Arthritis Rheum* 1997;40:1725.
96. Pons-Estel, BA, Catoggio, LJ, Cardiel, MH, et al. The GLADEL multinational Latin American prospective inception cohort of 1214 patients with systemic lupus erythematosus: Ethnic and disease heterogeneity among "Hispanics." *Medicine (Baltimore)* 2004;83:1.
97. Citera G, Wilson WA. Ethnic and geographic perspectives in SLE. *Lupus* 1993;2:351.
98. Johnson AE, Cavalcanti FS, Gordon C, et al. Cross-sectional analysis of the differences between patients with systemic lupus erythematosus in England, Brazil and Sweden. *Lupus* 1994;3:501.
99. Lawrence RC, Helmick CG, Arnett FC, et al. Estimates of the prevalence of arthritis and selected musculoskeletal disorders in the United States. *Arthritis Rheum* 1998;42:778.
100. Chakravarty EF, Bush TM, Manzi S, et al. Prevalence of adult systemic lupus erythematosus in California and Pennsylvania in 2000: Estimates obtained using hospitalization data. *Arthritis Rheum* 2007;56:2092.
101. Lau CS, Yin G, Mok MY. Ethnic and geographic differences in systemic lupus erythematosus: An overview. *Lupus* 2006;15:715-719.
102. Danchenko N, Satia JA, Anthony MS. Epidemiology of systemic lupus erythematosus: A comparison of worldwide disease burden. *Lupus* 2006;15:308.
103. Symmons DP. Frequency of lupus in people of African origin. *Lupus* 1995; 4:176.
104. Peschken CA, Esdaile JM. Systemic lupus erythematosus in North American Indians: A population based study. *J Rheumatol* 2000;27:1884-1891.
105. Serdula MK, Rhoads GG. Frequency of systemic lupus erythematosus in different ethnic groups in Hawaii. *Arthritis Rheum* 1979;22:328-333.
106. Lau CS, Mok MY. Lupus in Asia. *JAMA* 1998;14:5-7.
107. Segasothy M, Phillips PA. Systemic lupus erythematosus in Aborigines and Caucasians in central Australia: A comparative study. *Lupus* 2001;10:594-596.
108. New statistical report details state of women's health. *Health Care Financing Review* 2002;23:206-210.
109. Graciela A, Brooks K, Reveille JD, Lisse JR. *Do Patients of Hispanic and African-*

American Ethnicity with Lupus Experience Worse Outcomes than Patients with Lupus from Other Populations? The LUMINA Study. Rockville, MD, Lupus Foundation of America, 1999.

110. Ward MM, Studenski S. Clinical manifestations of systemic lupus erythematosus: Identification of racial and socioeconomic influences. *Arch Intern Med* 1990;150:849.
111. Reveille JD, Bartolucci A, Alarcon GS. Prognosis in SLE: Negative impact of increasing age at onset, black race, and thrombocytopenia, as well as causes of death. *Arthritis Rheum* 1990;33:37.
112. Callahan LF, Pincus T. Associations between clinical status questionnaire scores and formal educational levels in persons with systemic lupus erythematosus. *Arthritis Rheum* 1990;33:407.
113. Petri M, Perez-Gutthahn S, Longenecker JC, Hochberg M. Morbidity of systemic lupus erythematosus: Role of race and socioeconomic status. *Am J Med* 1991; 91:345.
114. Vlahakos DV, Foster, MH, Adams S, et al. Anti-DNA antibodies form immune deposits at distinct glomerular and vascular sites. *Kidney Int* 1992;41:1690.
115. D'Andrea DM, Coupaye-Gerard B, Kleyman TR, et al. Lupus autoantibodies interact directly with distinct glomerular and vascular cell surface antigens. *Kidney Int* 1996;49:1214.
116. Fernández M, Alarcón GS, Calvo-Alén J, et al. A multiethnic, multicenter cohort of patients with systemic lupus erythematosus (SLE) as a model for the study of ethnic disparities in SLE. *Arthritis Rheum* 2007;57:576-584.
117. Calvo-Alén J, Reveille JD, Rodríguez-Valverde V, et al. Clinical, immunogenetic, and outcome features of Hispanic systemic lupus erythematosus patients of different ethnic ancestry. *Lupus* 2003;12:377-385.
118. Ghaussy NO, Sibbitt W, Bankhurst AD, Qualls CR. Cigarette smoking and disease activity in systemic lupus erythematosus. *J Rheumatol* 2003;30:1215.

Scleroderma

119. Mayes M. Scleroderma epidemiology. *Rheum Dis Clin North Am* 1996;22:751-765.
120. Derk CT, Jimenez SA. Systemic sclerosis: Current views of its pathogenesis. *Autoimmun Rev* 2003;2:181-191.
121. Nietert PJ, Mitchell HC, Bolster MB, et al. Racial variations in clinical and immunological manifestations of systemic sclerosis. *J Rheumatol* 2006;33: 263-268.
122. Costner MI, Grau RH. Update on connective tissue diseases in dermatology. *Semin Cutan Med Surg* 2006;25:207-220.
123. Black CM. Scleroderma: Clinical aspects. *J Intern Med* 1993;234:115.
124. Grassi W, Medico PD, Izzo F, Cervini C. Microvascular involvement in systemic sclerosis: Capillaroscopic findings. *Semin Arthritis Rheum* 2001;30:397-402.
125. Steen VD. Clinical manifestations of systemic sclerosis. *Semin Cutan Med Surg* 1998;17:48-54.
126. Hawk A, English JC. Localized and systemic scleroderma. *Semin Cutan Med Surg* 2001;20:27-37.
127. Bombardieri S, Medsger TA Jr, Silman AJ, Valentini G. The assessment of the patient with systemic sclerosis: introduction. *Clin Exp Rheumatol* 2003;21: S2-4.
128. Charles C, Clements P, Furst DE. Systemic sclerosis: Hypothesis-driven treatment strategies. *Lancet* 2006;367: 1683-1691.

Liver Disease

129. Centers for Disease Control and Prevention, 2003, *www.cdc.gov/nchs/data/hus/tables/2003/03hus031.pdf*.
130. Bonkovsky H, Mehta S. Hepatitis C: A review and update. *J Am Acad Dermatol* 2001;44:159-179.
131. Farci P, Alter HJ, Wong D, et al. A long-term study of hepatitis C virus replication in non-A, non-B hepatitis. *N Engl J Med* 1991;325:98-104.
132. Barrera JM, Bruguera M, Ercilla MG, et al. Persistent hepatitis C viremia after acute self-limiting posttransfusion hepatitis C. *Hepatology* 1995; 21:639-644.
133. Rosen HR, Weston SJ, Im K, et al. Selective decrease in hepatitis C virus-specific immunity among African Americans and outcome of antiviral therapy. *Hepatology* 2007;46: 350-358.
134. Armstrong GL, Wasley A, Simard EP, et al. The prevalence of hepatitis C virus infection in the United States, 1999-2002. *Ann Intern Med* 2006;144:705-714.
135. Thomas DL, Astemborski J, Rai RM, et al. The natural history of hepatitis C virus infection: Host, viral, and environmental factors. *J Am Med Assoc* 2000; 284:450-456.
136. El-Serag HB, Mason AC. Rising incidence of hepatocellular carcinoma in the United States. *N Engl J Med* 1999;340:745-750.
137. Reddy KR, Hoofnagle JH, Tong MJ, et al. Racial differences in responses to therapy with interferon in chronic hepatitis C. Consensus Interferon Study Group. *Hepatology* 1999;30:787-793.
138. Conjeevaram HS, Fried MW, Jeffers LJ, et al. Peginterferon and ribavirin treatment in African American and Caucasian American patients with hepatitis C genotype 1. *Gastroenterology* 2006;131:470-477.
139. Muir AJ, Bornstein JD, Killenberg PG. Peginterferon alfa-2b and ribavirin for the treatment of chronic hepatitis C in blacks and non-Hispanic whites. *N Engl J Med* 2004;350:2265-2271.
140. Strader DB, Wright T, Thomas DL, et al. Diagnosis, management, and treatment of hepatitis C. *Hepatology* 2004;39:1147-1171.
141. Celona AF, Yu MC, Prakash M, et al. Hepatitis C in a Los Angeles public hepatitis clinic: Demographic and biochemical differences associated with race-ethnicity. *Clin Gastroenterol Hepatol* 2004;2:459-462.
142. Chung CM, Nunley JR. Overview of hepatitis C and skin. *Dermatol Nurs* 2006;18:425-430.
143. Scully C, el-Kom M. Lichen planus: Review and update on pathogenesis. *J Oral Pathol* 1985;14:431-458.
144. Jackson JM. Hepatitis C and the skin. *Dermatol Clin* 2002;20:449-458.
145. Soylu S, Gül U, Kiliç A. Cutaneous manifestations in patients positive for anti-hepatitis C virus antibodies. *Acta Dermatol Venereol* 2007;87:49-53.
146. Byrd JA, Davis MD, Bruce AJ, Drage LA, Rogers RS 3rd. Response of oral lichen planus to topical tacrolius in 37 patients. *Arch Dermatol* 2004;140:1508-1512.
147. Torti DC, Jorizzo JL, McCarty MA. Oral lichen planus. *Arch Dermatol* 2007;143: 511-515.
148. Byrd JA, Davis MD, Rogers RS 3rd. Recalcitrant symptomatic vulvar lichen planus: Response to topical tacrolimus. *Arch Dermatol* 2004;140: 715-720.
149. Lunel F, Musset L, Cacoub P, et al. Cryoglobulinemia in chronic liver diseases: Role of hepatitis C virus and liver damage. *Gastroenterology* 1994;106: 1291-1300.
150. Misiani R, Bellavita P, Fenili D, et al. Interferon alfa-2a therapy in cryoglobulinemia associated with hepatitis C virus. *N Engl J Med* 1994;330:751-756.
151. Ferri C, Marzo E, Longombardo G, et al. Interferon-alpha in mixed cryoglobulinemia patients: A randomized crossover-controlled trial. *Blood* 1993; 81:1132-1136.
152. Sansonno D, De Re V, Lauletta G, et al. Monoclonal antibody treatment of mixed cryoglobulinemia resistant to interferon alpha with an anti-CD20. *Blood* 2003;101:3818-3826.
153. Abdallah MA, Ghozzi MY, Monib HA, et al. Necrolytic acral erythema: A cutaneous sign of hepatitis C virus infection. *J Am Acad Dermatol* 2005;53:247-251.
154. Hivnor CM, Yan AC, Junkins-Hopkins JM, Honig PJ. Necrolytic acral erythema: Response to combination therapy with interferon and ribavirin. *J Am Acad Dermatol* 2004;50:S121-124.
155. Abdallah MA, Hull C, Horn TD. Necrolytic acral erythema: A patient from the United States successfully treated with oral zinc. *Arch Dermatol* 2005;141:85-87.
156. Robinson-Bostom L, DiGiovanna JJ. Cutaneous manifestations of end-stage renal disease. *J Am Acad Dermatol* 2000;43:975-986.
157. Shieh S, Cohen JL, Lim HW. Management of porphyria cutanea tarda in the setting of chronic renal failure: A case report and review. *J Am Acad Dermatol* 2000;42:645-652.
158. Ramsay CA, Magnus IA, Turnbull A, Baker H. The treatment of porphyria cutanea tarda by venesection. *Q J Med* 1974;43:1-24.

Toxic Epidermal Necrolysis (TEN)

159. Spies M, Sanford AP, Aili Low JF, et al. Treatment of extensive toxic epidermal necrolysis in children. *Pediatrics* 2001;108: 1162-1168.
160. Chia FL, Leong KP. Severe cutaneous adverse reactions to drugs. *Curr Opin Allergy Clin Immunol* 2007;7:304-309.
161. Roujeau JC, Kelly JP, Naldi L, et al. Medication use and the risk of Stevens-Johnson syndrome and toxic epidermal necrolysis. *N Engl J Med* 1995;333: 1600-1609.
162. Roujeau JC, Guillaume JC, Fabre JP, et al. Toxic epidermal necrolysis (Lyell

syndrome): Incidence and drug etiology in France, 1981-1985. *Arch Dermatol* 1990;126:37-42.

163. Rzany B, Mockenhaupt M, Stocker U, et al. Incidence of Stevens-Johnson syndrome and toxic epidermal necrolysis in patients with the acquired immunodeficiency syndrome in Germany. *Arch Dermatol* 1993;129:1059.
164. Mockenhaupt M, Kelly JP, Kaufman D, Stern RS. The risk of Stevens Johnson syndrome and toxic epidermal necrolysis associated with nonsteroidal anti-inflammatory drugs: A multinational perspective. *J Rheumatol* 2003;30: 2234-2240.
165. Trent JT, Kirsner RS, Romanelli P, Kerdel FA. Analysis of intravenous immunoglobulin for the treatment of toxic epidermal necrolysis using SCORTEN. *Arch Dermatol* 2003;139:39-43.
166. Letko GN, Papaliodis DN, Papaliodis GN, et al. Stevens-Johnson syndrome and toxic epidermal necrolysis: A review of the literature. *Ann Allergy Asthma Immunol* 2005;94:419-436.
167. Rzany B, Hering O, Mockenhaupt M, et al. Histopathologic and epidemiologic characteristics of patients with erythema exudativum multiforme major, Stevens-Johnson syndrome and toxic epidermal necrolysis. *Br J Dermatol* 1996; 134:710-714.
168. Chung WH, Hung SI, Hong HS, et al. Medical genetics: A marker for Stevens-Johnson syndrome. *Nature* 2004; 428:486.
169. Pereira FA, Mudgil AV, Rosmarin DM. Toxic epidermal necrolysis. *J Am Acad Dermatol* 2007;56:181-200.

Meningococcemia

170. Rosenstein NE, Perkins BA, Stephens DS, Popovic T, Hughes JM. Meningococcal disease. *N Engl J Med* 2001; 344: 1378-1388.
171. Hart CA, Cuevas LE. Meningococcal disease in Africa. *Ann Trop Med Parasitol* 1997;91: 777-785.
172. Manchanda V, Gupta S, Bhalla P. Menincococcal disease: History, epidemiology, pathogenesis, clinical manifestations, diagnosis, antimicrobial susceptibility and prevention. *Indian J Med Microbiol* 2006;24:7-19.
173. Rosenstein NE, Perkins BA, Stephens DS, et al. The changing epidemiology of meningococcal disease in the United States, 1992-1996. *J Infect Dis* 1999;180:1894-1901.
174. Schuchat A, Robinson K, Wenger JD, et al. Bacterial meningitis in the United States in 1995. *N Engl J Med* 1997;337 :970-976.
175. Harrison LH, Dwyer DM, Maples CT, Billmann L. Risk of meningococcal infection in college students. *J Am Med Assoc* 1999;281:1906-1910.
176. Centers for Disease Control and Prevention. Meningococcal Disease Technical Information, 2008, *www.cdc.gov/ncidod/dbmd/diseaseinfo/meningococcal_t.htm.*
177. Centers for Disease Control and Prevention. Travelers' Health: Yellow Book—Meningococcal Disease, 2008, *wwwn.cdc.gov/travel/yellowBookCh4-Menin.aspx.*
178. Shao Z, Li W, Ren J, et al. Identification of a new *Neisseria meningitidis* serogroup C clone from Anhui province, China. *Lancet* 2006;367:419-423.
179. Milonovich LM. Meningococcemia: Epidemiology, pathophysiology, and management. *J Pediatr Health Care* 2007; 21:75-80.
180. Wolf RE, Birbara CA. Meningococcal infections at an army training center. *Am J Med* 1968;44:243-255.
181. Carpenter RR, Petersdorf RG. The clinical spectrum of bacterial meningitis. *Am J Med* 1962;33:262-275.
182. Ramos-e-Silva M, Pereira AL. Life-threatening eruptions due to infectious agents. *Clin Dermatol* 2005;23:148-156.
183. Singh J, Arrieta AC. Management of meningococcemia. *Indian J Pediatr* 2004; 71: 909-913.
184. Fourrier F, Leclerc F, Aidan K, et al. Combined antithrombin and protein C supplementation in meningococcal purpura fulminans: A pharmacokinetic study. *Intensive Care Med* 2003;29:1081-1087.
185. Wong VK, Hitchcock W, Mason WH. Meningococcal infections in children: A review of 100 cases. *Pediatr Infect Dis J* 1989;8:224-227.
186. Algren JT, Lal S, Cutliff SA, Richman BJ. Predictors of outcome in acute meningococcal infection in children. *Crit Care Med* 1993;21:447-452.
187. Darmstadt GL. Acute infectious purpura fulminans: Pathogenesis and medical management. *Pediatr Dermatol* 1998;15:169-183.
188. de Kleijn ED, de Groot R, Hack CE, et al. Activation of protein C following infusion of protein C concentrate in children with severe meningococcal sepsis and purpura fulminans: A randomized, double-blinded,placebo-controlled, dose-finding study. *Crit Care Med* 2003;31:1839-1847.
189. White B, Livingstone W, Murphy C, et al. An open-label study of the role of adjuvant hemostatic support with protein C replacement therapy in purpura fulminans-associated meningococcemia. *Blood* 2000;96: 3719-3724.
190. Wheeler JS, Anderson BJ, De Chalain TM. Surgical interventions in children with meningococcal purpura fulminans: A review of 117 procedures in 21 children. *J Pediatr Surg* 2003;38:597-603.
191. Grubbauer HM, Dornbusch HJ, Dittrich P, et al. Ceftriaxone monotherapy for bacterial meningitis in children. *Chemotherapy* 1990;36:441-447.
192. Neu HC. Cephalosporins in the treatment of meningitis. *Drugs* 1987;34:135-153S.
193. Schaad UB, Krucko J, Pfenninger J. An extended experience with cefuroxime therapy of childhood bacterial meningitis. *Pediatr Infect Dis* 1984;3:410-416.
194. Centers for Disease Control and Prevention. Meningococcal Disease General Information, 2008, *www.cdc.gov/ncidod/dbmd/diseaseinfo/meningococcal_g.htm.*

Tuberous Sclerosis

195. Schwartz RA, Fernandez G, Kotulska K, Jozwiak S. Tuberous sclerosis complex: Advances in diagnosis, genetics, and management. *J Am Acad Dermatol* 2007; 57:189-202.
196. Webb DW, Clarke A, Fryer A, Osborne JP. The cutaneous feature of tuberous sclerosis: a population study. *Br J Dermatol* 1996;135:1-5.
197. Rose VM, Au KS, Pollom G, et al. Germline mosaicism in tuberous sclerosis: How common? *Am J Hum Genet* 1999; 64:986.
198. Kwiatkowska J, Wigowska-Sowinska J, Napierala D, et al. Mosaicism in tuberous sclerosis as a potential cause of the failure of molecular diagnosis. *N Engl J Med* 1999;340:703.
199. Verhoef S, Bakker L, Tempelaars AM, et al. High rate of mosaicism in tuberous sclerosis complex. *Am J Hum Genet* 1999; 64:1632.
200. van Slegtenhorst M, de Hoogt R, Hermans C, et al. Identification of the tuberous sclerosis gene *TSC1* on chromose 9q34. *Science* 1997;277:805.
201. The European Chromosome 16 Tuberous Sclerosis Consortium. Identification and characterization of the tuberous sclerosis gene on chromosome 16. *Cell* 1993; 75:1305.
202. Roach ES, Gomez MR, Northrup H. Tuberous sclerosis complex consensus conference: Revised clinical diagnostic criteria. *J Child Neurol* 1998;13:624-628.
203. Fischer K, Blain B, Zhang F, et al. Treatment of facial angiofibromas of tuberous sclerosis by shave excision and dermabrasion in a dark-skinned patient. *Ann Plast Surg* 2001;46:332-335.
204. Song MG, Park KB, Lee ES. Resurfacing of facial angiofibromas in tuberous sclerosis patients using CO_2 laser with flashscanner. *Dermatol Surg* 1999;25: 970-973.

Sickle Cell Disease

205. Bunn HF. Pathogenesis and treatment of sickle cell disease. *N Engl J Med* 1997; 337:762-769.
206. Centers for Disease Control and Prevention. Sickle Cell Disease Data and Statistics, 2008, *www.cdc.gov/ncbddd/sicklecell/hcp_data.htm.*
207. Saiki RK, Scharf S, Faloona F, et al. Enzymatic amplification of beta-globin genomic sequences and restriction site analysis for diagnosis of sickle cell anemia. *Science* 1985;230: 1350-1354.
208. Bhardwaj U, Zhang YH, Jackson DS, et al. DNA diagnosis confirms hemoglobin deletion in newborn screen follow-up. *J Pediatr* 2003;142:346-348.
209. Vernacchio L, Neufeld EJ, MacDonald K, et al. Combined schedule of 7-valent pneumococcal conjugate vaccine followed by 23-valent pneumococcal vaccine in children and young adults with sickle cell disease. *J Pediatr* 1998;133: 275-278.
210. Halasa NB, Shankar SM, Talbot TR, et al. Incidence of invasive pneumococcal disease among individuals with sickle cell disease before and after the introduction of the pneumococcal conjugate vaccine. *Clin Infect Dis* 2007;44:1428-1433.
211. Wong WY, Powars DR, Chan L, et al. Polysaccharide encapsulated bacterial infection in sickle cell anemia: A thirty

year epidemiologic experience. *Am J Hematol* 1992;39:176-182.
212. Falletta JM, Woods GM, Verter JI, et al. Discontinuing penicillin prophylaxis in children with sickle cell anemia. Prophylactic Penicillin Study II. *J Pediatr* 1995;127:685-690.
213. Wayne AS, Kevy SV, Nathan DG. Transfusion management of sickle cell disease. *Blood* 1993; 81:1109-1123.
214. Davies SC, Roberts-Harewood M. Blood transfusion in sickle cell disease. *Blood Rev* 1997;11:57-71.
215. David C. Rees , Ade D. Olujohungbe, Norman E. Parker , Stephens AD, Telfer P, Wright J. Guidelines for the management of the acute painful crisis in sickle cell disease. *Br J Haematol* 2003;120: 744-752.
216. Pearson HA, Cobb WT. Folic acid studies in sickle-cell anemia. *J Lab Clin Med* 1964;64:913-921.
217. Charache S, Terrin ML, Moore RD, et al. Effect of hydroxyurea on the frequency of painful crises in sickle cell anemia. *N Engl J Med* 1995;332:1317-1322.
218. Platt OS, Orkin SH, Dover G, et al. Hydroxyurea enhances fetal hemoglobin production in sickle cell anemia. *J Clin Invest* 1984;74:652-656.
219. Dover GJ, Humphries RK, Moore JG, et al. Hydroxyurea induction of hemoglobin F production in sickle cell disease: Relationship between cytotoxicity and F cell production. *Blood* 1986;67:735-738.
220. Charache S, Dover GJ, Moyer MA, Moore JW. Hydroxyurea-induced augmentation of fetal hemoglobin production in patients with sickle cell anemia. *Blood* 1987;69:109-116.
221. Serjeant GR, Serjeant BE, Mohan JS, Clare A. Leg ulceration in sickle cell disease: Medieval medicine in a modern world. *Hematol Oncol Clin North Am* 2005;19:943-956.
222. Eckman JR. Leg ulcers in sickle cell disease. *Hematol Oncol Clin North Am* 1996; 10:1333-1344.
223. Serjeant GR. Leg ulceration in sickle cell anemia. *Arch Intern Med* 1974;133: 690-694.
224. Nolan VG, Adewoye A, Baldwin C, et al. Sickle cell leg ulcers: Associations with haemolysis and SNPs in *Klotho, TEK* and genes of the TGF-_/BMP pathway. *Br J Haematol* 2006;133:570-580.
225. Serjeant GR, Galloway RE, Gueri MC. Oral zinc sulphate in sickle-cell ulcers. *Lancet* 1970;2:891-893.
226. Margraf HW, Covey TH Jr. A trial of silver-zincallantoinate in the treatment of leg ulcers. *Arch Surg* 1977;112:699-704.
227. Reindorf CA, Walker-Jones D, Adekile AD, Lawal O, Oluwole SF. Rapid healing of sickle cell ulcers treated with collagen dressing. *J Natl Med Assoc* 1989;81: 866-868.
228. Wethers DL, Ramirez GM, Koshy M, et al. Accelerated healing of chronic sickle-cell leg ulcers treated with RGD peptide matrix. *Blood* 1994;84: 1775-1779.
229. Heckler FR, Dibbell DG, McCraw JB. Successful use of muscle flaps or myocutaneous flaps in patients with sickle cell disease. *Plast Reconstr Surg* 1977;59:902-908.
230. Khouri RK, Upton J. Bilateral lower limb salvage with free flaps in a patient with sickle cell ulcers. *Ann Plast Surg* 1991; 27:574-576.
231. Spence RJ. The use of a free flap in homozygous sickle cell disease. *Plast Reconstr Surg* 1985;76:616-619.
232. Richards RS, Bowen CV, Glynn MF. Microsurgical free flap transfer in sickle cell disease. *Ann Plast Surg* 1992;29:278-281.
233. Aessopos A, Farmakis D, Loukopoulos D. Elastic tissue abnormalities in inherited haemolytic syndromes. *Eur J Clin Invest* 2002;32:640-642.
234. Bercovitch L, Terry P. Pseudoxanthoma elasticum 2004. *J Am Acad Dermatol* 2004;51:S13-14.
235. van Meurs T, van Hagen JM, van de Scheur MR, et al. Classic pseudoxanthoma elasticum in a patient with sickle cell disease. *J Am Acad Dermatol* 2007;56: 170-171.
236. Trent JT, Kirsner RS. Leg ulcers in sickle cell disease. *Adv Skin Wound Care* 2004; 17(8):410-416.

Neurofibromatosis Type I

237. Barkovich AJ, Kuzniecky RI. Congenital developmental, and neurocutaneous disorders, in Goldman L, Ausiello D (eds), *Cecil Textbook of Medicine,* 22nd ed. Philadelphia, Saunders, 2004, pp 2359-2363.
238. Tsao H. Neurofibromatosis and tuberous sclerosis, in Bolognia JL, Jorizzo JL, Rapini RP (eds), *Dermatology,* 2nd ed. New York, Elsevier, 2008, pp 825-839
239. Gutmann DH, Aylsworth A, Carey JC, et al. The diagnostic evaluation and multidisciplinary management of neurofibromatosis 1 and neurofibromatosis 2. *J Am Med Assoc* 1997;278:51-57.
240. Cawthon RM, Weiss R, Xu GF, et al. A major segment of the neurofibromatosis gene: cDNA sequence, genomic structure and point mutations. *Cell* 1990;62:193-201.
241. Wallace MR, Marchuk DA, Anderson LB, et al. Type 1 neurofibromatosis gene: Identification of a large transcript disrupted in three neurofibromatosis 1 patients. *Science* 1990;249:181-186.
242. Easton DF, Ponder MA, Huson SM, Ponder BA. An analysis of variation in expression of neurofibromatosis (NF) type I (NF1): Evidence for modifying genes. *Am J Hum Genet* 1993;53:305-313.
243. Lammert M, et al. Prevalence of neurofibromatosis 1 in German children at elementary school enrollment. *Arch Dermatol* 2005;141:71-74.
244. Friedman JM. Epidemiology of neurofibromatosis type 1. *Am J Med Genet* 1999;89:1-6.
245. [0]Cohen BH, Kaplan AM, Packer RJ. Management of intracranial neoplasms in children with neurofibromatosis type 1 and 2. *Pediatr Neurosurg* 1990-1991; 16:66-72.
246. Stiller CA, Chessells, JM, Fitchett M. Neurofibromatosis and childhood leukaemia/lymphoma: A population-based UKCCSG study. *Br J Cancer* 1994; 70:969-972.
247. Gutmann DH, Collins FS. Neurofibromatosis type 1, in Vogelstein B, Kinzler KW (eds), The Genetic Basis of Human Cancer. New York, McGraw-Hill, 1998, pp 423-442.
248. Cherqui A, Kim DH, Kim SH, Park HK, Kline DG. Surgical approaches to paraspinal nerve sheath tumors. *Neuro Surg Focus* 2007;22:E9.
249. Commens CA, Greaves MW. Cutis verticis gyrata due to an intradermal naevus with an underlying neurofibroma. *Clin Exp Dermatol* 1978:3:319-322.
250. Combs SE, Schulz-Ertner D, Moschos D, et al. Fractionated stereotactic radiotherapy of optic pathway gliomas: Tolerance and long-term outcome. *Int J Radiat Oncol Biol Phys* 2005;62: 814-819.

Internal Malignancy and Paraneoplastic Syndromes

251. American Cancer Society. Cancer Facts and Figures, 2008, *www.cancer.org/docroot/stt/stt_0.asp.*
252. Carey LA, Perou CM, Livasy CA, et al. Race, breast cancer subtypes, and survival in the Carolina Breast Cancer Study. *JAMA* 2006;295:2492-2502.
253. Miller BA, Hankey BF, Thomas TL. Impact of sociodemographic factors, hormone receptor status, and tumor grade on ethnic differences in tumor stage and size for breast cancer in women. *Am J Epidemiol* 2002;155:534-545.
254. Jemal A, Clegg LX, Ward E, et al. Annual report to the nation on the status of cancer, 1975-2001, with a special feature regarding survival. *Cancer* 2004;101:3-27.
255. Polite BN, Dignam JJ, Olopade OI. Colorectal caner model of health disparities: Understanding mortality differenes in minority populations. *J Clin Oncol* 2006;24:2179-2187.
256. Bach PB, Cramer LD, Warren JL, Begg CB. Racial differences in the treatment of early-stage lung cancer. *N Engl J Med* 1999;341:1198-1205.

SECTION 12

Cosmetic Dermatology

CHAPTER 69

Cosmetic Procedures in Skin of Color: Chemical Peels, Microdermabrasion, Hair Transplantation, Augmentation, and Sclerotherapy

Valerie D. Callender
Cherie M. Young

Key Points

- Ethnic and racial minorities underwent 21.7% of the cosmetic procedures performed in the United States in 2006.
- Hispanics accounted for 9.7% of those cosmetic procedures; African-Americans, 6.6%; Asians, 4.7%; and other non-Caucasians, 0.8%.
- With rising populations of people of color, dermatologic surgeons must understand and recognize the particular issues and needs relevant to those with darker skin.
- Among all patients of color, the most frequently obtained cosmetic procedures are chemical peels, microdermabrasion, and liposuction. Additionally, injections of toxins and fillers and hair transplantation are increasingly popular.
- Although photodamage is less of a concern in people of color, all races experience brow furrows, frown lines, and crow's feet from repeated facial muscle contractions that are amenable to improvement with botulinum toxin.
- Soft tissue augmentation with dermal fillers is used in the treatment and correction of fine lines, nasolabial folds, marionette lines, tear trough deformities, lip augmentation, volume loss, and acne scars in skin of color patients.
- Although the exact number of hair transplant procedures performed in persons of color is unknown, it is clear that as the awareness of alopecia in men and women grows, the numbers of hair transplantations in this group of patients will increase.

Cosmetic procedures are more popular now than ever before. The American Society for Aesthetic Plastic Surgery (ASAPS) reports that in 2006 alone, surgeons performed nearly 11.5 million cosmetic surgical and nonsurgical procedures in the United States.[1] The most frequently performed surgical cosmetic procedure was liposuction, followed by breast augmentation, eyelid surgery, abdominoplasty, and female breast reduction. The most popular nonsurgical procedures were botulinum toxin injections, hyaluroinc acid fillers, laser hair removal, microdermabrasion, and laser skin resurfacing. Over the past few years, the demand for such procedures has grown dramatically. Individuals are seeking cosmetic procedures that are less invasive with minimal downtime. According to the ASAPS, the overall number of procedures performed has increased 446% since 1997. This trend is likely to continue as new advances in surgical techniques and materials unfold.

Not only are more people turning to cosmetic dermatology for answers to their cosmetic needs, but also the group of patients who seek cosmetic procedures has become more diverse. In 2006, ethnic and racial minorities underwent 21.7% of the cosmetic procedures performed in the United States, representing an overall 2% increase from the year 2001.[1] Hispanics accounted for 9.7% of those procedures; African-Americans, 6.6%; Asians, 4.7%; and other non-Caucasians, 0.8%.

People of color represent the majority of the world and approximately one-third of the U.S. population. The U.S. Census Bureau estimated that in the year 2000, the resident population included 34 million African-Americans, 32 million Hispanic Americans, and 13 million Asian Americans, Pacific Islanders, and Native Americans.[2] The non-Caucasian population in the United States is projected to grow even more in years to come, with the Hispanic population showing the most significant increases.

With rising populations of people of color come increasing demands on cosmetic dermatologic surgeons, who must understand and recognize the particular issues and needs relevant to those with darker skin. Because the bulk of published data on cosmetic procedures thus far has focused on the Caucasian population, performing aesthetic procedures on patients with skin of color remains a challenge. Clearly, the medical community must expand its knowledge of the cosmetic issues relevant to this growing ethnic population.

COSMETIC PROCEDURES

Because people of color have unique cosmetic issues, they seek the procedures that best address their needs. Individuals with skin of color demonstrate less pronounced signs of photoaging when compared with whites.[3] Additionally, when the signs of photaging begin to manifest in darker-skinned individuals, it is at a later age. This is largely due to the photoprotective effects of melanin in more darkly pigmented skin.[4] Caucasian patients typically desire cosmetic procedures that diminish signs of photoaging—fine lines, rhytides, dyschromia, telangiectasias, and keratoses. In contrast, patients of color most often request cosmetic procedures for disorders of pigmentation, primarily postinflammatory hyperpigmentation.[5–8]

Intrinsic aging in patients of color typically manifests in the midfacial region.[9] Clinically, the malar fat pads descend, leading to a tear trough deformity, infraorbital hollowing, and deepening of the nasolabial folds (Figure 69-1). These classic signs of midface aging are a result of gravity-dependent sagging, volumetric

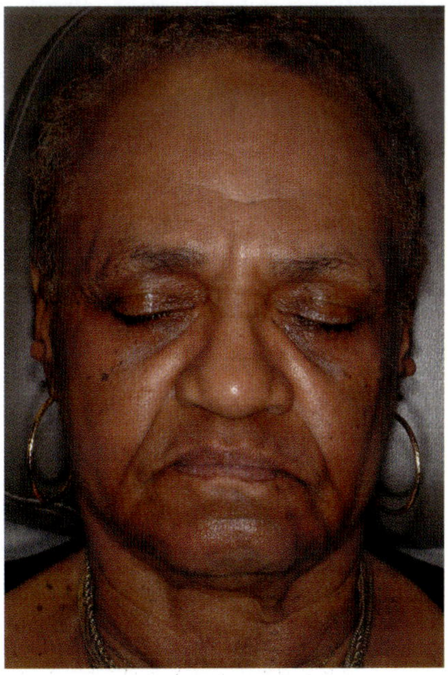

▲ **FIGURE 69-1** Signs of skin aging in patients of color. A 68-year-old African-American woman with infraorbital hollowing, tear trough deformity, descent of the fat pads, and deepening of the nasolabial folds.

loss, and soft tissue and skeletal alterations. Although facial rejuvenation and aesthetic improvement can be obtained by soft tissue augmentation, among all patients of color, the most frequently obtained cosmetic procedures are chemical peels, microdermabrasion, and liposuction.[5–8] These procedures and techniques may require modifications and special considerations when performed in patients of color. When used with understanding and caution, most cosmetic procedures are safe and effective for use in patients of color. In this chapter, the safety and efficacy of the following procedures in skin of color will be reviewed: chemical peels, microdermabrasion, hair transplantation, botulinum toxin injection, and soft filler augmentation and sclerotherapy.

CHEMICAL PEELS

Superficial and medium-depth peels may be performed safely on Fitzpatrick skin types IV–VI (Table 69-1). Chemical peeling is the process of applying one or more chemical agents to the skin for the purpose of exfoliating the epidermis or dermis, thus creating a wound that subsequently reepithelializes.

Chemical peels are performed using superficial, medium-depth, or deep peeling agents. Superficial peels, with agents such as glycolic acid (GA), salicylic acid (SA), Jessner's solution, and tricholoracetic acid (TCA) in concentrations of 10–30%, penetrate the stratum corneum to the papillary dermis. Medium-depth peels reach the upper reticular dermis and include TCA (35–50% concentration), Jessner's combined with TCA 35%, GA 70% combined with TCA 35%, and phenol 88%. Deep chemical peels using the Baker-Gordon phenol formula penetrate to the midreticular dermis.

Patient Selection

Primary indications for chemical peels in patients with Fitzpatrick skin types IV and IV are postinflammatory hyperpigmentation (PIH) and melasma unresponsive to topical bleaching agents.[10,11] Other indications in darker-skinned individuals are acne vulgaris, acne scarring, oily skin, rough skin texture, pseudofolliculitis barbae, solar lentigines, and periorbital rhytids.[12,13]

Indications

CHEMICAL PEELING FOR PIH This is often effective because the procedure removes excess pigment from the skin. Spot peeling specific sites of hyperpigmentation is a technique sometimes used in darker skin to establish how the skin will react to a particular agent. Peels are applied at 1-month intervals. All patients should be reminded that treatment of PIH takes an extended period of time, ranging up to 6 months, and that progress is made in small increments.

CHEMICAL PEELING FOR MELASMA This can be an effective method of removing excess epidermal pigment in the epidermal and mixed types of melasma (Figure 69-2). Dermal melasma is extremely difficult to treat, and attempting to treat this condition with deep chemical peels may result in scarring.[14] Within skin types IV–VI, ethnic groups vary widely in their responses to chemical peeling, and therefore, the type of peel must be selected carefully.

CHEMICAL PEELING FOR ACNE VULGARIS This improves the condition as well as acne-associated PIH. Staged peels, in which the patient returns for repeated treatments using the same concentration and formulation of a mild superficial peeling agent, are often used for skin of color. Both GA and SA have excellent safety profiles in patients with Fitzpatrick skin types IV–VI.[10,12,15] The choice of peeling agent depends on the physician's preference and/or experience.

Newer chemicals, such as the polyhydroxy acids, have been found to be extremely effective peeling agents for acne and pigmentary disorders in Asian skin.[14] Additionally, these agents are well tolerated in patients with dry, sensitive skin. Because the molecules in these agents are larger, they penetrate the epidermis more slowly, eliminating burning and irritation that sometimes occurs with α-hydroxy acid (AHA)–containing products.

CHEMICAL PEELING FOR SCARRING This is often beneficial in patients with skin of color, but hypertrophic scars do not usually respond well to the procedure. Medium-depth peels, which penetrate into the upper reticular dermis, are more effective peeling agents in the treatment of atrophic or crater-like acne scars and pitted or ice-pick scars that have a dermal component.[16]

Contraindications

There are several contraindications to chemical peeling in skin of color. These contraindications include

- Active herpes simplex infection or verrucae
- Atopic dermatitis
- Wounded, sunburned, or excessively sensitive skin
- Inflammatory rosacea
- Isotretinoin use within a year
- Salicylate allergy (SA peels)
- Pregnancy or active breast-feeding

Types of Peeling Agents

Many agents are available for use in chemical peeling. The choice of agent should depend in part on its established safety and efficacy profiles in individuals of color. Although few published studies have evaluated peeling in darker skin, we have experienced excellent results.

GLYCOLIC ACID GA, the most readily available peeling agent, belongs to a family of naturally occurring AHAs.[12] AHA peels have been used to treat a host of skin conditions, including melasma, hyperpigmentation disorders, photodamage, and acne. Improvement of these skin conditions has been observed with the use of AHA peels by their ability to thin the stratum corneum, diminish intercellular bonding,[17] promote epidermolysis, disperse basal layer melanin, and increase collagen synthesis within the dermis.[18]

A skin test always should precede treatment with GA peels in skin of color patients. Most chemical peeling is performed with GA concentrations ranging from a low of 30% to a high of 70%. Peeling with a 70% gel formulation delivers a high concentration of GA to the skin with a reduced risk of scarring.[12] Both superficial and medium-depth peeling are possible with GA; increased concentrations of GA and a lower pH produce deeper peels.

Asian skin in particular shows benefits with GA peels, which are used often to treat facial skin with PIH, ephelides, lentigines, and melasma.[14] Compared with other superficial peeling agents, GA may produce more benefit in darker skin that is dry and sensitive.[11]

SALICYLIC ACID SA is one of the older peeling agents and is used frequently. It belongs to the β-hydroxy acid family that occurs naturally in willow tree bark.[12] In 3–5% concentrations, SA is an effective keratolytic agent that improves the penetration of other peeling agents. One study assessing the keratolytic affect of SA in guinea-pig skin demonstrated a reduction in the intercellular cohesiveness of the horny cells.[19]

SA also has been found to be an effective comedolytic agent and is also used

TABLE 69-1
Studies Evaluating Chemical Peeling in Skin of Color

Author, Year	Skin Type/ Ethnicity/ Gender	Diagnosis	Topical Therapy	Type of Peel	Response	Adverse Events
Burns et al., 1997	19 IV–VI African-Americans	PIH	T 0.05% cream + 2% HQ/10% GA	GA 50% GA 68%	Decreased HASI by 50% in peel group vs 42% in controls	Erythema, superficial desquamation, and vesiculation
Lim, 1997	10 Asian women	Melasma, fine wrinkles	20% HQ and 10% HQ	GA 20–70%	NSS	20% redness burns and transient PIH
Wang, 1997	40 Asians	Acne	15% GA	GA 35% GA 50%	Significant resolution in acne	5.6% PIH, HSV flare, and mild skin irritation
Grimes, 1999	25 V–VI African-American and Hispanic women and men	Acne, PIH, melasma, oily skin, enlarged pores, and rough texture	4% HQ	SA 20% SA 30%	88% moderate to significant improvement	15% temporary crusting hypopigmentation, dryness, and hyperpigmenation
Javaheri, 2001	25 Indian women and men	Melasma	Sunscreen SPF 15, 10% GA, and oral acyclovir	GA 50%	46.7% epidermal 27.8% mixed 0% dermal	Hyperpigmentation
Al-Waiz, 2002	15 Dark-skinned women and men	Acne scars	RA cream in 3 patients	Jessner's solution + TCA 35%	6.6% significant 53.3% moderate 26.6% mild 6.6% minimal 6.6% no response	73.4% transient PIH
Sarkar, 2002	40 Indian patients	Melasma	HQ 5% + T 0.05% + HC 1% cream	GA peel in 20 patients	Decreased MASI in all patients, faster in peel group	Erythema, superficial desquamation, HSV, vesiculation, and PIH
Lee, 2003	35 Korean patients	Acne vulgaris	N/A	30% salicylic acid peels	Decrease in inflammatory and noninfla mmatory lesion counts	Tolerable
Khunger, 2004	10 Indian women	Melasma	N/A	Split-faced study: 1% tretinoin peel vs 70% GA	Significant decrease MASI; no difference between right vs left sides	Minimal
Kadhim et al., 2005	12 Dark-skinned women and men	Periorbital wrinkles (fine/ medium - sized	N/A	Jessner's solution + TCA 35%	33% Marked 25% Moderate 25% Mild 8% Minimal 8% No response	Mild

PIH = postinflammatory hyperpigmentation; T = tretinoin; HQ = hydroquinone; GA = glycolic acid; SPF = sun protection factor; RA = retinoic acid; HC = hydrocortisone acetate; SA = salicylic acid; TCA = trichloroacetic acid; HASI = Hyperpigmentation Area Severity Index; MASI = Melasma Area Severity Index; HSV = herpes simplex virus; NSS = not statistically significant.

in the treatment of acne. It has been formulated in a variety of vehicles. Ethanol solutions of SA produce excellent benefits for many conditions, including acne, melasma, and PIH, in dark-skinned patients.[15]

TRICHLOROACETIC ACID TCA is an inorganic compound found in crystalline form. TCA 10–30% solutions deliver a superficial peel; however, the risks of PIH and scarring increase with the use of higher concentrations in skin of color. TCA may be used alone or in combination with GA or SA. Used in combination with GA, it has been demonstrated to improve mottled facial pigmentation.[12] TCA is also an effective treatment for acne scarring in skin of color patients.

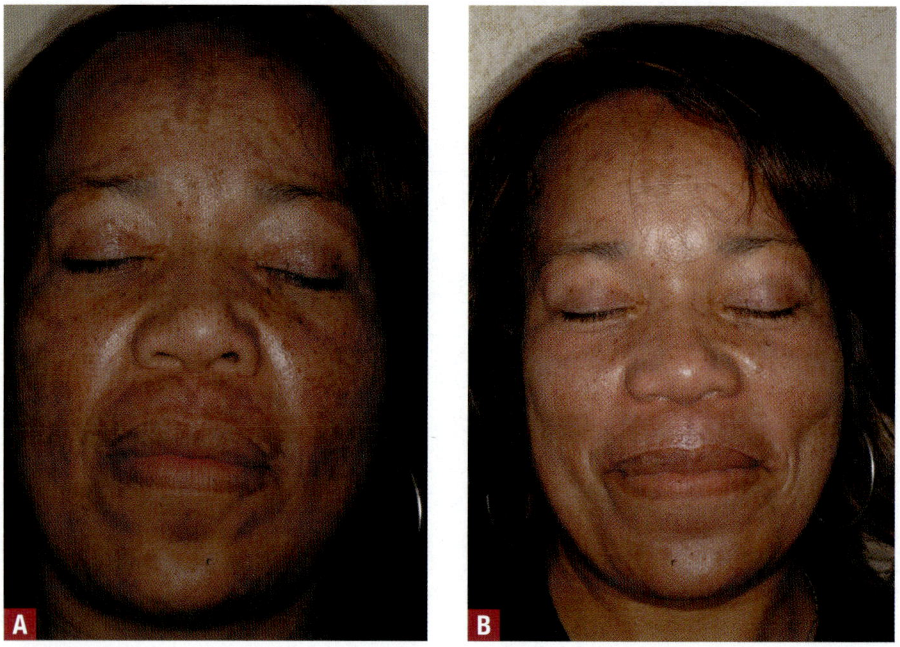

▲ **FIGURE 69-2** Before (**A**) and after (**B**) chemical peel for the treatment of melasma.

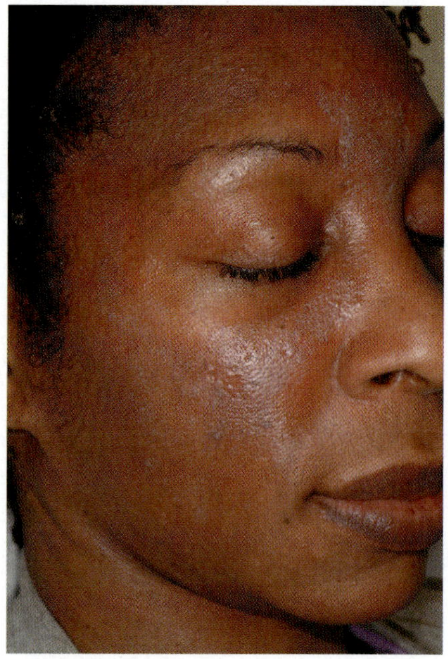

▲ **FIGURE 69-3** Patient undergoing a TCA peel showing the white frost indicating the endpoint of the peel.

JESSNER'S SOLUTION Jessner's solution has been in use as a superficial peeling agent for several decades and penetrates into the papillary dermis. It is a combination of resorcinol 14 g, salicylic acid 14 g, and lactic acid 14 g in ethanol 95%. The three keratolytic agents used together produce a synergistic effect.

Jessner's solution is well tolerated in Fitzpatrick skin types IV–VI, and an advantage of this agent is that it contains the phenolic skin-lightening agent resorcinol. Medium-depth peels using a combination of Jessner's solution followed by a 35% concentration of TCA have been found to be safe and effective in treating acne scars in patients with dark skin.[13]

Technique

Prior to treating a patient with a chemical peel, a careful history should be obtained and a thorough skin examination performed. Patients should avoid the following procedures 1 week prior to chemical peeling: electrolysis, waxing, use of depilatory creams, and laser hair removal. Two to three days prior to the procedure, patients should discontinue use of topical retinoids and products that contain retinol, AHA, β-hydroxy acid, or benzoyl peroxide. Prophylatic antiviral therapy should be given to patients with a history of herpes simplex infection. Prior to applying chemical peeling agents to the skin, all makeup should be removed, the eyes should be protected with moistened cotton pads or eye shields, and petrolatum should be applied to sensitive areas, such as the corners of the nose and lips.

For the treatment of pigmentary disorders, pre- and posttreatment hyperpigmentation therapy is essential and consists of treating the affected areas for 1 month prior to and after peeling with a combination skin-lightening agent containing hydroquinone. Peeling then can be performed using a 20–30% SA solution, 50–70% GA solution, Jessner's solution, or TCA 10–50%. The peel is applied with sponges or brushes for 3–5 minutes, neutralized when appropriate, and then rinsed off.

SA peels are also used to treat active acne and oily skin. A 20–30% solution is applied to the skin with a sponge applicator and to individual papules and pustules with a cotton-tipped swab. Pustules and papules are often unroofed in the process. Typically, 4–5 minutes of a tingling or burning sensation occurs before a white frost appears, signaling the end of the peel. This white frost of SA peels represents crystalline precipitation rather than protein agglutination associated with deep-peel frost. Patients are usually pleased with the results of this peel, and compliance remains high with the recommended three to six treatments. The number of peels performed is based on the severity of the acne. Patients usually tolerate the procedure well.

GA peels, available in many formulations and strengths, are also used for the treatment of acne. For skin of color, a partially buffered solution of 30–50% may be used.[12] The peeling agent contacts the skin for 2–4 minutes and then is rinsed off with cool water. Acne surgery performed with a comedone extractor on unroofed lesions often produces excellent results.

TCA peeling in skin of color patients must be performed cautiously beginning with low concentrations. After TCA peeling, a white frost usually marks the endpoint (Figure 69-3), and in some cases this frost is not desired in skin types V–VI because it is associated with higher risks of adverse effects.

A combination of 70% GA gel and 25% TCA also has been used successfully for peeling,[12] with the gel formulation limiting the harshness of the TCA. First, GA gel is applied generously; then TCA is applied over it. The peel remains on the face for 2–4 minutes before removal. The procedure is usually repeated in 4–6 weeks, and if tolerated well, the peel may be left on 1 or 2 minutes longer with subsequent treatments.

Outcome

Several studies have looked at the efficacy and safety of a variety of chemical peels used to treat conditions common to skin of color (see Table 69-1). Many of the studies have found this procedure to be safe with very minimal side effects in this population.

Serial GA peels appear to enhance the efficacy of a topical regimen when treating PIH in patients with dark skin. In a study of 19 patients with Fitzpatrick skin types IV, V, and VI and facial PIH, a control group was treated with 2% hydroquinone–10% glycolic acid twice daily and tretinoin cream 0.05% at night.[20] The active peel group received the same topical regimen plus a series of six serial GA peels. Greater improvement was noted in the chemical peel group, although this difference was not statistically significant between the two groups.

Several studies have assessed the efficacy of GA peels in the treatment of melasma in Indian patients. One study showed that serial GA peels with a topical regimen are an effective treatment for melasma in 40 dark-skinned Indian women with Fitzpatrick skin types III–V.[21] The women were divided into two groups; one received serial GA peels combined with a topical regimen, which was a modified Kligman's formula (hydroquinone 5%, tretinoin 0.05%, and hydrocortisone acetate 1% in a cream base). The other group received only Kligman's formula. At 21 weeks, the group that received the GA peels showed a trend toward significantly improved results. Few side effects were noted in the peel group.

Other investigators evaluated the safety and efficacy of GA peels in 25 Indian subjects with melasma.[22] Participants were asked to carry out a prepeel program of daily application of topical sunscreens and 10% GA lotion at night for 2 weeks. The women then were treated with a 50% GA facial peel once a month for three consecutive months. Results showed improvement in melasma in 91% of patients. Those with epidermal melasma had a better response than those with the mixed type. There were no significant side effects.

Another study compared the efficacy of GA peels versus tretinoin peels in the treatment of melasma in Indian women.[23] The results show that there was no statistically significant difference between the two agents, and both resulted in a significant decrease in melasma area severity index (MASI). The side effects were minimal in these subjects.

Several studies also have assessed the efficacy and safety of chemical peels in treating Asian skin. Asians and Asian-Americans have been found to respond well to staged GA peels.[24,25] A split-face study was performed that evaluated the safety and efficacy of GA peels in ten Asian women with melasma and Fitzpatrick skin types IV and V.[24] Each woman underwent eight peels and at least one peel with 70% solution. At the end of 26 weeks, GA peels lightened the skin in all women compared with baseline. Up to 33% lightening of melasma occurred in 6 patients, and as much as 66% in 4 patients. No patients suffered any scarring or worsening of their melasma. These results were not statistically significant, however, and the sample was small.

Forty Asian patients with acne vulgaris were treated with a series of GA peels (35–70%) with significant improvement in acne lesions.[25] There were several side effects experienced in 5.6% of the patients, which included PIH, herpes simplex virus reactivation, and mild skin irritation.

The efficacy and safety of SA peels also have been evaluated in skin of color. In a study that assessed the efficacy and safety of SA peeling in 25 patients (9 with acne, 5 with PIH, 6 with melasma, and 5 with rough, oily skin and enlarged pores) with skin types V and VI, the investigators found that superficial peels with 20% and 30% SA were safe and effective.[15] Side effects were mild or minimal and occurred in 16% of patients, with 3 experiencing transient hyperpigmentation that resolved in 7–14 days.

The efficacy and safety of SA peels in the treatment of acne vulgaris in Asian patients also have been assessed.[26] Thirty-five Korean patients with acne vulgaris were treated with 30% SA peels biweekly for 12 weeks. There was a decrease in both inflammatory and noninflammatory acne lesion counts, and there was no change in stratum corneum hydration, skin surface lipid, skin pH, and transepidermal water loss from baseline levels.[26] Side effects were tolerable, further demonstrating the safety and efficacy of SA peels in skin of color patients.

While the risk of transient hyperpigmentation with medium-depth peeling is high, at least one group of investigators has found medium-depth chemical peels to be safe and effective in dark-skinned Iraqi patients.[16] Treatment was mainly for crater-like and ice-pick scars and consisted of three sessions held 1 month apart. Moderate improvement was seen in 53.3%, significant improvement in 6.6%, and a mild response in 26.1%. Peeling was performed with a combination of Jessner's solution followed by 35% TCA. Of note is the fact that transient PIH developed in 73.4% of patients, but all pigmentary changes resolved within 3 months.

A study also was performed on darker-skinned patients for the treatment of periorbital wrinkling (fine to medium) using medium-depth peels. Twelve patients underwent two to four peeling sessions with a combination of Jessner's solution followed by 35% TCA; each session was performed 1 month apart.[13] On completing the study, 33% of the subjects showed marked, 25% moderate, 25% mild, and 8% minimal improvement of periorbital wrinkling. Eight percent of the patients revealed no response to treatment. The treatment was tolerated well, with mild side effects occurring in 33% of patients.

Although most of the studies performed in skin of color using chemical peels have had small sample sizes, these studies reveal that overall chemical peels are safe to use in skin of color and are very efficacious.

Complications

As with any cosmetic procedure, there is the risk of complications with the use of chemical peels in the skin of color population. However, the proper use of chemical peels in the properly selected patients significantly diminishes this risk. While superficial peeling agents, such as GA and SA, are generally well tolerated and safe in darker skin,[12,15] even superficial peeling may result in some scarring, hyperpigmentation, or hypopigmentation in susceptible individuals (Figure 69-4). Other complications include persistent erythema, milia

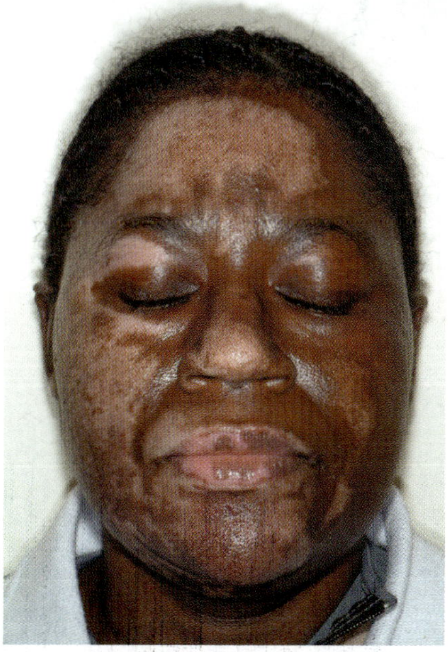

▲ **FIGURE 69-4** Patient with postinflammatory hypopigmentation from chemical peeling.

formation, and infection. For this reason, it is best to initiate peeling with agents at low concentrations and to perform skin testing prior to initiating a full procedure.

Time is an important variable when peeling with GA because this peel must be neutralized with water or 1% bicarbonate solution to discontinue keratolysis. Additionally, stronger solutions must be used cautiously because scarring has been reported following a 15-minute application of a 70% solution.[27,28]

Chemical peeling is not recommended for removal of dermal pigment in Fitzpatrick skin types IV–VI.[12] Peeling to the depth needed to reach this pigmentation carries increased risks for scarring and permanent depigmentation.

Although Jessner's solution is usually well tolerated in Fitzpatrick skin types V and VI, caution must be used with this peel because resorcinol also may produce depigmentation in Fitzpatrick skin types V and VI.[13]

Deeper peels, such as the Baker phenol peel, as a rule are not used in darker skin because they are associated with complications such as hyperpigmentation, hypopigmentation, scarring, and keloid formation.[29] This peel is also associated with cardiac, renal, and hepatic toxicity.

Follow-up and Patient Instructions

Following the peel, patients are instructed to wash the skin with gentle cleansers, apply emollients (e.g., Biafine) twice daily, and use daily sun protection (SPF 30). When treating disorders of pigmentation, an effective interval between superficial peels is 3–6 weeks. Following the last peel of the series, the patient is maintained on daily ultraviolet (UV) protection sunblock and often receives nightly application of hydroquinone-based bleaching agent for a 4- to 8-week period. Chronic melanocyte suppression can be accomplished by rotating the skin-lightening agents to avoid any of the adverse side effects of any one agent.[12] Topical retinoids or azelaic acid as maintenance therapy also can be used as an alternative to hydroquinone therapy.

MICRODERMABRASION

Microdermabrasion was first performed in Italy in 1985 by Marini and LoBrutto,[30] and since its introduction in the United States in 1996,[31] it has become one of the most popular cosmetic treatments among patients. Microdermabrasion is noninvasive, requires little or no recovery time, and may be performed safely on all Fitzpatrick skin types.[30]

Patient Selection

Microdermabrasion is an excellent option for the patient who is unable to tolerate peels or for whom extensive recovery time is not an option. It is felt to be equivalent in efficacy to a superficial chemical peel and is less invasive than the CO_2 or Er:YAG laser.[30] Indications for microdermabrasion are similar to those for chemical peels and include acne, acne scarring, hyperpigmentation, photodamage, facial rejuvenation, enlarged pores, textural changes, and striae.[30,31]

Contraindications

There are several relative contraindications to performing microdermabrasion:

- Active skin infections (e.g., herpes simplex, viral warts, and impetigo)
- Acute skin inflammation (e.g., atopic dermatitis, rosacea, and pustular acne)
- Koebnerizing skin conditions (e.g., psoriasis, lichen planus, and vitiligo)

Equipment and Technique

Most microdermabrasion systems use aluminum oxide crystals, which are angular and create microtrauma from high crystal flow and numerous passes.[31,32] Other machines employ less abrasive sodium chloride and sodium bicarbonate crystals that also minimize the pulmonary risks associated with chronic aluminum exposure.[33] Other units that are available use a diamond wand and are crystal-free.

A typical microdermabrasion procedure, which does not require topical anesthesia, consists of superficially abrading the skin with either a diamond chip or fine crystals, which are simultaneously delivered to and vacuumed off the skin. The number of passes in a session varies with the patient's tolerance and desired effect, but most patients require two or three passes. Depth of ablation depends on the amount of force used to spray the crystals onto the skin, the flow rate of the crystals, the crystal size, and the angle at which the crystals are applied to the skin.[34]

Three levels of microdermabrasion may be used in the treatment of the skin[34]:

- Level one produces a superficial abrasion of the epidermis.
- Level two is more aggressive, extends to the papillary dermis, and is used to treat superficial scars, striae, and fine wrinkles.
- Level three is most aggressive, extends to the level of the papillary and upper reticular dermis, and is used to treat striae.

Levels two and three must be used with caution in skin of color owing to an increased risk of hyperpigmentation.

Outcome

The benefits of microdermabrasion are proven for the treatment of acne and acne scarring. Investigators demonstrated the efficacy of the procedure in 25 patients with grade II or III acne.[35] The patients received eight treatments at weekly intervals. Overall, 96% of the patients were pleased with their results and reportedly would recommend this procedure to others.

The efficacy of microdermabrasion was accessed in 28 patients ranging in age from 40–75 with Fitzpatrick skin types I–IV by Shim and colleagues.[30] Of those enrolled, there were 14 patients with photoaging, 11 with comedonal acne or milia, and 3 with severe acne scarring. Following 12–14 weeks of treatment, microdermabrasion produced statistically significant improvement in skin roughness, mottled pigmentation, and overall skin appearance, but not in rhytids. Some acne scarring improved, but most patients required deeper ablation. Results in melasma were inconsistent, perhaps owing to the fact that dermal pigmentation was not affected. However, it is felt that the procedure should improve the penetration of other adjuvant topical medications, such as hydroquinone, used in the treatment of melasma. Adverse events, namely, PIH, did not occur.[30] Of note, some investigators have found that dual therapy consisting of microdermabrasion and combination lightening agents has benefits in melasma, but additional research is needed.[36]

Microdermabrasion is also useful for other types of facial scarring. In a study that evaluated 41 Asian patients with scars (16 acne scars, 18 traumatic scars, 3 surgical scars, 2 chicken pox scars, 1 burn scar, and 1 other scar) that were treated with microdermabrasion over a 2-year period in a Taiwan hospital. All patients reported good to excellent clinical results.[37] Mean frequencies of treatment were 19 treatments for acne scars, 4 for traumatic scars, 4 for surgical scars, and 5.5 for chicken pox scars.

Histologically, significant epidermal changes have been demonstrated after microdermabrasion treatment. Hernandez-Perez and Ibitt performed biopsies before and after microdermabrasion treatments. After five sessions, there was an increase in epidermal thickness ranging from 0.01–0.1 mm.[38] Freedman and colleagues also revealed epidermal thickening in their study. After three passes of microdermabrasion, epidermal thickness, as well as papillary dermal thickness, increased significantly.[39]

Changes in epidermal barrier function, such as transepidermal water loss, hydration, pH, and sebum production, may be responsible for the improved texture and overall appearance of the skin following microdermabrasion.[31,32] A study was performed in eight patients, three of whom were African-American and two Hispanic. This was a split-face study where half the face was treated with aluminum oxide microdermabrasion and the other half with sodium chloride microdermabrasion. Each patient received three passes. Transepidermal water loss, stratum corneum hydration, skin pH, and sebum production were measured, and it was revealed that microdermabrasion enhanced skin hydration and improved epidermal barrier function.[31]

An animal study was performed looking at enhanced penetration of hydrophilic and lipophilic substances following microdermabrasion.[40] It was found that after partially ablating and homogenizing the stratum corneum with microdermabrasion, there was increased penetration of hydrophilic substances into the skin.

A recent study examining the changes in lipid levels in the stratum corneum following microdermabrasion did result in changes in ceramide levels.[41] A statistically significant increase in the ceramide level was observed after two microdermabrasion treatments. Following the third and fourth sessions, the ceramide level returned to baseline. This study provides the first evidence of changes in the lipid barrier following microdermabrasion treatments.

Complicatons

Very few complications have been observed with the use of microdermabrasion. Following treatment, patients may experience mild erythema. Other complications may include development of petichiae, purpura, or skin wounding if the vacuum suction power is increased, which, in turn, may result in PIH.[37]

Ocular complications from the crystals may occur; therefore, it is recommended that patients keep their eyes closed or apply disposable eye shields during the procedure. Patients with a history of herpes simplex also should be treated with antiviral prophylaxis prior to microdermabrasion because the procedure can cause reactivation of the virus.[42]

Follow-up and Patient Instructions

Folllowing a treatment with microdermabrasion, patients are instructed to use mild cleansers, emollients, and sun protection (SPF 30). For maximal results, microdermabrasion is recommended 2–4 weeks apart for four to six treatments until desired results have been achieved.

HAIR TRANSPLANTATION

Hair transplantation techniques have evolved and improved tremendously over the years. Follicular unit transplantation (FUT) was developed to provide a more naturally appearing cosmetic result in males with androgenetic alopecia.[43,44] Since then, hair transplantation has become more popular and has expanded to include women and ethnic groups interested in correcting their hair loss. According to the International Society of Hair Restoration Surgery Practice Census, there were approximately 168,155 hair transplant procedures performed worldwide in 2005, and of these, half were performed in the United States.[45] Although the exact number of hair transplant procedures performed in persons of color is unknown, it is clear that as the awareness of alopecia in men and women grows, the numbers of hair transplantations in this group of patients will increase.[46] Thus there are several racial differences in hair morphology, surgical instrumentation, and surgical technique in hair transplant surgery that will be discussed (Table 69-2).

FUT involves removing follicular groups or follicular units (FU) from the permanently hair-bearing rim hair (donor area) and inserting them into tiny incisions produced in the area of hair loss (recipient area). Racial variations in the hair characteristics of individuals is by far the most important difference in hair transplant surgery. Patients of African descent have extremely curly hair and a curved hair follicle (Figure 69-5) compared with the straight hair and straight hair follicle in Caucasian and Asian patients. Larger grafts typically are used in patients of color because of this distinct curl pattern within the dermis. There are major concerns that exist during donor harvesting and graft preparation, mainly transection of the hair, which can affect graft survival.

Differences in hair densities between the races exist. Patients of African descent exhibit lower densities when compared with other races,[44,47] and this lower density results in a lower number of donor grafts needed for a hair transplantation procedure.

Patient Selection

The most common indication for hair transplantation is for the management of androgenic alopecia (AGA) in men with male-pattern baldness (MPB). Adjunctive medical therapy with topical minoxidil 5% or finasteride is recommended in younger patients to slow the progression of MPB before considering a hair transplantation procedure. The medical and surgical treatment of AGA in black men[48,49] is similar to that in other racial groups, but black men who wear their hair closely shaved in a "fade hair cut" will have difficulty in camouflaging the resulting donor scar produced by hair transplantation surgery.

Women also suffer from hair loss. The most common type of alopecia in women is female-pattern hair loss (FPHL), or androgenic alopecia, affecting 13% of premenopausal women and 37% of postmenopausal women.[50] In women, hair loss is characterized by a diffuse thinning of the hair over the crown and frontal scalp with preservation of the anterior hairline. In all ethnicities, topical minoxidil 2% is the mainstay of medical therapy for FPHL, but an increasingly popular option for women with FPHL is hair transplantation.[51]

Hair transplantation surgery is an effective treatment for traction alopecia, or traumatic alopecia marginalis, in

TABLE 69-2
Hair Transplantation Differences in Persons of Color

	Blacks	Caucasians	Asians
Hair shape	Curly	Straight, wavy	Straight
Hair follicle	Curved	Straight	Straight
Hair density*	0.6 FU/mm^2	1 FU/mm^2	1 FU/mm^2
Hair groupings*	Three	Two	Two
Indications	AGA, TA, CCCA	AGA	AGA
Recipient sites	>1.2 mm	<1.2 mm	<1.2 mm
Keloid risk	High	Low	Moderate

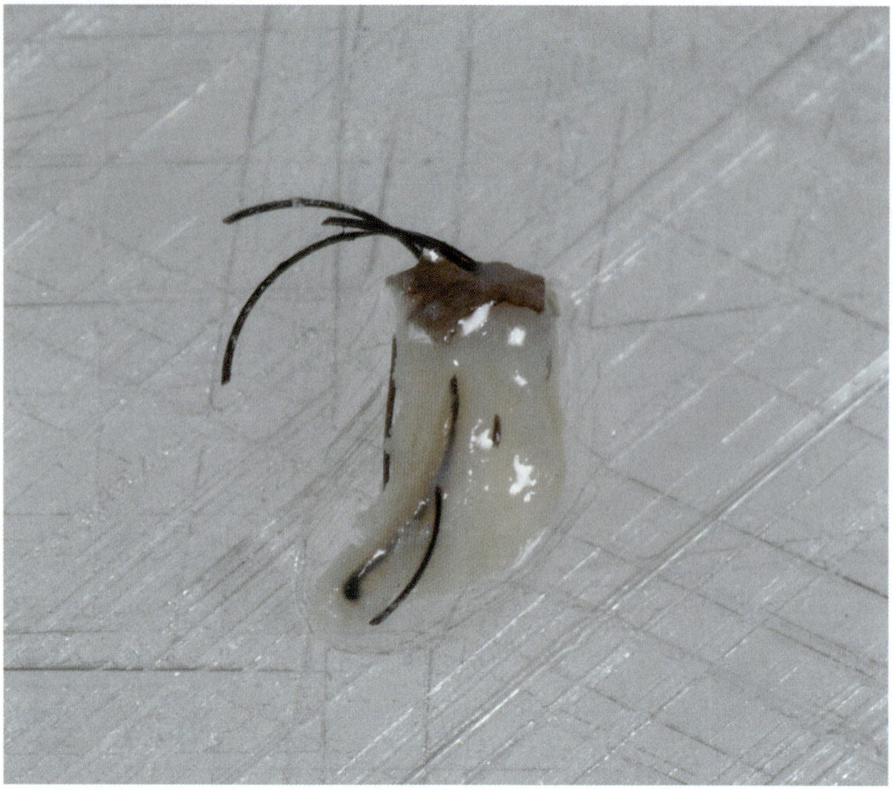

▲ **FIGURE 69-5** Hair follicles from an African-American patient demonstrating the curly nature of African-American hair.

black women[46,47,52,53] (Figure 69-6). Surgical correction in these patients can take the form of either multi–follicular unit grafts or flap rotations. Each method is effective and has advantages and disadvantages. The choice of surgical treatment is usually individualized to the patient depending on the severity of hair loss, the patient's desires, and the flexibility of the scalp. In many cases, a combination of techniques is the best choice.

Central centrifugal cicatricial alopecia (CCCA) is the term used to describe the crown and vertex scarring forms of alopecia that primarily affect black women.[54] Previous terminology includes *hot-comb alopecia*,[55] *chemically induced alopecia*,[56] and *follicular degeneration syndrome*.[57] CCCA develops in a roughly circular patch on the crown or vertex of region of the scalp, with the area of inflammation and scarring increasing in circumference as the condition progresses.[53] The scalp is often smooth and shiny with loss of follicular ostia. The hair remaining in the scarred zone is short and brittle. The cause of CCCA is unknown. Treatment consists of aggressive anti-inflammatory treatments, such as corticosteroids and oral antibiotics, to address the symptoms and stop progression. Inflammation may be decreased with high-potency topical corticosteroids used daily, with special attention to the vehicle and the patient's hair grooming practices. Intralesional corticosteoid therapy performed monthly using triamcinolone acetonide at a concentraion of 2.5–5.0 mg/mL suppresses dermal inflammation. Surgical correction with hair transplantation surgery is also an option after 9 months or more of medical therapy and a biopsy-proven noninflamed scalp.[46,58]

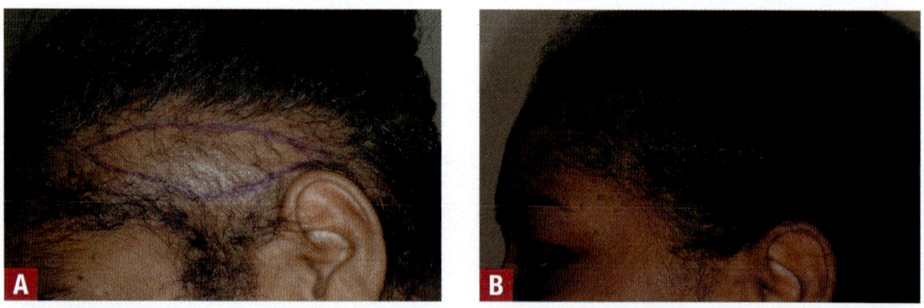

▲ **FIGURE 69-6** **A.** Patient with traction alopecia prior to hair transplantation. **B.** Twelve months after hair transplantation.

Contraindications

The contraindications for hair transplantation are similar in all racial groups, but patients of color have a higher incidence of keloid and hypertrophic scarring.[59] A careful and detailed history of keloid formation along with a physical examination to check for other scars should be performed.

Surgical Technique

Performing hair transplantation in patients with curly hair is challenging, and steps to avoid transection of the hair follicle within the grafts demand special attention and skill. The surgical equipment required to perform hair transplantation is listed in Table 69-3. Anesthesia is obtained by infiltrating 1% or 2% lidocaine with epinephrine for both donor and recipient areas. In addition, normal saline is injected into the donor area prior to excision of the donor strip to provide maximum skin turgor and to straighten the hair and hair follicles, thus allowing for less transection while harvesting the donor strip. There are four steps in performing a hair transplantation procedure that will be discussed: donor harvesting, graft preparation, recipient-site creation, and graft placement.

TABLE 69-3
Hair Transplantation Equipment

1. Aluminum rattail comb
2. Hair densitometer
3. Hibiclens solution
4. Gauze
5. Lidocaine with epinephrine
6. Normal saline for skin turgor
7. Scalpel with No. 15 blade
8. Tissue clamps
9. Hyfrecator and disposable sterile tips
10. 3-0 or 4-0 Prolene suture material
11. Stereomicroscope or loupe magnification
12. Cutting board with fiberoptic box lighting
13. Persona blade (DermaBlade)
14. Jeweler's forceps—straight, curved
15. Petri dishes with saline
16. Nokor needles—16 and 18 gauge
17. Spearpoint blades—Nos. 90 and 91
18. Punches—2 to 4 mm
19. Spray bottle with saline

DONOR HARVESTING This initial step involves excising a single strip of donor tissue from the occipital area of scalp in such a way that transection of hair follicles is limited and the resulting scar is undetectable. The length and width of the harvested tissue are determined by the hair density of the individual and the number of grafts needed to cover the area of hair loss. Trichophytic closure[60] is a new technique currently used to minimize the scar by trimming the epidermis of one edge of the wound before suturing the wound margins together. Undermining the wound margins, which results in less tension, and limiting the width to less than 1 cm also aid in minimizing the size of the donor scar.

GRAFT PREPARATION During this step, the donor strip is converted into individual grafts of different sizes. Caution must be taken with curly hair to avoid transection of the hair follicle, so a curved blade is often used to match the curvature of the hair. The grafts that are created contain one to four hair follicular units and are placed in saline until they are ready to be inserted into the recipient sites.

RECIPIENT-SITE CREATION AND GRAFT PLACEMENT A number of surgical instruments can be used to create recipient sites in areas of hair loss. We select instrumentation based on the degree of curl of the hair—the greater the curl, the larger is the recipient site. Typically, the recipient site ranges from 1.2–2.0 mm in size in patients with a significant curl pattern (Figure 69-7).

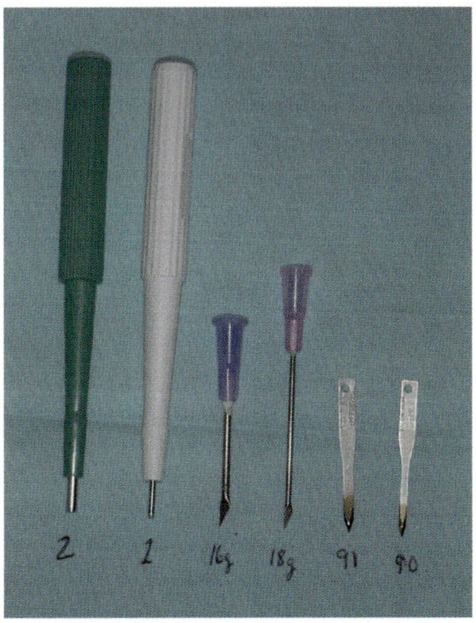

▲ **FIGURE 69-7** Hair transplantation: surgical instruments for recipient sites.

Complications

Most African-American patients have excellent cosmetic results from hair transplantation surgery and experience a low risk of keloidal scarring. However, at least one case of a large keloidal scar following hair transplantation has been reported. This was a 60-year-old African-American man with male-pattern alopecia and no previous history of keloidal scarring.[61] The scar developed over a large portion of the patient's scalp. This represents a significant potential complication, particularly in African-American and Asian patients with a history of scarring. To avoid this complication, test grafting is recommended in some patients before a hair transplantation procedure.[62,63] If normal healing occurs in the donor area and recipient site after 3 months, the patient is a good candidate for a full transplantation procedure.

BOTULINUM TOXIN

Although photodamage is less of a concern in people of color, all races experience the brow furrows, frown lines, and crow's feet that repeated facial muscle contractions produce over time. Botulinum toxin A (BTX-A) is an effective treatment to reverse these effects by temporarily relaxing the muscles in the upper face, resulting in smoother skin and a more relaxed, youthful appearance.

Botulinum neurotoxins are derived from various strains of *Clostridium botulinum*. Currently, there are seven serotypes of botulinum toxin—A, B, Cα, D, E, F, and G[64]— of which serotypes A and B are available commercially. Botulinum toxin works by inhibiting the exocytosis of the neurotransmitter acetylcholine from the nerve into the synaptic space of the neuromuscular junction. Within the nerve cytoplasm exists the SNARE (soluble *N*-ethylmaleimide-sensitive factor attachment protein receptor) protein complex that is responsible for the exocytosis of acetylcholine. The cleavage sites on the SNARE complex differ between the serotypes—BTX-A cleaves synaptosome-associated membrane protein 25 (SNAP-25), whereas botulinum toxin B cleaves vesicle-associated membrane protein (VAMP). This cleavage results in the inhibition of acetylcholine exocytosis and chemodenervation of the nerves that stimulate that muscle or eccrine sweat gland.

BTX-A is available in a crystallized form, which may be reconstituted with sterile nonpreserved 0.9% saline before injection. It is injected intramuscularly in small amounts with a tuberculin syringe. Benefits first become noticeable within 3–5 days following treatment, with peak effects occurring at 1–3 weeks. These effects last an average of 3–6 months. For many patients, repeated injections maintain longer-lasting effects.

Indications

- Glabellar brow furrow "frown lines" [Food and Drug Administration (FDA)–approved indication]
- Horizontal frontalis forehead lines
- Periocular crow's feet
- Axillary hyperhidrosis [Food and Drug Administration (FDA)–approved indication]
- Palm and sole hyperhidrosis
- Platysmal banding of the neck
- Perioral rhytides
- Marionette lines

Treatment

GLABELLAR BROW FURROW BTX-A injections are administered into the procerus muscle and corrugators with a 30-gauge needle and a tuberculin or diabetic syringe (Figure 69-8). There are usually five separate injection points.[65] Based on the muscle mass, 25–30 units of BTX-A is injected intramuscularly. Topical anesthesia is usually not required. Patients are instructed not to massage or manipulate the area of injection and to remain upright for at least 2–4 hours.

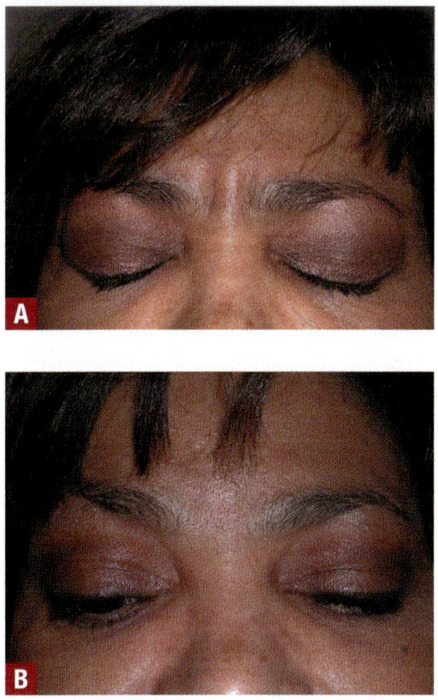

▲ **FIGURE 69-8** Before (**A**) and after (**B**) BTX-A injections for glabellar brow furrows.

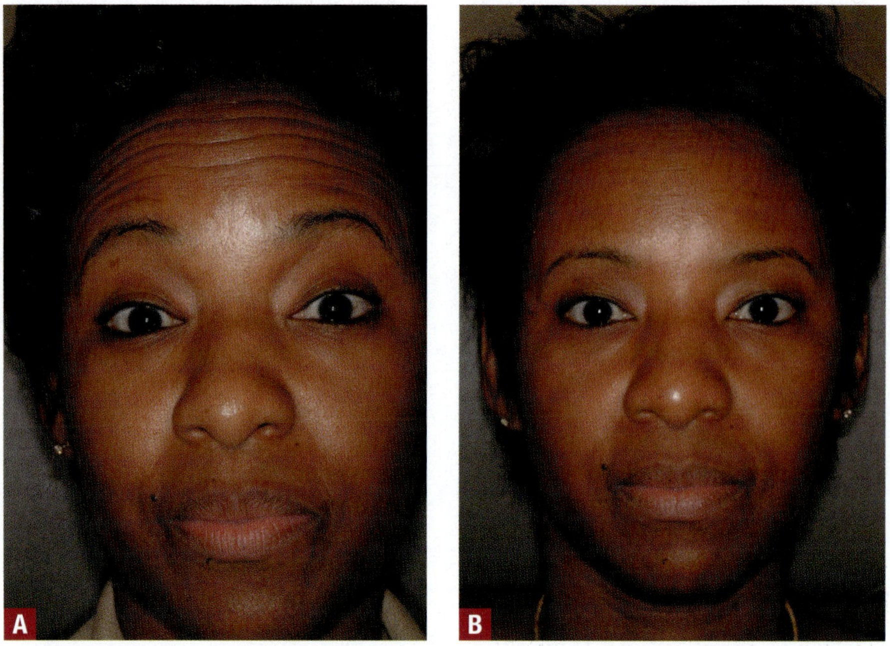

▲ **FIGURE 69-9** Before (**A**) and after (**B**) BTX-A injections for horizontal forehead lines.

HORIZONTAL FOREHEAD LINES The dose of BTX-A varies from 12–20 units based again on muscle mass (Figure 69-9). The lower third of the frontalis muscle is avoided in order not to produce brow ptosis. In a patient who has not been injected before, it is best to inject the glabellar brow area first and wait 2 weeks before injecting the forehead area.[66]

CROW'S FEET The injection point for the crow's feet area (orbicularis oculi muscle) is approximately 1 cm lateral to the lateral canthus.[67] This injection is performed intradermally as a "wheal" in one to three injection points and then gently massage laterally. The dose of BTX-A varies from 2–5 units per site and 10–18 units per side.

HYPERHIDROSIS BTX-A can be used to treat focal axillary hyperhidrosis.[68] Performing a Minor's starch-iodine test prior to the injections helps to demonstrate the area of axillary sweating. Topical anesthesia is recommended. Intradermal injections at doses between 2.5–4.0 units of BTX-A are placed into the skin 1–2 cm apart. A total of 50 units of BTX-A is used for each axilla. Results are expected in 2–4 days and can last up to 12 months.

Palmar hyperhidrosis also can be treated with BTX-A. Anesthesia is obtained by the use of a topical anesthetic under occlusion; regional block of the median, ulnar, and radial nerves; ice; or high-intensity vibration. Each palm requires 100 units of BTX-A, and the technique consists of multiple intradermal injections of 2–3 units each spaced approximately 1–2 cm apart. Results may vary, from 6–12 months of anhydrosis is common.

Outcome

As of yet, few studies have evaluated the safety and efficacy of botulinum toxin injections in skin of color, although the efficacy of BTX-A in Asian patients has been studied.[69,70] A 4-month randomized, double-masked dosing study for treatment of glabellar lines in women with skin types V and VI was performed to access efficacy of two dosing regimens of BTX-A—20 units versus 30 units. Both dosing regimens were found to be well tolerated.[71]

Complications

Local skin reactions can occur with BTX-A, such as swelling, erythema, and bruising. Most are mild and transient. Mild headache and flulike symptoms have been reported as well. A small percentage of patients experience transient ptosis that usually resolves within 2–4 weeks. Treatment with apraclonidine eye drops stimulates Muller's muscles to lift the eyelids. Injection of a minimally dilute solution 1 cm or more above the brow and postinjection counseling to emphasize the importance of remaining upright for 6 hours after the injection without massaging or manipulating the injected site help to minimize the risk of ptosis.

SOFT TISSUE AUGMENTATION

Soft tissue augmentation with dermal filler is used in the treatment and correction of fine lines, nasolabial folds, marionette lines, tear trough deformities, lip augmentation, volume loss, and acne scars. According to the ASAPS 2005 statistics, there were 1.2 million hyaluronic acid filler injections, 221,000 collagen injections, 91,000 autologous fat injections, 40,000 calcium hydroxy apatite injections, and 35,000 L-polylactic acid injections.[1] Hyaluronic acid fillers are used most often in soft tissue augmentation owing to their longer duration of action and excellent safety profile compared with collagen fillers. There are several fillers available (Table 69-4). Currently available dermal fillers will be reviewed, and special considerations in patients of color will be discussed (Table 69-5).

Bovine Collagen

Since 1981, bovine-derived collagen fillers were the "gold standard" in the correction of fine lines and wrinkles, acne scars and in lip augmentation. The available agents include Zyderm I, Zyderm II, and Zyplast, and they typically last 2–6 months. Zyderm I contains mainly type I collagen, 3.5% bovine collagen by weight, and is injected into the papillary dermis. Zyderm II contains mainly type I collgen, 6.5% collagen by weight, and is injected slightly deeper into the dermis. Zyplast contains 3.5% bovine collagen by weight and is cross-linked by glutaraldehyde, so it lasts longer than Zyderm I and II. It is injected into the deep dermis and lasts longer. All three bovine fillers contain 0.3% lidocaine. Treatment may be associated with allergic and nonallergic reactions; some 3–5% of patients experience allergic reactions on the pretreatment site,[72,73] thus requiring preprocedure skin testing. In people of color, skin irritation or a positive skin test result may present as hypopigmentation or hyperpigmentation[8] rather than erythema. In one unpublished report of two African-American patients, an intradermal injection of bovine collagen induced postinflammatory hypopigmentation on the forearms within 48–72 hours of test application. Given these reactions, the patients' nasolabial fold lines were left

TABLE 69-4
Features of Soft-Tissue Fillers

Filler	Uses	Type	Placement	Complications	Longevity
Zyderm I	Treatment of fine lines	Bovine collagen	Papillary dermis	Allergic reaction, misplacement	2–4 mo
Zyderm II	Treatment of medium lines, acne scars	Bovine collagen	Mid-dermis	Allergic reaction, misplacement, lumps	3–5 mo
Zyplast	Treatment of medium to deep folds, lips, acne scars	Bovine collagen	Deep dermis	Allergic reaction, misplacement, lumps	3–6 mo
CosmoDerm	Treatment of fine lines	Human-derived collagen	Papillary dermis	Allergic reaction, misplacement	2–4 mo
CosmoPlast	Treatment of medium to deep folds, lips, acne scars	Human-derived collagen	Deep dermis	Allergic reaction, misplacement, lumps	3–8 mo
Restylane	Treatment of medium to deep folds, lips, acne scars, periorbital hollows	Non–animal-derived stabilized hyaluronic acid	Mid to deep dermis	Allergic reaction or inflammation, blue discoloration, misplacement, lumps	5–8 mo
Perlane	Treatment of deep folds, lips, scars; facial contouring	Non–animal-derived stabilized hyaluronic acid	Deep dermis or superficial subcutis	Allergic reaction or inflammation, blue discoloration, misplacement, lumps	6–12 mo
Juviderm	Treatment of medium to deep folds, lips, acne scars	Non–animal-derived stabilized hyaluronic acid	Mid to deep dermis	Allergic reaction or inflammation, blue discoloration, misplacement, migration, lumps	5–8 mo
Radiesse	Treatment of deep folds, nipple reconstruction, nasal reconstruction, jawline augmentation	Calcium hydroxylapatite	Deep dermis to superficial subcutis	Nodules (especially in lips and periorbitally), misplacement with demarcation of product	6–? mo
Sculptra	Treatment of HIV lipoatrophy, cheek and temple hollows	Poly-L-lactic acid	Deep dermis to superficial subcutis	Visible and palpable papules	2 yr or longer
Autologous fat	Pan-facial filling, especially periorbital area	Autologous fat	Subcutaneous tissue	Bumps, vascular occlusive events with injudicious placement	5 yr or longer
Silikon 1000	Treatment of scars, HIV lipoatrophy, lips, deep folds	Silicone oil	Deep dermis	Delayed granuloma formation, migration	Permanent

HIV = human immunodeficiency virus.

untreated, and the dyspigmentation from the skin testing resolved within 2–4 weeks.[8] Although uncommon, this reaction may preclude the use of bovine collagen injections in those with darker skin. However, little clinical data on skin of color are available on the potential risk of PIH from injection of bovine collagen.

Human Collagen

There are two bioengineered forms of human collagen: autologous and allogenic. Autologous collagen is prepared from the patient's own tissue. As a result, this type of collagen is not allergenic and does not transmit exogenous infection. Because it contains intact dermal collagen fibers, it may be more resistant to enzymatic degradation. Two examples of autologous collagen are Autologen and Isolagen.[74] Autologen is no longer available. Isolagen preliminary phase III data were introduced in 2005, but the product remains unavailable in the United States. This dermal filler had to be injected into the patients within 48 hours of leaving the laboratory. In one study of 12 patients injected with autologous human fibroblasts, two showed significant sustained clinical improvement and the nasolabial fold region was the most responsive to treatment.

Allogenic collagen is provided from cadaver skin specimens and from discarded skin specimens obtained during plastic and reconstructive surgery.[75] Cosmoderm and Cosmoplast are derived from human collagen (foreskin). They have a low incidence of cross-reactivity, so skin testing is not required. Cosmoderm contains 35 mg/mL collagen and is injected into the superficial rhytides (perioral) and acne scars. Cosmoplast also contains 35 mg/mL collagen but in addition is cross-linked with glutaraldehyde and is injected into the middle to deep dermis (nasoloabial folds). They both contain 0.03% lidocaine, so they are contraindicated in patients who have a lidocaine allergy. Overcorrection is required, and results lasts 3–4 months.

TABLE 69-5
Fillers in Skin of Color: Available Clinical Data on Safety

Restylane
Perlane
Juvederm
Radiesse

Hyaluronic Acid Fillers

Hyaluronic acid (HA) fillers may be the agents of choice for soft tissue augmentation in patients with darker skin (Figure 69-10). Compared with bovine collagen, these agents carry a significantly lower risk of allergic hypersensitivity reaction. As a result, preliminary skin testing is not required. HA is a glycosaminoglycan consisting of alternating units of D-glucuronic acid and

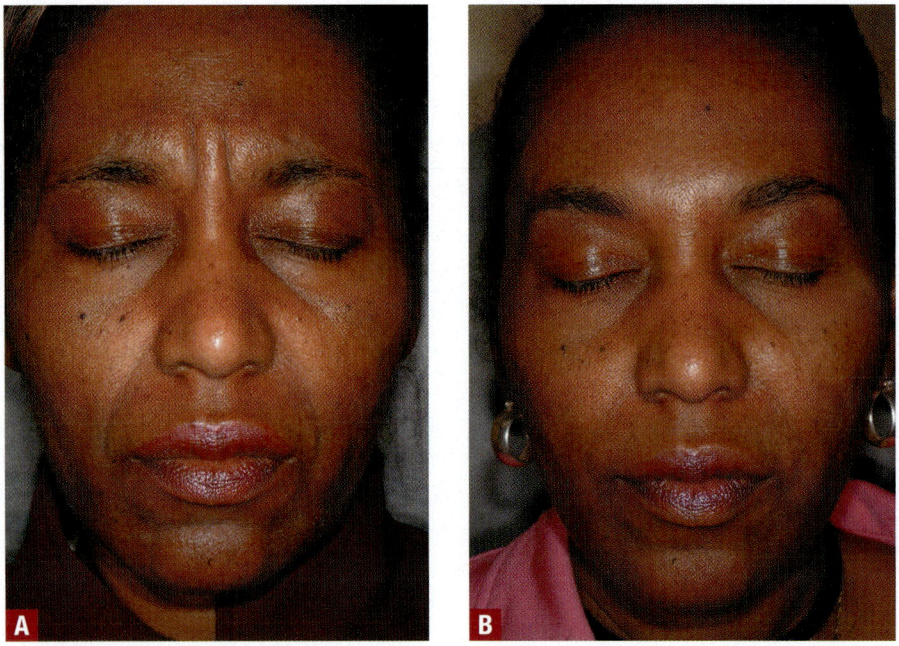

▲ **FIGURE 69-10** Before (**A**) and after (**B**) HA filler treatment for nasolabial folds and BTX-A injections for glabellar brow furrows.

N-acetyl-D-glucosamine disaccharides. It is found in the extracellular matrix of connective tissue in the skin, vitreous humor, synovial fluid, umbilical cord, and the capsules of certain microorganisms. Hypersensitivity secondary to trace amounts of proteins in the HA raw material or impurities of bacterial fermentation have occurred, but the introduction of more purified forms has reduced the incidence of this reaction. HA is a hydrophilic substance that attracts and holds water. Once injected into the skin, it attracts water and hydrates the skin. It is stabilized in the skin by cross-linking, which provides a longer duration than collagen fillers.

There are several HA fillers available in the United States, but only Restylane, Perlane, and Juvederm have clinical data on efficacy and safety in skin of color.

RESTYLANE AND PERLANE Restylane and Perlane are derived from nonanimal streptococcal bacteria. They both contain 20 mg/mL HA and are cross-linked using butane-diol-diglycidyl ether (BDDE). They differ in the gel bead size—Restylane 250 μm, 100,000 units/mL, compared with Perlane 1000 μm, 10,000 units/mL. Both are FDA approved for the treatment of moderate to severe facial rhytids, and the duration of effect is 6–12 months.[76]

A multicenter, prospective, randomized (split-face), patient-blinded comparative study was performed to evaluate the safety and efficacy of Perlane and Restylane in the treatment of moderate to severe nasolabial folds in 150 subjects with skin types IV–VI.[77] Most of the patients were African-American, and the Fitzpatrick skin types included 30% skin type IV, 45% skin type V, and 25% skin type VI. The results demonstrated duration of effect of at least 6 months with both Restylane (73%) and Perlane (70%), and PIH occurred in 5–7% of injection sites. These adverse events were considered mild to moderate and resolved within 12 weeks. No keloidal or hypertrophic scarring was seen during the study.

JUVEDERM ULTRA AND JUVEDERM ULTRA PLUS Juvederm Ultra and Juvederm Ultra Plus are derived from nonanimal streptococcal bacteria. They are formulated with Hylacross technology to allow a higher concentration of cross-linked HA.

A multicenter, double-blind, randomized, within-subject controlled study was performed to examine the efficacy and safety of a HA-based fillers (Juvederm family) and cross-linked bovine collagen.[78] Subjects received nasolabial fold treatment of HA filler on one side and bovine treatment on the contralateral side. There were 423 subjects who completed the 24-week study, of whom 26% were non-Caucasian. Subject demographics included 12% Hispanics, 11% African-Americans, and 2% Asians. All Fitzpatrick skin types (I–VI) were involved in the study, which included 20% type IV, 13% type V, and 3% type VI. The results demonstrated that the HA fillers resulted in longer-lasting clinical results than the bovine collagen, and the efficacy was similar for Caucasians and non-Caucasian subjects. In addition, there was no increased incidence of hyperpigmentation or hypertrophic scarring in the non-Caucasian subjects compared with the Caucasian subjects.

POLY-L-LACTIC ACID (SCULPTRA) Poly-L-Lactic Acid (PLLA) is FDA approved to treat acquired lipodystrophy in patients with human immunodeficiency virus (HIV) infection[79] and treated with highly active antiretroviral therapy (HAART). The injectable PLLA is biodegradable and biocompatible and produces a gradual and significant increase in skin thickness, improving the appearance of folds and sunken areas by fibroplasia.

PLLA is immunologically inert, so pretreatment skin testing is not required. Each vial contains a freeze-dried PLLA powder that is reconstituted with 3 mL sterile water and allowed to stand for at least 2 hours. Prior to injecting, 1–2 mL of 1% lidocaine is added to the suspension and then shaken. Additional anesthesia can be used if necessary and includes topical agents, local infiltration, and nerve blocks.

Multiple treatment sessions are required at 4- to 6-week intervals, with the effects lasting up to 2 years.[80] Results are not immediate, and touch-ups may be required. Vigorous massage of all injected areas is performed immediately after treatment and in some cases for 5 days after treatment. This step is extremely important to ensure proper distribution of the material and to decrease the possible formation of nodules. Although not FDA approved for cosmetic use, PLLA has been used for voluminizing and sculpting the face and hands. Currently, there are no clinical studies evaluating the safety of PLLA in skin of color.

CALCIUM HYDROXY APATITE (CaHA, RADIESSE) Radiesse is a semipermanent filler that, once injected into the deep dermis, forms a scaffold on which collagenesis occurs. It is used in the correction of nasolabial folds, marionette lines, jowls, cheeks, and chin. CaHA is not recommended for the lips, and the longevity varies from 3–12 months.

A postapproval open-label clinical study was initiated to assess adverse effects of Radiesse in persons of color.[81] One hundred subjects with Fitzpatrick skin types IV–VI whose nasolabial folds were treated with subdermal injections of

Radiesse were followed for 6 months. Subject characteristics included 85 blacks, 12 Hispanics, 2 Asians, and 1 other with Fitzpatrick skin types as follows: 24 skin type IV, 35 skin type V, and 41 skin type VI. At the end of the study, results showed no reports of hypertrophic scarring, keloid formation, or dyspigmentation.

DERMICOL-P35 COLLAGEN (EVOLENCE)
Evolence is composed of porcine collagen that has been processed by enzymatic digestion to eliminate the antigenic portions of the molecule. This fibrous gel filler is immunologically compatible with human collagen, so no skin testing is required. It is cross-linked with ribrose (Glymatrix technology), which has been shown to decrease its resorption rate, allowing for a longer duration of effect than bovine and human collagen fillers. It has been used in Europe since 2004 and Canada and Israel since 2005, in South Korea since 2006, and currently is awaiting FDA approval in the United States.

In a randomized, split-face, multicenter study involving 149 subjects, Evolence was compared with NASHA gel for the correction of nasolabial folds.[82] The results demonstrated that both dermal fillers showed statistical improvement in the Modified Fitzpatrick Wrinkle Scale scores with efficacy maintenance up to 6 months. There were differences in adverse events between the two groups. Subjects experienced more swelling, bruising, and pain on the NASHA-treated side, whereas subjects had more induration on the Evolence-treated side. Clinical data in patients is lacking.

SCLEROTHERAPY

Varicose veins are a very common cosmetic complaint and are observed in a large majority of the population. In fact, 41% of women in the fifth decade of life have varicose veins, whereas 72% have varicosities in the seventh decade.[83] Sclerotherapy for varicose and spider veins is a common procedure performed in dermatologic practices and has been used by dermatologists since the 1980s.[84,85] It is a first-line therapy for treatment of small varicose veins.

Patient Selection

A detailed history and physical examination should be performed on all patients with varicose veins considering sclerotherapy. Based on an individual's history and physical examination, a noninvasive diagnostic test of the venous system may be necessary.[86] The "gold standard" of this testing is duplex ultrasound, which assesses for blood clots within the veins. After the patient has been deemed a good candidate, informed consent is obtained.

Contraindications

- Reflux at the saphenofemoral junction
- Patients confined to bed
- Severely restricted arterial flow to legs
- History of deep venous thrombosis
- Allergy to sclerosing agents
- Obesity
- Pregnancy

Types of Sclerosing Agents

Numerous classes of sclerosing agents are available (Table 69-6). The selection of an agent depends on factors such as the size and location of the vessel undergoing treatment. There are three major classes of sclerosing agents, and they

TABLE 69-6
Comparison of Commonly Used Sclerosing Agents

Sclerosing Solution	Category	Advantages	Disadvantages	Vessels Treated	Concentrations
Sodium tetradecyl sulfate (Sotradecol)	Detergent	FDA approved Painless—unless injected extravascularly	May cause breakdown rarely—found to be equivalent to polidocanol in clinical studies	All sizes	0.1%–0.2% telangiectasias 0.2%–0.5% reticular 0.5%–1.0% varicose 1.0%–3.0% axial varicose
Polidocanol	Detergent	Painless Low ulceration risk at low concentrations	Not FDA approved	Small to medium	0.25%–0.5% telangiectasias 0.5%–1.0% reticular 1.0%–3.0% varicose
Hypertonic saline	Hyperosmolar	Low risk of allergic reactions	Ulcerogenic Painful to inject	Small	23.4%–11.7% telangiectasias 23.4% reticular
Hypertonic saline + dextrose (Sclerodex)	Hyperosmolar	Low risk of allergic reaction Mild stinging Low ulcerogenic potential	Not FDA approved Relatively weak sclerosant	Small	Undiluted—telangiectasias Undiluted—reticular
Sodium morrhuate (Scleromate)	Detergent	FDA approved	Allergic reactions highest	Small	Undiluted—telangiectasias Undiluted—reticular
Chromated glycerin (glycerin with 6% chromium salt; Scleremo)	Chemical irritant	Low skin ulcer potential	Not FDA approved Very weak sclerosant	Smallest	Undiluted to one-half strength—telangiectasias
Glycerin—plain	Chemical irritant	Painless, low risk of allergic reaction, decreased risks of pigmentation and matting	FDA approved for reduction of cerebral edema	Smallest	50%–72%
Polyiodinated iodine (Varigloban)	Chemical irritant	Highly corrosive—allows treatment of largest veins	Not FDA approved Avoid in iodine-allergic patients	Largest	1%–2% for up to 5-mm veins 2%–6% for the largest veins

FDA = U.S. Food and Drug Administration.

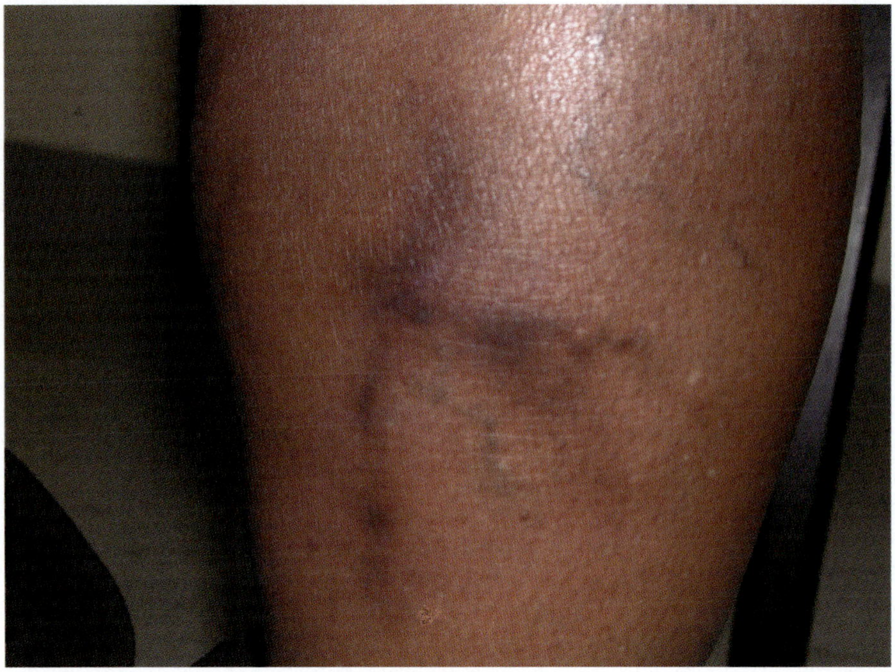

▲ **FIGURE 69-11** Postsclerotherapy hyperpigmentation.

TABLE 69-7
Sclerosing Agents Associated with Hyperpigmentation

Chromated glycerin (glycerin with 6% chromium salt)
Hypertonic saline
Hypertonic saline + dextrose
Polidocanol
Polyiodinated iodine
Sodium tetradecyl sulfate

include osmotic, detergent, and corrosive agents. Osmotic solutions are milder and less capable of initiating a cascade of inflammation, which could result in PIH, a common side effect of sclerotherapy in patients with skin of color (Figure 69-11).

Hypertonic saline is used in different concentrations ranging from 10–30%. Although allergenicity is low with this solution, it may cause skin necrosis if extravasation occurs at the injection site.

The hypertonic saline and dextrose solution contain a mixture of dextrose, sodium chloride, propylene glycol, and phenethyl alcohol. It is predominately marketed in Canada and used for treatment of smaller vessels.

Polidocanol is a detergent-based sclerosing agent that contains hydroxypolyethoxydodecane dissolved in distilled water with 5% ethanol. Injection with this agent is relatively painless, and it has a low incidence of cutaneous necrosis.

Sodium tetradecyl sulfate is considered a detergent and is a very effective sclerosing agent. In high doses, this agent has been reported to cause an increased incidence of posttreatment pigmentation.

Sodium morrhuate consists of a 5% solution of salts of saturated and unsaturated fatty acids in cod liver oil. This agent has an increased potential for cutaneous necrosis and is used rarely for treatment of varicose veins owing to its side effects. Fatalities owing to anaphylaxis from this agent have been reported.[87]

Chromated glycerin is considered a chemical irritant and is not approved by the FDA. It is a weak sclerosing agent but does have the ability to destroy the endothelium.

Polyiodinated iodine is also a chemical irritant and a strong sclerosing agent. It has a very toxic effect on the endothelium, and it is not approved by the FDA.

Technique

Sclerotherapy is performed beginning with treatment of the largest proximal varicosities and extending to the smaller distal vessels. Injection is performed using a 30-gauge needle that is inserted at a 10- to 30-degree angle with the bevel up. Initial treatment of telangietatic webs begins with the lowest concentration of sclerosing agents. The agents used most commonly are 0.1% sodium tetradecyl sulfate or 0.2% polidocanol. Sclerosing usually occurs 1–6 months after the procedure is done, and if it is not successful, the concentration is increased during subsequent treatments.

Compression foam sclerotherapy consists of a detergent sclerosing agent that is combined with air and is found to be more potent than liquid sclerosing agents.

Complications

Postsclerotherapy hyperpigmentation occurs at a rate of 0.3–10% and up to 30% in some studies.[88] The cause of this complication appears to be multifactorial and includes type and concentration of the sclerosing agent (Table 69-7), technique used, intravascular pressures, and postslerotherapy care.[89] Initially, this pigmentation is due to deposition of hemosiderin, and eventually the hemosiderin is replaced by melanin.[89] Within 6 months, the hyperpigmentation clears in 70% of patients.[89] For more persistent cases of hyperpigmentation, various treatments, including hypopigmenting agents, chemical peeling, and lasers, which have demonstrated limited success.

Other complications of sclerotherapy include telangiectatic matting, cutaneous necrosis and ulceration, superficial thrombophlebitis, and pulmonary embolism.

Patient Instructions and Follow-up

Four to eight weeks are usually allowed between subsequent treatments if needed. Patients are instructed to wear compression stockings for at least 2 weeks following treatment with sclerotherapy. Graduated 20–30 or 30–40 mmHg support hose are recommended after treatment of larger veins, and over-the-counter 15 mmHg compression stockings are recommended for smaller veins. In a study that evaluated postsclerotherapy compression with class II (30–40 mmHg) stockings in 37 women who underwent sclerotherapy for leg telangiectasia, hyperpigmentation decreased from 40.5–28.5%.[90] Edema in the ankle and calf also was reduced.

CONCLUSION

Individuals with skin of color and Fitzpatrick skin types IV–VI can undergoing cosmetic procedures safely and effectively as long as cosmetic dermatologic surgeons understand and recognize the particular issues and needs relevant to those with darker skin. Because most of the published data on cosmetic procedures thus far have focused on the Caucasian population, performing aesthetic procedures on patients with skin of color remains in some respacts a challenge.

REFERENCES

1. American Society for Aesthetic Plastic Surgery (ASAPS). 2006 Statistics on Cosmetic Surgery; available at *www.surgery.org/press/statistics-2006.php;* accessed October 28, 2007.
2. United States Census Bureau. *www.census.gov;* accessed August 2007.
3. Halder RM, Richards GM. Photoaging in patients of skin of color, in Rigel DS, Weiss RA, Lion HW, et al (eds), *Photoaging*. New York, Marcel Dekker, 2004, pp 55-63.
4. Kaidbey KH, Agin PP, Sayre RM, et al. Photoprotection by melanin: A comparison of black and Caucasian skin. *J Am Acad Dermatol* 1979;1:249-260.
5. Taylor SC. Cosmetic problems in skin of color. *Skin Pharmacol Appl Skin Physiol* 1999:12:199-143.
6. Grimes PE. Skin and hair cosmetic issues in women of color. *Dermatol Clin* 2000:18:659-665.
7. Grimes PE. Skin of color: Disease and cosmetic issues of major concern. *Cosmet Dermatol* 2003;16:1-4.
8. Callender VD. Cosmetic surgery in skin of color. *Cosmet Dermatol* 2003:16:53-56.
9. Harris MO. The aging face in patients of color: Minimally invasive surgical facil rejuvenation—A targeted approach. *Dematol Ther* 2004;17:206-211.
10. Grimes PE. Agents for ethnic skin peeling. *Dermatol Ther* 2000;13:159-164.
11. Grimes PE. Glycolic acid peels in blacks, in Moy R, Luftman D, Kakita LS (eds), *Glycolic Acid Peels*. New York, Marcel Dekker, 2002, pp 179-186.
12. Roberts WE. Chemical peeling in ethnic/dark skin. *Dermatol Ther* 2004;17: 196-205.
13. Kadhim KA, Al-Waiz M. Treatment of periorbital wrinkles by repeated medium-depth chemical peels in dark-skinned individuals. *J Cosmet Dermatol* 2005;4:18-22.
14. Kakita LS. The use of chemical peels in Asian skin, in Moy R, Luftman D, Kakita LS (eds), *Glycolic Acid Peels*. New York, Marcel Dekker, 2002, pp 141-153.
15. Grimes PE. The safety and efficacy of salicylic acid chemical peels in darker racial-ethnic groups. *Dermatol Surg* 1999;25: 18-22.
16. Al-Waiz M, Al-Sharqi AI. Medium-depth chemical peels in the treatment of acne scars in dark-skinned individuals. *Dermatol Surg* 2002;28:383-387.
17. Van Scott EJ, Yu RJ. Hyperkeratinization, corneocyte cohesion, and alpha hydroxy acids. *J Am Acad Dermatol* 1984;11: 867-879.
18. Tung RC, Bergfeld WF, Vidimos AT, Remzi BK. (-Hydroxy acid-based cosmetic procedures: Guidelines for patient management. *Am J Clin Dermatol* 2000;1:1-88.
19. Huber C, Christophers E. "Keratolytic" effect of salicylic acid. *Arch Dermatol Res* 1977;257:293-297.
20. Burns RL, Prevost-Blank PL, Lawry MA, et al. Glycolic acid peels for postinflammatory hyperpigmentation in black patients: A comparative study. *Dermatol Surg* 1997;23:171-175.
21. Sarkar R, Kaur C, Bhalla M, et al. The combination of glycolic acid peels with a topical regimen in the treatment of melasma in dark-skinned patients: A comparative study. *Dermatol Surg* 2002;28: 828-832.
22. Javaheri AM, Handa S, Kaur I, et al. Safety and efficacy of glycolic acid facial peel in Indian women with melasma. *Int J Dermatol* 2001;40:354-357.
23. Khunger N, Sarkar R, Jain RK. Tretinoin peels versus glycolic peels in the treatment of melasma in dark-skinned patients. *Dermatol Surg* 2004;30:756-760.
24. Lim JT, Tham SN. Glycolic acid peels in the treatment of melasma among Asian women. *Dermatol Surg* 1997;23:177-179.
25. Wang CM, Huang CL, Hu CT, et al. The effect of glycolic acid on the treatment of acne in Asian skin. *Dermatol Surg* 1997;23:23-29.
26. Lee HS, Kim IH. Salicylic acid peels for the treatment of acne vulgaris in Asian patients. *Dermatol Surg* 2003;29: 1196-1199.
27. Brody H. *Chemical Peeling*. St Louis, MO, Mosby-Year Book, 1992.
28. Atzore L, Brundu MA, Orru A, et al. Gylcolic acid peeling in the treatment of acne. *J Eur Acad Dermatol Venereol* 1999;12:119-122.
29.
30. Shim EK, Barnette D, Hughes K, et al. Microdermabrasion: A clinical and histopathologic study. *Dermatol Surg* 2001;27:524-530.
31. Rajan P, Grimes PE. Skin barrier changes induced by aluminum oxide and sodium choloride microdermabrasion. *Dermatol Surg* 2002;28:390-393.
32. Jackson BA. Cosmetic considerations and nonlaser cosmetic procedures in ethnic skin. *Dermatol Clin* 2003;21:703-712.
33. Masalkhi A, Walton SP. Pulmonary fibrosis and occupational exposure to aluminum. *J Ky Med Assoc* 1994;92:59-61.
34. Lim JT. Microdermabrasion, in Grimes PE (ed), *Aesthetic and Cosmetic Surgery for Darker Skin Types*. Philadelphia, Lippincott Williams & Wilkins 2008, pp 147-153.
35. Lloyd J. The use of micordermabrasion for acne: A pilot study. *Dermatol Surg* 2001;27:329-331.
36. Dual regimen for facial melasma. *Dermatol Times* 2003;24:47.
37. Tsai RY, Wang CN, Chan HL. Aluminum oxide crystal micordermabrasion: A new technique for treating facial scarring. *Dermatol Surg* 1995;21:539-542.
38. Henandez-Perez M, Ibiett V. Gross and microscopic findings in patients undergoing micodermabrasion for facial rejuvenation. *Dermatol Surg* 2001;27: 637-640.
39. Freedman BM, Rueda-Pedraza E, Waddell SP. The epidermal and dermal changes associated with microdermabrasion. *Dermatol Surg* 2001;27:1031-1034.
40. Lee WR, Tsai RY, Fang CL, et al. Microdermabrasion as a novel tool to enhance drug delivery via the skin: An animal study. *Dermatol Surg* 2006;32: 1013-1022.
41. Lew BL, Cho Y, Lee MH. Effect of serial microdermabrasion of the ceramide level in the stratum corneum. *Dermatol Surg* 2006;32:376-379.
42. Warmuth IP, Bader R, Scarborough DA, et al. Herpes simplex infection after microdermabrasion. *Cosmet Dermatol* 1999;12:13.
43. Bernstein RM, Rassman WR, Szaniawski W, et al. Follicular transplantation. *Int J Aesthet Rest Surg* 1995;3:119-132.
44. Bernstein RM, Rassman WR. The aesthetics of follicular transplantation. *Dermatol Surg* 1997;23:785-799.
45. International Society of Hair Restoration Surgery. 2005 Practice Census, *www.ishrs.org;* accessed March 2006.
46. Callender VD. Hair transplantation for pigmented skins, in Halder RM (ed), *Dermatology and Dermatological Therapy of Pigmented Skins*. London, Taylor and Francis, 2006, pp 245-257.
47. Sperling LC. Hair density in African-Americans. *Arch Dermatol* 1990;135: 656-658.
48. Pierce HE: The uniqueness of hair transplantation in black patients. *J Dermatol Surg Oncol* 1997;3:533-535.
49. Earles RM. Hair transplantation, scalp reduction, and flap rotation in black men. *J Dermatol Surg Oncol* 1986;12:87-91, 95-96.
50. Olsen EA. Female pattern hair loss. *J Am Acad Dermatol* 2001;45:S70-80.
51. Unger WP, Unger RH. Hair transplanting: An important but often forgotten treatment for female pattern hair loss. *J Am Acad Dermatol* 2003;49:853-860.
52. Earles RM Harland CC, Bull RH, et al. Surgical correction of traumatic alopecia marginalis or traction alopecia in black women. *J Dermatol Surg Oncol* 1986;12: 78-82.
53. Callender VD, McMichael AJ, Cohen GF. Medical and surgical therapies for alopecias in black women. *Dermatol Ther* 2004;17:164-176.
54. Sperling LC. A new look at scarring alopecia. *Arch Dermatol* 2000;136:235-242.
55. Lopresti P, Papa CM, Kligman AM. Hot comb alopecia. *Arch Dermatol* 1968;98: 234.
56. Nicholson AG, et al. Chemically induced cosmetic alopecia. *Br J Dermatol* 1993;128:537.
57. Sperling L, Sau P. The follicular degeneration syndrome in black patients: Hot comb alopecia, revisited and revised. *Arch Dermatol* 1992;128:68-74.
58. Callender VD. Alopecias and hair restoration in women, in Grimes PE (ed), *Aesthetic and Cosmetic Surgery for Darker Skin Types*. Philadelphia, Lippincott Williams & Wilkins, 2008, pp 287-295.
59. Shaffer J, Taylor S, Cook-Bolden F. Keloidal scars: A review with a citical look at therapeutic options. *J Am Acad Dermatol* 2002;46:S41-62.
60. Marzola M. Trichophytic closure of the donor area. *Hair Transplant Forum Int* 2005;15:113-116.
61. Brown MC, Johnson T, Swanson NA. Extensive keloids following hair transplantation. *J Dermatol Surg Oncol* 1990;16:867-869.
62. Pierce HE. Hair replacement surgery in black patients, in Pierce HE (ed), *Cosmetic Plastic Surgery in Non-White Patients*. New York, Grune & Stratton, 1982, pp 70-75.

63. Meyer M. Hair restoration in patients of African descent, in Unger W, Shapiro R (eds), *Hair Transplantation,* 4th ed. New York, Marcel Decker, 2004, pp 595-602.
64. Aoki KR. Pharmacology and immunology of boulinum toxin serotypes. *J Neurol* 2001;248:3S.
65. Carruthers JA, Lowe NJ, Menter MA, et al. A multicentre, double-blind, randomized, placebo-controlled study of efficacy and safety of botulinum toxin type A in the treatment of glabellar lines. *J Am Acad Dermatol* 2002;46:840-849.
66. Carruthers A, Carruthers J. Clinical indications and injection technique for the cosmetic use of botulinum A exotoxin. *Dermatol Surg* 1998;24:1189-1194.
67. Lowe NJ, Lask G, Yamauchi P, et al. Bilateral, double-blind, randomized, comparison of three doses of botulinum toxin type A and placebo in patients with crow's feet. *J Am Acad Dermatol* 2002;47: 834-840.
68. Lower NJ, Glaser DA, Eadie N, et al. Botulinum toxin type A in the treatment of primary axillary hyperhydrosis: a 52-week multicenter double-blind, randomized, placebo-controlled study of efficacy and safety. *J Am Acad Dermatol* 2007;56: 604-606.
69. Ahn KY, Park MY, Park DH, et al. Botulinum toxin A for the treatment of facial hyperkinetic wrinkle lines in Koreans. *Plast Reconstr Surg* 2000;205: 778-784.
70. Lew H, Yun YS, Lee SY, et al. Effect of botulinum toxin A on facial wrinkle lines in Koreans. *Ophthalmologica* 2002;216: 50-54.
71. Grimes PE. A four month randomized, double-masked evaluation of the efficacy of botulinum toxin type A for the treatment of glabellar lines in women with skin types V and VI. Poster presentation submitted for the AAD Annual Meeting, Washington, DC, 2004.
72. Lowe NJ, Maxwell CA, Patnaik R. Adverse reactions to dermal fillers: A review. *Dermatol Surg* 2005;31:1616-1625.
73. DeLustro F, Mackinno V, Swanson NA. Immunology of injectable collagen in human subjects. *J Dermatol Surg Oncol* 1988;14:S49-55.
74. West TB, Alster TS. Autologous human collagen and dermal fibroblasts for soft tissue augmentation. *Dermatol Surg* 1998;24:510-512.
75. Baumann L. Cosmoderm/Cosmoplast (human bioengineered) for the aging face. *Facial Plast Surg* 2004;20:125-128.
76. Narins RS, Brandt F, Leyden J, et al. A randomized, double-blind, multicenter comparison of the efficacy and tolerability of Restylane versus Zyplast for the correction of nasolabial folds. *Dermatol Surg* 2003;29:588-595.
77. Callender VD, Taylor SC, Burgess CM. Assessment of adverse experiences, keloid formation and pigmentary changes in subjects with Fitzpatrick skin types 4, 5, or 6 injected with hyaluronic acid gel dermal fillers. Presented at the *L'Oreal Institute for Ethnic Hair & Skin Research 4th International Symposium,* Miami, FL, November 11, 2007.
78. Grimes PE, Thomas JA, Murphy DK, et al. Efficacy and safety of novel hyaluronic acid-based fillers and cross-linked bovine collagen in Caucasians and persons of color. Poster presented at the AAD Annual Meeting, San Diego, CA, July 2006.
79. Valantin MA, Aubron-Olivier C, Ghosn J, et al. Polylactic acid implants (New-Fill) to correct facial lipoatrophy in HIV-infected patient: Results of the open-label study VEGA. *AIDS* 2003;17:2471-7.
80. Burgess CM, Quiroga RM. Assessment of the safety and efficacy of poly-L-lactic acid for the treatment of HIV-associated facial lipoatrophy. *J Am Acad Dermatol* 2005;52:233-239.
81.
82. Narins RS, Brandt FS, Lorenc ZP, et al. A randomized, multicenter study of the safety and efficacy of Dermicol-P35 and non-animal-stabilized hyaluronic acid gel for the correction of nasolabial folds. *Dermatol Surg* 2007;33:S213-221.
83. Engel A, Johnson ML, Haynes SG. Health effects of sunlight exposure in the Unites States: Results from the first national health and nutrition examination survey 1971-1974. *Arch Dermatol* 1988;124:72.
84. Weiss RA, Weiss MA. Sclerotherapeutic agents used for treatment of spider and varicose veins: Update 2002. *J Drugs Dermatol* 2002;1:53-59.
85. Duffy DM. Small vessel sclerotherapy: An overview. *Adv Dermatol* 1988;3:221.
86. Weiss RA. Vascular studies of the legs for venous or arterial disease (review). *Dermatol Clin* 1994;12:175.
87. van Haarst EP, Liasis N, Van Ramshorst B, et al. The development of valvular incompetence after deep vein thrombosis: A 7-year follow-up study with duplex scanning. *Eur J Vasc Endovasc Surg* 1996;12:295.
88. Goldman MP. Sclerotherapy treatment for varicose and telangiectatic leg veins, in Coleman WP, Hanke WK, Alt TH, Asken S (eds), *Cosmetic Surgery of the Skin.* Philadelphia, BC Decker 1991, p 197.
89. Weiss RA, Weiss MA. Resolution of pain associated with varicose and telangiectatic leg veins after compression sclerotherapy. *J Dermatol Surg Oncol* 1990;16: 333.
90. Goldman MP. How to utilize compression after sclerotherapy. *Dermatol Surg* 2002;28:860-862.

CHAPTER 70

Cosmetic Products

Cheryl M. Burgess

Key Points

- There has been over $1 billion in general business growth for ethnic hair care, beauty, and cosmetics.
- The term *cosmeceuticals* describes a product category that is intermediate between cosmetics and pharmaceuticals.
- The cosmeceutical market is driven by the antiaging market. Baby boomers comprise the largest market share.
- The cosmetic industry is governed by the Food, Drug, and Cosmetic Act and voluntary regulatory programs such as the Cosmetic, Toiletry and Fragrance Association (CTFA) and the Cosmetic Ingredient Review (CIR).
- The process of cosmeceutical product develop involves formulation, vehicle, active ingredient, and preservative considerations.

ABBREVIATIONS

AHA	α-hydroxy acid
CoQ10	coenzyme Q10
CIR	Cosmetic Ingredient Review
CTFA	Cosmetic, Toiletry, and Fragrance Association
FDA	Food and Drug Administration
FDCA	1938 Food, Drug, and Cosmetic Act
OPC	oligomeric proanthocyanidins
OTC	over the counter
SC	stratum corneum
TEWL	transepidermal water loss

OVERVIEW

For the past 50 years, the cosmetics industry has surpassed revenue expectations as one of the fastest-growing and most profitable market sectors in the United States. By all accounts, it appears that the new millennium will continue this record-breaking trend, and today, the growth continues as many companies expand into overseas markets and capitalize on new market segments, such as the fast-growing cosmeceuticals market.[1]

This chapter discusses several aspects of cosmetics use, beginning with an overview of the industry. The discussion includes the impact of cosmeceuticals, significant changes in the marketing of cosmetics, historical milestones in the development and use of cosmetics, the development of federal regulations, the formation of trade associations, and the chemical formulation of cosmetics. After discussing the industry, the chapter reviews various cosmetics products and ingredients, including antioxidants, growth factors, sunscreens, botanicals, and cosmoleculars.

Impact of Cosmeceuticals

Almost 30 years ago, Albert Kligman introduced the term *cosmeceuticals* to describe a burgeoning product category that was intermediate between cosmetics and pharmaceuticals.[2] Loosely defined, *cosmeceuticals* are any cosmetic, skin care, hair care, body care, foot care, or other products that treat or prevent a medical condition even as they beautify.[3] The market impact of cosmeceuticals is staggering: While the United States saw a 1% annual increase in the sales of skin care products in 2003, sales of cosmeceutical brands had an incredible 83% increase.[4] According to the Fredonia Group, cosmeceutical revenues in the United States are projected to top $5.1 billion by 2007.[5] Today, hundreds of products include vitamin supplements, antioxidants, and growth factors.

Marketing of Cosmetics

The marketing of today's cosmetics is no longer restricted to the pharmacy and department store. In fact, sales in the traditional big retailers have been in a decline. In contrast, cosmeceutical products are now widely available from diverse marketers, including mass, prestige, and alternative distribution channels[5] (Table 70-1).

TABLE 70-1
Places to Purchase Cosmetics[5]

Mass-market retailers
Direct-market retailers
Prestige retailers
Specialty stores
Health spas
Beauty salons
Health clubs and gyms
Physician's offices (including plastic surgeons, dermatologists, ophthalmologists, internists, dentists)
Internet boutiques
Infomercials

VERTICAL STRUCTURE The cosmetics industry is composed of large conglomerates that use *forward vertical integration* to manufacture and market products. According to this structure, large companies set up subsidiaries that distribute or market cosmetics to a variety of markets. What appears to the consumer as a host of different product lines is, in reality, a collection of products distributed from a single research and development source. Most cosmetics manufacturers do not use the practice of outsourcing development and production. In order to respond to quickly changing demands of consumers, production facilities must continually adjust the production processes. Outsourcing the production process would increase the time to bring a new product to market.[6]

THE CONSUMER Marketing strategies are also changing in response to changing consumer demographics and consumer demands. America's aging baby boomers, numbering 78 million, traditionally have driven the market for antiaging or other cosmeceutical products. However, today's market is driven by a new segment of nontraditional consumers as well. For example, increased discretionary spending by growing middle-class populations in Russia and Asia is also driving sales. In addition, the children of baby boomers, generations X, Y, Z, etc., are also fueling the sale of cosmeceuticals, and males 18–30 years of age are now targeted as another key growth segment.[5]

As today's consumers grow more knowledgeable about the physiology of their own skin, these consumers seek more science in personal care products and demand scientific data to back up marketing claims. As a result, clinical studies are often cited, regardless of the quality of scientific data, and doctors are increasingly becoming the spokespersons for skin care brands, adding to the credibility of these brands in the marketplace. Mass marketers are not only aligning with physicians to compete with doctor-owned brands, but the industry is also experiencing buyouts of smaller, doctor-driven brands by the larger companies. In addition to wanting sophisticated products with stable, efficacious active ingredients, consumers are asking for nonsurgical, noninvasive treatments that can be accomplished without visiting a clinic. To this end, several products have been positioned as a less drastic approach and an alternative to the dermatologist's office.[5]

ETHNIC MARKETS Another growth area in cosmetics is specialized ethnic populations, evidenced by the large success of products targeting the African-American, Hispanic, and Asian-American markets. According to market predictions, general business growth for the ethnic hair care, beauty, and cosmetics market will reach $40 billion by 2011. Products expected to grow in the ethnic markets include fade creams and gels, cleansers, toners, astringents, soaps, emollients, moisturizers, and antiwrinkle products. In the ethnic market, products that target skin discoloration are experiencing the best consumer response.[7]

For African-American consumers, uneven skin tone, sensitive skin, and acne-prone skin are the most problematic areas. Products targeting the African-American market have been most successful when sold at the mass-market and drugstore levels, as demonstrated by the success of certain ethnic products sold in Walgreen's and Wal-Mart stores. Ethnic skin care lines are handled more often through distributors compared with general-market products. This is so because successful marketing of ethnic products requires careful use of finely tuned distribution channels. Cofounder Dr. Cheryl Burgess and representatives of U.S. Black Opal note the success of distributors with operations in the United Kingdom, including destinations in the Caribbean, Botswana, Brazil, and Zaire.[7]

Certain ingredients are extremely popular among African-Americans, including α-hydroxy acid (AHA) and cocoa butter—AHA reduces the ashy appearance of skin in some African-Americans by speeding up the natural process of sloughing off dead skin cells, and cocoa butter has helpful emollient properties.[7]

Another indicator of the success of products targeting ethnic populations is the acquisition of cosmetics companies in non-Western countries, for example, L'Oreal's purchase of Yue Sai Kan Cosmetics and Carson, Inc.[7]

PERVASIVE MARKETING VERSUS HEALTHY COSMESIS The continued growth of the cosmetics industry is not terribly difficult to understand given America's obsession with perfect physicality and perfect beauty. Whether from Hollywood, the cosmetics industry, or even the medical health profession, Americans receive a steady dose of media images and messages *instructing* consumers to obtain physical perfection. Richard Fried writes, "Healthy cosmesis lies midway between total self-neglect and extreme makeover."[8] He notes that the dermatologist can play an integral role in the patient's decision-making process, providing clarity in a market that is permeated with unsubstantiated claims.[8]

Marketing claims tout the miracle-like effects of cleansers, moisturizers, skin supplements, and antiaging products. However, clinical studies that support these claims of miracle-like efficacy are often absent, flawed, or based on very small study populations, and many times the only clinical data are available from the product's manufacturer.[4]

HISTORY OF SKIN CARE PRODUCTS

Development of the Cosmetics Industry

Cosmetics were used for religious, medical, and personal care purposes by ancient societies that included the Egyptians, Chinese, and Indians. Based in part on ancient Egyptian pharmacopeia, the growth of cosmetics continued to develop in Rome and Greece. For several centuries, Rome remained a center of important cosmetic development, evidenced by the formulation of the first cold cream by Galen (AD 130–200). The Islamic culture encouraged the development of the beauty culture and contributed great advances in the use of botanical treatments for cosmetology. The thirteenth century marked the beginning of a divergence between formalized medicine and the science of cosmetology.[9] Moving forward, the cosmetics industry increasingly focused on the science of beauty, leaving behind medicine. Cosmetic products would not share medical status again until the flourishing of cosmeceuticals in the 1980s. Indeed, the debut in 1983 of these hybrid products—merging the research interests of science, medicine, and beauty—marked the birth of the modern cosmeceuticals industry.[10]

By the eighteenth century, most cosmetics were formulated in private homes from ingredients purchased at pharmacies. By the nineteenth and twentieth centuries, several important developments in the formal regulation of the industry helped to shape the modern-day cosmetics industry.[5] With the advent of formal regulation, the industry began gaining consumer confidence through improved safety, efficacy, and product stability. Today, many companies conduct cosmetics research with the same safety and testing methods used by pharmaceutical research and development.[5]

Development of Cleansers and Moisturizers

Some of the earliest cosmetic therapies were introduced by Galen, a Roman physician/cosmetician who invented cold cream, an emulsion of olive oil and beeswax. Much later, in the early 1900s, Paul Gersen Unna introduced Unna's boot, essentially a zinc oxide paste that is still the therapy of choice for stasis ulcers. Petrolatum was introduced in 1872 and has been hailed as the moisturizer *par excellence* without a serious rival in more than 100 years.[2]

REGULATORY AGENCIES

History of Regulation

Unlike the long history behind the development of the cosmetics industry, the passage of government regulations to establish the safety of cosmetics is a fairly recent historical development. The passage of the Food, Drug, and Cosmetic Act (FDCA) in 1938 marked the beginning of legislation to protect the consumer from unsafe cosmetic formulations.[1]

Beginning in the 1800s, a growing problem with tainted medications and food preservatives led to grass roots groups such as the Pure Food Movement, which helped to generate support for regulatory reforms that were made law by the Pure Food and Drug Act of 1906 (PFDA). However, the far-reaching legislation was stripped of its main powers of enforcement prior to becoming law.[9]

Concerns for consumer protection continued to fulminate in the 1900s, mainly at the state level. Politicians, recognizing a populist cause, exploited the horror stories (partly true, partly tall tale) illustrating the terrible harms caused by unregulated medications and cosmetics. The reform movement also was aided by a series of highly publicized books that demonized the practices of the food, drug, and cosmetics industry. These events eventually culminated in formulation of the 1938 Food, Drug, and Cosmetic Act.[1]

Provisions of the act addressed both adulteration and misbranding controversies. For example, the act states that a cosmetic is considered adulterated if it "contains any poisonous or deleterious substance that may render it injurious to users under customary conditions of use." In addition, the misbranding provisions prohibit labeling that is "false or misleading in any particular way."[11] Labeling provisions required by the FDA for the cosmetics industry include (1) proper cosmetic labeling, (2) declaration of ingredients, (3) label warnings, (4) tamper-resistant packaging, (5) contents quantity, and (5) the name and address of the manufacturer, packer, and distributor. The FDA defines *cosmetics* as articles "intended to be rubbed, poured, sprinkled, or sprayed on, introduced into, or otherwise applied to the human body or any part thereof for cleansing, beautifying, promoting attractiveness, or altering the appearance" while maintaining the structure and function.[11]

Throughout the 1900s, regulation of cosmetics was further defined, amid a continuing battle between consumers, manufactures, trade organizations, politicians, and the government—culminating in establishment of a voluntary regulatory program (discussed below).

COSMECEUTICALS: REGULATORY DILEMMA The dual nature of cosmeceuticals presents new challenges to lawmakers for classifying and regulating these products. The challenges range from fundamental questions to practical concerns. For example, should regulators reclassify drugs as cosmetics when manufacturers remarket products—not for their original therapeutic effect—but for newly discovered cosmetic side effects? Could drug vehicles themselves—absent any active ingredients—be given drug status based on their therapeutic effects as occlusive agents? In some cases, regulators have attempted to distinguish drugs from cosmetics based on the concentration of an active ingredient. However, no scheme is without drawbacks. Consider that the efficacy of AHA is more dependent on the design of the vehicle than on the concentration of AHA. As the cosmeceutical market grows, the regulatory difficulties are certain to be compounded.[12]

Cosmetic, Toiletry, and Fragrance Association (CTFA)

The CTFA was founded in 1894 as the Manufacturing Perfumes Association. The first decade of the association's existence was devoted primarily to furthering the industry's interests by helping to repeal several major tariffs and taxes. The association was very active in the 1920s as the cosmetics industry, boosted by the emerging flapper look in place of the more reserved Victorian style, experienced an explosion of growth. In 1937, the organization—renamed the American Manufacturers of Toilet Articles—gave support to the basic tenets of the legislation that would lead to the 1938 Food, Drug, and Cosmetic Act and lobbied for federally standardized regulations in place of a patchwork of state laws.[1]

In the 1970s, the CTFA worked closely with the FDA to establish a system of voluntary regulation, in which the industry provided regular registration of manufacturing establishments, submission of data on finished products, and reporting of consumer complaints. In the 1970s era of consumer and environmental concerns, the CTFA's program of voluntary regulation demonstrated the industry's willingness to supply information to the FDA while discouraging congressional legislation at the same time.[1] Today, about 40% of manufacturers voluntarily register their products with the FDA.[13]

In 1973, the first edition of the *Cosmetic Ingredient Dictionary* was published. The publication eventually gained international acceptance and would later provide an instrument for proper cosmetic ingredients labeling.[1]

The 1970s saw continued pushes for increased regulation of cosmetic ingredients labeling. Although the CTFA opposed the attempts to remove the voluntary regulation program, the CTFA eventually found itself working with the FDA to establish legislation, and in 1976, it supported further regulations on ingredient labeling. Manufacturers were required to substantiate the safety of their products or include a warning statement that the safety of the product had not been determined.[1]

Also evolving in the 1970s was the creation of another landmark volunteer regulatory program, the Cosmetic Ingredient Review (CIR). The CIR was established as a voluntary program to evaluate published and unpublished data on cosmetic ingredient safety. Today, the Expert Panel of the CIR is composed of scientists from the disciplines of dermatology, pharmacology, chemistry, and toxicology who have been publicly nominated by consumer, scientific, industry, and government agencies. The CIR program provides an open forum to present safety information and encourages congressional and public discourse.[1]

The CTFA is also responsible for *Cosmetic Industry ON CALL,* a publication created for industry members, government officials, medical professionals, and consumers to provide timely alerts regarding important ingredient safety information.[1]

Throughout the last quarter-century, the CTFA has helped industry, government, and consumers steer through many difficult social and legal challenges in cosmetics; for example, efforts to work with animal rights groups, safety testing of color additives, and regulation of volatile organic compounds, to name a few.[1]

The CTFA founded Look Good Feel Better—an initiative to advance the awareness and special use of cosmetics by cancer patients—and launched several initiatives to create funding for the program. Look Good Feel Better is funded by the cosmetics industry through the CTFA foundation to help female cancer patients overcome the appearance-related side effects and help to improve patients' self-esteem.

INTERNATIONAL COSMETIC INGREDIENT DICTIONARY The desire to normalize the process of describing botanical ingredients began in the United States. In the 1990s, an explosion of interest in botanicals drove the earliest rules for identifying and labeling botanical ingredients. At first, ingredients were labeled intuitively, for example, from a common name, such as apple or orange. However, as ingredients became increasingly more specialized, it became apparent that new rules for assigning names would be required. In addition, the intuitive terms developed in the United States were of little use internationally. With the help of the CTFA International Nomenclature Committee, several meetings were held in the United States and internationally. As a result of the meetings, the CTFA recommended that new rules recognize scientific terminology, using Latin genus and species names, as the basis for botanical-derived ingredients in nomenclature. In 1995, the sixth edition of CTFA's *International Cosmetic Ingredient Dictionary* introduced the labeling of botanical ingredients, showing both Latin and common botanical names.[1]

GENERAL BACKGROUND

Product Development

FORMULATIONS The formulation of a dermatologic product must satisfy certain requirements that include bioavailability of an agent, chemical and physical stability, freedom from contamination, and patient acceptability. Satisfaction of these requirements becomes a complex challenge when designing a delivery vehicle in conjunction with a specific target site for products applied to the skin. Cosmetic products may target the skin surface, the horny layer, sweat ducts, or living skin cells. To reach one of these targets, a vehicle must be individually designed to accommodate the specific needs of a therapeutic agent and a specific therapeutic target. Therefore, product formulation and vehicle design are almost synonymous.[14]

DERMATOLOGIC VEHICLE Dermatologic vehicles include topical liquids (lotions or liquid emulsions), anhydrous and hydrous semisolids, patches and tapes, liposomes, and microparticles. Some basic questions in the development of a delivery system may be answered early on. For example, what degree of occlusion will be needed, or will a penetration enhancer be required? Occlusion affects the percutaneous absorption of a product by changing the hydration of the SC and raising skin temperature. Penetration enhancers change the normal resistance of the SC.[14]

PRESERVATIVES Cosmetics can suffer degradation through oxidation and hydrolysis. Microbial growth can produce enzymes that cause degradation of active ingredients and change pH. Preservatives are generally required for any topical product containing water. Preservatives prevent or limit fungal and bacterial growth and contamination—after the product is manufactured, during storage, and in the hands of the consumer.[14] Vitamin E (tocopherol) and ethylenediaminetetraacetic acid (EDTA) are common preservatives in cosmetics.[1]

ACTIVE INGREDIENTS The use of generic drugs has helped the health care and health insurance systems to extend therapies to many patients who, without generic pricing, would not be able to sustain prescription drug costs. However, these benefits are not afforded without a tradeoff. In several cases, the interchangeability of products leads to therapy failure. This can be the result of (1) failure of a vehicle to deliver enough active ingredient or (2) patient noncompliance that results when inert ingredients in the vehicle cause adverse effects. Most disturbing is the misinterpretation by a clinician that an active ingredient has failed when the culprit actually may be the generic's vehicle.[15]

Generic Evaluation The interchangeability of two formulations is evaluated by three measures: (1) pharmaceutical or chemical equivalence, (2) bioequivalence of the active ingredient, and (3) therapeutic equivalence. For topical formulations, measuring bioavailability is more involved because active ingredients are present in very low concentrations in these formulations. The low concentrations are problematic because they lead to difficulties in accurately measuring the concentration of active ingredient in blood, and blood levels are often not representative of the concentration at the target site—the skin. As shown in Table 70-2, generics are allowed significant variation from brand-name drugs. Even small modifications to a product vehicle cause significant changes in therapeutic efficacy. This may call into question any assumptions of true equivalence.[15]

LABEL TERMS THAT MISLEAD The marketing of cosmetics often relies on the use of promotional terms such as *fragrance-free* and *hypoallergenic* to suggest that a product has special characteristics. These product claims often cause consumers to form grand assumptions about product ingredients. Unfortunately, these promotional terms have very imprecise meanings and may mislead consumers about the actual qualities and ingredients of a cosmetic. In many cases, consumers simply jump to conclusions, such as the assumption that "natural" products are superior. In other cases, federal standards or definitions are entirely absent, leaving claims about ingredients unchallenged, with regard to actual ingredients or scientific basis. A few of these terms are presented below.

Alcohol-Free Cosmetics that are labeled "alcohol-free" are sometimes chosen by consumers because they believe that alcohol will dry out their skin or hair. However, alcohol-free only pertains to the absence of ethyl alcohol. Cosmetic products, including those labeled "alcohol-free," still contain other alcohols, such as cetyl, stearyl, or lanolin alcohol. These alcohols, known as *fatty alcohols,* have a variety of effects quite different from those of ethyl alcohol.[16]

Hypoallergenic When cosmetics are labeled "hypoallergenic" or "allergy tested," many consumers assume that ingredients contained in the product are gentler to the skin or safer than nonhypoallergenic cosmetics. However, both dermatologists and the FDA say the term has very little meaning. Indeed, the FDA states that "almost all cosmetics can cause allergic reactions in certain individuals."[17] The FDA provides no federal standards or definitions to govern the use of the term, and manufacturers of cosmetics labeled "hypoallergenic" are not required to substantiate their claims. Not surprisingly, the FDA found that a majority of cosmetics labeled "hypoallergenic" contained the same ingredients as nonhypoallergenic cosmetics.[17]

Natural or All Natural Many consumers also believe that "natural" or "all natural"

TABLE 70-2
Terminology of Generic Drug Evaluation[15]

Term	Comment	
Therapeutic equivalence	A comparison of the therapeutic efficacy and toxicity profile of two different drugs given by the same dosage regimen to patients being treated.	
Bioavailability	The rate at and the extent to which an active ingredient is absorbed from the site of administration and reaches the systemic circulation.	
Bioequivalence	A comparison of the relative bioavailability of two different drug products in the same test population.	
Pharmaceutical equivalence	***Constant***	***Variable***
	Active ingredient Strength	Inert ingredients (binders, fillers, excipients)
	Route of administration	Color
	Dosage form (tablet vs capsule)	Flavor
		Shape
		Scoring
		Configuration
		Packaging
		Shelf life
		Manufacturing process

ingredients are better for the skin. However, the FDA warns that the implied superiority of natural ingredients is based neither in fact nor in scientific legitimacy. Moreover, there is no official government definition for *natural* or *all natural*.[18] "All natural" products contain plant-derived substances that are conducive to microbial growth, causing them to have an unusually short shelf life. Consumers and manufacturers should carefully consider the risk of contamination in products that contain nontraditional preservatives or no preservatives at all.[13]

Fragrance-Free and Unscented Cosmetics labeled "fragrance free" or "unscented" suggest that a product contains no fragrance or that no fragrance has been added. However, fragrance-free products may contain fragrance ingredients in small quantities to mask offensive odors caused by various ingredients, for example, the fatty odor of soap. Most manufacturers list these small quantities of fragrance among their ingredients, even though the FDA requires no such labeling.[19]

Preservative-Free Consumers also believe a product is superior, natural, or less harmful to skin if labeled "preservative free." However, most cosmetic preparations require preservation to prevent spoilage owing to microbial action or to retard oxidative deterioration, particularly that of fats and oils. Many of the components of cosmetics can serve as substrates for microbes, and contamination of a cosmetic, usually from airborne bacteria or fungi, can cause partial or total deterioration of the product.[20] There are no regulations requiring cosmetic manufactures to indicate the shelf life on the labels of their products. However, voluntary shelf-life guidelines have been developed by the cosmetics industry. For example, products used in the area of the eye have a shorter recommended shelf life. Accordingly, industry experts recommend replacing mascara 3 months after purchase.[13]

Some products labeled as "preservative free" actually may contain preservatives. This is so because manufactures can exploit loopholes in the regulations to make preservative-free claims. Manufactures can exclude preservatives from the ingredients label if raw material used in the product was preserved unnecessarily or if a raw material is overpreserved using any preservative, whether synthetic or natural.[21]

In 2004, concerns about the possible connection between parabens and breast cancer caused significant ramifications in the preservative industry and led some manufacturers to seek preservative-free systems to control microbial growth and prevent product deterioration. However, industry efforts have not yielded a satisfactory solution that is readily adaptable to current manufacturing requirements.[21]

In Japan, a different approach has been taken by the Fancl Corp. In 1999, Fancl built a $45 million manufacturing facility to execute the company's 25-year-long preservative-free philosophy. The new facility adopted a novel manufacturing process that eliminated the need for adding preservatives to cosmetics. Much of this is accomplished through automated processes that take place in bacteria-free environments. The company uses clean rooms, air filtration, and vigilant quality control to keep products from becoming contaminated with bacteria. Many of the processes meet medical and pharmaceutical manufacturing standards.[22]

COSMETIC PRODUCTS

Cleansers

Cleansers generally fall into two categories: soap and synthetic detergents. Soap, the most common known cleanser, damages skin because it fails to distinguish between unwanted dirt and important intercellular lipids. Certain lipids in the SC contribute to the water-holding function of the SC.[23–25] The water content in the SC is largely responsible for the flexibility and amount of shedding in this layer. The uptake of water and water-holding capacity, in turn, depends primarily on the quantity of natural moisturizing factor (NMF)—the water-soluble hydroscopic and surface-active materials present in the SC.[26,27] When soap disrupts the NMF, it reduces the skin's capacity to retain water, and transepidermal water loss (TEWL) leads to dry skin.

Soap causes the pH of skin to change and strips away valuable humectant agents, resulting in irritant contact dermatitis.[28] An alternative to soap is *syndets* (synthetic detergents). Although syndets remove less unwanted dirt, syndets spare more intercellular lipids, and the pH remains adjusted.[28] The use of syndets leaves the skin more capable of retaining moisture and thus avoids drying the skin out.

It is important to avoid certain additives in cleansers, especially if there is a history of sensitive skin. Examples include detergents such as sodium lauryl sulfate, parabens, and fragrances.[28] Table 70-3 lists several types of cleansers and their main attributes.

TABLE 70-3
Cleansers[28]

Type of Cleanser	Formulation Comments
Soap	Composed of anionic surfactants Drying and irritating to skin Raises pH of skin (neutral to alkaline)
Superfatted soap and beauty bars	Composed of anionic surfactants Drying and irritating to skin Causes follicular plugging Raises pH of skin (neutral to alkaline) Emollient may be added to reduced dryness
Dermatologic bars/cakes	Composed of amphoteric, anionic, and nonionic surfactants May raise pH of skin Emollient added to reduced dryness and irritation
Cosmetic liquid cleansers	Composed of amphoteric, anionic, and nonionic and silicone surfactants Can be mild and less irritating to skin Generally have pH similar to skin Generally have emollients and humectants added
Antiseptic and antibacterial washes	Composed of amphoteric, anionic, and nonionic surfactants May raise pH of skin Emollients added to reduced dryness and irritation Adjunct to acne treatment May help control bacteria, not believed to penetrate follicle Potentially less irritating and drying than topical bactericide.

TABLE 70-4
Moisturizer Ingredients[28]

Type of Ingredient (Function)	Examples	Side Effects and Problems
Occlusive agents (block water loss in the stratum corneum)	Lanolin, mineral oil, petrolatum	Messy Some can cause folliculitis May clog pores May cause contact dermatitis (lanolin) Can block hair follicles and cause pustules (folliculitis) or boils Can aggravate acne or cause an unsightly facial rash, perioral dermatitis
Humectants (hydroscopic substances that attract moisture)	α-Hydroxy acids, amino acids, collagen, elastin, glycerin, glycogen, glycosphingolipids, glycosaminoglycans, hyaluronic acid, lecithin, phospholipids, polysaccharides, proteins, pyrrolidone carboxylate (NaPCA), sodium hyaluronate, sorbitol, sugars, and urea	Some may cause irritation (urea, lactic acid)
Emollients (smooth and soften skin by failing the spaces between skin flakes)	Cholesterol, fatty acids, myristates, palmitates, squalene, stearates, and triglycerides	Not always effective May cause allergic reaction
Anti-irritants (reduce itching and irritation)	Allantoin, bisabolol, glycyrrhetinic acid, and vitamin C	Not always effective May cause allergic reaction
Antioxidants (may aid in cell turnover and healing and may reduce dehydration)	Selenium, superoxide dismutase, vitamin A (retinyl palmitate and retinol), vitamin C, ascorbyl palmitate and magnesium ascorbyl palmitate, β-glucan, vitamin E (α-tocopherol, tocotrienol), curcumin, coenzyme Q10, and α-lipoic acid	Not always effective May be irritating

Moisturizers

Moisturizers assist in skin repair by creating a suitable environment for healing. Moisturizers accomplish this by reducing the loss of water and creating a barrier on the skin. Moisturizer ingredients can be broken into three basic categories: (1) occlusive agents, (2) humectants, and (3) emollients[28] (Table 70-4).

OCCLUSIVE AGENTS Occlusive agents are defined by their ability to stop or retard water loss. Petrolatum is the superior choice of occlusive agents.[29] Other choices include lanolin, silicones, and mineral oils. It is highly recommended to apply occlusive agents right after cleansing to trap the maximum quantity of water in the skin[28] (see Table 70-4).

HUMECTANTS Humectants can improve the overall hydration of the skin by attracting moisture. However, when using high levels of humectants, an occlusive agent also should be used to help prevent water loss from surrounding cells. Without an occlusive agent to trap moisture, the skin actually could dry out even further.[28,29] Examples of common humectants include AHAs, amino acids, collagen, elastin, glycerin, glycogen, glycosphingolipids, glycosaminoglycans, hyaluronic acid, lecithin, phospholipids, polysaccharides, proteins, pyrrolidonecarboxylate, sodium hyaluronate, sorbitol, sodium principal component analysis (PCA), sugars, and urea. Some of these may cause irritation (e.g., urea and lactic acid)[28] (see Table 70-4).

EMOLLIENTS Emollients provide a soft, smooth feeling that consumers desire. The smooth feeling is actually achieved by filling in spaces between skin flakes. Emollients are classified according to their composition. Hydrogel emollients are either surface-active, providing a thin layer at the surface, or they are carbomer gels, which penetrate deeper into the skin. Oil-in-water emollients come in the form of lotions or creams. These emollients posses a hydrophilic external phase with superb absorption rates. Emollients can be incorporated easily into products.[28,30] On the other hand, water-in-oil emollients have a lipophilic external phase. Since these emollients mainly include petrolatum and/or paraffin oil, they are aesthetically less pleasing and usually are used in more chronic disease situations[30] (see Table 70-4).

Examples of common emollients found in moisturizers include cholesterol, fatty acids, myristates, palmitates, squalene, and triglycerides[28] (see Table 70-4). The most effective moisturizers are anhydrous lanolin and petrolatum, which have very little water and probably act by retarding loss of water.[29]

To replace diminished moisturizing and barrier properties in cases of deficit sebum production, future moisturizers will contain optimal molar ratio of skin surface lipids that mimic synthetic molecules, such as pseudoceramides. Other products under development include the acrylate polymer, a spherical microparticle that absorbs and binds sebum.[31]

Sun Protection

Terrestrial sunlight consists of ultraviolet B radiation (UVB, 280–320 nm), UVA radiation (320–400 nm), visible light (400–800 nm), and infrared (IR) radiation (800 nm and above). To protect human skin from free-radical generation, skin has a sophisticated antioxidant system that includes superoxide dismutase, glutathione reductase, and glutathione peroxidase. However, UV light damages skin throughout life because the cutaneous antioxidant system is less than 100% effective. In addition, these cutaneous antioxidant

TABLE 70-5
FDA Sunscreen Final Monograph Ingredients[33]

Drug Name	Concentration %	Absorbance
Aminobenzoic acid	≤15	UVB
Avobenzone	2–3	UVA
Cinoxate	≤3	UVB
Dioxybenzone II	≤3	UVB, UVA
Homosalate	≤15	UVB
Menthyl anthranilate	≤5	UVA
Mexoryl	≤8	UVA
Octyl methoxycinnamate	≤7.5	UVB
Octisalate	≤5	UVB
Oxybenzone	≤5	UVB
Padimate O	≤8	UVB
Phenylbenzimidazole sulfonic acid	≤4	UVB
Sulisobenzone	≤10	UVB, UVA
Titanium dioxide	2–25	Physical
Trolamine salicylate	≤12	UVB

systems themselves experience continuous damage from the sun, compromising their effectiveness.[32] For many years, scientists have known that UVB causes sunburn and serves as a surrogate for more serious skin disorders, including cancer. However, scientists have come to believe that UVA also may contribute to skin disorders, including photoaging and skin cancers.[32]

Sunscreens traditionally have been categorized as chemical absorbers, physical blockers, or both. Chemical sunscreens generally have aromatic compounds that absorb high-density UV rays, causing excitation to a higher energy state (Table 70-5). When the molecules return to the ground state, the energy absorbed in the photochemical process causes the emission of longer, safer wavelength radiation. Physical blockers are opaque compounds that reflect the sun's light. Recent research indicates that the newer micronized forms of physical blockers also may function in part by absorption.[33]

UVA SUNSCREENS Although benzophenones are primarily UVB absorbers, oxybenzone absorbs through UVA, making it a broad-spectrum absorber. It significantly augments UVB protection when used in a given formula. The anthranilates are weak UVB filters that absorb mainly in the near-UVA portion of the spectrum, making them less effective than benzophenones. Butyl methoxydibenzoylmethane provides superior protection through a greater portion of the UVA range. Although it is a significant addition to true broad-spectrum UV protection, concerns have been raised regarding its photostability and potential to degrade other sunscreen ingredients.[33]

It is recommended that all skin types and ethnic groups be advised and encouraged to use daily sun protection. The level of protection from sunscreen is indicated using the sun protection factor (SPF). Although consumers readily understand the meaning of the number—the higher the number, the greater the protection—studies show that people often mistake the higher SPF number as meaning that they can stay in the sun longer. Indeed, studies have shown that using higher SPF sunscreens has led to increased sun exposure by consumers. In addition to consumers misusing the SPF information, other problems exist. Consumers fail to correctly apply sunscreens—applying too little, too infrequently—perhaps as a result of labeling confusion. Descriptors such as "sun block," "all-day protection," "broad spectrum," "waterproof," and "water resistant" are misleading, especially since all sunscreens allow some portion of damaging UV radiation to penetrate the skin.[33]

Many of the organic chemicals commonly used in sunscreen products have not been tested for long-term safety. For example, titanium dioxide– and zinc oxide–based sunscreens have been promoted on the assumption that they are less harmful than organic sunscreen absorbers. However, the use of titanium dioxide as a sunscreen also has no long-term safety data.[33]

There is a growing interest in botanicals for sun protection, and research has found that some plant oils contain natural sunscreens. For example, sesame oil resists 30% of UV rays, whereas coconut, peanut, olive, and cottonseed oils block out about 20%. Although mineral oil does not resist any UV rays, it helps to protect skin by dissolving the sebum secreted from oil glands, thus assisting evaporation from the skin. Tea tree oil is a popular component of sunscreen formulations that relieves sunburn by increasing blood flow in capillaries and bringing nutrients to damaged skin.[33]

Evidence is growing that the addition of antioxidants to sunscreen formulations can protect human skin against UVB, UVA, and IR irradiation. In a study of 30 patients, Muizzuddin and colleagues[32] demonstrated significant protection from a cocktail of antioxidants. Results indicated protection from UVB, UVA, and IR irradiation.

Today, the addition of antioxidants is common among cosmeceuticals, especially for the purpose of treating photodamaged skin. However, the investigations of antioxidant use for preventing damage are in the very early stages of research and development.[34]

Clothing should not be overlooked as an integral part of sun protection. Wide-brimmed hats should be worn, and clothes should be chosen carefully with an appropriate fabric. Loosely woven fabrics may still transmit UV, up to 30% of UV with wet fabrics such as swimsuits. In addition, a white T-shirt has an SPF of 5–9, and UV-protective fabrics raise the SPF to 30.[33]

Antiaging Formulations: Overview

Just as antiaging products overtook the vitamin and supplements industry in the 1990s, antiaging products, referred to as *cosmeceuticals* are flooding the cosmetics marketplace. However, because the therapies are not classified or marketed as drugs, cosmeceuticals lack FDA oversight, and many claims go unsubstantiated. Before recommending antiaging therapies, dermatologists should seek clinical data on the efficacy of a product in a scientific, peer-reviewed journal independent of the manufacture's data. At a minimum, dermatologists should determine whether an ingredient has been shown to penetrate the skin and whether the proposed effects have been documented histologically, biochemically, or at the molecular level. In particular, dermatologists should warn patients that encouraging data from in vitro studies might prove irrelevant if an agent fails to penetrate human skin.[35] The first generation of antiaging cosmetics, mostly antioxidants, has been followed by a second generation of antiaging cosmetics comprised mainly of

TABLE 70-6
Partial List of Cosmeceutical Agents[4]

First-Generation Cosmeceuticals	
Vitamin A (retinoids, retinoic acid, retinol)	
Vitamins C, B, E	
Coenzyme Q10	
Idebenone	
α-Lipoic acid	
Grape seed extract	
Green tea	
Superoxide dismutase	
Second-Generation Cosmeceuticals	
Copper peptides (Cu + glycyl-L-histidyl-L-lysine)	
Growth factor-containing preparations:	
	TNS Recovery Complex
	4% Skin Growth Factor from placental extract
	Recombinant EGF
	Recombinant TGF-β1
Pal-KTTKS (palmitoyl pentapeptide)	

growth factors[4] (Table 70-6). Experts are now evaluating the use of hormone therapy in skin care products,[35] for example, synethetic peptides such as Argireline to relax muscle and dimethylaminoethanol (DMAE) to reduce fine lines and wrinkles.

Exfoliants

AHAs are naturally occurring organic carbolic acids found in numerous cosmetics. AHAs are found in food sources, including fruit, sour milk, molasses, honey, and sugar cane, and can be synthesized as well.[36] Glycolic acid and lactic acid are the two most common AHAs used in cosmetics, although many others are used in combination.[37] AHAs diminish skin scales (exfoliate), remove excess skin oil, and moisturize the skin. In addition, studies suggest that AHAs and β-hydroxy acids (BHAs) also may assist in the rejuvenation of photodamaged skin.[36–38] These compounds reduce corneocyte cohesion by modulating the secretion of cytokine- and keratinocyte-derived growth factors, possibly leading to the disruption of ionic bonds between corneocytes. AHAs reduce skin thickness, resulting in greater flexibility of the skin and reduced cracking and fissuring at the skin surface.[36,39]

Although AHAs initially gained interest in skin therapy because of the capacity to treat ichthyosis, the use of AHAs dates back to ancient times, when wine and sour milk were sometimes used to rejuvenate skin.[36] At the proper concentration, AHAs can be used as peeling agents.[37] Elsewhere, glycolic acid was demonstrated to be effective for treating pseudofolliculitis barbae,[39] and salicylic acid has been successful in treating hyperkeratosis.[36,39–42]

Unlike true keratolytics, AHAs exert influence at lower, newly forming levels of the SC.[36] Many patients experience irritation from using products containing AHAs. While prescription and OTC products differ only in pH and concentration, studies have shown that efficacy depends more on pH than on concentration.[38] Chemical peels have nearly all been replaced with AHA-containing products.[37]

Skin Supplements and Nutrients

VITAMIN C Since skin uses endogenous antioxidants to protect itself from photodamage, the potential to use cosmetics containing antioxidants for additional protection is not unexpected.[43] Antioxidants applied topically have been shown to be effective in stabilizing free radicals on the skin, but absolute proof as to the clinical value has not yet been provided.[44] Because proof is still lacking, the FDA limits the labeling of cosmetics to only the chemical name—for instance, ascorbic acid instead of vitamin C—so that consumers do not automatically assume that a cosmetic will provide the commonly understood benefits of vitamin C taken orally.[45]

Vitamin C is a free-radical scavenger and a cofactor for the hydroxylation of procollagen. In addition, pretreatment with vitamin C has been shown to reduce sunburn cells in porcine and human skin exposed to UV light. As an ascorbic acid, vitamin C is very unstable, causing manufacturers often to replace it with ascorbyl palmitate. However, only L-ascorbic acid significantly increases vitamin C levels in the skin. Very few human studies have demonstrated the potential photoprotective properties of vitamin C.[46] However, a few studies are worth noting. Vitamin C was shown to reduce wrinkling in a double-blind, vehicle-controlled clinical investigation with 19 participants.[35] In addition, a recent 6-month double-blinded, randomized trial showed a highly significant increase in the density of skin microrelief and a decrease in furrows.[47]

VITAMIN E Vitamin E is a well-known antioxidant that contains mixed tocopherols, a class of very strong antioxidants.[48] Many studies have shown that vitamin E can help to decrease the effects of psoriasis and erythema and may help in reducing the risk of skin cancer. Vitamin E also has been shown to help in the reduction of scarring from wounds and to help reduce the appearance of stretch marks.[35]

Vitamin E *acetate* is often used instead of vitamin E in skin care products because it lacks the free phenolic hydroxyl group. However, vitamin E acetate is biologically inactive. Despite this, the addition of vitamin E acetate to skin care products appears to protect skin against the harmful affects of sunlight after topical application. This is so because vitamin E acetate is a provitamin that is converted to the active vitamin by hydrolysis in the skin.[49]

Recently, Nakayama found that α-tocopherol-6-*O*-phosphate provided protection against UVB-induced damage in cultured mouse skin. In the study, which compared α-tocopherol-6-*O*-phosphate with α-tocopherol acetate, the water-soluble provitamin E provided greater protection that α-tocopherol acetate against sunburn cell formation, DNA degradation, and lipid peroxidation.[50]

α-LIPOIC ACID α-Lipoic acid is a naturally occurring dithiol compound known as an *essential cofactor* for mitochondrial energy production via the citric acid cycle.[51,52] α-Lipoic acid scavenges hydroxyl radicals, singlet oxygen, and nitric oxide and has been afforded "superantioxidant" status because it is both water- and lipid-soluble.[53] To direct antioxidant activity, α-lipoic acid protects vitamins E and C and downregulates the transcription factor NFκB.[53] In addition, the powerful antioxidant prevents lipid peroxidation in the cell membrane by reducing glutathione.[54]

α-Lipoic acid is under investigation as a possible agent to treat pathophysiologies of many chronic diseases. It improves polyneuropathies and glycemic control in association with diabetes and mitigates toxicities of heavy metals.[51] In vitro studies have shown α-lipoic acid to have anti-inflammatory properties. It has recently become a popular additive in cosmetics designed to treat benign photodamage.[54] However, only limited data on efficacy are available. Although α-hydroxy acid has been shown to penetrate into subcutaneous tissues,[55] properly designed clinical trials are still needed to demonstrate the efficacy of manufacturers' claims.[52]

COENZYME Q10 Reactive oxygen species, formed in the mitochondrial respiratory chain, have been implicated in a number of diseases and in the natural aging process.[56] Coenzyme Q10 (ubiquinone, CoQ10) is a naturally occurring antioxidant that quenches free-radical formation in the mitochondria. Coenzyme Q10 originally gained interest as a potential cancer treatment when investigators discovered that cancer patients experienced reduced levels of the enzyme. Although initial studies of using CoQ10 as a potential cancer treatment were encouraging, well-designed studies with definitive results are still lacking.[57]

Investigation of CoQ10 in treating human skin conditions also has been promising. In vitro studies found that topical CoQ10 reduced UV-induced expression of collagenase in cultured fibroblasts and provided antioxidant activity in human skin. In addition, a small 6-month controlled trial found a modest improvement in periorbital lines following 10 weeks of treatment with twice-daily topical CoQ10.[4]

IDEBENONE Idebenone is a short-chain biosynthetic analogue of CoQ10 containing the antioxidant properties of CoQ10 but with greater capacity to quench free-radical generation.[56] The drug was developed originally for the treatment of cerebral ischemia–induced lesions. However, the results of treating neurologic disease with idebenone have not been encouraging.[58]

The potential for using idebenone to treat skin conditions has been demonstrated in several in vitro and in vivo studies and at least one clinical study. In an assay designed to screen for potential treatments of common neurodegenerative disorders—involving reactive radicals and oxidative stress—idebenone provided protection from endogenous oxidative stress in skin fibroblasts derived from Friedreich ataxia patients.[58] In addition, in vitro studies indicated greater antioxidant capacity, compared with CoQ10, vitamins E and C, kinetin, and α-lipoic acid. Moreover, clinical photographs showed an appreciable improvement in periorbital lines, and immunostaining confirmed downregulation of MMP expression.[4]

FURFURYLADENINE N_6-Furfuryladenine is a plant-derived growth hormone known to have senescence-retarding effects in plants.[59] This cytokinin's antiaging effects—notably, antioxidant properties protecting DNA and protein from oxidative and a glycoxidative damage—have been demonstrated effectively in several in vitro and in vivo studies using plants, cultured human skin cells, and fruit flies.[59,60] Unfortunately, there are only a limited number of studies testing its efficacy in humans. The studies in humans, sponsored by manufacturers of furfuryladenine, have indicated that furfuryladenine may be equivalent or superior in effectiveness to Retin A. Manufacturers also reported that treatment with furfuryladenine produced few side effects.[61]

COPPER PEPTIDES The role of copper in stimulating angiogenesis has been acknowledged for over two decades, and copper peptides have exhibited dermal wound-healing properties in several studies.[62,63] For example, copper sulfate induced expression of vascular endothelial growth factor (VEGF) in primary and transformed human keratinocytes, and topical copper sulfate accelerated wound healing in murine dermal skin.[64] Copper peptides have been shown to (1) stimulate collagen[63] and elastin[4] formation, (2) stimulate the formation of glycosaminoglycans,[65] (3) increase blood vessel formation and oxygenation within the skin,[64] and (4) provide potent antioxidant protection.[4]

Important studies include a well-designed 12-week study that demonstrated increased skin density in 67 patients. Copper peptides also have enhanced healing of postoperative wounds and diabetic foot ulcers.[4]

GROWTH FACTORS Growth factors, important in wound healing, are present in a number of cosmeceuticals. Among the growth factors found in new cosmeceutical products, trandforming growth factor β (TGF-β) is the most important collagen-stimulating growth factor. TNS Recovery Complex by SkinMedica is a tissue-repairing complex containing growth factors derived from cultured fibroblasts of neonatal foreskin. The growth factors contained in TNS Recovery Complex help to repair sun-damaged skin by stimulating the epidermal thickening and deposition of collagen. TNS Recovery Complex also contains antioxidants, matrix proteins, and soluble collagens.[4]

Efficacy of the product has been demonstrated in a single small study conducted by the manufacturer, in which 79% of patients showed clinical improvement, as measured by optimal prophylimetry and investigator grading.[4]

However, significant questions exist about whether these large molecules cross the SC and whether it is even necessary for these molecules to cross the SC to stimulate collagen production. Large clinical studies are still needed.[4]

GREEN TEA Green tea contains polyphenols known to have superior antioxidant activity.[66] In cosmetic science, the term *green tea* does not refer to common herbal tea. Instead, *green tea* refers to the product of a careful process in which the leaves of the plant *Camellia sinensis* are processed, taking care to avoid oxidation and polymerization of the polyphenolic components. In green tea, the most powerful of these polyphenols is (–)-epigallocatechin-3-gallate (EGCG).[66]

Preclinical studies in mouse models have provided evidence that green tea polyphenols provide protection against UVB-induced immunosuppression and the generation of reactive oxygen species. Topical application to mice demonstrated protection against several tumorigenic agents and was associated with the inhibition of several biochemical markers of chemical carcinogenesis. In other studies, topical application to both mice skin and human skin demonstrated that green tea may have the potential to reduce UV-induced oxidative stress-mediated skin diseases in humans.[66]

Recent reports also suggest that EGCG reactivates dying cells. According to Dr. Stephen Hsu, old skin cells found in the upper layer of the skin appear to start dividing after exposure to EGCG. It also was reported that exposure to EGCG accelerates the differentiation process among new cells.[67]

Liao and Hiipakka[68] have shown that green tea polyphenols are potent inhibitors of type 1,5-α-reductase, suggesting the potential use of green tea polyphenols in the treatment of androgen-mediated skin disorders such as androgenetic alopecia.

Presently, numerous products are supplemented with green tea, even though the concentration of active polyphenols in these products is unknown, and controlled clinical trials have not been conducted.[66]

GRAPE SEED EXTRACT Grape seed extract contains polyphenols, mainly flavonoids, including oligomeric proanthocyanidins (OPCs), which have antioxidant capabilities 20 times greater than vitamin E and 50 times greater than vitamin C.[69,70] Studies suggest that grape seed extract binds to collagen, where its antioxidant effects promote youthful skin, elasticity, and flexibility.[71] Studies also show that OPCs help to protect the body from several age-related diseases, including cardiovascular disease and cancer.[71,72]

TABLE 70-7
Plant Derivatives for Cosmetic Use[75]

Skin Care Property	Plant Derivative
Astringent	Witch hazel, Hawthorne
Emollient	Allman oil, hazelnut oil, sesame oil, wheat germ oil
Moisturizer	Aloe vera, jojoba, Shea butter
Refreshing	Camphor, hypericum, cypress
Softening	Geranium, licorice
Soothing	Aloe vera, avocado oil, chamomile (bisabolol), Linden flower, lotus, seaweed
Toner	Elder, horsetail, marjoram, sage
Miscellaneous:	
Decreases skin edema	Marigold
Anti-irritant	Allantoin
Strengthens nails	Myrrh

OPC flavonoids have been shown to strengthen and repair connective tissue.[71] Grape seed extract may aid wound healing in two ways. Studies show that grape seed extract helps the body make more VEGF for angiogenesis to regenerate damaged blood vessels, and it also decreases the amount of free radicals in the wound site.[71,73]

PEPTIDES Oligo-, penta- and hexapeptides such as retinoids improve the appearance of photodamaged skin by stimulating collagen production, resulting in thickening of the skin. Palmitoyl pentapeptide (pal-KTTS) is a procollagen pentapeptide fragment showing efficacy in several well-designed studies for improving photoaged skin, including wrinkle appearance, age spots, and skin firmness. Histologic assessments in studies showed positive changes to elastin and collagen IV.[74] In addition, palmitoyl pentapeptide was comparable with significantly higher concentrations of retinol in reducing fine lines and wrinkles and improving hyperpigmentation and dark circles. The pentapeptide was less irritating, did not cause redness or barrier damage, and had no effect on TEWL.[4]

BOTANICALS It is likely that plant-derived ingredients were among the very first cosmetics. Ingredients used since ancient times include colorants, plant juices (for soothing and protection from insects), and fragrant oils. Several plant derivatives are purported to have various skin care properties, as seen in Table 70-7.[75] Caution must be observed because plants can cause serious allergic reactions in certain individuals.[54]

RETINOLS In 2004, retinol was reportedly a component of at least 60 cosmeceutical products.[4] However, the prominence of retinol in consumer skin care products should not be viewed without substantial attention to the differences between prescription-strength retinoids and retinols in consumer skin care products. Topical retinoids are prescription-strength drugs with the ability to help normalize hyperkeratinization and provide anti-inflammatory effects. In contrast, all-*trans*-retinol is a parent form of vitamin A and has limited efficacy.[76] Some experts propose that the benefits of the parent form of retinol are due to the oxidation of all-*trans*-retinol to the active retinoid after absorption into skin cells.[77] Retinol is present in consumer skin care products in widely varying categories. Some retinol products are efficacious,[78] some are present below clinically effective concentrations,[4] and other consumer skin care products contain biologically inactive retinol forms.[79] However, the lower concentrations make these products less irritating than prescription-strength retinoids. Retinol has been combined with other products, including AHAs, to improve results.[4]

Topical all-*trans*-retinoic acid protects the skin against damage from UVA and UVB rays by facilitating the ability to prevent collagen loss and the ability to stimulate new collagen formation within the capillary dermis of sun-exposed skin.[80,81] These protective properties form the basis for its use in minimizing the appearance of fine wrinkle lines.

NEW AND INNOVATIVE APPLICATIONS FOR SOY IN SKIN CARE The soybean, with its broad spectrum of components, including proteins, essential fatty acids, phytosterols, isoflavonoids, lecithins, and saponins, has long been known to have skin care benefits from its use in traditional Chinese medicine. Scientists have identified several possible applications in skin care, and current research is successfully uncovering the mechanisms behind these skin care applications. Potential applications include (1) providing oil control, (2) providing moisturization, (3) delaying hair regrowth, (4) enhancing skin elasticity, and (5) reducing the appearance of pigmentation and UV-induced erythema and pigmentation.[82,83]

Scientists have determined that small soybean proteins [soybean trypsin inhibitor (STI) and Bowman Birk inhibitor (BBI)] can reduce hyperpigmentation through regulation of the protease-activated receptor 2 (PAR-2) pathway.[84] Cosmetic formulations containing these proteins have been shown clinically to help even out skin tone and smooth skin texture.[82,83]

Cosmetic scientists also found that a natural soy formulation could effectively reduce the appearance of unwanted facial hair above the upper lip area while improving the overall skin appearance and skin condition.[85]

The Future of Cosmeceuticals

One of latest technologies in development is the use of spin traps. These are the very newest antioxidants, which catch or trap an aberrant electron as it starts to spin out of control and returns it to its orbit before it can do any damage. Although the use of spin traps in dermatology is in its infancy, these compounds have shown a great deal of promise in the field of dermatology.[86]

Spin traps were used originally as a way to measure free-radical activity both in vivo and in vitro through their ability to form stable complexes. The most well-known spin trap is phenyl butyl nitrone (PBN).[86]

CONCLUSION

The cosmetic industry is an ever-changing, ever-growing market that promises to continue providing novel agents for maintaining healthy skin. The true clinical efficacy of some of these products remains to be proven. However, many products are known to provide clinically relevant results. In time, clinical efficacy and safety data will be supplied.

The development and tremendous growth in cosmeceutical sales are a response to consumer demands for more scientific and sophisticated cosmetic products. The first generation of cosmeceuticals provided supplements and antioxidants. The second generation of cosmeceuticals focused on growth factors to help stimulate repair of photoaged skin. While the twentieth century brought the development of cosmeceuticals, the twenty-first century will mark the introduction of new skin care technology in the form of Cosmoleculars—designer molecules in cosmetics products.[86]

REFERENCES

1. CTFA History. *Cosmetic, Toiletry, and Fragrance Association.* Available at *www.ctfa.org;* accessed September 23, 2004.
2. Kligman AM. Why cosmeceuticals? *Cosmetics Toiletries* 1993;108:37-38.
3. Dowd T. Cosmeceuticals take on new personalities. *Cosmetic Packaging and Design.* Available at *www.cosmeticpackaginganddesign.com;* accessed September 9, 2004.
4. Farris P. Aging and appearance. Paper presented at Clinical Symposia Advances in Dermatology 2004, Amelia Island, FL, 2004.
5. Lewis W. Scientific research produces advanced skincare products. *Aesthetic Buyers Guide* 2004:77-80.
6. How does collaboration with supply-chain partners play a role in new product success? Cass Business School. Available at *www.cass.city.ac.uk;* accessed September 21, 2004.
7. *Global Cosmetic Industry News,* January 2, 2008.
8. Fried R. Extreme makeover: In a world of misguided strivings for eternal youth, dermatologist can help patients find a balance. *Skin Aging* 2004;June: 58-59.
9. Epstein HA. Cosmetic science regulation. *Skinmed* 2004;3:160-162.
10. MD Formulations. Company profile. Available at *www.mdformulations.com ;* accessed September 15, 2004.
11. FDA. *Cosmetic Handbook.* Available at *www.cfsan.fda.gov;* accessed September 16, 2004.
12. Vermeer BJ, Gilchrest BA. Cosmeceuticals: A proposal for rational definition, evaluation, and regulation. *Arch Dermatol* 1996; 132:337-340.
13. Tips for safe keeping and use of cosmetics. Medical College of Wisconsin Healthlink, November 29, 2000. Available at *http://healthlink.mcw.edu;* accessed September 21, 2004.
14. Zatz J. The formulation of dermatologic vehicles. *Cutis* 1995;55:17-27S.
15. Piacquadio D. Generic drug substitution in dermatology: clinical implications. *Cutis* 1995;55:28-36S.
16. FDA. Alcohol free. U S. Food and Drug Administration, Center for Food Safety and Applied Nutrition, Office of Cosmetics and Colors Fact Sheet, March 7, 2000. Available at *http://vm.cfsan.fda.gov/~dms/cos-227.html;* accessed September 20, 2004.
17. FDA. Hypoallergenic cosmetics. U.S. Food and Drug Administration, Center for Food Safety and Applied Nutrition, Office of Cosmetics and Colors Fact Sheet, October 18, 2000. Available at *http://vm.cfsan.fda.gov/~dms/cos-224.html;* accessed September 20, 2004.
18. Lewis C. Clearing up cosmetic confusion. FDA Consumer, May-June 1998. Available at *www.fda.gov/fdac/features/1998/398_cosm.html;* accessed September 20, 2004.
19. FDA. Fragrance free and unscented. U.S. Food and Drug Administration, May 1995. Available at *http://vm.cfsan.fda.gov;* accessed September 20, 2004.
20. Preservation of cosmetics. Perfume and Cosmetic World, 2001. Available at *www.a-world-of-perfumes-cosmetics.com/cosmetics_preservation.htm;* accessed September 21, 2004.
21. A preservative update. Household and Personal Products Industry, May 2004. Available at *www.happi.com;* accessed September 21, 2004.
22. Delaers J. A preservative-free process. Available at *www.thecosmeticsite.com;* accessed May 19, 2004.
23. Imokawa G, Kuno H, Kawai M. Stratum corneum lipids serve as a bound-water modulator. *J Invest Dermatol* 1991;96: 845-851.
24. Imokawa G, Hattori M. A possible function of structural lipids in the water-holding properties of the stratum corneum. *J Invest Dermatol* 1985;84:282-284.
25. Elias PM, Menon GK. Structural and lipid biochemical correlates of the epidermal permeability barrier. *Adv Lipid Res* 1991; 24:1-26.
26. Jacobi OK. About the mechanism of moisture regulation in the horny layer of the skin. *Toilet Goods Association* 1959: 22-24.
27. Rawlings AV, Scott IR, Harding CR, Bowser PA. Stratum corneum moisturization at the molecular level. *J Invest Dermatol* 1994;103:731-741.
28. Krivda M. Making the choice: Tips for selecting appropriate cleansers and moisturizers for patients who have special skincare needs. *Skin Aging* 2004;June: 64-71.
29. Kligman AM. Regression method for assessing the efficacy of moisturizers. *Cosmetics Toiletries* 1978;93:27-35.
30. Fluhr: Basic emollient classification, in Leyden JJ, Rawlings AV (eds), *Skin Moisturization.* New York, Marcel Dekker, 2002, pp 224-225.
31. Abramovits W, Gonzalez-Serva A. Sebum, cosmetics, and skin care. *Dermatol Clin* 2000;18:617-620.
32. Muizzuddin N, Shakoori AR, Marenus K. Effect of antioxidants and free radical scavengers on protection of human skin against UVB, UVA and IR irradiation. *Skin Res Technol* 1999;5:260-265.
33. Mufti J. UV Protection. Household and Personal Products Industry, June 2003; available at *www.happi.com/current/June032.htm;* accessed September 23, 2004.
34. Bryant R. Popular sunscreen seeks U.S. approval. *Dermatol Times* 2004;September: 19-25.
35. Ghadially R. Do anti-aging creams really work? *Cosmet Dermatol* 2000;XX: 13-17.
36. Van Scott EJ, Yu RJ. Hyperkeratinization, corneocyte cohesion, and alpha hydroxy acids. *J Am Acad Dermatol* 1984;11: 867-879.
37. Ramos-e-Silva M, de Castro MC, da Silva Carneiro SC, Lambert WC. Alpha-hydroxy acids: Unapproved uses or indications. *Skinmed* 2004;3:141-148.
38. Vidt DG, Bergfeld WF. Cosmetic use of alpha-hydroxy acids. *Cleve Clin J Med* 1997;64:327-329.
39. Perricone NV. Treatment of pseudofolliculitis barbae with topical glycolic acid: A report of two studies. *Cutis* 1993;52: 232-235.
40. Roberts DL, Marshall R, Marks R. Detection of the action of salicylic acid on the normal stratum corneum. *Br J Dermatol* 1980;103:191-196.
41. Davies M, Marks R. Studies on the effect of salicylic acid on normal skin. *Br J Dermatol* 1976;95:187-192.
42. Marks R, Davies M, Cattell A. An explanation for the keratolytic effect of salicylic acid *J Invest Dermatol* 1975; 64: 283.
43. Pinnell SR. Cutaneous photodamage, oxidative stress, and topical antioxidant protection. *J Am Acad Dermatol* 2003;48: 1-19.
44. Keller KL, Fenske NA. Uses of vitamins A, C, and E and related compounds in dermatology: A review. *J Am Acad Dermatol* 1998;39:611-625S.
45. Foulke J. Cosmetics industry: Understanding the puffery. *FDA Consumer Magazine,* 1995. Available at *www.fda.gov/fdac/reprints/puffery.html;* accessed September 23, 2004.
46. Chiu A, Kimball AB. Topical vitamins, minerals and botanical ingredients as modulators of environmental and chronological skin damage. *Br J Dermatol* 2003;149:681-691.
47. Humbert PG, Haftek M, Creidi P, et al. Topical ascorbic acid on photoaged skin: Clinical, topographical and ultrastructural evaluation—Double-blind study vs placebo. *Exp Dermatol* 2003;12:237-244.
48. Ricciarelli R, Zingg JM, Azzi A. Vitamin E 80th anniversary: A double life, not only fighting radicals. *IUBMB Life* 2001;52: 71-76.
49. Beijersbergen van Henegouwen GM, Junginger HE, de Vries H. Hydrolysis of RRR-alpha-tocopheryl acetate (vitamin E acetate) in the skin and its UV protecting activity (an in vivo study with the rat). *J Photochem Photobiol B* 1995;29:45-51.
50. Nakayama S, Katoh EM, Tsuzuki T, Kobayashi S. Protective effect of alpha-tocopherol-6-*O*-phosphate against ultraviolet B–induced damage in cultured mouse skin. *J Invest Dermatol* 2003;121: 406-411.
51. Smith AR, Shenvi SV, Widlansky M, et al. Lipoic acid as a potential therapy for chronic diseases associated with oxidative stress. *Curr Med Chem* 2004;11: 1135-1146.
52. Alpha lipoic acid skin care: What is all the fuss about? *Smartskincare.com.* Available at *www.smartskincare.com/treatments/lipoic.html;* accessed September 22, 2004.
53. Guttman C. Cosmeceutical market expanding rapidly while scientific support lags. *Dermatol Times,* June 1, 2004.
54. Draelos ZD. Cosmetic conundrums. *Dermatol Times,* September 1, 2003.
55. Perricone NV. Topical alpha-lipoic acid for anti-aging. *Skin Aging* 1998;May: 17-19.
56. Lenaz G, Bovina C, D'Aurelio M, et al. Role of mitochondria in oxidative stress and aging. *Ann NY Acad Sci* 2002;959: 199-213.
57. Coenzyme Q10: Questions and answers. National Cancer Institute, June 12, 2002. Available at *www.cancer.gov/cancerinfo/*

pdq/cam/coenzymeQ10; accessed September 16, 2004.
58. Jauslin ML, Wirth T, Meier T, Schoumacher F. A cellular model for Friedreich ataxia reveals small-molecule glutathione peroxidase mimetics as novel treatment strategy. *Hum Mol Genet* 2002; 11:3055-3063.
59. Rattan SI, Clark BF. Kinetin delays the onset of ageing characteristics in human fibroblasts. *Biochem Biophys Res Commun* 1994;201:665-672.
60. Olsen A, Siboska GE, Clark BF, Rattan SI. *N*(6)-Furfuryladenine, kinetin, protects against Fenton reaction–mediated oxidative damage to DNA. *Biochem Biophys Res Commun* 1999;265:499-502.
61. Todorov G. Furfuryladenine (kinetin and kinerase) for skin rejuvenation. *Smartskincare.com;* accessed August 1, 2004.
62. Canapp SO Jr, Farese JP, Schultz GS, et al. The effect of topical tripeptide-copper complex on healing of ischemic open wounds. *Vet Surg* 2003;32:515-523.
63. Buffoni F, Pino R, Dal Pozzo A. Effect of tripeptide-copper complexes on the process of skin wound healing and on cultured fibroblasts. *Arch Int Pharmacodyn Ther* 1995;330:345-360.
64. Sen CK, Khanna S, Venojarvi M, et al. Copper-induced vascular endothelial growth factor expression and wound healing. *Am J Physiol Heart Circ Physiol* 2002;282:H1821-1827.
65. Simeon A, Wegrowski Y, Bontemps Y, Maquart FX. Expression of glycosaminoglycans and small proteoglycans in wounds: modulation by the tripeptide-copper complex glycyl-L-histidyl-L-lysine-Cu^{2+}. *J Invest Dermatol* 2000;115: 962-968.
66. Katiyar SK, Ahmad N, Mukhtar H. Green tea and skin. *Arch Dermatol* 2000;136: 989-994.
67. Hurley-Deriso C. Green tea research translates into skin-care products. Medical College of Georgia. Available at *www.mcg.edu/news/2003NewsRel/hsu.html;* accessed September 23, 2004.
68. Liao S, Hiipakka RA. Selective inhibition of steroid 5-alpha-reductase isozymes by tea epicatechin-3-gallate and epigallocatechin-3-gallate. *Biochem Biophys Res Commun* 1995;214:833-838.
69. Bagchi D, Sen CK, Ray SD, et al. Molecular mechanisms of cardioprotection by a novel grape seed proanthocyanidin extract. *Mutat Res* 2003;523-524:87-97.
70. Bagchi D, Bagchi M, Stohs S, et al. Cellular protection with proanthocyanidins derived from grape seeds. *Ann NY Acad Sci* 2002;957:260-270.
71. Shi J, Yu J, Pohorly JE, Kakuda Y. Polyphenolics in grape seeds: Biochemistry and functionality. *J Med Food* 2003;6:291-299.
72. Bouhamidi R, Prevost V, Nouvelot A. High protection by grape seed proanthocyanidins (GSPC) of polyunsaturated fatty acids against UV-C induced peroxidation. *C R Acad Sci III* 1998;321:31-38.
73. Sen CK, Khanna S, Gordillo G, et al. Oxygen, oxidants, and antioxidants in wound healing: an emerging paradigm. *Ann NY Acad Sci* 2002;957:239-249.
74. Guttman C. Studies demonstrate value of procollagen: Pal-KTTKS shows positive changes, improves wrinkle appearance without causing irritation. *Dermatol Times* 2002;23.
75. CTFA. Important notice about cosmetic ingredient names, in Curry A, McEwen G (eds), *Cosmetics Industry On Call.* Washington, Cosmetic, Toiletry, and Fragrance Association, 2002, pp iii-iv.
76. Actinic keratoses net. American Academy of Dermatology. Available at *www.skincarephysicians.com/actinickeratosesnet/treatment.htm;* accessed September 21, 2004.
77. Prystowsky JH. Topical retinoids, in Wolverton S (ed), *Comprehensive Dermatologic Drug Therapy*. Philadelphia, Saunders, 2001, pp 578-594.
78. Legenne S. Personal communication: Retinol clinical research by Johnson & Johnson, internal document, 2004.
79. Baumann LS. Topical treatments for photodamage: New directions in the uses of retinoid therapy in cosmetic dermatology. *Skin Allergy News* 2003.
80. Francz PI, Conrad J, Biesalski HK. Modulation of UVA-induced lipid peroxidation and suppression of UVB-induced ornithine decarboxylase response by all-*trans*-retinoic acid in human skin fibroblasts in vitro. *Biol Chem* 1998;379: 1263-1269.
81. Griffiths CE. The role of retinoids in the prevention and repair of aged and photoaged skin. *Clin Exp Dermatol* 2001;26: 613-618.
82. Liu J-C, Seiberg M, Miller J et al. Soy: Potential applications in skin care. Poster presented at: 59th Annual Meeting of the American Academy of Dermatology, Washington, DC, March 2-7, 2001.
83. Liu J-C, Wu J, Payonk G, Summer B, Kollias N. Clinical evaluation of a total soy formulation in improving appearance of skin tone in phototype VI populations. Poster presented at: 60th Annual Meeting of the American Academy of Dermatology, New Orleans, LA, February 22-27, 2002.
84. Seiberg M, Paine C, Sharlow E, et al. The protease-activated receptor 2 regulates pigmentation *via* keratinocyte-melanocyte interactions. *Exp. Cell Res.* 2000;254:25-32.
85. Greenspan AH, Nebus J, Wallo W, et al. Effectiveness of a natural soy preparation in reducing the appearance of unwanted facial hair. Poster presented at the 61st Annual Meeting of the American Academy of Dermatology, San Francisco, CA. March 21-26, 2003.
86. Graf J. Personal communication: MD Dermatologic Formula, Cosmeceuticals, Great Neck, NY, 2004.

CHAPTER 71

Skin and Lip Typology

Diane Baras
Laurence Caisey

Key Points

- Diversity of skin color covers a large and continuous color space where different racial or ethnic groups overlap each other.
- Racial or ethnic origin and cultural background play a major role in self-perception of skin tone and undoubtedly influence makeup strategy.
- There emerged four main makeup strategies.
- The lip color space is as large as the skin color space.

The ideal makeup is a tailor-made product that respects a woman's individuality. Individual uniqueness can be characterized by biophysical as well as psychological features. A thorough understanding of a woman based on her own characteristics entails these two dimensions.

The diversity of women comes from the various types of skin tone, lips, and eyelashes, all of which could be enhanced, corrected, or transformed by makeup according to the user's expectations.

These expectations are linked to self-perception of the biophysical properties of the face. A women's features and concerns about skin tone, lips, and lashes strongly depend on racial or ethnic origin, as well as on the cultural and geographic environment. There may be a discrepancy between self-perception and objective assessment.

Objective assessments are provided by instrumental measurements of physical and biophysical properties of the face. Several characteristics are recorded, such as color and unevenness of skin tone and morphologic and biomechanical hydration properties of the lips. Such measurements emphasize the diversity among different racial or ethnic groups as well as within each racial or ethnic group.

This chapter expands on the main results of our dual approach, combining qualitative assessments and quantitative measurements in women with different skin of color and cultural background. It focuses on the two main cosmetic supports of the facial appearance: skin complexion and lips through their colorimetrical features.

THE COLOR OF THE SKIN

For most women, applying a "colored" makeup to the skin is the first step of the makeup routine. It is the foundation. A woman is free to enhance her face by matching or changing the color of the skin. To better understand how a woman thinks up her makeup strategy and how the latter is influenced by skin color, racial or ethnic origin, and living place, a dual qualitative and quantitative approach was required on a large panel of women from different racial or ethnic groups. The method consisted in (1) exploring the various skin colors to define worldwide skin color space, to show the differences between racial or ethnic groups, and to observe the diversity within each group, (2) exploring how women self-perceived facial skin complexion, what ideal skin tone they were longing for, how they managed to achieve it, what they did, and how much they were satisfied with makeup results, and (3) assessing makeup results by colorimetric measurements and comparing data with a woman's feelings as verbalized. Integrating such data should allow the level of agreement between results to be assessed and both a woman's makeup strategy and final perception to be estimated.

We carried out two main studies. In 2003, color measurements were done on 507 women from different racial or ethnic groups before and after applying the foundation. Measurements were followed by in-depth interview to record self-description of the face and satisfaction level. Data were crossed to bring out the needs of women. On the other hand, since 1999, we have started a study to progressively involve the largest diversity of women's skin colors in different places in the world. To date, 3721 women living in nine countries have been included.

Skin Tones: A High Diversity

A number of papers have explored the differences in skin color among different racial or ethnic groups. However, they often do not provide information about the diversity and mixing of involved populations. The scale of most of these studies was too small, and the places where measurements were made were too limited to reflect the large range of skin tones within each racial or ethnic group and to reveal the overlapping of skin color range between groups.[1–7] Since 1999, we have conducted a study that progressively included 3721 women living in nine countries. The color of the skin was measured and classified independently of racial or ethnic origin to emphasize the diversity and overlap.

PANEL A total of 3721 female volunteers from six different racial or ethnic origins and living in nine different geographic locations were involved. They were in the age range 18–65 years and included 1993 Asians, 160 Indians, 1120 Caucasians, 219 Hispanics, 127 French Africans, and 102 African-Americans (Table 71-1). None suffered from disease that might impair or change color or facial skin condition.

METHODS The color of forehead and cheeks was measured using a spectroradiometer inside a Chromasphere. The Chromasphere, developed and patented by L'Oreal Research,[8] is a stable, reliable,

TABLE 71-1
Racial or Ethnic Group and Living Place of the 3721 Female Volunteers Involved in the Study

Ethnic Groups	Living Places	Frequency
African-American	USA	102
Asian	China, Japan, Korea, Thailand	1993
Caucasian	France, Russia, USA	1120
French African	France	127
Hispanic	Brazil, USA	219
Indian	India	160

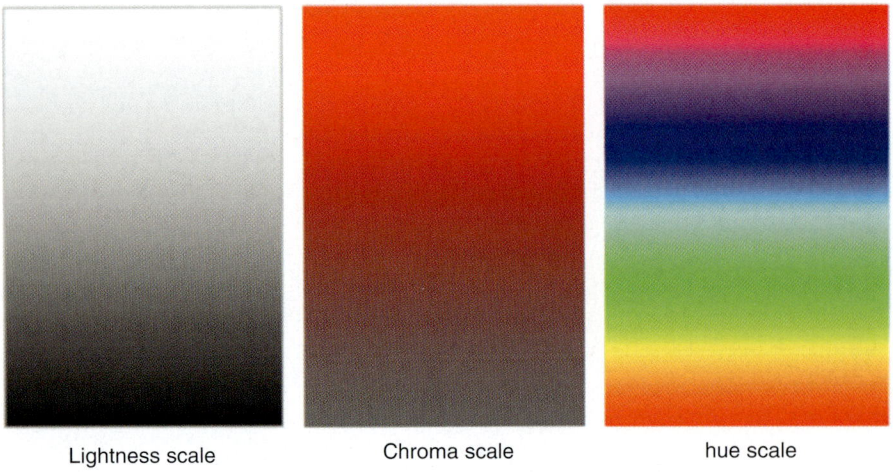

▲ **FIGURE 71-1** Scales of lightness, chroma, and hue. When the chroma/saturation is low, the color appears gray.

and diffuse lighting system that faithfully mimics natural daylight (CIE illuminant D65). The volunteer placed her face into the Chromasphere. Such a device avoids contact measurements that alter blood flow by applying pressure on the skin and thus alter skin color. Moreover, standardized cameras were used to acquire pictures of the face.[9] The unevenness of skin color then could be assessed through image analysis. In the present study, we used a spectroradiometer that measured the reflectance of forehead and cheeks in the visible field from 400–700 nm every 4 nm. The recorded spectrum was expressed in the CIE 1976 standard colorimetric space L^*C^*hD65/10°, where each color is described through three coordinates that reflect perception by human eye: h for hue angle (angular coordinate), C^* for chroma (radius coordinate), and L^* for lightness (z axis) (Figure 71-1). The hue h is the approximate psychosensorial translation of the dominant wavelength. This is why the hue is that aspect of a color described with names such as *red, yellow.* etc. The chroma C^*, or saturation, refers to the pureness or vividness. A highly colorful skin is vivid and intense, whereas a less colorful skin appears more muted, even close to gray. The lightness L^*, or brightness, coordinate grades skin color (more or less light, more or less dark) using a gray scale.

STATISTICS The significant differences between racial or ethnic groups were demonstrated using univariate analysis on L^*, C^*, and h data on both forehead and cheek. The diversity of skin tones was described using principal component analysis (PCA) from L^*, C^*, and h data on forehead and cheek of subjects. PCA brought out the significant components on which a *hierarchical ascending classification* was carried out to classify skin tones from different ethnic groups.

RESULTS From measurements performed in 3721 volunteers, a huge color space could be defined (Figure 71-2). The darkest skin tones are found in African-American, French-African, and Indian women. At the opposite end, Caucasians significantly show the lightest complexions. They also have the reddest cheeks. On the other hand, Asian and Indian women significantly show the most yellowish skin (Figure 71-3). Interestingly, Caucasian, Asian, and Hispanic women cover the same lightness range, Caucasian and Hispanic women the same chroma (saturation) range, and African-American and Caucasian women the same range of hue (see Figure 71-3). It is the first type of information that highlights the diversity. However, such analyses do not shed light on the diversity within each racial or ethnic group, which motivated us to distinguish classes in the skin color space.

The classification emphasized six groups of skin tones (Figures 71-2 and 71-4). The first group encompasses the darkest and the less saturated skin tones (L^* = 42.0; C^* = 19.4 on forehead; see Figure 71-3), including African-American, French-African, Brazilian, and Indian women. The second group is composed of significantly lighter skin than group 1 but still significantly darker than in the other groups (L^* = 54.4 on forehead; see Figure 71-3). It includes not only some African-American, French-African, and Indian women but also some Asian (living in Thailand) and Hispanic (living in Brazil and the United States) women. Even among dark skin, there is high level of diversity.

Compared with the second group, the third group gathers significantly lighter and the most saturated skin (L^* = 61.2 and C^* = 26.5 on forehead; see Figure 71-3). These skin tones could be named *tanned skins.* They come from a great number of racial or ethnic groups

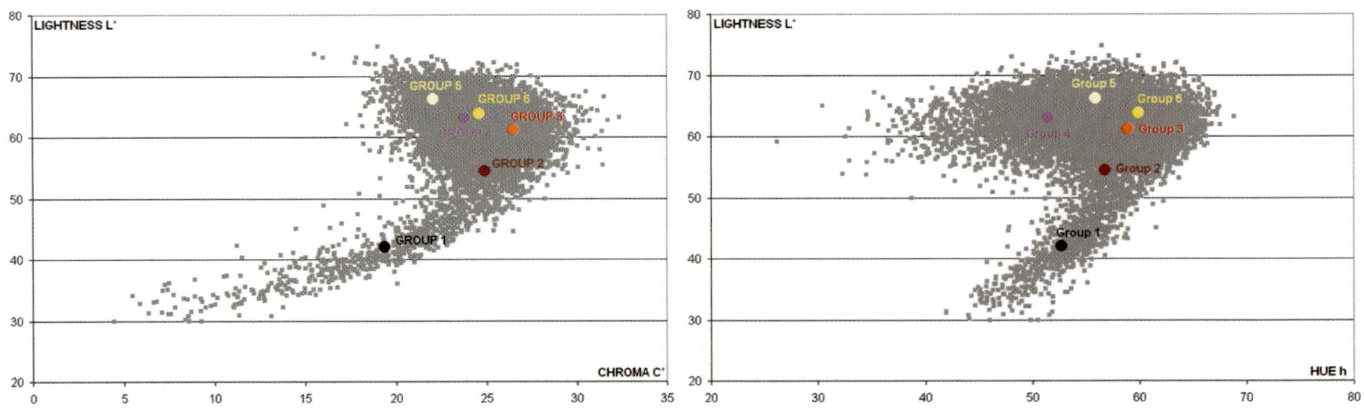

▲ **FIGURE 71-2** The worldwide skin color space depicted in two dimensions: (*a*) C^*, L^*, (*b*) h, L^*.

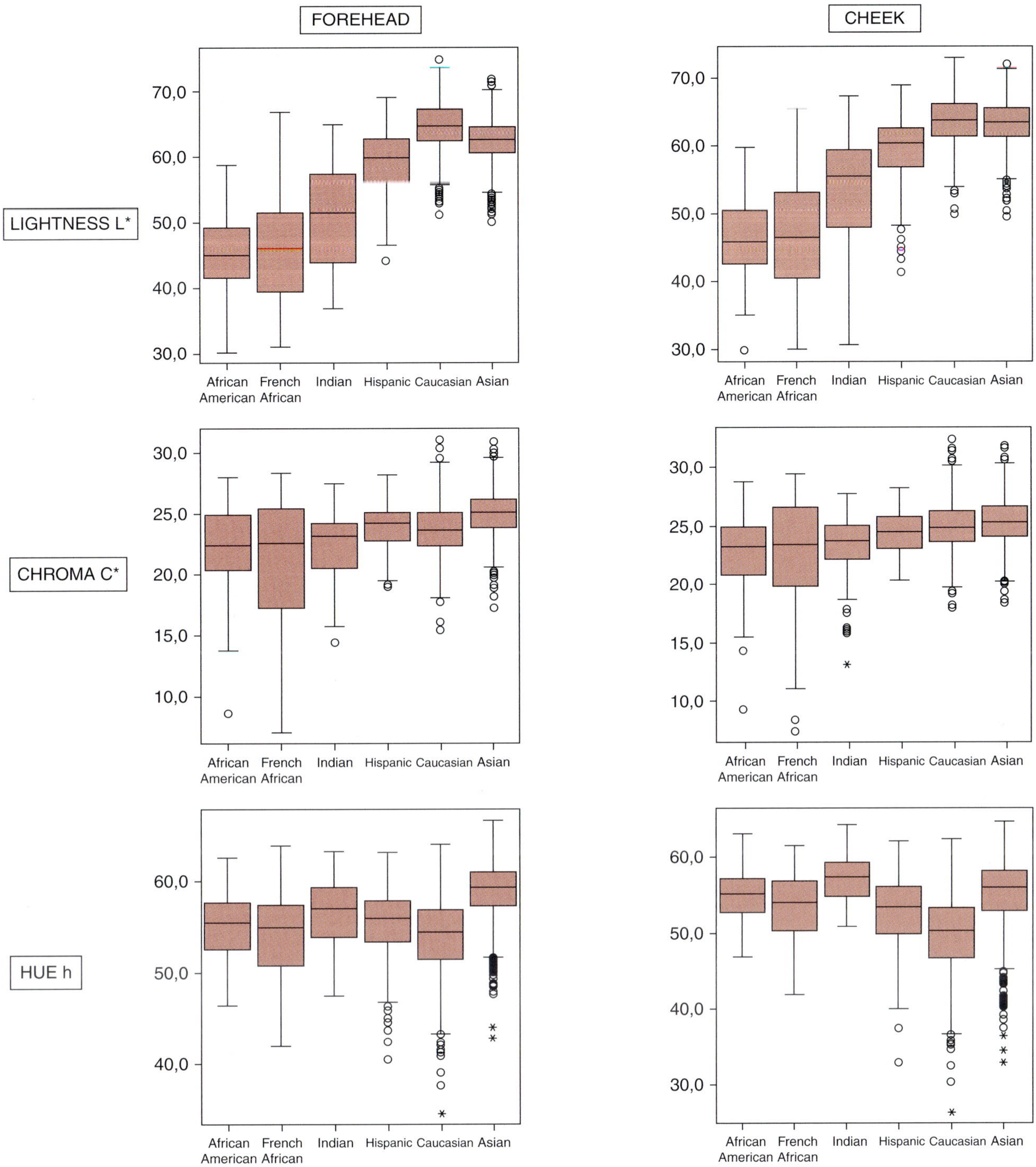

▲ **FIGURE 71-3** Boxplots bringing out the ranges of lightness, chroma, and hue of the different racial or ethnic groups on the forehead and cheek, respectively. It is interesting to note that Caucasian and Asian women practically cover the same lightness range, Caucasian and Hispanic women the same chroma range, and French-African and African-American women the same hue range.

we have studied. This group is the meeting point where many racial or ethnic groups (e.g., Caucasian, Asian, Hispanic, and French African) overlap each other. The fourth group is significantly the reddest (h = 51.4 and 46.3 on forehead and cheek, respectively; see Figure 71-3). It is mainly composed of Caucasian women, but some Asian and Hispanic women also show such "pink" skin tones. Group 5 is the lightest one, with a good balance between red and yellow components and a low saturation level that reinforces the white visual appearance of the skin (L^* = 66.2, C^* = 22.1, and h = 55.9 on the forehead; see Figure 71-3). Except French Africans, African-Americans, and Indians, all the racial or ethnic groups are found in group 5. The last group, that is, group 6, is significantly the most yellow (h = 59.9 on forehead; see Figure 71-3). Contrary to prejudgment, group 6 includes not only Asian but also Caucasian and Hispanic women in not insignificant proportion.

It is essential to note that these results show a tremendous diversity of skin color covering a large and continuous color space where different racial or ethnic groups overlap each other.

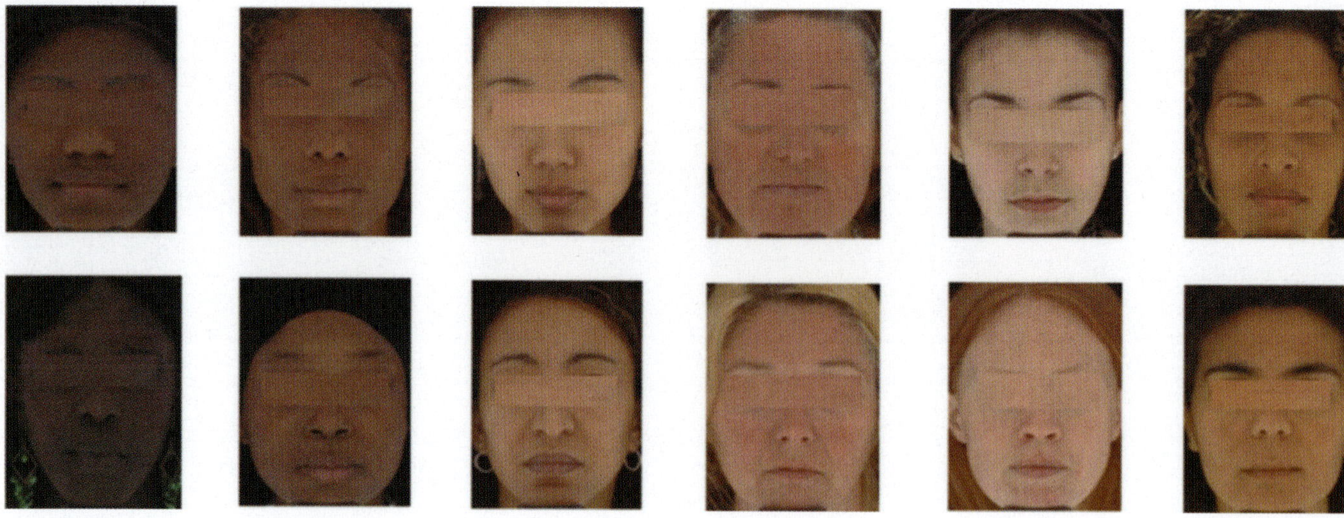

Group 1 Group 2 Group 3 Group 4 Group 5 Group 6

▲ **FIGURE 71-4** The six groups of skin tones reflecting the diversity.

Self-Perception and Satisfaction Level of Skin Color before and after Applying Foundation Makeup.

In 2006, we reported a study[10] on self-perception of facial skin by women from different racial or ethnic groups, showing how it was influenced by skin color, racial or ethnic origin, and living place.

PANEL The study involved 507 healthy women from distinct racial or ethnic groups using foundation on a daily basis and living in different geographic locations, that is, 112 French Caucasians in Paris, 107 American Caucasians in New York, 118 Japanese in Tokyo, and 75 African-Americans and 95 Hispanic Americans in New York. The volunteers were from 25 to 65-years-old, including 170 women in the age range 25–35 years, 174 women in the age range 36–45 years, and 163 women in the age range 46–65 years, respectively.

METHODS Fourteen women selected from each group were involved in semi-directive in-depth interviews based on a specific guideline to establish self-perception about their skin complexion. The interviewer belonged to the same specific racial or ethnic group in each case. The interviews were designed to explore self-perception and description of skin complexion and skin tone by the volunteers and their expectations from liquid foundation.

RESULTS For the African-American women, skin color was an important part of their identity. They described themselves as "people of color." In general, dark skin complexion was well regarded by the African-American community. It was reflected in the use of positive expressions to describe their skin tone, such as "dark chocolate" and "mahogany" to depict dark skin and "toast" or "pecan" for lighter hues. None of the women used negative words about color itself. While women appeared to be fairly satisfied with their skin tone, they were yet concerned about color and texture unevenness. Subjects frequently complained about light/dark color variations and visible texture irregularities, for example, dark marks or scars and skin blemishes such as pimples, wrinkles, rough skin, large pores, and facial hair. The major issue addressed when applying foundation was to provide evenness by covering up blemishes. Makeup application resulted in shades darker than the natural skin tone. Women in this group chose shades at least as dark as their darkest skin area to even face color. They also expected shades that brought glow and clarity from dullness. They use "vibrant" shades, dark but not dull, such as "ebony," or with a slightly reddish undertone, such as "mahogany." A few individuals chose to lighten darker areas with a light foundation. Thus African-American women have a positive self-perception of their own color. Although they declared themselves not satisfied with their usual foundation product because appropriate foundation shades were not available in stores, they managed to improve evenness by mixing several products.

Two independent groups of Caucasian women were involved in the study; one included women in Paris, France, and the other one was made up of American women living in New York. We noticed a clear similarity between the results obtained from these two groups. The range of color used to depict skin included descriptors such as "beige," "medium beige," and "bronze-like." Skin defects most commonly mentioned included pimples, acne, blackheads, and wrinkles. They were often described as "redness" by the French subjects and as "dark blotches" by the American group. However, as a general observation from the in-depth interviews, we noted that Caucasian women were the least concerned group about skin unevenness. Ideal facial skin complexion was depicted as a healthy look with even color and radiance. Most women chose a shade slightly darker than their skin tone. It allows them to look "healthy" ("*bonne mine*"), provide a better coverage by covering the darkest areas or skin imperfections, and thereby obtain evenness. They selected colors that impart a "healthy" look, such as "tan" or "bronze-like" colors—"sun tan," "gold," "sand on the beach." Otherwise, they selected "rosy-orangy" (the French group) and "blush pink" (the American group) that enhances a glowing look.

In this study, Asian skin was represented by Japanese women. It is worth noting that Japanese women described their skin complexion using a skin tone scale: pink, ocher, and beige. Some of them described themselves as "yellow." Japanese women did not describe their yellow skin color as a source of dissatisfaction. They seemed to be more concerned by unevenness of their skin color because of the presence of pigment spots. Makeup strategies in this group consistently focused on improving skin evenness, irrespective of age or skin tone subgroup. Interestingly, the Japanese women were the only racial or ethnic group that expected a "lightly tinted," "white," lucid and bright skin. They chose "white peach," "boiled egg," and "chinaware" shades or a color not different from the bare skin of the neck. To achieve this, they "played with color" by blending different foundation shades and by balancing powder and foundation shades.

Unlike the preceding groups, Hispanic Americans originate from a wide range of geographic areas that may result in specific cultural characteristics. The Hispanic group included women from Puerto Rico, Dominica, Cuba, Venezuela, and Mexico, and many were recent immigrants. In contrast to the African-American group, we found that some Hispanic-American women tended not to enhance their own skin color by using descriptors such as "olive" and "dull." They complained about the "yellow tone" of their skin, which had a negative association with conditions such as jaundice and other types of sickness. Furthermore, they commented on uneven color, notably beneath the eyes, and reddish marks. The perception of skin color influenced makeup strategy. They expected color evenness with "one color all over the face" and a "healthy" skin color. This means enhancing the yellow skin using shades that bring radiance, such as "golden bronze," "sun kissed," and "honey." The approach to cosmetics undoubtedly also was influenced by the fact that the Hispanic-American group included women having a wide range of cultural backgrounds, which likely contribute to a certain discrepancy between skin makeup result and declared cosmetic approach. Even when subjects verbally described a consistent desire to seek darker skin tones with a view to achieve a "sun kissed" skin color and to resolve perceived unevenness, the result was either lightened or darkened or reddened skin.

To clarify our conclusions, a new qualitative study was carried out on self-perception and makeup expectations of women according to native country. The in-depth interviews took place in Los Angeles, Miami, and New York. Women involved in the study in Los Angeles originated from Mexico, Honduras, Guatemala, and Nicaragua with an equal number of light/medium/dark complexions according to the self-perception to get a wide range of skin tones. Women involved in Miami originated from Cuba, Colombia, Venezuela, and Argentina with the same distribution over the lightness scale. Women involved in New York were native of Puerto Rico and the Dominican Republic with an equal number of light/medium/dark complexions too. Age range was from 25–65 years. This study confirmed that the self-perception and approach of Hispanic Americans to cosmetics is undoubtedly influenced by lightness of skin complexion and native country. Those with the lightest skins were the least satisfied with skin complexion, except for women of Cuban and Mexican origin. A too light skin tone was referred to as "pale," "yellowish," "illness," and "sickly." A medium skin complexion was much more appreciated, especially in women from the Dominican Republic, Puerto Rico, and South America. Although not unsatisfied with medium complexions, Cuban and Mexican women expressed preference for lighter complexions. The darkest skin tones were very well appreciated and referred to tanned skins that are robust to the sun and not sickly. But the level of satisfaction depended on social background and native country. The darkest skin complexions were hard to come to terms with for Mexican and Central America women, whereas the lightest skin tones were reported to be "less discriminating," "more elegant," and "cleaner." Women from Puerto Rico and the Dominican Republic were much more satisfied with their dark complexions, particularly because they were living in New York, where the high level of mixing makes the complexion not a source of concern. Cuban women living in Miami belonged to a large community. This could explain why they pretty well accepted dark complexions. They did, however, express appeal for "rosy" tones. Women from South America living in Miami often came from favored social backgrounds and so assumed their dark skin tone. All in all, the ideal color was a "tanned," "bronze" skin tone that brings radiance to the face. To achieve such a complexion, women with fair skin tones chose darker shades, especially those native of the Dominican Republic and except for those originating from Mexico and Cuba, who preferred to slightly lighten the skin with "rosy" or "bronze" shades that corrected the disliked "yellow" component. Most of those with medium complexions looked for a matching foundation. However, they preferred to slightly darken the face if they could not get the appropriate shade, except for Cuban, Mexican, and some Puerto Rican women, who rather would like to slightly lighten the skin. Those with the darkest skin tones liked to match their own skin tones, but because of uneven skin color, they finally decided to darken the face and achieve a homogeneous result.

Regarding the colorimetric overlap of the different racial or ethnic groups, it is obvious that racial or ethnic origin and cultural background play a major role in self-perception of skin tone and undoubtedly influence makeup strategy.

The Color of the Skin after Applying Makeup: Main Strategies, Specificities, and Common Strategies

The second stage of the large study carried out since 1999 was to colorimetrically assess and to classify the makeup strategies. Women were asked to apply their usual and most preferred foundation with their own makeup routine. Measurements were done before (see the first part of the study) and after making up. The difference was computed for each color coordinate L^*, C^*, and h on both forehead and cheek to evaluate makeup strategy.

PANEL The trial involved 2047 women in the age range 18–65 years from five different racial or ethnic origins and living in five different geographic locations: 1319 Asians (living in China and Japan), 432 Caucasians (living in France, Russia, and the United States), 98 Hispanics living in the United States, 112 French Africans, and 86 African-Americans.

STATISTICS Makeup strategies were investigated from the differences in L^*, C^*, and h coordinates (ΔL^*, ΔC^*, and Δh, respectively) on the forehead and cheek using PCA. PCA brought out the significant components on which a hierarchical ascending classification was carried out to classify the strategies.

RESULTS There emerged four main strategies involving the three attributes lightness L^*, saturation C^*, and hue h (Table 71-2 and Figure 71-5). The first strategy made the skin darker, with most of the women making the skin

TABLE 71-2
Percent of Each Makeup Strategy in Different Racial or Ethnic Groups

	Makeup Strategies			
	"Golden Look"	"Matching"	"Glow Look"	"Whitening"
French Caucasian	**54%**	20%	20%	6%
Russian Caucasian	**32%**	**54%**	14%	0%
American Caucasian	**33%**	**31%**	**28%**	8%
African-American	**35%**	14%	**46%**	5%
French African	**36%**	20%	**38%**	6%
American Hispanic	**32%**	19%	**41%**	8%
Chinese	2%	14%	**48%**	**37%**
Japanese	6%	22%	**46%**	**26%**

Note: The percents higher than 25% are highlighted in boldface.

more saturated and/or redder at the same time ($\Delta L^* = -1.6$, $\Delta C^* = +1.3$, $\Delta h = -2.1$ on forehead and $\Delta L^* = -1.9$, $\Delta C^* = +1.3$, $\Delta h = -1.6$ on cheek). We named it the "golden look." The second main strategy did not change the color, that is, matched the skin tone. We named it "matching." The third main strategy made the skin redder and slightly less saturated ($\Delta h = -2.0$, $\Delta C^* = -1.1$, on forehead, $\Delta h = -1.6$, $\Delta C^* = -1.0$ on cheek). We named it the "glow look." The last strategy made the skin highly less saturated to mute the color, most of the women making the skin redder and lighter at the same time ($\Delta C^* = -3.0$, $\Delta h = -3.2$, $\Delta L^* = +1.4$ on forehead and $\Delta C^* = -2.7$, $\Delta h = -2.5$, $\Delta L^* = +1.3$ on cheek). We named it "whitening."

A lot of the African-American women (35%; see Table 71-2 and Figure 71-5) made their skin darker, which shows good consistency with the qualitative study. Many of the women explained that a darkening strategy was the easiest way to homogenize and/or the way to get a vibrant dark complexion. However, 46% preferred the "glow look," which doesn't alter the lightness, and 14% made up the skin without changing skin tone. We found only 5% that made the skin strongly less saturated and at the same time lighter and redder. This extreme strategy could be considered as a "whitening" strategy. The weak percentage confirms that most of the African-American women are not willing to lighten their skin tone.

Most of the Chinese and Japanese women (85% and 72%, respectively; see Table 71-2 and Figure 71-5) made their skin less saturated. More detailed analysis showed that 37% and 26%, respectively, obtained a visible "white" appearance by strongly unsaturating the skin and making it lighter and redder. Only 14% of the Chinese and 22% of the Japanese women decided not to change their skin tone. It is worth noting that skin complexion in Asia strongly influences makeup strategy. Women who decide to strongly unsaturate skin

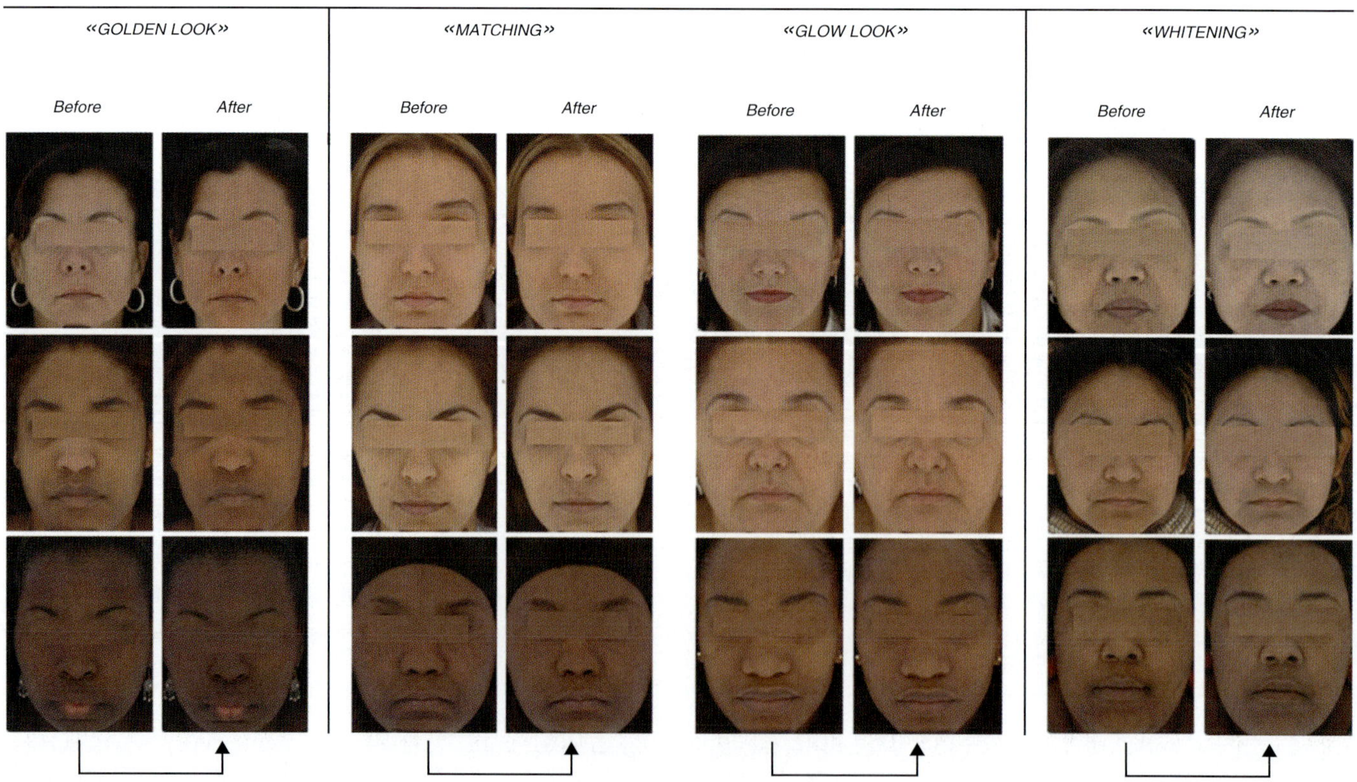

▲ **FIGURE 71-5** The four main strategies of women from different racial or ethnic groups.

have a bare skin tone significantly darker and more saturated, and women who decide to match their skin tone have significantly less saturated and redder skin, which means a pinkish complexion. Cross-correlating all data, we may suggest that the ideal Asian skin tone is a fair, not too saturated and pink-ochre skin complexion.

In good agreement with their expectations, most Caucasian women made the skin darker (54% among French, 32% among Russians, and 33% of American Caucasians, respectively; see Table 71-2 and Figure 71-5). Between 20% and 31% of the French and American women, respectively, preferred to match their skin tone. The percentage increased to 54% in Russian Caucasians. Still consistent with the in-depth interview, 20% and 28% of the French and American women, respectively, brought a glow look to their faces. Few women decided to lighten the skin. Six percent of the French and 8% of the American women, respectively, made the skin highly less saturated principally to mute a too vivid color.

As detailed in the qualitative study, the makeup strategies are much more varied in Hispanic women depending on native country and skin complexion. Nevertheless, 41% preferred to get a "glow look," and 32% darkened the skin to get a "tanned," "bronze" complexion as desired (see Table 71-2 and Figure 71-5). And 19% chose to match their skin tone. When looking deeper, only 8% strongly unsaturated the skin to get an apparent whitening/lightening effect.

There is a real diversity of makeup strategies. The matching strategy is transversal across different racial or ethnic groups. It is the way to enhance a well-appreciated skin color by hiding unevenness. The darkening strategy is either a way to homogenize the face or a way to make the skin more "tanned" and "radiant." The brightening strategy that goes through the unsaturation of color is either a way to mute a too vivid color or a cultural routine to get a brightened fair skin.

CONCLUSION

A woman's uniqueness is striking with regard to the diversity of skin tones and various perceptions, expectations, and makeup strategies. Taking into account this diversity is of prime importance when formulating a makeup foundation range. It also means that proper advice should be provided to women to help them in selecting the most appropriate shade, which entails using their own words to meet their expectations.

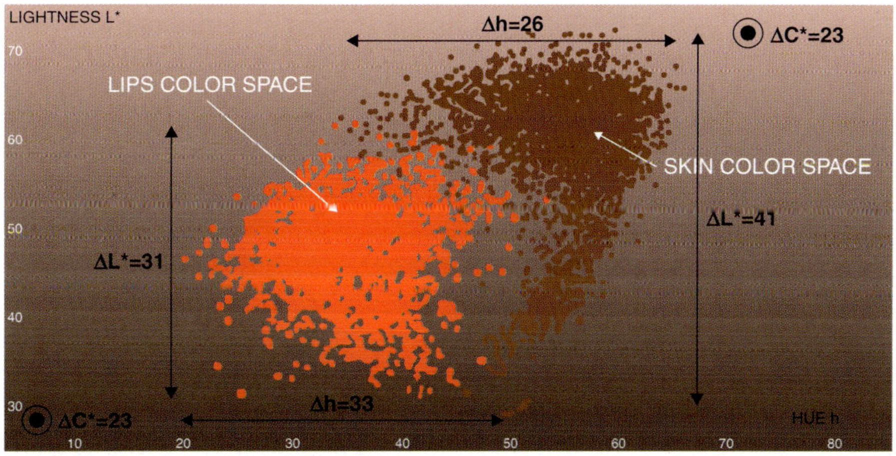

▲ **FIGURE 71-6** The lip and skin color spaces.

THE LIPS

Lip makeup has a special place in the makeup routine. It could be the overall finish of the makeup routine or a way to enlighten skin tone. Unlike skin tone makeup, lip makeup is highly diversified in terms of color ranges and optical effects from matte to extreme shiny. Anatomically, lips are composed of the upper and lower vermilion borders and the perilabial skin that includes the area from the nose to the chin. Our approach consisted in defining the color space of the vermilion border, juxtaposing it to the skin color space, enlightening various contrasts, and determining the differences between different racial or ethnic groups.

PANEL The colorimetric study included 1940 subjects—166 French-Caucasian, 169 Russian-Caucasian, 292 Chinese, 315 Japanese, 409 American-Caucasian, 416 African-American, and 160 Indian women.

METHODS Colorimetrical measurements were done inside the Chromasphere using a spectroradiometer as described earlier.

STATISTICS The significant differences between racial or ethnic groups were demonstrated using univariate analysis on L^*, C^*, and h data. The limit for significance was $p < 0.05$.

RESULTS Surprisingly, the lip color space is as large as skin color space (Figure 71-6). Some differences between racial or ethnic groups were brought out. Indian and African-American women have the darkest and less saturated lips ($L^* = 42.9$ and 43.1, $C^* = 17.7$ and 18.5, respectively; see Figure 71-7), whereas the Asian and Caucasian women showed the lightest and most saturated lip complexions ($L^* = 50.0$ and 50.6, $C^* = 23.3$ and 23.4, respectively; see Figure 71-7). However, the hue distinguished Caucasian and Asian women. Caucasian women have redder lips than Asian women, and Indian women have the most yellowish lips ($h = 32.4$, 37.5, and 39.1, respectively; see Figure 71-7).

Comparison of the vermilion border and perilabial skin color refers to colorimetric contrasts. Indeed, lips can be likened to a color object placed on a colored background, that is, the skin tone. The resulting contrast effect may change our visual perception of the color of the lips in relation to the color of skin tone. This issue was documented by the following study.

PANEL A total of 914 women were involved in a colorimetric study using the same devices as described earlier to characterize the contrast between vermilion border and perilabial skin—238 African-American, 238 American-Caucasian, 225 French-Caucasian, and 213 Japanese women equally distributed in the thre age ranges—18–35, 36–50, and 51–65.

STATISTICS Comparison between the vermilion border and the perilabial skin was carried out using the Student t test if normal distribution and nonparametric Wilcoxon test if not. The difference was significant if $p < 0.05$.

RESULTS Measurements show widely varying contrasts between the vermilion border and the perilabial skin from sharp

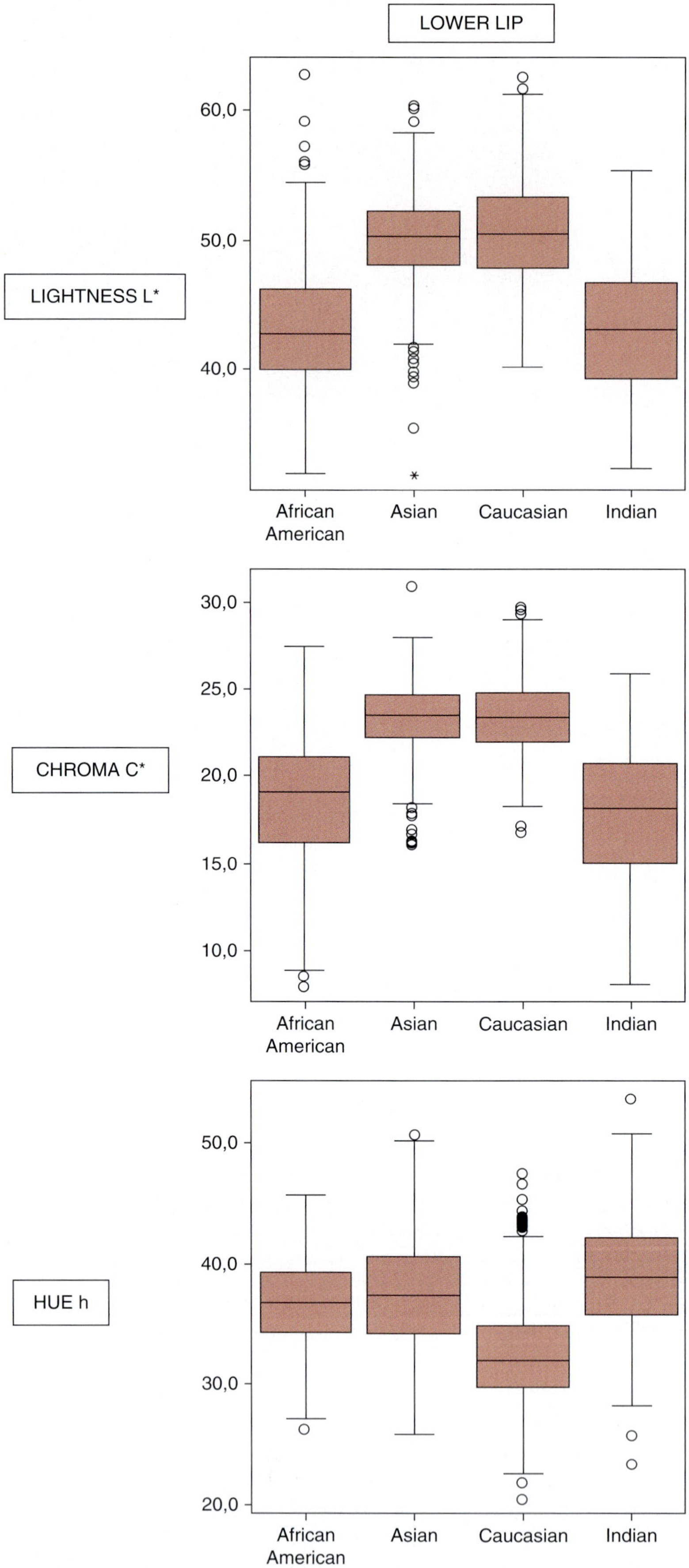

▲ **FIGURE 71-7** Boxplots bringing out the ranges of lightness, chroma, and hue of the different racial or ethnic groups on the lower lip. It is interesting to note that Caucasian and Asian women practically cover the same lightness and chroma ranges but are distinguished by the hue. African-American and Indian women also have the same lightness and chroma ranges, but Indian lips are significantly more yellowish.

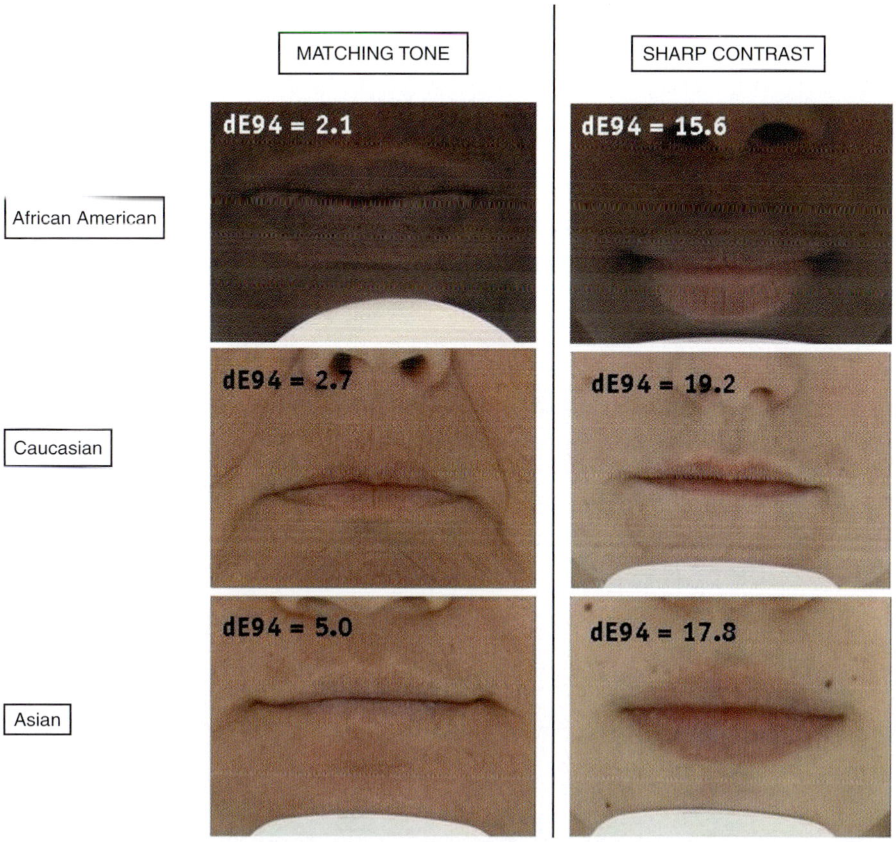

▲ **FIGURE 71-8** Various contrasts between the vermilion border and the perilabial skin expressed by the dE94 value.

differences to matching tones (Figure 71-8). In all the racial or ethnic groups, except African-American women, lips were significantly darker than perilabial skin (Figure 71-9). In African-American women, the vermilion border may be lighter or darker, which has an impact on the contrast (Figure 71-10). Not surprisingly, the lips of women are significantly redder than the perilabial skin. However, some women show matching tones between lips and skin that decreases lip highlighting visually. In each racial or ethnic group, there was no significant difference in saturation between the lips and perilabial skin. Consequently, lips could be either more saturated or less saturated than the skin.

CONCLUSION

The great number of contrasts between skin and lips offers a new perspective to enhance either skin tone or lip color or both. New studies should be conducted to explore which are the most appreciated contrasts for women. Other lip characteristics could be investigated, such as morphologic, biomechanical, and hydration properties. Women express various concerns about these characteristics that also strongly depend on racial or ethnic origin, as well as on the cultural and geographic environment.

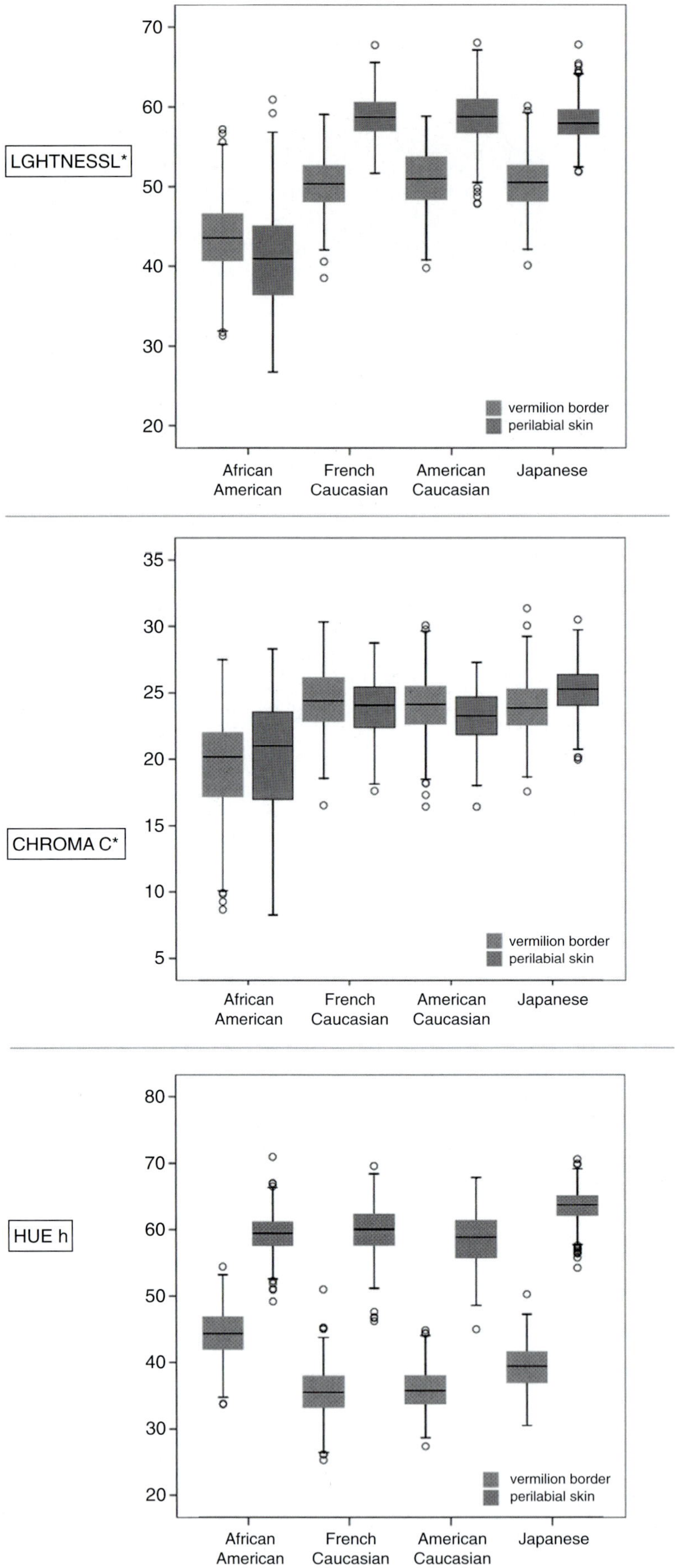

▲ **FIGURE 71-9** Boxplots bringing out the differences of lightness, chroma, and hue between the vermilion border and the perilabial skin.

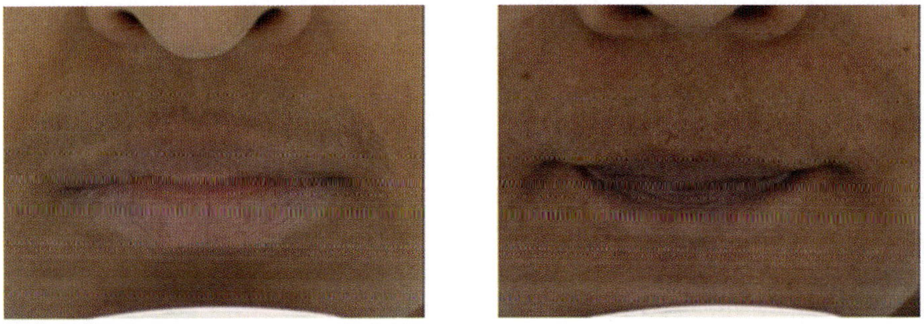

▲ **FIGURE 71-10** Two extreme contrasts.

REFERENCES

1. Sonoda I, Hirai Y, Okabe N, et al. On the preference of the color of makeup products related to the skin color in Japanese women. *J Soc Cosmet Chem* 1987;21: 219-224;
2. Lee KY, Shimagami K, Sato M, Miyazaki Y. Measurement of the color for bare skin and foundation-applied skin in women in their 20s: Comparison of Japanese and Korean. *J Physiol Anthropol Appl Hum* 2001;20:301.
3. Richards GM, Oresajo CO, Halder RM. Structure and function of ethnic skin and hair. *Dermatol Clin* 2003;21:595-600.
4. Morizot F, Jdid R, Dheurle S, et al. Features related to skin pigmentation: Differences between Japanese and French women. *Skin Res Technol* 2005;11:76-77.
5. Minami J, Minami T. Designing the color of cosmetic foundations: Analysis on consumers' opinions about changing face color and measurement of colorimetric properties of foundation layers. *FRAGR J* 1999;27:21-26.
6. Chardon A, Cretois I, Hourseau C. Skin colour typology and suntanning pathways. *Int J Cosmet Sci* 1991;13:191-208.
7. Liu Wei, Wang Xuemin, Lai Wei. Skin color measurement in the Chinese female population: Analysis of 407 cases from four cities of China. *Int J Dermatol* 2007;46:835-839.
8. Giron F. Dispositif d'acquisition d'au moins une image d'au moins une partie du visage ou de la chevelure d'une personne. French patent 0111215. Paris, France, L'Oréal, 2001.
9. Caisey Bluteau L, Aubert J. Procédé et dispositif de mesure de la couleur. French patent 9606425. Paris, France, L'Oréal, 1996.
10. Caisey L, Grangeat F, Lemasson A, et al. Skin color and makeup strategies of women from different racial or ethnic groups. *Int J Cosmet Sci* 2006;28:427-437.

CHAPTER 72

Dermatosis Papulosa Nigra

Marcia J. Glenn

Key Points

- Common skin finding in many skin of color patients
- Benign pigmented papules of face, neck, and trunk
- Genetic predilection
- Rare in childhood
- Increased number and size with age
- Pathology similar to seborrheic keratosis
- Chronic progressive course
- Elective therapy

SYNONYMS AND RELATED KEYWORDS

- DPN
- Pigmented papules
- Seborrheic keratosis

Dermatosis papulosa nigra (DPN) refers to benign pigmented papules appearing primarily on the face, neck, and trunk of women and men with skin of color worldwide.[1] The incidence of DPN is reported to be as high as 70% in the African-American population and up to 50% among their family members.[2,3] A retrospective study of 1000 African-Caribbean subjects ranked DPN as a common finding.[4] In Africa, 40% of the population over age 30 has DPN.[5] Similar lesions are described in Asians (e.g., Fillipinos and Vietnamese) and less frequently in Mexicans and Native Americans.[2] The development of DPN, while rare in children, is chronic and progressive in adults.[6] Although DPN is generally asymptomatic, treatment is often pursued to enhance cosmetic appearance.

ETIOLOGY AND PATHOGENESIS

Castellani reported the first case of DPN in 1925.[2] The exact etiology remains uncertain. It is speculated that DPN is derived from an epidermal nevus or a hamartoma with follicular origin or a nevoid developmental defect of the pilosebaceous follicles.[7–9] The preponderance of DPN within certain families suggests a strong genetic predilection.[3] Niang suggests that the sun may be an etiopathogenic factor in the increase in lesions in the African population.[10]

CLINICAL FINDINGS

DPN may begin as early as the first decade of life.[6] However, these small, darkly pigmented papules usually begin in adolescence and progress slowly over years, peaking in number in the sixth decade.[1] DPN has been reported to have a 1:1 to 2:1 female-to-male incidence.[1,2] Family history of DPN is reported by at least 50% of those with DPN.[3] While most people with DPN are generally asymptomatic and present primarily with a cosmetic dilemma, some individuals pursue removal because of symptoms, including pruritus, burning, and tenderness.[11]

Darker and deeper skin hues evidence more DPN.[1] Lesions are seldom or not described at all on "white skin" and less frequently described in lighter black skin than on darker skin.[1,3,12] These pigmented papules become more numerous, may enlarge, and often flatten in occluded areas (see Figures 72-3 and 72-5). In a prospective study of DPNs in Dakar, Senegal, 67% of patients had 50 to 100 lesions, and 27% coalesced to form plaques.[10] Some papules are smooth and round, and others are filliform, projectile, or keratotic (Figures 72-1 through 72-6). The face is the most common location of DPN, predominating in the malar and temple areas (see Figures 72-1 and 72-2). The neck and the trunk are also frequently affected areas[9] (see Figures 72-4 and 72-6). Scaling, crusting, and ulcerations are not features of DPN.[13]

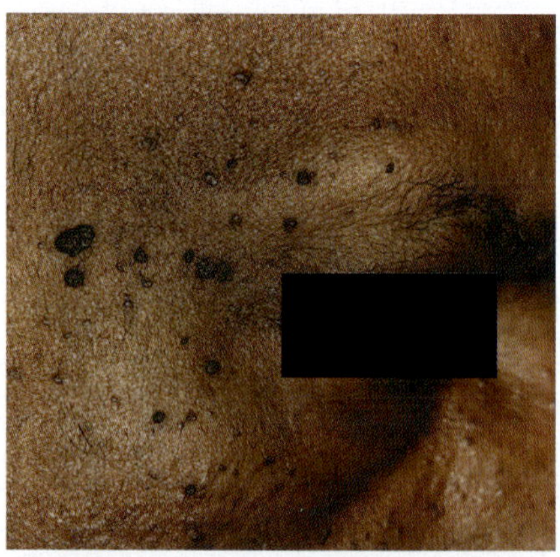

▲ **FIGURE 72-1** Skin type VI man with periocular and temple pigmented papules.

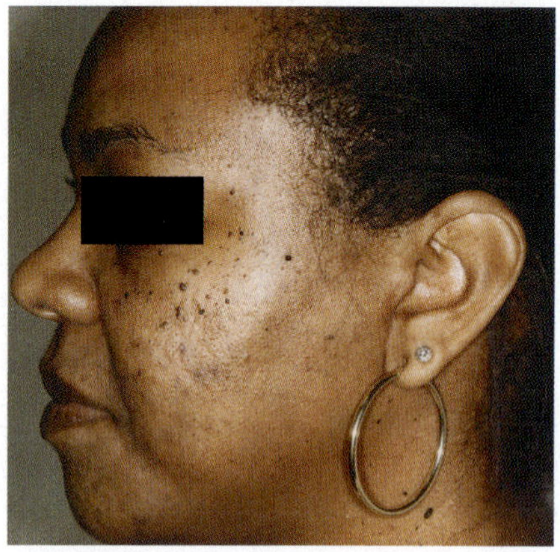

▲ **FIGURE 72-2** African-American woman with scattered 0.5- to 1-mm pigmented papules predominately in the photoexposed malar area.

An explosive eruption of DPN was reported in a 42-year-old black woman coincident with symptomatic iron-deficiency anemia. Lesions quickly progressed from her face to her trunk. Remarkable was the Christmas tree pattern of pigmented papules on her back. Subsequent workup revealed an ascending colon adenocarcinoma.[14] Biopsy was consistent with the diagnosis of DPN.

PATHOLOGY

The histopathology of DPN is similar to seborrheic keratosis. Hyperkeratosis, irregular acanthosis, and marked hyperpigmentation of the basal layer are char-

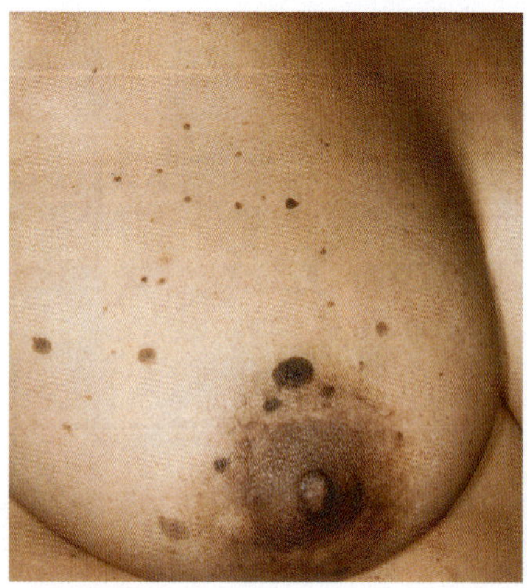

▲ **FIGURE 72-3** Small, medium, and large pigmented papules on breast usually covered by a bra.

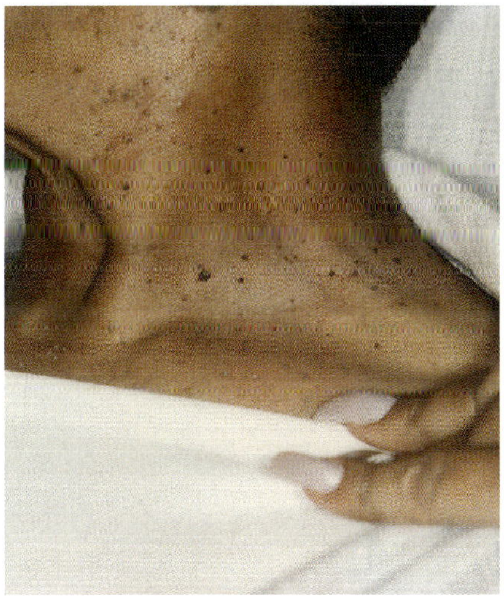

▲ **FIGURE 72-4** Small to medium-sized smooth pigmented papules on the lateral neck.

acteristic.[3,13] Keratin-filled invaginations of the epidermis are present.[13] DPN usually has an acanthotic pattern with thick interwoven tracts of epidermis, but it also may have a reticulated pattern consisting of a double row of basaloid cells.[13]

LABORATORY AND OTHER TESTS

The sign of Lesser-Trelat is the association of malignancy with numerous eruptive seborrheic keratoses.[14] Routine cancer screening, especially for colon and breast cancer, may be advisable with sudden onset and large numbers of DPN lesions, as seen with seborrheic keratosis and referred to as the sign of Lesser-Trelat.[14,15]

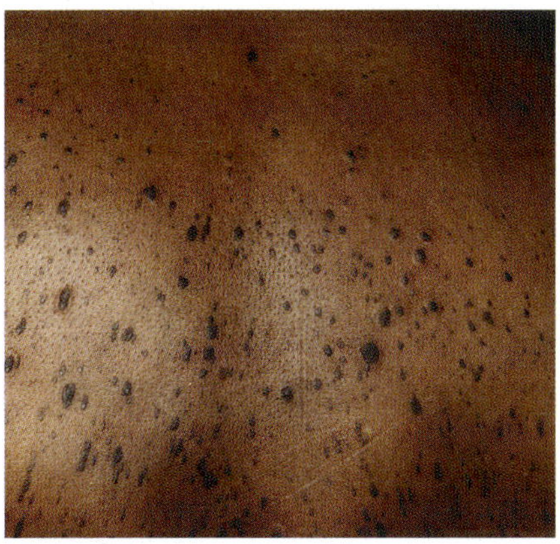

▲ **FIGURE 72-5** Individual and confluent pigmented papules on the trunk of an African-American man.

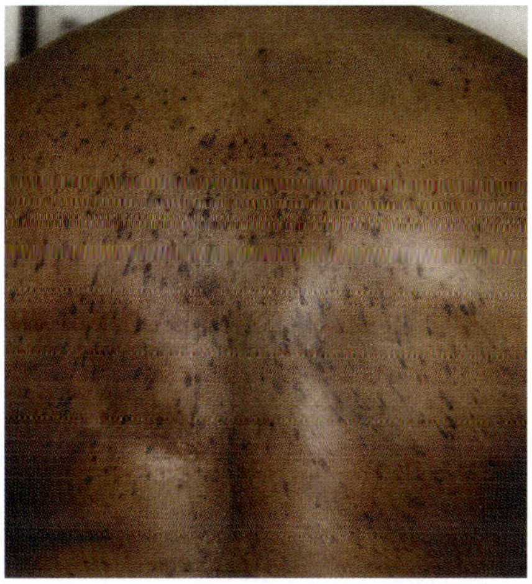

▲ **FIGURE 72-6** Christmas tree distribution of pigmented papules on the trunk of man with dark skin.

DIFFERENTIAL DIAGNOSIS

DPN is generally a clinical diagnosis. Biopsy may be helpful in differentiating melanocytic nevus.

- Achrochordons
- Seborrheic keratosis
- Verruca vulgaris
- Melanocytic nevi

COMPLICATIONS

DPN is cosmetically offensive when papules obscure clear complexions and facial features as they increase in number and even size in some instances. If one theorizes that the lesions are a variant of seborrheic keratosis in patients with skin of color, large and sudden eruptions may foretell internal malignancy, and patients with this history should be worked up appropriately.[14,15]

PROGNOSIS/PREVENTION

The lesions of DPN increase in number and sometimes size with age, peaking in the sixth decade.[1] A positive family history is likely in 50–90% of those affected.[3,10] Because the lesion itself is benign, our medical intervention should not provide more risk than the disease process itself. In a prospective study done at the Department of Dermatology in Senegal, lesions were primarily photodistributed and implicate sun as a provocateur.[10] With the aforementioned possible exception, preventative measures do not exist.

TABLE 72-1
Dermatosis Papulosa Nigra Treatment Options

First-Line Therapy
- Electrodesiccation—depletes water and blood supply to lesion by electrical generation of heat
- Scissor/shave excision—slices a surface growth off
- Cryotherapy—spraying of liquid nitrogen to freeze skin

Second-Line Therapy
- Laser—CO_2, Er:YAG, 532 diode, Aura ktp—light-specific destruction of tissue
- Curettage—scraping off unwanted skin

TREATMENT

Treatment of DPN is elective, and a conservative approach minimizes dyschromia (i.e., hyperpigmentation or hypopigmentation) and scarring (i.e., hypertrophic or keloidal) resulting from aggressive therapy.[13] EMLA (lidocaine-prilocaine cream), LMX (topical lidocine cream), or intralesional 1% lidocaine with or without epinephrine provides simple and uncomplicated anesthesia for the procedures outlined as first or second line[16–19] (Table 72-1). First-line therapies are inexpensive and efficient surgical options for medical providers practiced in the treatment of pigmented skin, which includes gradle or iris excision, electrodesiccation, and cryosurgery with liquid nitrogen.[13,18] Second-line therapies such as laser are more costly but may have a benefit in patient comfort.[17,18] Treatment expectations should be managed. Multiple treatments are often needed because of new lesions or incomplete resolution of any particular lesion(s). A conservative approach avoids disfigurement caused by therapy. Too aggressive electrodesiccation and/or curettage may create permanent change in pigment or scar formation. On darkly pigmented skin, loss or deposition of color may result from liquid nitrogen. Risk of hypertrophic scarring or keloid formation should be assessed before any cold steel ablation.

CONCLUSION

DPN is a common benign skin finding in darker complexions worldwide. The diagnosis is made clinically by appearance and distribution of small, darkly pigmented papules on the face, neck, and trunk. Onset is usually after childhood, and lesions have a famililal predilection. The course is chronic and progressive. An eruptive variant may correlate with malignancy. DPN is rarely symptomatic, and most surgical interventions are elective because of cosmetic concerns.

REFERENCES

1. Grimes PE, Arora S, Minus HR, et al. Dermatosis papulosa nigra. *Cutis* 1983;32:385-386, 392.
2. Castellani A. Observations on some diseases of Central America. *J Trop Med Hyg* 1925:28:1-14.
3. Shaheedi M, Ghafoori-Naseh H. Dermatosis papulosa nigra in a white female and her family members, *www.ams.ac.ir/aim/0253197.*
4. Dunwell P, Rose A. Study of the skin disease spectrum occurring in an Afro-Caribbean population. *Int J Dermatol* 2003;42:287-289.
5. van Hees C, Naffs B. *Common Skin Disease in Africa: An Illustrated Guide.* 2001, p 75.
6. Barboapour R, Leachslevy H. Dermatosis papulosa nigra in a young child. *Pediatr Dermatol* 1993;10:356-358.
7. Michael JC, Seale ER, et al. Dermatosis papulosa nigra. *Arch Dermatol Syphilol* 1929;20: 629-639.
8. Harter P. Dermatosis papulosa nigra de Castellani a percu chinigne et geographigne. *Bull Soc Fr Dermatol Syphilol* 1963;70:532-535.
9. Champion RH, Burton JL, Ebling F, et al. *Rook/Wilkinson/ Eblings Textbook of Dermatology,* 6th ed. Oxford, UK, Blackwell Publishing, 1998, pp 2413-2415.
10. Niang SO, Kane A, Diallo M, et al. Dermatosis papulosa nigra in Dakar, Senegal. *Int J Dermatol* 2007;46: 4522-4527S.
11. Woodhouse JG, Tomecki KJ. Common Benign Growths of the Skin. The Cleveland Clinic Foundation, 2005, *www.celevlandclinicmede.com/meicalpubs/diseasemanagement/dermatology.*
12. Morand JJ, Lightburn EE. Characteristics of genetically pigmented skins. *Bull Soc Pathol Exot* 2003;96:394-400.
13. Nowfar-Rad M. Dermatosis papulosa nigra. eMedicine Specialities, December 2006, *www.eMedicine.com.*
14. Schwartzberg J. Eruptive dermatosis papulosa nigra as a possible sign of internal malignancy. *Int J Dermatol* 2007;46: 186-187S.
15. Bailin A. Seborrheic keratosis. eMedicine Specialities, July 2006, *www.eMedicine.com.*
16. Kauh YC, McDonald JW, Rapaport JA, et al. A surgical approach for dermatosis papulosa nigra. *Int J Dermatol* 1983;22:590-592.
17. Joshi S, Ki-Young S, Roopal V, et al. Comparison of electrodessication and KTP laser for treatment of dermatosis papulosa nigra. *J Am Acad Dermatol* 2008; 58(2):135:2800.
18. Jackson B. Lasers in ethnic skin: A review. *J Am Acad Dermatol* 2003;8(6):5134-5138.
19. Carter EL, Coppola CA, Baranti FA. Formulation prior to eletrodesiccation of dermatosis papulosa nigra. *Dermatol Surg* 2006;32:1-6.

CHAPTER 73

The Use of Lasers for Treatment of Skin of Color Patients

Lori M. Hobbs

Key Points

- The use of lasers in persons of color requires an understanding of laser physics and laser tissue interactions.
- Dermatologic lasers can be used in all persons regardless of color depending on the proper selection of the laser wavelength (device) and laser parameters.
- Test spots are highly encouraged when treating people with darker phototypes.
- Realistic expectations and goals need to be discussed with the patient prior to treatment.
- To minimize unwanted side effects, aggressive parameters are discouraged.
- Multiple treatments are necessary in people with darker phototypes in comparison with those with lighter phototypes.
- Older classic laser devices such as the PDL, Q-switched laser, and long-pulsed Nd:YAG systems are reliable, reproducible, and efficacious in people with darker phototypes.
- IPL devices have a high learning curve and should be reserved for use on people with phototype IV or lighter.
- Nonablative long-wavelength devices, although safer for people with darker phototypes, are less reproducible in their clinical effects.
- Newer devices, such as the fractional photothermolysis and radiofrequency devices, show promise.
- Newer ablative devices are contraindicated in people with phototypes V and VI.
- More studies need to be conducted with newer ablative devices to determine the true efficacy on people with phototype IV.

With an estimated three-fourths of the world's population being of color, there is a growing and diverse segment of the international population demanding health care specific to its needs. This group comprises individuals who are of various shades of yellow, tan, olive, brown, and black hue. Despite the overwhelming worldwide number of people of color, these persons are often marginalized as "ethnic," "non-Caucasoid," or "minority."

Within the United States, the fastest-growing population is Hispanic. They comprise 13% of the U.S. population, with African-Americans and Asians following at 12.7% and 4%, respectively.[1] From April 2000 to July 2003, the U.S. population grew 2.5%. Hispanics accounted for half this national increase.[1] Owing to the increased number of persons of color, there is and will be a continual demand for dermatologic laser therapy.

To date, most dermatologic laser treatments are best suited for lighter-skinned individuals. Most dermatologic laser surgeons are comfortable with treating Fitzpatrick's phototypes I–III. However, when treating pigmented skin, phototypes IV–VI, the dermatologic laser surgeon is challenged with delivering reproducible, efficacious, and safe outcomes. Patient selection, the choice of laser, appropriate parameters, understanding of skin optics, tissue response, and early treatment of untoward events are the keys to successfully treating people of color.

Lasers (an acronym for *l*ight *a*mplification by the *s*timulated *e*mission of *r*adiation) were introduced in 1960. The principle of lasers is based on Einstein's quantum theory of radiation.[2] In general, atoms and electrons are usually in a resting state or lowest energy level. When an electron absorbs the energy of a photon of light, the electron becomes excited and is raised to a higher energy level. The excited electron then can give up its energy by emitting a photon of light identical to the photon that it absorbed. This process is called *spontaneous emission.* If a photon collides with another excited electron, the electron will return to its resting state, emitting two photons. This is called *stimulated emission* of radiation. To ensure the occurrence of stimulated emission, more excited electrons must be present in comparison with electrons in a lower energy state. This is called *population inversion.* Thus photons have a greater chance of encountering excited electrons and stimulating more emission of photons with the same energy.

Lasers are made up of a pumping system, which is the power supply or energy source. The lasing medium, which supplies the electrons needed for the stimulated emission of radiation, determines the wavelength of light. The lasing medium can be gaseous, liquid, or solid. The optical cavity is made up of parallel mirrors. The photons of light are reflected off the mirrors, producing laser light. One of the mirrors is partially reflective, allowing some of the energy of light to leak from the chamber in the form of a laser beam.

The light that is emitted from the laser beam is monochromatic (single color or of narrow wavelength band), coherent (spatially and temporally in phase), collimated (traveling parallel), and high energy (high-intensity light). Laser light can be delivered onto the skin in a continuous, quasi-continuous, or pulsed mode. This is determined by the amount of time the laser light is on the skin. Continuous lasers emit a beam of light that is continuously on the skin and at a constant energy. Quasi-continuous lasers emit a series of beams of light that are so closely spaced together that they appear to be continuous. Pulsed lasers emit a beam of light on the skin in pulses which can be long (milliseconds) or short (nanoseconds) duration on the skin.

As the laser light hits the skin, it can be reflected, scattered, transmitted, or absorbed. According to the Grothus-Draper law, light absorption is required for a tissue effect.[3] Simply stated, if there is no absorption of light, there is not a tissue effect. Reflected and transmitted light does not cause a clinical effect. Reflected light occurs primarily within the epidermis. Transmission of light occurs when light is transmitted straight through the target tissue without causing any chemical effect. Scattering of light occurs predominately within the dermis and can occur in all directions. Forward and sideways scattering will decrease the power density of light within the tissue. Backscattering will increase the power density of the beam of light within the tissue. With longer wavelengths, there is less scattering.

Laser light is absorbed by chromophores, which are "light loving" substances within the skin. There are three main endogenous chromophores of the skin: hemoglobin (oxyhemoglobin), melanin, and water. Each chromophore has specific peak absorption wavelength in the electromagnetic spectrum (Figure 73-1). Tattoo ink is considered an exogenous chromophore.

In order to determine the desired clinical laser effect, one must choose a

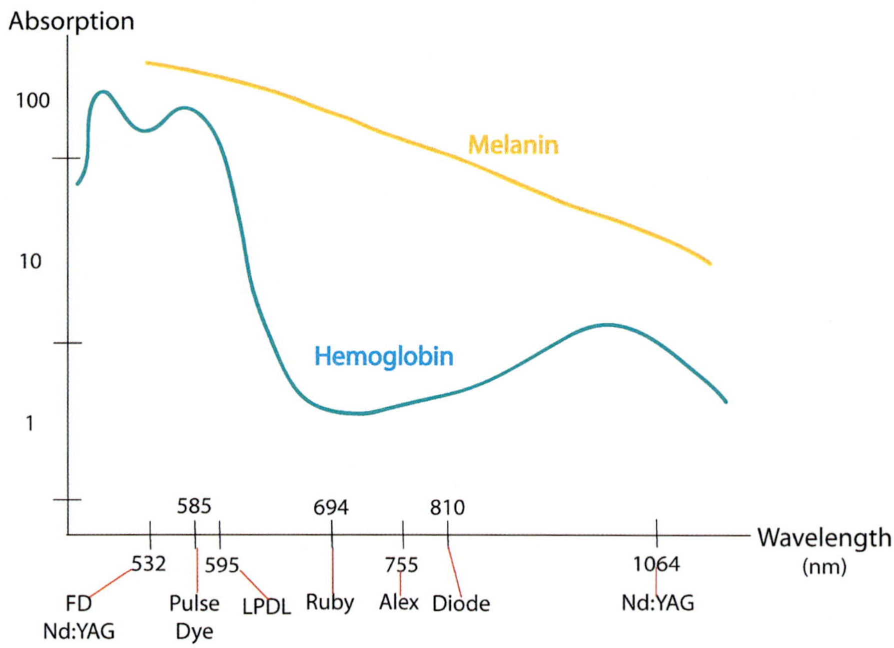

▲ **FIGURE 73-1** Absorption spectrum of hemoglobin and melanin with commonly used lasers.

specific wavelength that will be absorbed by the intended chromophore and also choose an appropriate pulse duration. When light is absorbed by the target, heat loss occurs by conduction to surrounding tissue. This is called *thermal relaxation*. The *thermal relaxation time* is defined as the time necessary for the target tissue to cool down to half the temperature to which it was heated. Thus the thermal relaxation time varies according to the size of the target. Smaller objects cool faster than larger objects.

If an object is heated for longer than its thermal relaxation time, there is enough time for thermal diffusion of heat to the surrounding area, causing damage to nontargeted tissue. If an object is heated for less than its thermal relaxation time, the heat is confined to the target without damaging the surrounding tissue. Therefore, the theory of selective photothermolysis states that selective heating of a target chromophore is achieved when the appropriate laser light is absorbed, and heat is confined within the target chromophore when the pulse duration is equal to or shorter than the thermal relaxation time.[4]

Energy fluence is the measurement of pulsed lasers. It is the amount of energy absorbed by the lesion. This is measured in joules (laser power times the pulse duration) per square centimeter (laser beam cross-sectional area). Irradiance is used for continuous-wave lasers because there is not a fixed pulse duration. Irradiance is measured in watts (joules per second or laser power output) per square centimeter (laser beam cross-sectional area).

THE CHALLENGE OF PIGMENTED SKIN

Melanin lies within the basal layer of the skin. In light-skinned individuals, there are a few small melanin granules seen on hematoxylin and eosin (H&E) stain within the basal layer. However, in darker-skinned individuals, numerous melanin granules are present within the basal layer. Additionally, in pigmented skin, moderate numbers of melanosomes are found throughout the epidermis. However, the melanocyte density of distribution (melanocytes per unit area of skin) shows no difference between lighter-skinned individuals and darker-skinned individuals. Nevertheless, in pigmented skin, the large quantity of melanin within the epidermis provides the ultimate and fundamental challenge for laser surgeons.

The main principle in treating darker skin tones lies in knowledge of the absorption spectrum of melanin. Melanin absorbs light in the range of 250–1200 nm. This wide absorption spectrum of melanin is the target of all visible and near-infrared dermatologic lasers. The problem arises when treating pigmented skin. The high density of melanin within the epidermis acts as a competitive chromophore with the intended dermal chromophore(s). The laser light gets absorbed by the epidermal melanin before ever reaching the dermis. Laser light is converted to heat within the epidermis, causing nonselective thermal injury. Blistering, crusting, scarring, and pigmentary discoloration can ensue that sometimes is permanent. In addition, owing to the competitive absorption by epidermal melanin, there is a limited amount of laser light that can penetrate to the necessary dermal target(s). The reduction of laser light reaching the intended chromophore decreases the efficacy of the laser treatment.

SUMMARY

- Melanin lies in the basal layer of skin.
- Melanosomes are located throughout the epidermis.
- Melanocyte density is the same for all skin colors.
- Melanin has an absorption spectrum between 250–1200 nm.
- In darker skin types, epidermal melanin acts as a competitive chromophore:
  - This limits the amount of light reaching the dermal target(s).
  - There is the potential to absorb light in the form of heat within the epidermis.
  - This causes nonselective epidermal thermal damage.
  - The result is crusting, scarring, and dyspigmentation that can be permanent.

LASER VARIABLES NECESSARY FOR TREATING SKIN OF COLOR

Some of the newer-generation lasers can treat pigmented skin safely. Longer wavelengths, longer pulse durations, and efficient cooling devices have been revolutionary in the use of lasers on skin of color.

The use of longer wavelengths is one of the parameters that is necessary to treat skin of color safely. With melanin having a wide absorption range, there is less melanin absorption as the wavelength increases. The longer wavelengths penetrate deep through the heavily melanized epidermis, reaching dermal targets. Longer wavelengths help to spare heat within the epidermis.

Second, longer pulse durations allow for efficient cooling of the epidermis by gently heating it. Delivering the laser heat over a longer duration of time allows the epidermal melanin to absorb the light in the form of heat much more slowly. Reducing the speed of absorption of light by the epidermal melanin slows the heating of the epidermis. This gentle heating enables the epidermis to cool more efficiently. Thus the longer pulse durations help to minimize direct melanosome destruction. With the thermal relaxation time of the melanosome being less than 1 μs (250–1000 ns), the melanosome is directly spared when using pulse durations in the millisecond range.

Efficient cooling is imperative to directly protect the epidermis from untoward events such as blistering, crusting, burning, and dyspigmentation. The common types of cooling devices are contact and noncontact. Contact cooling devices touch the skin directly. An example of a contact cooling device is a sapphire cooling tip. The tip is chilled and is in direct contact with the skin. Noncontact cooling devices do not come in contact with the skin. These can be a spray of water, air, or gas. An example of a noncontact cooling device is a cryogen spray. Cryogen sprays can reach temperatures as low as –26.2°C.

It must be stressed that excessive cooling, especially with noncontact cooling devices, can harm darker skin by producing a thermal burning that usually results in postinflammatory altered pigmentation.

Conservative fluences are crucial in treating darker skin tones. Aggressive fluences are not optimal. High fluences cause too much heat within the epidermis and surrounding dermal tissues. The ideal fluence produces no side effects to obtain the desired clinical outcome. To determine the appropriate fluence, test spots are performed. Test spots should be placed in a representative area that is the most inconspicuous. For example, when treating the cheek, test spots should be performed laterally, not medially. Immediate tissue response from the test spot can be determined. This may take 5–15 minutes to see the immediate tissue effect. To determine the clinical outcome or delayed response of the test spot site, the patient can be reevaluated in 1 month. At this time, the laser surgeon can evaluate the latent tissue response as well as the clinical outcome for most dermatologic laser procedures.

It is important to note, when performing laser procedures on darker skin types, that the laser parameters, especially fluence, are adjusted individually. It is crucial to choose the appropriate laser settings by determining the appropriate tissue response. Guidelines from the manufactures are often based on the Fitzpatrick skin types. The problem is that Fitzpatrick phototyping is not precise for non-white individuals. Therefore, laser manufacturer guidelines are helpful but are not 100% reliable. Thus test spots are encouraged. Often the laser surgeon will need to wait for a delayed response of the test site. It is not uncommon to have the patient return in a month to check the latent response as well as the clinical outcome.

SUMMARY

- Test spots are important to determine clinical outcome and potential adverse events.
- They should be done in a representative but inconspicuous area.
- Immediate responses can be seen within 5–15 minutes.
- The clinical outcome and/or delayed response (such as dyspigmentation and scarring) typically can be seen within 1 month.
- The information from the test spot can be used to determine the appropriate fluence.

VASCULAR LASERS

Port-Wine Stain

Port-wine stains affect 0.3–0.5% of newborns.[5] Occurring less often in African-Americans, there is an equal frequency in males and females. The most common location is the face, with only one third of port-wine stains occurring on nonfacial areas. Laser treatments offer a twofold effect. They attenuate the color and size of the port-wine stain, which, in turn, improves the psychological impact on the patient.

Unlike hemangiomas, which tend to regress with time, port-wine stains get darker and worsen over time. Usually by the fifth decade of life, approximately two-thirds of all patients develop nodularity or hypertrophy of the lesion. Port-wine stains have an average vessel size of 10–100 μm. The ectatic vessels within port-wine stains are increased in diameter but are not increased in number. The prognosis is poor for patients over 50, those with phototypes V and VI skin, and those with larger lesions or nonfacial port-wine stains.[6,7]

The pulsed-dye laser, with wavelengths of 585 or 595 nm, is efficacious in the treatment of port-wine stains in patients with pigmented skin. The pulsed-dye laser uses the principle of selective photothermolysis. By selecting a specific wavelength that targets hemoglobin, and by using a pulse duration that is equal to or less than the thermal relaxation time to blood vessels, there is selective damage of blood vessels with minimal damage to the surrounding tissues.

Phototypes IV–VI have epidermal melanin that acts as a competitive chromophore against hemoglobin. Epidermal melanin has a higher absorption coefficient than hemoglobin in the range of pulse-dye laser (see Figure 73-1). As a result, there is a risk of epidermal injury such as blistering, crusting, and dyspigmentation. In addition, because melanin acts as a competitive chromophore, less light is able to reach the targeted blood vessels. Intuitively, higher fluences may be necessary to produce the desired clinical response. However, fluences that are too high or aggressive will injure the heavily melanized epidermis. By decreasing the fluence appropriately to protect the epidermis from unwanted thermal sequelae, and by performing multiple treatments, one can achieve a cosmetically acceptable clinical improvement in pigmented skin. Interestingly, in a study with the shorter-wavelength 577-nm pulsed-dye vascular laser, Tong and colleagues[8] found epidermal injury in phototype V individuals with melanosomes appearing morphologically normal.

The 585-nm wavelength penetrates to a depth of 1.2 mm. The slightly longer wavelength of the 595 nm allows deeper penetration into the dermal ectatic vasculature of the port-wine stain. However, the absorption coefficient of oxyhemoglobin is three times higher at 585 nm than at 590 nm, which makes the 585-nm laser more selective to the ectatic vasculature.[9] For this reason, the 585-nm laser may have a slight advantage in treating port-wine stains.[10,11]

The thermal relaxation time of blood vessels is important in determining the appropriate pulse duration. Larger vessels require longer pulse durations, and depending on the depth of the ectatic vessels, possible longer wavelengths are required for deeper penetration. For vessels 20 μm in diameter, a pulse duration of 450 μs is adequate.[12] For vessels with a larger diameter, say, 30–150 μm, the pulse duration should be approximately 1–10 μs.[13] Port-wine stains of predominately smaller vessels generally respond better with the 585-nm pulsed-dye laser that has a pulse duration of 0.45 μs.[10]

Nevertheless, both the 595-nm and the 585-nm pulsed-dye lasers are excellent devices in the treatment of port-wine stains. Both lasers can be used for fair-complexioned phototype IV ethnic skin. Longer-wavelength pulsed-dye lasers should be used on darker phototypes, such as V and VI. Likewise, longer pulse durations with darker skin types are safer. Depending on the fluence chosen, pulse durations of 0.45–10 ms are better suited for lighter phototypes (IV) than for darker phototypes (V and VI), which tend to require 10 ms or longer in most clinical situations. In addition, using a larger spot size allows for deeper penetration and a smaller decrease in fluence within the tissue.[10]

It is generally believed for the treatment of port-wine stains that the earlier and more aggressive the treatments, the better will be the clinical outcome with fewer treatments. However, this presents a challenge in treating pigmented skin. Too aggressive fluences can damage the epidermis. Therefore, test spots are crucial in determining the appropriate fluence for port-wine stains. Initially, a test spot should be performed by delivering several juxtaposed pulses onto the lesion. This should be performed in a nonconspicuous yet representative area. Depending on the skin color and pulse duration, the typical purple discoloration may or may not be clinically apparent. The laser surgeon should wait a sufficient amount of time to determine tissue response. This may take 5–15 minutes. If there is no immediate vesiculation, intense erythema, extreme purpuric color, profound edema, or gray discoloration, more pulses can be delivered for an adequately sized test spot area. There should be varying fluences to determine the best clinical outcome. Pulses should be placed with a minimum overlap of 10% to prevent a cobblestone effect. The patient can return in 1 month to check the clinical outcome before undergoing treatment of the entire lesion.

The fluence chosen should be the highest possible with no clinical side effects to ensure cutaneous safety to the patient. However, when initially treating a large port-wine stain in patients with darker phototypes, it is not uncommon to err on the side of safety and use the most modest fluence from the test spot area. It is important to remember that a test spot is only a guide. It will not determine with 100% accuracy that there will be no untoward effects, especially when treating a large lesion. Therefore, reduction in fluence and choice of longer pulse durations when initially treating larger port-wine stains are efficacious in persons of color.

With the pulsed-dye laser, a transient violaceous discoloration of the treated area is normal. How long it lasts depends on the pulse duration selected, the skin complexion, and the amount of chromophore. With a pulse duration of 1.5 ms or less, the violaceous discoloration can last for a few days to a couple of weeks. With longer pulse durations, the purple discoloration is transitory, lasting a few hours to a few days. Limiting sun exposure and exercise is important for postlaser care.

Few side effects are encountered when fluences are determined based on the outcome of the test spots. In addition, longer pulse durations and sufficient cooling will ensure safety. As the port-wine stain lightens (decreasing number of chromophores) with subsequent laser treatments, higher fluences are necessary. Multiple treatments are performed monthly or every 2 months. The exact number of treatments necessary to improve color and texture of a port-wine stain is unknown in skin of color. This is due to the many variables such as skin color, fluence, spot size, pulse duration, site of lesion, and size of the lesion, including vessels size.

Side effects are minimal. Transient hyperpigmentation has been reported to be as high as 44–46% of patients.[11,14] Transient or permanent hypopigmentation, and scarring are rarely encountered.

The intense pulsed light (IPL) is a broad-band light source emitting noncoherent light between the wavelengths of 500 and 1200 nm. The IPL provides an option for treatment of port-wine stains. In treating pigmented skin, the broad-band light source is best suited for phototypes IV or less. Because of the range of wavelengths, the IPL potentially can treat vessels that are larger and of varying depths. Multiple treatments are necessary to achieve a suitable outcome. Ho and colleagues[15] were able to achieve a 25–50% clearance with five to seven treatments every 3–4 weeks in patients who were phototype IV.

The IPL tissue response is erythema and mild edema that can last from a few hours to a few days. Adequate cooling is crucial. Dyspigmentation is often a transitory side effect. Blistering, vesiculation, and scarring, although rare, can occur. The broad range of wavelengths can affect the absorption of melanin not only in the skin but also within hair follicles. Permanent reduction of hair is a risk with the IPL system. Unlike the pulsed-dye laser system, which is user-friendly, the IPL system has a higher learning curve. To decrease unwanted side effects in pigmented skin, it requires expertise and knowledge of subtleties of this system.

Lastly, another common vascular laser device that is used for port-wine stains in pigmented skin is the variable-pulse 532-nm laser. This laser is best used on skin types IV and lighter. The inherent difficulty with the use of this laser is that the shorter wavelength competes more strongly with melanin, and therefore, sufficient cooling is necessary to prevent untoward events. The shorter wavelength carries more risk of epidermal injury such as pigmentary changes, blistering, and crusting. The appropriate tissue response is generally immediate blanching of the vasculature with simultaneous development of erythema and edema. Nevertheless, the longer vascular wavelengths are preferable alternatives for the treatment of port-wine stains.

SUMMARY

- Although rare in persons of color, port-wine stains get darker with time and can be cosmetically disfiguring.
- For the treatment of port-wine stains, laser treatments often require aggressive parameters.
- These are difficult to achieve in persons of color owing to the competitive chromophore melanin.
- To ensure cutaneous safety, test spots are crucial.
- The highest fluence without cutaneous side effects should be used initially, except when treating larger port-wine stains.
- Larger lesions are best treated with modest fluences and longer pulse durations.
- However, the laser surgeon will not be at fault if low fluences are employed initially in persons of color to ensure patient safety.
- With improvement of the lesion, the fluence may need to be adjusted upward owing to the decreased amount of chromohpores.
- Nevertheless, in choosing the optimal fluence, the key is tissue response.

Hemangiomas

Capillary hemangiomas are the most common vascular tumor. They are present in 2.6% of newborns.[5] Hemangiomas are more common in Caucasians than in African-Americans, affecting 8–12% of Caucasian infants by age 1.[5] There is a female predominance. Premature infants are more at risk. Hemangiomas improve over time. The general rule of thumb is that by the age of 5, 50% of hemangiomas improve, 70% improve by age 7, and 90% improve by age 9.[16] Since most hemangiomas will improve cosmetically with time, laser treatments are best indicated for lesions that are proliferating or ulcerated and for postinvolution lesions with residual vasculature. Additionally, hemangiomas compromising vital structures should undergo laser intervention.

There is controversy regarding early laser treatment of uncomplicated hemangiomas. Some experts believe that the inherent risk of the laser procedure itself (i.e., scarring and pigmentary alterations) outweighs the benefit of treatment at. Waiting for the lesion to improve over time is a more prudent approach to managing hemangiomas. In addition, the limited depth of 1.2 mm with the 585-nm pulsed-dye laser will minimally help hemangiomas that are raised and thick.

Nevertheless, early intervention is helpful for ulcerated hemangiomas, hyperproliferating hemangiomas, or hemangiomas that are compromising a vital structure or function. Multiple treatments are necessary and can be performed every 2–3 weeks if necessary. Pulsed-dye laser systems are ideal for treating hemangiomas in skin of color. The possibility of using the newer long-pulsed Nd:YAG lasers for hemangiomas seems promising, but studies are pending.[17]

Leg Veins

The "gold standard" for treating leg veins is sclerotherapy, but lasers can be used for patients in whom sclerotherapy has failed, patients with postsclerotherapy matting, patients who are needle phobic, and patients who are allergic to the sclerosing agent. Owing to the high fluences needed to achieve successful closure of leg vessels, patients with ethnic skin types beyond phototypes IV are not suitable. There are no published studies for the treatment of leg veins in patients with phototype VI and very few for patients with phototype V in the literature. It should be stated that phototype V skin should be treated with caution owing to the high side effects that potentially can be encountered. Treating leg veins in phototype VI patients is not recommended.

Among the variables that should be considered when treating leg veins, skin type is the most important. As noted above, patients with phototypes I–III can be treated with greater efficacy and fewer complications than patients with phototype IV or higher. Another important variable is the vasculature, including size, depth, and color. (oxygenated and deoxygenated). Class I superficial reddish telangiectasias are easier to treat than class II and III deeper bluish venulectases.

For class I telangiectasias (vessels 0.2–1 mm in diameter), shorter-wavelength lasers such as the 532-, 585-, and 595-nm lasers absorb the chromophore oxyhemoglobin. Depending on the size of the vessel, the pulse durations can be adjusted, for example, shorter pulse durations for smaller vessels and longer pulse durations for larger vessels. Longer wavelengths, such as 810 and 1064 nm, are more specifically absorbed by the deoxygenated bluish vessels with deeper penetration of the laser light to the targeted chromophore. Longer pulse durations are necessary to thermocoagulate the entire vessel adequately. The largest spot size should be used to penetrate deeper into the tissue and to optimize the fluence delivery into the vasculature.

In treating pigmented skin, the pulsed-dye laser systems work best for the treatment of class I leg veins, especially those measuring 0.1 mm in diameter or smaller.[18] Lower fluences of 10 J/cm^2 or less with appropriate pulse durations (ranging from 1.5–20 ms) depending on vessel size are recommended when using the 595-nm pulsed-dye laser. Multiple treatments are necessary with intervals of 2–3 months between treatments depending upon the development of side effects. Double pulsing is highly discouraged with pulse-dye lasers. The pulse-dye systems can leave expected purpura lasting for weeks depending on the pulse duration and phototype of the skin.

Postinflammatory hyperpigmentation can be seen in more than half the patients with darker skin types. Hypopigmentation occurs less frequently, ranging from 15–50% of patients. Kono and colleagues[18] treated 14 patients with skin phototypes III–V with 38 vascular leg veins. Patients received two treatments at 2-month intervals. The authors reported 100% clearance of type IA vessels, 78.3% clearance of type I vessels, and only 22.2% clearance of type II vessels. For vessels measuring less than 0.2 mm in diameter (type IA), pulse durations of 1.5–3 ms were used; for vessels measuring 0.2–1 mm in diameter (type I), pulse durations of 3–10 ms were used; and for vessels measuring 1.1–2.0 mm in diameter (type II), pulse durations of 10–20 ms were used in the study. Fluence remained fixed at 10 J/cm^2. Transient postinflammatory hyperpigmentation was seen in 57.9% of treated sites.

The 800-nm diode laser has been used recently to treat leg veins. Based on the small peak of hemoglobin absorption in the 700- to 900-nm range, the long-pulsed diode laser has been used to treat larger-caliber leg veins. Phototype IV is the darkest skin type in the literature analyzed for the treatment of leg veins. The longer wavelength works best on larger vessels with a diameter of 1–4 mm. The near-infrared wavelength penetrates deeper into the skin with less interference with melanin absorption. Trelles and colleagues[19] treated 10 women with leg veins measuring 1–4 mm in diameter. Of the 10 patients, 4 were phototype IV. Patients received a maximum of three treatments 2 months apart. The authors used a 3-mm spot, a 50-ms pulse duration, and a 50-ms delay. The pulses were stacked (5–8 stacked pulses with each pulse 42 J/cm^2), reaching a cumulative fluence that ranged from 210–336 J/cm^2. Since the thermorelaxation time for blood vessels in this study was 500 ms, pulse stacking attempts were made to reach this thermal relaxation time with minimum collateral heat damage to the surrounding tissues. At 6 months, most of the patients had a good to very good improvement of their leg veins both subjectively and objectively. Side effects included transient erythema in all patients. Blistering and pruritus were experienced infrequently. Postinflammatory hyperpigmentation was seen in two of the four patients who were phototype IV. This resolved by 6 months. Owing to the small sample size, more studies need to be conducted in patients with skin phototypes IV and higher to determine the true efficacy and safety profile of this laser.

The long-pulsed Nd:YAG laser with its long wavelength of 1064 nm and pulse durations of up to 100 ms treats vessels larger than 1 mm in diameter more efficiently.[20,21] However, high fluences are required to cause adequate thermocoagulation of the vasculature. To date, there are no published studies on the use of this laser system in darker skin types. The fluences are too great to protect the epidermis from unwanted injury.

Likewise, use of the IPL system with its broad-band light source and deep penetrance has not been reported in the literature in darker skin types.

Showing promise in the treatment of leg veins is the combination diode and radiofrequency system. The Electro-optical Synergy (ELOS) technology combines bipolar radiofrequency with optical energy of either the diode laser or the IPL source. The two forms of energy may act synergistically to achieve selective photothermolysis of the target chromophore. There are no published data on the use of this system in the treatment of leg veins in pigmented skin beyond phototype IV. In a study of 50 women with skin phototypes II–IV with leg veins 1–4 mm in diameter, approximately 75% of patients had greater than 50% improvement in their vessels. Side effects were minimal. The side effects were prolonged erythema, which subsided in 2 weeks, tolerable discomfort, and transient hyperpigmentation that did not correlate with skin type.[22] Future studies are pending.

Hypertrophic Scars and Keloids

Unlike hypertrophic scars, which are confined to the borders of injury, keloids extend beyond the borders of injury. Both can be challenging to treat. African-Americans have the highest incidence of keloids, which is reported as high as 16%.[23] Intralesional steroids injections, cryotherapy, 5-fluorouracil (5-FU), radiotherapy, and interferon have been used to help improve keloids. With surgical removal of keloids, the recurrence rate ranges from 45–100%.[23] The nonablative pulsed-dye laser offers some degree of clinical improvement for keloids and hypertrophic scarring.[24] Especially for patients with skin phototype VI, low subpurpuric fluences are typical, with multiple treatments performed monthly to every 2 months. However, some laser experts advocate aggressive fluences and purpuric pulse durations in the treatment of hypertrophic scars and keloids. These parameters are best suited for patients with skin phototypes IV and V.

The pulsed-dye laser demonstrates a clinical and more profound histologic improvement of collagen remodeling. Early laser intervention is the key, and it often can begin on the day of suture removal. Concomitant intralesional injections of steroids and/or 5-FU immediately after laser therapy, when the tissue is more edematous, allows easier injection and a faster cosmetic and symptomatic improvement.[25] However, in most cases, especially for keloids, the clinical outcome is less than satisfactory.

Either the pulsed-dye 585-nm laser or the long pulsed-dye 595-nm laser is acceptable in treating scars and keloids in persons with darker skin tones. Lighter-complexioned skin types can use the 585-nm pulsed-dye system. If there is a choice, for darker skin types, the 595-nm laser is ideal.

Skin Rejuvenation with Vascular Lasers

The aging process is dynamic and ongoing. It is well established in the literature that cutaneous histologic improvement of skin can be achieved with use of the pulsed-dye laser. Zelickson and colleagues[26] demonstrated improvement with the pulsed-dye laser of collagen types I and III as well as elastin within the dermis. Collagenase and procollagen were increased.

With the pulsed-dye system, the best patient for this procedure is one who does not have severe rhytides. Low subpurpuric fluences are used for nonablative skin rejuvenation. The entire face typically is treated. Test spots can be performed before the full facial treatment. The pulses should be slightly overlapped by 30%. Multiple treatments are necessary. The patients can expect mild improvement of dyspigmentation and wrinkle improvement.[27–29]

The results for skin rejuvenation with the pulsed-dye laser are not often dramatic. To enhance the pulsed-dye treatments, nonlaser therapeutic modalities are encouraged. For the best outcome, concomitant use of sunscreens, topical agents, chemical or mechanical peels, injectable chemodenervation substances, and filler substances, when appropriate, aid in the battle against aging.

The IPL system has been used to improve skin texture. Negishi and colleagues[30] demonstrated improvement in pigmentation in 90%, telangiectasias in 83%, and skin texture in the 65% of 97 Asian patients with skin phototypes IV and V. Cutoff filters for shorter wavelengths were used. Multiple treatments were performed. Their second study revealed a 60% improvement in 80% of patients. There were no reports of scarring or changes in pigmentation. However, transient erythema and blistering were noted.[31] Hernandez-Perez and Ibiett[32] treated five Hispanic women with five sessions with the IPL system. The group noted a moderate to very good improvement in their patients' skin, including mild rhytides and dilated pores. Histologically, there was a statistically significant difference in epidermal thickness, suggesting not only dermal improvement but also epidermal textural improvement.

Psoriasis

Pulsed-dye and excimer lasers are both used in the control of psoriasis vulgaris. The dermal vasculature is increased in psoriatic plaques. There is increased blood flow through the dilated and elongated blood vessels. These aberrant vessels are a good target for the pulsed-dye laser. There seems to be no difference bewteen short pulsed-dye laser systems (450 ms) or long pulsed-dye laser systems (1500 ms).[33] Although Hacker and colleagues[34] achieved improvement after one treatment using the 585-nm laser, multiple treatments are necessary. Lanigan and colleagues,[35] in a small series of patients, saw improvement of psoriasis after three treatments. de Leeuw and colleagues[36] used the pulsed-dye laser with topical calcipotriol and/or salicylic acid for palmar plantar psoriasis, with up to five treatments every 4–6 weeks, and noted improvement in 76% of patients. Side effects included the transient purpura, nonsevere pain, transient hyperpigmentation, and rarely, transient hypopigmentation.

The result in skin of color has not been consistent. This may be due to the competitive chromophore in darker phototypes. In order to enhance treatment with the pulsed-dye laser, it is best to remove scale prior to treatment. Conservative fluences and multiple treatments every 2–4 four weeks are necessary.

The excimer laser has a wavelength of 308 nm. Its mechanism of action is thought to be similar to narrow-band (311-nm) ultraviolet B (UVB). The excimer laser produces photons from an unstable excited gas dimer of xenon chloride that produces the wavelength of 308 nm. This laser has its advantage when treating localized disease. There is a lower cumulative dose of UV light with a lower risk for carcinogenicity. The excimer laser has a 20- to 40-ns pulse width with a rate of 200 Hz. Multiple treatments are necessary when using lower doses. However, one study suggests that with single high blistering doses, one treatment can yield a remittent effect for months. The excimer laser works best for truncal psoriasis, for which fluence seems to be the most single important variable in determining clinical clearing.[37]

SUMMARY

- Common hemangiomas do not need to be treated with lasers because they have a high rate of involution.
- Complicated hemangiomas such as those that are ulcerated, hyperproliferating, or compromising vital structure or function should undergo laser treatment.
- Sclerotherapy and not laser therapy is the "gold standard" for treating leg veins.
- Leg veins in patients with skin phototype VI should not be treated with lasers.
- Hypertrophic scars and keloids in patients with skin phototype VI should be treated with subpurpuric fluences at monthly intervals.
- Skin rejuvenation can be achieved with vascular lasers.
  - The clinical results are often not dramatic.
  - Multiple treatments are necessary.

PIGMENTED LESIONS

The Q-switched lasers are best suited to treat persons of color for a variety of pigmented dermatologic disorders. The three Q-switched laser systems are, in order of increasing wavelengths: the Q-switched ruby (694 nm), alexandrite (755 nm), and Nd:YAG (1064 nm) lasers. The Q-switched ruby laser is best suited for phototype IV or less. The Q-switched alexandrite laser is best suited for phototype V or less. The Q-switched Nd:YAG laser can be used for all skin types. This is due to the absorption coefficient of melanin. It decreases as wavelength increases. Thus epidermal melanin absorbs approximately four times as much energy with the 694-nm Q-switched ruby laser as when exposed to the 1064-nm Q-switched Nd:YAG laser.[38]

In Summary

- Q-switched lasers are best suited to treat persons of color.
  - Q-switched ruby (694 nm) laser: Best suited for phototype IV or less.
  - Q-switched alexandrite (755 nm) laser: Best suited for phototype V or less.
  - Q-Switched Nd:YAG (1064 nm) laser: Good for all skin types.

The mechanism of action of Q-switched laser systems is not fully understood. It is believed that the melanosomes or target chromophore undergoes a photoacoustic (light and sound) effect. A typical melanosome (1 μm) has a thermorelaxation time of between 0.5 to 1.0 μs. The high peak power of fluence delivered in nanoseconds appears to create a shock wave and/or cavitation damage to the melanosome. Melanin absorbs the high-intensity light, which creates a temperature gradient between the melanosome and its surrounding tissue. This gradient leads to thermal expansion and the generation as well as propagation of acoustic waves, hence the photoacoustic effect.

The IPL system, with its broadband wavelengths, has been helpful in the treatment of a number of pigmentary disorders. The IPL system emits a polychromatic noncoherent light. The wavelengths range from 500–1200 nm. There are many different adjustable parameters that determine the clinical outcome. These parameters are pulse duration, pulse delay, fluence, wavelength, cutoff filters, and spot size (which can be fixed). With the use of cutoff filters, the treatment can be individualized based on the desired targeted chromophore and skin type. Specific cutoff filters are chosen to reduce the absorption of melanin and are best suited for persons of darker skin tones. In addition, wavelength determines not only the absorption behavior of the targeted chromophore but also the depth of penetration of the light. The pulse duration of the IPL system can vary from less than 1 ms to as long as 200 ms depending on the manufacturer. Single and multiple pulses are possible. High fluences can be divided into multiple pulses. The interval between pulses, or pulse delay, can be chosen. The pulse delay is important to allow the epidermis and smaller vessels to cool while the heat is being retained in larger targets, such as hair follicles. Expected erythema rarely lasting a few days and edema are common side effects. Microcrust lasting 2 weeks can be seen in areas where there were hyperpigmented lesions. Crusting, blistering, and transient hyperpigmentation and hypopigmentation have been reported.

There are limited published studies of use of the IPL system in the treatment of various pigmentary disorders in persons of color. Expertise and comfort with use of the IPL system, as well as use of longer wavelengths and long pulse durations, are important when treating pigmented skin types. Of the ethnic skin types, patients with skin phototype IV can be treated with greater ease than those with phototype V, which has to be treated cautiously with the IPL system.

Lentigines

Often a sign of aging and sun damage, lentigines are cosmetically undersirable for most persons, especially when they occur on the face and dorsum hands. The Q-switched lasers are best used for patients with skin phototype IV or higher. For fair-complexioned individuals, the Q-switched ruby laser is efficacious. In addition, the frequency-doubled 532-nm Q-switched Nd:YAG laser is an alternative when used at the lowest possible fluence. Usually one or two treatment sessions are needed. The greatest risk is pigmentary alteration. Postinflammatory hyperpigmentation is common in patients with skin phototype IV and higher. Postinflammatory hypopigmentation is more common with the use of lower-wavelength Q-switched lasers. Typically, a frostlike whitening is observed. It is important to have the patient avoid excessive sun exposure while healing from the laser treatment (Figures 73-2 and 73-3).

The IPL system has been used to treat lentigines. Kawada and colleagues[39] treated 66 Japanese patients with facial lentigines and ephelides. The patients had three to five treatments. Forty-eight percent of patients had more than a 50% improvement, with 20% of patients experiencing more than 75% clearing. The expected mild crusting seen with pigmented lesions was experienced in over half the patients. One patient experienced a burn. The authors postulated that this was due to the darker lesion and darker skin tone. They stated that caution should be used in patients with darker skin phototypes. Wang and colleagues,[40] in comparing the IPL system and the Q-switched alexandrite laser for the treatment of ephelides and lentigines in Asian women, found a preference for the IPL system for lentigines and the Q-switched alexandrite laser for ephelides.

Nevus of Ito and Ota

These dermomelanocytic lesions are best treated with Q-switched laser systems. Multiple treatments are necessary to achieve a clinically acceptable outcome. On average, treatments range

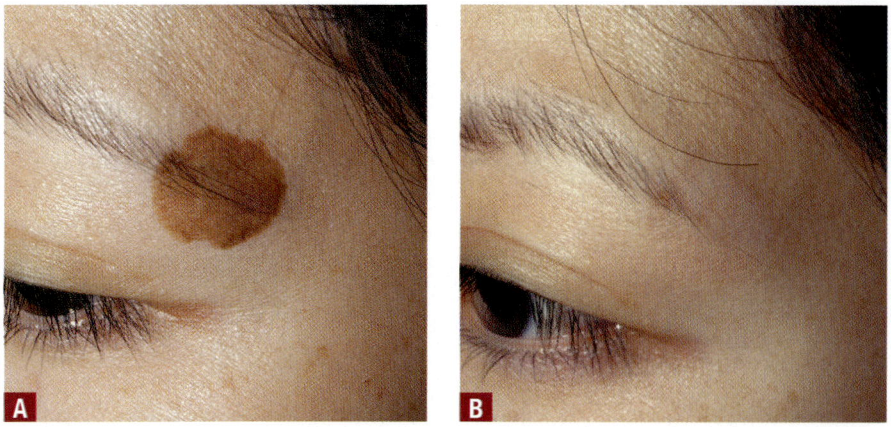

▲ **FIGURE 73-2** Q-switched ruby laser. Lentigo near the eyebrow before (**A**) and after (**B**) treatment. Courtesy of H. Lui, M.D.

from four to eight sessions and can be performed every 1–2 months. It is believed that 2-month intervals may reduce the overall number of treatments over time. Watanabe and Takahashi,[41] with their 114 Asian patients, found good to excellent results after three or more treatments with the Q-switched ruby laser. As previously stated, the choice of device should be based on the patient's phototype: the Q-switched ruby lazor for type IV, the Q-switched alexandrite laser for types IV and V, or the Q-switched Nd:YAG laser for all types.

In addition, depending on the clinical response and the depth of the dermal melanocytes, laser systems may need to be interchanged. The longer-wavelength lasers are better suited for the more deeply situated dermal melanocytic cells. Chan and colleagues[42] found that the Q-switched Nd:YAG laser was more effective than the Q-switched alexandrite laser after three or more treatments. The most common side effect was transient postinflammatory altered pigmentation (Figure 73-4).

Melasma

Q-switched laser systems are not recommended for the treatment of melasma. The results are disappointing, with clearing rare. Initially, epidermal and dermal injury with extracellular melanin is noted. Subsequently, there are focal increased dermal macrophages. Postinflammatory altered pigmentation is the major side effect with these systems.[43]

The IPL system has been reported to be helpful in reducing melasma in patients with skin phototype IV. Wang and colleagues[44] reported improvement in 31 patients (phototypes III–IV) with refractory melasma. Patients were treated with four sessions with the IPL system and hydroquinone. Thirty-five percent had more than 50% improvement of their melasma. There was an average of 40% improvement of the relative melanin index compared with controls. More than half the patients experienced the typical microcrust, which appeared 2– 3 days after treatment and dissipated over 2 weeks. Smaller subject studies are reported in the literature. Moreno Arias and colleagues[45] treated two patients with epidermal melasma. After two treatments, there was a clearance rate of 76–100%. Three patients with mixed melasma were treated. After four sessions, there was a less than 25% improvement. Post-IPL induced transient hyperpigmentation was noted.

Interestingly, the IPL system has been reported in the literature to exacerbate subclinical melasma when aggressive fluences are used. Negishi and colleagues[46] postulated that patients with latent melasma detected by UV photography should be treated with mild IPL parameters to avoid erythema. IPL-induced erythema should last only a few minutes and not hours. The longer the IPL-induced erythema lasts, the greater is the chance of melasma-like hyperpigmentation. The group postulated that postinflammatory melasma-like hyperpigmentation was a result of erythema induced by the IPL system.

Nonablative lasers are helpful in improving melasma in patients with skin phototypes IV–VI. The nonablative 1064-nm laser has been noted in unpublished reports to improve melasma as well as postinflammatory altered pigmentation. The exact mechanism is unclear. However, there appears to be dermal remodeling with the release of cytokines that enhances the quality of skin. As with the other nonablative devices, multiple treatments every 3–4 weeks are necessary. Adjunctive treatments with topical retinoids, sunscreens, and hydroquinone, as well as the use of chemical or mechanical peels, are helpful to improve the condition. The laser parameters with the long-pulsed 1064-nm laser are a 5-mm spot size, 0.3 ms, and 5 Hz, with an average fluence of 13 J/cm^2.

In addition, fractional photothermolysis, a nonablative laser technique, is helpful in controlling melasma. It is approved for all skin types, but there are few reports of its use in patients with skin phototype VI. Fractional photothermolysis creates tiny microscopic wounds that are small enough to repair themselves quickly without extensive cutaneous thermal damage. These tiny wounds are called *microscopic treatment zones* (MTZs). The MTZs have a 5:1 depth-to-width ratio. These are long columns of thermal injury zones that

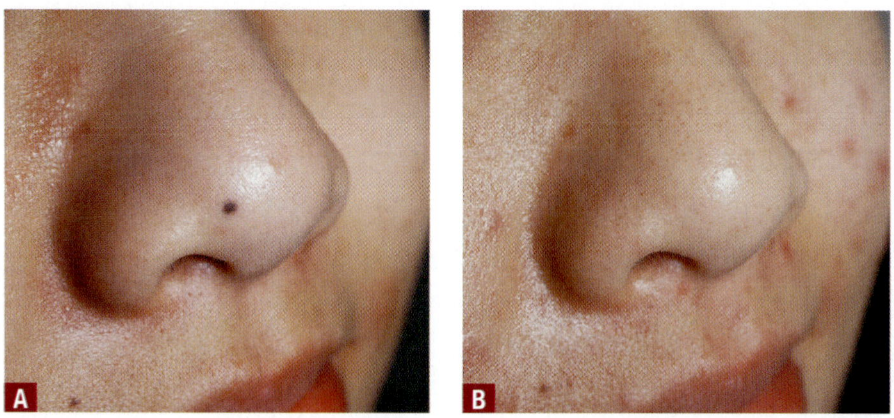

▲ **FIGURE 73-3** Q-switched ruby laser. Blue nevus on the tip of the nose before (**A**) and after (**B**) one treatment. Courtesy of H. Lui, M.D.

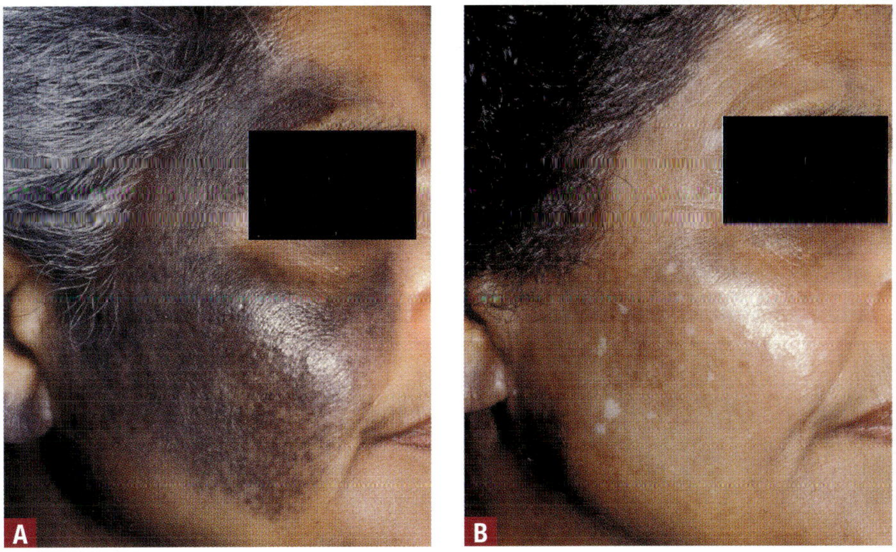

▲ **FIGURE 73-4** Q-switched ruby laser. Nevus of Ota before (**A**) and after (**B**) several treatments. Note the mild transient hypopigmentation but excellent clearance. Courtesy of H. Lui, M.D.

can be, on average, 100 μm in diameter (usually less than 250 μm). The adjustable depth up to 1 mm is based on the pulse-energy setting in millijoules. The density of the MTZs is variable. Parameters are based on the energy and the density of these MTZs. For the treatment of melasma with fractional photothermolysis, it is not uncommon to have patients with darker skin phototypes use hydroquinone for at least a month prior to treatment. Prophylaxis with an antiviral agent is routine. Test spots should be performed and reevaluated in 4 weeks before a full treatment is performed. Melasma has been reduced with the use fractional photothermolysis. Some laser surgeons, in treating persons of color, will regionally treat the affected areas. Low energy and low densities are appropriate parameters for the initial treatment. There are few published reports of the use of photothermolysis in patients with darker skin phototypes. Multiple treatment (average three to five) should be given 6–8 weeks apart, and patients may require touch-up treatments months to years later. Topical anesthesia is necessary. Postinflammatory changes are side effects that often are transitory and rarely permanent. The exact incidence of permanent postinflammatory changes is not reported in the literature. The etiology of the postinflammatory pigmentary changes is unclear. Thus it is important to educate the patient and to set realistic goals with melasma patients of darker phototypes undergoing fractional photothermolysis. The treatment endpoint should be a reduction in the appearance of melasma, not clearance or eradication (Figure 73-5).

Tattoos

Tattoos can be exogenous (e.g., decorative or amateur) or traumatic (e.g., asphalt, gravel, etc.). The Q-switched laser systems work best to improve tattoos. Laser-assisted tattoo removal is considered the "gold standard" for treatment of tattoos. Before the advent of lasers, unwanted tattoos were removed via surgery, salabrasion, cryosurgery, or chemical peels. These techniques often left a visible scar. With laser-assisted tattoo removal, there is decreased risk of scarring and pigmentary alteration. Professional tattoos generally require more treatments than amateur tattoos. And traumatic tattoos often can be cleared after only a few treatments.

The Q-switched laser systems with their nanosecond pulse duration destroy the small tattoo particles so that the tiny fragmented particles are eliminated transepidermally and/or are engulfed by scavenger cells and brought to the local lymph nodes to be eliminated or picked up by residing macrophages. Depending on the ink's absorption spectrum, a particular wavelength can be chosen. Red inks are best treated with the 532-nm laser, green or teal inks are best treated with the 755-nm laser, and black ink, which is absorbed throughout the visible to near-infrared spectrum, can be treated with the 694-, 755-, and 1064-nm lasers. However, the 1064-nm laser has been used most frequently to remove black tattoo ink.

In general, the longer-wavelength Q-switched laser systems work best for pigmented skin. Use of the 1064-nm laser produces less interference with cutaneous melanin. The longer wavelength penetrates deep into the skin to reach the tattoo pigment with less damage to the epidermal melanocytes. It is the wavelength of choice when treating pigmented skin.[47] With use of shorter Q-switched laser wavelengths, such as 694 and 755 nm, there is more risk of hypopigmentation for patients with skin of color tones. The risk of transient hyperpigmentation is common and is usually seen with darker-complexioned individuals. Textural irregularities and pruritus are sometimes encountered.

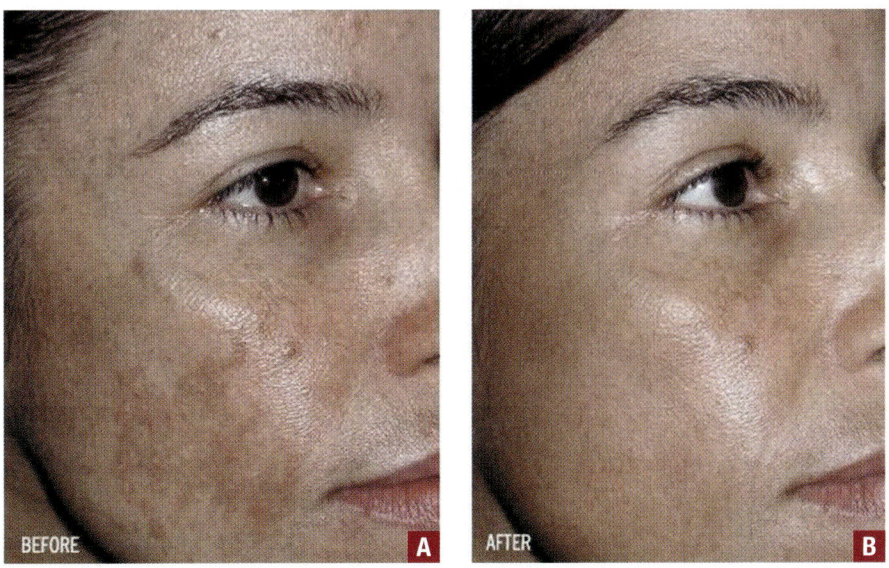

▲ **FIGURE 73-5** Fraxel by Reliant for the treatment of melasma before (**A**) and after (**B**) four treatments at 7 mJ, treatment level 5 (14% coverage). Courtesy of Howard Conn, M.D.

There are few contraindications to laser tattoo removal. The most severe is an allergy to the tattoo ink. When patients exhibit a localized allergic reaction to a specific tattoo ink, Q-switched lasers are not recommended. These Q-switched laser systems fragment the tattoo ink particles, dispersing the allergen within the body and causing a potential anaphylactic response. Instead, the tattoo ink should be either surgically removed or vaporized with an ablative laser. Second, cosmetic tattoos that are flesh tones or white may undergo immediate pigment darkening with Q-switched lasers. This occurs when the ferric oxide in the inks is reduced to ferrous oxide by the Q-switched laser. This black-colored reaction product cannot always be removed successfully. A test spot is recommended when flesh-tone or cosmetic tattoos are encountered. Third, keloid formers should be treated with caution.

Not all tattoos are removed completely. Large decorative tattoos may be better left alone depending on the size and colors. Bright colors, especially red, are often difficult to remove in pigmented skin because shorter-wavelength Q-switched laser systems are necessary to eradicate the ink. These shorter-wavelength lasers often cause hypopigmentation that can be transient in most cases and rarely permanent.

For the initial treatment, it is not unusual to perform a test spot. There is associated discomfort with treatments. Patients often remark that laser tattoo removal hurts more than placement of the tattoo. If necessary, a topical anesthetic is helpful in reducing the pain. The laser pulses should be placed with a 0–10% overlap. There is usually slight edema and a whitish debris with minimal bleeding. If there is significant epidermal debris and bleeding, the fluence should be lowered. With each treatment, higher fluences are needed because of the decreased number of chromophores and more deeply situated tattoo particles (Table 73-1).

TABLE 73-1
Commonly Used Q-Switched Laser-Assisted Tattoo Removal

Wavelength	Color of Tattoo Ink
532 nm	Red, orange, yellow
585 nm	Sky blue
650 nm	Green
694 nm	Black, blue, green
755 nm	Blue, teal, green
1064 nm*	Black, blue

*The 1064-nm Q-switched laser is ideal for skin of color. Shorter wavelengths are likely to cause transient to permanent hypopigmentation.

SUMMARY

- Q-switched lasers are safe and can be used on darker phototypes for lentigines, nevus of Ito and O-ta, and tattoos.
- Melasma is not treated with Q-switched lasers.
- Fractional photothermolysis shows promise in the control of melasma in patients with darker skin phototypes.
- The IPL broad-band light source has a high learning curve.
- The IPL system can be used for a number of skin conditions, for example, lentigines, melasma, and skin rejuvenation in patients with darker skin phototypes, often routinely limited to phototypes IV and V.
- Laser-assisted tattoo removal is the "gold standard" form of treatment.
- Not all tattoos can be completely removed.
- Bright colors are difficult to remove.
- Red inks are best treated with the 532-nm laser.
- Green or teal inks are best treated with the 755-nm laser.
- Black ink may be treated with the 694-, 755-, and 1064-nm lasers, but the 1064-nm laser is most reliable to treat a black ink tattoo.
- Flesh-tone tattoos should be treated with caution owing to the immediate pigment-darkening effect.
- Specific tattoo ink demonstrating a cutaneous allergy (edema and/or erythema) should never be treated with the Q-switched laser owing to release of the allergen into the system, causing a potential anaphylactic attack.
- Colored tattoo ink should be ablated or removed surgically.

NONABLATIVE LASERS

Laser resurfacing is highly effective in improving photoaging, especially rhytides, dyschromia, and telangiectasias. It is best suited for fair-complexioned phototypes. Ablative resurfacing vaporizes the epidermis and a portion of the dermis, creating a controlled cutaneous thermal destruction with resulting reepithelialization and neocollagenesis with new elastic fibrils. It is associated with a prolonged healing process and a significant number of potential adverse events, including scarring, hyperpigmentation, and erythema. In patients with skin phototypes IV–VI, ablative laser resurfacing carries a profound risk of cosmetically unacceptable scarring and pigmentary alteration.

To overcome the challenges of ablative laser resurfacing, nonablative laser resurfacing emerged. Although the results are not as impressive clinically as with laser resurfacing, nonablative lasers have provided a treatment modality to improve skin texture and dyschromia while leaving the epidermis intact. Thus there is little risk of scarring and dyspigmentation with the associated downtime.

Because the absorption coefficient of melanin decreases as wavelength increases, near-infrared and infrared wavelengths bypass melanin within the epidermis and penetrate deep within the dermis. With the use of cooling devices, which help to protect the epidermis, infrared light devices can deliver high fluences to the dermis. Within the dermis, there is increased fibroblast activity and increased collagen production.[48]

There are several devices that help to improve skin texture and hence rejuvenate the skin. The 1320-nm Nd:YAG laser is one of the most commonly used lasers for skin rejuvenation. This laser induces changes within the dermis and possibly the epidermis depending on the pulse duration by heating dermal water at 50–300 μm. The 1320-nm Nd:YAG laser produces collagen enhancement by scattering the thermal energy throughout the dermis owing to its nonspecific absorption of water within the papillary and midreticular dermis. In addition, there is epidermal spongiosis and edema of the basal cell layer, suggesting subclinical epidermal injury, which helps to improves skin texture.[49,50] Fatemi and colleagues[50] suggest that mediators and cytokines released from the injured epidermis contribute to fibroblast formation and collagen remodeling. The histologic results are impressive, with clinical outcomes often lagging behind. Trelles and colleagues[51] found that treatment with the nonablative 1320-nm laser, although safe, resulted in low patient satisfaction for improvement of facial rhytides after eight sessions. However, when Trelles reevaluated the patients months later, there was clinical improvement.[52] Nevertheless, clinical results are often subtle, and multiple treatments may be necessary. It appears that better improvement may be had with the 1320-nm Nd:YAG laser with fluence and skin cooling adjusted to a T_{max} of 45–48°C and multiple passes to a total of three. There are no published reports on use of the 1320-nm Nd:YAG laser in patients with skin phototype VI with the aforementioned parameters.[50]

Chan and colleagues[49] were the first to study the effectiveness of this laser in wrinkle reduction and the treatment of acne scarring. Twenty-seven women received three passes that were performed every 4–6 weeks for a total of five to six treatments. Fluence was adjusted so that the skin temperature reached 42–45°C immediately after laser exposure for the precooling pass and less than 40°C degrees for the postcooling pass. Patients noted on a scale of 0–9.8 a 4.9 improvement of wrinkle reduction and on a scale from 0–10 an improvement of 4 for acne scarring. Mild to moderate improvement of collagen production was seen in most patients. Unexpectedly, the epidermal thickness increased in fewer than half the patients. This may suggest more epidermal improvement than was previously thought. Side effects encountered were infrequent but included blistering in five patients and postinflammatory hyperpigmentation in three.

The 1320-nm Nd:YAG laser has shown little improvement on dyschromia. However, the IPL system for nonablative skin rejuvenation achieves reduction in pigmentary alterations. The broad-band polychromatic light allows penetration to varying depths within the skin, thereby targeting multiple chromophores including melanin. The use of cutoff filters allows the elimination of shorter wavelengths of the visible spectrum to limit melanin absorption. Pulse widths are determined to match the thermal relaxation time of the targets. Collagen stimulation has been noted and the are some reports of improvement of elastic fiber proliferation. Phototype IV patients are suitable. Caution should be used when treating phototype V patients. Phototype VI patients should be avoided. As has been noted, there is a significant learning curve with the IPL system, owing to the multiple Parameters that are adjustable. The novice laser surgeon should be at ease with treating patients with skin phototypes I to III before performing the procedure on darker-skinned patients. Mild fluences, appropriate cutoff filters to block shorter wavelengths, and longer pulse widths and delay are imperative when treating skin of color types. Depending on the complexion of the individual, erythema may not be obvious. Excessive erythema, vesiculation, and graying of the skin are tissue effects that indicate too aggressive parameters.

Negishi and colleagues[30] investigated use of the IPL system in Asians for skin rejuvenation. After three to six treatments 2–3 weeks apart, the 97 patients experienced 90% improvement in pigmentation, 83% improvement in telangiectasias, and 65% improvement in texture. Blistering and erythema were experienced by four patients.

The long-pulse 1064-nm laser and, in some reports, the Q-switched 1064-nm laser help to rejuvenate the skin and reduce acne scarring.[53] The long infrared wavelength penetrates deep into the dermis to remodel collagen. There is histologic improvement with both systems. The long-pulse Nd:YAG laser is used frequently. The mechanism of action remains unclear. However, dermal heating with subsequent cytokines release and stimulation of fibroblast proliferation induces collagen remodeling.

Combination Approach

A combination and synergistic approach for skin rejuvenation is advantageous. Lee and colleagues[54] treated 150 patients with the long-pulsed KTP 532-nm laser and the long-pulsed Nd:YAG laser either separately or in combination depending on phototype. Patients were treated monthly ranging between three and six times and observed up to 18 months after the last treatment. All patients were noted to have mild to moderate improvement in skin tone, texture, erythema, and pigmentation. The combined use of the KTP and Nd:YAG lasers was superior to either laser alone. Trelles and colleagues[55] reported improvement with the synergistic action of the 595-nm laser with the 1450-nm laser for skin rejuvenation. The 595-nm laser's targeting of melanin and hemoglobin improves skin texture and dyspigmentation. The 1450-nm laser's targeting of water and penetration deep within the dermis to a level of 644 μm in the skin stimulates collagen formation. The two lasers together augment the often subtle clinical results of the use of one laser alone. The darkest participating phototype was IV.

Nevertheless, this combination synergistic approach for skin rejuvenation using nonablative lasers offers the best therapeutic modality for improving skin texture and quality in pigmented skin types. With one type of laser for skin rejuvenation, the clinical outcome is often subtle. The dual-laser approach with two synergistic lasers (an appropriate shorter-wavelength device coupled with a longer-wavelength device) may be the wave of the future in treating darker skin types for skin rejuvenation and acne scarring.

A new device that combines radiofrequency with either the diode laser or the IPL system has been developed to improve skin quality, including rhytides and laxity. The radiofrequency technology generates heat as a result of tissue impedance and depends on the electrical properties of tissue, not melanin. Thus radiofrequency is chromophore-independent. The mechanism of action of this combined technique is called *selective radiophotothermolysis.* The optical energy preheats the target chromophore. The temperature gradient that is created helps to conduct the radiofrequency component of the system. Higher temperatures produce a lower impedance, and the electric current will flow through a path of least resistance. The heat generated lowers the impedance at the target, which allows easy conduction of radiofrequency to the target chromophore. The combination of the two energy sources damages the target chromophore. The thermal destruction sets up a cascade for dermal remodeling. With the use of these two systems, the optical energy can be lowered, which decreases the risk of the laser or broad-band light portion of the device. Thus this pulsed light or diode laser in the same pulse profile with the conduction of bipolar radiofrequency generates an Electro-optical Synergy (ELOS). This technology can be used on all skin types.

Most reported cases in the literature have been on skin phototypes I–IV.[56,57] There are no specific studies in the literature of the use of this technology on skin phototypes IV–VI. However, there are unpublished reports of its use on darker phototypes. For skin rejuvenation with the ELOS, multiple passes are necessary. There is little patient discomfort. Transient mild erythema and edema are common. The clinical achievements are skin tightening and delayed collagen remodeling. It is theorized that the optical energy helps with the superficial aspect of skin rejuvenation, for example, dyschromia and telangiectasias. The radiofrequency aspect of this device is responsible for heating the dermis to implement neocollagenesis.

Fractional Photothermolysis

Fractional photothermolysis is one of the newest nonablative laser treatments for facial rejuvenation. As with the other nonablative lasers, when there is dermal remodeling, there is improvement in acne scarring. Unlike the other nonablative devices that do not have direct epidermal improvement, fractional photothermolysis improves skin texture, which may lead to improvement in certain pigmentary dermatologic disorders such as melasma. Fractional photothermolysis uses a midinfrared laser for which the chromophore is water. Fractional photothermolysis produces tiny intentional wounds within the skin called *microscopic treatment zones* (MTZs) of thermal injury to improve skin tone and quality. These tiny columns of MTZs have a depth-to-width ratio of 5:1. The typical diameter is 150–200 μm with a depth of typically up to 1 mm. The stratum corneum stays intact, thus allowing for rapid healing and decreased risk of infection.

These intentionally created wounds (MTZs) are confined and self-contained without affecting the surrounding tissue. With an intact stratum corneum, a repair phase is initiated within the epidermis with reepithelialization and dermal remodeling. This nonablative technique delivers aspects of a mild clinical ablative resurfacing with nonablative dermal remodeling.

Histologically, there is complete epidermal and dermal necrosis that is confined to the MTZs. There is no confluent epidermal or dermal injury. These tiny submillimeter-size zones are likened to pixels in a digital photograph.

Healing time is rapid, with reepithelialization occurring in 24 hours. This allows the opportunity for multiple treatments to achieve a cosmetically acceptable outcome. Side effects are usually transient. Erythema, edema, xerosis, and flaking can be expected.

Although indicated for all skin types, most of the studies in the literature have been in skin phototypes I–IV. Studies for skin rejuvenation, acne scarring, and melasma will need to be conducted in darker-complexioned persons. The creation of MTZs with their epidermal injury causes legitimate concerns about potential postinflammatory hyperpigmentation and scarring for patients with darker skin phototypes, such as phototype VI. However, when performed cautiously in appropriate patients, this laser technique shows promise with skin phototypes IV–VI.

A test spot can be performed in persons with darker complexions. The posterior auricular location offers the best advantage. One can start with a test spot of initially a low density and low energy setting with varying degrees of increasing energy settings and number of passes (usually one to four depending on the dermatologic disorder). Waiting 1 month to determine the clinical outcome is necessary before a full facial treatment is done. It is not uncommon to treat regionally in patients with darker skin phototypes for the treatment of melasma and acne scarring. Prophylaxis with hydroquinone for a minimum of 1 month and the use of antiviral agents are prudent. Contraindications are tanned skin, oral retinoid use, and a history of keloids. Currently, the laser is being investigated to treat acne scarring in patients with darker skin phototypes.

SUMMARY

- Nonablative lasers are used to treat a variety of skin disorders ranging from superficial rhytides, to acne scarring, to textural irregularities and pigmentary and vascular dermatologic disorders.
- Numerous treatments are necessary.
- Clinical results vary and often are perceived as subtle.
- Fractional photothermolysis offers the best promise in treating a variety of dermatologic disorders in all skin types.

LASER-ASSISTED HAIR REMOVAL DEVICES

Laser-assisted hair removal achieves a permanent reduction of hair. With the advent of longer wavelengths, longer pulse durations, and efficient cooling devices, all skin types can experience a permanent reduction of hair with few or no side effects. By exploiting the competition of melanin in the epidermis with the use of longer wavelengths, there is less epidermal injury. Melanin absorption decreases as wavelength increases. The longer wavelengths penetrate deep into the dermis to the intended chromophore, melanin, within hair follicles. Longer pulse durations help to gently heat the intended chromophore while protecting the epidermis. With the slow delivery of light in the form of heat to the intended follicular chromophore, the epidermis heats up slowly, resulting in less thermal damage. In addition, efficient cooling devices further protect the epidermis from injury. Cooling devices can be contact or noncontact. Regardless, appropriate cooling helps to protect the epidermis. However, excessive cooling in pigmented skin can result in epidermal injury in the form of hyperpigmentation.

There are two lasers that were approved initially by the Food and Drug Administration (FDA) for laser-assisted hair removal in pigmented skin (phototypes IV–VI): the diode laser (810 nm) and the Nd:YAG laser (1064 nm). Both lasers with multiple treatments achieve a cosmetically acceptable permanent reduction of hair with few side effects. With each treatment, a patient can expect up to a 20% decrease in hair, with the remaining hair appearing finer or lighter in color. The tissue response is perifollicular edema that can last for a few minutes to hours and often results without pigmentary sequelae. It is important to note that in patients with darker skin tones the perifollicular edema may not be evident clinically. In addition, the hairs may singe during treatment, but nonsinged hairs are not the clinical endpoint. Excessive pain, frank erythema, and/or graying of the skin indicate too high a fluence. Blistering should not be encountered.

Test spots should be performed to determine the appropriate fluence and pulse duration. Test spots usually are placed in a representative area that has been shaven or clipped. Excessive hairs on the skin act as "hot coals" and potentially can cause epidermal injury. Immediate tissue response should be noted. Patients can return in 1 month to determine the latent tissue response and best clinical effect.

The IPL system for laser hair removal has been documented in the literature to achieve a permanent reduction of hair. These devices are not approved by the FDA for laser-assisted hair removal, however.

The ELOS technology is one of the newest approved devices for hair reduction. It combines bipolar radiofrequency with optical energy using either the diode laser or IPL source. The radiofrequency component of the system is not dependent on melanin to selectively heat the target, and the energy is not absorbed by melanin within the epidermis. Thus a lower level of optical energy can be used to make it safe for darker skin types. Published reports document its use for phototype VI. It is suggested that with ELOS-assisted hair removal, regardless of skin color, results are determined predominately by the level of radiofrequency and less so by the optical energy. Saddick and colleagues[58] reported after four treatments 6–8

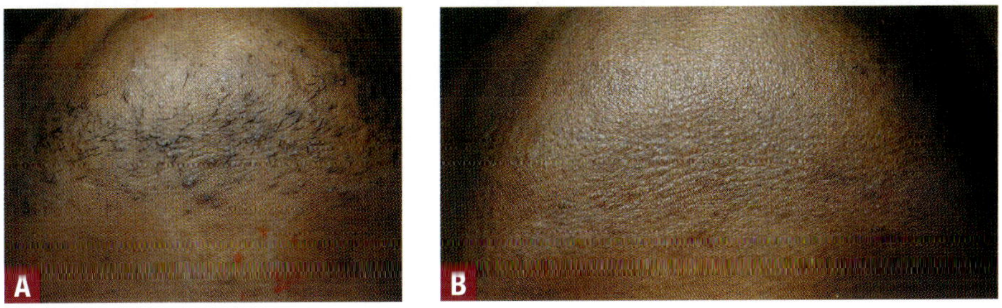

▲ **FIGURE 73-6** Laser-assisted hair removal by Cutera before (**A**) and after (**B**) 1064-nm long-pulsed laser removal at 30–35 J/cm², 10 mm spot, four treatments. Courtesy of Samuel Lederman, M.D.

weeks apart a 64–84% reduction of hair. Laughlin and colleagues,[59] in their study of 10 patients (phototypes V and VI), reported a mean hair loss of 30.2%. No blistering was seen. Yaghmai and colleagues,[60] in a multicentered study, enrolled 87 patients. Sixty-nine patients completed the study. Twenty-one patients were phototypes IV–VI. The patients received one treatment. There was an average of 46% reduction of hair counts from baseline, with 43% of patients having a 50% or greater reduction at 90 days. The authors concluded that the combination of optical energy and radiofrequency delivered simultaneously achieves effective hair reduction in all skin types. Transient scaliness and crusting were seen in two patients. Transient hyperpigmentation was noted in three patients, as well as transient hypopigmentation in one patient who was skin phototype III.

Hirsutism/Hypertrichosis

Unwanted hairs or excessive hairs are cosmetically unappealing. Hair on the face in women is the most challenging area to treat. With laser-assisted hair removal, terminal black hairs respond better than intermediate and fine hairs. Brown and light brown hairs are difficult and challenging to treat. Red, blonde, white, and gray hairs do not respond. The long-pulsed diode laser (100 ms or greater) can safely and effectively treat patients with skin phototypes V and VI.[61] Long-pulsed Nd:YAG lasers (30 ms or greater) were able to achieve a greater than 50% reduction in facial hairs in 6 months in patients with skin phototypes V and VI.[62] Multiple treatments every 1–2 months are necessary to achieve a cosmetically acceptable outcome. Side effects such as scarring, dyspigmentation, infection, and increased hair growth are rare. Increased hair growth, although extremely rare, can be frustrating to both the laser surgeon and the patient (Figure 73-6).

This phenomenon appears to be most common in persons of Mediterranean descent with ill-defined hairlines within the temporal region of the face. When encountered, multiple treatments are necessary, and if possible, changing the laser-assisted hair removal device is helpful (Table 73-2).

Pseudofolliculitis Barbae

Laser-assisted hair removal is considered the "gold standard" in the treatment of pseudofolliculitis barbae. Laser-assisted hair removal should be used only in patients who are willing to experience a permanent reduction in hair at the treatment site. When treating the bearded area, the laser surgeon needs to be aware of the *bridging effect*. The dense, thick terminal bearded hairs retain a greater amount of heat, which can lead to scarring. Therefore, it is important to decrease the fluence and increase the pulse duration when treating areas of high density. The long-pulsed Nd:YAG laser is best suited for pseudofolliculitis barbae.[63,64]

Acne Keloidalis Nuchae (AKN)

Laser-assisted hair removal is an adjunctive therapy for AKN. It works best when used in combination with standard therapies. Entrapped and tufted hairs are often difficult to treat even with laser systems. Milder cases that are more papular in nature are better suited for laser-assisted hair removal.

TABLE 73-2
Two Common Laser-Assisted Hair Removal Devices for Skin of Color

Wavelength	Pulse Width
800- to 810-nm diode	5–400 ms
1064-nm long-pulsed Nd:YAG*	0.1–300 ms

*The 1064-nm long-pulse device is ideal for skin of color, especially darker skin tones.

SUMMARY

- Laser-assisted hair removal is a permanent reduction in hair.
- Multiple treatments are necessary.
- Gray, blond, white, red, and light brown hairs have either no response or little response to laser-assisted hair removal.
- Thick black hairs are best treated.
- Side effects are rare.
- Aberrant induction of hair growth is an uncommon side effect of laser hair removal, occurring in persons most commonly of Mediterranean descent.
- Anecdotally, the phenotype of fine to intermediate hairs located within the temple area or the lateral forehead is at a greater risk of this phenomenon.
- The increased hair growth is often difficult to treat and requires multiple treatments and sometimes alternative laser-assisted hair removal devices.

LASERS FOR ACNE VULGARIS AND ACNE SCARRING

Although ablative resurfacing offers the most dramatic results in acne scarring, with improvement ranging from 30–50%, it is associated with significant downtime, a high side-effect profile, and limitations of its use on patients with darker skin phototypes. These reasons make it an uncommon therapeutic option. Nonablative lasers do play a role in improving acne scarring. The pulsed-dye laser, the 585-, 595-, and 1064-nm Nd:YAG lasers, the 1320-nm Nd:YAG laser, the 1450-nm diode laser, the 1540-nm erbium-glass laser, and the fractional nonablative (1550-nm) resurfacing laser help to improve acne scarring and skin textural irregularities. Acne scarring responds better to infrared wavelengths that target dermal water to stimulate collagen formation. These longer wavelengths penetrate deep to alter the structure of the sebaceous gland and promote neocollagenesis of the surrounding dermal tissues, thus improving acne scarring. The pulsed-dye laser, 1064-nm Nd:YAG laser, 1320-nm Nd:YAG laser, and the fractional laser all have been discussed previously in this text.

The 1450-nm laser has a penetrating wavelength that is absorbed by dermal water. It heats 300–400 μm below the skin surface to alter the structure of the sebaceous gland. Histologically, there is rupture of the pilosebaceous units. Although temporary, this alteration of the sebaceous gland hypothetically causes a reduction in the sebum secretion.[65] This alteration in sebaceous gland helps in the control of acne. In addition, there is dermal improvement of collagen, which aids in improving acne scarring.

With use of the 1450-nm laser, there is patient discomfort. Erythema and edema are expected, with erythema sometimes lasting more than 24 hours. Postinflammatory hyperpigmentation is sometimes encountered in patients with darker skin phototypes. Multiple treatments are necessary to achieve decreased lesional counts and control of acne.[66] Friedman and colleagues[67] were the first to report improvement of inflammatory back acne with the 1450-nm diode laser by showing decreased lesional counts after three treatments. Side effects of transient edema and erythema were minimal. Topical anesthetics were recommended for the associated discomfort.

Chua and colleagues[68] were among the first to report use of the 1450-nm diode laser in the treatment of facial acne scarring in patients with skin phototypes IV and V. The study enrolled 57 patients who received four to six treatments at 4-week intervals. Thirty-nine percent of patients reported significant scar improvement of between 11% and 20%, and 21% reported very significant improvement of between 21% and 50%. No one had over 50% improvement. Side effects included discomfort, with most patients reporting minimal to moderate pain. Postinflammatory hyperpigmentation was reported in 39% of patients. The authors felt that the increased percentage was due to aggressive cooling.

Tanzi and colleagues[69] compared the 1320-nm laser and the 1450-nm laser in 20 patients with facial acne scarring. Both systems improved the facial acne scarring, but the 1420-nm laser demonstrated greater improvement. The phototypes included in this study were I–V. After 6 months, there was modest improvement of facing acne scarring. Histologically, neocollagenesis was reported at 6 months but did not extend to 12 months. Postinflammatory erythema was more prolonged with the 1450-nm laser, and postinflammatory hyperpigmentation was seen in twice as many patients as those treated with the 1,320-nm laser. Patients did note concerns about lack of significant improvement.

The erbium-glass 1540-nm laser is used to treat inflammatory acne. The long infrared wavelength absorbs very little melanin and penetrates deep to the sebaceous gland and surrounding tissue to temporarily shrink and alter the gland. There is also dermal remodeling, which helps with acne scarring. Multiple treatments are necessary. Patient discomfort is minimal. Transient erythema is expected. Side effects are minimal. More studies are necessary to determine thes true efficacy of this system in the control of acne vulgaris in patients with darker skin phototypes.

Laser Resurfacing (LSR)

Laser resurfacing is largely a skilled dermatologic procedure that is best suited for patients with skin phototypes I and II. The ablative procedure using the CO_2 and/or erbium laser dramatically improves photoaging, including rhytides, hyperpigmentation, and lentigines. The procedure vaporizes the epidermis, requiring meticulous wound care. Erythema, edema, oozing, and crusting are common for the first week, with decreasing erythema and repithelialization over the next several weeks. Side effects are scarring, hyperpigmentation, hypopigmentation, and infection, with pigmentary alterations the greatest in patients with skin phototypes III and IV.

The CO_2 laser offers the most dramatic results in comparison with the Er:YAG laser. Both the CO_2 (10,600 nm) and the Er:YAG (2940 nm) infrared wavelengths are absorbed by water. The CO_2 laser heats and vaporizes intracellular water, resulting in tissue destruction. The heat generated denatures and shrinks collagen, causing a visible tightening of the skin during the procedure. There is tissue vaporization with nonselective thermal damage.

The erbium laser is a gentler alternative to the CO_2 laser. The Er:YAG wavelength is close to the absorption peak of water, which is 16 times greater than that of the CO_2 laser (a higher water absorption coefficient, 12,800/cm, compared with the CO_2 laser's water coefficient of 800/cm). The shallower absorption depth allows less residual thermal damage and faster healing time in comparison with the CO_2 laser. However, the clinical results with the erbium laser are less impressive than those with the CO_2 laser.

Although laser resurfacing has been performed on pigmented skin, the numbers treated are few. When performed correctly on lighter-complexioned phototypes, the results are superb. However, the great risk of scarring and dyspigmentation, the prolonged hyperpigmentation lasting for months, and the associated downtime make LSR an impractical option for skin of color rejuvenation.

In order to decrease the unacceptable side effects of scarring, expected transient hyperpigmentation, and the risk of permanently altered pigmentation, patient selection and counseling are crucial. Lighter-complexioned individuals will fare better than darker-skinned individuals. Experts have found that reducing prolonged erythema and inflammation (<2 weeks) will help to reduce unwanted pigmentary side effects.[70] Thus one-pass techniques with the CO_2 laser, gentle removal of desiccated tissue between passes to minimize erythema, and good perioperative (e.g., hydroquinones, tretinoin, sunscreens, mechanical and chemical peels, etc.) and postoperative regimens (e.g., reducing sun exposure, trauma, infection, etc.) will help to limit the unwanted side effects.[71] No overlapping or stacked pulsing is strongly recommended. To avoid lines of demarcation, it is recommended that no treatment be given to regional or focal areas. Pilnikorn and colleagues[72] laser resurfaced 50 patients (phototypes III and IV) with the Er:YAG laser for a myriad of dermatologic conditions. His group found improvement in all patients, with no reports of scarring. Ho and colleagues[73] treated patients with skin phototypes III and IV with acne scarring and facial rhytides with the CO_2 laser. All patients were treated pre- and postoperatively with hydroquinones, tretinoin, and desonide 0.1% in addition to sunscreens postoperatively. There was a 25–50% improvement with acne scarring and rhytides. These resurfaced focally first to specific problematic areas with one to four passes, followed by one laser pass to the entire cosmetic unit, or vice versa.

New ablative devices such as the variable-pulsed Er:YAG resurfacing laser, the 1540- and 1420-nm fractional Er:YAG resurfacing laser, and the fractional 10,600-nm CO_2 resurfacing laser show a significant decrease in edema, erythema, downtime, and scarring with a faster healing time for the patient in comparison with conventional ablative CO_2 lasers. Multiple treatments are necessary. In comparison with traditional

CO_2 resurfacing, the clinical results are not as dramatic in the reduction of rhytides and the improvement of photoaging. Unfortunately, these newer devices are not indicated in patients with darker skin phototypes. There are limited reports in the literature on the use of these fractional ablative devices in patients with skin phototype IV. Studies are still needed to determine its true efficacy in persons of color.

Laser resurfacing can be achieved in lighter individuals with skin of color (phototype IV) with caution. With the advent of nonablative lasers, laser resurfacing should be reserved for select patients for whom the benefits outweigh the risks. Darker-skinned patients (phototypes V and VI) should be strictly avoided. Postinflammatory hyperpigmentation is expected and can last for months. The procedure should be reserved for experts. Patients should be counseled in detail on the side effects, which can be transient or permanent. Postoperative monitoring with strict sun avoidance is crucial.

SUMMARY

- Laser resurfacing should be reserved for patients with skin phototypes I–III.
- Patients with skin phototypes IV–VI should be treated cautiously.
- Patient selection is the key.
- Prophylaxis and meticulous postlaser care are crucial for a successful outcome.
- The benefits should outweigh the risks.
- Owing to the high risk of scarring in persons with pigmented skin and the risk of permanent hypopigmentation, laser resurfacing should not be conducted by novice laser surgeons but should be reserved for those who are true experts in the field.

CONCLUSION

With the advent of new lasers and light sources, never before has there been a better time for the dermatologic laser surgeon. Research in the laser subspeciality of pigmented skin is slowly evolving. Clearly, much more is needed. With the increasing demand for the use of lasers for people of color, the laser surgeon is and will be constantly challenged. However, with a firm understanding of laser and skin optics, one can efficaciously treat all skin types for a variety of dermatologic disorders.

REFERENCES

1. US Census Bureau, 2003, *www.usatoday.com/news/nation/census/2003-06-18-census_x.htm.*
2. Einstein A. Zurguantentheorie der strahlung. *Physik Z* 1917;18:121-128.
3. Anderson RR, Parrish JA. The optics of human skin. *J Invest Dermatol* 1981;77:13-19.
4. Anderson RR, Parrish JA. Selective thermolysis:precise microsurgery by selective absorption of pulsed radiation. *Science* 1983;220:524-527.
5. Jacobs HA, Walton RG. The incidence of birth marks in the neonate. Pediatrics 1976;58:218-222.
6. Morelli JG, Weston WL, Huff JC, Yohn JJ. Initial lesion size as a predictive factor in determining the response of port-wine stains in children treated with pulsed dye laser. *Arch Pediatr Adolesc Med* 1995;149:1142-1144.
7. Ho WS, Chan HH, Ying SY, Chan PC. Laser treatment of congenital facial port wine stains: Long term efficacy and complication in Chinese patients. *Lasers Surg Med* 2002;30:44-47.
8. Tong AK, Tan OT, Eng JB, et al. Ultrastructure: effects of melanin pigment on target specificity using a pulsed dye laser (577 nm). *J Invest Dermatol* 1987;6:747-752.
9. Van Kampen EJ, Zijlstra WG. Determination of hemoglobin and its derivatives, in Sobotka H, Stewart CP (eds), *Advances in Clincial Chemistry,* Vol 8. New York, Academic Press, 1965, pp 158-187.
10. Scherer, K, Lorenz, S, Wimmershoff, M, et al. Both the flashlamp-pumped dye laser and the long pulsed tunable dye laser can improve results in port-wine stain therapy. *Br J Dermatol* 2001;145: 79-84.
11. Chang CJ, Kelly KM, van Gemert MJ, Nelson JS. Comparing the effectiveness of 585 nm vs 595 nm wavelength pulsed dye laser treatment of port wine stains in conjunction with cryogen spray cooling. *Lasers Surg Med* 2002;31:352-358.
12. Anderson RR. Laser-tissue interactions in dermatology, in Arndt KA, Dover JS, Olbricht SM (eds), *Lasers in Cutaneous and Aesthetic Surgery.* Philadelphia, Lippincott-Raven, 1977, pp 25-51.
13. Dierickx CC, Casparian JM, Venugopalan V, et al. Thermal relaxation of port-wine stain vessels probed in vivo: the need for 1-10 millisecond laser pulse treatment. *J Invest Dermatol* 1995;105: 709-714.
14. Sommer S, Sheehan-Dare RA. Pulsed dye lser treatment of port-wine stains in pigmented skin. *J Am Acad Dermatol* 2000;42:667-671.
15. Ho WS, Ying SY, Chan PK, Chan HH. Treatment of port wine stains with intense pulsed light: A prospective study. *Dermatol Surg* 2004;30:887-891.
16. Bowers RE, Graham EA, Tomlinson KM. The natural history of the strawberry nevus. *Arch Dermatol* 1960;82:667-680.
17. Mariwalla K, Dover JS. The use of lasers in the pediatric population. *Skin Ther Lett* 2005;8:7-9.
18. Kono T, Takashi Y, Erocen AR, et al. Treatment of leg veins with the long pulse dye laser using variable pulse durations and energy fluences. *Lasers Surg Med* 2004;35:62-67.
19. Trelles MA, Allones I, Alvarez J. The 800 nm diode laser in the treatment of leg veins: Assessment at 6 months. *J Am Acad Dermatol* 2006;54:282-289.
20. Goldman M. Laser treatment of leg veins with 1064 nm long-pulsed lasers. *Cosmet Dermatol* 2000;5:27-30.
21. Weiss RA, Dover JS. Laser surgery of leg veins. *Dermatol Clin* 2002;20:19-36.
22. Saddick N, Trelles MA. A clinical, histological and computer-based assessment of the Polaris LV, combination diode, and radiofrequency system, for leg veins. *Lasers Surg Med* 2005;36:98-104.
23. Craft N. Keloids: Current concepts in pathogenesis and treatment. *Cosmet Dermatol* 2002;15:35-39.
24. Alster T, Williams CM. Treatment of keloid sternotomy scars with 585 nm flashlamp-pumped pulsed dye laser. *Lancet* 1995;13:1198-1200.
25. Manuskiatti W, Fitzpatrick RE. Treatment response of keloidal and hypertrophic sternotomy scars: Comparison among intralesional corticosteroid, 5-FU (5-fluorouracil) and 585 flashlamp-pumped pulsed dye laser treatments. *Arch Dermatol* 2002;138: 1149-1155.
26. Zelickson BD, Kilmer SL, Bernstein E. Pulsed dye laser therapy for sun damage skin. *Lasers Surg Med* 1999;25:229-236.
27. Tanghetti E, Sherr MS, Alvarado SL. Multiple treatment of photodamage using the pulse dye laser. *Dermatol Surg* 2003;29:686-691.
28. Bjerring P, Clement M, Heickendorff L, et al. Selective nonablative wrinkle reduction by laser. *J Cutan Laser Ther* 2000; 2: 9-15.
29. Hsu TS, Zelickson B, Dover JS, et al. Multicenter study of the safety and efficacy of a 585 nm pulsed-dye laser for the nonablative treatment of facial rhytides. *Dermatol Surg* 2005;31:1-9.
30. Negishi K, Tezuka Y, Kudshikata N, Wakamatsu S. Photorejuvenation for Asian skin by intense pulsed light. *Dermatol Surg* 2001;27:627-632.
31. Negishi K, Wakamatsu S, Kushikatat N, et al. Full-face photorejuvenation of photodamage skin by intense pulsed light with integrated contact cooling: Initial experiences in Asian patients. *Lasers Surg Med* 2002;30:298-305.
32. Hernandez-Perez E, Ibiett E. Gross and microscopic findings in patients submitted to nonablative full face resurfacing using intense pulsed light: A preliminary study. *Dermatol Surg* 2001;27:627-632.
33. Zelickson BD, Mehregan DA, et al. Clinical and histologic evaluation of psoriatic plaques treated with a flash lamp pulsed dye laser. *J Am Acad Dermatol* 1997;35:64-68.
34. Hacker SM, Rasmussen JE. The effect of flashlamp-pulsed dye laser on psoriasis. *Arch Dermatol* 1992;128:853-855.
35. Lanigan SW, Katugampola GA. Treatment of psoriasis with the pulsed dye laser. *J Am Acad Dermatol* 1997;37:288-289.
36. de Leew J, Tank B, Bjerring P, et al. Concomitant treatment of psoriasis of the hands and feet with pulsed dye laser and topical calcipotriol, salicylic acid or both: A prospective open study in 41 patients. *J Am Acad Dermatol* 2006;54: 266-271.

37. Asawononda P, Anderson RR, Chang Y, et al. 308-nm excimer laser for the treatment of psoriasis: A dose-response study. *Arch Dermatol* 2000;136:619-624.
38. Macedo O, Alster TS. Laser treatment of darker skin tones: a practical approach. *Dermatol Ther* 2000;13:114-126.
39. Kawada A, Shiraishi H, Mutsuyo A, et al. Clinical improvement of solar lentigines and ephelides with an intense pulsed light source. *Dermatol Surg* 2002;28: 504-508.
40. Wang CC, Sue YM, Yang CH, Chen CK. A comparison of Q switched alexandrite laser and intense pulsed light for the treatment of freckles and lentigines in Asian persons: A randomized, physician-blinded, split face comparison trial. *J Am Acad Dermatol* 2006;54:804-810.
41. Watanabe S, Takahashi H. Treatment of nevus of ota with the Q-switched ruby laser. *N Engl J Med* 1994;331:1745-1750.
42. Chan HH, Ying SY, Ho WS, et al. An in vivo trial comparing the clinical efficacy and complications of Q-switched alexandrite and Q-switched 1064 nm Nd:YAG lasers in the treatment of nevus of Ota. *Dermatol Surg* 2000;26:919-922.
43. Taylor C, Anderson RR. In effective treatment of refractory melasma and postinflammatory hyperpigmentation by Q switched ruby laser. *J Dermatol Surg Oncol* 1994;20:592-597.
44. Wang CC, Hui CY, Sue YM, et al. Intense pulsed light for the treatment of refractory melasma in Asian persons. *Dermatol Surg* 2004;30:1196-1200.
45. Moreno Arias GA, Ferrando J. Intense pulsed light for melanocytic lesions. *Dermatol Surg* 2001;27:397-400.
46. Negishi K, Kushikata N, Tezuka Y, et al. Study of the incidence and nature of "very subtle epidermal melasma" in relation to intense pulsed light treatment. *Dermatol Surg* 2004;30:881-886.
47. Kilmer S. Laser treatment of tattoos. *Dermatol Clin* 1997;15:409-417.
48. Menaker GM, Wrone DA, Williams RM, Moy RL. Treatment of facial rhytides with a nonablative laser: A clinical and histologic study. *Dermatol Surg* 1999;25(6): 440-444.
49. Chan HH, Lam L, Wong DS, et al. Use of 1,320 nm Nd:YAG laser for wrinkle reduction and the treatment of atrophic acne scarring in Asians. *Lasers Surg Med* 2004;34:98-103.
50. Fatemi A, Weiss MA, Weiss RA. Short-term histologic effects of nonablative resurfacing: Results with a dynamically cooled millisecond domain 1,320 nm Nd:YAG laser. *Dermatol Surg* 2002;28: 172-176.
51. Trelles MA, Allones I, Luna R. Facial rejuvenation with a nonablative 1,320 nm Nd:YAG laser: A preliminary clinical and histologic evaluation. *Dermatol Surg* 2001; 27:111-116.
52. Trelles MA. Short and long term follow up of nonablative 1,320 nm Nd:YAG laser facial rejuvenation. *Dermatol Surg* 2001;27:781-782.
53. Lipper G, Perez M. Nonablative acne scar reduction a short pulsed 1064 nm Nd:YAG (Abstract). American Society of Laser Medicine and Surgery, 2002 (Abstract 290).
54. Lee M. Combination 532 nm and 1064 nm lasers for noninvasive skin rejuvenation and toning. *Arch Dermatol* 2003;139: 1265-1276.
55. Trelles MA, Allones I, Levy JL, et al. Combined nonablative skin rejuvenation with the 595 nm and 1,450 nm. *Dermatol Surg* 2004;30:1292-1298.
56. Saddick N. Electro-optical synergy in aesthetic medicine: Novel technology, multiple applications. *Cosmet Dermatol* 2005;18:201-206.
57. Doshi SN, Alster TS. Combination radiofrequency and diode laser for treatment of facial rhytides and skin laxity. *J Cosmet Laser Ther* 2005;7:11-15.
58. Saddick N. Combination radiofrequency and light energies:electo-optical synergy technology in aesthetic medicine. *Dermatol Surg* 2005;31:1211-1217.
59. Laughlin SA. *Epilation in Dark Skin (Types V and VI) with Integrated Radio-Frequency and Optical Energy (data onfile).* Yokneam, Israel, Syneron Medical Ltd, 2008.
60. Yaghmai D, Garden J, Bakus A, et al. Hair removal using a combination radio-frequency and intense pulsed light source. *J Cosmet Laser Ther* 2004;6:201-207.
61. Battle E, Suthamjariya K, Alora M, et al. Very long pulse (20-200 ms) diode laser for hair removal on all skin types (abstract). *Lasers Surg Med* 2000;2:21S.
62. Alster TS, Bryan H, Williams CM. Long-pulsed Nd:YAG laser assisted hair removal in pigmented skin: A clinical and histological evaluation. *Arch Dermatol* 2001;137:885-889.
63. Ross EV, Cooke L, Overstreet K, et al. Treatment of psedofolliculitis barbae in very dark skin with long pulse Nd:YAG Laser. *J Natl Med Asso* 2002;94:888-893.
64. Weaver SM, Sagaral EC. Treatment of pseudofolliculitis barbae using the long pulsed Nd:YAG laser on skin types V and VI. *Dermatol Surg* 2003;29:1187-1191.
65. Doshi S, Alster TS. 1450 nm long pulsed diode for nonablative skin rejuvenation. *Surg Dermatol* 2005;31;1223-1226.
66. Jih MH, Friedman PM, Goldberg LH, et al. The 1450 nm diode laser for facial inflammatory acne vulgaris: Dose response and 12 month follow-up study. *J. Am Acad Dermatol* 2006; 55:80-86.
67. Friedman PM, Jih MH, Kimyasi-Asadi A, Goldberg LH. Treatment of inflammatory facial acne vulgaris with the 1450 nm diode laser: A pilot study. *Dermatol Surg* 2004;30:147-151.
68. Chua SH, Ang P, Khoo LS, Goh CL. Nonablative 1450 nm diode laser in the treatment of facial atrophic acne scars in type IV to V Asian skin: A prospective clinical study. *Dermatol Surg* 2004;30: 1287-1291.
69. Tanzi El, Alster T. Comparison of a 1450 nm diode laser and a 1320 nm Nd:YAG laser in the treatment of atrophic facial scars: A prospective clinical and histologic study. *Dermatol Surg* 30;2:152-157.
70. Esparza JR, Lupton JR. Laser resurfacing of darkly pigmented patients. *Dermtol Clin* 2002;20:113-121.
71. David L, Ruiz-Esparza J. Faster healing after laser skin resurfacing: The minmal mechanical trauma technique. *Dermatol Surg* 1997;23:395-361.
72. Pilnikorn N, Goldberg D, Suwanchinda A, Weng S. Erbium:YAG laser resurfacing in Asians. *Dermatol Surg* 1998;24: 1303-1307.
73. Ho C, Nguyen Q, Lowe N, et al. Laser resurfacing in pigmented skin. *Dermatol Surg* 1995;21:1035-1037.

CHAPTER 74

Liposuction

Ella L. Toombs

Key Points

- The ideal cosmetic liposuction is in a healthy adult of any age who is not overweight, has good skin elasticity, and has isolated areas of fat that do not respond to diet and exercise.
- There are ethnic differences in regard to body habitus. In addition, patients of different ethnicities will have different desired outcomes of liposuction.
- The areas treated most often with cosmetic liposuction are submandibular/neck, male breasts, abdomen, hips, flanks/lateral thighs, and medial thighs.

Liposuction surgery is a sculpting technique designed to eliminate localized areas of cosmetically unwanted adipose tissue in order to achieve a more slender silhouette. Innovations in anesthesia, equipment, and technique have elevated the surgical removal of fat to a level of safety, precision, and predictability that epitomizes the philosophy of cosmetic surgery. Statistics compiled by the American Society for Aesthetic Plastic Surgery (representing dermatologists, otolaryngologists, and plastic surgeons) rank liposuction as the most frequently performed cosmetic surgical procedure in both males and females. Over 380,000 liposuctions were completed in the United States in 2003—a 125% increase over 1997 (170,000); non-Caucasians as a group represented 20% of patients on whom cosmetic surgery was performed.[1] According to the American Society of Plastic Surgeons, 6%, 5%, 3%, and 3% of Hispanics, African-Americans, Asians, and "other non-Caucasians" underwent cosmetic surgical procedures in 2003.[2]

HISTORICAL PERSPECTIVE

Charles Dujarrier is credited with the earliest attempt at localized fat removal.[3] In 1921, he used a uterine curette to remove adipose tissue from the knees and calves of a dancer. Injury to one of the femoral arteries resulted in loss of one of the treated legs. Forty years later, in 1964, Schrudde tried to remove fat from the leg through incision and curettage. The postoperative course was complicated by the development of hematomas and seromas.[4] Also, in the 1960s, Pitanguy performed resection of skin and fat of the thigh; visibility of the incisions made the outcome less than ideal.[5] In 1976, Arpad and Fisher of Italy described the use of suction attached to blunt-tipped cannulas, which were inserted into 5-mm skin incisions, enabling suction of unwanted adipose tissue.[6] Later, Fournier in Paris developed the *dry technique;* Illouz, also in Paris, preferred the *wet technique.* Both became leaders in the field.[3,7] American dermatologists, otolaryngologists, and plastic surgeons traveled to Europe to learn this new cosmetic surgical procedure. Julius Newman, an American otolaryngologist, coined the term *liposuction,* taught the first liposuction course in the United States, and formed the American Society of Liposuction Surgery in 1982. Liposuction became part of the core curriculum in dermatology at Tulane University School of Medicine in 1987, the same year that dermatologist Jeffrey Klein described *tumescent anesthesia.*[3,8] The tumescent technique completely revolutionized liposuction surgery and has been used subsequently in other dermatologic surgical procedures such as hair transplants and dermabrasion.[9,10] The American Academy of Dermatology became the first society to publish guidelines for liposuction in 1991.[11] The American Society for Dermatologic Surgery published guidelines for liposuction in 2000.[12] Smaller cannulas were developed, aspirators became more efficient, and finally, before the turn of the century, power liposuction was introduced.[13–15]

PATIENT SELECTION

The goal of liposuction is removal of localized areas of excess adipose tissue that results in loss of inches and a more desirable body contour. The ideal candidate is a nonoverweight, healthy adult of any age with good skin elasticity who has isolated areas of fat that are unresponsive to diet and exercise. Bilateral full-skin-thickness "pinch tests" from the proposed site provide the surgeon and patient with an estimate of the amount of removable fat, quality of skin tone, and symmetry and an assessment of underlying muscle integrity. Cutaneous abnormalities such as striae, hyperpigmentation, and cellulite should be pointed out to the patient. Hypertrophic scars and keloids involving skin other than the earlobes are relative contraindications. During the consultation, patients are given the surgical consent form in order to ensure that they understand the benefits, limitations, and risks associated with liposuction.

Serum chemistry, complete blood counts, clotting times, and human immunodeficiency virus (HIV) evaluations are performed on all patients. Electrocardiograms and chest x-rays are ordered on patients over 40 years of age. Abnormalities require clearance by the primary care physician.

EQUIPMENT

Basic equipment for liposuction includes an infiltration system for tumescent fluid infusion, an aspirator (and backup) with disposable containers, and blunt-tipped cannulas of varying lengths, diameters, and styles. A cardiac monitor (with pulse oximetry, blood pressure, pulse, and respiration readings) is advisable. For emergencies, a "crash cart" with oxygen/oxygen mask, IV kit, atropine, diazepam 5 mg/ml, Solu-Cortef 125 mg/ml, epinephrine 0.1 mg/ml, and lidocaine 50 mg/5 ml should be readily available.

TECHNIQUE

Anesthesia

Tumescent (*tumesc,* "balloon up") anesthesia is a drug-delivery system designed to optimize the anesthetic effect of lidocaine at the target tissue site, minimize lidocaine absorption, while maximally expanding the defined compartment. Tissue expansion serves as a buffer zone, preventing trauma to the underlying tissue, and provides the additional benefit of local hydrostatic pressure, which in conjunction with epinephrine decreases bleeding.[9,10,16] The use of tumescent anesthesia in liposuction eliminates the need for general anesthesia and its attendant risks. Patients walk in for surgery and walk out after surgery. Depending on the area treated, many patients return to work the next day.

Studies support the average safe dose of lidocaine to be 45–60 mg/kg; men may be more sensitive and require a

TABLE 74-1
Inhibitors of Cytochrome P450-3A4*

Clarithromycin	Erythromycin	Fluconazole
Ketoconazole	Cimetidine	Diazepam
Isoniazid	Itraconazole	Nifedipine
Sertraline	Ritonavir	Metronidazole
Diltiazem	Acetozolamide	Omeprazole

*This list is not all-inclusive.

15% dosage reduction.[9,10] It is important to note that lidocaine is metabolized by the cytochrome P450 isozyme 3A4; therefore, it is recommended that other drugs metabolized by the same isozyme be used with caution in patients undergoing tumescent liposuction[17] (Table 74-1).

General

Prophylactic oral antibiotics and antimicrobial skin cleansers are started 48 hours before the procedure; the former is continued for 8 days after surgery. With the consent of the primary care physician, drugs that inhibit cytochrome P450-3A4 are discontinued in the perioperative period to minimize possible lidocaine toxicity. Prior to infiltration of tumescent anesthesia, vital signs and measurements are recorded, digital photographs are taken, and areas to be suctioned are marked and agreed on by the patient. After sterile prepping and draping, incisions are strategically placed in locations where they are least noticeable (e.g., submental, umbilical, lateral thorax, and groin) and provide the most direct subcutaneous tissue access. The lowest effective and safe concentrations and volumes of tumescent anesthesia are used. Tumescence is adequate when the tissue is firmly ballooned. Cannulas with diameters of 4 mm or less are preferred. The cannula, parallel to the skin's surface with the apertures directed toward the fascia, is inserted into the deep layers of fat. The nondominant hand rests on the skin overlying the cannula and serves as a guide. During suctioning, the pinch test is performed frequently in order to ensure symmetry. On completion, incision sites are dressed and/or sutured, and compression garments are worn for 7–14 days depending on the area.[12,13]

Ethnic Considerations

Approximately 40% of our liposuction patients are non-Caucasian, and 60% are men. In my experience, the primary ethnic differences in regard to body habitus are as follows:

- African-Americans tend to have larger buttocks.
- Asians tend to have more lower than upper abdominal fat.
- Hispanic women tend to have more prominence of the lateral thighs and hips.

Furthermore, there are differences in the desired outcome. In general, African-American woman are seemingly content with their gluteal dimensions (even if disproportionate) but do not like saddlebags. I have also noted ethnic differences in the texture of the subcutaneous tissue, with the subcutaneous and truncal fat of African-American men being more fibrous than that of other ethnic groups in whom I have performed liposuction. The same area in East Indian men is less fibrous than in other groups. I am unaware of any studies comparing the morphology of subcutaneous fat in different groups, but there are data suggesting racial differences in visceral-to-subcutaneous-fat ratios. African-Americans, Hispanics, and Asians seem to have more subcutaneous fat than age-matched Caucasians.[18–25]

AREAS MOST FREQUENTLY TREATED WITH COSMETIC LIPOSUCTION

Submandibular/Neck (Figure 74-1)

Neck sculpting is very rewarding for the patient and the surgeon. Removal of small quantities of adipose tissue (35–100 ml) results in an immediately noticeable improvement in the patient's profile. Familiarity with cutaneous anatomic landmarks and experience in liposuction are prerequisites.

A 3-mm horizontal submental crease incision provides cannula access from the angle of the mandibles laterally to the arch of the cricoid cartilage inferiorly. Suctioning is completed external to the platysma and medial to the sternocleidomastoid muscle using 1.5- to 3-mm-diameter nonaggressive standard cannulas. Unique to this area, the dermis is gently abraded, thereby enhancing skin contraction. Care should be taken to avoid the marginal branch of the mandibular nerve by lifting the skin away from the mandible and orienting the cannula medially and inferiorly. Postoperative compression garments are worn for 7 days.

Male Breast (Figure 74-2)

Preoperatively, correctable causes of gynecomastia/pseudogynecomastia

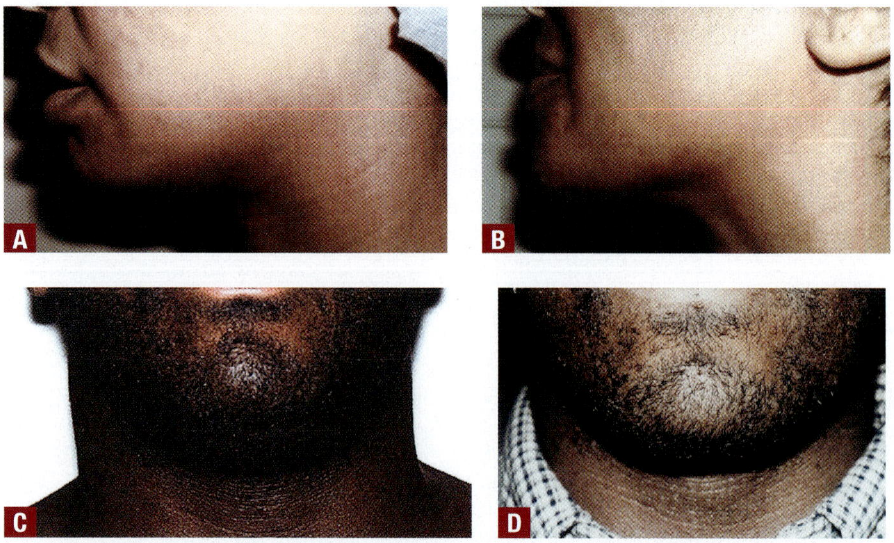

▲ **FIGURE 74-1** An African-American woman before *(A)* and after *(B)* liposuction of the neck and submandibular area. An African-American man before *(C)* and after *(D)* a similar procedure.

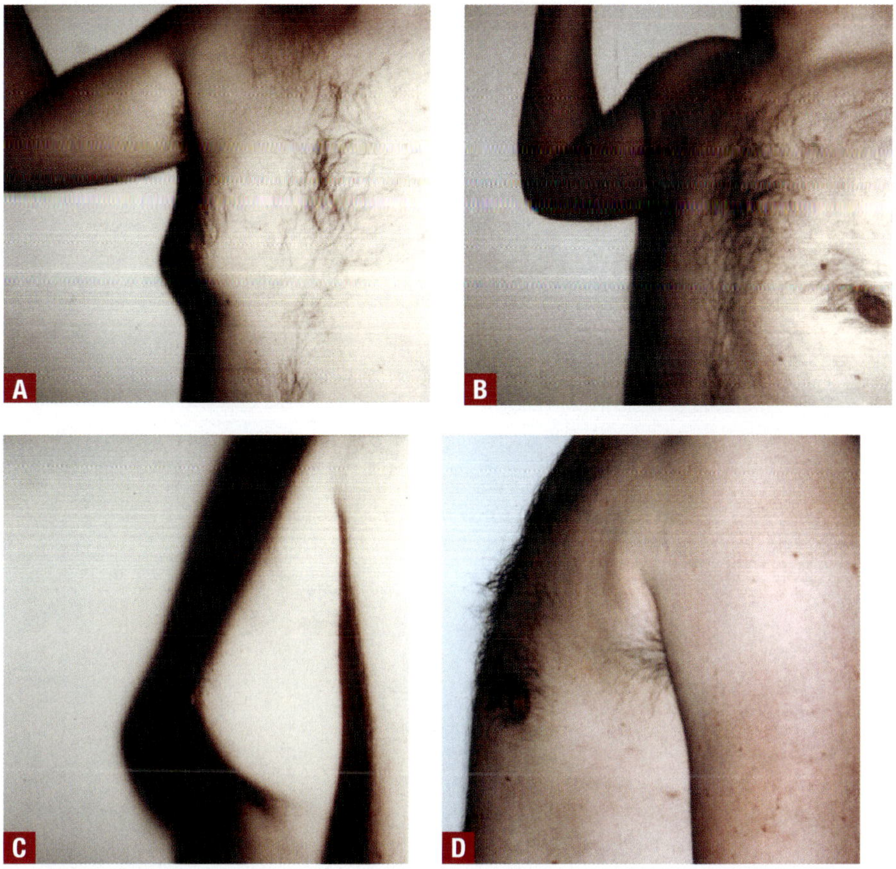

▲ **FIGURE 74-2** Liposuction of the male breast. Appearance before *(A, C)* and after *(B, D)* in a Hispanic man.

should be excluded by history (drugs) and physical examination (symmetry and masses)[26,27] (Table 74-2).

A 3- to 4-mm incision is made at the level of the serratus anterior in the anterior axillary line. Tissue debulking is completed simultaneous with mechanical tumescent solution infiltration (175–350 ml/breast). The goal of liposuction for enlarged male breasts is safe maximum tissue removal; therefore, aggressive grater and loop cannulas may be used, except under the areola and nipple. Suction is complete when the skin lies completely flat against the chest wall. Postoperative compression garments are worn for 3 weeks to ensure complete maximum skin contraction.

TABLE 74-2
Differential Diagnosis of Pathologic Gynecomastia

Testosterone Deficit	Increased Estrogen	Drugs
Congenital anorchia	Testicular tumors	Estrogen
Testicular feminization	True hermaphrodism	Ketoconazole
Kleinfelter syndrome	hCG-producing tumors	Metronidazole
Viral orchitis	Adrenal disease	Cisplatin
Trauma	Liver disease	Spironolactone
Castration	Malnutrition	Cimetidine
Granulomatous disease		Flutamide
Neurologic disease		Etomidate
Renal failure		Isoniazide
		Tricyclics
		Diazepam
		ACE inhibitors
		Heroin
		Marijuana

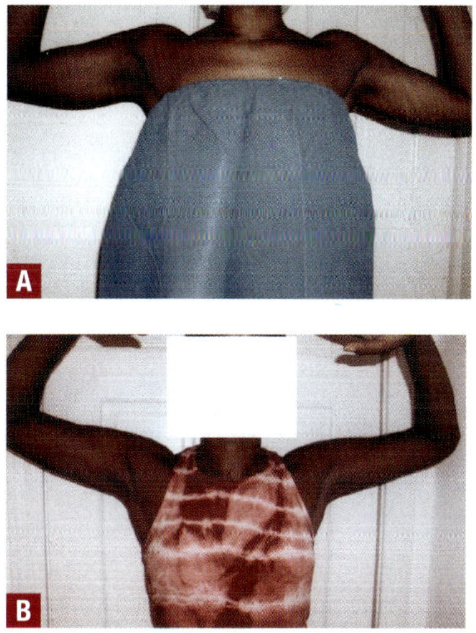

▲ **FIGURE 74-3** Liposuction of the upper arms. Appearance before *(A)* and after *(B)* in an African-American woman.

Upper Arms (Figure 74-3)

The skin of the upper arms is subject to dimpling and should be suctioned gently with nonaggressive cannulas. One 2- to 3-mm incision into the skin covering the olecranon fossa is sufficient for tumescent infusion and suction of the fat external to the triceps muscle. Nonaggressive long (22-cm) 3-mm or less manual cannulas and reciprocating power liposuction can be useful. The thin skin of the upper arm is subject to irregularities and may not contract well; therefore, err on the side of removing less. Proper positioning of the patient's arm when approaching the axilla avoids injury to the eighth cervical and first thoracic nerves of the brachial plexus. The patient is asked to wear the compression garment for 2 weeks postoperatively.

Abdomen (Figure 74-4)

Anecdotally, clinical variations in ethnic fat distribution and texture of the abdomen are discernible. African-Americans and Latinos tend to accumulate fat in the upper and lower abdomen. Asians and East Indians have greater fat accumulations in the lower abdomen. Asian and African-American women tend to have smaller waist-to-hip ratios than Latinos.

Suctioning of the lower abdomen can be completed successfully through incisions in the umbilicus (leaving no visible scar) and groin (midway between the femoral canal and the anterosuperior iliac spine). Treatment of the upper

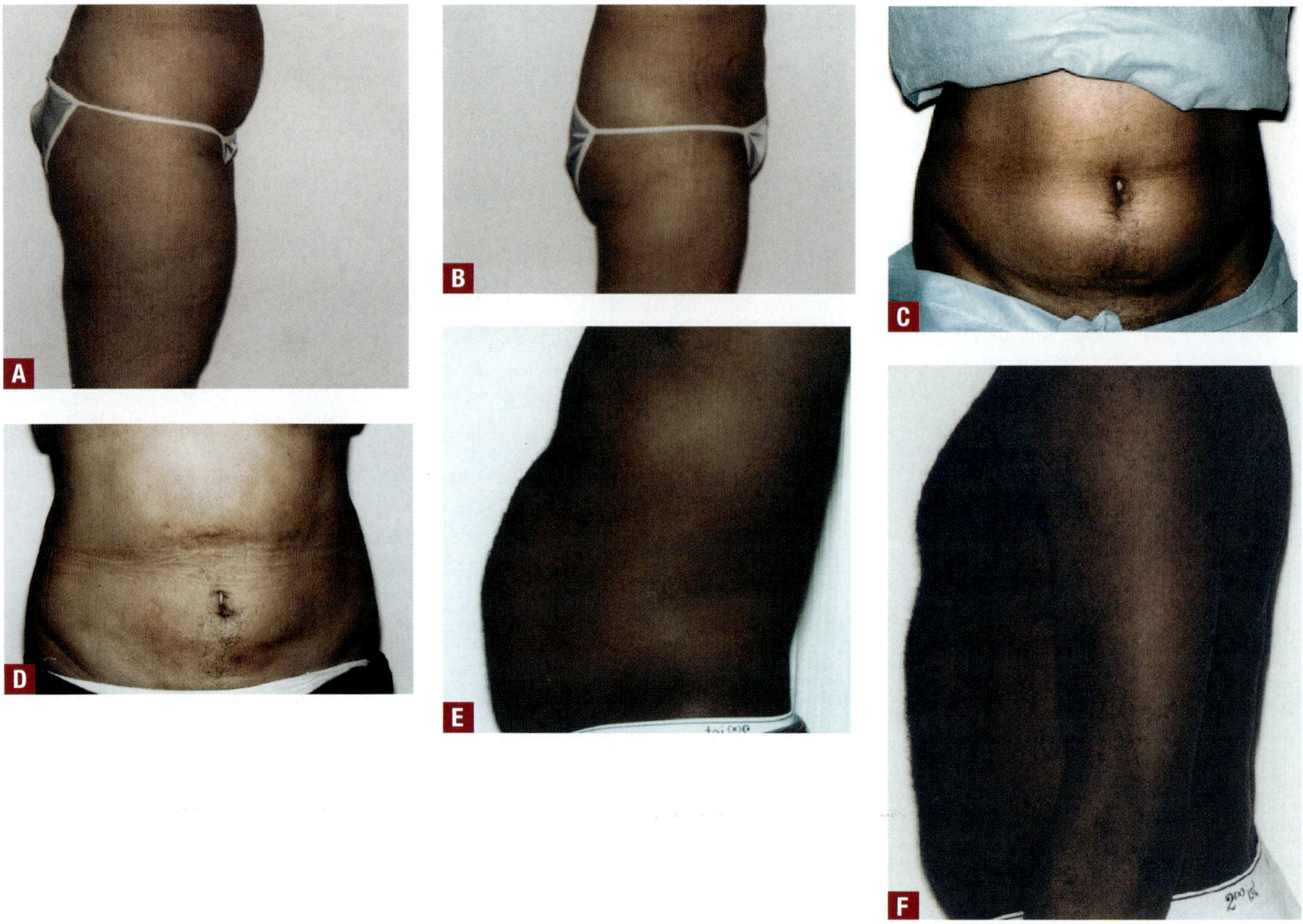

▲ **FIGURE 74-4** Liposuction of the abdomen. Appearance before *(A)* and after *(B)* in an African-American woman. Appearance before *(C)* and after *(D)* in another African-American woman. Appearance before *(E)* and after *(F)* in an African-American man.

abdomen requires additional incisions. Placing incisions asymmetrically in moles or inframammary creases is favored. Tumescent fluid infusion volumes (1.5–4 L) should be titrated to patient comfort levels. Suctioning is performed in the deep fat planes using vertical to-and-fro strokes with moderately aggressive short (15-cm) followed by long manual and power cobra cannulas whose apertures are directed away from the skin surface. Power sculpting significantly decreases physician fatigue and is soothing to the patient. Frequent pinching of the skin ensures symmetry. The tunnels created in the subcutaneous tissue should be drained after the fat has been removed by suctioning of residual tumescent fluid in order to decrease postoperative drainage. Patients should be instructed to gently message the skin toward the incision in lukewarm showers with each dressing change. Male patients should be informed of possible scrotal swelling; females may experience vulvar swelling. In both cases, resolution occurs in less than 7 days without sequelae. Wearing a compression garment for 2 weeks ensures that skin contraction will be excellent.

Flanks (Figure 74-5)

The surgeon is physically challenged by liposuction of the male flank. African-American and Hispanic men, regardless of age, seem to have more dense flank tissue than their age-matched East Indian and Asian counterparts. Aggressive debulking and suctioning with pinto and candy cane cannulas effectively remove the fibrofatty tissue in this area. Powered cannulas may be helpful; however, the thickness of the skin precludes their use exclusively.

One incision in the skin overlying the tubercle of the iliac crest is adequate for tumescence and suctioning small to medium flanks (350 mL or less). The tiny scar is barely perceptible. Larger flanks require an additional incision in the skin overlying the tenth rib in the midaxillary line. These sites also provide

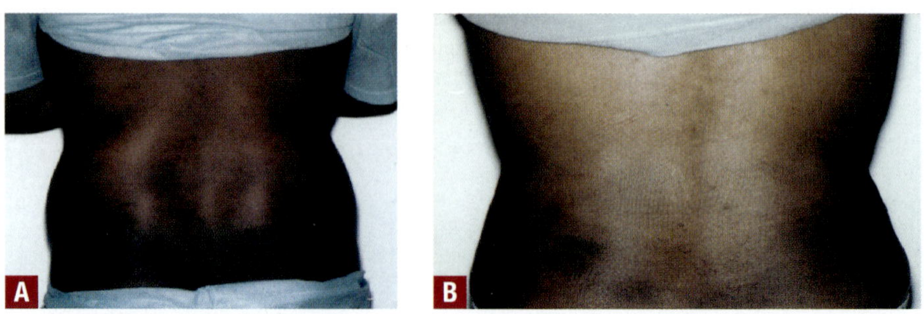

▲ **FIGURE 74-5** Liposuction of the flank. Appearance before *(A)* and after *(B)* in an East Indian man.

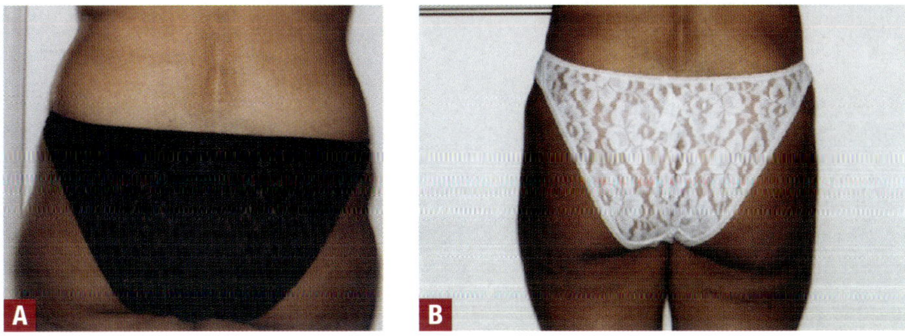

▲ **FIGURE 74-6** Liposuction of the hip and lateral thigh. Appearance before *(A)* and after *(B)* in a Hispanic woman.

access to the lower back and waistline without visible scarring. Two weeks of postoperative compression is generally well tolerated. The skin of the flanks is forgiving, and contraction is excellent.

Hip/Lateral Thigh (Figure 74-6)

Clinically, the quality of the subcutaneous tissue of the lateral thigh and hip is similar. Cosmetically, the contour of both can be disconcerting, even for otherwise slender women, and both areas may be suctioned in concert. Lower concentrations of xylocaine in the tumescent solution are well tolerated (150–300 ml/hip or thigh). Most patients want to attain or maintain the soft downward slope from the waistline to the hip and the gentle curve of the lateral thigh, and less aggressive suctioning preserves this balanced silhouette. Contouring of the hip is achieved by nonaggressive suction with a two-port standard cannula through an anterior gluteal incision. An infragluteal crease incision hides the scar of lateral thigh suctioning. A benefit of tumescent anesthesia is that patients can stand up during the procedure, allowing the surgeon to check for symmetry. Power sculpting works well in both areas. Hip and lateral and medial thigh compression for 10 days postoperatively helps to ensure good contraction.

Medial Thigh (Figure 74-7)

In contrast to the lateral thigh, the skin of the medial thigh, similar to the skin of the upper arm, is not forgiving. The skin is thin and more sensitive, and the fat is deep. Tumescence can be achieved with 75–150 ml of fluid infused into the inferomedial border of the protuberance, and 2-mm standard reciprocating cannulas are a good choice for this area. Suctioning should be less aggressive and confined to the deeper plane to avoid the "doll" medial thigh appearance.

OUTCOMES FOR PEOPLE OF COLOR

African-Americans, Asians, Africans, East Indians, Hispanics, and other non-Caucasians comprise about 20% of the patients undergoing cosmetic procedures. For procedures interrupting the skin of these individuals, adverse effects could include the development of keloids and/or hyperpigmentation. Regarding the former, I consider a history of keloids (other than earlobe) a contraindication for liposuction. Despite the large number of people of color on whom I have performed liposuction, I have never had a patient develop a keloid or a hypertrophic scar. Postoperative hyperpigmentation of the incision scar and skin overlying the surgical site are additional possible adverse events in patients of color. Although the incision sites for liposuction are small (2–4 mm), I have seen hyperpigmentation in scars. The response to compounded hypopigmenting creams and/or a single low dose of intralesional triamcinolone has been excellent. Dyspigmentation of skin overlying the suctioned site has not been seen. Excluding the neck, the cannulas are kept away from the dermis.

Tissue density is another factor that expresses ethnic variation. The density and fibrous component of the subcutaneous tissue seem greater in African-Americans, Africans, and Hispanics compared with East Indians, Asians, and Caucasians. No difference has been noted in healing or outcome.

Finally, and most important, body habitus, that is, contours and fat distribution, differs in various ethnic groups. Beauty is culturally defined. The surgeon should respect these differences in performing liposuction surgery.

COMPLICATIONS

All surgical procedures may have resulting complications. Complications from liposuction can include scarring, seromas, infections, pulmonary emboli, perforations, and death. Dermatologists performing liposuction have an excellent safety record.[25, 28–30] The risk is decreased by adherence to established guidelines, including physician training, patient selection, proper technique, separating multiple procedures, limiting the amount and type of anesthesia, and pre-, intra-, and postoperative monitoring/care.

CONCLUSION

The surgeon with an artistic eye and proper technique will find that the results of liposuction are excellent. Patients are pleased with their new, improved contour and the positive effect it has on their lifestyle.[31] The most important considerations include patient selection, patient communication, and individualizing the technique.

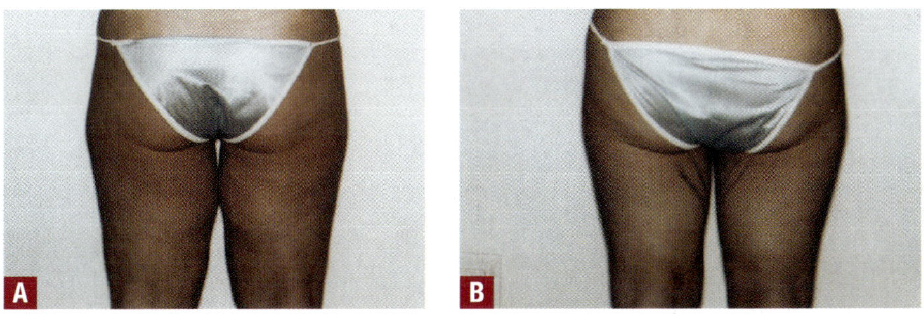

▲ **FIGURE 74-7** Liposuction of the medial thigh. Appearance before *(A)* and after *(B)* in an Asian woman.

REFERENCES

1. American Society of Aesthetic Plastic Surgery. *Report of 2003 Patient Statistics*, 2004.
2. American Society of Plastic Surgeons. *2003 Quick Facts on Cosmetic and Reconstructive Surgery*, 2004.
3. Coleman WP. The history of liposculpture. *J Dermatol Surg Oncol* 1990;16:1086.

4. Schruddle J. Lipexheresis for body conturing. *Clin Plastic Surg* 1982;11:445-456.
5. Pitanguy I. Trochanteric dystrophy. *Plast Reconstr Surg* 1964;34:280.
6. Fisher A, Fisher G. First surgical treatment for molding body's cellulite with three 5-mm incisions. *Bull Int Acad Cosmet Surg* 1976;3:35.
7. Fournier PF. Reduction syringe liposculpturing. *Dermatol Clin* 1990;8:539-551.
8. Klein JA. The tumescent technique for liposuction surgery. *Am J Cosmet Surg* 1987;4;263-267.
9. Lillis PJ. Liposuction surgery under local anesthesia: Limited blood loss and minimal lidocaine absorption. *J Dermatol Surg Oncol* 1988;14:1145-1148.
10. Ostad A, Kageyama N. Tumescent anesthesia with a lidocaine dose of 55 mg/kg is safe for liposuction. *Dermatol Surg* 1996;22:921-927.
11. Guidelines/Outcomes Committee. *Guidelines of Care for Liposuction.* Dermatology World Symposium, October 2000.
12. Task Force on Liposuction. American Society for Dermatologic Surgery guidelines of care for liposuction. *Dermatol Surg* 2000;26:265-269.
13. Weber PJ, Wulc AE. Warning: Traditional liposuction cannulas may be dangerous to your patient's health. *J Dermatol Surg Oncol* 1988;14:1136-1143.
14. Collins PS. Selection and utilization of liposuction cannulas. *J Dermatol Surg Oncol* 1988;17:1139-1143.
15. Coleman WP. Powered liposuction. *Dermatol Surg* 2000;26;315-318.
16. Hagerty T, Klein P. Fat partitioning of lidocaine in tumescent liposuction. *Ann Plast Surg* 1999;42:372-375.
17. Taro DS. Cytochrome P450 enzyme drug interactions. *Drug Newsletter* 1995;14: 59-61.
18. Deurenberg P, Bhaskaran K. Singaporean Chinese adolescents have more subcutaneous adipose tissue than Dutch Caucasians of the same age and body mass index. *Asia Pacific J Clin Nutr* 2003; 12:261-265.
19. Huang TT, Johnson MS. Growth of visceral fat, subcutaneous fat, and total body fat in children. *Obes Res* 2001;9: 283-289.
20. Okosun IS, Liao Y. Impact of birth weight on ethnic variations in subcutaneous and central adiposity in American children aged 5–11 years. *Int J Obes Relat Metab Disord* 2000;24:479-484.
21. Lovejoy JC, Smith RC. Comparison of regional fat distribution and health risk factors in middle aged white and African-American women. *Obes Res* 2001;9: 10-16.
22. Wolanski N. Comparison of growth patterns of subcutaneous fat tissue in Mexican and Polish with US and Peruvian populations. *Ann Hum Biol* 1998;25:467.
23. Goran MI, Nagy TR. Visceral fat in white and African-American prepubertal children. *Am J Clin Nutr* 1997;65:1703-1708.
24. Lovejoy JC, de la Bretonne JA. Abdominal fat distribution and metabolic risk factors: Effects of race. *Metabolism* 1996;45:1119-1124.
25. Yu TC, Perez MI, Dermatologic liposuction: Safety record and techniques. *Cosmet Surg* 2004;17:2009-2012.
26. Braunstein GD. Glassman HA. Gynecomastia. *Curr Ther Endocrinol Metab* 1997;45:401-404.
27. Thompson DF, Carter R. Drug-induced gynecomastia. *Pharmacotherapy* 1993; 13:37.
28. Housman SH. The safety of liposuction: Results of a national survey. *J Am Soc Dermatol Surg* 2002;28:971-978.
29. Coldiron B. Office surgical incidents: 19 months of Florida sata. *Dermatol Surg* 2002;28:710-713.
30. Perez EH, Ibiett EV. Analysis of liposuction related complications and mortality in the United States and Latin America. *Cosmet Dermatol* 2000;15:23-28.
31. Goyen MR. Lifestyle outcomes of tumescent liposuction surgery. *Dermatol Surg* 2002;28:459-462.

CHAPTER 75

Rhinoplasty

Jimmy J. Brown
Gina D. Jefferson
Lorenzo Brown

Key Points

- The nose of a skin of color patient has innate features of weak supporting cartilages and prominent subcutaneous fibrofatty tissue and does not lend itself to the aggressive narrowing or lengthening techniques often employed in rhinoplasty procedures for Caucasian patients.
- Tip modification and management of the lower lateral cartilages may be accomplished with most standard techniques, but the external rhinoplasty approach allows for access to address the unique challenges accompanying rhinoplasty in a skin of color patient.
- Prolonged postoperative edema is a more frequent occurrence in rhinoplasty in a skin of color patient and is a result of thicker skin and more pronounced tissue reaction to the trauma of surgery. Kenalog injection may serve to reduce prolonged postoperative edema.
- The surgeon who intends to do rhinoplasty surgery in skin of color patients as a part of his or her practice must seek out expert mentorship from the few surgeons with experience in this practice area because there is a dearth of information and knowledge among clinicians trained in cosmetic and plastic surgery for this patient population.

It is an accepted fact that a study of our population today would unearth substantial variability in aesthetic dimensions among the groups classified as non-Caucasian. For example, the so-called typical Negroid nose did not typify the common aesthetic features demonstrated by a large group of African-Americans' nasal configuration studied.[1] Also, some non-Caucasian groups consider certain salient features to be distinguishing and desire to preserve these as defining features while accentuating others. In the past, many authors believed that non-Caucasian patients who sought aesthetic nasal surgery desired to achieve Caucasian features. It was Pitanguy in 1972 who clearly outlined the ideals that the nose should match the face, taking into consideration the race of the patient.[2]

PATIENT SELECTION

Non-Caucasian patients requesting nasal surgery in order to achieve an aesthetically pleasing nose and who possess an understanding that their racial characteristics may impose certain surgical challenges are considered the ideal patients desiring rhinoplasty. In general, the nasal features of the non-Caucasian, African-American nose, which present a challenge for surgeons to address, are a broad, flat dorsum and nasal bones[1,2]; a broad, flat, amorphous nasal tip owing to thick skin and a prominent subcutaneous fibrofatty pad[3]; a dorsum that lacks projection[4]; a poorly developed nasal spine that causes an acuteness in the nasolabial angle[5]; very wide, round nasal openings and wide alae; and so-called weak nasal cartilages.[6] Figure 75-1 demonstrates some of the salient characteristics of the non-Caucasian nose.

The common goal of surgeon and patient is to achieve physical

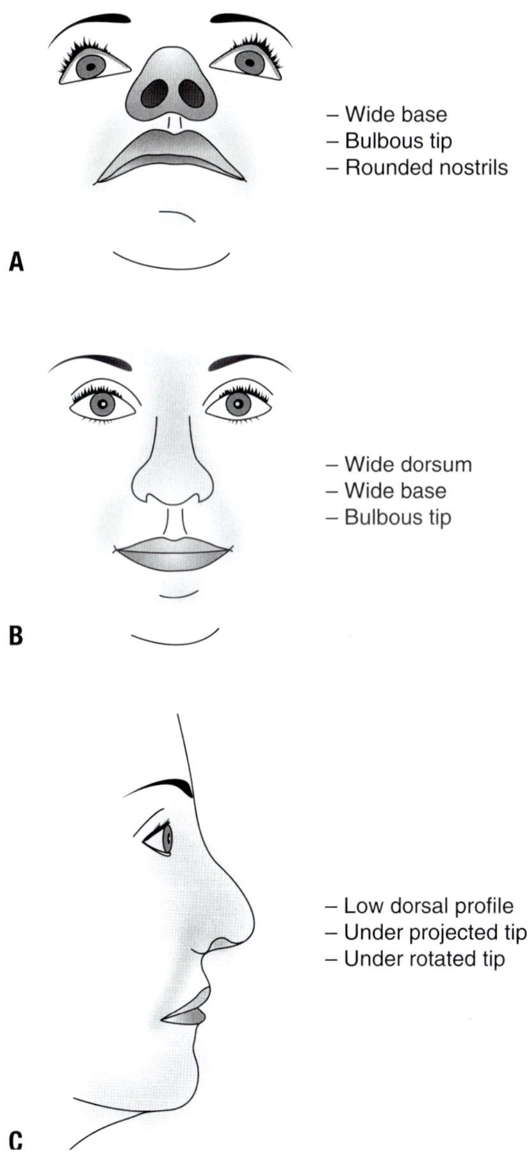

▲ **FIGURE 75-1** Characteristic features of the non-Caucasian nose. *A.* Basal view shows a wide nasal base with bulbous tip and rounded nostrils. *B.* Frontal view shows a wide dorsum, wide base, and bulbous tip. *C.* Lateral view shows a low dorsal profile, underprojected tip, and underrotated tip.

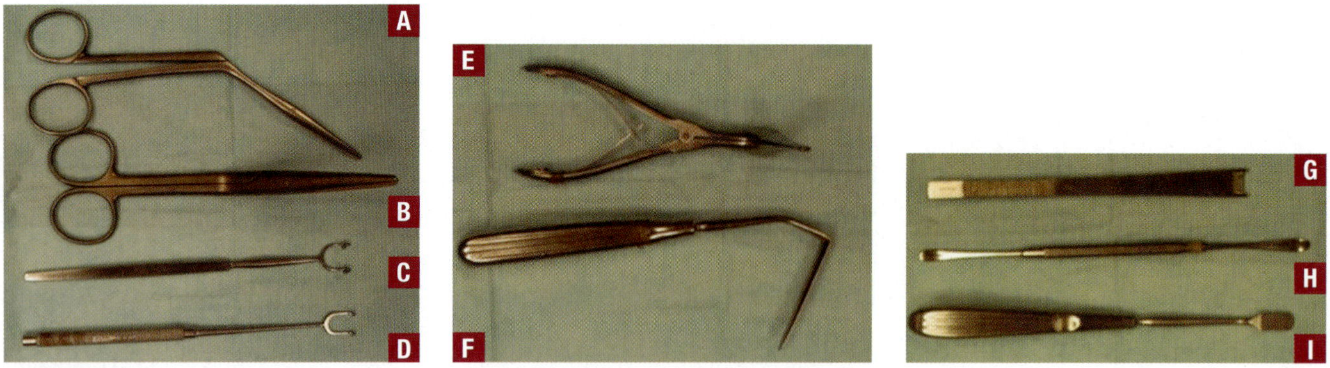

▲ **FIGURE 75-2** *A.* Lakeside scissors. *B.* Foman curved nasal scissors. *C.* Double-ball retractor. *D.* Double-prong skin hook. *E.* Nasal speculum. *F.* Aufricht retractor. *G.* Wide guarded osteotome. *H.* Freer elevator. *I.* Rasp.

improvement surgically while maintaining harmony with the remaining facial features and preservation of function. In particular, Asian and African-American patients will not benefit from the aggressive techniques to narrow or lengthen the nasal framework frequently used in Caucasian rhinoplasty.

RISKS AND PRECAUTIONS

- Edema
- Septal hematoma or perforation
- Nasal obstruction
- Deformity
- Implant migration or extrusion
- Hypo- or hyperpigmentation
- Stitch abscess/columellar base infection
- Nostril notching
- Complete loss of ethnic characteristics

PATIENT POSITIONING

The patient is positioned on the operative table supine with his or her head oriented toward the anesthesiologist. Flexing the operative table at the patient's waist approximately 30 degrees facilitates the surgeon's intermittent reassessment of surgical progress and intraoperative decision making because this position is more natural with respect to the effect of gravity.

EQUIPMENT

- Headlight
- Various-length nasal specula
- Double-ball retractors/double-prong hooks
- Various scissors
- Aufricht retractor
- No. 15 blade scalpel
- Freer and Cottle elevators
- Various-sized osteotomes and mallet
- Various-sized rasps
- Bayonet forceps
- Either 4% cocaine solution or oxymetolazone (Afrin) nasal spray
- Surgical pledgets, 3 in long by 1/2 in wide

Figure 75-2 depicts some of the common instruments used in performing rhinoplasty procedures. There are a wide variety of instruments used, but the selection of particular instruments is surgeon-dependent. The instruments in Figure 75-2*A* and *B* are indispensable to any rhinoplasty procedure. The nasal speculum and Aufricht retractor depicted in Figure 75-2*B* provide for superior exposure and examination of the nasal deformity to be addressed. The instruments in Figure 75-2*C*, an osteotome, freer elevator, and rasp, are particularly suited to the management of the wide dorsum frequently encountered as a feature of the non-Caucasian nose.

TECHNIQUE

There are three basic approaches for tip modification and management of the lower lateral cartilages. These techniques include cartilage delivery, cartilage splitting, and external rhinoplasty approaches. The selection of any given technique may be driven by the complexity of the case presented. Some authors believe that the challenges inherent in African-American or other non-Caucasian rhinoplasty lend themselves well to the external approach. The concern that the transcolumellar incision may result in a prominent scar or even keloid has not borne out in several series.[1,3,4]

Cartilage Delivery Approach

The cartilage delivery approach is accomplished via intranasal, intercartilaginous, and marginal incisions. This technique allows visual presentation of the alar cartilages as bipedicled chondrocutaneous flaps for further analysis and modification. Aggressive reduction of the alar subunit is ill-advised in most non-Caucasian rhinoplasty procedures. The following steps encompass nasal cartilage delivery for surgical treatment and refinement of the non-Caucasian nose:

1. Volume reduction (cephalic trim) of the medial portion of the lateral crus is accommodated while maintaining a complete strip at least 5 mm in width.
2. Further tip refinement may be accomplished with the purpose of narrowing a bulbous tip by performing transdomal suturing of the complete strips with horizontal mattress sutures of 5-0 PDS.
3. In addition, significant defatting of the tip can be performed to enhance tip definition and projection by using a variety of rhinoplasty scissors. Figure 75-2*A* depicts a selection of rhinoplasty scissors and retractors for exposure of the nasal tip.
4. Tip projection also can be increased, particularly in patients with thick nasal tip skin, via suture fixation of elongated medial crura developed by borrowing from the lateral crura (lateral crural steal).
5. Tip rotation can be further accentuated by shortening the caudal septum or placing cartilage plumping grafts on the anterior nasal spine, thereby increasing the nasolabial angle.

This technique does not lend itself to manipulation of the nasal dorsum, which in non-Caucasian patients often requires augmentation.

Cartilage-Splitting Approach

The cartilage-splitting approach is advantageous because these incisions are not in close proximity to an alloplastic dorsal implant and provide reasonable access for management of tip and columellar problems:

1. Cartilage-splitting incisions are made to meet the transfixion incision at an acute angle, joining the two incisions.
2. Lateral crura of the lower lateral cartilages are trimmed at the cephalic margins and set aside in saline solution for use later as a free graft.
3. Soft tissues of the dorsum are elevated preserving as thick a flap as possible using an Aufricht retractor, as seen in Figure 75-2*F,* for exposure and scissors to accomplish the elevation of the flap.
4. The inferior aspect of the transfixion incision is addressed, severing the depressor septi muscle and its fibrous attachments from the anterior nasal spine and septum. A double-ball retractor, as shown in Figure 75-2*C,* is used for exposure, and scissors and a Freer elevator are used to sever the fibrous attachments; an inferior tunnel is thereby created in the premaxilla/nasal spine region.
5. If septal surgery is required, it is performed at this stage in the operation. A unilateral mucoperichondrial flap is created by using a Freer elevator, as illustrated in Figure 75-2*H,* to elevate the mucosa with the mucoperichondrium oriented anteriorly and the mucoperiosteum oriented posteriorly, exposing the bony septum. Septal cartilage along the nasal floor is resected from a posterior to anterior direction measuring approximately 3–5 mm in width and 12–15 mm in length and is set aside in saline solution for later use as a columellar strut.
6. The columella is now addressed in an attempt to orient the nostril more vertically, increase columellar length, and improve tip projection. The fibrous tissue attachments between the domes of the lower lateral cartilages and where the medial crura diverge inferiorly are severed using curved iris scissors. The domes and diverging medial crura are coapted using Vicryl mattress sutures. The previously resected portions of the lateral crura of the lower lateral cartilages are incised in their midline while leaving the dorsal perichondrium intact so that the cartilage is hinged, approximately 4 by 4 mm. These hinged portions of cartilage are placed anterior to the nasal spine and are held in place by the previously created premaxillary inferior tunnels. The columellar base is pinched using bayonet forceps while superiorly retracting the columella using a 10-mm double-ball retractor to indicate the intent of narrowing the inferior flare via the following surgical maneuvers. A Brown-Adson forceps is positioned where the bayonet was previously located to create impressions where the small stab incisions on either side of the columella are next made. A mattress suture is placed using a Keith needle and 4-0 Vicryl suture, first passing through one stab incision and then exiting the incision on the opposite side of the columella. The Keith needle is reinserted into the stab wound from which it exited and is passed through the dermis approximately 2–4 mm posterior to the transfixion incision where the needle again exits and is placed into the mucosal septal cartilage and exits through the mucosa on the opposite side of the columella, traversing the septum at a slightly higher level to achieve a subtle increase in columellar height. The suture then is tied, thereby narrowing the inferior flare and closing the tunnels with the prespinal cartilage grafts.
7. The superior aspect of the columella is similarly addressed using a Keith needle to pass 4-0 Vicryl suture approximately 2–3 mm posterior to the columellar rim and passing the return suture superior to the first pass and approximately 6 mm deep to the rim, thereby narrowing the superior flare.
8. A columellar strut is next inserted via a 5- to 6-mm incision made on the lateral side of the columella and carried through the skin, perichondrium, and medial crus on that side. A pocket is created in the intercrural space with a curved iris scissors, taking care not to disrupt previously placed mattress sutures that mark the superior and inferior limits of the pocket. The septal cartilage graft previously harvested is now trimmed appropriately and placed in the pocket for columellar augmentation. The pocket incision is closed using running or interrupted 5-0 chromic suture.
9. The nasal dorsum is now addressed, where most often the non-Caucasian patient requires augmentation rather than dorsal hump removal. Medial osteotomies may be required to provide a better base for the dorsal implant, or it may be necessary in conjunction with lateral osteotomies for narrowing of the bony pyramid and increasing dorsal height. Here, 3-mm osteotomes produce little tissue trauma and preserve a significant amount of investing periosteum, which enhances stability. Various implant materials can be selected for use in augmentation, and the material selected is contoured appropriately and secured with 4-0 Vicryl suture. The transfixion and cartilage-splitting incisions are closed with absorbable 4-0 suture.
10. Alar base surgery is best accomplished with incisions and resections in the nasal sill and inferior alar crease so as to camouflage the incisions.

External Rhinoplasty Approach

The external rhinoplasty approach is the technique of choice for adequate exposure and surgical modification of the non-Caucasian nose. This technique achieves the necessary exposure for accurate placement of augmentation grafts and for appropriate nasal contouring.[1]

1. An inverted gull-wing incision is made along the narrowest part of the columella or along a prominent columella-labial groove.
2. The gull-wing incision is extended anteriorly along the margin to the tip cartilages and then partially along the alar cartilage margin.
3. Using a blunt-tipped scissors, the skin envelope is dissected off the columella over the tip cartilages and extending up to the dorsum. This is done just under the subcutaneous tissue to allow defatting of the tip and dorsal nasal skin.
4. The fibrofatty tissue in the midcolumella region is dissected up and carried up over the tip and alar cartilages to its insertion in the supratip region and is discarded.
5. The medial crura are separated down to the anterior nasal spine and premaxilla. A small pocket is made in

the premaxilla region to accommodate multiple plumper implants.

6. A straight, thin strut is fashioned from cartilage and is positioned between the medial crural cartilages and stabilized with interrupted 5-0 Monocryl sutures. The sutures are placed beginning at the nasolabial angle and moving toward the nasal tip, incorporating some lateral crural steal. Additional support can be attained using a 4-0 Prolene dome-binding suture.
7. A large nasal dorsum implant, with or without the tip component, depending on the amount of augmentation desired, is then carved to the appropriate shape using a No. 10 blade scalpel. The ideal size and shape of the implant may be determined by positioning the implant along the dorsum under the skin envelope to see if it provides the desired contour. A sheet of AlloDerm can be wrapped around the top of the implant to camouflage any minor irregularities. Placement of an infratip lobule shield graft provides a smooth contour with the columella and may be obtained from septal cartilage. The shield graft is secured with 6-0 Prolene suture.
8. The transverse columellar incision is closed with interrupted 5-0 Vicryl in the deep layer, followed by interrupted 6-0 nylon sutures for skin closure. The marginal incisions are closed with 5-0 chromic sutures.
9. The nasal apertures can be narrowed by precise resection of nasal alae tissue, or Weir incisions. For the non-Caucasian nose, this likely will be an important technique to reduce nostril shape and size. Excising nasal vestibular skin narrows the nostril size, whereas excising skin along the cutaneous alar margin will reduce nasal base width and flare. A medial skin flap should be created during excision of the vestibular skin to safeguard against nasal sill notching.

Excision of a segment of alar base and floor of the nostril produce a moderate reduction in width of the nose, as depicted in Figure 75-3. There are other variations to this technique.

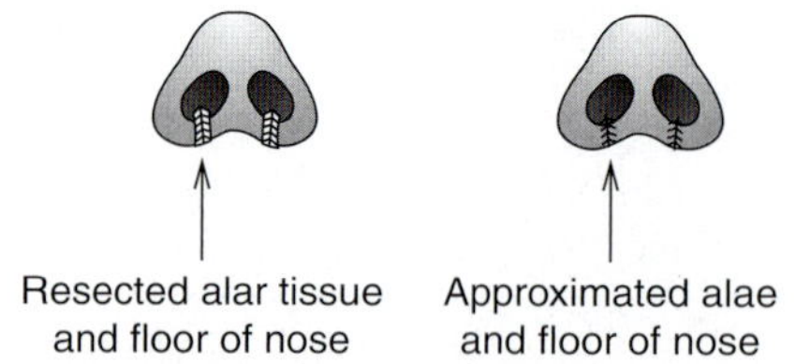

▲ **FIGURE 75-3** Excision of a segment of alar base and floor of the nostril produces a moderate reduction in the width of the nose.

1. Lateral osteotomies can be performed through the nasal base incisions for further definition of the nasal dorsum. The alae are then exactingly reapproximated using 5-0 Vicryl deep sutures and interrupted 6-0 nylon sutures for the skin. Skin closure begins at the superior-most lateral edge of the incision to hide any irregularities of closure within the medial intranasal portion of the incision.
2. External nasal tape is applied to reduce postoperative edema, followed by a cast. Silastic sheeting is applied along the septum bilaterally and anchored anteriorly with a 4-0 through-and-through nylon suture. This assists in coaptation of the mucoperichondrial flap and allows for healing of any mucosal tears. Merocel sponges impregnated with antibiotic ointment are positioned anteriorly to decrease postoperative oozing.
3. The Merocel sponges are removed on postoperative day 1 or 2. The Silastic sheeting and nasal cast are removed on postoperative day 5 or 7.

Figure 75-4 demonstrates characteristic postoperative changes in a non-Caucasian patient.

OUTCOMES

Using techniques of external rhinoplasty, as described by Romo and

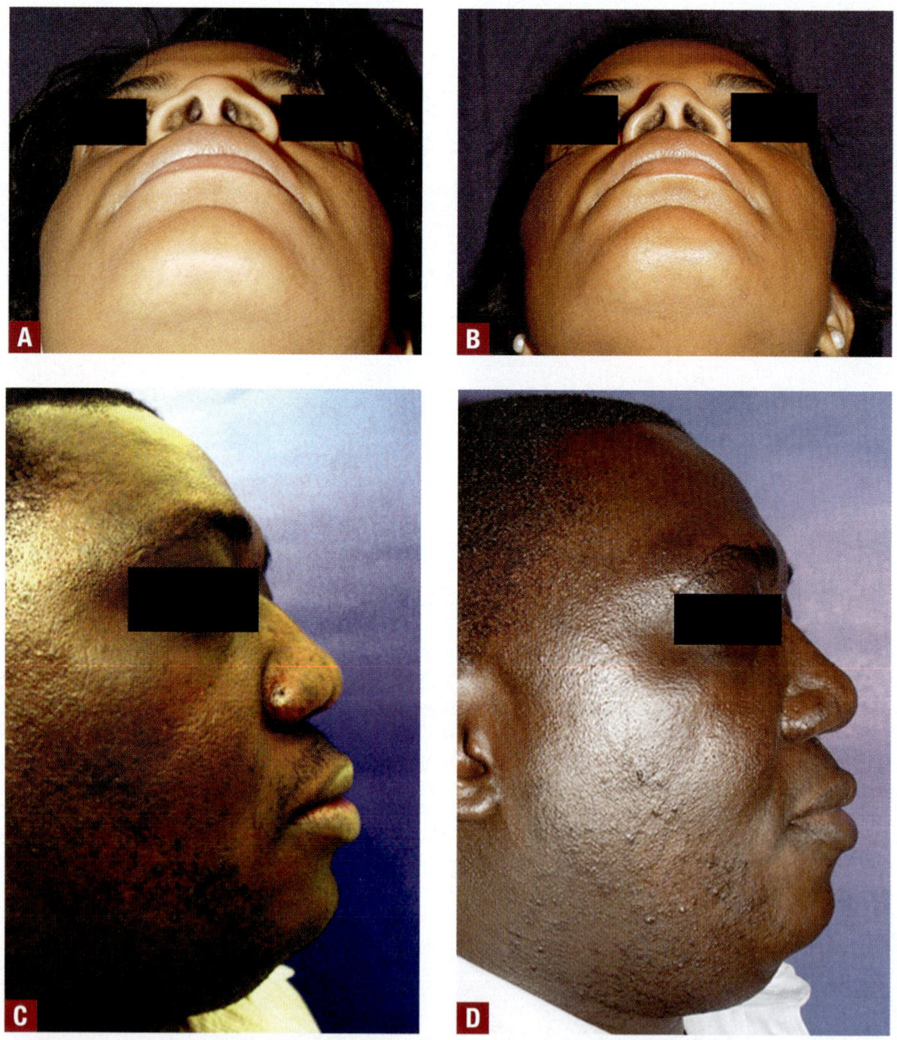

▲ **FIGURE 75-4** Characteristic postoperative changes in a non-Caucasian nose. *A.* Basal view shows a more narrowed base, better-defined tip, and more oval nostrils. *B.* Frontal view shows a narrowed dorsum, narrowed base, and more well-defined tip. *C.* This shows the improved dorsal profile, increased tip projection, and increased tip rotation.

Abraham, the vast majority of non-Caucasian patients undergoing the procedure are happy with the result of surgery.[1] Romo and Shapiro reported 100% satisfaction with cosmesis in 75 patients 2–7 years following ethnic rhinoplasty using autogenous cartilage grafts and the techniques described at that time.[3] These types of results also depend on appropriate patient selection and patient understanding of the limitations of the procedure.

COMPLICATIONS

In ethnic rhinoplasty, prolonged edema is often seen as a result of having thicker skin. Early pressure taping can be helpful, and triamcinolone (Kenalog) injections may be useful every 6–8 weeks as needed.

Keloid formation on the face is rare. Conchal cartilage harvest results in keloid formation less than 10% of the time and may be treated with Kenalog injection as needed. In alar base wedge resection, irregular scar formation may result in the alar groove. This may be avoided by placing an incision 2 mm above the alar groove. Careful suturing of the columellar incision will prevent alar rim notching,[6] which is usually difficult to correct.

Potential late complications of any rhinoplasty include nasal obstruction, septal perforation, deviation and irregularities of the nasal dorsum, saddle nose, pollybeak deformity, tip distortion, tip ptosis, columella retraction, and implant distortion or extrusion.[7] Specifically regarding the external rhinoplasty approach, a technique particularly amenable to the challenges of the non-Caucasian nose, an unsightly transcolumellar scar may occur, especially in patients at risk for hypertrophic or keloid scar formation. The surgical exposure achieved via the external rhinoplasty approach far outweighs the risk of unsightly scar formation, which the surgeon can manage conservatively.

FOLLOW-UP CARE

Postoperative care begins with application of adequate internal and external nasal dressings. Goals of internal nasal dressing, that is, Merocel sponges, include good tissue reapproximation, prevention of septal hematomas/swelling/bleeding, prevention of synechiae, and prevention of displacement. However, packing applied too tightly or for too long prevents adequate venous and lymphatic drainage. Septal suturing to reappose the mucoperichondrial flap(s) also can help to circumvent development of superperichondrial hematomas. In general, this intranasal packing may be removed 24–48 hours postoperatively.

Goals of external nasal dressings are the following: to fix the skin–soft tissue envelope to the bony dorsum, thus reducing dead space and preventing hematoma; limitation of edema; prevention of bony framework displacement; and prevention of widening of the lateral walls by intranasal edema. The external splint is removed after 1 week.

Patients are encouraged to keep their follow-up appointments at 6 months, 1 year, and 2 years. This facilitates surgeon learning from their patients' outcomes and ensures patient satisfaction.[8]

PATIENT INSTRUCTIONS

After intranasal splint removal, 5 days of topical intranasal vasoconstrictor may enhance comfort. Nasal irrigations with saline will assist in removal of postoperative crusts. Antibiotic prophylaxis is indicated when a nasal implant is placed and while intranasal packing is in place. Patients avoid strenuous activity for 3–4 weeks, as well as any contact sport activity.

REFERENCES

1. Romo T, Abraham MT. The ethnic nose. *Facial Plast Surg* 2003;19:269-277.
2. Pitanguy I. The Negroid nose, in Conley J, Dickinson J (eds), *First International Symposium on Plastic and Reconstructive Surgery of the Face and Neck*. New York, Grune and Stratton, 1972, pp 147-152.
3. Romo T, Shapiro AL. Aesthetic reconstruction of the platyrrhine nose. *Arch Otolaryngol Head Neck Surg* 1992;118:837-841.
4. Stucker, FJ. Non-Caucasian rhinoplasty and adjunctive reduction cheiloplasty. *Otolaryngol Clin North Am* 1987;20:877-894.
5. Tardy ME, Hendrick D, Alex J. Refinement of the nasal tip, in Bailey BJ, et al (eds), *Head & Neck Surgery–Otolaryngology*. Philadelphia, Lippincott Williams & Wilkins, 2001, pp 2255-2271.
6. Trenite GJN. Considerations in ethnic rhinoplasty. *Facial Plast Surg* 2003;19:239-245.
7. Johnson CM, Toriumi DM. Surgical anatomy and physiology of the nose, in Johnson CM, Toriumi DM (eds), *Open Structure Rhinoplasty*. Philadelphia, Saunders, 1990, pp 9-22.
8. Wang T. Non-Caucasian rhinoplasty. *Facial Plast Surg* 2003;19:247-255.

CHAPTER 76

Adjunctive Reduction Cheiloplasty

Gina D. Jefferson
Jimmy J. Brown
Lorenzo Brown

Key Points

- A simultaneous reduction cheiloplasty may assist in maintaining facial harmony in patients undergoing rhinoplasty for the purpose of decreasing a broad nose.
- Patients who undergo adjunctive reduction cheiloplasty, particulary black patients, are at risk for hypertrophic scarring, hyperesthesias, and asymmetry of the lips.
- Underresection is a common complication for surgeons until a few procedures are performed, which improves the surgeon's preoperative/intraoperative judgment of adequate reduction.

A pair of full lips is currently a desired feature sought after by a fair number in the public eye, as well as ordinary citizens. Excessively prominent lips, or macrocheilia, however, affect facial harmony and even may compromise function. The causes are multiple and may be iatrogenic from overzealous augmentation, a common procedure performed today. Some of the more common causes of macrocheilia include ethnicity, as seen among the non-Caucasian population and more commonly among blacks, congenital conditions such as double lip, neoplasm, various syndromes, and acquired conditions related to trauma, infection, neoplasm development, and glandular hypertrophy.

Most patients seeking reduction cheiloplasty are motivated by aesthetic concerns. Frequently, embarking on other aesthetic facial surgical procedures will accentuate an already prominent set of lips. Therefore, for some non-Caucasian patients, in particular black patients, performing an adjunctive reduction cheiloplasty during rhinoplasty, for example, will be paramount to achieving facial harmony.

PATIENT SELECTION

In considering patients for reduction cheiloplasty as an adjunctive procedure to the patient's prospective rhinoplasty procedure, the overall goal is to achieve facial harmony. Macrocheilia is a feature associated most commonly with patients of non-Caucasian ethnicity; these patients typically seek correction for cosmetic reasons. Non-Caucasian patients planning rhinoplasty often desire improvement of a broad, flat nasal dorsum, an underprojected nasal dorsum, an acute nasolabial angle, and flared nasal alae (Figure 76-1). With reduction of this nasal phenotype, a simultaneous reduction cheiloplasty likely would contribute to overall facial harmony about 50% of the time.[1]

RISKS AND PRECAUTIONS

- Asymmetric lips
- Hypertrophic scarring
- Hyperesthesia

PATIENT POSITIONING

There is a single surgical preparation and draping of the patient where the performance of tandem procedures flows from the most sterile procedure. Surgery therefore is initiated with performance of the rhinoplasty. The same patient position used during rhinoplasty is also ideal for performance of the reduction cheiloplasty. That is, the patient is supine and flexed at the waist for an upright head position of 30 degrees. This position facilitates the surgeon's intermittent reassessment of surgical progress and intraoperative decision making because this position is more natural with respect to the effects of gravity.

EQUIPMENT AND ANESTHESIA

- Headlight
- No. 15 blade scalpel
- Side-cutting bone cutter or a Satinsky vascular clamp
- 1% lidocaine with 1:100,000 epinephrine

TECHNIQUE

The lips are injected with approximately 5 ml of the lidocaine solution to assist with hemostasis and immediate postoperative pain control. Care is taken to avoid overinjecting the local anesthetic solution, which can distort the tissue, thereby making it more difficult to perform an accurate resection.[2]

For horizontal reduction, the amount of excised tissue and the grade of planned inversion are determined individually by first clamping the amount to be excised using the side-cutting bone cutter or a Satinsky vascular clamp. The clamping device is left in place for 5 minutes. Care must be taken to plan the resection within the confines of or posterior to the wet line of the lip. In addition, the area of Cupid's bow should not

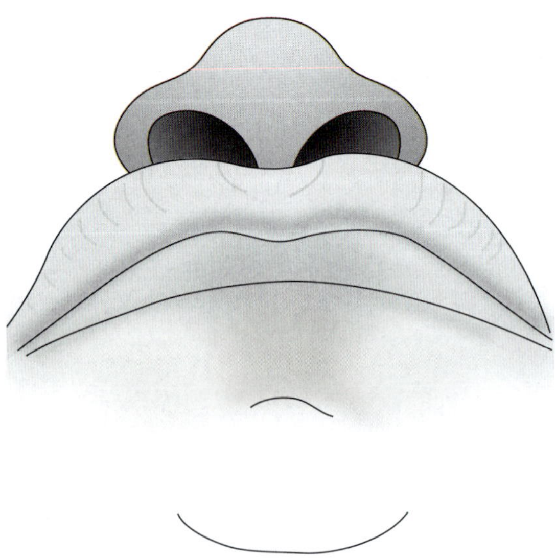

▲ **FIGURE 76-1** Basal view of nose showing relation of nose and overly prominent upper lip.

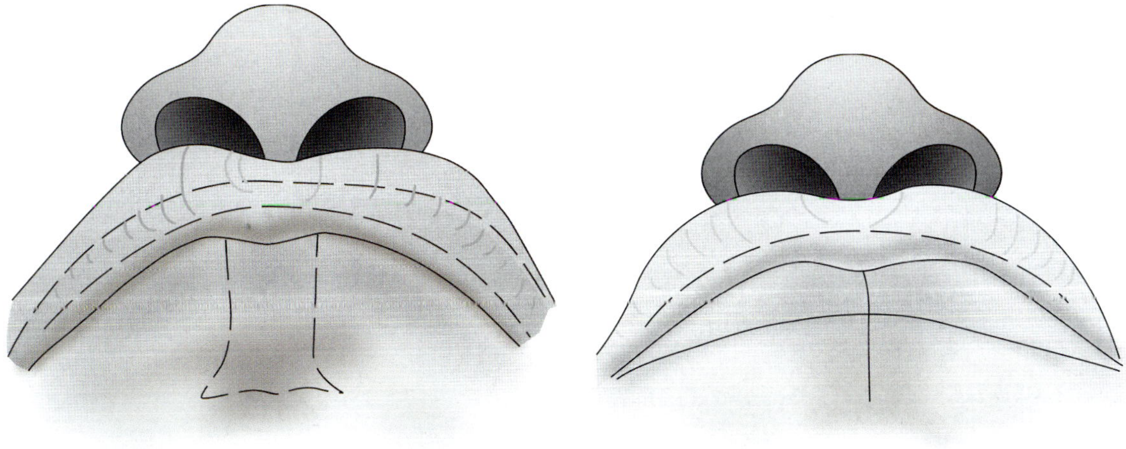

▲ **FIGURE 76-2** *A.* Depiction of horizontal reduction of upper lip and vertical reduction of lower lip. *B.* Illustration of well-healed upper and lower lips after cheiloplasty. Lines of closure are accentuated for descriptive purposes.

be directly altered. It is useful to actually perform this step prior to injection of the local anesthetic if the procedure is performed under general anesthesia.

The lip is grasped at the commissure and everted. The previous mucosal markings created by the clamping device are reemphasized using a marking pen after drying the lip surface. The strip of mucosa excised includes submucosal glandular tissue while leaving the orbicularis oris muscle intact and unaffected. This strip of excised tissue is at least 1–2 cm in width in order to achieve the desired effect.

The incisions are approximated at the midline first, without undermining; then the right and left halves are closed with 4-0 silk sutures. The philtrum identifies the center of the upper lip incisions. The frenulum is used for midline identification and closure of the lower lip incisions.

For vertical reduction of either the upper or the lower lip, the area of planned resection is outlined before injection of the lidocaine solution. After the appropriate amount of lidocaine is injected, the lip is grasped with a moist raytec, and full-thickness reduction is achieved following the previously placed lines.

To achieve the most effective approximation, the orbicularis oris muscle must be sought and approximated separately at its cut ends, followed by subcutaneous approximation and finally skin closure (Figure 76-2).

OUTCOMES

Stucker reports that reduction cheiloplasty is straightforward, is accomplished in 20 minutes time, and produces consistently good results.[2] There is no large series with outcome data currently available in the English literature.

COMPLICATIONS

Underresection is common until one has done several cases. Lip seal is usually unachievable for the patient initially and may persist for 7–10 days postoperatively; therefore, drooling during sleep is a common postoperative occurrence, and patients should be forewarned preoperatively.[2] A variable degree of lip edema also occurs and is relative with respect to the patient. Theoretically, mucocele formation may occur but is rarely seen in practice.[3]

FOLLOW-UP

In order to ensure mucosal integrity in a wet and mobile environment, the sutures remain in place until postoperative day 10. The initial postoperative appointment is within 24–48 hours, as is traditional after rhinoplasty to remove intranasal packing. If cheiloplasty is performed as a single procedure, initial assessment is recommended after 48 hours to ensure that no excessive postoperative edema exists, which may indicate hematoma formation.

PATIENT INSTRUCTIONS

The patient is instructed to follow a liquid or soft diet during the first 5 postoperative days, both for comfort and to avoid undue stress on the suture lines. Routine ice pack application directly to the lip for the first 48 hours, applied every hour while awake for 20 minutes at a time, will lessen postoperative edema and provide some degree of additional patient comfort.

REFERENCES

1. Stucker FJ. Non-Caucasian rhinoplasty and adjunctive reduction cheiloplasty. *Otolaryngol Clin North Am* 1987;20:877-894
2. Stucker FJ. Reduction cheiloplasty: An adjunctive procedure in the black rhinoplasty patient. *Arch Otolaryngol Head Neck Surg* 1988;114:779-780.
3. Lip reduction. eMedicine, 2006, *www.emedicine.com/plastic/topic66.htm*.

CHAPTER 77

Other Head and Neck Surgical Procedures

Jimmy J. Brown
Gina D. Jefferson

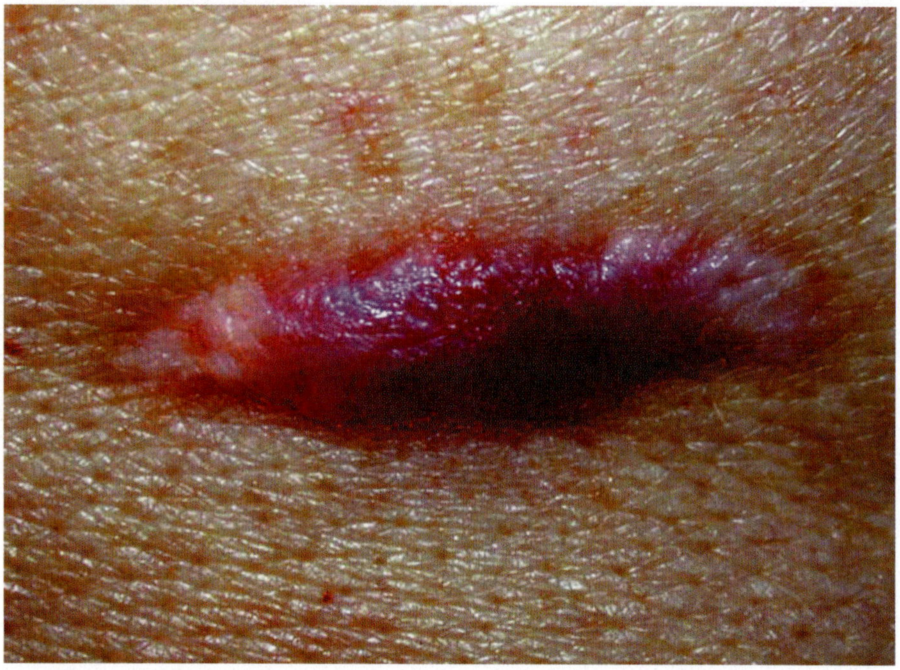

▲ **FIGURE 77-1** The appearance of a keloid scar after thyroidectomy surgery.

Key Points

- Skin of color requires special care when subjected to surgical procedures because all surgeries encompass trauma.
- Today, more patients with skin of color are seeking to have elective head and neck surgical procedures that place them at risk for untoward outcomes.
- Careful patient selection in those with skin of color is warranted for any elective head and neck surgical procedure.
- When operating on patients with skin of color, pay particular attention to preoperative and intraoperative measures that will optimize scar outcomes.
- Ensure that patients understand their risks for poor scar outcome and that there may be a need for multiple revision surgeries.

The head and neck surgeon is faced with the challenges of planning aesthetically acceptable surgical incisions, atraumatically manipulating tissues, and performing adjunctive skin treatments when indicated because the head and neck operative site is exposed to public view and scrutiny. An unsightly operative outcome most likely will result in patient dissatisfaction and possibly a loss of self-confidence. Patients of color are particularly susceptible to untoward aesthetic results, at times related to improper planning and placement of surgical incisions and traumatic tissue handling. Skin of color has a proclivity for dyspigmentation changes and abnormal wound healing compared with Caucasian skin.

Some of the more common untoward outcomes associated with the performance of surgery on skin of color include keloid formation, hypertrophic scar formation, abnormal scar contracture, and the previously mentioned problem with dyspigmentation, Thyroidectomy, parotidectomy, neck dissection, and rhytidectomy (face lift) are common elective head and neck surgical procedures in which complications of wound healing may result in conspicuous or grossly unsightly scars. Other head and neck operative procedures frequently done as adjuncts to the aforementioned surgical procedures include dermabrasion, chemical peel, laser skin resurfacing, and laser depigmentation.

COMMON HEAD AND NECK SURGICAL PROCEDURES

Patients of color undergoing the procedure of thyroidectomy are at particular risks to develop an unsightly anterior neck scar postoperatively. Many patients will not have remembered the original indications for their surgery, which frequently include a neoplastic condition, but will focus their attention to their skin and the surgical scar. In our practice, based in an ethnically diverse community with predominantly African-Americans and Latinos, we have frequently employed special measures to reduce the risk of unsightly scar formation. These include, along with the usual tissue-handling cares, injection of steroid preparations intraoperatively and the use of a soft cervical collar for 6–8 weeks during the immediate postoperative period. We have found that this measure prevents widening of the scar and keloid formation in up to 95% of our at-risk patients (Figure 77-1).

Other scenarios, such as benign masses located in the lateral superior neck requiring surgical intervention, are best handled with hidden incisions. For example, we have predominantly employed a modified face lift incision instead of the conventional modified Blair incision for most surgical access to the parotids. The modified Blair access incorporates an unsightly incision in the upper neck that may be prone to keloid formation. The modified face lift incision therefore is used when performing surgery in this vicinity on a majority of our patients of color. These incisions are partially hidden in the hairline and behind the auricle and can be readily camouflaged or concealed (Figure 77-2).

Operative radical neck dissections for surgical management of head and neck malignancies use a wide variety of incision designs. It is interesting to note, however, that none of these designs save for one, the MacFee approach, take into consideration patients' postoperative cosmetic outcomes. The MacFee approach for neck dissection uses two horizontal incisions, one in the upper neck and a second in the lower neck. The incisions are parallel and follow the relaxed skin tension lines, avoiding any vertical component, a common feature

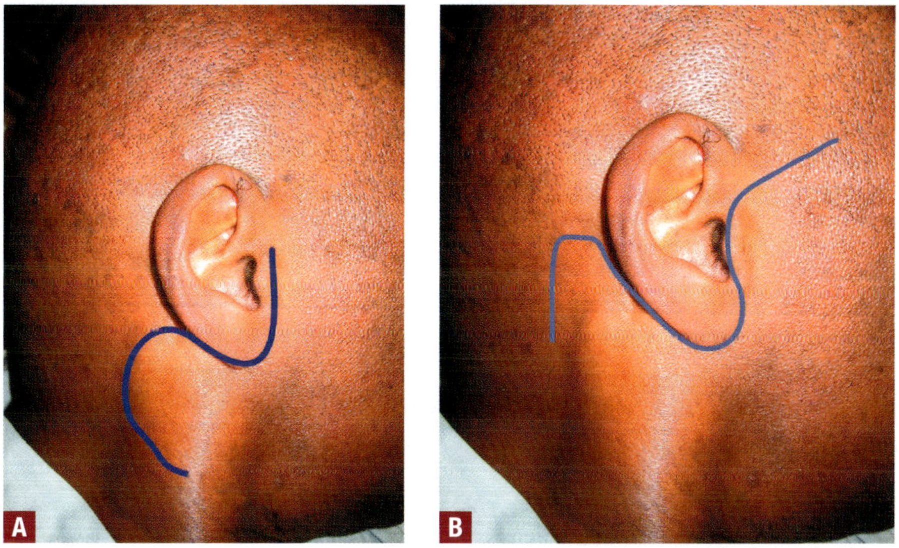

▲ **FIGURE 77-2** **A.** Modified Blair incision for parotid surgery. **B.** Modified face lift incision for parotid or removal of neck masses in the upper neck. Incisions are concealed at the hairline and behind the ear.

of other surgical approaches to the neck currently used.[1] The vertical component incision of the customary designs frequently results in significant scar contracture and keloid formation and is not suited to patients of color who are at risk (Figure 77-3). Patients today are concerned with their quality of life, even in the setting of a grave prognosis for their malignancies, and frequently their desires require modifications of standard approaches.

ADJUNCTIVE SKIN PROCEDURES

Dermabrasion, chemical peels, and laser resurfacing are common adjunctive skin procedures performed in patients undergoing rhytidectomy or in the management of the aging skin. Performance of these procedures in patients with Fitzpatrick skin types IV, V, and VI, the so-called skin of color, was thought initially to frequently result in skin hypopigmentation; however, several studies have demonstrated that postinflammatory hyperpigmentation (PIH) is a more frequent occurrence.[2,3]

Dermabrasion is mechanical abrasion of the epidermis that creates a mechanical wound at the papillary and reticular dermis, thereby stimulating synthesis of a new layer of skin. This, in essence, will result in removal all sun-damaged skin cells, superficial scars, and premalignant lesions above the reticular dermis, which subsequently reepithelializes.[4,5] Laser therapy and chemical peels essentially do the same. The problem, however, is the response to these inflammation-inducing procedures, which is highly unpredictable in skin of color. Laser therapy using tissue chromophores is somewhat different and poses a different problem in skin of color. For example, the pulsed-dye laser (PDL) uses hemoglobin within tissues as a chromophore to mediate its effects. In skin of color, there are melanosomes, which are chromophores, and they compete with the intended chromophores of the PDL or other lasers using this technique and essentially make this process less effective.

PREVENTION AND MANAGEMENT OF WOUND COMPLICATIONS

As with any surgical intervention, prevention of complications is the best approach to the operative management of patients, especially those at increase risk. With this in mind, the careful and meticulous surgeon will relish a practice with infrequent postoperative complications and sustain a satisfied patient population. Appropriate patient selection is of utmost importance, especially in the setting of elective surgical procedures. Perhaps this is of even greater importance when one considers ethnic population groups in which wound healing is inherently more apt to suboptimal results given the higher propensity to aberrant scar formation.

Performing surgical operative procedures on patients with skin of color requires exquisite technique and special atraumatic tissue-handling maneuvers. The surgeon should avoid holding wound skin edges with forceps of any kind. He or she should avoid excessively stretching the wound edges, as is customary when attempting to access distant structures or pathologic entities through minimal invasive approaches. Liberal debridement of traumatized skin edges just before wound closure is of utmost importance in improving scar outcomes.

Selection of the appropriate suture materials plays a vital role in the eventual outcome of the scar and specifically its aesthetic appearance. A number of suture materials are available from which to choose in the closure of any given defect. For example, in the closure of a cutaneous facial incision, a surgeon may choose to close the skin edges with a fast-absorbing gut suture or opt instead to use a subcutaneous synthetic monofilamentous suture type such as Monocryl, which will elicit less tissue reaction than the polybraided varieties such as Vicryl and Dexon. The patient of color may benefit from wound closure with Monocryl in light of its less inflammatory tissue reaction. The fast-absorbing gut suture is absorbed via a proteolytic enzymatic process that inherently elicits an inflammatory response and may contribute to aberrant scar formation. The

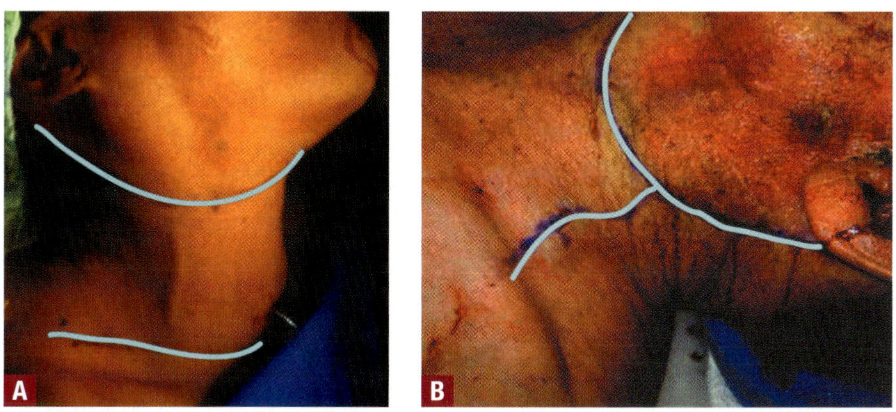

▲ **FIGURE 77-3** **A.** Design of MacFee incisions for aesthetic neck dissection. **B.** Standard utility incision with vertical component for easy surgical access.

monofilament synthetic sutures are absorbed via the process of hydrolysis and thus are less inflammatory in nature and less likely to lead to aberrant scar formation. Although many patients will object to it, metallic staples will elicit the least tissue reaction and, if removed at the appropriate time, can result in a cosmetically pleasing scar.

Wound tension is also a known contributing factor to aberrant scar formation, particularly among patients of color. Wound tension in large surgical wound defects or in surgical wounds involving large skin flaps is lessened by the placement of subcutaneous anchoring sutures as needed. However, the least amount of suture material present in the wound, the least amount of foreign material available to potentially incite an exuberant tissue inflammatory response, forming an aberrant scar.

The application of silicone sheeting to surgical incisions has been employed with moderate success in lessening exuberant scar formation in some patients of color. The exact mechanism of action remains unknown, but some studies have demonstrated increased water content within the scar microenvironment.[6] The increased hydration theoretically enhances orderly proteoglycan matrix deposition and collagen architecture, thereby decreasing the likelihood of aberrant scar formation.[7] A shortcoming of this prophylactic measure is its dependence on steadfast patient compliance. Also, it may prove difficult to maintain adherence of the silicone sheet to the incision site in some patients with oily skin. The silicone sheet also can result in the development of a rash with subsequent wound dehiscence in a small number of patients.[7]

The management of hypertrophic or keloid scars frequently involves injection with the steroid preparation triamcinolone both intraoperatively and in the early postoperative period. Triamcinolone increases the activity of the enzyme collagenase as its main mechanism of action.[2,7] Triamcinolone does not decrease the number of cells producing collagen or the amount of collagen synthesized in the healing wound. Intraoperative steroid injection is considered in patients with a significant history of aberrant scar formation with the patient's informed consent regarding the potential for hypopigmentation.

FOLLOW-UP CARE

Exquisite postoperative care is a most important aspect of wound management, ensuring a favorable scar outcome. Patients follow-up care should be accelerated when the surgeon anticipates an untoward outcome in the at-risk patient of color. The patient should be reassured and an initial conservative management approach instituted. Instructions to patients should be reviewed and reinforced. Once conservative measures have failed and it is clear that the scar will not improve, then surgical revision should be contemplated.

CONCLUSION

Skin of color provides unique challenges in the management of postoperative changes. Patients with skin of color are at an increase risk of developing complications of surgery. One should not approach these skin types casually. These patients should be given detailed informed consents with respect to potential untoward outcomes. The surgeon should be versed in information with respect to prevention and subsequent management of complications in skin of color before embarking on making this group a part of his or her practice.

REFERENCES

1. Myers EN, Suen JY, Myers JN, Hanna EYN. *Cancer of the Head and Neck,* 4th ed. Philadelphia, Saunders, 2003.
2. Taylor SC, Burgess CM, Callender VD, et al. Postinflammatory hyperpigmentation: Evolving combination treatment strategies. *Cutis* 2006;78:6-19S.
3. Lin JY, Chann HH. Pigmentary disorders in Asian skin: Treatment with laser and intense pulsed light sources. *Skin Ther Lett* 2006;11:8-11.
4. Coleman WP, Hank CS, Alt TH, Asken S (eds). *Cosmetic Surgery of the Skin: Principles and Techniques,* 2nd ed. St Louis, MO, Mosby–Year Book, 1997.
5. Johnson BL, Moy RL, White GM (eds). *Ethnic Skin: Medical and Surgical,* 1st ed. St Louis, MO, Mosby, 1997.
6. O'Brien L, Pandit A. Silicone gel sheeting for preventing and treating hypertrophic and keloid scars. *Cochrane Database Syst Rev* 2006.
7. Zuruda JM, Kriegel D, Davis IC. Topical treatments for hypertrophic scars. *J Am Acad Dermatol* 2006;55:1024-1031.

SECTION 13

Pediatric Dermatology

CHAPTER 78

Pediatric Dermatology

Andrea Trowers

Key Points

- Learn the differences in treatment, pigmentary changes, and precautions necessary for pediatric patients.
- Recognize that by the year 2050, 15% of all dermatology visits will be for conditions affecting pediatric patients with skin of color.
- Understand that pigmentary effects of seborrheic dermatitis can be severe but are reversible.
- Remember to treat asymptomatic carriers in households with a patient afflicted by tinea capitis.
- Consider high-potency topical steroids for short term use when initiating therapy for atopic dermatitis.
- Consider sequelae prior to doing a biopsy.

There are several diagnoses unique to pediatric patients with skin of color, and there are common conditions that differ in presentation when afflicting such children. The inherent characteristics of skin of color, especially children with darker skin, are pigment lability and an increased tendency to scar. When treating pediatric patients, this must be combined with concerns regarding percutaneous absorption. These are additional challenges to be considered when treating these younger patients.

Currently, 10% of all pediatrician visits are due to primary skin complaints, and 30% of dermatology appointments are for pediatric patients.[1] By the 2050, 47% of the U.S. population will be non-Caucasian, making familiarity with treating this patient group essential. In the future, almost 15% of all dermatology visits will be for conditions affecting pediatric patients with skin of color.

The conditions to be discussed in this chapter will be separated by those more commonly seen in infants versus children, with the expectation that patients do not always mirror published prevalence rates. The presentation characteristics that differ from Caucasian skin are stressed, in addition to specific therapeutic considerations in this patient population.

INFANTILE CONDITIONS

When any parent bring their infant in for evaluation of a skin condition, their main concern is that it is not life-threatening. The look of concern and tense body posture do not resolve until hopefully the words "This is nothing bad" come out of the doctor's mouth. Only then is the parent really able to actually hear what you are saying. Fortunately, most of the conditions that present frequently in infants of color are benign. However, the inability to recognize these conditions can result in undue stress for the parents and physicians until the correct diagnosis is made.

Mongolian Spots

Mongolian spots are benign blue-gray patches that are typically found on the lower trunk and buttocks at birth. In one study of 437 newborns, the lesions were present in 96% of African-Americans, 46% of Hispanics, and 9.5% of Caucasians.[2] Resolution over time is to be expected. However, extensive Mongolian spots have been associated with inborn errors of metabolism, such as GM1 gangliosidosis and Hurler syndrome.

Transient Neonatal Pustular Melanosis

This is a benign pustular eruption that can occur in utero or on the first day of life. Lesions consist of pustules that dry, leaving a collarette of scale and a hyperpigmented macule in their wake that resolves over 4–6 weeks.

Lesions typically involve the sacrum and buttocks but can involve any region of the body. Sometimes infants can be born with only the hyperpigmented macules because all of the pustules resolved in utero. About 4% of newborns are afflicted, and most of them are African-American males. The reason for racial preference of the condition is unknown.

Acropustulosis of Infancy

This condition occurs at birth or during infancy. Crops of intensely pruritic vesicles and pustules occur on the soles, palms, and dorsal surfaces of acral sites. The lesions will resolve within a few days, leaving a hyperpigmented macule that can be more difficult to discern in pigmented skin. New crops recur within a few weeks. The condition is rare but typically affects African-American infants. A scabies prep always must be done prior to making the diagnosis because the two conditions have very similar presentations. Therapeutic options include strong topical steroids, antihistamines, and in severe cases, dapsone.

Seborrheic Dermatitis (Figure 78-1)

Seborrheic dermatitis is a very common condition in infants. It is commonly known as "cradle cap" and can affect the scalp, face, ears, neck, and skin folds. The condition consists of dry yellow scale and the underlying skin can be unaffected, or at times slightly inflammed and erythematous. When skin folds are involved, there also can be accompanying maceration. In patients with skin of color, the inflammation caused by seborrheic dermatitis can cause significant hypopigmentation. It is often misdiagnosed as vitiligo. The pigmentary changes can be significant but resolve rapidly once the primary condition has been treated. It is important to vocalize to parents that this is not vitiligo, even if they have not expressed this fear. Treatment options include hydrocortisone 2.5% cream mixed with equal parts of ketoconazole cream to be applied twice daily. Severe cases may require the additional use of ketoconazole shampoo for cleansing the areas. Pimicrolimus (Elidel) cream also can be used twice a day. The scaling of the condition and the pigmentary changes usually resolve with 3 weeks of initiating therapy.

CHILDHOOD CONDITIONS

Tinea Capitis (Figure 78-2)

Tinea capitis is a dermatophyte infection that involves the hair on the scalp and is characterized by scaling and patchy alopecia. Currently, the most common pathogen in the United States causing this condition is *Trichophyton tonsurans,* which is an endothrix infection. This means that the spores proliferate within the hair shaft. However, *Microsporum canis,* which is responsible for a minority of cases of tinea capitis, is a small spore ectothrix that produces

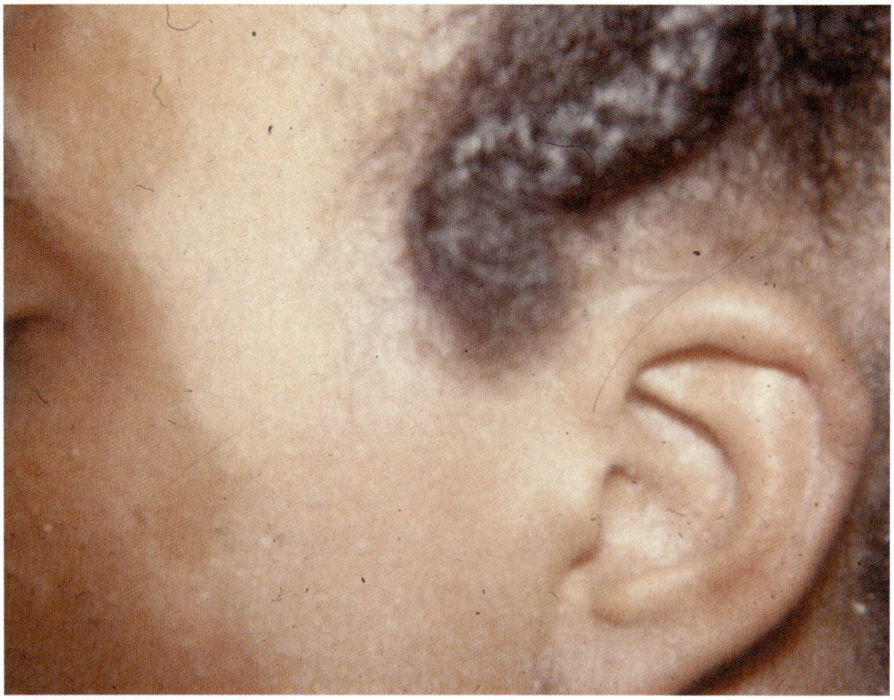

▲ **FIGURE 78-1** Seborrheic dermatitis with hypopigmentation on a child.

fluorescent pteridines. As a result, tinea capitis cases caused by *M. canis* fluoresce under a Wood's light, whereas those caused by *T. tonsurans* do not.

Frequently, parents of black children are unaware that their child is suffering from this condition and believe instead that their child suffers from a "dry scalp." Sometimes they may complain that frequent greasing of their child's scalp has failed to resolve the condition. Therefore, it is the responsibility of the physician to examine the scalps of all children who come to their office for this condition because it is extremely contagious. Infections after puberty are rare, and it hypothesized that this is due to "a higher content of fungistatic fatty acids in the sebum of postpubertal individuals."[3]

The incidence of tinea capitis is much greater among African-American children than among children of other races. A study conducted in San Francisco from 1984–1993 showed that the rate of grsieofulvin (Grifulvin V, Gris-Peg) use in African-American children was 5.8 times the mean rate for all other races in 1984 and 13.9 times the mean rate in 1993.[4] Some practitioners have proposed that the high rate of tinea capitis among African-American children is due to infrequent washing, traction resulting from tight hairstyles, and the use of pomades,[5,6] but these theories lack supportive evidence.[7] The most likely explanation lies in the fact that "epidemics of tinea capitis have always been in poorer communities" in which crowded living conditions enable the spread of infection.[4,8]

Most patients with tinea capitis are treated with oral griseofulvin for 6 weeks. The standard dose is griseofulvin 20–25 mg/kg for 6 weeks. It is important to remember that this is not the dosing published in the Harrison's pediatric handbook, which is 10–15 mg/kg. This increased dose is required owing to dermatophyte's acquired resistance to lower dosing. Terbinafine (Lamisil) also can be used to treat tinea capitis, but it is important to remember that it is not effective for infections caused by *M. canis*. The dosing is one quarter a 250-mg tablet for children weighing 0–20 kg, one half of a tablet for 20–40 kg, three quarters of a tablet for 40–60 kg, and 1 tablet for children 60 kg and over to be taken for 2 weeks.[9] Side effects with griseofulvin are rare, and baseline testing is not required. However, there is a possible cross-reactivity in penicillin patients. Lamisil does carry a risk of hepatotoxicity, so in children a baseline hepatic profile can be repeated after the course of medication is completed. The pill can be pulverized without affecting its effectiveness, but the taste is very unappealing, making it difficult to administer. One option is to mix it with the filling of an Oreo cookie to cover the taste.

Secondary bacterial infections require treatment with oral antibiotics. Severely, inflamed nodules with loose hairs, known as kerions, should be treated with short term oral prednisone.

In addition to oral therapy, ketoconazole (Nizoral) or selenium sulfide shampoo (Head & Shoulders) should be used.

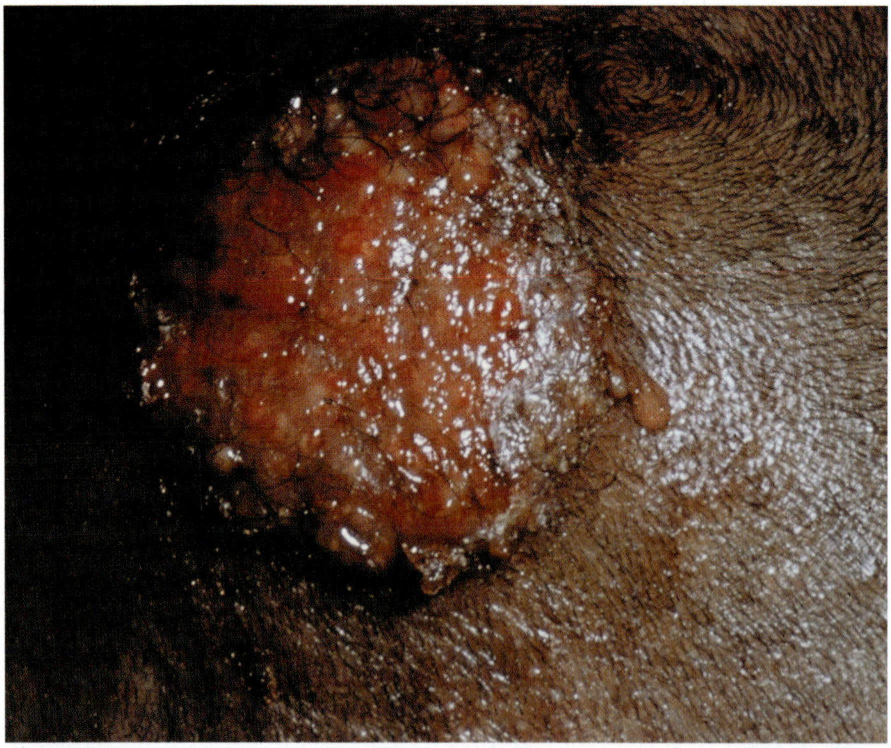

▲ **FIGURE 78-2** Kerion (inflammatory mess) of tinea capitis.

This treatment regimen is based on studies showing that the use of a sporacidal shampoo, such as selenium sulfide, twice weekly or ketoconazole shampoo used daily reduces the number of viable arthroconidia and negatively affects transmission.[0] However, washing an Africa-American child's hair two times a week and especially daily can be extremely difficult. The nature of most of their hair is kinky, thick, and dry, requiring washing only once weekly. Some children may have their hair washed more or less frequently depending on the texture. Hair washing and combing can be difficult and in some cases even a little traumatic. Most people with thick hair have at least one memory of trying to run away from the brush that was used to tame their curls.

A valid option is to use an antifungal cream, lotion, or gel (based on patient or parent preference) daily and to wash weekly with a ketoconazole or selenium sulfide shampoo. Although no studies have been performed on this combination therapy, it is logical to assume that this approach would immobilize spores, which would inhibit transmission.[8] By using this method of therapy, it is my belief that parents, siblings, and physicians will all benefit. Physicians who were previously unaware of the difficulties of daily washing will have increased compliance, which may have been playing a role in prior treatment failures.

Also, because there have been reports of asymptomatic carrier rates as high 63%,[9] other children in the household should also use topical therapies and shampoos, even if they have no signs of infection. In addition, any other child who accompanies the patient should be examined for infection. Parents should be shown the clinical signs that raise suspicion of infection so that siblings that are not in the office can be examined at home. All contacts should be started on the medication at the same time in order to break a chronic cycle of reinfection.

Atopic Dermatitis (Figure 78-3)

Atopic dermatitis affects all races. However, experience shows that the sequelae are more cosmetically disfiguring in ethnic skin. A number of children with severe dyschromia and adults with permanent pigmentary changes are the direct result of insufficiently aggressive treatment. When developing a treatment plan for atopic dermatitis, always address the three I's—itch, infection, and inflammation. The itch of the itch, scratch cycle must be eliminated or else topically applied medications will not have a chance to work. Some physicians prefer sedating medications such as hydroxyzine and in very severe cases doxepin. These can be prescribed on a fixed schedule for the first week of therapy and then on an as-needed basis. It is important to stress to parents that these medications are not addictive or else they may fail to use them. If there is also a history consistent with allergic rhinitis, cetirizine (Zyrtec), loratadine (Claritin), or fexofenadine (Allegra) should be prescribed for use every morning.

Patient's with atopic dermatitis are frequently carriers of *Staphylococcus aureaus*. Secondary impetiginization results in worsening of the disease, but the constant use of oral antibiotics can lead to bacterial resistance. If there are obvious signs of infection, such as open, oozing fissures or yellow crusted erosions, oral antibiotics should be used. Cephalexin can be the first choice, but it is important to culture these patients because resistance is common. Also, if longer courses are required, minocycline and tetracycline (if the patient is 9 years of age or older) or erythromycin (if the patient is younger than 9 years of age) can be used depending on the sensitivity profile of the culture. It is important to recall that antibiotics have an anti-inflammatory effect as well that can be beneficial even if an active infection is not present.

The sooner antibiotics can be eliminated from the patient's regimen, the better. Bleach baths are an excellent way to achieve this and have been a phenomenal success with some patients (once their parent's get over the shock of using it). For mildly to moderately affected patients, I typically start them on a bath with ¼ cup of bleach each night until their first follow-up appointment at 3 weeks. For small babies, 1 tablespoon of bleach is added to the little tubs that fit into the sink. Dr. Adelaide Herbert's regimen, based on the poster by Browning, Levy, Rosseau, and colleagues, is as follows: ⅛ cup of bleach to every 8 inches of water; do not immerse face in water; soak for 20 minutes; then rinse off or shower.

High-potency topical steroids can be used to treat flares of severe atopic dermatitis initially. The plan is to hit hard initially and then to ease up with the intensity of the steroid used. Many physicians are fearful of using high-potency topical steroids in children. However, using mild topical steroids for an extended period of time will not result in clearing and will result in much longer time periods of steroid use. Studies have been done using class 1 topical steroids in pediatric patients for up to 2 weeks without cutaneous or systemic side effects.[10–12] However, it is important to limit the amount of medication prescribed and the number of refills allowed. After using a class 1 topical steroid for 5–10 days, the patient can be tapered down to a middle-potency topical steroid. An ointment base is frequently beneficial. In some cases, patients will clear not by changing the class of steroid but prescribing the same medication in an ointment formulation rather than a cream.

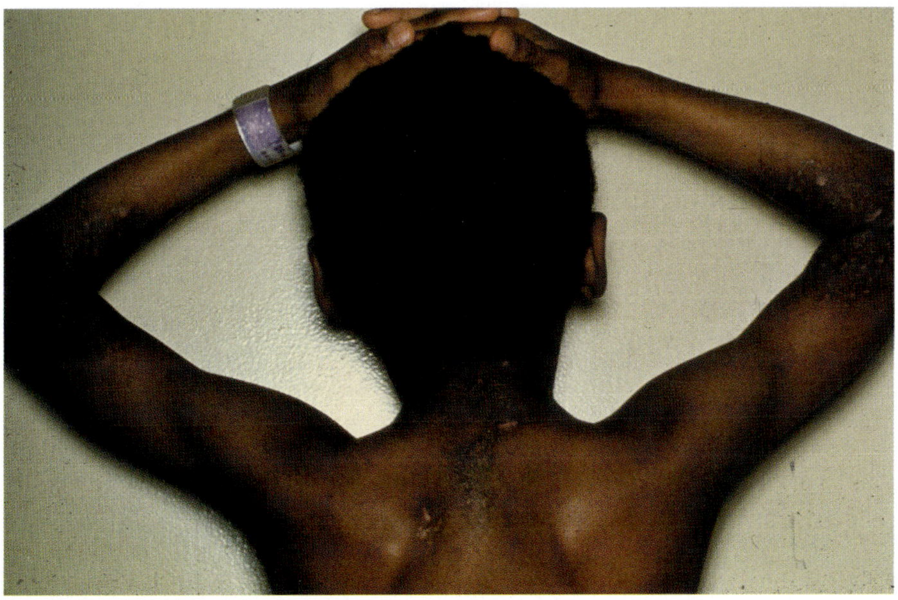

▲ **FIGURE 78-3** Atopic dermatitis with pigmentary changes.

When using potent topical steroids on pediatric patients it is important to limit application to 5% of the body surface area, owing to the pediatric patient's high ratio of body surface area (BSA) to body weight. Topical immunomodulators are also useful for patients who continue to flare. Interestingly, the initial studies showed that tacrolimus (Protopic) 0.1% was more effective in African-American patients than in whites.

The importance of quality soaps and lotions also cannot be underestimated; all over-the-counter products are not equal. Parents must be educated about this or the clearing achieved by medications will not be maintained. Cocoa butter is very popular among people of color, but standardized studies have not upheld its mythical powers. Also, cost may prevent some parents from buying brand names. Crisco lard chilled in the refrigerator is an excellent emollient and is very soothing when applied to inflammed skin. Petrolatum is greasy but can be applied copiously at night following a shower or bath for minimal cost.

Psorasis, like atopic dermatitis, is another skin disease found in pediatric patients.

Vitiligo

Vitiligo carries a huge psychosocial burden for children.[13] However, it possibly has a greater effect on children with skin of color. In many fair Caucasian children it sometimes can be very difficult even to see the areas of involvement. In children with skin of color, the areas are clearly evident and are in a sharp contrast to the normally pigmented skin.

This contrast is compounded in sunny areas because the child's natural skin color is darkened by chronic sun exposure. Try to show parents the comparison of the inner aspect of the child's one arm with the outer aspect of the other, or have them take a look at the patient's buttocks to stress the effect of the sun on the child's pigmentation. By using a sunscreen with a skin protection factor (SPF) of at least 30 and containing a physical blocker such as zinc and/or titanium dioxide, the contrast of involved and uninvolved skin can be lessened dramatically.

Other options for therapy include phototherapy (depending on age), calcipotriene (Dovonex), topical retinoids, and topical immunomodulators. The option of makeup cover-ups (or color creams, as I prefer to refer to them when discussed with male patients) also should be reviewed because we as physicians cannot determine in a few minutes the psychosocial effect of the condition on our younger patients, but they may bring up this option later with their parents if it is discussed at the time of the visit. Makeup companies have made huge strides during recent years in recognizing the variety of colors present in the population. However, my preferred brand for vitiligo patients is Dermablend owing to camoflauge abilities, reasonable price for the number of applications provided, and wide range of colors available. The product is available online, but it should be recommended that patients visit a makeup counter where a salesperson who has been trained by the company is available because color mixing may be required.

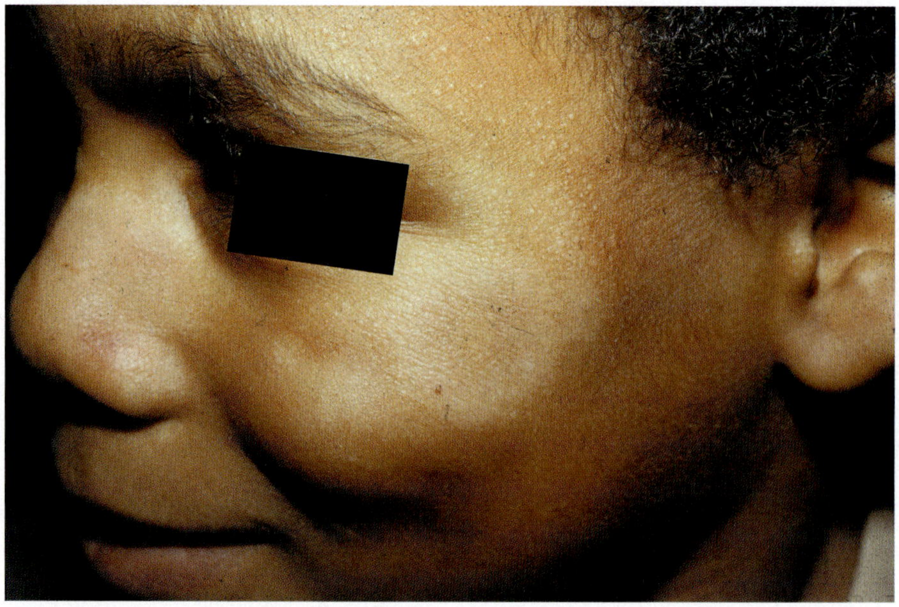

▲ **FIGURE 78-4** Pityriasis alba.

Pityriasis Alba (Figure 78-4)

Pityriasis alba is a benign condition characterized by hypopigmented patches with ill-defined borders. At times, the lesions can be scaly. Histologically, there is spongiosis and acanthosis. The disorder is typically defined as a "subclinical dermatitis resulting in postinflammatory hypopigmentation."[14]

This condition afflicts atopic and nonatopic patients. Typical areas of involvement include the face, arms, and upper trunk. The condition typically is noted during the summer months when tanning of the surrounding skin makes the lesions more noticeable and year round in sunny climates. The condition is especially distressing to patients with skin of color and their parents because it is more noticeable in these patients.

It is important to reassure parents that this is not vitiligo. It is also important to stress to them what a significant role sun exposure plays in this condition. Patients with skin of color often do not realize how easily they and their children tan. Demonstrate to them an area of their child's body that is not sun-exposed such as the buttocks or axillae and show them that it is the same color as the lesions of pityriasis alba. Then explain that the inflammation of the lesions prevent tanning and that this is actually the child's true skin color.

If scaling is present within the lesions of pityriasis alba, it can be treated with a low-potency topical steroid such as hydrocortisone 2.5% or a topical immunomodulator such as pimicrolimus (Elidel) or tacrolimus (Protopic). More severe cases, especically if scaling is present, may require short term use of a moderate strength topical steroid. If no scaling is present, consider treating only with strict photoprotection with an SPF equal to or greater than 30 containing zinc oxide and/or titanium dioxide. Tinted sunscreens or those containing microionized zinc oxide will be more cosmetically acceptable to your patients with skin of color. Daily use and reapplication every two hours must be stressed.

Acne

Acne affects all races, but postinflammatory hyperpigmentation is unique to patients with skin of color. In a study of the incidence of common dermatoses in a predominately black dermatologic practice, pigment disorder was the third most common complaint in 2000 black patients.[15]

Frequently, when teenage patients with skin of color present with acne, their main complaint is the hyperpigmented macule that remains for months after their pimple has disappeared. Some may say that postinflammatory macules is a misnomer in a patient with comedonal acne and hyperpigmented macules because comedones are known to be noninflammatory. However, in a study done in 1996 by Kelly,[16] comedones, papules, and pustules were biopsied from African-Americans and surprisingly defied the accepted teachings in the dermatology community by showing comedones with marked inflammation of infiltrates of polymorphonuclear leukocytes. As a result, physicians should consider being more aggressive when treating acne in ethnic skin. For example, one should consider prescribing oral antibiotics even if there is only mild acne in order to speed resolution.

Treatment of hyperpigmentation must be included in the treatment plan. Compounded bleaching cream starting at a minimum of 8% hydroquinone and containing 0.025% tretinoin always should be prescribed to speed the resolution of hyperpigmentation. This must be localized to areas of hyperpigmentation using a toothpick or cotton swab for application. Even when care is taken with application, there is the risk of a hypopigmented halo developing around the area of hyperpigmentation. In such cases, or simply to speed resolution overall, chemical peels with salicylic and retinoic acids should be used. Daily photoprotection with sunscreens with a minimum SPF of 30 and containing physical blockers such as titanium dioxide and/or zinc oxide must be stressed to assist in clearing.

Acanthosis Nigricans

Acanthosis nigricans presents as velvety brown plaques. It is located most frequently on the neck but can involve any body fold. Cases involving the face and hands also have been reported. It is typically associated with an above-normal body mass index (BMI), and patients should be evaluated for insulin resistance. One study of 618 children ages 7–17 years found that 19% were African-Americans with the disease with BMIs greater or equal to the 98th percentile.[17] There are multiple reported therapies but no proven cure. Weight loss can result in resolution.

THERAPEUTIC CONSIDERATIONS

Molluscum

This condition is caused by the poxvirus and is characterized by pearly white umbilicated papules. Some articles report its resolution without treatment within a year, but in clinical practice, lesions have persisted longer while multiplying. The question of 'to treat or not to treat' becomes more complicated in patients with atopic dermatitis, who are at greater risk for secondary infection of the lesions. It is also challenging to treat the condition during swimming season because the lesions are known to spread in water.

Some of the treatments for these lesions are destructive and include canthardrin and liquid nitrogen. However, in skin of color, these therapies can result in significant disfigurement owing to secondary pigmentary changes. The parent who presented initially to complain about the molluscum on his or her child can return for follow-up appointments for months to years to complain about the hyperpigmentation resulting from your treatment.

Imiquimod cream and tretinoin cream/gels do not seem to be effective despite a number of trials. Success is possible with tazoratene (Tazorac) 0.05% cream that parents apply at night with a toothpick. This medication is category X and should not prescribed if the mother is pregnant or planning to become pregnant during the treatment course. It is important to stress to parents several times the use of a toothpick because use of a Q-tip or finger will result in additional areas being treated and thus irritated. Repeat to parents several times that the reason the medication works is because it causes inflammation, and as a secondary result, the molluscum clears. If any lesions remain at the follow-up appointment in 3 weeks and the parent does not want to continue topical therapy, the remaining lesions can be curetted. Bathing and swimming must be discontinued, and only showering is allowed. Some scaling and erythema of the treated areas is normal, but if the patient becomes extremely uncomfortable or complains of the irritation, a low-potency topical steroid can be used twice daily for 4–5 days.

Biopsies

Biopsies of pediatric patients are always difficult because no one likes inflicting pain on an individual who is too young to understand the explanation for why it is being done. The additional consideration when performing a biopsy on a pediatric patient with skin of color is that the child may be left with a lifelong hypertrophic keloid scar, or pigmentary change (Figure 78-6).

Prior to doing a biopsy on an ethnic patient, the physician should consider if this is a life or death matter. If it is, a

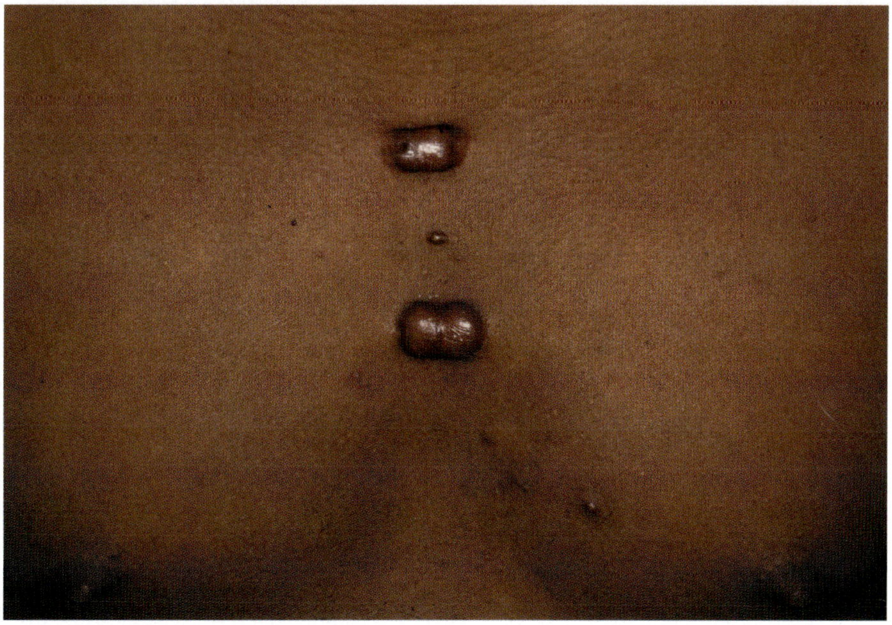

▲ **FIGURE 78-6** Keloidal biopsy scar on a child.

biopsy should be done. If it is only to satisfy intellectual curiosity and will make no difference in the therapy prescribed, consider that the biopsy should not be done. Also, a short trial of one medication to be quickly followed by another if there is no response also may be an option. By considering these alternatives, you can avoid making your permanent mark on a patient. Explaining this to parents is also helpful and involves them in the decision. Keloids are also a risk from biopsies in pediatric patients.

CONCLUSION

Physicians must recognize that by 2050, 15% of all dermatology visits will be for conditions affecting pediatric patients with skin of color. Familiarity with condition affected this group of patients will result in correct and rapid diagnosis.

REFERENCES

1. Schachner LA, Hansen RG. Preface, in Schachner LA, Hansen RC (eds), *Pediatric Dermatology,* 2nd ed. New York, Churchill-Livingstone, 1995, p IX.
2. Mendez HM, Pinto LI, Paskulin GA, Ricachnevsky N. Is there a relationship between inborn errors of metabolism and extensive mongolian spots? *Am J Med Genet,* 1993;87(3):276-277.
3. Kligman AM. Tinea capitis due to *M. audouinii* and *M. canis:* II. Dynamics of host-parasite relationship. *Arch Dermatol* 1955;71:313-337.
4. Lobato MN, Vugia DJ, Frieden IJ. Tinea capitis in California children: A population-based study of a growing epidemic. *Pediatrics* 1997; 99:551-554.
5. Reid BJ, Shimkin MB, Blank P. Study of tinea capitis in Philadelphia using cases and control groups. *Public Health Rep* 1968;83:497-502.
6. Provost B. The rise and fall of fluorescent tinea capitis. *Pediatr Dermatol* 1983;1:127-133.
7. Sharma V, Silverberg NB, Howard R, et al. Do hair care practices affect the acquisition of tinea capitis? A case-control study. *Arch Pediatr Adolesc Med* 2001;155:818-821.
8. Bonnie Elewski, personal communication, 2003.
9. Vargo K, Cohen BA. Prevalence of undetected tinea capitis in household members of children with disease. *Pediatrics* 1993;92:155-157.
10. Herz G, Blum G, Yawalkar S. Halobetasol propionate cream by day and halobetasol propionate ointment at night for the treatment of pediatric patients with chronic localized plaque psoriasis and atopic dermatitis. *J Am Acad Dermatol* 1991;25:1166-1169.
11. Wolkeistorfer A, Strobos MA, Glazenburg EJ, et al. Fluticasone propionate 0.05% cream once daily versus clobetesone butyrate 0.05% cream twice daily in children with atopic dermatitis. *J Am Acad Dermatol* 1998;39:226-231.
12. Boner AI, Richelli C, De Stefano G, et al. Adrenocortical function during prolonged treatment with clobetasone butyrate in children with chronic atopic dermatitis and elevated IgE levels. *Int J Clin Pharmacol Res* 1985;5:127-131.
13. Hill-Beauf A, Porter JD. Children coping with impaired appearances: social and psychololgic influences. *Gen Hosp Psychiatry* 1984; 6(4):294-301.
14. Schachner LA, Hansen RC (eds), *Pediatric Dermatology,* 2nd ed. New York, Churchill-Livingstone, 1995, p 691.
15. Henderson Al. Skin variations in blacks, *Cutis* 1983;32:388-392.
16. Kelly AP. Nuances of black skin. Presented at the NMA Section on Dermatology, New Orleans, LA, 1974.
17. Brickman WJ, Binns HJ, Jovanovic BD, et al. Acanthosis nigricans: a common finding in overweight youth. *Pediatr Dermatol* 2007; 24:601-606.

SECTION 14

International Dermatology

CHAPTER 79

Common Skin Diseases and Treatment in Africa

Edith Nkechi Nnoruka
Felix D. Oresanya
Osumane Faye

Key Points

- Africa is the second largest continent with 53 individual countries and a population of 877, 500,000 in 2006. Skin diseases are a common and important cause of ill health in Africa. Most of the population has Fitzpatrick skin types IV, V and VI.
- Africa has a lower incidence of skin cancers and less pronounced photo aging attributed to melanin content and melanosome distribution.
- With great differences in ethnicity, culture, hygiene, nutrition and socioeconomic status, as well as genetic factors, common dermatologic conditions seen in one part of Africa may be different from those seen in other parts.
- Some skin disorders that are showing a rising trend of prevalence throughout Africa similar to those in the Western world are eczemas, acne vulgaris, and blistering disorders.
- The most common diseases are infectious disorders, in particular, the superficial fungal infections.
- Less common are deep mycoses, cutaneous tuberculosis, cutaneous leshmaniasis, yaws, and Buruli ulcers.
- The emergence of HIV and AIDS, whose impact has been greatest in Sub-Saharan Africa, have altered the pattern of skin diseases in all of Africa.

Africa is the second largest continent of the planet, 30,065,000 km^2 (11,608,000 mi^2) with a coastline of 30,539 km (18,976 mi). Africa occupies 20.2% of earth's land with 53 individual countries. It contains the world's largest desert, the Sahara, and the world's longest river, the Nile. The population was 877,500,000 in 2006. Africa has people of diverse cultures and practices and is endowed with lots of natural and human resources.

Most of the African population has Fitzpatrick skin types IV, V, and VI, which rarely or never burn on sun exposure and readily tan, whereas a small proportion has skin types II and III. These properties are based on the skin phototype (SPT) system, developed by Fitzpatrick, which is predicated on the reactions or vulnerability of various types of skin to sunlight and ultraviolet (UV) radiation.[1] In addition, darker skin is known to differ from Caucasian skin not only in its reactivity but also in disease presentation. The darker shade of skin is attributable to the increased amount of melanin in the skin. Melanin protects the skin from sunlight, slows down the aging process, and plays a part in the younger appearance of dark-skinned versus white-skinned people. The lower incidence of all skin cancers and less pronounced photoaging in blacks is attributed to increased melanin content and melanosome distribution.[2–4] On the contrary, dark skin can become greatly problematic by triggering excess melanin (resulting in postinflammatory hyperpigmentation) or excess collagen production (resulting in keloids/hypertrophic scars). Ethnic differences in skin properties also may explain racial disparities seen in dermatologic disorders and provide insight into appropriate differences in the management of these disorders.

Skin diseases are a common and important cause of ill health in Africa. Their burden within Africa varies extensively, accounting for as high as 60% in some rural communities and up to 30% of consultations in the urban settings.[5,6] While mortality rates are generally insignificant, the fact that morbidity is significant—either through disfigurement, disability, or symptoms such as intractable itch—makes identification of common and prevalent skin diseases for each region an important public health goal. When care is taken to make the proper diagnosis and to institute proper treatment, the management of skin diseases often results in great improvement and satisfaction for the affected individuals, thereby improving the quality of life.

Within Africa, there are great differences in ethnicity, culture, hygiene, nutrition, and socioeconomic status, as well as genetic factors, with the result that common dermatologic conditions seen in one part of Africa may be different from those seen in other parts. There are, however, some skin disorders that are showing a rising trend of prevalence throughout Africa similar to what holds in the Western world, for example, eczemas, acne vulgaris, and blistering disorders. In addition, there are other disorders that are seen more commonly in Africa, such as infectious disorders, in particular, the superficial fungal infections (e.g., dermatophytosis, pityriasis versicolor, and candidiasis), pyodermas, and parasitic disorders such as scabies and onchocerciasis. Other disorders peculiar to Africa include lichen planus, pseudofolliculitis, acne kelodalis nuchae, keloids, and dermatologic disorders related to cultural practices. There are as well some disorders that occur less commonly in various parts of Africa, such as the deep mycoses (e.g., histoplasmosis, sporothricosis, chromoblastomycosis, and mycetomas), cutaneous tuberculosis, cutaneous leshmaniasis, yaws, and Buruli ulcers. Moreover, the emergence of the human immunodeficiency virus (HIV) and the acquired immune deficiency syndrome (AIDS) pandemic in the last 25 years, whose impact has been greatest in sub-Saharan Africa, also has altered the pattern of skin and sexually transmitted diseases in all of Africa,[7] Table 79-1 shows the common skin diseases seen in Africa.

INFECTIOUS SKIN DISORDERS

Superficial Fungal Infections

Key Points

- The hot, humid climate for most of Africa, the tropics and substropics, favors the high prevalence of these infections in these areas.
- Consists mainly of dermatophytosis, pityriasis versicolor, and candidiasis.

Dermatophytosis

Key Points

- Synonyms include tineas and ringworm.
- Filamentous fungi that thrive only on nonviable keratinized tissues of the skin (e.g., stratum corneum, nails, and hair).
- Presents with very certain distinctive features that are characteristic of that particular site, but the most common are scaling plaques or patches with a serpiginous border.

- Pruritus is common and is often the chief complaint.
- Tinea corporis, tinea capitis, tinea cruris, tinea pedis, tinae faciale, and tinea incognito are the most common presentations.
- Children have more of tinea capitis, whereas adult males present commonly with either tinea pedis or tinea cruris.

TABLE 79-1
Common Skin Disorders in Africa

Infectious Disorders
Fungal
Dermatophytosis
Pityriasis versicolor
Candidiasis
Parasitic
Scabies
Insect-bite allergy (papular urticaria)
Myasis
Cutaneous larva migrans
Onchocerciasis
Pediculosis
Bacterial
Impetigo
Folliculitis
Pyodermas
Excemas/dermatitides
Atopic dermatitis
Seborrheic dermatitis
Contact dermatitis
Exfoliative dermatitis
Acne/Acnieform Disorders
Acne
Acne keloidalis nuchae
Dermatitis papulosa nigra
Keloids
Spontaneous keloid
Hypertrophic scars
Papulosquamous Disorders
Lichen planus
Pityriasis rosacea
Psoriasis
Pigmented Disorders
Exogenous ochronosis
Albinism
Vitiligo
STDs/HIV/AIDS
Drug Reactions
Fixed drug eruptions
Steven Johnsons syndrome
Toxic epidermal necrosis
Dermatoses Secondary to Cultural Practices
Tribal marks
Scarification marks
Traction alopecia
Central centrifugal cicatricial alopecias

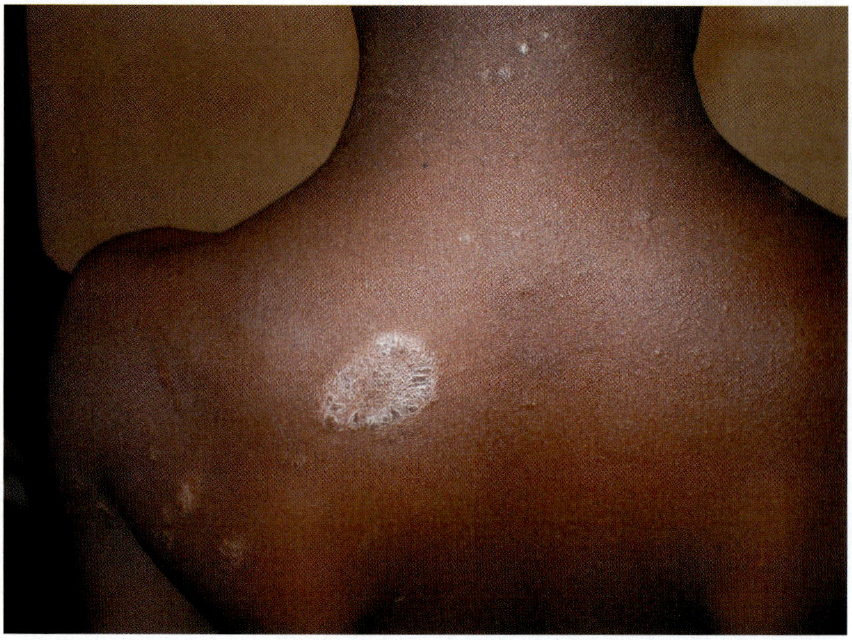

▲ **FIGURE 79-1** Typical macular lesion of tinea corporis with central clearing and serpiginous border.

Dermatophytosis is very prevalent in African countries. just as in other tropical and subtropical countries.[8–10] Adults and children are affected, with children having more of tinea capitis. The three principal genera that cause dermatophytosishere as elsewhere are (1) *Microsporum,* (2) *Trichophyton,* and (3) *Epidermophyton.* Dermatophyte infection in Africa may be acquired via three sources: human to human (anthropophilic), from animals (e.g., dogs, cats, or cattle; zoophilic), and from the soil (geophilic). Immunosuppressed individuals and diabetics undergo a higher incidence of intractable dermatophytoses.

CLINICAL FEATURES Patients often present with scaly rash. Pruritus is common and often the chief complaint. Various clinical lesions can result, but the most common are scaling, papules, plaques, and patches that often have irregular or serpiginous borders (Figure 79-1). The actual clinical presentation also depends on the anatomic site and the strain of fungus involved.

Tinea Capitis

Key Points

- Most common type of dermatophytosis occurring in children in Africa.
- May present as a solitary, well-defined scaly patch of hair loss, as small patches of gray scaly and broken strands, as a seborrhoid pattern studded with scattered pustules, or as a kerion.

- Sharing of combs and caps, rubbing of heads together while playing at school, and pets are the main sources of infection.

In most African countries, it is a very common disease affecting 5–10% of primary school children.[11–13] The causative organisim varies from county to country, with *Trichophyton violeceum* and *Microsporum ferrugineum* in East Africa[8,14] and *T. soudanense, M. audonii,* and *T. gourvilli* in West Africa.[8,15–17] In parts of equatorial and South Africa, particularly Mozambique and the Democratic Repulic of Congo, *T youndaei* is most common. Tinea capitis may present as a sharply delinated, pruritic scaly ring (Figure 79-2) or as small patches of gray scaly and broken hair strands (Figure 79-3). It also may present as a kerion (Figure 79-4), a boggy swelling inflammation with pustulations, often so fierce that a bacterial infection may be suspected. This is often associated in ringworm of the scalp acquired from animals (*M. canis*). Hair loss occurring in kerion formation is often permanent. Enlarged occipital lymph nodes also may occur, and extensive lesions may give rise to an id eruption.

Tinea favousa (favus), resulting from infection with *T. schoenleinii,* is widespread in North Africa and Eurasia, where it shares with *T. violaceum* a place of predominance among the agents of tinea capitis.[8,18] It produces a scarred type of hair loss distinguished by the formation of scutula, which consist of yellow crust surrounding and matting many scalp hairs together.

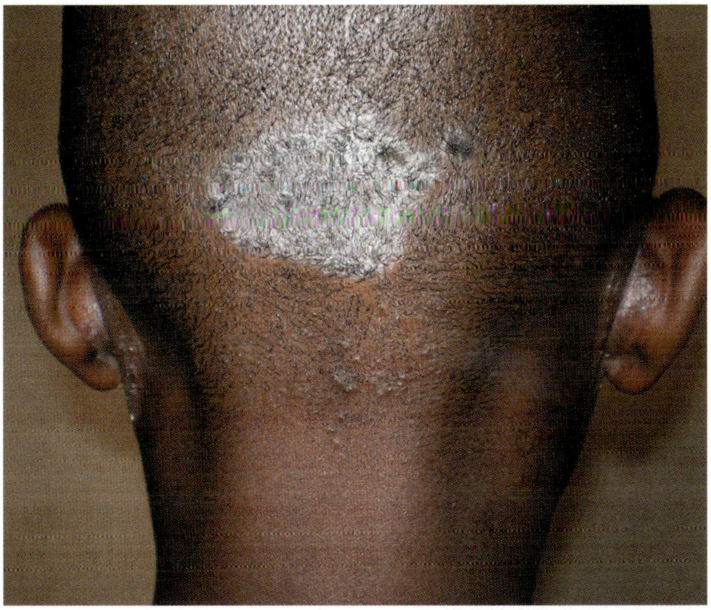

▲ **FIGURE 79-2** ▲ Tinea capitis in a 9-year-old boy.

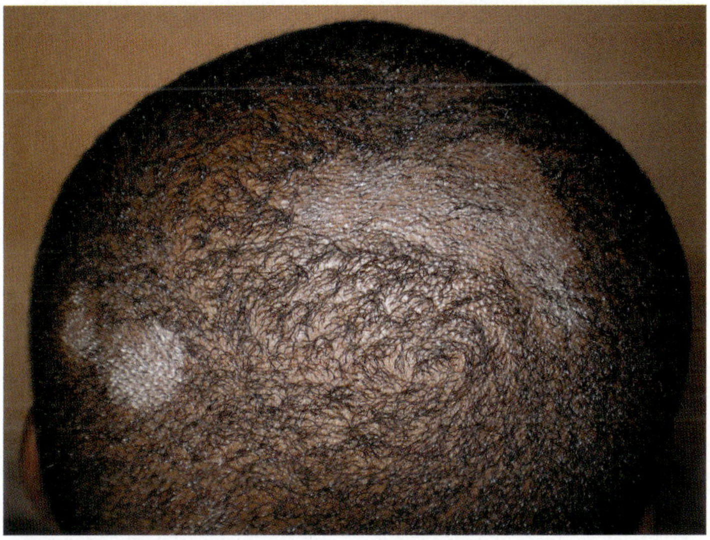

▲ **FIGURE 79-3** Tinea capitis—gray scaly patches of alopecia.

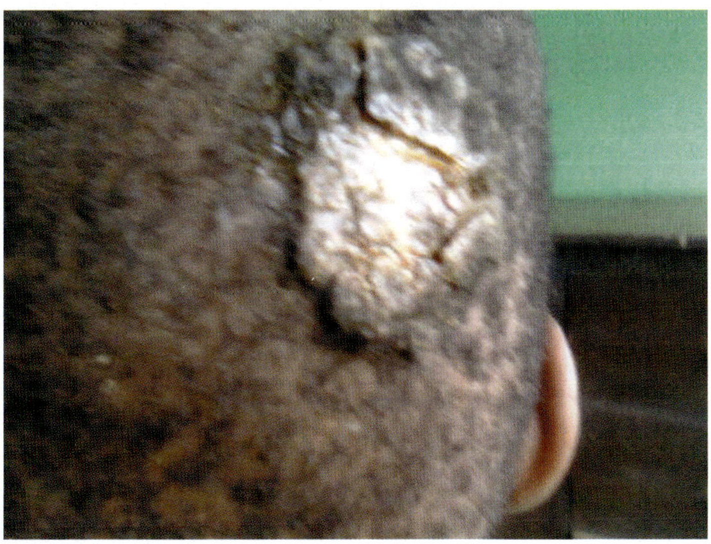

▲ **FIGURE 79-4** Broken kerion.

Tinea Pedis (Athletes Foot)

Key Points

- Most common type of dermatophyte infection in men.
- The three common clinical forms encountered in Africa include (1) soggy interdigital scaling, (2) diffuse scaly soles of the feet, and (3) vesiculopustulation usually along on the instep.
- Onychomycosis usually occurs with tinea pedis.
- Coal miners, communal users of showers by various residents living in low-income buildings or gyms, swimming pools, occlusive and tight-fitting shoes.

Tinea pedis is the most common type of infection in men. Constant heat and humidity, as well as maceration between the toe webs enhanced by tight-fitting/occlusive shoes, lead to this disorder. Individuals who sweat excessively on the soles of the feet are particularly vulnerable. The earliest sign of tinea pedis is maceration (Figure 79-5), followed by scaling and, at times, fissuring of the toe webs of the little toes.

Tinea Corporis

Key Points

- Most common form occurs as anular lesions with raised serpiginous borders and central clearing.
- Tinea corporis is the classic ringworm.
- Multiple annular lesions also may be observed, occurring as a diffuse area of fine scaling without inflammation.

Tinea corporis can present as an active annular lesion with advancing borders and scaliness, and a few vesicles and pustules may be seen within them (Figure 79-6). The lesions expand slowly, and healing in the center leaves the classic ringlike pattern. Tinea corporis has to be differentiated from discoid excema and pityriasis rosea within Africa.

Tinea Cruris

Key Points

- Common infection in men.
- Presents as an itchy groin.
- Asymmetric patch with a serpiginous border.
- Factors predisposing to maceration of the groin include humidity and tight-fitting nylon or crepeline underpants.

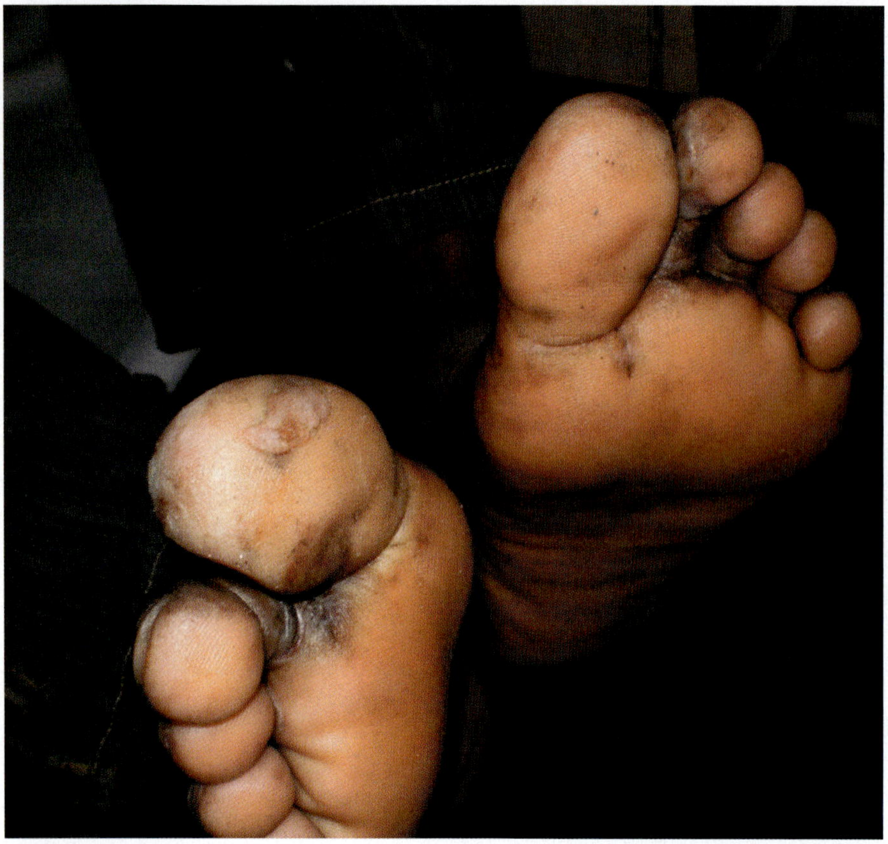

▲ **FIGURE 79-5** Tinea pedis—fissures and wet, soggy toe webs.

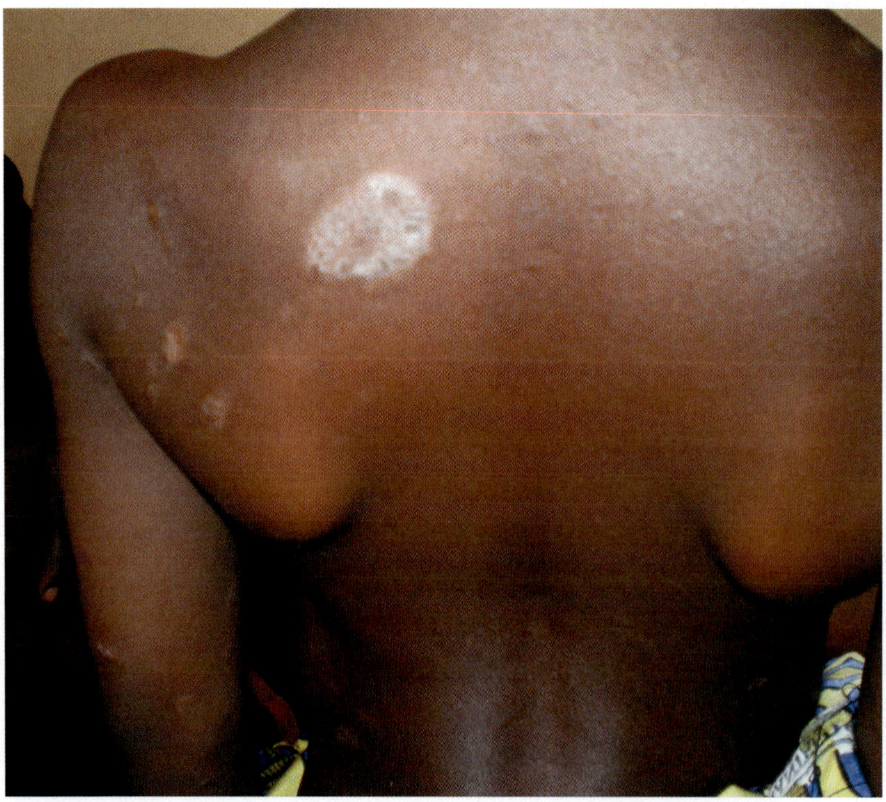

▲ **FIGURE 79-6** Tinea corporis.

This is a common groin rash that affects mostly men. It presents as a macerated patch with raised edges. The initial rash is indolent and spreads within months to years. Humidity, excessive perspiration, and the use of tight-fitting nylon/crepeline underpants are the common predisposing factors. Often prolonged or intermittent use of anti-inflammatory corticosteroid preparations results in a groin that is simply sore and red. Intertrigo, candidiasis, and seborrhoeic dermatitis are differential diagnoses. Erythrasma is a notable differential diagnosis of tinea cruris that is caused by a diptheriod, *Corynebacterium minutissimum,* athough the rash is dry.

Tinea Incognito

Key Points

- Prevalence is high in Africa because of the misuse of steroids.
- Atypical rash with ill-defined borders.

Tinea incognito is a term used to describe a dermatophyte infection that has been rendered clinically atypical by the misuse of corticosteroid preparations. Prevalence is high in most African countries.[19–21] A high index of suspicion is required (Figure 79-7), as well as mycologic studies, to confirm the diagnosis.

Tinea Unguium

Key Points

- Infection of the nails
- Trauma
- Both dermatophytes and nondermatophyte molds have been implicated as causes of onychomycosis in Africa.

Infection of the nails often commences at the distal lateral free edges of the nail plates. Toe nail infection is usually associated with tinea pedis. Subungal hyperkeratosis (Figure 79-8), separation of the nail plate with dyschromia, has been associated with infections such as *T. soudanense* and *T. rubrum* and nondermatophyte molds such as *Pseudomonas, Aspergillus,* and *Cladosporium* in Africa.[22]

Tinea Manum

This is usually asymmetric and often is associated with tinea pedis. It usually may present as a diffuse scaling patch on the palmar surface of only one hand

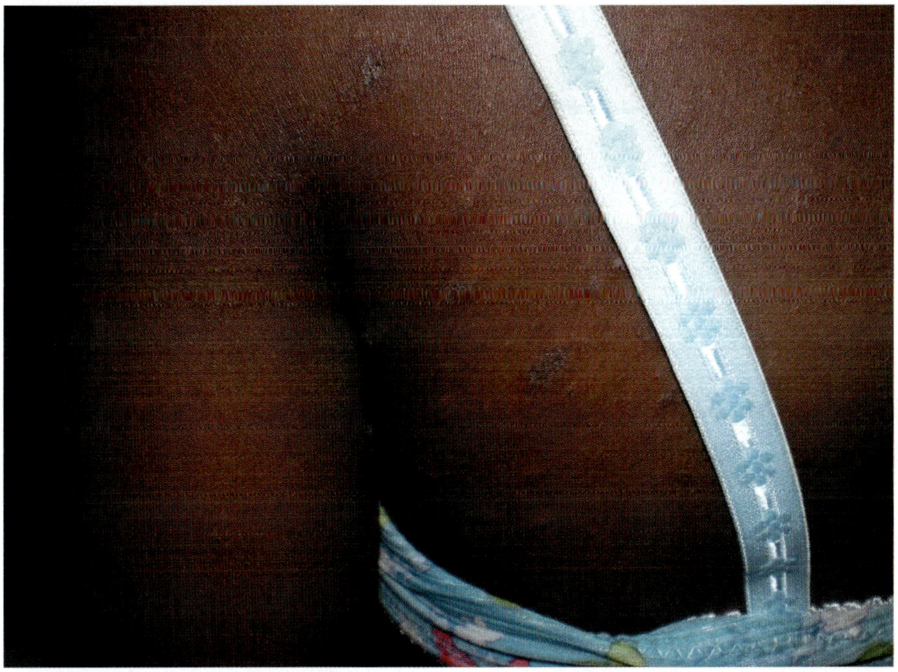

▲ **FIGURE 79-7** Tinea incognito.

(Figure 79-9). Overall, this dermatopyte infection is not very common.

Diagnosis

LABORATORY TESTS FOR DERMATOPHYTE INFECTIONS

- Potassium hydroxide (KOH) mount must be carried out for all scaly rashes in Africa.
- Direct microscopy is perfomed on the mounted sample, which could be a skin scraping, a nail clipping, or a hair.
- A low illumination ×10 is used initially to scan the entire coverslip, looking for branching hyphae.
- Culture is performed next using Sabouraud dextrose agar or the dermatophyte test medium for confirmation of diagnosis.
- Culture reports may take up to 4 weeks.
- Wood's light examination may be carried out (where facilities are available). Examination of the scalp, stump of hair, or face is done in a dark room using the Wood's lamp (an ultraviolet source of light). A green fluorescence is seen with *M. audonii* and *M. canis* infection.

Treatment

Therapy may be topical or systemic for dermatophyte infection. Topical therapy is effective for localized and limited infections, but for tinea capitis or tinea unguium or extensive dermatophytosis, systemic therapy is the mainstay, although shampoos may be used as adjunct therapy for tinea capitis.

- Topical therapy includes Witfield ointment, azoles (e.g., miconazole and clotrimazole), imidazoles (e.g., ketoconazole), or allylamines (e.g., terbinafine or naftifine cream); these are applied twice daily for 4 weeks.
- Systemic therapy includes the use of griseofulvin for adults, 250–500 mg bid, and for children, 10–20 mg/kg per day. Headaches often may be a significant side effect. Other newer drugs available include ketoconazole, 200 mg/day (adults); terbinafine, 250 mg/day (adults) and 125 mg/day (children weighing 20–40 kg); triazole (Itranox), 200 mg/day (adults) and 100 mg/day (children weighing 20–40 kg).
- For tinea capitis in children, treatment requires the use of griseofulvin, 10–20 mg/kg of body weight for 8–12 weeks. Where newer antifungals are available, treatment is for 4–6 weeks. Adjunctive treatment for 2–3 weeks with selineum sulfide shampoo or Nizarol shampoo further shortens the time course of the infection.

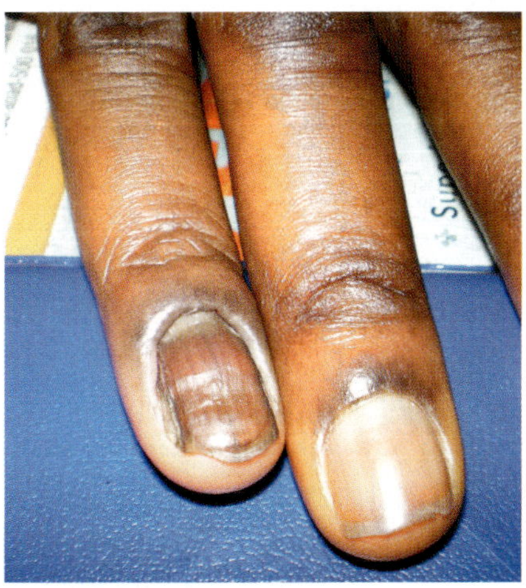

▲ **FIGURE 79-8** Tinea unguium.

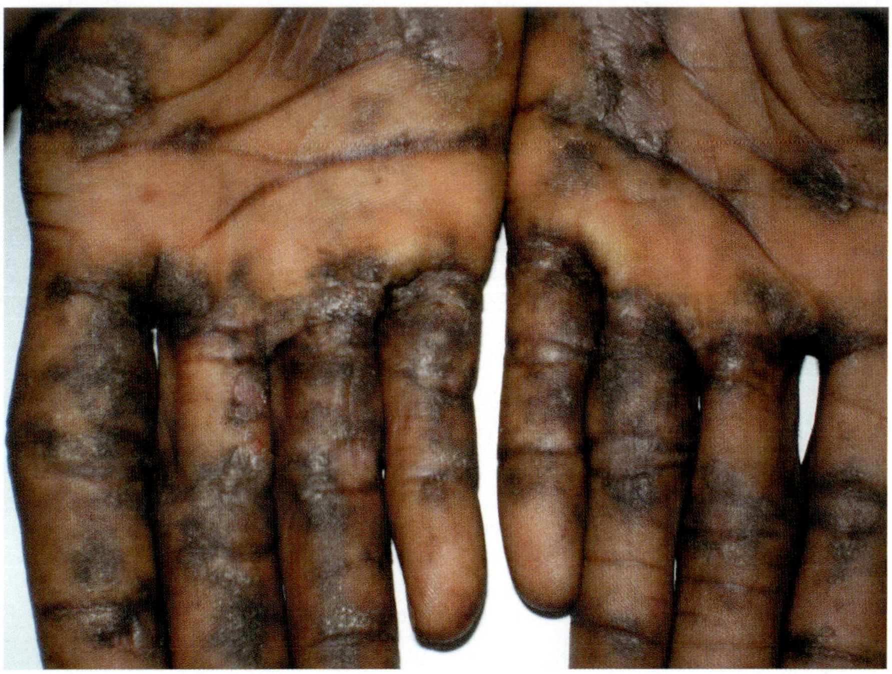

▲ **FIGURE 79-9** Tinea manum.

- For tinea unguium, grisefulvin is given in a dose of 500 mg/day (adults) and 20 mg/kg of body weight twice daily (children) for 4–9 months. Alternatively, terbinafine, 250 mg/day for 6–12 weeks; itraconazole, 200 mg twice daily for 1 week of each month for 3 months; or itraconazole, 200 mg/day for 3 months, may be used.

Pityriasis Versicolor

Key Points

- Also a common superficial fungal infection in Africa, as in other tropical climates.
- Affects all age groups, although more common in adults.
- Individuals who sweat profusely, immuno-suppressed patients, or those on systemic corticosteroids.
- Lesions of pityriasis versicolor can be of various colors—hypopigmented or hyper-pigmented patches with fine scales.
- Face, neck, chest wall, upper back, and shoulders are the predominant sites.
- KOH preparation of pityriasis versicolor gives the diagnostic "spaghetti (short hyphae) and meatballs (spores)" appearance.

Pityriasis versicolor is quite prevalent in warm, humid climates, affecting mainly the very young and middle-aged adults. This infection is caused by *Malassezia furfur,* and the fungal enzymes act on surface lipids to produce dicarboxylic acids that diffuse into the epidermis. These acids inhibit tyrosinase, the enzyme in melanocytes that is responsible for melanin production. Initially, the rash starts off as pinhead-sized areas of macular hypopigmentation that gradually coalesce together to form irregularly shaped macules scattered over the trunk, face, neck, chest wall, and upper arms (Figure 79-10).

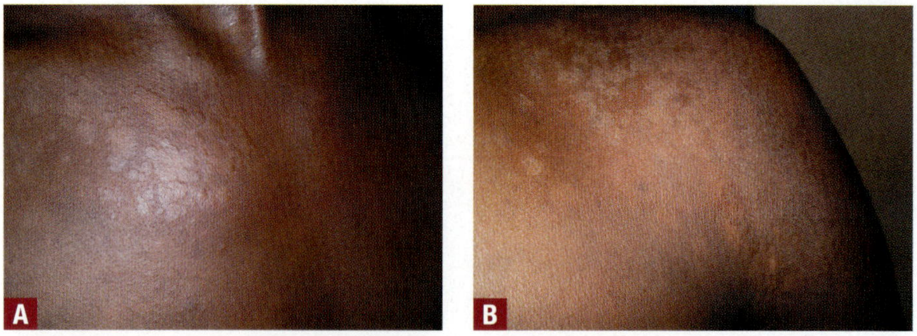

▲ **FIGURE 79-10** Pityriasis versicolor macules scattered on (**A**) chest wall and (**B**) shoulders.

Diagnosis

The diagnosis rests on KOH examination because the organism cannot be grown on routine fungal culture. Direct microscopic examination of scrapings usually reveals short hyphae that are often mixed with spores, thus giving the "spaghetti and meatballs" appearance. Biopsies reveal a lot of fungal organisms in a hyperkeratotic stratum corneum.

Treatment

TOPICAL TREATMENT Treatment consists of application of topical selenium sulfide, ketoconazol, or Head and Shoulders shampoo over affected areas for 10 minutes, after which it is washed off; washing the scalp and face twice daily for 2–4 weeks with the same agent is helpful, particularly for recurrent lesions. Topical imidazole creams (e.g., ketoconazole or miconazole) may be used applying twice daily for 4 weeks, or salicylic acid 5% plus sulfur 5% ointment may be used overnight for 2–4 weeks.

SYSTEMIC TREATMENT Ketoconazol, 200 mg/day for 2 weeks, or itraconazole, 200 mg once daily for 1 week, or fluconazole, 200 mg weekly for two to three doses, may be used for severe recurrent cases. Recurrences can be further prevented by twice-weekly or once-monthly preventive treatment with any of the preceding topical treatments.

Candidiasis

Key Points

- A common infection among debilitated individuals with lowered immunity.
- Candida albicans is the cause of the infection.
- Moisture predisposes to candidiasis.

Mucocutaneous candidiasis is caused by a yeast infection. Usually, *Candida albicans* and *C. tropicalis* are the common offending culprits. Patients at any age may be affected. It usually occurs in moist cutaneous sites and mucosal linings, as occurs in individuals who sweat excessively. It is often refered to as "excema" by the laypeople within most African communities.[19] Predisposing factors include moisture; underlying systemic conditions; diabetes mellitus; pregnancy; obesity; wet work (people who immerse their hands in water during work); oral contraceptive, oral antibiotic, and oral or topical corticosteroid use; polyendocrinopathies; HIV/ AIDS; and chronic debilitating conditions (e.g., malignancies, particularly patients on chemotherapy). Candidiasis may present as interdigital or intertriginous candidiasis (Figure 79-11), paronychial candidiasis, chronic cutaneous candidiasis, vulvovaginitis, balanoposthitis, or mucosal candidiasis. In children, it also may present as diaper candidiasis.

Treatment

Treatment involves the use of topical and/or systemic antifungal agents depending on the extent of the disease.

TOPICAL THERAPY

- Nystatin paint/ointment/cream/powder
- Clotrimazole
- Miconazole
- Ketoconazole

SYSTEMIC THERAPY

- Ketoconazole, 200 mg/day
- Fluconazole cream, 100 mg/day
- Griseofulvin is not effective against candidiasis and has no place in its management.

PARASTIC INFECTIONS

Key Points

- These infections are caused mainly by ectopararasites.
- Although a major group of tropical dermatoses, they are not confined to the tropics only.
- Itching is usually prominent.
- A wide range of skin reactions is provoked by these parasites.
- They include scabies, pediculosis, onchocerciasis, insect-bite allergy, and cutaneous larva migrans.

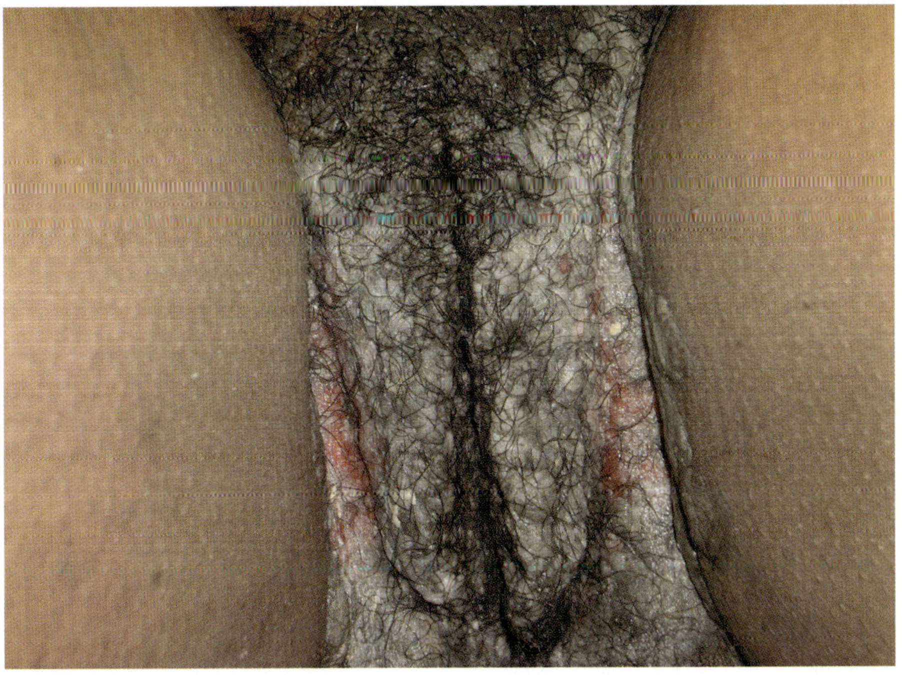

▲ **FIGURE 79-11** Vulvovaginal candidiasis.

Scabies

Key Points

- Parasitic infection caused by *Sarcoptes scabei* var. *hominis.*
- Highly contagious and affects all ages.
- Transmitted by mainly by close contact with an infected person.
- Intractable pruritus that is worse at night is typical.
- Burrows are pathognomic and mainly spotted at the edges/interdigital webs of the hands and feet.
- Family members, friends, and classmates often also itch.

Scabies occurs worldwide.[23–25] It is an infestation of the epidermis caused by the itch mite *Sarcoptes scabei* var. *hominis.* Scabies also may be transmitted by formites and sexual contacts. The incidence of scabies is greater in overcrowded African environments, particularly among school children, prison or psychiatric hospital inmates, and people living in barracks and refugee camps. Debilitated patients, immobilized elderly individuals, HIV/AIDS patients, and people with Down syndrome are prone to infestations with high mite counts, often referred to as *Norwegian scabies.* This condition is also associated with crusted, oozing plaques and is often misdiagnosed as eczema, psoriasis, or exfoliative dermatitis.

Clinical Features

Scabies presents with severe pruritus that is usually worse at night. A history of other family members or close personal contacts with scabies is often elicited. The burrows, which are often difficult to pick out in dark skin, are found at the sides of affected hands or feet (Figure 79-12). Common sites of predilection are the finger webs, toe webs, sides of hands and feet, flexural surfaces of the wrists, extensor surfaces of the wrists and knees, axillae, inframamary sites, phallus, and buttocks. In children, the face, neck, soles of the feet, and palms are also affected. Inflammatory papules associated with secondary bacterial infection often lead to the formation of multiple pustules, whereas with prolonged scratching, excematization and lichenification occurs. In long-standing cases, nodules and even blisters may be found. Several complications also may develop from impetiginized scabies, and these include cellulitis, pyoderma, lymphangitis, acute glomerulonephritis, and delusions of parasitosis. The inflammatory itching and inflammation are believed to be the result of a hypersensitivity reaction to the mites, eggs, and feces. This takes about 1–2 weeks to subside after treatment.

Diagnosis

Diagnosis is made based on a tiny black speck that is often seen at the end of a trail/burrow; this may be lifted with a needle. The burrow ink test[26] is another method used for identifying the mites, eggs, and feces.

Treatment

- Topical or systemic medications may be chosen.
- For severely excoriated scabies, ivermectin is preferable.
- All family members and close personal contacts must be treated.
- Clothing and bedding must be washed in hot soapy water and ironed once treatment has begun.
- Antihistamines and antibiotics also may be added in impetiginized scabies.

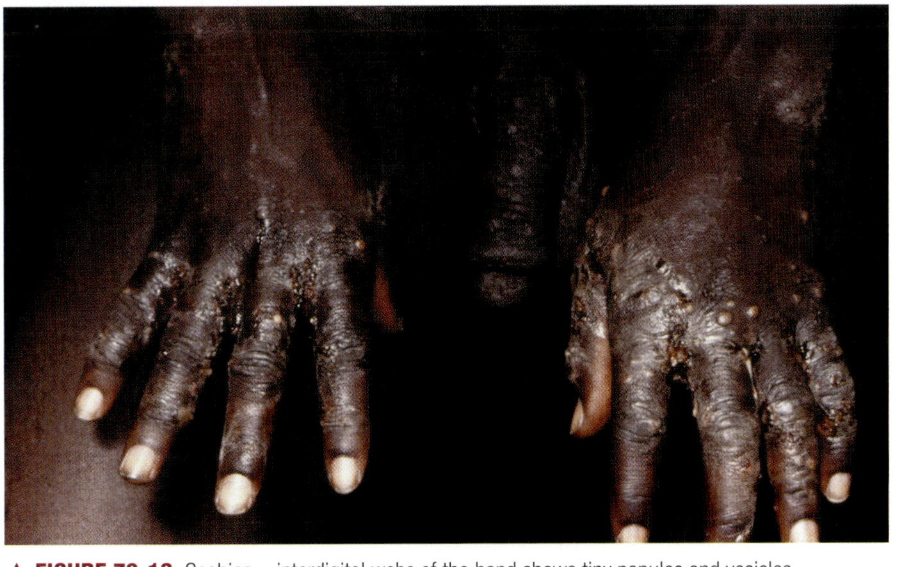

▲ **FIGURE 79-12** Scabies—interdigital webs of the hand shows tiny papules and vesicles.

TOPICAL THERAPY

Benzyl Benzoate. Benzyl benzoate 25% is applied from the neck down to the toes and allowed to say on for 24 hours for 3days. This is washed off each day for 3 days using monosulfiram BP (Tetmosol) soap. For children, a dilution of 1:1 or 12.5% benzyl benzoate is used.

Permethrin. Overnight application of 5% permethrin cream, repeated 1 week later, is effective.

Lindane. The same overnight application, repeated 1 week later, is effective.

Whichever treatment option is selected, it is recommended for the entire household and contacts at the same time.

SYSTEMIC THERAPY Oral ivermectin has been used successfully for treating scabies in a single dose at 0.1– 0.2 mg/kg. In Africa, compliance with topical medications is poor because of the pain associated with the application of benzyl benzoate, for instance. Ivermectin thus is given in a single dose of 3–12 mg.

FURTHER SUPPORTIVE THERAPY

- Antihistamine
- Antibiotics for secondary bacterial infection
- Tetmosol (monosulfiram BP) for bathing affected individuals, family members, and close contacts

Papular Urticaria

Key Points

- Also known as insect-bite allergy.
- Common disorder, particularly among children.
- Confined mainly to exposed areas, especially the limbs.
- Bites from sandflies, mosquitoes, fleas, or bedbugs may cause papular urticaria.
- Healed lesions leave a lot of postinflammatory hyperpigmented patches.
- May present a similar picture to papulopruritc itch of HIV/AIDS.
- Treatment includes the use of insect repellent and covering up exposed parts of the body most times.

Papular urticaria, also known as *insect-bite allergy,* is a common disorder among children and occasionally in susceptible adolescents and adults.[27,28] Reactions to insect bites vary according to the degree of sensitivity of the individual. The disorder presents with urticarial papules, vesicles, or lumps and is persistently itchy. It occurs repeatedly in affected individuals. In most cases, it is believed to be a hypersensitivity reaction to contact with the insect, its bite, or its vomitus. Not every family member is affected. It may become weepy, crusted, and secondarily infected. Healing leaves a lot of postinflamatory hyperpigmented patches scattered on the limbs (Figure 79-13); this is often confused with the papulopruritic itch of HIV/AIDS.

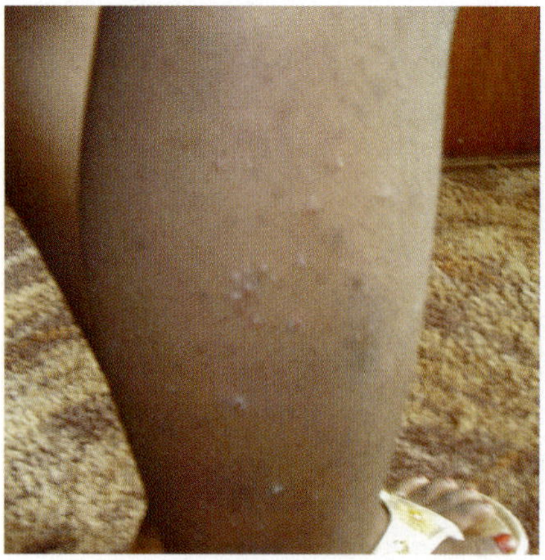

▲ **FIGURE 79-13** Papular urticaria.

Treatment

Antihistamines are given to break the itch-scratch cycle. Antibiotics may be used in patients with secondary bacterial infection. Topical steroids may be applied. To prevent repeated attacks, insect repellents are used, and patients are advised to wear clothing that covers exposed areas, particularly in the evening.

Myasis

Key Points

- Presents with painful or stinging boils.

This is the development of larva of some species of fly within a human being as one of several possible hosts. Commonly caused by the Tumbu fly, *Cordylobia anthropophaga,* in Africa. The skin lesions may look like boils, but movement may be detected within and is usually associated with a lot of pain. The diagnosis is verified by incising the nodule and extracting the larva. Postextrusion antibiotics may be neccasary.

Cutaneous Migrans Larva

This usually presents with migratory, pruritc, serpiginous lesions owing to unchecked movement within the superficial layer of the skin of larval parasites (Figure 79-14). Humans are not the definitive host and hence the wandering movement. Common causes of this condition include larva of *Strongyloides, Ancylostoma braziliensis, A. canum,* and *Gnathostoma.* Favored sites include the feet and buttocks and any site for children who play on the ground naked.[29]

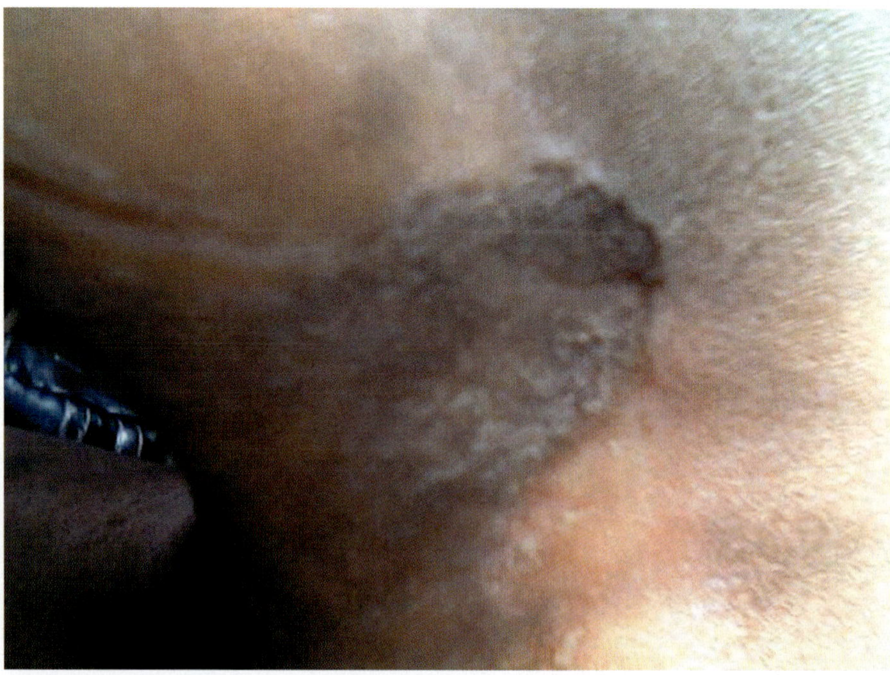

▲ **FIGURE 79-14** Cutaneous larva migrans.

Treatment

Treatment involves application of topical thiabendazole cream every 12 hours or a single dose of albendazole (400 mg) or ivermectin (150–200 μg/kg).

Pediculosis

Key Points

- This is also known as lice infestation.
- Pediculosis capitis, pediculosis corporis, and pubic lice are all variants of lice infestation.
- Caused by *Pediculus humanus capitis, Pediculus humanus corporis,* and *Phthrius pubis.*
- Poverty, neglect, and poor personal and community hygiene.

This infestation is found mainly among unkempt persons, socially deprived people, and asylum and prison inmates in Africa. There are three main variants—pediculosis capitis, pediculosis corporus, and pubic lice. The main features of all lice infestations are severe itching, followed by scratching and secondary infection. On the scalp, the eggs for pediculosis capitis are seen easily and are found stuck to the hair shafts at the sides and back of the scalp. While the body louse looks similar to the scalp louse, it lays its eggs in the seams of clothing in contact with skin. Pubic lice are usually spread by sexual contact.

Treatment

Treatment involves use of specific pediculocides such as 5% malathion or Carbary lotion applied to the scalp and left on for 12 hours. Permethrin 1% or Lindane cream are alternatives that can be used. Treatment should be repeated after the first week. All family members or groups should be treated at the same time.

BACTERIAL INFECTIONS

Key Points

- Common infections.
- Skin bacteria include *Staphylococcus epidermidis,* diptheroids, and streptococci deeper down.
- Impetigo commonly affects children.

Bacterial infections are also common infections within African countries.[25,30,31] Many of these infections are established through the hair follicles. These infections include folliculitis, sycosis, furunculosis, and carbuncles. These are localized infections often caused by staphylococci, whereas deeper infections such as erysipelas, cellulitis, and lymphangitis are caused by streptoccoci.

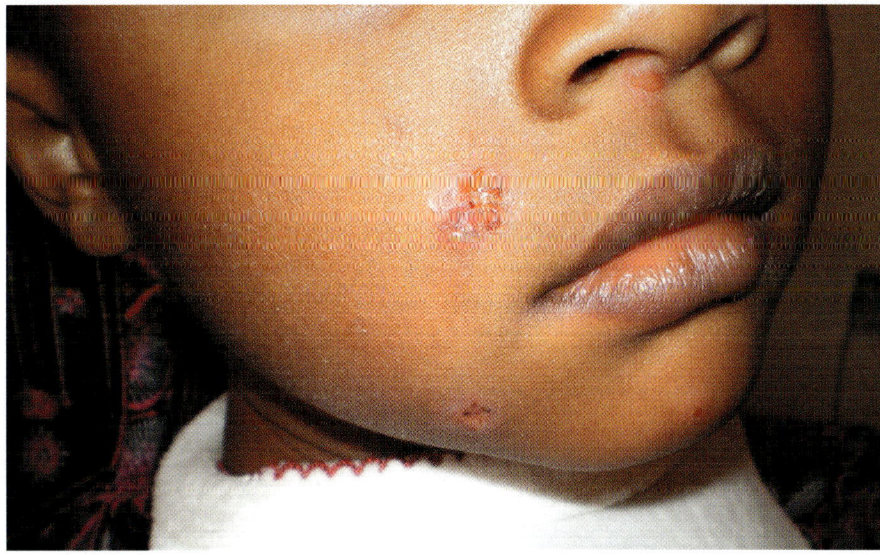

▲ **FIGURE 79-15** Crusted lesions of impetigo scattered on the face.

Impetigo

This is a common, highly contagious infection affecting mainly children. This condition may be caused by staphylococci, streptococci, or both together. The bullous type is usually caused by *Staphylococcus aureus,* whereas the crusted ulcer type is caused by β-hemolytic strains of streptococci. Rupture of pustules or blisters often leads to honey-colored exudates that quickly spread to adjacent areas by contact, resulting in new lesions. The face is the most affected site (Figures 79-15 and 79-16). Spread may

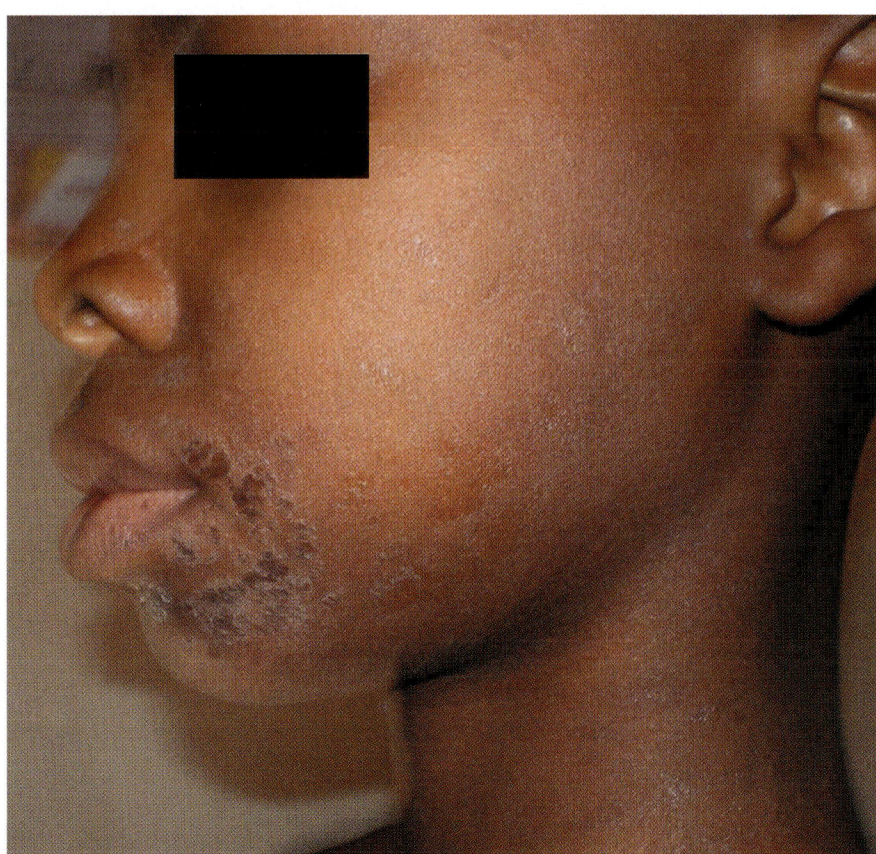

▲ **FIGURE 79-16** Healing impetigo.

be through a family member or classmates. Variants of impetigo include impetigo neonatorium, bullous impetigo, and a follicular type of impetigo known as *superficial folliculitis*.

Treatment

TOPICAL THERAPY Cleanse the affected areas with astringents such as potassium permanganet or betadine lotion, and then apply mupiricin ointment twice daily. This is done mainly for mild cases. Use of antibacterial soaps (e.g., Dettol soap, Carat or Dial) is helpful.

SYSTEMIC THERAPY Systemic broad-based antibiotics may be needed for severe cases and include flucloxacillin and erythromycin or doxycyline.

Folliculitis

This is a bacterial infection of the hair follicle and tends to occur at the level of the hair follicle orifice. *S. aureus* is the most common cause. Clinically, it appears as a pustule with centrally placed hairs. The scalp is a common site, especially in children, but in adults, the face, beard, and extremities may be involved. Involvement of the deeper part of the hair follicle results in a condition referred to as *sycosis*. Mineral oils, plasters, and other chemicals often clog the orifice of the hair follicle, resulting in folliculitis (Figure 79-17).

Treatment

A broad-spectrum antibiotic is used, as well as antisceptic cleansers such as betadine.

Pyodermas

These present as multiple skin abscesses. Clincally, they present with yellow crusts with dirty sores and pustules. In diabetics, they may be recurrent.

Treatment

Treatment involves the use of oral antibiotics (broad spectrum). Also, cleanse affected areas with potassium permanganent solution or 10% povodine-iodine.

DERMATITIS

Key Points

- Dermatitis is currently gaining ground in African countries.
- *Eczema* and *dermatitis* are synonyms.
- Dermatitis may be idiopathic or may have specific causes.
- It may present acutely with weeping and vesiculations, subacutely, or chronically with lichenification and hyperpigmentation.

Eczemas are currently gaining ground in African countries. This is probably a result of the increased urbanization and industrialization, as well as corresponding changes in diet, exposure to irritants and pollutants, and increased levels of sanitization and hygiene. As predicted by earlier authors, there has been a 10% increase in their overall incidence, reaching the levels recorded in developed countries.[32] Dermatitis currently has a prevalence of between 5% and 21% in Africa.[33] Atopic eczema, seborrheic dermatitis, and contact dermatitis are the main dermatides that have seen significant increases in African countries.[34–36] Each of these may present in the acute, subacute, or chronic phase.

Dermatitides are noninfective conditions and may be defined as a reaction pattern to endogenous or exogenous stimuli. They can present acutely with weeping vesiculations or subacutely or chronically with lichenification and hyperpigmentation (Figure 79-18).

Atopic dermatitis is common throughout the world and currently tops the list in a rising trend for Africa. It occurs commonly in individuals with a generic predisposition and a family or personal history of atopy. However, environmental factors also play a prominent role.[37,38] The natural history is that of a chronic disorder that waxes and wanes spontaneously or in

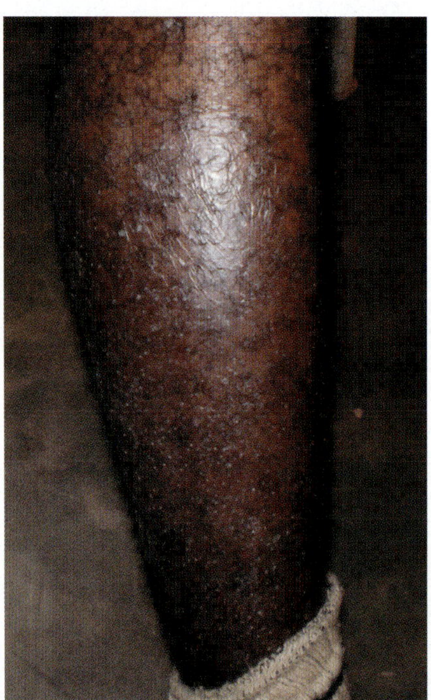

▲ **FIGURE 79-17** Sycosis cruris,

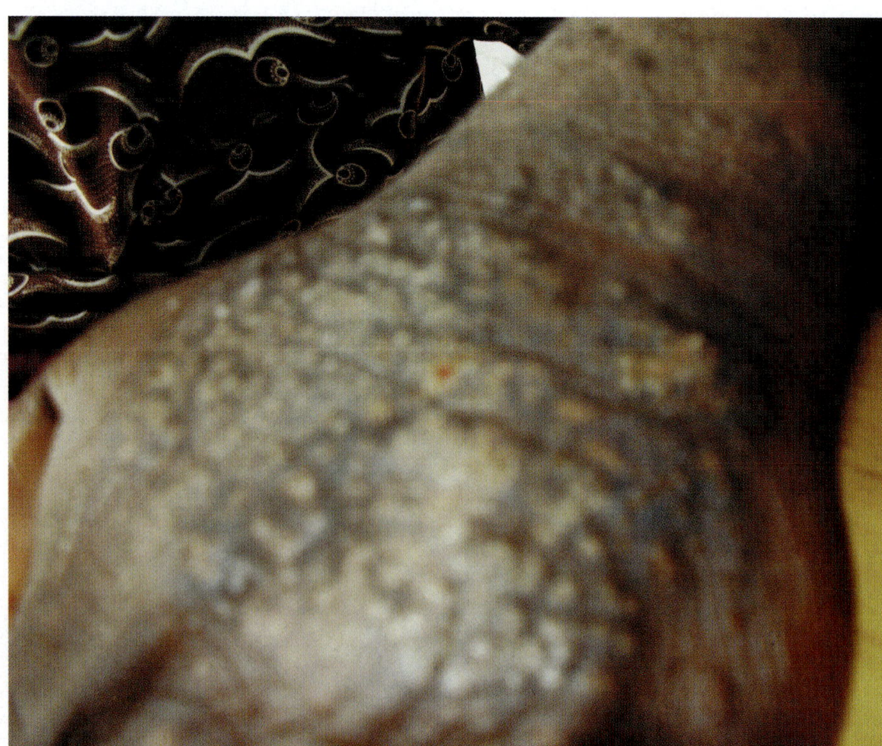

▲ **FIGURE 79-18** Chronic eczematous plaque over the dorsum of the hand.

response to changes in the weather. Children or adults may be affected. In infancy, the rash is widespread and nonspecific in distribution. Gradually, it affects the flexures, neck, elbows, and knees (Figure 79-19). In later childhood, an extensor presentation of lesions may be one of the features peculiar to blacks (Figure 79-20), whereby the extensor surfaces and pressure areas are affected more than the flexures. Affected infants are usually restless, itching, irritated, and scratching the entire body, with the result that parents have sleepless nights. Widespread excoriations, lichenification, fissuring, and secondary bacterial infection become common complications. Hyperpigmentation is a feature following constant rubbing and scratching.

Atopic dermatitis in adult life may start de novo, or it may be a carry-over from adolescence. The skin remains dry and sensitive and prone to lichenification, lichen simplex chronicus, hand eczema, and pompholyx.

Treatment

- Counsel parents for a child to avoid irritants (e.g., extremes of temperature, woolen clothes, harsh soaps, and food allergens such as peanuts, eggs, milk, and shellfish/crayfish).
- If weeping, cleanse/soak affected areas in a 1:10,000 dilution of potassium permanganate.
- Regular application of emollient (aqueous cream, Diprobase, emulsifying ointment, or white soft parafin).
- Twice-daily topical application of medium- to potent-strength topical steroids (e.g., Eumovate or Betnovate), rapidly tapering it down within 2 weeks to a mildly potent steroid (e.g., hydrocortisone).
- Nothing stronger than 1% hydrocortisone should be used on the face.
- For chronic cases, 2% tar ointment with salicylic acid may be used.
- Use of sedating antihistamines such as chlopheniramine, terfenadine, and ketotifen (Zaditen) has been very helpful as well.
- Use broad-spectrum antibiotics particularly to reduce the high rate of colonization of the skin with *S. aureus.*
- Immumodulants (e.g., azathioprine or cyclosporine).
- Antifungals are used when there is a secondary fungal infection.

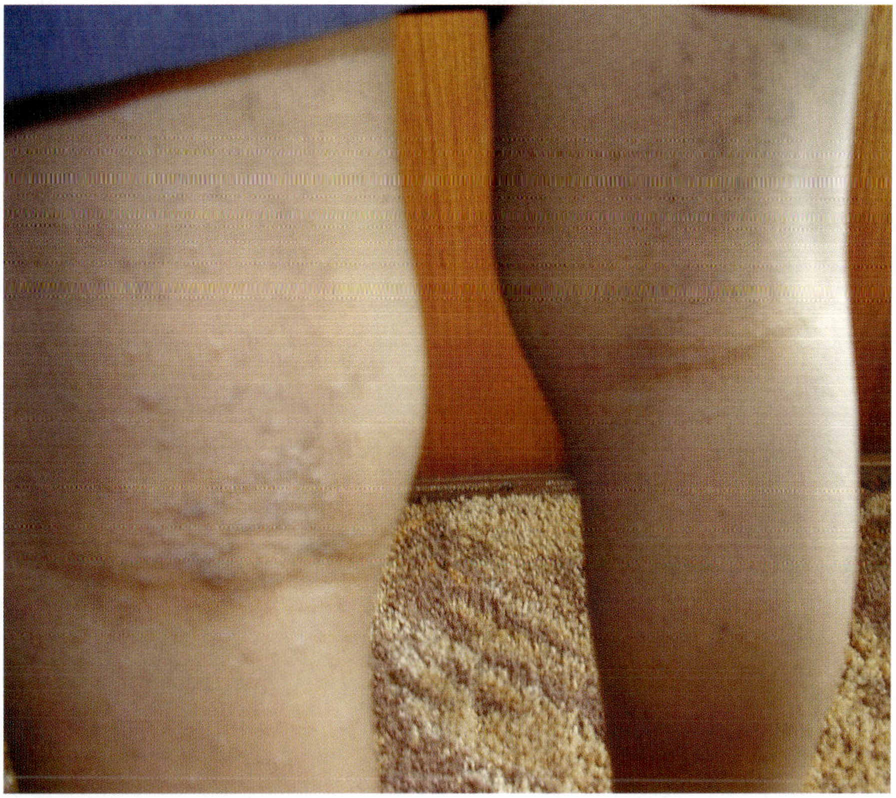

▲ **FIGURE 79-19** Atopic dermatitis.

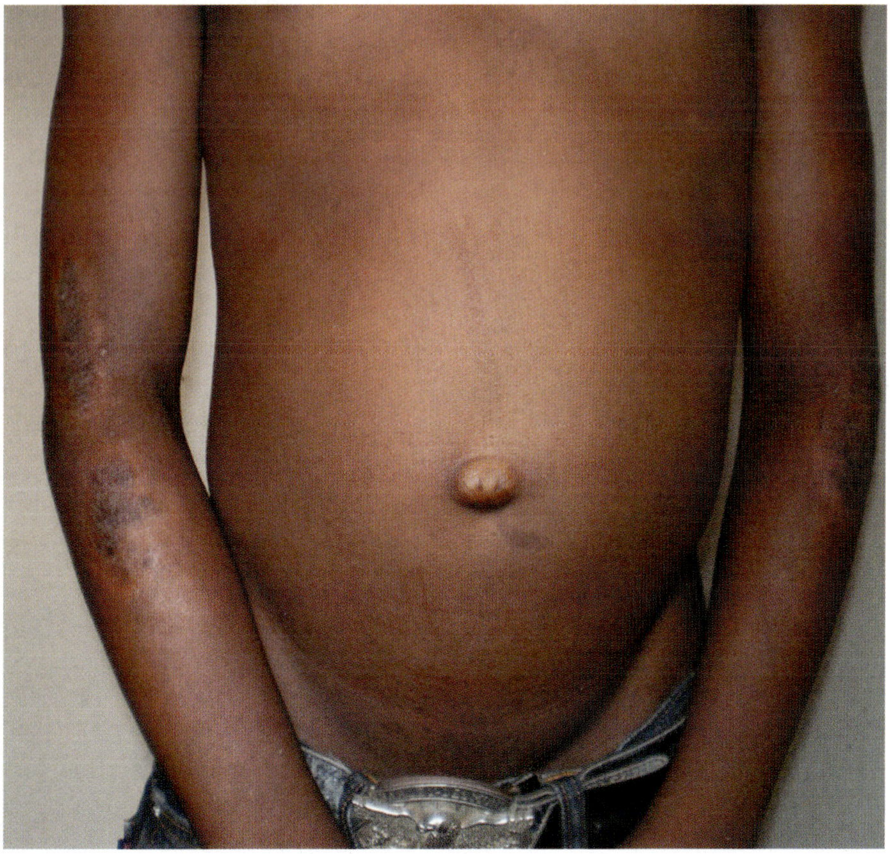

▲ **FIGURE 79-20** Atopic dermatitis lesions revealing an extensor surface distribution.

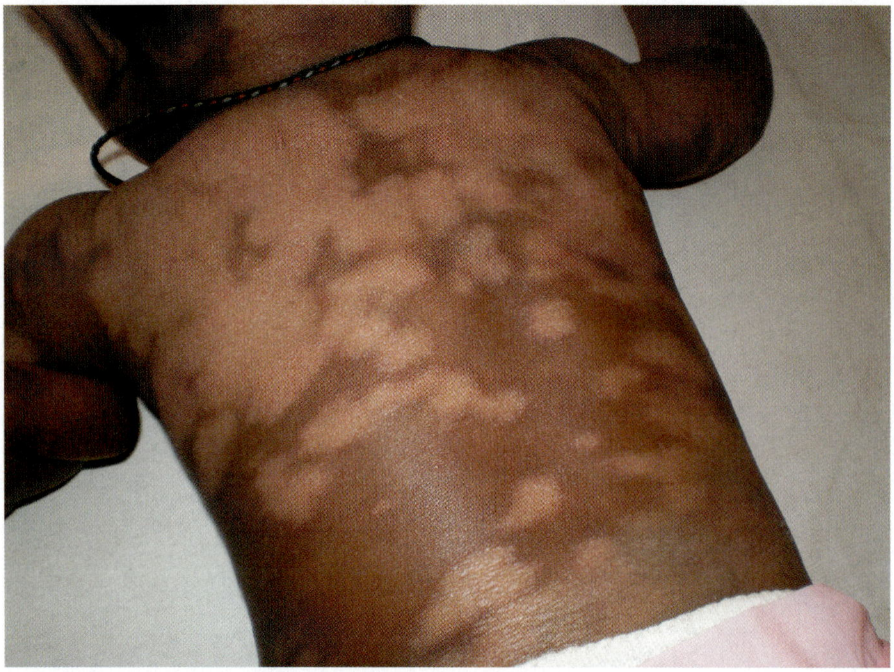

▲ **FIGURE 79-21** Seborrhoeic dermatitis in an 6-month-old baby.

Seborrhoheic Eczemas

This is a chronic inflammatory process affecting the hairy areas of the skin. It may present in infancy (Figure 79-21), childhood, adolescence, or adult life (Figure 79-22) and at times runs in families. The etiology is unclear, and the condition is unrelated to seborrhea. *Pityrospoum ovale* may contribute to the cause of seborrhoiec dermatitis.

In adults, the course is unpredictable. It may be recurrent, and in some it may be very stubborn and recalcitrant. In children, it clears readily with treatment.

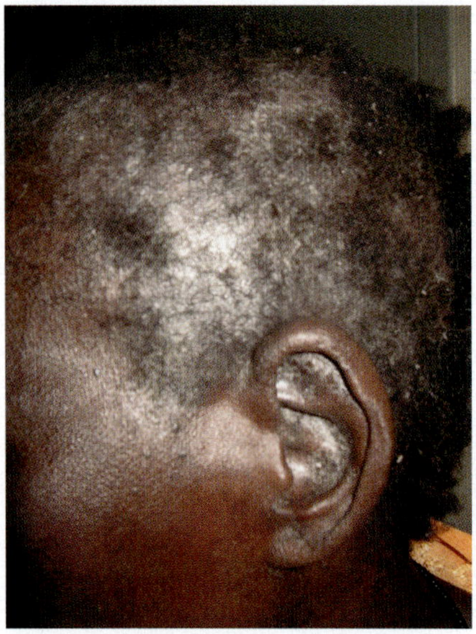

▲ **FIGURE 79-22** Seborrhoeic dermatitis.

Severe cases have been reported in patients with HIV/AIDS.

Clinical Features

- The rash is often bilateral and has a predilection for hairy areas such as the scalp, eyebrows, eyelids, nasolabial creases, ears, chest wall, intertreginous areas, axilla, and groin. However, the face and scalp are commonly affected.
- May present as dry, scaly petaloid lesion on the chest and interscapular area. There also may be extensive follicular papules or pustules on the trunk (i.e., seborrheic folliculitis or *Pityrisporum* folliculitis).
- In its mildest form, it presents as dandruff with fine scales.
- The patches and plaques of seborrheic dermatitis have indistinct borders with greasy scales.

Treatment

TOPICAL THERAPY

- Apply Nizarol shampoo or selenium sulfide or zinc pyrithione shampoo and allow to stay on for 3–5 minutes twice daily for 2 weeks and then three times per week.
- Also, 2% sulfur ointment and 2% salicylic acid in aqueous cream are often helpful and avoid the problem of topical steroids.
- Low-strength steroids (1% or 2.5% hydrocortisone cream) may be used for inflammatory seborrheic dermatitis. High-potency steroids must be avoided in this condition.

SYSTEMIC THERAPY For severe cases, oral itraconazole, 100 mg/day for 2 weeks, may be used or weekly doses of fluconazole, 200 mg, in combination with 2–5% salicylic acid and tar ointment applied twice daily to the face or 1% hydrocortisone or Betnovate RD cream/ointment applied twice daily over the affected areas.

Contact Dermatitis

Over the years, with rapid urbanization and westernization, the prevalence of contact dermatitis also has increased in Africa. Contact dermatitis results from the contact of the skin with an offending agent, which could be an irritant or an allergen. This sets off the inflammatory process, which could be acute or chronic. Contact dermatitis worldwide is divided into two broad types, namely, allergic contact dermatitis and irritant contact dermatitis. Common causes of irritant dermatitis within Africa are from locally made caustic soda soaps, detergents, fuel and related products, alcohol, and other chemical reagents (Figure 79-23).

Allergic contact dermatitis is associated with an initial sensitization phase following prior exposure to the allergen. This takes place before the actual elicitation phase. Several allergens have been implicated in our environment and include the following: shoe and clothing allergens, medicinal allergens, jewelry (particularly costume jewelry), and occupational and environmental allergens. A patch test is often carried out to determine the offending allergen group.

Photoallergic contact dermatitis is another form of contact dermatitis in which the skin is exposed to a photoallergen.

Treatment

First, for contact dermatitis, identification and avoidance of the identified group of allergens (products) is very important to help contain the illness. If the dermatitis is acute and weeping, affected areas should be soaked twice daily with 1:10,000 potassium permanganate in lukewarm water for the first 3–5 days, and then an emolient should be applied, as well as a medium-strength to potent topical steroid twice daily and then rapidly trailed off.

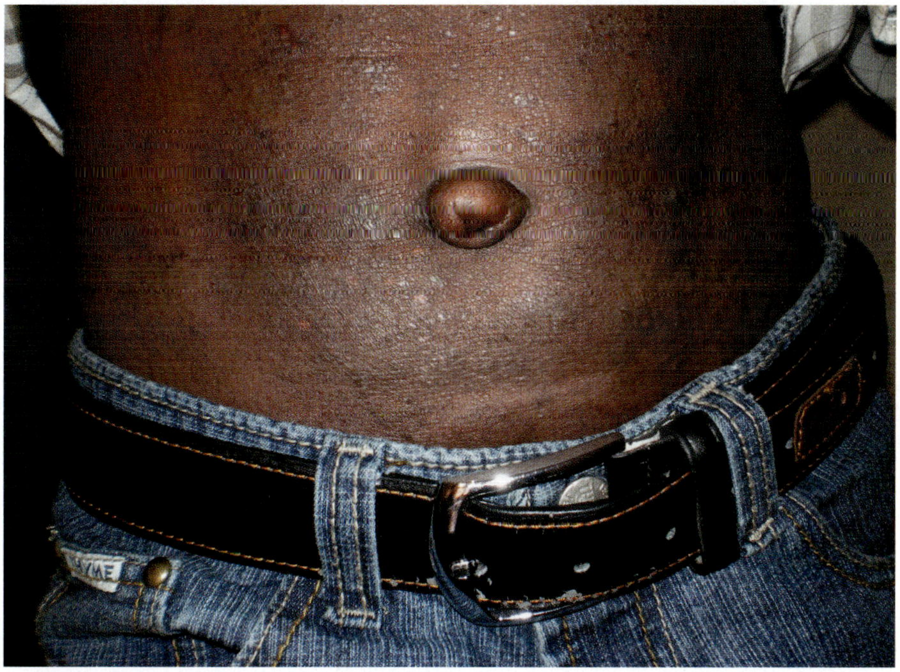

▲ **FIGURE 79-23** Contact dermatitis from a belt.

TABLE 79-2
Cultural Practices and Dermatosis

Procedure	Disorders
Tribal marks	Scar, keloids Also may be associated with lichen planus, sarcoidosis, hepatitis
Scarification marks	Scar, keloids Also may be a portal for transmission of hepatitis, HIV/AIDS if nonserilized instruments are used
Traction alopecia	Hair care practices, use of tight headgears
Central centrifugal cicatricial alopecias	Hair care practices
Pomade acne	Topical application of occlusive oils/pomade

In chronic situation, a keratolytic such as 5–10% salicylic acid and potent-strength steroids are applied twice daily. Antihistamines (e.g., promethazine, terfenadine, loratidine, citerazine, or ketotifen) may be used. Antibiotics also may be used if there is evidence of secondary bacterial infection.

If the patient has photoallergic contact dermatitis, avoidance of sunlight is very important, as well as the use of sunblock creams/lotions or sprays.

DERMATOSIS SECONDARY TO CULTURAL PRACTICES

This is an aspect that has generated a lot of interest in recent times. There are certain practices, listed in Table 79-2, that are prevalent in certain parts of Africa based on traditional or cultural beliefs.

REFERENCES

1. Fitzpatrick TB.The validity and practicality of sun reactive skin type I through VI. *Arch Dermatol* 1988;124:869-871.
2. Kaidbey KH, Agin PP, Sayre RM, Kligman A. Photoprotection by melanin: A comparison of black and Caucasian skin. *J Am Acad Dermatol* 1979;1:249-260.
3. Halder RM, Bridgeman-Shan S. Skin cancer in African-Americans. *Cancer* 1995;75:667-673.
4. Herzberg AJ, Dinehart SM. Chronologic aging in black skin. *Am J Dermatopathol* 1989;11:319-328.
5. Figueroa JI, Fuller LC, Abraha A, Hay RJ. Dermatology in southwestern Ethiopia: Rationale for a community approach. *Int J Dermatol* 1998;37:752-758.
6. Mahe A, N'Diaye T, Bobin P. The proportion of medicalconsultaions motivated by skin diseases in the health centers of Bamako (Republic of Mali). *Int J Dermatol* 1997;36:185-186.
7. UNAIDS. *2005 Report on the Global AIDS Epidemic*. Geneva: UNAIDS, 2005.
8. Rebell G, Taplin D. *Dermatophytes: Their Recognition and Identification*, 4th ed. Miami, University of Miami Press, 1979, pp 1-79.
9. Woldeamanuel Y, Mengsitu Y, Chryssanthou E, Petrini B. Dermatophytosis in Tulugudu Island, Ethiopia. *Med Mycol* 2005;43:79-82.
10. Nwogu AC, Otukunefor TV. Epidemiology of dermatophytosis in a rural community in eastern Nigeria and review of literature from Africa. *Mycopathologica* 2007;164:149-158.
11. Robertson VJ, Wright S. A survey of tinea capitis in primary school children in Harare, Zimbabwe. *J Trop Med Hyg* 1990;93:419-422.
12. Figueroa JI, Hawranek T, Abraha A, Hay RJ. Tinea capitis in southwestern Ethiopia: A study of risk factors for infection and carriage. *Int J Dermatol* 1997;36: 661-666.
13. Olumide YM..Superficial fungal infections as seen in LUTH (local factors in Managemen). *Niger Med J* 1977;3:284.
14. Verhagen AR. Distribution of dermatophytes causing tinea capitis in Africa. *Trop Geogr Med* 1974;26:101-120.
15. Nweze EI. Etiology of dermatophytoses among children in northeastern Nigeria. *Med Mycol* 2001;39:181-184.
16. Nnoruka EN, Ndu AC, Ohanu ME, et al. Patchy hair loss in school children: Tinea capitis reassed. *J Pediatr Infect Dis* 2007;2:147-151.
17. Menan EI, Zongo-Bonou O, Rouet F, et al. Tinea capitis in schoolchildren from Ivory Coast (western Africa): A 1998-1999 cross-sectional study. *Int J Dermatol* 2002;41:204-207.
18. Ayaya SO, Kamar KK, Kakai R. Aetiology of tinea capitis in school children. *East Afr Med J* 2001;78:531-535.
19. Olumide YM. *A Pictorial Self-Instructional Manual on Common Skin Diseases (Where There Is No Dermatologist)*. Nigeria, Heinmann Educational Books, 1993 pp 15-26.
20. Nnoruka EN, Okoye OP. Topical steroid abuse: Its use as a depigmenting agent. *J Natl Med Assoc* 2006;98:934-939.
21. Ly F, Soko AS, Dione DA, et al. Aesthetic problems associated with the cosmetic use of bleaching products. *Int J Dermatol* 2007;46:15-17.
22. Omar AA. Importance of mycological confirmation of clinically suspected cases of tinea corporis, tinea pedis, and tinea cruris. *J Egypt Public Health Assoc* 2004:79:43-58.
23. Landwehr D, Keita SM, Ponnighaus JM, Tounkara C. Epidemiologic aspects of scabies in Mali, Malawi, and Cambodia. *Int J Dermatol* 1998;37:588-590.
24. Hegazy AA, Darwish NM, Abdel-Humid IA, Hamma SM. Epidemiology and control of scabies in an Egyptian village. *Int J Dermatol* 1999;38:291-295.
25. Canizares O, Harman RM. *Clinical Tropical Dermatology*, 2nd ed. Oxford, England, Blackwell Scientific, 1992.
26. Woodley D, Saurat JH. The burrow ink test and the scabies mite. *J Am Acad Dermatol* 1981;4:715-722.

27. Hernandez RG, Cohen BA. Insect bite-induced hypersensitivity and the SCRATCH principles: A new approach to papular urticaria. *Pediatrics* 2006;118: e189-196.
28. Naafs B. Allergic skin reactions in the tropics. *Clin Dermatol* 2006;24:158-167.
29. McCrindle CM, Hay IT, Kirkpartick D, et al. A primary health care approach to an outbreak of cutaneous larva migrans. *J South Afr Vet Assoc* 1996;67:133-136.
30. Belcher DW, Afoakwa SN, Osei-Tutu E, et al. Endemic pyoderma in Ghana: A survey in rural villages. *Trans R Soc Trop Med Hyg* 1977;71:204-209.
31. Mahe A, Faye O, Thiam N'Diaye H, et al. Definition of an algorithm for the management of common skin diseases at primary health care level in sub-Saharan Africa. *Trans R Soc Trop Med Hyg* 2005;99: 39-47.
32. Steele K. Primary dermatologic care in general practice. *J R Coll Gen Pract* 1984; 34:22-24.
33. The International Study of Asthma and Allergies in Childhood (ISAAC) Steering Committee. Worldwide variation in prevalence of symptoms of asthma, allergic rhinoconjunctivitis, and atopic eczema. *Lancet* 1998;351:1225-1232.
34. Sheshibi D. Pattern of skin diseases at the Ethio-Swedish Pediatric Hospital, Addis Ababa, Ethiopia. *Pediatr Dermatol* 2000;17: 337-359.
35. Nnoruka EN. Current epidemiology of atopic dermatitis in southeastern Nigeria. *Int J Dermatol* 2004;43:739-744.
36. Ogunbiyi AO, Owaje EM, Ndahi A. Prevalence of skin diseases in school children in Ibadan, Nigeria. *Pediatr Dermatol* 2005:226-210.
37. Beyer K, Wahn U. Is atopic dermatitis predictable? *Pediatr Allergy Immunol* 1999: 10:7-10.
38. Kjellman NI. Predictive value of high IgE levels in children. *Acta Paediatr Scand* 1976:65: 465-471.

CHAPTER 80

Common Skin Diseases and Treatment in Asia

Joyce Teng-Ee Lim
Yuin-Chew Chan

Key Points

- Asia is the largest continent in the world and has many different geographic terrains. It extends from countries in the temperate zones, the Far East (including Japan, Korea. and China) to countries in the tropics, the South and Southeast Asian countries (including Singapore, Malaysia, the Philippines, Indonesia, Thailand, Vietnam, Cambodia, Laos, and Myammar) and to the countries in the subtropics (including the Indian subcontinent and countries in the Middle East).
- Most of the Asian population has Fitzpatrick skin phototypes III, IV, and V, whereas a small proportion has skin phototypes II and VI.
- There is a wide variety of differences in ethnicity, culture, hygiene, nutrition, and socioeconomic status.
- It is common that dermatologic conditions seen in one part of Asia may be different from those seen in another part.
- There are, however, some skin disorders that are common throughout Asia as well as other parts of the world, for example, eczema, and acne vulgaris.
- Other skin disorders more commonly seen in Asia are lichen amyloidosis or Nevus of Ota/Ito.

Asia is the largest continent in the world and has many different geographic terrains. It extends from countries in the temperate zones, the Far East (including Japan, Korea, and China) to countries in the tropics, the South and Southeast Asian countries (including Singapore, Malaysia, the Philippines, Indonesia, Thailand, Vietnam, Cambodia, Laos, and Myanmar) and to countries in the subtropics (including the Indian subcontinent and countries in the Middle East). Most of the Asian population has Fitzpatrick skin phototypes III, IV, and V, whereas a small proportion has skin phototypes II and VI. There is a wide variety of differences in ethnicity, culture, hygiene, nutrition, and socioeconomic status. Hence it is common that dermatologic conditions seen in one part of Asia may be different from those seen in another part. There are, however, some skin disorders that are common throughout Asia as well as other parts of the world, for example, eczema and acne vulgaris; there are others that are more seen commonly in Asia, for example, lichen amyloidosis or nevus of Ota. Table 80-1 shows the common skin diseases seen in Asia.

TABLE 80-1
Common Dermatoses in Asia

Eczematous Dermatosis
Atopic dermatitis
Contact dermatitis
Contact dermatitis to topical plants
Contact dermatitis to topical medicament
Acne vulgaris
Eosinophiilic pustular folliculitis
Pigmentary Disorders
Melasma
Acquired bilateral neavus of Ota–like macules (ABNOMs)
Postinflammatory hyperpigmentation
Mongolian spot
Naevus of ota
Vitiligo
Infections
Leprosy
Cutaneous tuberculosis
Miscellaneous
Dermatosis owing to cultural practices
Chronic arsenic toxicity
Lichen amyloidosis

ECZEMATOUS DERMATOSES

Atopic Dermatitis

Summary

- Common skin disorder in Asia and around the world.
- Papular eczema and prurigo nodularis are common manifestations in Asia.
- Postinflammatory hypopigmentation and pityriasis alba are great social handicaps because they are very prominent on pigmented skin.

Atopic dermatitis is one of the top 10 conditions seen in any dermatologic clinics in Asia. Most patients develop the condition before they reach 10 years of age, whereas in some communities late onset is often seen.[1] The prevalence rate among school children in Asia varies from 3.1% to over 20%.[2–9] A higher prevalence is seen in Singapore (20.8%) and Taiwan (18.0%), with a much lower prevalence in the Middle East. With the exception of Taiwan, recent studies show that there is no increase in the prevalence rate in Asia.[5–9]

CLINICAL FEATURES The condition may present as acute, subacute, or chronic skin reaction patterns with characteristic distribution of the rash in infants, children, and adults. The clinical presentation of eczema in Asians resembles that seen in the rest of the world. Papular eczema is seen commonly (Figure 80-1). The itch can be intense, and the constant scratching often results in postinflammatory or hypopigmentation (Figure 80-2). In children, patches of hypopigmentation with fine scales and indistinct borders are often seen on the face, a condition referred to as *pityriasis alba* (Figure 80-3). This is often seen after sun exposure when the surrounding normal skin becomes tanned, accentuating the contrast. Chronic rubbing results in prurigo nodules (Figure 80-4). The most common infective complication is bacterial (e.g., impetigo, folliculitis, and furuncles), followed by viral (e.g., herpes simplex infection and molluscum contagiosum).

TREATMENT Patient education is important because many myths abound in Asia. Trigger factors must be avoided and frequent baths discouraged. Patients living in the humid tropics often find it uncomfortable to use emollients. They should be encouraged to use moisturizers after bathing. Moisturisers and topical steroids (titrated to disease activity) are the mainstay of therapy. Second-line therapeutic modalities such as topical calcineurin inhibitors, phototherapy, and oral immunosuppresants such as cyclosporine and azathioprine are available in the big cities but not the rural areas. A survey of dermatologists in Southeast Asia revealed that familiarity with diagnostic criteria, the early and judicious use of moisturizers and topical corticosteroids, and the treatment of *Staphylococcus aureus* superinfection with penicillinase-stable antibiotics should be emphasized in this region.[10] There is a

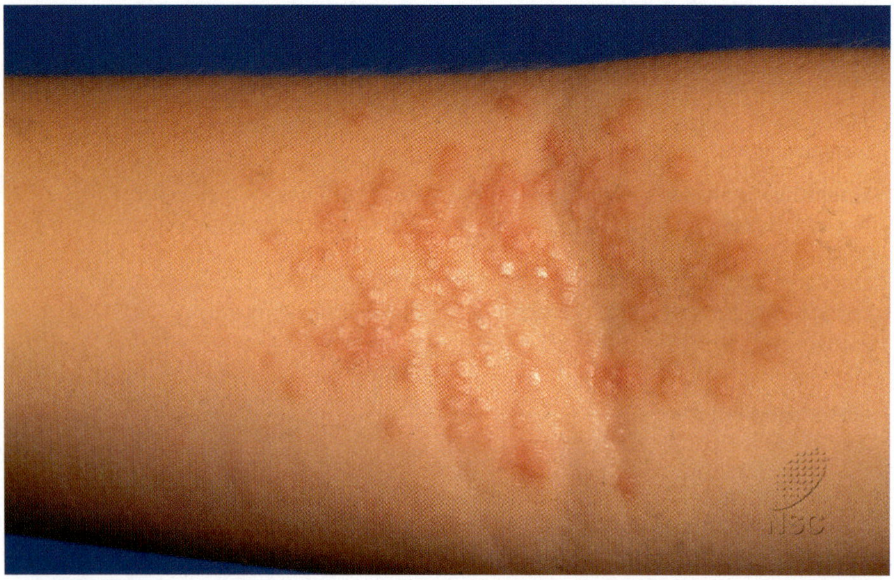

▲ **FIGURE 80-1** Papular eczema. Itchy papules on the cubital fossa of a Chinese girl. Courtesy of National Skin Centre, Singapore.

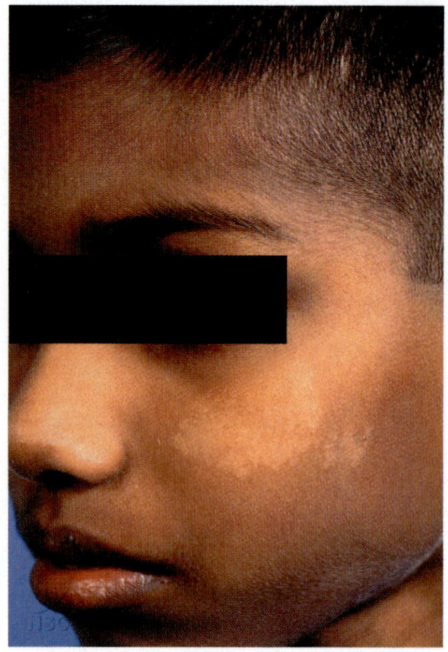

▲ **FIGURE 80-3** Pityriasis alba. Hypopigmented patches on both cheeks of an Indian boy. Courtesy of National Skin Centre, Singapore.

tendency in many Asian communities to use indigenous remedies, some of which may contain potent steroids.

Contact Dermatitis

Summary

- Traditional folk medication is widely used in Asia.
- Investigation of contact dermatitis to these preparations is often hindered by the lack of clear labeling.
- Plants belonging to the Anacardiaceae and Compositae families are notorious for causing allergic contact dermatitis.

CONTACT DERMATITIS TO TOPICAL MEDICAMENTS

Traditional Folk Medications Traditional folk medications are still used widely in Asia. Investigation of contact dermatitis to these preparations can be difficult because ingredients may not be clearly labeled, and herbal preparations often do not come in standardized concoctions.[11]

Topical traditional Chinese medicaments are one example of such medications and include the following preparations:

1. *Wind oils.* These are used for the relief of headaches and abdominal pain. They contain menthol, camphor, and essential oils. The essential oils may cause allergic contact dermatitis.
2. *Rheumatism oils.* These are used for joint and muscle aches. They contain methyl salicylate, menthol, camphor, and essential oils.
3. *Oils and bonesetter's herbs.* These are used for musculoskeletal injuries such as sprains, contusions, and fractures. These contain mastic and myrrh, which are potential allergens.

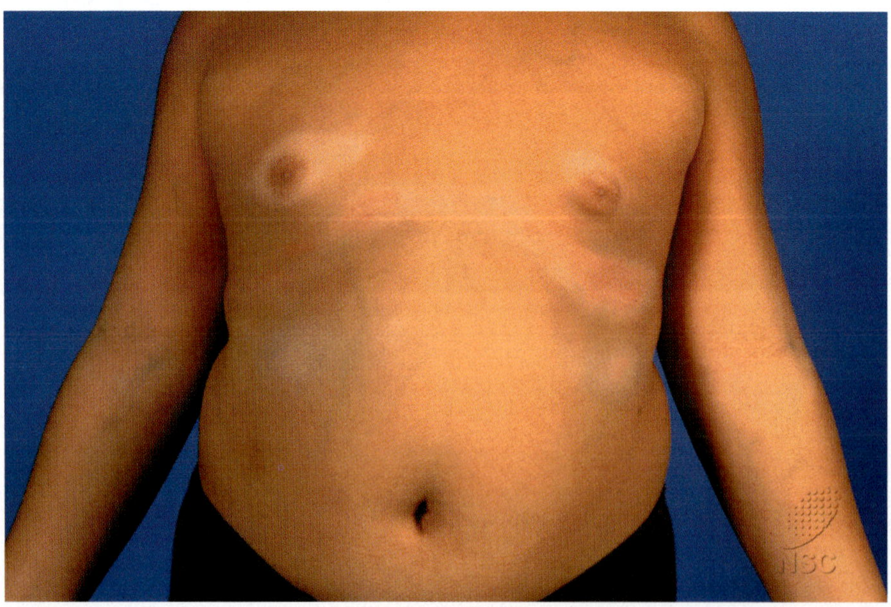

▲ **FIGURE 80-2** Postinflammatory hypopigmentation. Atopic dermatitis on the nipples, chest, and upper abdomen of a Chinese boy, healing with hypopigmented patches. Courtesy of National Skin Centre, Singapore.

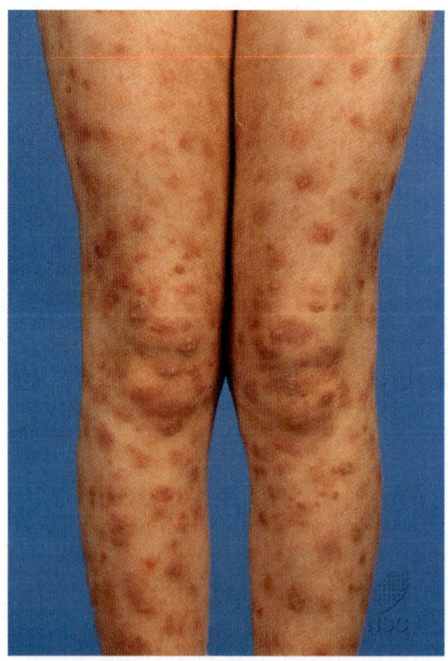

▲ **FIGURE 80-4** Prurigo nodularis. Itchy erythematous nodules on the lower limbs of a Chinese man, some of which have healed with postinflammatory hyperpigmentation on the thighs. Courtesy of National Skin Centre, Singapore.

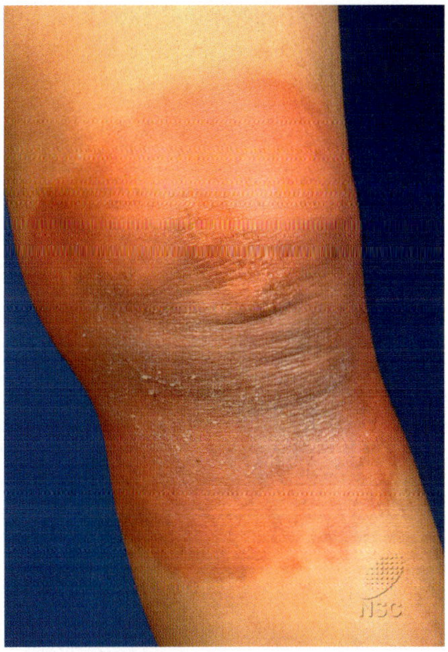

▲ **FIGURE 80-5** Allergic contact dermatitis to topical traditional Chinese medicament (TCM). An itchy erythematous patch on the knee of a Chinese woman after application of a TCM plaster for knee pain. Note the clearly demarcated edge of the dermatitis, which corresponds to the edge of the plaster. Courtesy of National Skin Centre, Singapore.

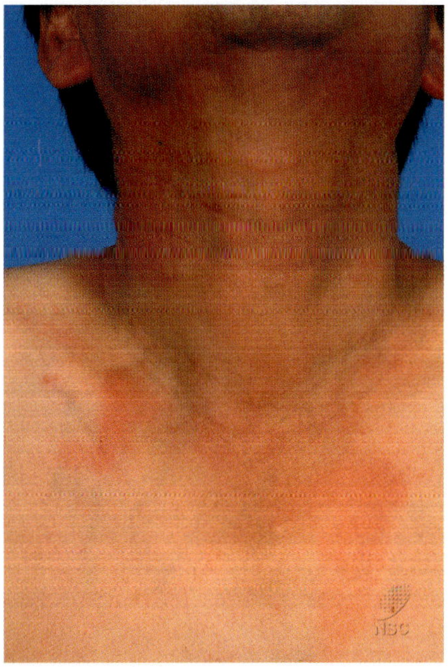

▲ **FIGURE 80-6** Allergic contact dermatitis to mango sap. Erythematous blotches and streaks resulted from mango sap dripping on the neck and upper chest of a Chinese man while harvesting the fruit. Courtesy of National Skin Centre, Singapore.

4. *Medicated creams, balms, and plasters* (Figure 80-5).

PROFLAVINE Proflavine, or flavine, is a common over-the-counter antiseptic. It is a yellow solution that can cause severe allergic contact dermatitis, including vesiculobullous, purpuric, and erythema-like reactions. It has a propensity for secondary spread.

LIME In Malaysia, lime has been used in traditional herbal baths and massage oils. Photocontact dermatitis to the psoralen in lime juice may occur.

CONTACT DERMATITIS TO PLANTS Plants belonging to the Anacardiaceae and Compositae families are notorious for causing allergic contact dermatitis.[11]

Anacardiaceae Family

- The sap of the mango (*Mangifera indica*) may cause allergic dermatitis, which may be erythema multiforme–like, in mango pickers (Figure 80-6).
- Rengas (*Gluta rengas*) is a hardwood indigenous to Malaysia and Indonesia. It is a potential allergen in woodworkers.
- Black exudates from the fruit of the marking nut tree (*Semecarpus anacardium*) are used traditionally to mark laundry in Sri Lanka and India. Dermatitis to the laundry mark is known as *dhobie mark dermatitis* in these countries.
- The Thai lacquer tree (*Melanrrhoea usitata*) and the Japanese lacquer tree (*Rhus verniciflua*) contain the resins thitsiol and urushiol, respectively. The resins may cause allergic contact dermatitis in lacquer workers.
- Cashew (*Anacardium occidentale*) nut oil derived from the shells may cause irritant and allergic contact dermatitis in cashew nut workers.
- Many species of the Anacardiaceae family are known to cross-react with poison ivy and poison oak.

Compositae Family

- *Parthenium hysterophorus* is an important cause of allergic contact dermatitis in India. The allergen is a sesquiterpine lactone called *parthenin* that is present in all parts of the plant.
- The wild sunflower (*Tithonia diversifolia*) is a perennial shrub in Sri Lanka with bright yellow flowers that may cause an allergic contact dermatitis.

CONTACT DERMATITIS TO COSMETICS The bindi or kumkum is a colorful circular disc or spot applied to the central forehead of Hindu women. The adhesive or azo dye used may lead to allergic contact dermatitis, chemical leukoderma, or pigmented contact dermatitis[11] (Figure 80-7).

Acne Vulgaris

Summary

- Common dermatosis in adolescents and young adults.
- Postinflammatory hyperpigmentation owing to acne and/or treatment is common in Asians.
- Photosensitivity owing to tetracycline therapy is uncommon in Asians.

Acne vulgaris, a multifactorial disorder of the pilosebaceous unit, is very common among adolescents in Asia.

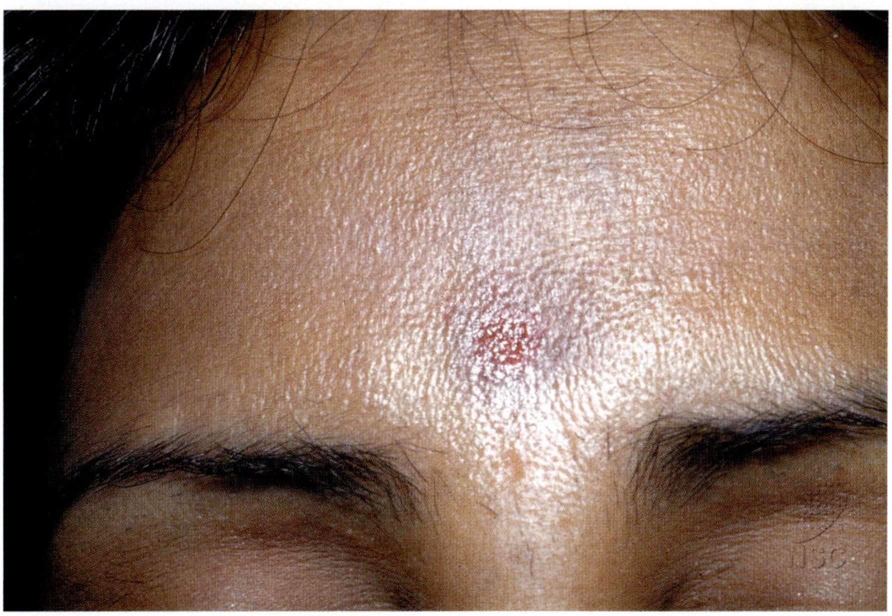

▲ **FIGURE 80-7** Allergic contact dermatitis to azo dye. Itchy subacute eczema on the central forehead of an Indian woman who had applied a bindi (or kum kum) there. Courtesy of National Skin Centre, Singapore.

The prevalence among young people between the ages 15 and 25 years may be as high as 90%.[12]

CLINICAL FEATURES Both inflammatory and noninflammatory lesions are seen in Asians. In some rural communities where acne is often viewed as a passage of adolescence and something that does not require medical treatment, it is not uncommon for patients to present late with nodulocystic acne and/or acne scars.

TREATMENT The treatment options for acne are the same for all skin types. However, Asian patients have a higher risk of developing postinflammatory hyperpigmentation and acne keloid scars. In initiating therapy, physicians must choose between aggressive, effective treatments and the risk of skin irritation, which may lead to pigmentation. Topical treatments that are known to irritate the skin must be introduced slowly and titrated to response and skin irritation. A combination of medical and procedural treatments is often used (Table 80-2).

Topical Treatment For comedonal and mild inflammatory acne, patients often self-medicate with over-the-counter preparations containing benzoyl peroxide, salicylic acid, sulfur, or traditional herbs or oil.[13,14] For most physicians, topical retinoids and topical antibiotics are the mainstay of treatment. Generally, topical retinoids are well tolerated,[15] although patients may complain of a burning sensation on sun exposure. Other topical agents are azelaic acid, glycolic acid, and retinaldehyde.[16–18] These topical agents can improve postinflammatory hyperpigmentation and therefore have an added advantage for use in Asian patients.

TABLE 80-2
Treatment for Acne/Acne Scars

Medical Treatment for Acne
- Topical
  - Benzoyl peroxide
  - Sulfur, resorcinol
  - Tretinion
  - Adapalene
  - Antibiotics, e.g., clindamycin, erythromycin
- Oral
  - Antibiotics, e.g., doxycycline, minocycline, erythromycin
  - Antiandrogen hormones
  - Isotretinion

Procedural Treatment for Acne
- Chemical peels
- Microdermabrasion
- LED laser
- Laser

Treatment for Acne Scars
- Surgery
- Chemical peels
- Microdermabrasion
- Laser

Oral Treatment Oral antibiotics are given for moderate to severe inflammatory acne. The drug of choice is often doxycycline, 100–200 mg/day, because phototoxicity is not a problem for most Asian patients. Minocycline, 100 mg/day, on the other hand, is less popular because blue-black pigmentation sometimes is seen on acne scars, and some patients may have an overall darkening of their facial skin. Resistant strains of *Propionibacterium acnes* to antibiotics follows the same pattern as those in Europe. In a study in Singapore,[19] resistance of *P. acnes* to erythromycin was seen most commonly, and this is associated with cross-resistance to clindamycin. The minimum inhibitory concentration (MIC) of *P. acnes* isolates to tetracycline was higher than that for doxycycline, and this is, in turn, higher than that for minocycline. In the same study, antibiotic resistance rate increases with duration of antibiotic usage—more resistant isolates were found when antibiotics were taken for more than 16 weeks.

Oral isotretinoin is the treatment of choice for nodulocystic acne, although it is often used for other, less severe forms acne. Because of cost constraints, there is a tendency to start the treatment late and for patients to stop treatments early, at the first sign of clinical improvement. The efficacy and relapse rates among Asian patients are comparable with those elsewhere.[20–23] In one study, a dose of 0.5 mg/kg for 4 months was found to be effective for most patients, with a relapse rate of 5%.[22] Hormonal therapy in the form of oral contraceptive pills containing cyproterone acetate is available in Asia and effective for women with premenstrual acne flares or acne along the jawline.

Procedural Treatment Besides medical treatment, procedural treatments are popular because they not only clear the acne lesions but also improve the acne sequelae as well. Chemical peels are effective in treating both inflammatory and comedonal acne.[24–27] These peels are done at fortnightly intervals for a total of 5–10 sessions. Glycolic acid, Jessner's solution, or salicylic acid peels are equally effective and safe in Asian patients.[25–27] However, some physicians prefer glycolic acid to Jessner's solution because the latter is associated with more exfoliation.[27] In addition to improving the acne lesions, chemical peels also improve the overall skin texture, lighten skin pigmentation, and improve pore size. However, there is no effect on sebum secretion.[28]

Phototherapy using a combination of blue (415 nm) and red (630–660 nm) LED lights can improve inflammatory acne[29,30] by destroying *P. acnes*. Treatment is given twice a week, 3 days apart, for a total of eight sessions. Acne lesions start to clear within 4 weeks, and this is thus a useful alternative for patients with inflammatory acne who are unable or reluctant to take oral antibiotics. Aminolaevulinic acid photodynamic therapy (ALA-PDT) is another useful option.[31–33] A photosensitiser, aminolaevulinic acid, is applied to the acne lesions for a period of time ranging from 45 minutes to 3 hours under occlusion and then irradiated. The light source can be a broad-band light source (550–700 nm), red light from a diode laser (635 nm), or a pulsed-dye laser (595 nm). Acne lesions cleared after ALA-PDT and remained clear for more than 5 months after the treatment. Side effects were minimal, with transient erythema and pain being the most common.

Lasers have been used in the treatment of inflammatory acne.[34–37] It is suggested that lasers may act on the sebaceous glands or that they improve acne by reducing inflammation.[37] The diode laser can improve lesion counts by a third after one treatment, and treated areas are almost clear after three treatment sessions.[37] Treatment-related pain was well tolerated, and adverse effects were limited to transient erythema and edema at treatment sites. The pulsed- dye laser has been reported in some studies to be beneficial, but there was a controlled study that showed no significant improvement.[36]

Treatment of Acne Scars

One of the main aims of acne treatment is to prevent scarring. However, scarring may occur owing to delay in seeking treatment, suboptimal control, or disease severity. Various treatment options are available to improve acne scars depending on the type of scar.

For pitted scars, the most effective treatment is punch excision, whereby the scars are individually punched out and sutured. For boxcar scars, subcision, whereby the fibrous attachments below the scars are surgically released, followed by a variety of resurfacing methods, is helpful. Rolling scars can be improved with filler injections or resurfacing procedures.

The common resurfacing procedures are chemical peels,[38,39] laser resurfacing,[40–44] microdermabrasion,[45] dermabrasion, and fractional resurfacing. Chemical peels are popular because they improve acne and concomitant acne scars.[38,39] Most physicians prefer to use superficial chemical peels because there is little risk of complications. However, such peels may not be as effective for the deeper acne scars. Medium-depth peels are better for deeper scars and, if done carefully, are safe on darker skin types.[28] Ablative laser resurfacing gives the best results[43,44] but is usually accompanied by prolonged erythyma and postinflammatory hyperpigmentation in Asian patients. Nonablative laser resurfacing is safer and useful for rolling acne scars.[40–42]

Eosinophilic Pustular Folliculitis

Summary

- Recurrent pruritic follicular papulopustules.
- Mainly on face, trunk, and arms.
- Infundibular eosinophilic pustules on histology.

Eosinophilic pustular folliculitis or Ofugi disease (Figure 80-8) was first reported more than 40 years ago by Ise and Ofugi in 1965.[46] Most of the reports are from Japan, and the disease affects mainly adult males. However, a recent study from Singapore showed a predilection for females.[47]

CLINICAL FEATURES The condition is characterized by recurrent episodes of grouped follicular papulopustules on the face, back, and extensor surfaces of the arms, the same areas where acne vulgaris lesions are seen. Pustules also have been reported to occur on the palms and soles. These lesions are itchy, but the patient is otherwise well. The papulopustules tend to spread outward on an erythematous plaque, leaving an area of central clearing. Each crop of pustules lasts for a week or two and recurs every 3–4 weeks. This condition is seen in people with normal immune status and must be distinguished from the immunosuppression-associated [mostly human immunodeficiency virus (HIV)–related] and infancy-associated eosinophilic folliculitis.[48]

DIAGNOSIS Diagnosis is made from the clinical presentation and is confirmed by histology. Pathology of involved follicles shows the presence of eosinophils and lymphocytes within the sebaceous glands and extending into the infundibular portion of the sebaceous duct.

TREATMENT Topical and oral corticosteroids are sometimes helpful. Oral indomethacin (50–75 mg/day) is an effective treatment. Minocycline, 100 mg twice daily; dapsone, 50–100 mg twice daily; and ultraviolet B (UVB) phototherapy have been used with some success.[49]

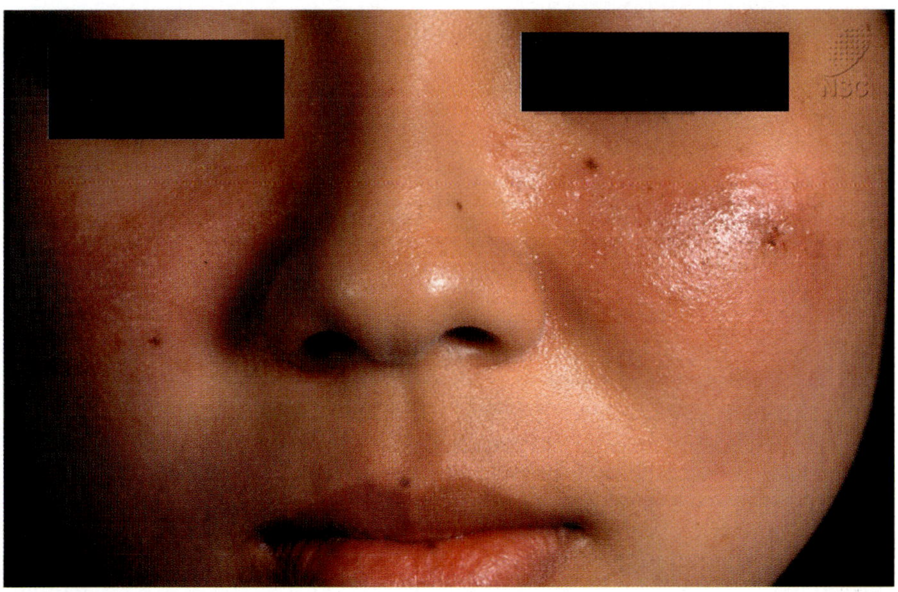

▲ **FIGURE 80-8** Eosinophilic pustular folliculitis (Ofuji disease). Follicular papules and pustules on the cheeks of a young Chinese woman. Courtesy of National Skin Centre, Singapore.

PIGMENTARY DISORDERS

Melasma

Summary

- Common acquired hyperpigmentary condition.
- Affects mainly women.
- Present on face and occasionally sun-exposed areas.
- Combination treatment gives better results.
- Recurrence is common.

Melasma is the most common acquired hyperpigmentary condition affecting Asian patients and is among the top 10 conditions presenting to dermatologists. It is more common in women than in men.[50] Melasma usually develops in the third to fourth decades of life,[50] although it may start earlier in some darker racial groups. Several factors have been implicated in the pathogenesis of this disorder, including pregnancy, oral contraceptive use, sun exposure, genetic factors, cosmetics, and race.[50–53] A positive family history is common, and more than half of patients will have a family history.[50,51] Individuals who work under the sun or in a hot environment tend to have worsening of their melasma The same clinicopathologic factors are seen in both males and females.[52,53]

PATHOGENESIS The main pathologic findings are in the epidermis. There is increased melanin in all layers of the epidermis. Melanosomes numbers are also increased, and melanosomes are more widely dispersed in the keratinocytes. Epidermal melanocytes and staining intensity are also increased. There is no change in keratonocytes proliferation. In the superficial and middermis, melanin or melanophages are seen, but these findings are not present in all patients.[54,55] Flattening of the epidermis and solar elastosis are usually present, suggesting an association of melasma with sun exposure. It is still controversial whether the number of melanocytes is increased.[54,55] Kang and colleagues[54] reported an increase in melanocyte number as well as activity of melanocytes in facial melasma skin compared with adjacent normal skin. These melanocytes have more mitochondria, Golgi apparatus, rough endoplasmic reticulum, and ribosomes in their cytoplasm. A dihyhroxyphenylalanine reaction was apparent in the cisternae and vesicles of the trans-Golgi network. The melanoyctes showed an increase in active protein synthesis and DOPA-reactive tyrosinase formation,

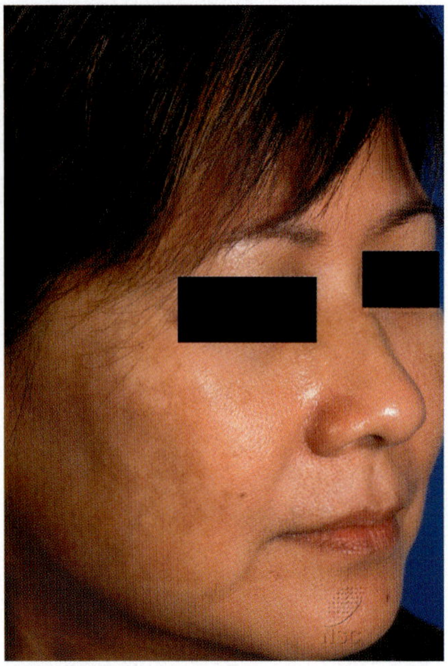

▲ **FIGURE 80-9** Melasma. Bilateral blotchy pigmentation on the cheeks and nasal bridge of a Chinese woman. Courtesy of National Skin Centre, Singapore.

suggesting that they are responsible for the formation of melasma.

CLINICAL FEATURES Melasma is seen on the face and, occasionally, on the arms, which are areas of sun exposure (Figure 80-9). The lesions are light to dark brown and occasionally may be gray. They are distributed symmetrically in three major patterns. In the centrofacial pattern, the most common presentation, melasma is seen on the forehead, nose, upper lip, chin, and cheeks. In the malar pattern, the next most common presentation, melasma is confined to the cheeks and the nose, whereas in the mandibular pattern, melasma is seen on the skin overlying the mandible. Centrofacial melasma usually accounts for more than half the melasma seen,[50,54] although in some communities the malar pattern may be more common.[51] Using Wood's light, melasma can be further classified into epidermal, dermal, or mixed type depending on location of the pigment.

TREATMENT In Asia, melasma is considered by most patients as a medical problem rather than a cosmetic nuisance. Some seek treatment for sociocultural reasons because the presence of melasma is often associated with "bad luck" for the patient, the family, or the family business. Treatment goals include removal or lightening of existing lesions and prevention of new pigment formation. Treatment is difficult because most modalities target epidermal pigment, and there is no effective treatment for dermal melasma. Effective treatment is made difficult by the long-standing nature of the problem and the high rate of recurrence once treatment is discontinued. Usually, a combination of topical and procedural treatments is employed for good results.

Medical Treatment Patients should minimize sun exposure by using a broad-spectrum sun block during the day. The sun block should be reapplied after 2–4 hours, especially if the patient is outdoors. In addition, patients should use physical protection in the form of broad-brimmed hats, sunglasses, umbrellas, or protective clothing when outdoors. For added protection, an oral sun block containing *Polypodium leucotomos* (a fern extract marketed as Helioblock) can be taken before sun exposure. This oral sun block is both an antioxidant and an immune modulator that prevents actinic erythema and increases the skin's tolerance to the effects of UV radiation.[56]

The presence of increased melanin and melanosomes in all layers of the epidermis[54] suggests an increased synthesis of melanosomes in the melanocytes and increased transfer and decreased degradation of melanosomes in the keratinocytes. Medical therapy of melasma includes topical agents that decrease synthesis of melanosomes (e.g., tyrosinase inhibitors), agents that prevent the transfer of melanosomes to keratinocytes, and agents that accelerate cell turnover in the epidermis (Table 80-3).

A common formulation used in Asia is that proposed by Kligman and Willis in 1975, which combined hydroquinone 5%, tretinoin 0.1%, and dexamethasone 0.1%[57] or variations of the original formulation, with dermatologists substituting different corticosteroids and modifying the concentrations of tretinoin and hydroquinone. Using this formula, Kligman and Willis were able to lighten the skin of African-American volunteers almost completely within 5–7 weeks. None of the agents used singly resulted in more than slight skin lightening, and omitting one component greatly reduced the level of therapeutic efficacy.[57,58] Hydroquinone blocks melanogenesis by competitive tyrosinase inhibition, inhibits DNA and RNA synthesis in melanotic cells, degrades melanosomes, and destroys melanocytes.[59] Tretinoin causes dispersion of pigment granules in keratinocytes, interferes with pigment transfer, accelerates epidermal transfer, and accelerates cell turnover in the epidermis. It also decreases the rate of transfer of melanosomes to the keratinocytes. The steroid suppresses the biosynthetic and secretory function of melanocytes, thus suppressing melanin production without destroying the melanosomes.[58,60] In the triple combination, tretinoin overrides the atrophy—promoting an antimitotic effect of the corticosteroid and facilitating epidermal penetration of hydroquinone, also preventing its oxidation. The corticosteroid antagonizes the thinning effect of tretinoin and reduces tretinoin-induced irritation.

A more stable formulation which is approved by the Food and Drug Administration (FDA) for treatment of melasma (Triluma cream) contains hydroquinone 4%, tretinoin 0.05%, and fluocinolone acetonide 0.01%. In two multicenter studies that enrolled 641 patients with mild to moderate facial melasma, 78% achieved complete or near-complete clearing in 8 weeks.[61] Treatment-related adverse events seen at 8 weeks were erythema, desquamation, burning, dryness, and pruritus. Only one patient had skin atrophy. The number of patients who achieved complete or near-complete clearing at 12 months increased to 81%, and the adverse events remained low.

Another combination therapy that is used is sequential therapy with clobetasol propionate 0.05% for 8 weeks followed by azelaic acid 20% for 16 weeks. A total of 70% of patients had more than

TABLE 80-3
Treatment for Melasma

Medical Therapy
Sunprotection
Agents that inhibit tyrosinase
Hydroquinone
Azelaic acid
Kojic acid
Arbutin
Licorice extracts
Mulberry, bearberry
Agents that Prevent the Transfer of Melanosomes to Keratinocytes
Nicotinic acid
Niacinamide
Soy
Tretinoin
Agents that Accelerate Cell Turnover in the epidermis
Alphahydroxyacids
Betahydroxyacids
Tretinoin
Procedural Therapy
Chemical peels
Microdermabrasion
Intense pulsed light
Lasers

66% clearance of their melasma compared with 3% in the group using azelaic acid alone.[62] When azelaic acid, in concentrations of 15% and 20%, was combined with glycolic acid, it was as effective as 4% hydroquinone.[63] Azelaic acid can be irritating, and this may lead to postinflammatory hyperpigmentation.

Kojic acid is a common ingredient found in many over-the-counter cosmetic lightening products in Asia. Combined with glycolic acid and 2% hydroquinone, it helps to lighten melasma.[64] Another popular over-the-counter lightening agent is niacinamide, which works by inhibiting melanosome transfer from melanocytes to keratinocytes. In clinical studies, it significantly decreased hyperpigmentation and increased skin lightness compared with vehicle alone after 4 weeks of use.[65]

Procedural Therapy Melasma is a therapeutic challenge for the dermatologist. Since most Asian patients with melasma have both epidermal and dermal pigmentation, topical therapy alone is often insufficient to clear their melasma. Chemical peels, microdermabrasion, lasers, and intense pulsed light are often used in combination with topical therapy.

Chemical peels can improve or clear melasma. Among these agents are glycolic acid, trichloroacetic acid, Jessner's solution, lactic acid, salicylic acid, phenol, and tretinoin. In treating melasma in an Asian skin type, it is safer to use only superficial peeling agents and to start with lower concentrations to avoid the risk of causing postinflammatory hyperpigmentation. Glycolic acid peels (20–70%) performed every 3 weeks on one-half the face to a total of eight peels improved melasma among Singapore Chinese women when compared with the side that did not receive any peeling.[66] Combining glycolic acid peels with a topical regimen, modified Kligman's formula, results in a more rapid and greater improvement than when peels are used alone.[67] Another peeling agent that is useful for treating melasma is trichloroacetic acid. However, this has a higher risk of postpeel hyperpigmentation in Asian skin. In order to reduce this risk and increase the effect of the chemical peel, the skin must be primed at least 2 weeks prior with either hydroquinone or tretinoin, with hydroquinone being more superior as a priming agent.[68] Tretinoin 1% peels are as effective as glycolic acid 70% peels in lightening moderate to severe melasma in Indian women. The peels were performed weekly for 12 weeks.[69]

Microdermabrasion is a safe and effective procedure in lightening melasma in Asian skin types. It is done at 1- to 2-week intervals for a total of six treatments. Patients can continue with their topical lightening agents. In treating Asian skin, overly aggressive microdermabrasion may lead to worsening of the skin pigmentation.

Intense pulsed light has been used to treat melasma in Asian persons with some success.[70,71] Treatment is given at 4-week intervals for four sessions. Patients noted improvement in melasma as well as in skin texture. However, there is a low risk of transient postinflammatory hyperpigmentation. In some patients, "very subtle epidermal melasma" not noticed initially may be "unmasked" during intense pulsed light treatment.[72]

There are conflicting reports on the use of lasers for melasma. Although there are reports of melasma improving after treatment with Q-switched pigment-specific lasers, postinflammatory hyperpigmentation is a complication in Asians.[73,74] Results from laser treatment are better when there is an associated dermal component of melasma or in the presence of acquired bilateral nevus of Ota–like macules. Ablative lasers have been used to treat melasma[75,76] with some success, and the rationale is the ablation of abnormal clones of melanocytes causing the melasma. For therapy-resistant melasma, fractional resurfacing using the Fraxel laser is effective for both epidermal and dermal melasma.[77,78]

Controversial Treatment In some Asian countries, oral medications such glutatamic acid, tranexamic acid, and grapeseed extract[79] are used in combination with topical treatment. Recently, intradermal injections of tranexamic acid was reported be effective in lightening melasma.[80] Another popular treatment is the use of vitamin C iontophoresis in melasma.[81] Further studies are warranted to determine the long-term efficacy and safety of these treatments.

Acquired Bilateral Nevus of Ota–Like Macules

Summary

- Also known as *Hori's nevus* and *nevus fuscoceruleus zygomaticus.*
- Bilateral bluish macules on the zygoma in an Asian adult.
- No mucosal involvement.
- May coexist with melasma.
- Melanocytes present in dermis.

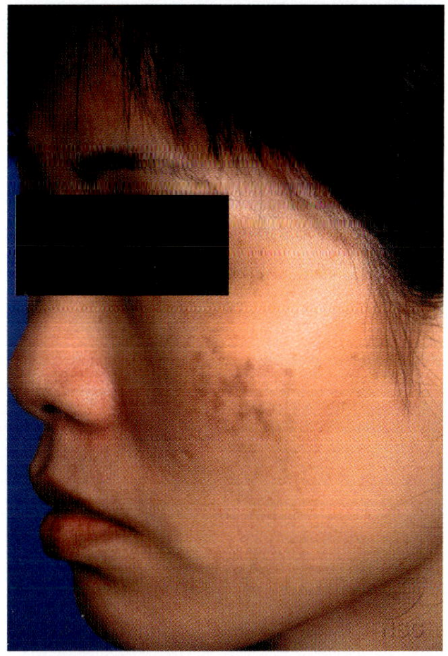

▲ **FIGURE 80-10** Acquired bilateral nevus of Ota–like macules (Hori's nevus): Cluster of pigmented macules on both upper cheeks of a Chinese woman. Courtesy of National Skin Centre, Singapore.

Acquired bilateral nevus of Ota–like macules (ABNOMs) or nevus fuscoceruleus zygomaticus was first described by Hori and is often referred to as *Hori's nevus*. It is often seen together with melasma and often mistaken for melasma. Sometimes ABNOMs may not be present clinically, but dermal melanocytes are visible on histology.[54]

CLINICAL FEATURES The pigmentation initially starts as brown macules and later become darker and confluent (Figure 80-10). Onset is usually in the third to fourth decades and is more common among Chinese and Japanese women. There is usually a family history.[82] ABNOMs are distinguished from nevus of Ota by the late onset, the bilateral involvement of the zygoma, and the absence of mucosal involvement.

PATHOLOGY Histology shows the presence of melanocytes in the dermis. The intradermal melanocytes are clustered in groups and dispersed perivascularly in ABNOMs, unlike those in nevus of Ota, where they are scattered evenly throughout the dermis. This is one reason why the incidence of postinflammatory hyperpigmentation after laser treatment is higher in ABNOMs than in nevus of Ota.[83]

TREATMENT Unlike melasma, ABNOMs do not respond to topical agents or chemical peels. They can be cleared almost completely with dermabrasion.[84] Lasers are used to treat ABNOMs with relative success and few side effects. The common lasers used for Asians are the Q-switched Nd:YAG laser[85–87] and the Q-switched alexanderite laser.[88] The Q-switched Nd:YAG laser can clear ABNOMs completely, and the lesion remains clear at 3–4 years of follow-up.[88] A significant number of patients will develop postinflammatory hyperpigmentation (which needs to be addressed using topical lightening agents) or hypopigmentation, which will resolve spontaneously over time. There are no textural changes from the laser treatments. The number of treatment sessions varies from 2–11. Good results also were seen by combining an ablative laser prior to using a Q-switched ruby laser[89] or by using topical lightening agents with a Q-switched ruby laser.[90]

Postinflammatory Hyperpigmentation

Summary

- Common acquired hyperpigmentation in Asians.
- Seen after inflammation or injury.
- More severe in darker skin types.
- Due to increased melanin in epidermis or dermis,

Postinflammatory hyperpigmentation (PIH) is common in Asians, especially in darker individuals such as the Indians or Malays.

CLINICAL FEATURES PIH is characterized by asymptomatic, irregular localized or diffuse macules of brown to gray-blue pigmentation on the sites of previous inflammation or trauma to the skin.[91,92] The pigmentation surfaces after the inflammation resolves. There is a strong correlation between the degree of inflammation and the resulting pigmentation.[93] It is often seen after an episode of acne, eczema, or insect-bite reaction and is made worse by constant picking or scratching at the lesion. PIH often follows interface dermatitis or lichenoid dermatitis. Exposure to UV rays tends to darken the areas of pigmentation.[91].

Diagnosis is usually made when there is a history of a preceding skin injury or skin inflammation, which may be iatrogenic, for example, after a laser procedure. Diagnosis may be difficult if the cutaneous inflammation is transient or mild, escaping the patient's notice. Histology shows an increased number of pigmented granules in the keratinocytes and the presence of melanin-laden macrophages in the upper dermis and around blood vessels.[91]

TREATMENT Treatment of PIH is difficult in Asians. It often lasts for months and even up to a year. The currently available treatment modalities are often not effective. Minimizing sun exposure is important.

Topical agents using tyrosinase inhibitors tretinoin[94] or glycolic acid can reduce PIH, especially the epidermal component. However, some patients may experience irritation from the treatment. In such instances, the addition of a low- to middle-potency topical steroid can reduce the risk of further PIH. Azelaic acid has been shown to be useful in treating patients with both acne and PIH from acne.[95]

Procedural therapy is often used in an attempt to reduce dermal PIH. Options include chemical peels,[96,97] microdermabrasion, intense pulsed light, and lasers. These must not be done too aggressively in order to prevent further PIH. The use of lasers is controversial; improvement is seen initially, but recurrence or worsening may occur as a result of trauma to the epidermis.[74,98,99]

Mongolian Spot

Summary

- Present at birth.
- Seen in 90–100% of Asian infants.
- Blue or gray-blue pigmentation commonly on buttocks or lumbosacral region.
- Spontaneous regression in childhood.

Mongolian spot, or dermal melanocytosis, is common among Asian infants, with an incidence of 90–100%. It is present at birth, and most will regress in childhood.

CLINICAL FEATURES The blue or gray-blue patches are seen commonly on the buttocks or lumbosacral region and sometimes on the trunk and limbs (Figure 80-11).

TREATMENT No treatment is needed because the majority of lesions will regress spontaneously during childhood. Some may persist, and these have to be distinguished from nevus of Ota or nevus of Ito. For persistent lesions, laser treatment is helpful.

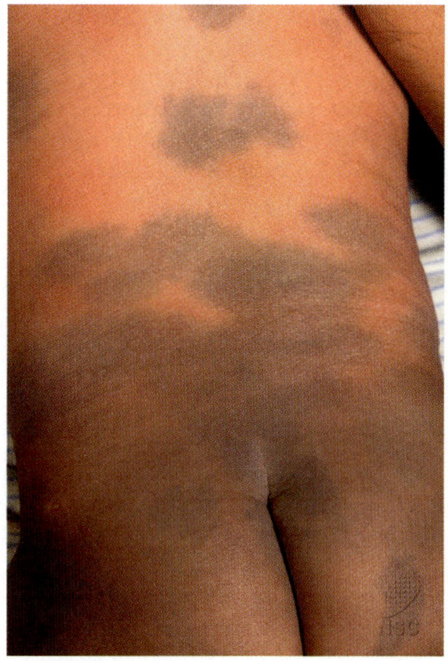

▲ **FIGURE 80-11** Mongolian spot. Congenital blue-gray patches on the buttocks and back of an infant. Courtesy of National Skin Centre, Singapore.

Nevus of Ota

Summary

- Present in infancy or during puberty.
- Unilateral facial lesion.
- Often affects ipsilateral sclera.
- Effectively treated by laser.

Nevus of Ota, or nevus fuscoceruleus ophthalmomaxillaris, is common among the Japanese and Chinese and affects 0.014–0.034% of the Asian population.[100] It is present in infancy for most patients; a third will present around puberty. Late onset in adults is rare.[101]

PATHOGENESIS The hyperpigmentation is due to the presence of melanocytes in the upper or middle dermis. These melanocytes appear in the dermis during fetal life and fail to migrate to the epidermis.

CLINICAL FEATURES Nevus of Ota presents as pigmentated patches varying from a few centimeters to larger ones that cover almost half the face (Figure 80-12). It appears as shades of brown to blue-black. The lesion is usually unilateral (different from ABNOMs) and follows the distribution of the first two branches of the trigeminal nerve, that is, the periorbital region, temple, malar region, forehead, nose, and pre- and retroauricular regions. The infraorbital

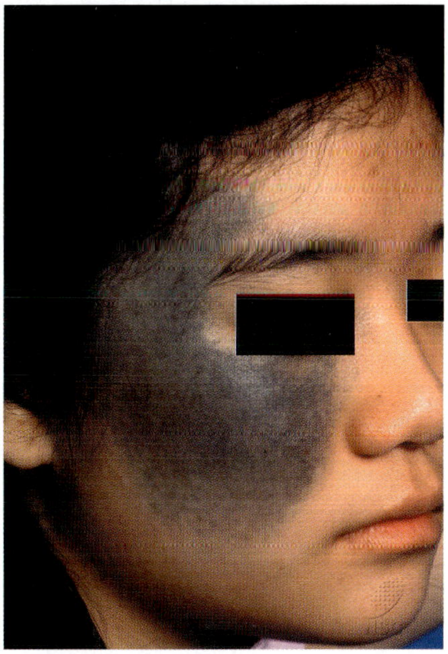

▲ **FIGURE 80-12** Nevus of Ota. Unilateral congenital blue-gray patch involving the right temple, cheek, and sclera of a young Chinese woman. Courtesy of National Skin Centre, Singapore.

area is the most frequent site of involvement.[101] Extracutaneous involvement has been reported, especially ocular involvement. In two-thirds of patients, the ipsilateral sclera is involved. Other sites of involvement include the eye and the optic nerve, the tympanum and external auditory canal, the nasal mucosa, the lips, the palate, and the pharynx. Complications are rare. There are reports of associated glaucoma and optic melanomas, but these are rare in Asians.

TREATMENT The treatment of choice for nevus of Ota is the Q-switched laser. Previous treatment using cryotherapy and microsurgery was associated with scarring.[102,103] The Q-switched ruby laser, Q-switched alexandrite laser, and Q-switched Nd:YAG laser can effectively lighten nevus of Ota without significant side effects.[101,104–108] Treatment response depends on the age of the patient, the predominant color of the lesion, the thickness of the lesion, and the number of treatments. The mean number of treatments to achieve significant clearing is much fewer when treatment is started in a child as compared with starting treatment in a adult.[109] Fewer treatment sessions are needed to clear brown lesions (average of three) than violet-blue or blue-green lesions (average of four to five sessions).[110] Lesions with a depth of 1 mm or less have a better treatment outcome.[111] Better results are obtained for patients with unilateral lesions and in patients who received more treatment sessions.[101] Complications are few, but transient hyperpigmention or hypopigmention is common. Scarring or textural change is rare.[112] In children, epidermal cooling (either contact or air cooling) can be incorporated to reduce the pain.[113]

Vitiligo

Summary

- Hypopigmentation is more visible in Asian skin.
- Source of great cosmetic concern.
- Mistaken for the hypopigmented lesions of leprosy in parts of Asia.
- Preservation of follicular melanocytes is important for therapeutic success.

Vitiligo has great social and cosmetic concern in certain parts of Asia, such as the Indian subcontinent. The hypopigmentation is more visible in the Asian skin because the contrast is more striking than in Caucasians. It may be mistaken for the hypopigmented lesions of leprosy in countries where this dreaded illness is endemic.

EPIDEMIOLOGY Vitiligo is an acquired macular depigmentation with a prevalence of 0.1–2% in different populations. In a population study of 15,685 people in Calcutta, India, the prevalence was 0.5%, with a mean age of onset of 22 years.[114]

PATHOGENESIS The key pathogenetic event is the loss of melanocytes by melanocytoxicity or possibly melanocytorrhagy. Many hypotheses, including genetics, autoimmunity, and neural and autocytotoxicity, have been proposed. These mechanisms may occur independently or in combination.

GENETICS There is familial clustering, and studies done in India, South Korea, and China supported a polygenic inheritance.[115–117] Genome-wide linkage analysis of Chinese families showed minimal overlap between the linkage results in the Chinese population and the results of previous analyses in Caucasians, suggesting great genetic heterogeneity between ethnic populations.[118]

CLINICAL FEATURES Vitiligo can begin at any age but is hardly ever present at birth. It can present on any part of the body as nonscaly depigmented macules or patches with well-demarcated borders. It is usually symmetric, but one clinical variant, segmental vitiligo, is unilateral (Figure 80-13). Areas of predilection include the periorificial regions of the face, neck, flexures, elbows, hands, knees, and feet. Generalized vitiligo is slowly progressive. In a study of 400 Korean patients, those with a positive family history, nonsegmental vitiligo, Koebner phenomenon, or mucous

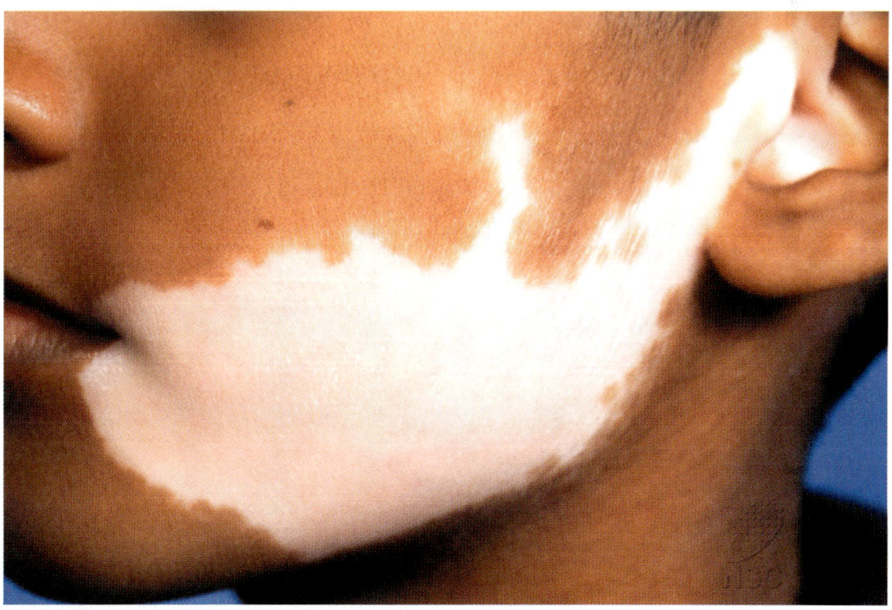

▲ **FIGURE 80-13** Segmental vitiligo. An acquired unilateral depigmented patch with well-demarcated borders on the mandibular region of the face in an Indian boy. Courtesy of National Skin Centre, Singapore.

membrane involvement showed more progression of vitiligo.[119] In contrast, segmental vitiligo is rapidly progressive and then remains stable and is not expected to progress to generalized vitiligo.

TREATMENT Spontaneous partial repigmentation is common in isolated spots but rarely sufficient cosmetically. Preservation of follicular melanocytes is important for therapeutic success. Topical therapy (e.g., potent corticosteroids and tacrolimus), phototherapy (e.g., narrow-band ultraviolet B), photochemotherapy (e.g., psoralen and ultraviolet A or natural sunlight), excimer laser, and autologous skin graft have been used in Asia with variable success. The hands and feet show poor response to therapy. Segmental vitiligo is less responsive to topical and phototherapy, but autologous grafting has been successful.

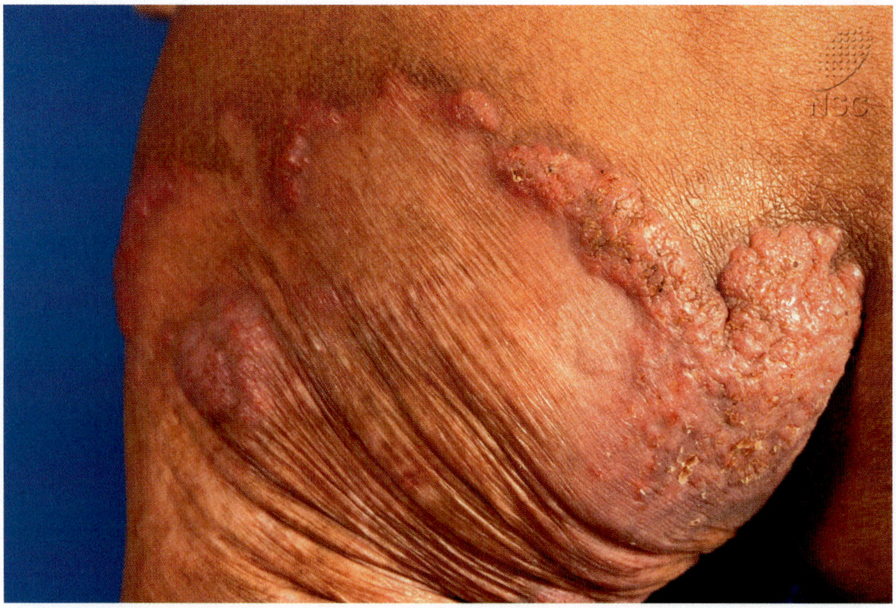

▲ **FIGURE 80-14** Tuberculosis verrucosa cutis. A chronic annular plaque on the buttock of an elderly Chinese man with warty papular borders and central hypopigmented clearing. Courtesy of National Skin Centre, Singapore.

SKIN INFECTIONS

Cutaneous Tuberculosis

Summary

- Presents as a spectrum of skin changes.
- Common variants in Asia: tuberculosis verrucosa cutis, scrofuloderma, lupus vulgaris, and erythema induratum.
- A standard 6-month regimen is recommended.

EPIDEMIOLOGY Pulmonary tuberculosis is endemic in many Asian countries, but cutaneous tuberculosis is relatively uncommon. *Mycobacterium tuberculosis* causes a spectrum of skin changes depending on the route of infection and host immunity. In India, the most common variants in children and adults are scrofuloderma and lupus vulgaris, respectively.[120] In data from a tertiary referral center in Pakistan, scrofuloderma was the most common clinical presentation, followed by lupus vulgaris and tuberculosis verrucosa cutis.[121] The most common forms in Hong Kong are erythema induratum, lupus vulgaris, and tuberculosis verrucosa cutis.[122] The incidence of cutaneous tuberculosis in Japan is decreasing and shows a shift toward older generations.[123]

CLINICAL FEATURES The most common forms of presentation in Asia are described. Tuberculosis verrucosa cutis is an indolent warty plaque owing to inoculation of mycobacteria into the skin of a patient with moderate to high degree of immunity (Figures 80-14 and 80-15). Sites of predilection are the knees, ankles, and buttocks. Scrofuloderma is caused by breakdown of the skin overlying a focus of tuberculosis, which may be a lymph node, an infected bone or joint, or a lacrimal gland or duct. This may present as a bluish red nodule or an undermined ulcer. Lupus vulgaris usually occurs as a chronic reddish brown plaque, which occurs in people with a moderate to high degree of immunity. There are multiple clinical forms of lupus vulgaris depending on the host response to the mycobacteria. Besides contiguous, hematogenous, or lymphatic spread from a focus of infection, it also can develop after exogenous inoculation or as a complication of bacille Calmette-Guérin (BCG) vaccination. Erythema induratum is a nodular tuberculide that usually occurs on the legs as recurrent nodules and ulcers secondary to tuberculosis elsewhere in the body. This disease has a predilection for women.

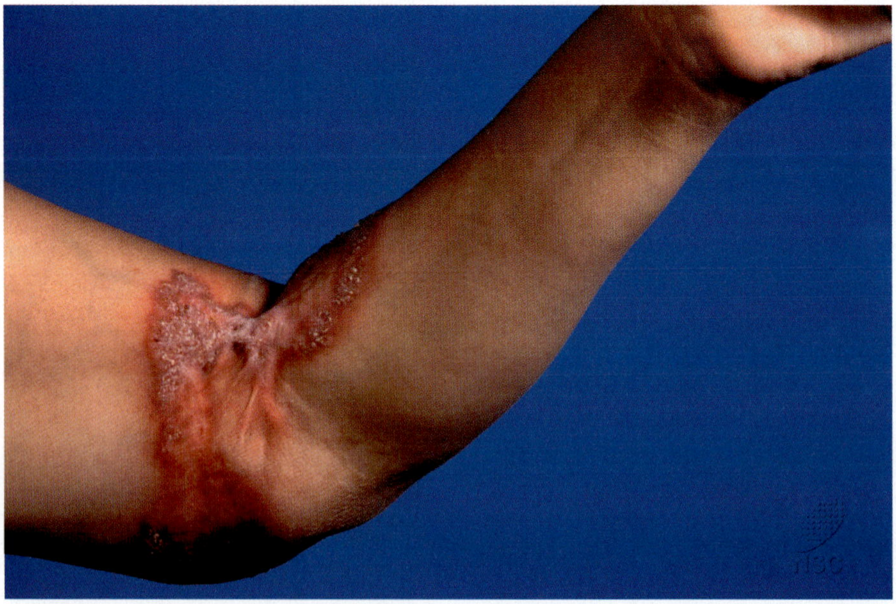

▲ **FIGURE 80-15** Tuberculosis verrucosa cutis. Chronic warty red plaques on the cubital fossa with fibrotic bands leading to elbow contracture. Courtesy of National Skin Centre, Singapore.

DIAGNOSIS A positive culture of *M. tuberculosis* or identification of its DNA by polymerase chain reaction (PCR) from the skin lesion confirms the diagnosis. Presence of active tuberculosis elsewhere in the body, acid-fast bacilli in the skin lesion, infective granuloma on histopathology, positive tuberculin reaction, and/or a good response to antituberculosis therapy support the diagnosis.

TREATMENT The American and British thoracic societies recommend a standard 6-month regimen for adults[124,125]:

- Isoniazid 300 mg daily for 6 months
- Rifampicin 450–600 mg daily for 6 months (The higher dosage is given for adults weighing more than 50 kg.)
- Pyrazinamide 1.5–2.0 g daily for the first 2 months (The higher dosage is given for adults weighing more than 50 kg.)
- Ethambutol 15 mg/kg daily for the first 2 months

Leprosy

Summary

- Affects the skin and peripheral nerves.
- Often results in social stigmatization.
- Permanent neurologic disability if untreated.
- Treatment with multidrug combination for 6–24 months.

Leprosy is a chronic infectious disease caused by Mycobacterium leprae. The cutaneous manifestations of leprosy and neurological deformities are responsible for social stigma in many societies.

EPIDEMIOLOGY Over the past 20 years, the global caseload has decreased by almost 90%. There were 405,147 new cases of leprosy detected in Southeast Asia during the year 2003.[126] This region accounts for the major burden of leprosy worldwide, with most of the cases attributed to India, Indonesia, and Myanmar. The mode of transmission is believed to occur via nasal droplet infection. The incubation period is long, usually about 2–5 years for paucibacillary cases and 8–12 years for multibacillary cases. The peak age of onset is early adulthood, commonly 20–30 years of age.

CLINICAL FEATURES It often affects the skin and peripheral nerves. Leprosy is classified as paucibacillary or multibacillary depending on the bacillary load. Paucibacillary leprosy, for example, tuberculoid leprosy, is milder, characterized by a few (up to five) hypopigmented or erythematous anesthetic dry hairless patches or plaques (Figure 80-16). In multibacillary leprosy, for example, lepromatous leprosy, there are multiple (more than five) nodules or plaques; other organs, such as the mucosa, eyes, and testes, may be involved (Figures 80-17 and 80-18). Involvement of peripheral nerves leads to loss of function, resulting in numbness, paralysis, loss of sweating, and xerosis.

Lucio leprosy is a variant of lepromatous leprosy characterized by loss of hair, diffuse scleroderma-like thickening of the skin, and peripheral neuropathy.

Type 1 reaction occurs in borderline disease, usually after starting treatment, and results in acute neuritis and acutely inflamed skin (Figure 80-19). Type

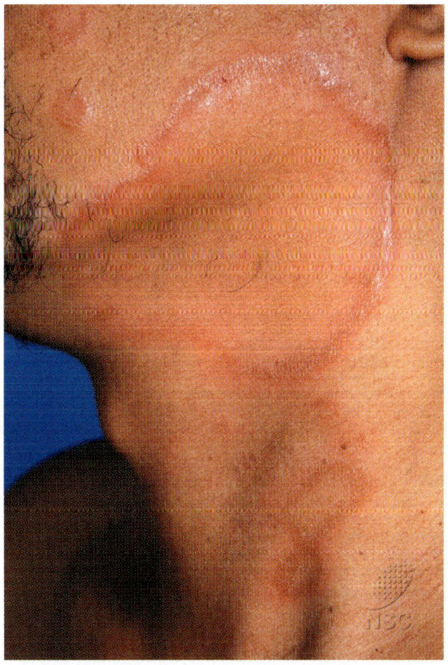

▲ **FIGURE 80-16** Borderline leprosy. Annular anesthetic erythematous plaques on the face and neck of a Malay man. Courtesy of National Skin Centre, Singapore.

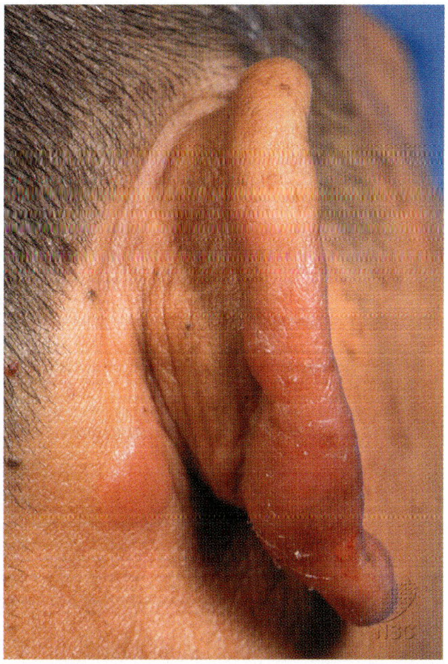

▲ **FIGURE 80-18** Lepromatous leprosy (same patient as Figure 80-17). Red nodules on the ear helix and earlobe, a classic site. There is another nodule just behind the ear. Courtesy of National Skin Centre, Singapore.

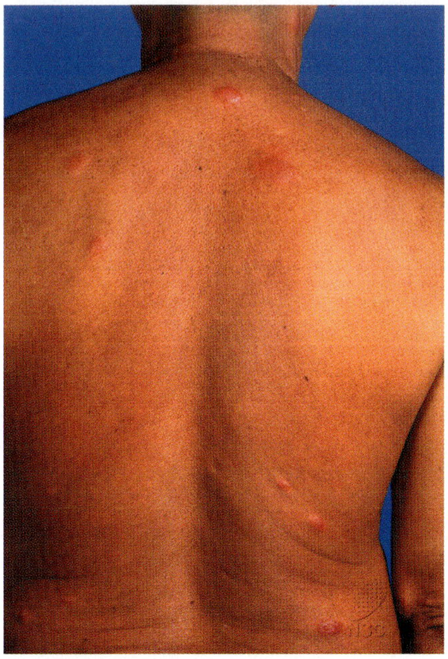

▲ **FIGURE 80-17** Lepromatous leprosy. Multiple red plaques and nodules on the neck and back of a Chinese man. Courtesy of National Skin Centre, Singapore.

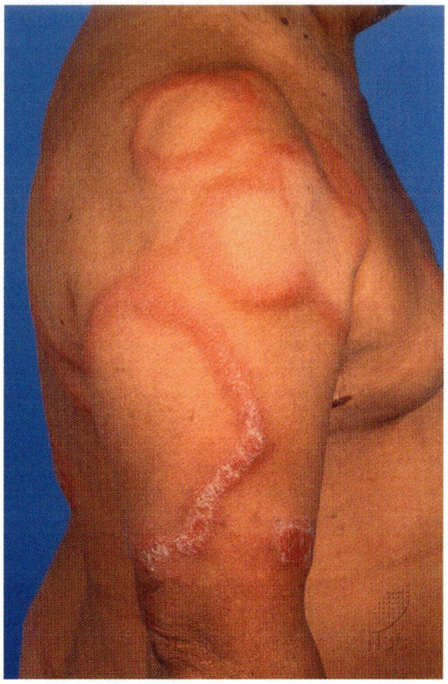

▲ **FIGURE 80-19** Type 1 reaction in borderline leprosy. Existing annular plaques became acutely tender, erythematous, and swollen in a Chinese man. Courtesy of National Skin Centre, Singapore.

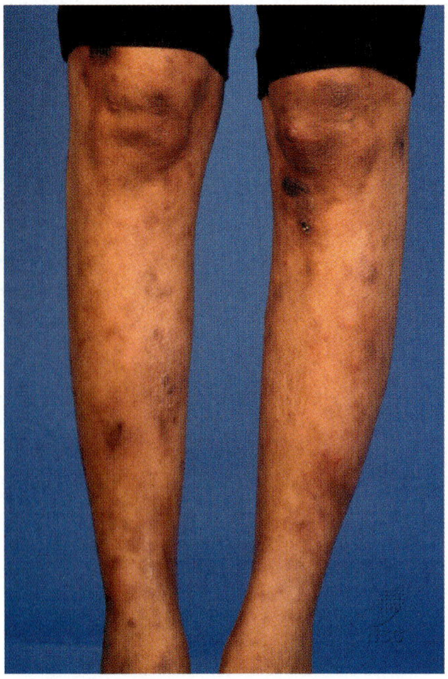

▲ **FIGURE 80-20** Type 2 reaction (erythema nodosum leprosum) in lepromatous leprosy. Painful red nodules on extensor surfaces of the legs of an Indonesian woman. Courtesy of National Skin Centre, Singapore.

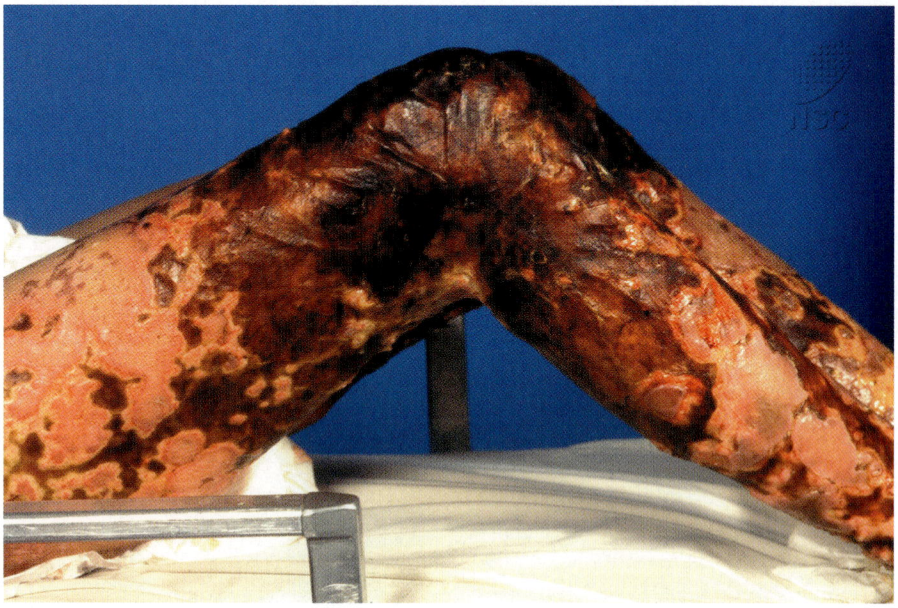

▲ **FIGURE 80-21** Lucio reaction. Extensive painful ulcers and necrotic plaques on the lower limbs of an elderly Chinese man with untreated Lucio leprosy. Courtesy of National Skin Centre, Singapore.

2 reaction occurs in multibacillary leprosy, either spontaneously or while on treatment. It presents commonly as painful red nodules on the face and extensor surfaces of limbs (Figure 80-20). Fever may be associated with uveitis, dactylitis, arthritis, neuritis, lymphadenitis, myositis, and orchitis. The Lucio reaction is a complication of Lucio leprosy owing to deep cutaneous vasculitis. The vasculitis leads to infarction, manifesting clinically as bullae, necrotic plaques, and deep, painful ulcers (Figure 80-21). Reactions must be recognized early and treated aggressively to prevent nerve and organ damage.

DIAGNOSIS In rural parts of Asia, the diagnosis is usually made clinically on the basis of typical skin lesions, anesthesia, and/or thickened nerves. Presence of acid-fast bacilli on slit-skin smears and/or histology typical of leprosy strongly support the diagnosis.

TREATMENT Antibacterial treatment for leprosy is effective but needs to be taken over many months. The multidrug regimen recommended by the World Health Organization (WHO) is shown in Table 80-4. Ofloxacin, minocycline, and clarithromycin are established second-line drugs. Prednisolone and thalidomide are used to treat reactions. BCG vaccination confers some protection against the disease.

DERMATOSIS OWING TO CULTURAL PRACTICES

Summary

- Characterized by purpura and hemorrhagic blisters.
- Produced by cupping, skin scraping or coin rubbing, and moxibustion,
- Can masquerade as physical abuse, child abuse, or bleeding disorders.

Cupping

This is a common practice in traditional Chinese medicine that is used to treat patients with febrile illnesses.[127] A cup is warmed and applied to the patient's back. Suction is produced when the cup cools, resulting in a round purpuric patch and occasionally hemorrhagic blisters.

Skin Scraping and Coin Rubbing

This is another practice in traditional Chinese medicine that is used to treat many complaints. The coin, or occasionally a spoon, is scraped over the skin until redness or purpura is produced. Pinching or pulling of the skin often accompanies this. The nasal bridge, glabella, neck, intercostal spaces, and cubital and popliteal fossae are common sites.

Moxibustion

Moxibustion has been a part of acupuncture practice for centuries. It includes direct moxibustion, in which moxa sticks are burned at acupuncture points on the skin, and indirect moxibustion, in which monkshood cakes or ginger or garlic slices are used to insulate the skin from burning moxa cones (Figure 80-22).

The skin changes produced by cupping, skin scraping, and moxibustion

TABLE 80-4
WHO treatment regimen for leprosy

Type of Leprosy	Monthly Supervised	Daily Self-Administered	Duration of Treatment	Duration of Follow-up
Paucibacillary	Rifampicin 600 mg	Dapsone 100 mg	6 months	2 years
Multibacillary	Rifampicin 600 mg Clofazimine 300 mg	Clofazimine 300 mg Dapsone 100 mg	24 months	5 years

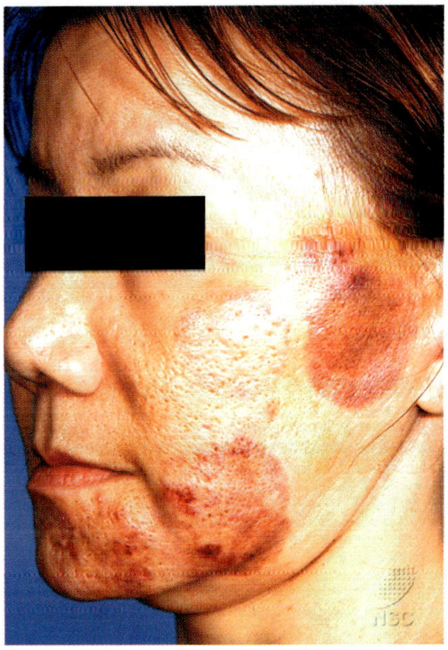

▲ **FIGURE 80-22** Moxibustion. Discoid purpura on the face of an Indonesian woman that developed after she was treated by a traditional healer with acupuncture and moxibustion for a facial rash. Courtesy of National Skin Centre, Singapore.

can masquerade as physical abuse, child abuse, or bleeding disorders.[128–130]

CHRONIC ARSENIC TOXICITY

Summary

- Associated with ingestion of contaminated well water and contaminated traditional Chinese medications.
- Multisystemic disorder.
- May lead to cutaneous and visceral malignancy.

Exposure to arsenic in Asia occurs owing to ingestion of contaminated well water or contaminated traditional Chinese medications.[131] Areas of Asia in which the former has occurred include West Bengal, Bangladesh, South Calcutta, Vietnam, and Taiwan.[132–134]

Clinical Features

Symptoms of chronic arsenic toxicity usually develop after 6 months to 2 years of exposure. The time of onset depends on the arsenic concentration in the drinking water, cumulative intake, and the health status of the individual. Chronic arsenic toxicity is a multisystem disorder.

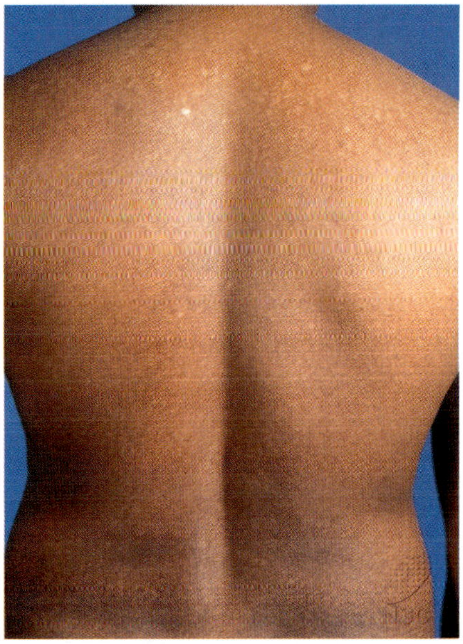

▲ **FIGURE 80-23** Chronic arsenic toxicity. Guttate hypopigmentation on the back of a Malay man. Courtesy of National Skin Centre, Singapore.

Areas of hyperpigmentation interspersed with hypomelanotic macules (the so-called raindrops on a dusty road) are seen on the trunk, axillae, and groin (Figure 80-23). Other cutaneous manifestations include palmoplantar punctate keratoses (arsenical keratosis), guttate hypopigmentation, and skin neoplasms such as Bowen disease, squamous cell carcinoma, and basal cell carcinoma (Figure 80-24). The mucosa is not involved. Arsenical keratosis may progress to squamous cell carcinoma. Bowen disease occurs within 10 years of exposure and invasive carcinomas within 20 years.[135]

Patients may suffer from generalized weakness, loss of appetite and weight, anemia, sensory neuropathy, and other symptoms. Besides skin cancer, malignancies of the lung, liver, kidney, and bladder may develop.

Treatment

There is no effective treatment for chronic arsenic toxicity. Oral retinoids, currettage, and cryosurgery have been used to reduce arsenic keratoses, but these treatments are anectodotal or based on small series.[136] Treatment is mainly to detect and treat skin neo plasms as and when they arise.

LICHEN AMYLOIDOSIS

Summary

- Localized primary cutaneous amyloidosis.
- Common in Southeast Asia.
- Persistent pruritic papules on shin.

Lichen amyloidosis is a common localized primary cutaneous amyloidosis seen in Southeast Asia.[137]

Clinical Features

The lesions appear initially as discrete, firm pigmented papules on extensor surfaces of the extremities (Figure 80-25).

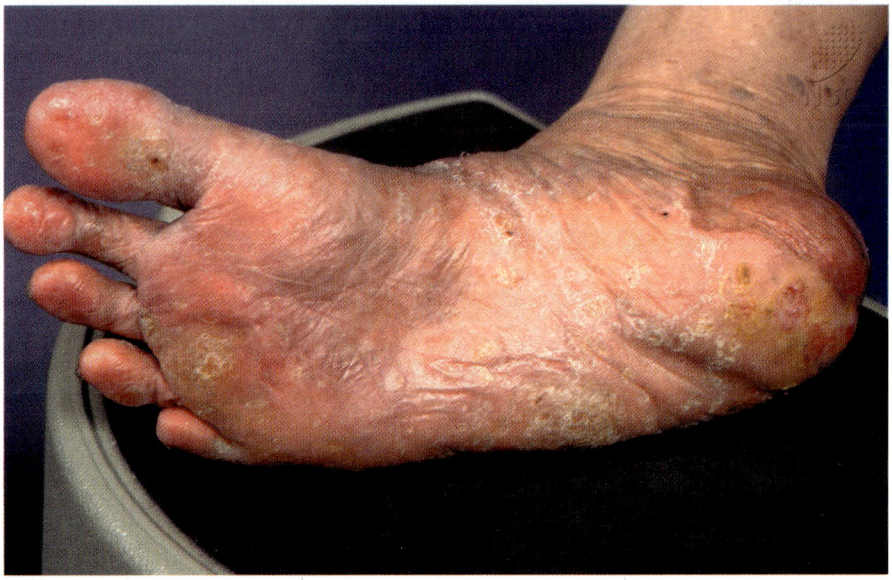

▲ **FIGURE 80-24** Chronic arsenic toxicity. Arsenical keratosis (punctate keratoses on the sole) and Bowen disease (eroded plaques) on the heel. This Malay woman had lived in a mining area during her childhood. Courtesy of National Skin Centre, Singapore.

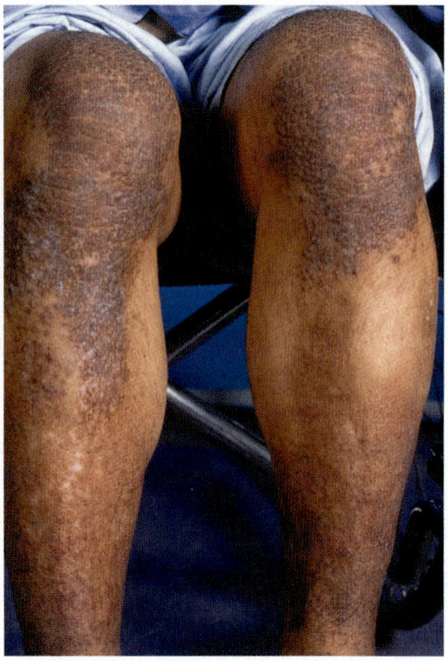

▲ **FIGURE 80-25** Lichen amyloidosis. Firm pigmented papules in a ripple pattern on the knees and legs of a Malay man. Courtesy of National Skin Centre, Singapore.

The legs are affected most frequently, followed by the arms and then the back. When the upper extremities are affected, the lower extremities are usually involved. Initially, an asymmetric distribution may be seen.[138] The papules become larger and confluent over time, forming plaques that have a rippled pattern. Pruritus is the main symptom. Large papules resembling prurigo nodules may develop as a result of persistent scratching. The condition persists through life. The differential diagnoses include hypertropic lichen planus and lichen simplex chronicus.

Pathology

Amyloid deposits are seen mainly in the papillary dermis and less often in the subpapillary layer and the upper reticular dermis. The overlying epidermis is acanthotic and hyperkeratotic.

Treatment

There is no effective treatment for lichen amyloidosis. Treatment is mainly to relieve the pruritus and to improve appearance. Patients are advised to refrain from scratching or rubbing the lesions because these may aggravate the lesions. Potent topical steroids, with or without occlusion, used together with salicylic acid, may help to relieve the itch and improve the appearance. Dimethylsulfoxide, dermabrasion, and laser resurfacing have produced significant improvement in some patients.

REFERENCES

1. Alakloby OM. Pattern of skin diseases in eastern Saudi Arabia. *Saudi Med J* 2005;26:1607-1610.
2. Tay YK, Khoo BP, Goh CL. The profile of atopic dermatitis in a tertiary dermatology outpatient clinic in Singapore. *Int J Dermatol* 1999;38:689-692.
3. Tay YK, Kong KH, Khoo L, et al. The prevalence and descriptive epidermiology of atopic dermatitis in Singapore school children. *Br J Dermatol* 2002;146:101-106.
4. Al-Saeed WY, Al-Dawood KM, Bukhari IA, et al. Prevalence and pattern of skin disorders among female schoolchildren in eastern Saudi Arabia. *Saudi Med J* 2006;27:227-234.
5. Yan DC, Ou LS, Tsai TL, et al. Prevalence and severity of asthma, rhinitis and eczema in 13-14 year-old children in Taipei, Taiwan. *Ann Allergy Asthma Immunol* 2005;95:579-585.
6. Liao ME, Huang JL, Chiang LC. Prevalence of asthma, rhinitis and eczema from the ISAAC survey of schoolchildren in Central Taiwan, part I. *Asthma* 2005;42:833-837.
7. Teeratakulpisarn J, Wiangnon S, Kosalaraksa P, Heng S. Surveying the prevalence of asthma, allergic rhinitis and eczema in school-children in Khon Kaen, northeastern Thailand using the ISSAC questionnaire, part III. *Asian Pacific J Allergy Immunol* 2004,22:175-181.
8. Quah BS, Wan-Pauzi I, Ariffin N, Mazidah AR. Prevalence of asthma, eczema and allergic rhinitis: Two surveys, 6 years apart, in Kota Bharu, Malaysia. *Respirology* 2005;10:244-249.
9. Sugiura H, Umemoto N, deGuchi H, et al. Prevalence of childhood and adolescent atopic dermatitis in a Japanese population: Comparision with the disease frequency examined 20 years ago. *Acta Dermatol Venereol* 1998;78:293-294.
10. Chan YC, Tay YK, Sugito TL, et al. A study on the knowledge, attitudes and practices of Southeast Asian dermatologists in the management of atopic dermatitis. *Ann Acad Med Singapore* 2006; 35:794-710.
11. Ng SK, Goh CL (eds). *The Principles and Practice of Contact and Occupational Dermatology in the Asia-Pacific Region.* Singapore, World Scientific Publishing Company, 2001.
12. Yeung CK, Teo LH, Xiang LH, et al. A community-based epidemiological study of acne vulgaris in Hong Kong adolescents. *Acta Dermatol Venereol* 2002;82:104-107.
13. Sharquie KE, Al-Turfi IA, Al-Shimary WM. Treatment of acne vulgaris with 2% topical tea lotion. *Saudi Med J* 2006; 27:83-85.
14. Chomnawang MT, Surassmo S, Nukoolkarn VS, Gritsanapan W. Antimicrobial effects of Thai medicinal plants against acne-inducing bacteria. *J Ethnopharmacol* 2005;101:330-333.
15. Tu P, Li GQ, Zhu XJ, et al. A comparison of adapalene gel 0.1% vs tretinoin gel 0.025% in the treatment of acne vulgaris in China. *J Eur Acad Dermatol Venereol* 2001;15:31-36S.
16. Spellman MC, Pinus SH. Efficacy and safety of azelaic acid and glycolic acid combination therapy compared with tretinoin therapy for acne. *Clin Ther* 1998;20:711-721.
17. Dreno B, Nocera T, Verriere F, et al. Topical retinaldehyde with glycolic acid: Study of tolerance and acceptability in association with anti-acne treatments in 1709 patients. *Dermatology* 2005;210:22-29S.
18. Poli F, Ribet V, Lauze C, et al. Efficacy and safety of 0.1% retinaldehyde/6% glycolic acid (diacneal) for mild to moderate acne vulgaris: A multicentre, double-blind, randomized vehicle-controlled trial. *Dermatology* 2005;210:14-21S.
19. Tan HH, Goh CL, Yeo MG, et al. Antibiotics sensitivity of *Propionibacterium acnes* isolates from patients with acne vulgaris in a tertiary dermatological referral centre in Singapore. *Ann Acad Med Singapore* 2001;30:22-25.
20. Profile of acne patients in the Philippines requiring a second course of oral isotretinoin. *Int J Dermatol* 2005;44:999-1001.
21. Isotretinoin in acne vulgaris: A prospective analysis of 160 cases from Kuwait. *J Drugs Dermatolol* 2005;4:369-373.
22. Shahidullah M, Tham SN, Goh CL. Isotretiinoin therapy in acne vulgaris: A 10 year retopestive study in Singapore. *Int J Dermatol* 1994;33:60-63.
23. Ng PP, Goh CL. Treatment outcome of acne vulgaris with oral isotretinoin in 89 patients. *Int J Dermatol* 1999;38:213-216.
24. Atzori L, Brundu MA, Orru A, et al. Glycolic acid peeling in the treatment of acne. *J Eur Acad Dermatol Venereol* 1999; 12:119-122.
25. Wang CM, Huang CL, Hu CT, et al. The effect of glycolic acid in the treatment of acne in Asian patients. *Dermatol Surg* 1997;23:23-29.
26. Lee HS, Kim IH. Salicyclic acid peels for the treatment of acne vulgaris in Asian patients. *Dermatol Surg* 2003;29:1196-1199.
27. Kim SW, Moon SE, Kim JA, et al. Glycolic acid versus Jessner's solution: Which is better for facial acne patients? A randomized, prospective clinical trial of split-face model therapy. *Dermatol Surg* 1999;25:270-273.
28. Lee SH, Huh CH, Park KC. Effects of repetitive superficial chemical peels on the facial sebum secretion in acne patients. *J Eur Acad Dermatol Venereol* 2006;20:964-968.
29. Goldberg DJ, Russell BA. Combination blue (415 nm) and red (633 nm) LED phototherapy in the treatment of mild to severe acne vulgaris. *J Cosmet Laser Ther* 2006;8:71-75.
30. Papageorgiou P, Katsambas A, Chu A. Phototherapy with blue (415 nm) and red (660 nm) light in the treatment of acne vulgaris. *J Dermatol* 2000;142:973-978.
31. Pollock B, Turner D, Stringer MR, et al. Topical aminolaevulinic acid photodynamic therapy for the treatment of acne vulgaris: A study of clinical efficacy and mechanism of action. *Br J Dernatol* 2004;151:616-622.
32. Hongcharu W, Taylor CR, Chang Y, et al. Topical ALA-photodynamic therapy

for the treatment of acne vulgaris. *J Invest Dermatol* 2000;115:183-192.
33. Alexiades-Amenakas M. Long pulse dye laser-mediated photodynamic therapy combined with topical therapy for mild to severe comedonal, inflammatory, or cystic acne. *J Drugs Dermatol* 2006;5:45-55.
34. Friedman PM, Jih MH, Kimyai-Asadi A, et al. Treatment of inflammatory facial acne vulgaris with the 1450 nm diode laser: Pilot study. *Dermatol Surg* 2004;30:147-151.
35. Seaton ED, Charakida A, Moucer PE, et al. Pulsed-dye laser treatment for inflammatory acne vulgaris: Randomised, controlled trial. *Lancet* 2003;25:1347-1352.
36. Orringer JS, Kang S, Hamilton T, et al. Treatment of acne vulgaris with a pulsed dye laser: A randomized, controlled trial. *JAMA* 2004;291:2834-2839.
37. Seaton ED, Mouser PE, Charakida A, et al. Investigation of the mechanism of action of nonablative pulsed-dye laser therapy in the photorejuvenation and inflammatory acne vulgaris. *Br J Dermatol* 2006;155:748-755.
38. Erbagci Z, Akcali C. Biweekly serial glycolic acid peels vs long-term daily use of topical low-strength glycolic acid in the treatment of atrophic acne scars. *Int J Dermatol* 2000;39:789.
39. Al-Waiz MM, Al-Sharqi AI. Medium-depth chemical peels in the treatment of acne scars in dark-skinned individuals. *Dermatol Surg* 2002;28:383-387.
40. Chan HH, Lam LK, Wong DS, et al. Use of 1320 nm Nd:YAG laser for wrinkle reduction and the treatment of atrophic acne scarring in Asians. *Laser Surg Med* 2004;34:98-103.
41. Lipper GM, Perez M. Nonablative acne scar reduction after a series of treatments with a short-pulsed 1064 nm neodymium:YAG laser. *Dermatol Surg* 2006;32:998-1006.
42. Nonablative 1450 nm diode laser in the treatment of facial atrophic acne scars in type IV to V Asian skin: A prospective clinical study. *Dermatol Surg* 2004;30:1287-1291.
43. Woo SH, Park JH, Kye YC. Resurfacing of different types of facial acne scar with short-pulsed, variable-pulsed, and dual-mode Er:YAG laser. *Dermatol Surg* 2004;30:488-493.
44. Jeong JT, Kye YC. Resurfacing of pitted facial acne scars with a long-pulsed Er:YAG laser. *Dermatol Surg* 2001:27:107-110.
45. Tsai RY, Wang CN, Chang HL. Aluminum oxide crystal microdermabrasion: A new technique for treating facial scarring. *Dermatol Surg* 1995;21:539-542.
46. Ise S, Ofugi S. Subcorneal pustular dermatosis: A follicular variant? *Arch Dermatol* 1965;92:169-171.
47. Tang MB, Tan E, Chua SH. Eosinophilic pustular folliculitis (Ofuji's disease) in Singapore: A review of adult cases. *Australas J Dermatol* 2003;44:44-47.
48. Nervi SJ, Schwartz RA, Dmochowski M. Eosinophilic pustular folliculitis: A 40 year retrospect. *J Am Acad Dermatol* 2006;55:285-289.
49. Ellis E, Scheinfeld N. Eosinophilic pustular folliculitis: A comprehensive review of treatment options. *Am J Clin Dermatol* 2004;5:189-197.
50. Goh CL, Diova CN. A retrospective study on the clinical presentation and treatment outcome of melasma in a tertiary dermatological referral centre in Singapore. *Singapore Med J* 1999;40:455-458.
51. Moin A, Jabery Z, Fallah N. Prevalence and awareness of melasma during pregnancy. *Int J Dermatol* 2006;45:285-288.
52. Vazquez M, Maldonado H, Benmaman C, et al. Melasma in men: A clinical and histologic study. *Int J Dermatol* 1988;27:25-27.
53. Sarkar R, Jain RK, Puri P. Melasma in Indian males. *Dermatol Surg* 2003;29:204.
54. Kang WH, Yoon KH, Lee ES, et al. Melasma: Histopathological characteristics in 56 Korean patients. *Br J Dermatol* 2002;146:228-237.
55. Sanchez NP, Pathak MA Sato S, et al. Melasma: A clinical, light microscopic, ultrastructural, and immmunofluorescence study. *J Am Acad Dermatol* 1981;4:698-710.
56. Elmets CA, Singh D, Tubesing K, et al. Cutaneous photoprotection from ultraviolet injury by green tea polyphenols. *J Am Acad Dermatol* 2001;44:425-432.
57. Kligman AM, Willis I. A new formula for depigmenting human skin. *Arch Dermatol* 1975;111:40-48.
58. Menter A. Rationale for the use of topical corticosteroids in melasma. *J Drugs Dermatol* 2004;3:169-174.
59. Grimes PE. Melasma: Etiologic and therapeutic considerations. *Arch Dermatol* 1995;131:1453-1457.
60. Kanwar AJ, Dhar S, Kaur S. Treatment of melasma with potent topical corticosteroids. *Dermatology* 1994;188:170-172.
61. Taylor SC, Torok H, Jones T, et al. Efficacy and safety of a new triple-combination agent for the treatment of facial melasma. *Cutis* 2003;72:67-72.
62. Sarkar R, Bhalla M, Kanwar AJ. A comparative study of 20% azelaic acid cream monotherapy versus a sequential therapy in the treatment of melasma in dark-skinned patients. *Dermatology* 2002;205:249-254.
63. Fitton A, Goa KL. Azelaic acid: A review of its pharmacological properties and therapeutic efficacy in acne and hyperpigmentary skin disorders. *Drug* 1991;41:780-798.
64. Lim JTE. Treatment of melasma using kojic acid in a gel containing hydroquinone and glycolic acid. *Dermatol Surg* 1999;25:282-284.
65. Hakozaki T, Minwalla L, Ang JZ, et al. The effect of niacinamide on reducing cutaneous pigmentation and suppression of melanosome transfer. *Br J Dermatol* 2002;147:20-31.
66. Lim JTE, Tham SN. Glycolic acid peels in the treatment of melasma. *Dermatol Surg* 1997;23:177-179.
67. Sarkar R, Charandeep K, Bhalla M, et al. The combination of glycolic acid peels with a topical regimen in the treatment of melasma in dark-skinned patients: A comparative study. *Dermatol Surg* 2002;28:828-832.
68. Nanda S, Grover C, Reddy BS. Efficacy of hydroquinone (2%) versus tretinoin (0.025%) as adjunct topical agents for chemical peeling in patients of melasma. *Dermatol Surg* 2004;30:385-389.
69. Khunger N, Sarkar R, Jain RK. Tretinoin peels versus glycolic acid peels in the treatment of melasma in dark skinned patients. *Dermatol Surg* 2004;30:756-760.
70. Wang CC, Hui CY, Sue YM, et al. Intense pulsed light for the treatment of refractory melasma in Asian persons. *Dermatol Surg* 2004;30:1196-1200.
71. Negishi K, Tezuka Y, Kushikata N, et al. Photorejuvenation for Asian skin by intense pulsed light. *Dermatol Surg* 2001;27:627-632.
72. Negishi K, Kushikata N, Tezuka Y, et al. Study of the incidence and nature of "very subtle epidermal melasma" in relation to intense pulse light treatment. *Dermatol Surg* 2004;30:881-884.
73. Rusciani A, Motta A, Rusciani L, Alfano C. Q-switched alexandrite laser-assisted treatment of melasma: 2-year follow-up monitoring. *J Drugs Dermatol* 2005;4:770-774.
74. Kopera D, Hohenleutner U. Ruby laser treatment of melasma and postinflammatory hyperpigmentation. *Dermatol Surg* 1995;21:990-995.
75. Manaloto RMP, Alster T. Erbium:YAG laser resurfacing for refractory melasma. *Dermatol Surg* 1999;25:121-123.
76. Angsuwarangsee S, Polnikorn N. Combined ultrapulse CO. *Dermatol Surg* 2003;29:59-64.
77. Tannous ZS, Astner S. Utilizing fractional resurfacing in the treatment of melasma. *J Cosmet Laser Ther* 2005;7:39-43.
78. Rokhsar CK, Fitzpatrick RE. The treatment of melasma with fractional photothermolysis: A pilot study. *Dermatol Surg* 2005;31:1645-1650.
79. Yamakoshi J, Sano A, Tokutake S, et al. Oral intake of proanthocyanidin-rich extract from grape seeds improves chlosma. *Phytother Res* 2004;18:895-899.
80. Lee JH, Park JG, Lim SH, et al. Localized intradermal microinjection of tranexamic acid for the treatment of melasma in Asian patients: A preliminary clinical trial. *Dermatol Surg* 2006;32:626-631.
81. Huh CH, Seo KI, Park JY, et al. A randomized, double-blind, placebo-controlled trial of vitamin C iontophoresis in melasma. *Dermatology* 2003;206:318-320.
82. Ee HL, Wong HC, Goh CL, et al. Characteristics of Hori's naevus: A prospective analysis *Br J Dermatol* 2005;154:50-53.
83. Lee B, Kim YC, Wang WH, et al. Comparison of characteristics of acquired bilateral nevus of Ota-like macules and nevus of Ota according to therapeutic outcome. *J Korean Med Sci* 2004;19:554-559.
84. Kunachak S, Kunachakr S, Sirikulchayanonta V, et al. Dermabrasion is an effective treatment for acquired bilateral nevus of Ota-like macules. *Dermatol Surg* 1996;22:559-562.
85. Kunachak S, Leelaudomlipi P. Q-switched Nd:YAG laser treatment for bilateral nevus of Ota-like macule: A long-term follow-up. *Lasers Surg Med* 2000;26:376-379.
86. Suh DH, Han KH, Chung JH. Clinical use of the Q-switched Nd:YAG laser for the treatment of acquired bilateral nevus of Ota-like macules (ABNOM) in Koreans. *J Dermatol Ther* 2001;12:163-166.
87. Polnikorn K, Tanrattanakorn S, Goldberg DJ. Treatment of Hori's nevus with the

Q- switched Nd:YAG laser. *Dermatol Surg* 200;26:477-480.
88. Lam AY, Wong DS, Lam LK, et al. A retrospective study on the complications of Q-switched alexandrite laser in the treatment of acquired bilateral nevus of Ota-like macules. *Dermatol Surg* 2001; 27:937-941.
89. Manuskiatti W, Sivayathorn A, Leelaudomlipi P, et al. Treatment of acquired bilateral nevus of Ota-like macules (Hori's nevus) using a combination of scanned carbon dioxide laser followed by Q-switched ruby laser. *J Am Acad Dermatol* 2003;48:584-591.
90. Momosawa A, Yoshimura K, Uchida G. Combined therapy using Q-switched ruby laser and bleaching treatment with tretinion and hydroquinone for acquired dermal melanocytosis. *Dermatol Surg* 2003;29:1001-1007.
91. Nordlund JJ. Postinflammatory hyperpigmentation. *Dermatol Clin* 1988;6:185-192.
92. Nordlund JJ, Abdel-Malek ZA. Mechanisms for post-inflammatory hyperpigmentation and hypopigmentation. *Prog Clin Biol Res* 1988;256:219-236.
93. Takiwaki H, Shirai S, Kohnm H, et al. The degree of UVA-induced erythema and pigmentation correlate linearly and are reduced in a parallel manner by topical anti-inflammatory agents. *J Invest Dermatol* 1994;103:42-46.
94. Bulengo-Ransby SM, Griffiths CEM, Kimbrough-Green CK, et al. Topical tretinion (retinoic acid) therapy for hyperpigmentated lesions caused by inflammation of the skin in black patients. *N Engl J Med* 1993;328:1438-1443.
95. Lowe NJ, Rizk D, Grimes PE, et al. Azelaic acid 29% cream in the treatment of facial hyperpigmentation in darker-skinned patients. *Clin Ther* 1998;20:945-959.
96. Burns RL, Prevost-Blank PL, Lawry MA, et al. Glycolic acid peels for post-inflammatory hyperpigmentation in black patients: A comparative study. *Dermatol Surg* 1997;23:171-174.
97. Grimes PE. The safety and efficacy of salicylic acid chemical peels in darker racial-ethnic groups. *Dermatol Surg* 1999;25:18-22.
98. Dierickx C, Goldman MP, Fitzpatrick RE. Laser treatment of erythematous, hypertrophic, and pigmented scars in 26 patients. *Plast Reconstr Surg* 1995;95:84-90.
99. Taylor CR, Anderson RR. Ineffective treatment of refractory melasma and postinflammatory hyperpigmentation by Q-switched ruby laser. *J Dermatol Surg Oncol* 1994;20:592-597.
100. Chan HH, Kono T. Naevus of Ota: Clinical aspects and management. *Skinmed* 2003;2:89-96.
101. Suh DH, Hwang JH, Lee HS, et al. Clinical features of Ota's naevus in Koreans and its treatment with Q-switched alexandrite laser. *Clin Exp Dermatol* 2000;25:269-273.
102. Hosaka Y, Onizuka T, Ichinose M, et al. Treatment of naevus of Ota by liquid nitrogen cryotherapy. *Plast Reconstr Surg* 1995;95:703-711.
103. Hata Y, Matsuka K, Ito O, et al. Treatment of naevus of Ota: Combined skin abrasion and carbon dioxide snow method. *Plast Reconstr Surg* 1996;98: 1112-1113.
104. Watanabe S, Takahashi H. Treatment of naevus of Ota with the Q-switched ruby laser. *N Engl J Med* 1994;29: 1745-1750.
105. Chang CJ, Nelson JS, Achauer BM. Q-switched ruby laser treatment of oculodermal melanosis (nevus of Ota). *Plast Reconstr Surg* 1996;98:1784-1790.
106. Yang HY, Lee CW, Ro YS, et al. Q-switched ruby laser in the treatment of nevus of Ota. *J Korean Med Sci* 1996; 11:165-170.
107. Alster TS, Williams CM. Treatment of naevus of Ota by the Q-switched alexandrite laser. *Dermatol Surg* 1995;21: 592-596.
108. Lu Z, Fang L, Jiao S, et al. Treatment of 522 patients with naevus of Ota with the Q-switched alexandrite laser. *Chin Med J* 2003;116:226-230.
109. Kono T, Chan HH, Ercocen AR, et al. Use of Q-switched ruby laser in the treatment of nevus of Ota in different age groups. *Laser Surg Med* 2003;32: 391-395.
110. Ueda S, Isoda M, Imayama S. Response of naevus of Ota to Q-switched ruby laser treatment according to lesion colour. *Br J Dermatol* 2000;142:77-83.
111. Kang W, Lee E, Choi GS. Treatment of Ota's nevus by Q-switched alexandrite laser: The therapeutic outcome in relation to clinical and histological findings. *Eur J Dermatol* 1999;9:639-643.
112. Chan HH, Leung RS, Ying SY. A retrospective analysis of complications in the treatment of nevus of Ota with the Q-switched alexandrite and the Q-switched Nd:YAG lasers. *Dermatol Surg* 2000;26:1000-1006.
113. Chan HH, Lam LK, Wong DS, et al. Role of skin cooling in improving patient tolerability of Q-switched alexandrite laser in naevus of Ota treatment. *Lasers Surg Med* 2003;32:148-151.
114. Das SK, Majumder PP, Chakraborty R, et al. Studies on vitiligo: I. Epidemiological profile in Calcutta, India. *Genet Epidemiol* 1985;2:71-78.
115. Bhatia PS, Mohan L, Pandey ON, et al. Genetic nature of vitiligo. *J Dermatol Sci* 1992;4:180-184.
116. Kim SM, Chung HS, Hann SK. The genetics of vitiligo in Korean patients. *Int J Dermatol* 1998;37:908-910.
117. Zhang XJ, Liu JB, Gui JP, et al. Characteristics of genetic epidemiology and genetic models for vitiligo. *J Am Acad Dermatol* 2004;51:383-390.
118. Chen JJ, Huang W, Gui JP, et al. A novel linkage to generalized vitiligo on 4q13-q21 identified in a genomewide linkage analysis of Chinese families. *Am J Hum Genet* 2005;76:1057-1065.
119. Hann SK, Chun WH, Park YK. Clinical characteristics of progressive vitiligo. *Int J Dermatol* 1997;36:353-355.
120. Kumar B, Rai R, Kaur I, et al. Childhood cutaneous tuberculosis: A study over 25 years from northern India. *Int J Dermatol* 2001;40:26-32.
121. Yasmeen N, Kanjee A. Cutaneous tuberculosis: A three year prospective study. *J Pak Med Assoc* 2005;55:10-12.
122. Chong LY, Lo KK. Cutaneous tuberculosis in Hong Kong: A 10-year retrospective study. *Int J Dermatol* 1995;34:26-29.
123. Hamada M, Urabe K, Moroi Y, et al. Epidemiology of cutaneous tuberculosis in Japan: A retrospective study from 1906 to 2002. *Int J Dermatol* 2004;43: 727-731.
124. Chemotherapy and management of tuberculosis in the United Kingdom: Recommendations 1998. Joint Tuberculosis Committee of the British Thoracic Society. *Thorax* 1998;53: 536-548.
125. Blumberg HM, Burman WJ, Chaisson RE, et al. American Thoracic Society/ Centers for Disease Control and Prevention/Infectious Diseases Society of America: Treatment of tuberculosis. *Am J Respir Crit Care Med* 2003;167:603-662.
126. WHO global strategy for further reducing the leprosy burden and sustaining leprosy control activities. *Indian J Lepr* 2006;78:7-31.
127. Green A. Scarification, cupping and other traditional measures, with references to folk medicine in Greece and elsewhere. *Australas J Dermatol* 1971;12: 89-96.
128. Asnes RS, Wisotsky DH. Cupping lesions simulating child abuse. *J Pediatr* 1981;99:267-268.
129. Look KM, Look RM. Skin scraping, cupping, and moxibustion that may mimic physical abuse. *J Forens Sci* 1997;42: 103-105.
130. Overbosch D, Fibbe WE, Stuiver PC. Pseudo-bleeding disorder due to coin rubbing. *Neth J Med* 1984;27:16-17.
131. Yeh S. Skin cancer in chronic arsenicism. *Hum Pathol* 1973;4:469-485.
132. Rahman MM, Chowdhury UK, Mukherjee SC, et al. Chronic arsenic toxicity in Bangladesh and West Bengal, India: A review and commentary. *J Toxicol Clin Toxicol* 2001;39:683-700.
133. Mazumder DN, Das Gupta J, Chakraborty AK, et al. Environmental pollution and chronic arsenicosis in South Calcutta. *Bull WHO* 1992;70: 481-485.
134. Agusa T, Kunito T, Fujihara J, et al. Contamination by arsenic and other trace elements in tube-well water and its risk assessment to humans in Hanoi, Vietnam. *Environ Pollut* 2006;139: 95-106.
135. Miki Y, Kawatsu T, Matsuda K, et al. Cutaneous and pulmonary cancers associated with Bowen's disease. *J Am Acad Dermatol* 1982;6:26-31.
136. Piamphongsant T. Chronic environmentalal arsenic poisoning. *Int J Dermatol* 1999;38:401-410.
137. Tan T. Epidemiology of primary cutaneous amyloidosis in Southeast Asia. *Clin Dermatol* 1990;8:20-24.
138. Wang WJ. Clinical features of cutaneous amyloidosis. *Clin Dermatol* 1990;8: 13-19.

CHAPTER 81

Common Skin Diseases and Treatment in North America: Mexico

Ivonne Arellano-Mendoza
Amado Saúl

Key Points

- The ethnically diverse population of Mexico includes indigenous peoples (Indians), Caucasians from a variety of European countries, Mestizos (individuals derived from European and indigenous Indian ancestry), and individuals of African descent.
- Cutaneous diseases commonly seen in Mexico are quite varied and include those of infectious, malignant, pigmentary, and photocutaneous etiology.
- Mexico is geographically location adjacent to the United States, which has an impact on diseases observed by American dermatologists.
- The Hispanic population is the fastest-growing population in the United States, facilitated by immigration from Mexico, which necessitates an understanding of disorders that occur in Mexico.

Mexico, a country of approximately 103 million people, is racially and ethnically diverse. The Mexican population consists of indigenous Indians, Caucasians from a variety of European countries, Mestizos (individuals derived from European and indigenous Indian ancestry), as well as individuals of African decent. Cutaneous diseases commonly seen in Mexico are quite varied and include those of infectious, malignant, pigmentary, and photocutaneous etiology (Table 81-1). Since the Hispanic population is the fastest-growing population in the United States, facilitated by immigration from Mexico, it is important for dermatologists to have a working knowledge of common cutaneous diseases that occur in this country. This chapter reviews these common diseases.

TABLE 81-1
Common Dermatoses in Mexico

Solar dermatitis–prurigo
Ashy dermatitis
Melasma
Tokclau
Mycetoma
Sporotrichosis
Cutaneous tuberculosis
Leprosy
Mexican leishmaniasis
Cutaneous larva migrans
Nonmelanoma skin cancer
Melanoma

SOLAR DERMATITIS–PRURIGO

Solar dermatitis is one of the 10 most frequently occurring dermatoses in Mexico, representing approximately 3–5% of all cutaneous diseases. Also known as *solar dermatitis, actinic prurigo, luscitis, summer prurigo,* and *polymorphous light eruption,* it tends to predominate in people who live in higher elevations. Onset of solar dermatitis may occur during childhood, with improvement occurring during the adolescent years. It is seen primarily in Mestizo patients with darker skin color and occurs more often in women (2:1). Patients frequently seek dermatologic treatment during the third or fourth decade of life.

Solar dermatitis is induced by exposure to ultraviolet (UV) radiation, primarily UVB and less often UVA.[1,2] Hojyo and colleagues demonstrated that 92.8% of patients with actinic prurigo were HLA-DR4-positive. Eighty percent of the HLA-DR4-positive patients also were positive for the HLA-DRB1*0407 allele. HLA-A28 and HLA-B39 (B16) also were significantly increased, possibly explaining the higher frequency in the Mexican population.[3]

Actinic prurigo is a chronic photodermatosis present in sun-exposed areas, including the malar region, nose, upper lip, helix, neck, chest, and extensor aspects of upper limbs. The clinical presentation is variable and may include erythema, papules, eczematous dermatitis, lichenification, pinpoint scarring, hemorrhagic crusts, and hyperpigmentation. Cheilitis of the lower lip is a constant feature, and almost 45% of Mexican patients present with conjunctival hyperemia, epiphora, hyperpigmentation, and pseudopterygium formation[1,4,5] (Figure 81-1). Severe, long-standing pruritus is a hallmark of this disorder and is present year round. Eyebrow pseudoalopecia may be observed from chronic rubbing or scratching.

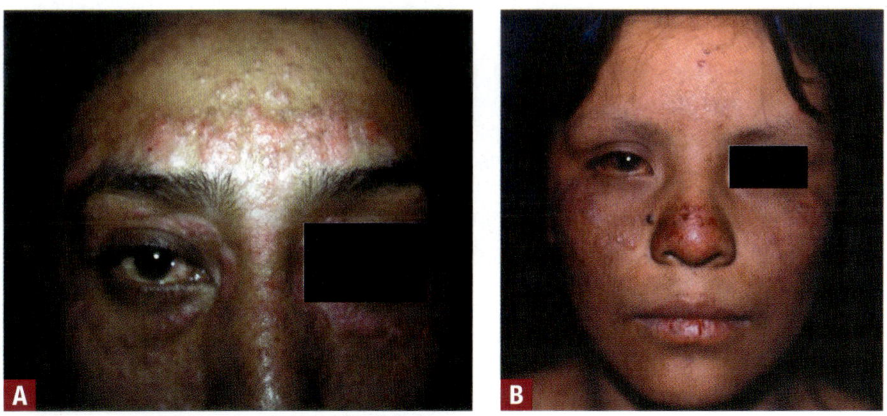

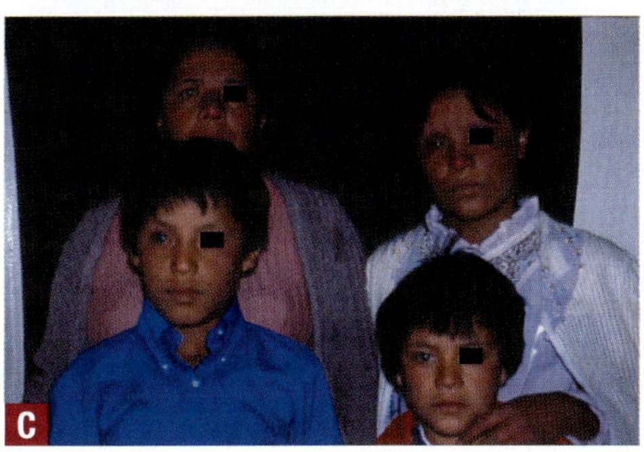

▲ **FIGURE 81-1** **A.** Solar dermatitis–prurigo. Note intense conjunctivits and chronic papular lesions. **B.** Solar dermatitis–prurigo. Note conjunctivitis, cheilitis, and scarring. **C.** Familial case of solar dermatitis–prurigo.

The diagnosis of solar dermatitis is based on clinical manifestations because abnormalities are not found on routine screening laboratory tests. Photopatch testing is negative and does not exclude diagnosis. Biopsy specimens demonstrate several findings, including[2,5]

- Epidermal hyperplasia (with or without parakeratosis)
- Spongiosis
- Vacuolar alteration of the basal cell layer
- Thickening of the basement membrane
- Dense lymphoid infiltrate in the dermis with formation of lymphoid follicles (particularly on the lips)
- Vasodilatation
- Dermal edema

Arrese and colleagues suggested that in genetically predisposed patients, UV radiation induces the production of tumor necrosis factor α (TNF-α) in significant amounts (which may explain the clinical benefits of treating this patients with thalidomide).

The differential diagnosis includes pellagra, lupus erythematosus, erythropoietic protoporphiria, and other photodermatoses. Contact dermatitis or secondary infection is frequently associated with solar dermatitis.

Treatment of solar dermatitis in Mexico is often successful but requires the institution of both preventative measures and aggressive therapy. One of the most important aspects of treatment is a full explanation of the disease to the patient, stressing the fact that even small amounts of sun exposure exacerbate this dermatosis. Sun protection with hats, eyeglasses, umbrellas, and a broad-spectrum sunscreen is mandatory. Emollients and mild cleansers should be applied as part of nightly adjuvant treatment. Sedating antihistamines are often necessary to control pruritus during exacerbations. Topical steroids are used occasionally to control acute eczematous lesions, but in severe or acute cases, oral treatment is preferred. The antimalarial agents chloroquine phosphate and hydroxychloroquine are used widely in Mexico for treatment of solar dermatitis. Antimalarial treatment necessitates ophthalmologic examinations at baseline and every 6 months until the drug is discontinued. Thalidomide has produced outstanding results and is prescribed in refractory or severe cases at 100 mg/day.[6] After remission of signs and symptoms, the dose is then tapered after several months. Special attention must be paid to the teratogenic effects of thalidomide, and contraceptives must be used once a negative pregnancy test is obtained. Although reported, these authors have not observed drug-induced neuropathy. Finally, oral photosensitizers should be avoided in patients with this condition.

ASHY DERMATOSIS

Ashy dermatosis, also known as *dermatosis cenicienta, erythema chronicum figuratum melanodermicum,* and *pintoid,* was first described by Dr. Oswaldo Ramírez in El Salvador in 1957. The name *erythema dyscromicum perstans* was suggested by Dr. Sulzberger in the early 1960s. This disorder is seen most commonly in Latin American and Asian patients, but there have been well-documented cases in patients of European and Turkish decent. There is a slight predominance in women.[8,9]

The etiology of ashy dermatosis is unknown, but associations include ingestion of ammonium nitrate, intestinal parasitosis, orally administered x-ray contrast media, and occupational cobalt allergy. The classic form of this chronic, asymptomatic disorder affects all body segments, sparing the scalp, palms, and soles. Clinical manifestations include symmetrically distributed 1- to 2-cm macules that become confluent and form large plaques. Characteristically, the macules and plaques are pigmented and have an erythematous halo at the periphery that later becomes hypopigmented and finally displays a gray "ashy" pigmentation.[10]

The differential diagnosis of ashy dermatosis includes lichen planus pigmentosus (LPP), which can be differentiated by its pruritic, brown-black macules that primarily affect the face and flexor folds. LPP may involve mucosal surfaces, unlike ashy dermatosis[11,12] (Figure 81-2).

Histologically, a biopsy of the erythematous border of ashy dermatosis demonstrates hyperkeratosis, thinned epidermis, hydropic degeneration of the basal layer, pigment incontinence, and perivascular lymphohistiocytic infiltrate. Colloid bodies can be seen. Immunologic findings include expression of CD36, ICAM-1, CD69, and CD94, which suggests activation of cytotoxic T cells.[8,13]

Treatment is generally unsatisfactory. However, in most of the cases, the disease progression stops, although the pigmentation may persist for years. The treatment that has proven most effective is clofazimine, 100 mg every other day (for patients weighing less than 40 kg) or daily (for those weighting 40 kg or more). Dapsone has been used with inconsistent results.[9,13]

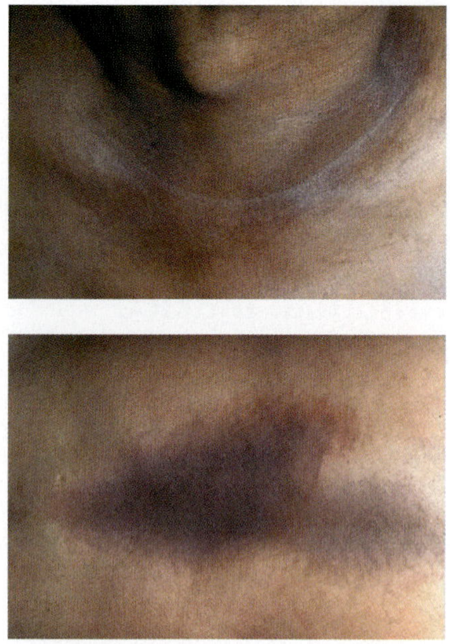

▲ **FIGURE 81-2** Ashy dermatitis. Note grayish color of pigmented lesions.

MELASMA

Although Mexico is geographically located in North America, most of its culture, ethnic roots, traditions, and diseases are similar to those described in Mesoamerica.[14] Melasma is one such disease, and this very common facial dyschromia is also known as *chloasma* or the *pregnancy mask*. In Hospital General de Mexico, it represents the third most frequent reason for dermatology consultation.

Melasma is seen most frequently in women, with men only 10% of patients. Several studies reveal that this disease is related to an increase in the number and functioning of melanocytes. Hormonal factors influence melasma, particularly pregnancy and in those receiving progesterone or estrogen therapies. Other triggering factors reported include the use of cosmetics and hair dyes and the ingestion of phototoxic and anticonvulsant drugs. However, 30% of patients have none of these precipitating factors.[15]

Melasma is an acquired facial pigmentation characterized by brown to gray-blue facial macules or patches. The pigmentation may be distributed in one of three patterns: malar, mandibular, or centrofacial (seen most frequently in the Mexican population).

Histologically, epidermal melasma is characterized by

- Increased melanin deposition in basal and suprabasal epidermal layers
- Highly dendritic melanocytes laden with pigment
- Vacuolar degeneration of basal cells
- Small numbers of melanophages in the papillary dermis

In dermal melasma, melanin deposition is observed in perivascular macrophages in superficial and deep dermal vessels with minimal focal perivenular lymphocytic infiltration; epidermal changes are not prominent.

The mixed pattern shares features of both the dermal and epidermal types.[16,17] The diagnosis of melasma is clinical, but a helpful aid in locating the depth of pigment is with Wood´s light illumination of the skin; epidermal pigment will be more apparent and appear brown or black, and dermal pigment will be less evident and appear bluish[18,19] (Figure 81-3).

Treatment will not be successful without daily photoprotection with sunblock. Patients should be advised that sun-protection measures not only include the use of a broad-spectrum sunscreen but also avoidance of direct sun exposure using a cap or a hat. A considerable number of topical lightening agents have been used, including[20]

- Tyrosinase inhibitors: hydroquinone, kojic acid, azelaic acid, and arbutin
- Inhibitors of melanin production: ascorbic acid and glutathione
- Direct melanocyte cytotoxics: ammoniated mercury, isopropylcatechol, and *N*-acetylcysteine
- Nonselective suppressors of melanogenesis: indomethacin and corticosteroids

Lightening agents may be formulated as single-ingredient, double-combination, or triple-combination formulas that the patient applies nightly. Recently, the efficacy and long-term safety of a triple-combination formula consisting of fluocinolone acetonide 0.01%, hydroquinone 4%, and tretinoin 0.05% have been reported.[21] Efficacy was demonstrated when the agent was used consistently until clearing of the melasma occurred, followed by a maintenance regimen to avoid relapse of the pigmentation. Recurrence after the discontinuation of therapy occurs consistently, thus necessitating intermittent therapy.[22] In addition to lightening agents, superficial chemical peels (30% salicylic acid) are also effective therapeutic modalities for melasma. Since multiple sessions may be required, patients should receive a full explanation of the long-term nature of this treatment.

Although asymptomatic, disorders of facial pigmentation have profound social and psychological impact in Mexican culture. Balkrishnan and colleagues demonstrated that effective treatment of melasma improves the quality of life of patients with melasma.[23]

TOKELAU (TINEA IMBRICATA)

Tinea imbricate, also known as *elegant* or *laced tinea,* is a chronic dermatophyte infection that involves hairless skin.[1,24] First observed among the natives of Polynesia, it is caused by an anthropophilic fungus, *Trichopyton concentricum,* that is transmitted form person to person through direct skin contact. Tinea imbricate is now found in Asia, Africa, and Central and South America. In Mexico, there are several endemic areas that include Guerrero, Puebla, and Chiapas (Lacandon ethnic group).[25] Tokelau has an equal sex predilection and affects individuals of all ages. Genetic and racial factors appear to determine its geographic distribution. Additionally, environmental factors, including heat and humidity, are strong determinants of distribution.[26,27]

Clinical lesions classically occur on hairless areas of the upper trunk, extremities, and face. The disorder is chronic, and slight itching is reported[1] (Figure 81-4). Lesions are characterized by erythema and scales that overlap like roof tiles to form extended polycyclic figures resembling a fence or lace. Diagnosis is made through direct mycologic examination, which reveals long intermixed filaments. Fungal culture confirms the causative agent, and

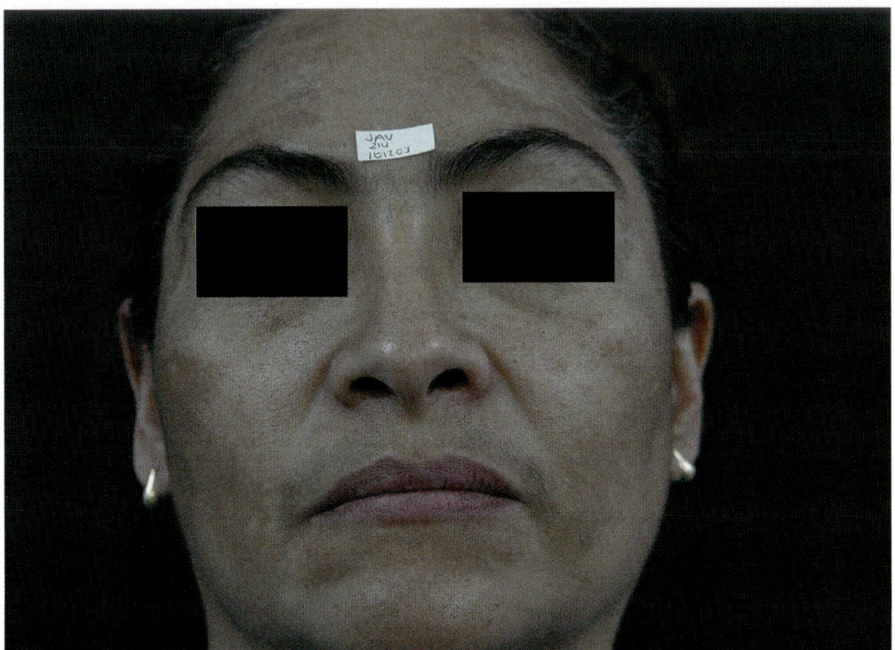

▲ **FIGURE 81-3** Melasma.

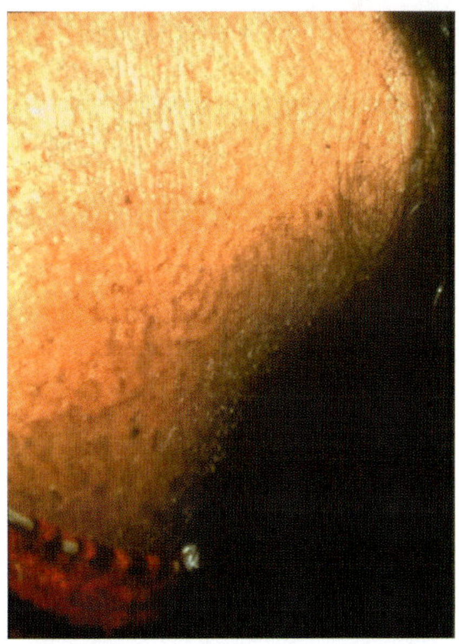

▲ **FIGURE 81-4** Tokelau. Note typical "laced" pattern.

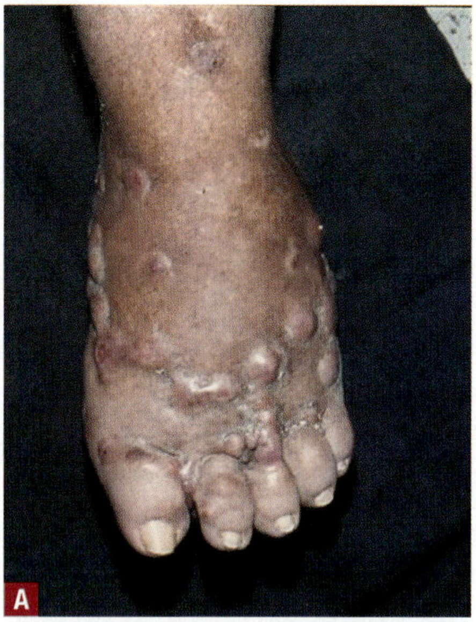

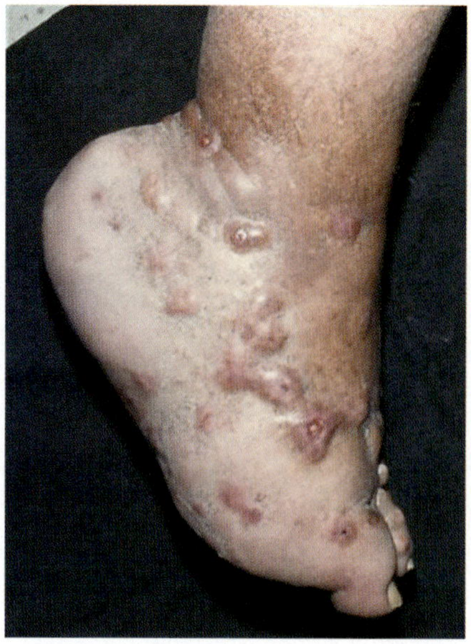

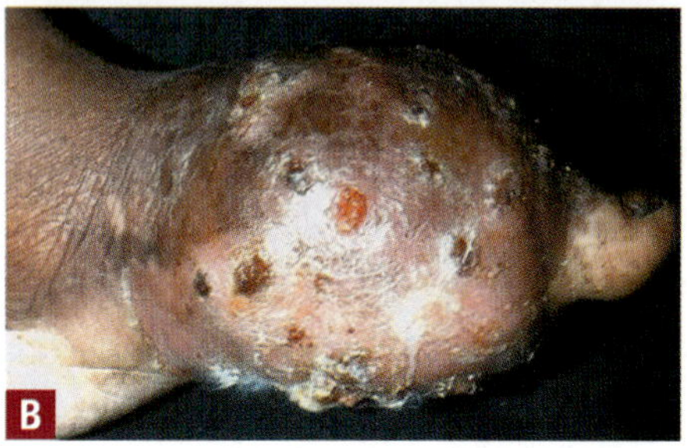

▲ **FIGURE 81-5** **A.** Mycetoma, typical long-standing lesions. **B.** Mycetoma in most frequent location.

further laboratory studies are not required.[24]

This superficial mycosis responds well to a variety of topical and systemic antimycotic agents. Griseofulvin, azoles, and terbinafine are rapidly acting agents, but resistance and relapses are observed frequently.[28]

MYCETOMA

Mycetomas are caused by either actinomycetes (bacteria) or eumycetes (fungi), aerobic agents that are distributed widely throughout nature. The most common actinomycetes are *Nocardia brasiliensis, Actinomadura madurae*, and *Streptomyces somaliensis*. The most common eumycetes are *Madurella mycetomatis, M. grisea, Leptosferia senegalensis, Pyrenochaeta romeroi*, and *Pseudoallescheria boydii*, as well as species of *Acremonium* and *Fusarium*.

These agents enter the body through cutaneous wounds from wood, thorns, or vegetables.[1] Mycetomas occur frequently in the tropical and subtropical countries of Asia and Africa and the Latin American countries of Mexico, Central America, Venezuela, Colombia, Brazil, and Argentina. In Mexico and Central America, mycetoma owing to actinomycetes predominates, whereas in South America, Asia, and Africa, eumycetoma is more frequent.[29]

Mycetoma is more common in males than in females (5:1) between the third and fifth decades of life. It is uncommon in children before puberty because it is believed that androgens influence the development of the disease.[29,30] Mycetoma commonly occurs on the lower extremities (i.e., feet, legs, knees, thighs, and hips), which are more susceptible to injury and inoculation (Figure 81-5). Person-to-person or site-to-site transmission does not occur.[31] In Mexico, it is seen primarily in peasants who wear sandals or walk barefoot or who carry wood on bare backs, where thoracic involvement occurs (Figure 81-6). Other less common areas of involvement include the hands, elbows, arms, shoulders, neck, and head.

Clinically, mycetoma is characterized by unilateral swelling, tissue deformity, and development of sinuses often surrounded by tissue growths known as *pseudonodules*. The sinuses drain filant exudates in which grains may be observed with the unaided eye (eumycetomas) or through microscopic examination (actinomycetomas).[1,31] The process can penetrate deeply and involve periostium, bone, and even viscera (particularly the lungs). Thoracic disease may lead to vertebral involvement with medullary compression and paraplegia.[1] Mycetoma is a chronic disease, and symptoms are often unrelated to the extent of clinical involvement.

Diagnosis is often obvious from the clinical presentation, but confirmation with mycologic examination is required. Direct examination of the exudate reveals the presence of grains that differ according to the species: *Nocardia* grains are 150- to 300-μm, round or bean shaped, colorless grains with clubs (Figure 81-7); *Actinomadurae madurae* are up to 1 mm in diameter, with geographic boundaries; *S. pelletieri* are red; and eumycetes are either white or black. Biopsy allows for better agent identification through affinity of the granules and evaluation of their morphology. Culture identifies the species, and in the case of *N. brasiliensis,* cultures grown in casein-enriched media are needed to differentiate it from other *Nocardia* species because only *N. brasiliensis* hydrolyzes casein.[24,32]

In addition to a complete examination of the patient, radiographic examination is required to determine the depth and aggressiveness of the disease. Prognosis depends on the location of the infection, the depth of involvement, and the etiologic agent.[1]

Treatment of actinomycetoma is achieved using several regimens, including

- Diaminodifenil-sulfone, 100 g/day, plus sulfamethoxazole-trimethoprim, 2 tablets per day

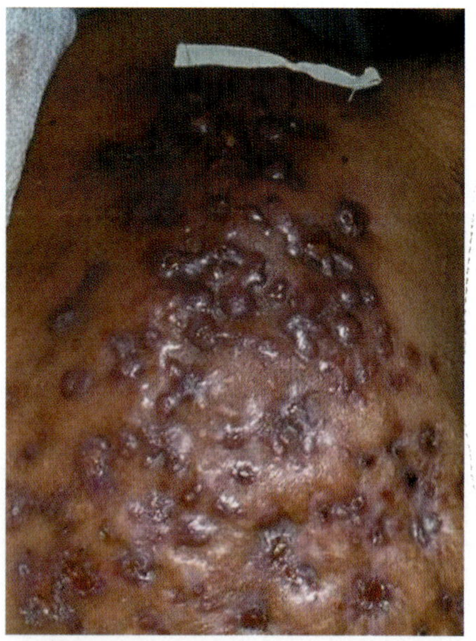

▲ **FIGURE 81-6** Advanced toracic mycetoma, inoculation secondary to carrying wood on the shoulders.

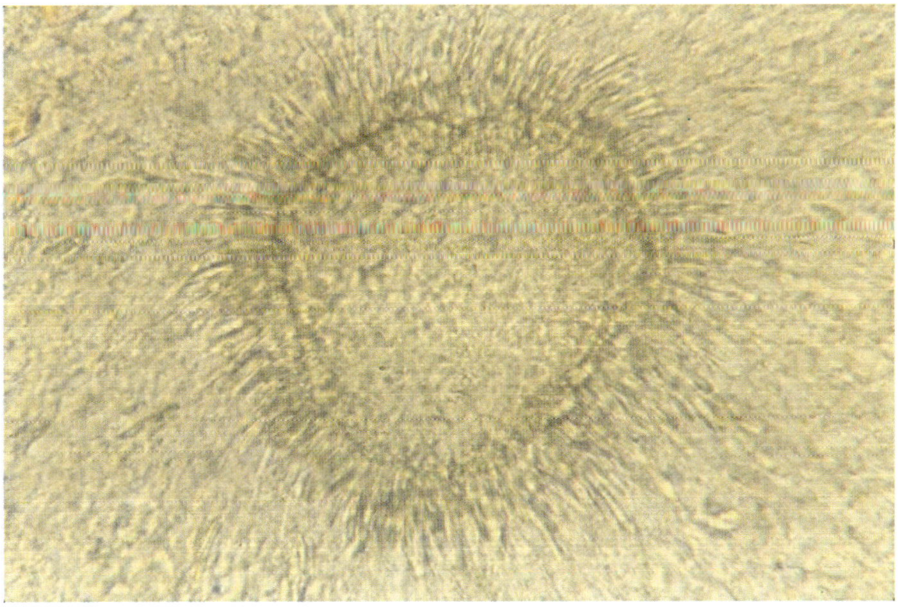

▲ **FIGURE 81-7** Nocardial grain.

- Severe long-standing cases require sulfamethoxasole-trimethoprim, 2 tablets per day, plus pulse therapy with amikacin, 15 mg/kg for 15–20 days (close follow-up of this regimen is required with audiometric and renal function monitoring)
- Amoxicilin-clavulanate plus sulfamethoxasole-trimethroprim for 3–6 months, with repeated treatments sometimes necessary[24,33,34]

Other drugs used for therapy include phosphomycin, streptomycin, rifampin, and imipenem.

Therapy for eumycetomas include itraconazole, fluconazole, and amphotericin B. In advanced cases, amputation may be required. Disease prevention includes education of agricultural workers about the disease and adequate protection with proper clothing and footware.[1]

SPOROTRICHOSIS

Sporotrichosis is caused by the ubiquitous fungus *Sporotrix schenckii,* which is found in vegetables, wood, straw, and flowers. Sporotrichosis occurs in tropical and subtropical regions of the world, although cases have been described in temperate and cold regions. In Mexico, it predominates in the central portion of the country. Men and women are equally affected, and it may be observed in any age group from childhood through to old age. In Monterrey, Mexico, sporotrichosis has been considered an occupational disease.[35]

Sporotrix penetrates the host's skin through an abrasion and then produces cutaneous manifestations that vary owing to the patient's immune response.[24] The clinical presentation may be divided into hyperergic and anergic forms. The two hyperergic forms, lymphangitic and fixed, are the most common, and these patients always have a positive intradermal reaction (sporotricin). The lymphangitic presentation accounts for 70% of patients, with nodules and gummas distributed along the lymphatic vessels of the face and upper or lower limbs.[12] The fixed form, which consists of only one lesion, is generally located on the face and is found in 25% of Mexican patients. The lesion may be a erythematous, nodular, infiltrated or limited plaque covered by thin scales. The course may be chronic and asymptomatic.[13]

Two to three percent of patients present with an anergic form of sporotrichosis, but it is increasingly diagnosed in association with acquired immune deficiency syndrome (AIDS). Several clinical forms are recognized, including superficial erythematous-squamous, nodular hematogenous, osteoarticular, and systemic (affecting mainly the lung). Patients with anergic forms of this disease have a negative sporotricin titer[36,37] (Figure 81-8).

The differential diagnosis of the fixed-plaque form of sporotricosis includes cutaneous tuberculosis (lupus vulgaris) and leishmaniasis.

Diagnosis is made via culture, in which a white colony is observed at 8

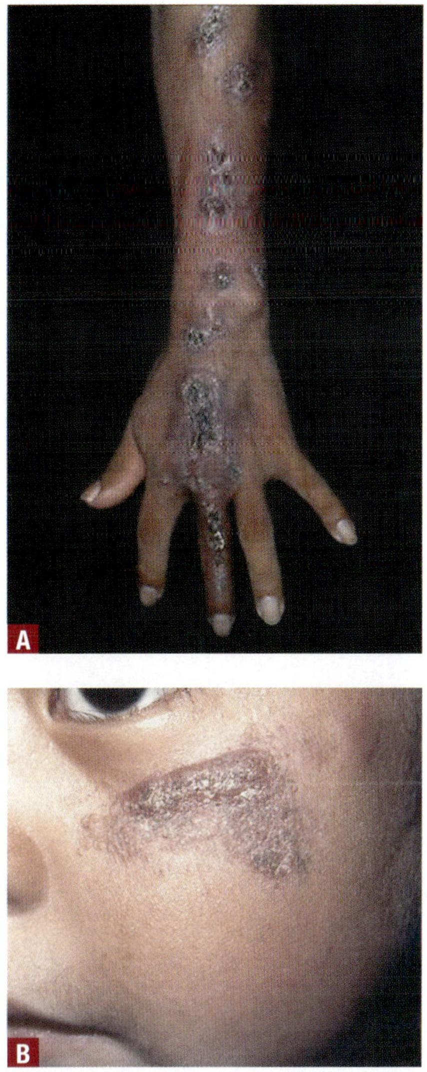

▲ **FIGURE 81-8** **A.** Lymphangitic sporotrichosis. **B.** Fixed-plaque sporotrichosis.

days that later turns black in color. Microscopic examination of the colonies show characteristic microconidial structures ("peaches in blossom" image). Direct smears are not useful diagnostically because it is difficult to visualize the levaduriform structures, with the exception of some anergic patients.

Histopathologic features of sporotrichosis include nonsuppurative granulomas, in which yeast and structures resembling stars, called *asteroid bodies,* can be found. Of note is the fact that asteroid bodies are not exclusive to sporotrichosis.

The intradermal reaction, sporotricin, read at 48 hours, is not diagnostic of sporotrichosis but identifies the immunologic response to this fungus and helps to classify the case as anergic or hyperergic.[38]

A very effective, well-tolerated, and inexpensive treatment for sporotrichosis is oral potassium iodide. In adults, this first-line treatment is administered at 3–6 g daily, and in children, the dosage is 1–3 g daily for 3 months. Other effective but more expensive medications include griseofulvin, itraconazole, terbinafine, and sulfametoxipiridazin and local heat. Amphotericin B is indicated for anergic forms of sporotrichosis.[39]

CUTANEOUS TUBERCULOSIS

There was a steady decline in the incidence of tuberculosis (TB) until 1985, when it began rising again in association with AIDS. In 1993, the number of cases of TB in New York surpassed those in developing countries, which prompted the World Health Organization (WHO) to declare a global emergency. By the year 2003, two million deaths were related to TB, with 80% of the patients being between 15 through 49 years of age.[40]

In Mexico, TB remains a public health concern, with an incidence of 16 cases per 100,000 inhabitants. Pulmonary tuberculosis is the most frequently observed type, followed by osteoarticular, genital, and digestive TB. Cutaneous tuberculosis represents the fifth most common clinical presentation, and 20% of patients seen are in people under 15 years of age.[41]

Primary cutaneous infection is extremely rare, but when it occurs, it may appear as a cutaneous nodule with associated lymphangitis and adenopathy. Most cases are considered reinfection, with patients having had pulmonary infection with *M. tuberculosis bovis* or *hominis* and a positive purified protein derivative (PPD) test. Patients can be reinfected endogenously from the original disease, or they may be reinfected from external sources. There are several classifications of the cutaneous forms of TB in Mexico, and the one described by Latapi, Escalona, and Estrada (based on observations from Dr. Foch, an outstanding Austrian dermatologist and director of the Lupus Hospital in Vienna, who spent his last years in Mexico) is commonly followed[1] (Table 81-2).

TABLE 81-2
Cutaneous Tuberculosis

Primary infection: rare
Reinfection: endogenous
Exogenous
I. Chronic forms (normergic)
   Colliquative tuberculosis, scrofuloderma: endogenous reinfection
   Verrucous tuberculosis (warty tuberculosis): endogenous reinfection
   Lupus tuberculosis, lupus vulgaris: endogenous and exogenous reinfection
   Orificial tuberculosis: endogenous reinfection
   Acute miliary tuberculosis: endogenous reinfection
II. Hematogenous forms (hyperergic)
   Deep nodular tuberculosis, erythema induratum of Bazin
   Nodular-necrotic tuberculosis, papulonecrotic
   Microdular or liquenoid tuberculosis, scrofulosus lichen

The first group consists of colliquative TB, verrucous TB, lupus vulgaris, orificial TB, and acute miliary TB. Patients have a normergic response to the *Mycobacterium* organism, and bacilli can be found in the lesions. These forms are chronic. The second group consists of the tuberculids, erythema induratum of Bazin, nodulonecrotic tuberculid, and lichen scrofulosum, in which the patient has a hyperergic response to the *Mycobacterium* antigens. Bacilli are not found in lesions.

Colliquative TB, also known as *scrofuloderma* or *scrofulosis,* is the most common form of cutaneous TB in Mexico. Affecting primarily children and young adults, it is usually secondary to ganglion, bone, or articular infection. Lesions occur in the supraclavicular, axillary, groin, elbow, knee, and malleolar regions, where bones are in close proximity to the skin. Clinically, nodules and gummas form that begin as small lesions, enlarge over several weeks, and become confluent and erythematous. The lesions subsequently become fluctuant and drain a yellow purulent material. Several lesions often evolve simultaneously until the entire region is affected with nodules, fistulas, and "cold abscesses." Scarring invariably occurs, which leads to restriction of movement and deformity of the affected area. Systemic symptoms include fever, malaise, and anorexia. Pulmonary infection may occur simultaneously, with cough, expectoration, thoracic pain, and dyspnea. The differential diagnosis includes cervicofacial actinomycosis, sporotrichosis, and mycetoma[1,42,43] (Figure 81-9).

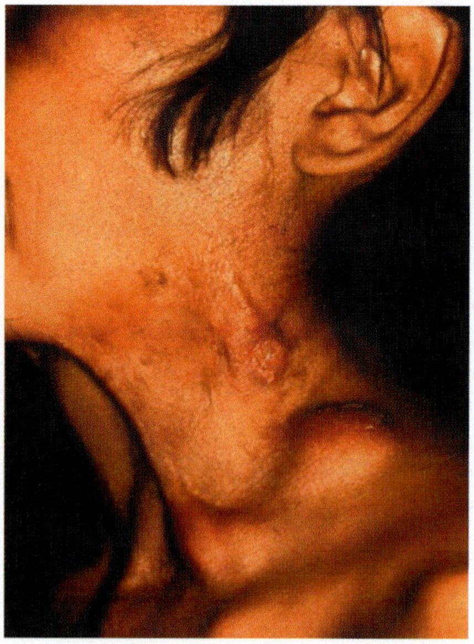

▲ **FIGURE 81-9** Coliquative tuberculosis in malnourished patient.

Verrucous TB (warty TB) results from the exogenous inoculation of the causal agent, generally as an occupational disease, in butchers and laboratory workers. Typically, verrucous TB affects the distal aspects of the hands and feet, although cases occurring in the gluteal area have been reported. A localized, asymptomatic, solitary verrucous nodule appears first and enlarges to form circular or oval, well-defined plaques with a rough surface. Some lesions heal centrally as they enlarge peripherally. Verrucous TB can affect lymphatic vessels, producing lymphestasis. The differential diagnosis includes chromomycosis, sporotrichosis, verrucous lymphestasis, and extensive verruca vulgaris.[44,45]

Lupus vulgaris is a clinical variant that generally occurs after endogenous inoculation. Lesions are located on the nose, cheeks, and ears. Lesions on the upper or lower extremitites have been described, as well as on conjunctival and nasal mucosae. The first lesion to appear is a nodule (lupoma) that progresses to an erythematous, verrucous, circular plaque with peripheral extension and central healing. When pressure is applied with a translucent glass on the lupoma, it has a classic "apple jelly" appearance. If left untreated, lupus vulgaris can produce extensive destruction and scarring.[42]

Orificial, miliary, vegetant, and fungous varieties of TB are extremely rare in Mexico[46] (Figure 81-10).

Darier was the first to use the term *tuberculids* to name a group of dermatologic diseases that he thought were related to active TB. Tuberculids always have been considered clinical manifestations of internal TB. They consist of symmetric, disseminated cutaneous nodules owing to hyperergic immune reactions to circulating bacillus or its

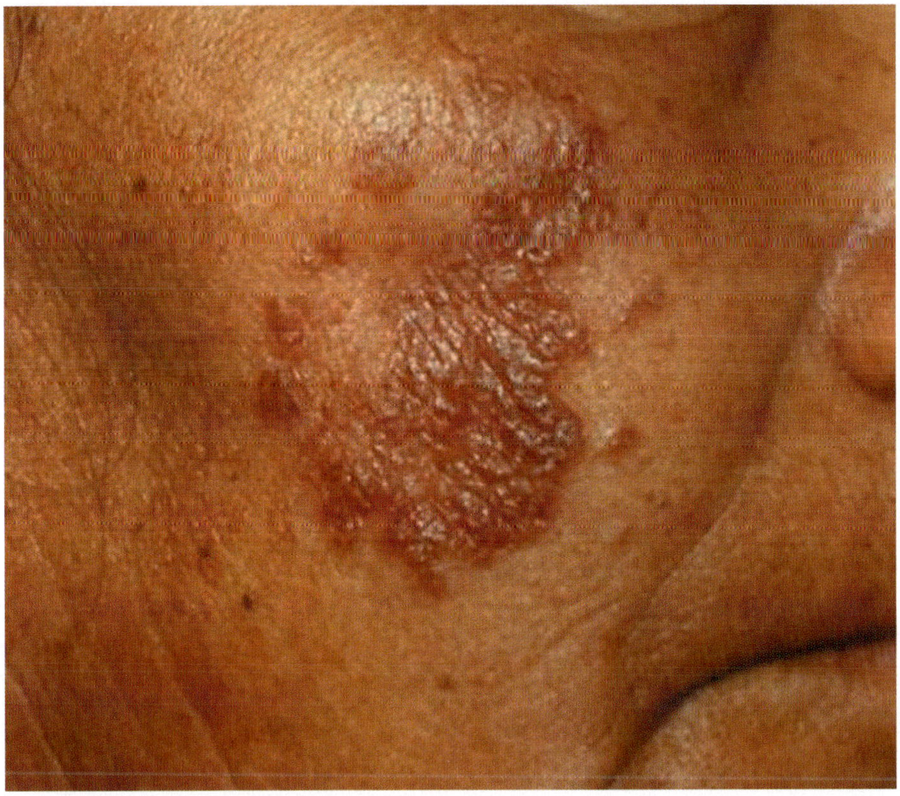

▲ **FIGURE 81-10** Typical lupus vulgaris of the cheek.

antigens in individuals with strong cell-mediated immunity.

Deep nodular TB was described by Bazin, and the diagnosis may be made in the presence of nodular vasculitis caused by *M. tuberculosis.* Characteristically affecting women, chronic painful nodules are present on the calves. They resolve with atrophic scars that may produce leg deformities. The lesions appear during the winter or after cold exposure, and lesions in different stages of evolution can be observed in the same patient. In chronic cases, lymphedema is present. When the nodules ulcerate, the term *Hutchinson form* is used.[47]

Nodule-necrotic TB, also termed *papulonecrotic TB,* occurs primarily on the elbows, knees, and gluteal area and rarely involves the face and earlobes. Morphologically, it presents as tiny nodules that ulcerate, crust, and heal with varioliform scars[48] (Figure 81-11).

Tuberculid in liquenoid or micronodular TB is extremely rare and is diagnosed infrequently. Characterized by plaques that can be several centimeters in size, it occurs in the lumbar or posterior thoracic regions. Several asymptomatic, confluent, 1- to 2-mm follicular nodules appear that are often misdiagnosed as keratosis pilaris or frinoderma. This form of TB usually presents along with scrofuloderma and was originally named *scrofulosus lichen*[49] (Figure 81-12).

The diagnosis of cutaneous TB and/or tuberculids is sometimes very difficult and is often achieved by the elimination of other disorders. A complete physical examination of the patient is mandatory, along with a chest radiograph, tuberculin test (PPD), and sputum and urine examinations (BAAR). A biopsy of the cutaneous lesion is often very helpful. A caseating tuberculoid granuloma may be found, and in rare instances, bacilli can be seen. Polymerase chain reaction (PCR) is another important tool in diagnosing cutaneous TB.[50–53]

The treatment of cutaneous TB is the same as for any other type of TB.[40] According to the World Health Organization (WHO), poorly supervised or incomplete treatment of TB is worse, from a public health perspective, than no treatment at all.

LEPROSY

Leprosy, or Hansen disease, was discovered by Armauer Hansen in Norway in 1872. It is an infectious disease of low transmissibility caused by *M. leprae.* This bacterium has not been cultured on artificial media and has only been inoculated successfully in the nine-band armadillo and a few species of monkeys.[54] Although it primarily affects the skin and peripheral nerves, leprosy is a systemic disease.[1]

Transmission of leprosy is from person to person through nasal droplets and possibly through cutaneous injuries. Intimate and continuous contact is required, as is a large inoculation, for

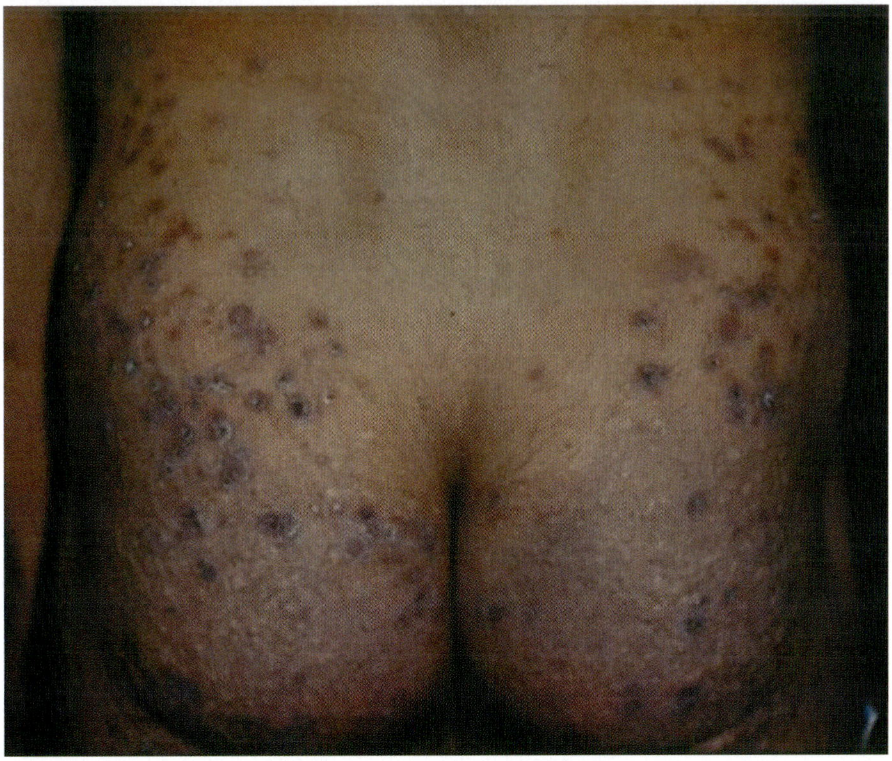

▲ **FIGURE 81-11** Nodular necrotic tuberculid. Note varioliform scarring.

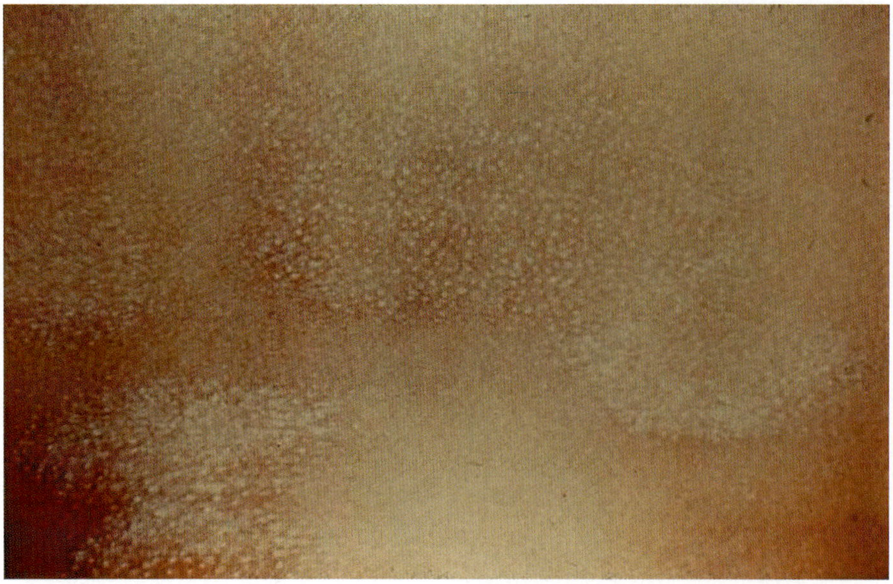

▲ **FIGURE 81-12** Liquenoid micronodular tuberculid (lichen scrofulorum).

successful transmission. However, only 5% of the population is susceptible to leprosy because a genetically acquired deficiency of cellular immunity to the bacillus is required to establish infection.[1,55] Transplacental transmission does not occur, nor does transmission through vectors.

The WHO estimates that there are 1.5 million people with the disease worldwide, distributed among the poorest countries of Asia, Africa, and Latin America. In Mexico, prevalence is estimated to be 0.4 cases per 10,000 persons, and according to the WHO, it is no longer a public health issue. However, there are areas of higher prevalence, such as the Mexican states of Sinaloa, Colima, and Guanajuato.[1,56]. Leprosy occurs more often among males and middle-aged persons, but it can be seen in children, including infants.

Leprosy may be classified as either lepromatous or tuberculoid. Lepromatous leprosy, in which the patient is anergic, is systemic, progressive, and transmissible. Tuberculoid leprosy is nonsystemic, reversible, and nontransmissible, and the patient is hyperergic. There are initial cases or indeterminate and dimorphic or interpolar cases that can be found in the middle of the immunologic spectrum. A lepromatous case will not shift to tuberculoid or vice versa. For treatment purposes, only two groups are considered: multibacillary and paucibacillary.[56]

Clinical features of leprosy depend on the cellular immune response to the bacillus. In lepromatous cases, there is involvement of the skin, peripheral nerves, eyes, upper airways, liver, spleen, and testicles.[1] Nodules, infiltrated plaques, or erythematous macules involving the ears, face, upper body, or limbs may occur. A diffuse myxedematous infiltrate of the entire body surface also may occur (diffuse cases of Lucio and Latapi described in Mexico)[1] (Figure 81-13). Involvement may include congestion, edema and bleeding of the nasal mucosa, iridocyclitis of the eyes, and alopecia of the eyebrows and eyelashes (madarosis). Nerves are usually thickened (e.g., cubital, auricular, and tibial), which leads to dysesthesia as well as motor and trophic disorders in the hands and feet (e.g., cubital claw, claw hand, equine foot, and malum perforans pedis) (Figure 81-14). Adenopathy and splenic enlargement may be observed.[56]

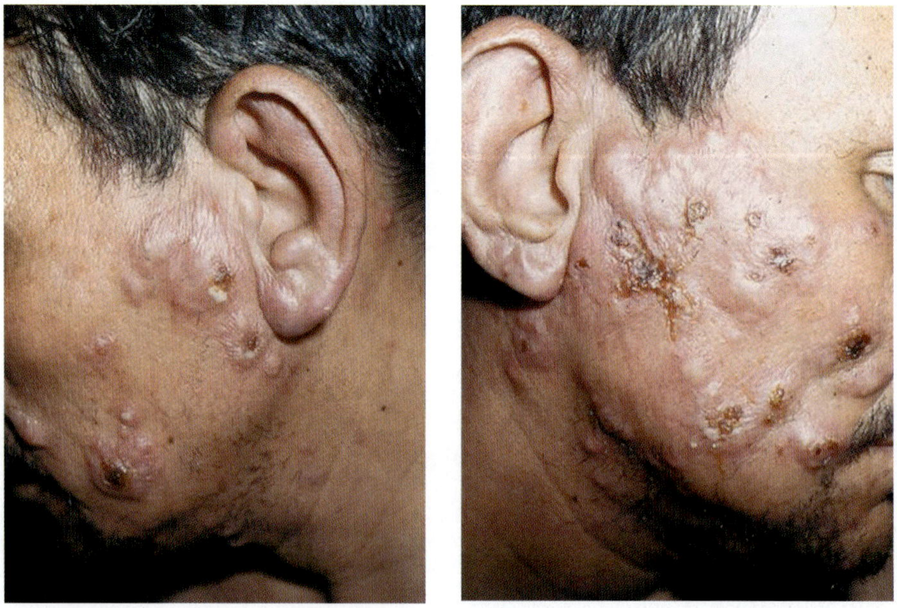

▲ **FIGURE 81-13** Leprosy, nodular case.

In tuberculoid cases, cutaneous and peripheral nerve involvement is present with scant erythematous infiltrated lesions. There is no involvement of the nose, eyes, or viscera (Figure 81-15). In indeterminate cases, hypochromic anesthetic lesions are present, as well as neural involvement, and in dimorphic cases, both lepromatous and tuberculoid cutaneous lesions can be present[1] (Figure 81-16).

In lepromatous leprosy, acute episodes known as leprous reactions may occur that are characterized by fever, malaise, iritis, neuritis, orchitis, multiform erythema, or erythema nodosum. In diffuse lepromatous leprosy, necrotic lesions can develop, known as *Lucio's phenomenon,* which worsens the prognosis.[1] In some lepromatous patients, the immunologic deficiency can reverse, with or without treatment, with the development of a reversal reaction. In these patients, edematous infiltrated lesions appear, accompanied by severe neural involvement of the hands and feet with irreversible facial palsy.[4]

For accurate diagnosis of lepromatous leprosy, identification of the bacillus in nasal mucosae as well as in lymphphatic drainage from cutaneous nodules is required. Biopsy of lepromatous cases reveals a histiocytic granuloma with abundant bacilli. In tuberculoid leprosy, dermal tuberculoid granulomas are formed. In indeterminate cases, nonspecific findings are present, and in dimorphic cases, there is a mixture of lepromatous and tuberculoid features. Intradermal reaction with lepromin,

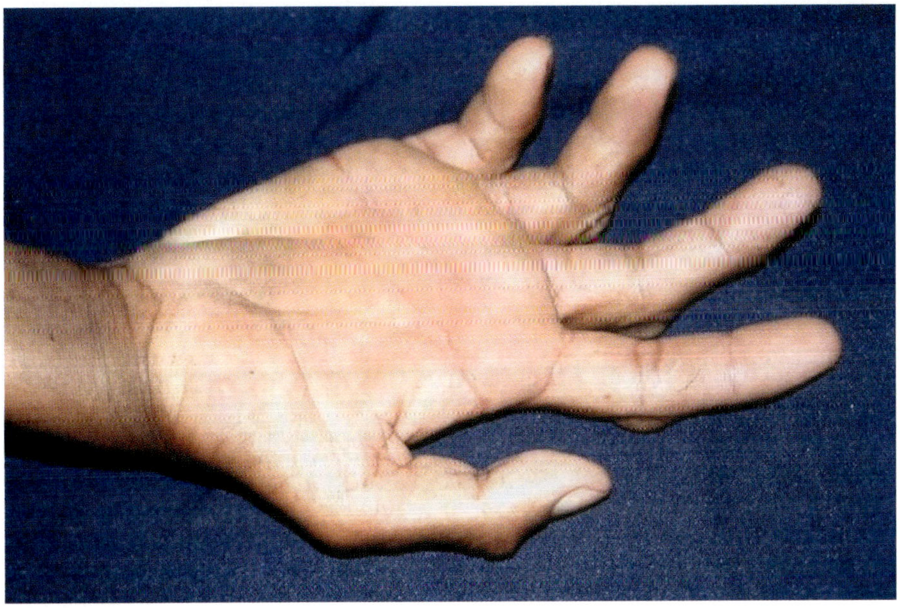

▲ **FIGURE 81-14** Leprosy, neuritis sequelae.

called *Mitsuda's reaction,* measures cellular immunity to the bacillus and is positive only in tuberculoid cases. Physical and emotional evaluation of patients is required because prejudice towards individuals with this disease abounds.[1]

Leprosy has been a curable disease since 1941. Currently, there are several effective drugs, including dapsone (DDS), rifampin, clofazimine, minocycline, and ofloxacin. Multibacillary cases require the use of at least two drugs: DDS, 100 mg/day, and rifampin, 600 mg each month, or clofazimine, 100 mg/day. Treatment of lepromatous cases must continue for at least 2 years, and tuberculoid, for 6 months. Low-dose steroids may be useful to prevent sequelae of neuritis.[56]

For the treatment of leprous reactions, thalidomide at doses of 200 mg/day is effective. Contraceptive measures must be used to avoid thalidomide's teratogenic effects. Pentoxifyline and clofazimine also can be useful in controlling acute episodes.[1,56]

Physical, psychological, and social rehabilitation is mandatory for the leprosy patient.[56] There is no longer a need for measures that were formerly used, such as isolation of the patients and their belongings.

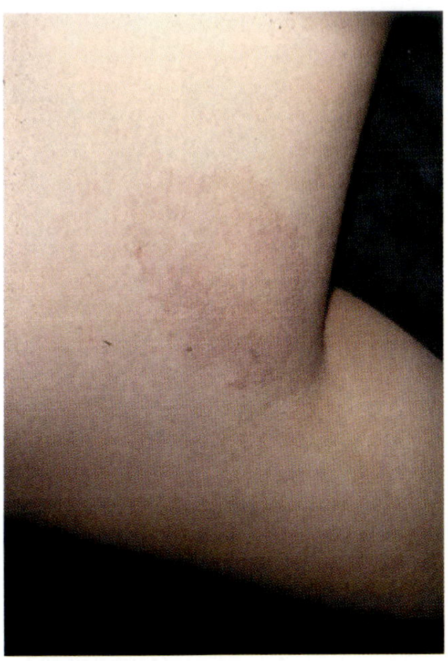

▲ **FIGURE 81-15** Leprosy, tuberculoid, single lesion.

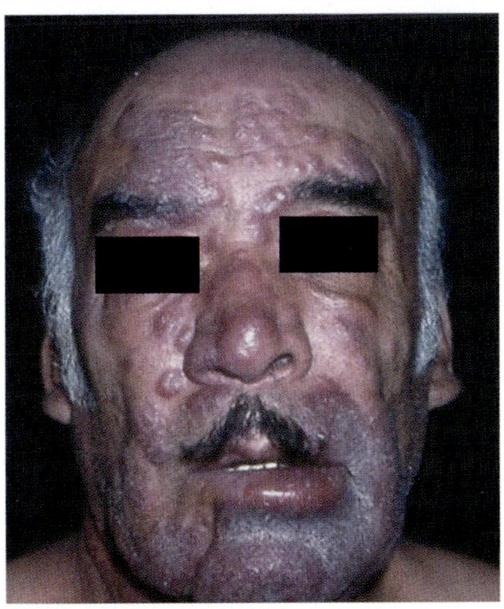

▲ **FIGURE 81-16** Leprosy, dimorphous case,

MEXICAN LEISHMANIASIS

Leishmaniasis is a parasitic disease caused by a protozoa from the *Leishmania* generum; several species exist depending on the region of the world. *L. donovani* causes kalaazar, frequently seen in Asia; *L. tropica* causes the disease in Mediterranean countries; *L. mexicana* complex is the causal agent from Texas down to Costa Rica; and *L.brasiliensis* and *L. peruviana* produce leishmaniasis in South America.[1] The infectious agent is inoculated through a bite from *Phlebotomus* or *Lutzomia* mosquitos that affects skin, mucosae, and viscera.

In Mexico, leishmaniasis is caused by *L. mexicana* that is transmitted by the mosquito *Lutzomia olmeca. L. olmeca* bites an infected patient and carries the amastigote, the nonflagellated form of the parasite, in its blood. The amastigote turns into the flagellated form, the promastigote. The insect then bites a healthy person or a reservoir (e.g., dogs, wolves, or foxes) and introduces the infecting form, the promastigotes, into this organism. The promastigote loses its flagellum and is phagocytosed by macrophages and subsequently invades other cells.[1] In Mexico, mucocutaneous cases are not seen.

In Mexico, the states most affected by leishmaniasis are Yucatan, Chiapas, Veracruz, and Oaxaca, but some cases have been reported in northern regions, such as Nuevo Leon, Coahuila, and Nayarit, and in the south of Texas.[1,57] The disease is frequently found in agriculture workers, men between the second and fourth decades of life who live in jungle or forest zones where gum and wood are exploited. Some cases have been described in the children and wives of agricultural workers who take their families to live with them in camps located in the zones where vectors exist.[58]

The most frequent clinical presentation of leishmaniasis is the so-called gummer ulcer, which is located asymmetrically mainly on the helix of ears, where the mosquito bites most often. A nodule appears and rapidly turns into an ulcer with purulence and well-demarcated and well-infiltrated borders. The disease then runs an asymptomatic and chronic course, enlarging and destroying the ear. Lesions on the ears do not heal spontaneously, in contrast to those on the nose, cheeks, and upper limbs, which tend to heal spontaneously[57] (Figure 81-17).

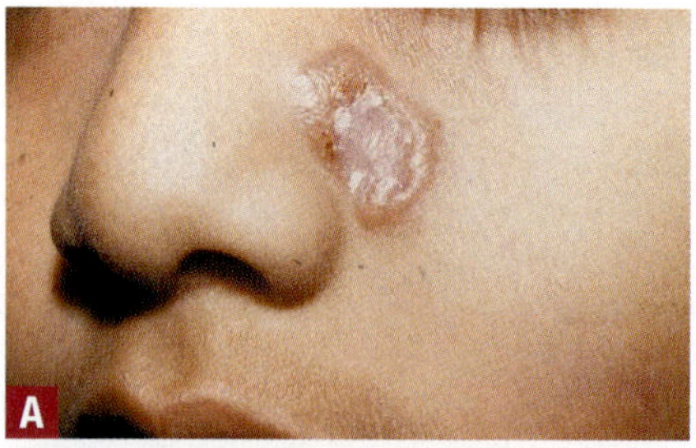

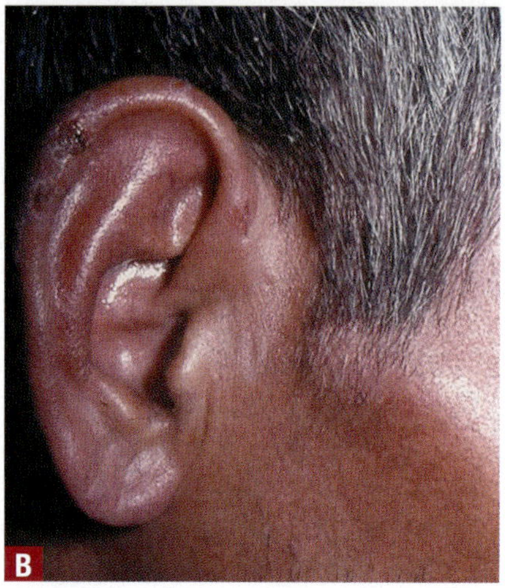

▲ **FIGURE 81-17** **A.** Leishmaniasis in the face. **B.** Gumma ulcer.

In hyperergic cases, leishmaniasis is very difficult to demonstrate on biopsy, occasionally being found as puntiform structures inside giant cells or macrophages in tuberculoid infiltrates. In these patients, Montenegro´s reaction, or *leishmanin,* is positive.

In Venezuela, a diffuse, anergic lepromatoid form of leishmaniasis that resembles a nodular lepromatous case has been described, and it also has been diagnosed in several patients in Mexico. These patients present with several disseminated ulcerated nodules affecting different parts of the body. Severe malaise is present. There is some controversy about these cases; some authors think that it is caused by a special kind of *Leishmania* called *L. pifanoi,* and others think that it is due to the immunologic status of the affected person.[57]

Intramuscular or intralesional pentavalent antimalarials are effective for treatment of leishmaniasis; chloroquin, ketoconazole, and itraconazole for 2–3 months also have been used with good results. The Mexican forms destroy the ear, which necessitates surgical reconstruction. The ulcers in other locations involute spontaneously after several months without treatment.[57]

CUTANEOUS LARVA MIGRANS

Cutaneous larva migrans is a disease caused by the larvae of nematodes that infect dogs and cats and occasionally can parasitize humans. It occurs frequently in tropical countries near the seashore or on riversides. The superficial form of cutaneous larva migrans is the most common and is caused by *Ancylostoma* larvae from *A. brasiliensis, A.caninum,* and *A. americanus.* The adult worm is a parasite in the gut of dogs and cats, and contaminated animal feces when deposited on the ground infects patients through bare skin. The larva penetrates the skin, often through hair follicles, and immediately digs a tunnel, attempting to reach the surface of the skin.

Cutaneous larva migrans occurs on the limbs and back, areas that commonly come into contact with infected sand. Lesions consist of linear "tracts" of different lengths that may assume a serpiginous form. Erythema, edema, and small vesicles may surround the lesions. Cutaneous larva migrans is an intensely pruritic disorder. Systemic symptoms do not occur because the larvae do not invade deeply. However, moderate eosinophilia may be observed[59,60] (Figure 81-18). Lesions resolve spontaneously once the larva dies, although the life span of the larva is several months.

The diagnosis of cutaneous larva migrans is made clinically. Histologic demonstration of larvae is very difficult because of constant migration. Oral treatment is effective and includes Iivermectin, 250 μg/kg in a single dose; albendazole, 400 mg in three doses; and thiabendazole. Preventative measures include wearing sandals and avoiding contact of bare skin with the sand in areas of disease prevalence.[59,60]

NONMELANOMA SKIN CANCER

Since 1998, the Mexican Histopathologic Registry of Malignant Neoplasm (NMSC) has reported that nonmelanoma skin cancer (NMSC), notably basal cell carcinoma (representing 70% of cases) and squamous cell carcinoma (representing 17% of cases), is the second most common malignant tumor after cervical-uterine cancer.[61,62] According to data published by Dr. Jorge Peniche of the Dermato-Oncology Unit, Hospital General de Mexico, the relationship of basal cell carcinoma to squamous cell carcinoma is 3–4:1. Analyzing a group of 2885 patients, basal cell carcinoma (BCC) occurred more frequently in women (2:1), and 80% of the patients were over 50 years of age. Most of the patients with BCC had signs of chronic sun exposure that was occupational (e.g., peasants, sailors, and salesmen). In this study, 88% of the BCCs were located on the face (i.e., nose 33.2%, eyelids 18.3%, cheek 14.7%, and frontal area 8.5%). Other locations included the torso, neck, scalp, and upper extremities.

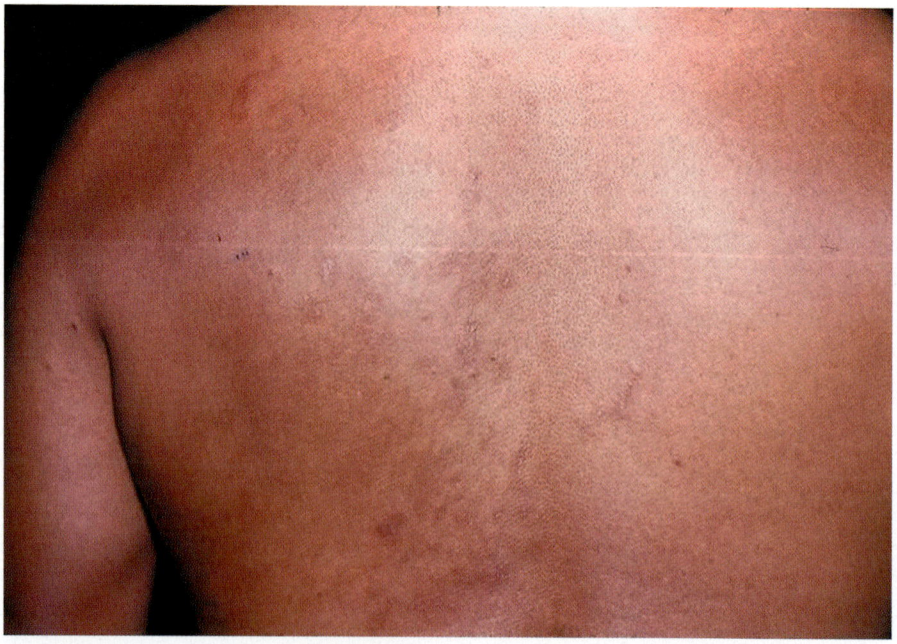

▲ **FIGURE 81-18** Cutaneous larva migrans, location on the back after sleeping in the sand.

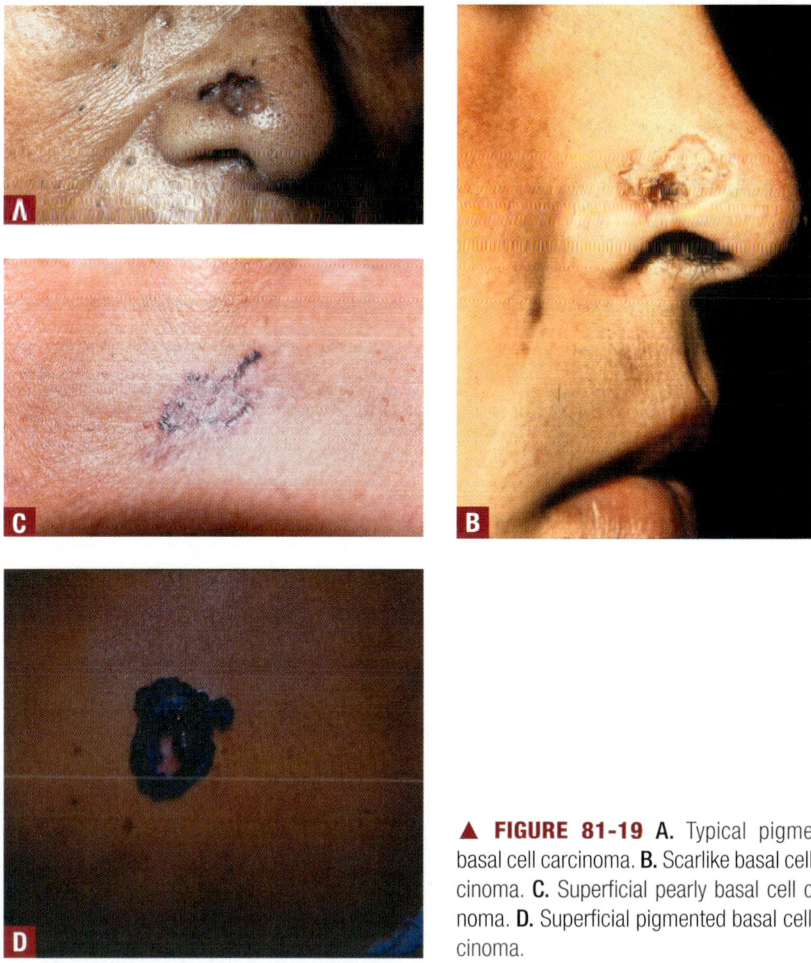

▲ **FIGURE 81-19** **A.** Typical pigmented basal cell carcinoma. **B.** Scarlike basal cell carcinoma. **C.** Superficial pearly basal cell carcinoma. **D.** Superficial pigmented basal cell carcinoma.

Clinically, the BCCs were classified as one of four types: exophytic (nodular and pseudocystic), flat (superficial or pagetoid, scleroatrophic with scarlike and morpheaform varieties), ulcerated (ulcerated and nodular-ulcerated variety), and pigmented. In this series, the predominant type was nodular (33%), followed by ulcerated (24%), flat scarlike (18%), and pigmented (15%). Nodular BCC presents as a smooth, elevated, firm, pearly translucent tumor with surface telangiectasias. Ulcerated BCC begins as an ulcerated lesion within infiltration and destruction of surrounding tissues. Scarlike BCC presents with flat, skin-colored, atrophic lesions limited by a pearly border. The pigmented subtype occurs relatively frequently in Mexico. Lesions may be nodular, flat, or ulcerated, although dark pigmentation always predominates[62] (Figure 81-19).

Histologically, BCCs consist of neoplastic, basaloid cells that derive from the epidermis or an adnexial structure. They are organized into lobules, islands, nests, or cords that display an orderly arrangement of the basaloid cell nuclei at their periphery termed a *palisading array*. In the dermis, there is stromal retraction or clefting around the neoplastic aggregates. Specific BCC histologic subtypes are recognized by their architectural pattern of tumor cell aggregates and the accompanying stromal reaction of the tumor.[63] In Mexico, the three most frequently observed histologic types are as follows: solid (33%), mixed solid-infiltrative (22%), infiltrative (8%), and pigmented (10%).

The diagnosis of BCC is made clinically, although histologic confirmation is essential. The differential diagnosis of BCC includes pigmented nevi, sebaceous hyperplasia, trichoepithelioma, and squamous cell carcinoma, to name a few. Treatment of this malignant neoplasm is selected according to the clinical and histologic type and age and health status of the patient. The standard of care for BCC is removal of the lesion via curettage, cryosurgery, simple excision, or Mohs surgery. Certain locations may necessitate treatment with radiation therapy. Recently, topical 5% imiquimod has been used for treatment of nodular or superficial BCC with good results after 16 weeks of treatment.[64]

In Mexico, squamous cell carcinoma (SCC) predominates in men in the 70-year age group, most of whom have a history of chronic and intense sun exposure. In addition to SCCs, actinic keratoses, solar lentigines, telangiectasias, and intense wrinkling may be present (Figure 81-20). In a series of 414 patients with SCC, 67.6% of the tumors were located on the face, 12% on the upper extremities, 8% on the lower extremities, 4.8% on the scalp, 3.6% in genital area, 2.1% on the torso, and 1.4% on the neck. Head lesions predominated, and of those located on the face, the cheeks, nose, and upper lip were the locations most often involved. Clinically, 36.4% of the SCCs were the ulcerated type, 25.8% nodular, 20.5% vegetant, 8.6% erythematous-squamous, and 8.4% hyperkeratotic.[61,65] Tumors located in mucosal areas were more aggressive than those in other locations (Figure 81-21).

Histologic features of SCCs include atypical cells that derive from the epidermis and spread to the dermis and nuclei that are enlarged and atypical. Mitotic activity is variable. Atypical mitotic figures and keratin pearls are present. Dyskeratotic and prematurely cornifying cells are seen. Inflammation is present in ulcerated forms. Perineural invasion should be documented.[66]

Treatment is individualized for each patient, including a complete physical examination, with evaluation of regional lymph nodes and a skin biopsy.

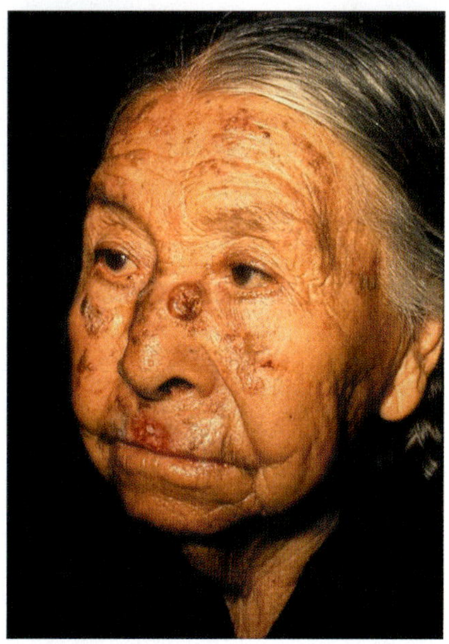

▲ **FIGURE 81-20** Chronic actinic damage.

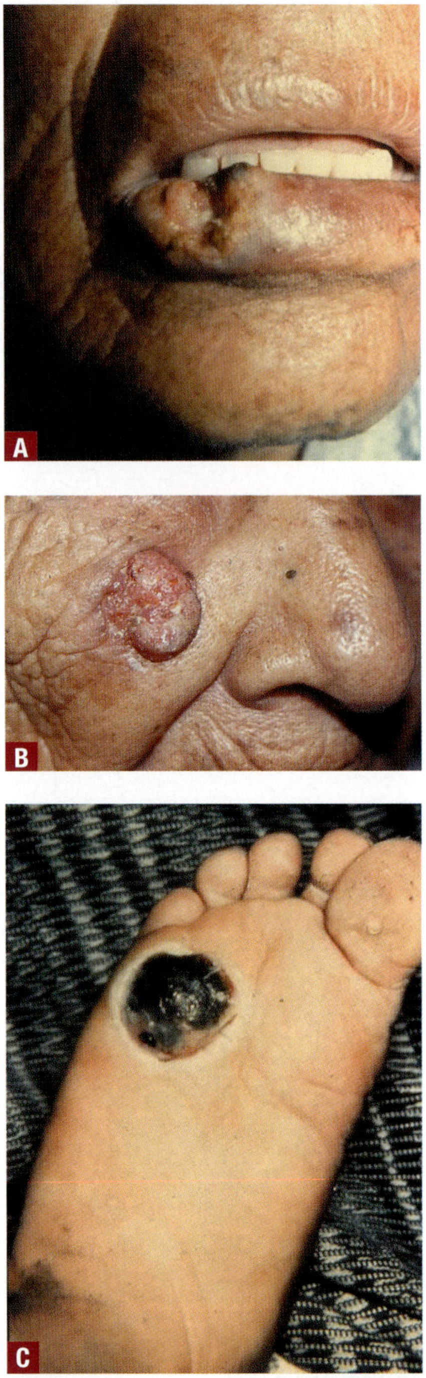

▲ **FIGURE 81-21** **A.** Squamous cell carcinoma of the lip. **B.** Squamous cell carcinoma of the cheek. **C.** Nodular distal melanoma of the sole.

The most common treatment modality for SCC is excisional surgery with margin assessment. For some lesions, radiation therapy is indicated. Cryosurgery or curettage in these tumors is not performed, and patients with clinically palpable lymph nodes are treated in conjunction with the oncologic surgeon. Patients with NMSC are followed yearly. Instruction regarding sun protection and early detection of new lesions is emphasized.

MALIGNANT MELANOMA

Although in some countries malignant melanoma (MM) is an important public health issue owing to the steady increase in incidence, the epidemiologic data in Mexico reveal a different situation. According to the data of the National Registry of Cancer and Histopathologic Registry of Malignant Neoplasia, the incidence of MM has remained at 1 per 100,000, with a mortality rate of 0.3 per 100,000.[62]

In Mexico, MM occurs slightly more often in women (58.4%). In 500 Mexican patients, MM was located as follows: 51.2% on the lower extremities, 15.8% on the head and neck, 14.8% on the upper extremities, 9.4% on mucosae, 7.6% on the torso, and 1.2% on the globe of the eye. Of the lesions located on the extremities, distal locations on the feet and hands predominated. These findings were consistent with series of patients in other hospitals in Mexico.[67–69] Nodular MM is the most frequent type of melanoma, representing 35% of the lesions in our series and 63% of the cases at the National Cancer Institute (INCan). Acral lentiginous melanoma is the second most common type of MM (30%), located on palms and soles and affecting subungual regions, primarily the first digit of the hands and feet. Of the less frequently seen forms of melanoma, superficial spreading MM represented 9% in our series and 15.6% in NCan's. Finally, lentigo maligna melanoma represented 5% in our series[67–72] (Figure 81-22).

Clinical characteristics of MM include an asymmetric pigmented lesion, often with irregular borders and pigmentation, that changes in a short period of time. Diagnosis is achieved via pathologic examination of incisional or excisional biopsy specimens. Patients are staged according to the TNM approved classification of 2001.[73] Successful treatment is surgical excision of early lesions. Unfortunately, most patients who seek medical consultation for MM have very advanced lesions, with in-transit metastasis present at diagnosis. Often patients have been misdiagnosed or initially treated inappropriately, thus necessitat-

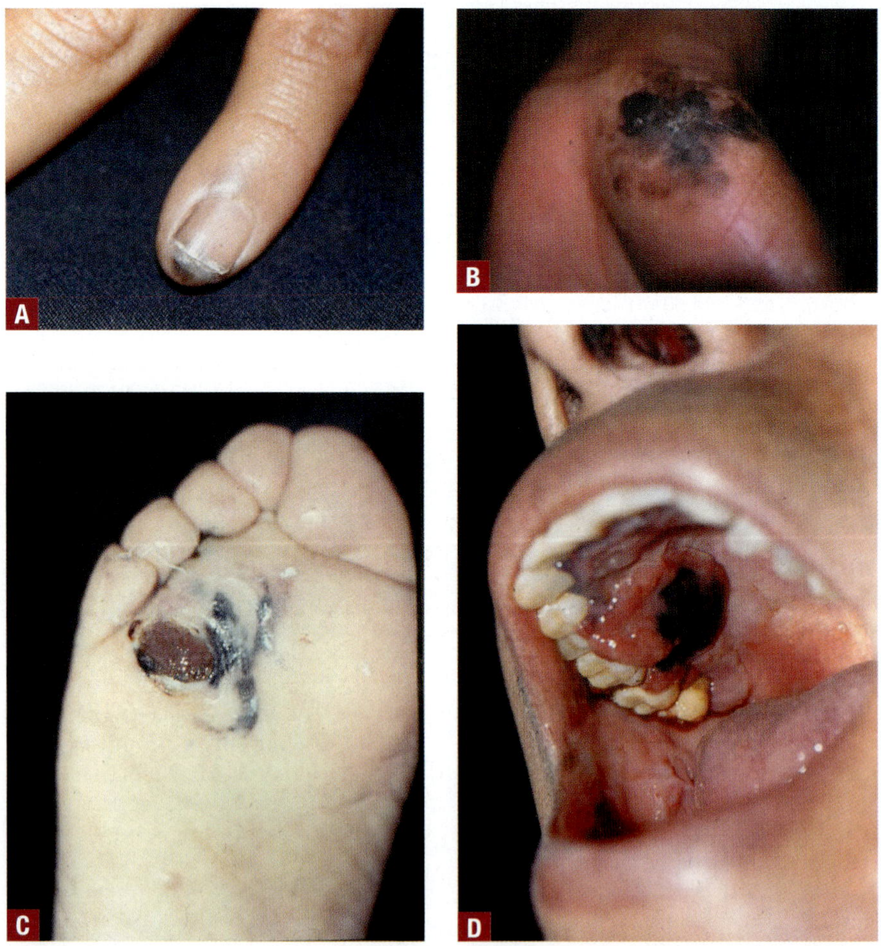

▲ **FIGURE 81-22** **A.** Acral lentiginous melanoma affecting the nail. **B.** Acral lentiginous melanoma distal palmar location. **C.** Acral advanced, ulcerated lentiginous melanoma. **D.** Mucosal oral melanoma.

ing referral to the oncology department. In Mexico, efforts are being made to assist patients in identifying and detecting suspicious pigmented lesions at early, treatable stages.

REFERENCES

1. Saúl A. *Lecciones de Dermatología.* Mexico City, Mendez Editores, 2001.
2. Hojyo-Tomoka T, Vega-Memije E, Granados J, et al. Actinic prurigo: An update. *Int J Dermatol* 1995;34:380.
3. Hojyo-Tomoka T, Granados J, Vargas-Alarcon G, et al. Further evidence of the role of HLA-DR4 in the genetic susceptibility to actinic prurigo. *J Am Acad Dermatol* 1997;36:935.
4. Dominguez-Cherit J, Vega-Memije E. Queilitis actínica: Estudio retrospectivo en 15 pacientes. *Dermatol Rev Mex* 1996; 40:27.
5. Arrese J, Domínguez-Soto L, Hojyo-Tomoka T, et al. Effectors of inflammation in actinic prurigo. *J Am Acad Dermatol* 2001;44:957.
6. Castañedo-Cazares, Moncada B, Lepe V, et al. Actinic prurigo. eMedicine Dermatology, 2004.
7. Moncada B, Baranda ML, González A, et al. Thalidomide effect on T-cell subsets as a possible mechanism of action. *Int J Lepr Other Mycobact Dis* 1985;53:201.
8. Ramírez CO, López L, Estado DG. Actual de la dermatosis cenicienta: Sinonimia-erytema discromicum perstans. *Med Cutan Ibero Lat Am* 1984; 12:11.
9. Schwartz R. Erythema dyschromicum perstans: The continuing enigma of Cinderella or ashy dermatosis. *Int J Dermatol* 2004;43:230.
10. Torres M, Castillo G. Amiloidosis queratinocitica pigmentada vs dermatitis cenicienta y pigmentación ideopática maculosa eruptiva. *Gaceta Dermatol Ecuator* 1999;2:1.
11. Vega ME, Waxtein L, Arenas R, et al. Ashy dermatosis versus lichen planus pigmentosus: A controversial matter. *Int J Dermatol* 1992;31:87.
12. Vega ME, Waxtein L, Arenas R, et al. Ashy dermatosis and lichen planus pigmentosus: A clincopathologic study of 31 cases. *Int J Dermatol* 1992;31:90.
13. Baranda L, Torres-Alvarez B, Cortes-Franco R, et al. Involvement of cell adhesion and activation molecules in the pathogenesis of erythema dyschromicum perstans (ashy dermatitis): The effects of clofazimine therapy. *Arch Dermatol* 1997; 133:325.
14. Saul A. La dermatología en los Paises Tropicales. *Dermatol Rev Mex* 1989;2:3.
15. Grimes P. Melasma: Etiologic and therapeutic considerations. *Arch Dermatol* 1995; 131:1453.
16. Im S, Hann S, Kang W. *New Concept of Melasma and Postinflammatory Hyperpigmentation.* Korea, 2002.
17. Katsambas A, Antoniou C. Melasma: Clasification and treament. *J Eur Acad Dermatol Venereol* 1995;4:217.
18. Gilchrest B, Fitzpatrick T, Anderson R, et al. Localization of melanin pigmentation in the skin with Wood's lamp. *Br J Dermatol* 1977;96:245.
19. Mosher D, Fitzpatrick T, Ortonne J-P, Hori Y. Hipomelanosis e hipermelanosis, in Fitzpatrick TB, et al (eds), *Dermatology in General Medicine.* Mexico City, Editorial Medica Panamericana, 2001, p 1045.
20. Piamphongsant T. Treatment of melasma: A review with personal experience. *Int J Dermatol* 1998;37:897.
21. Taylor SC, et al. Efficacy and safety of a new triple combination agent for the treatment of facial melasma. *Cutis* 2003; 72:67.
22. Kang WH, Chun SC, Lee S. Intermittent therapy for melasma in Asian patients with combined topical agents: Clinical and histological studies. *J Dermatol* 1998; 25:587.
23. Balkirshnan R, Kelly AP, McMichael A, et al. Improved quality of life with effective treatment of facial melasma: The Pigment Trial. *J Drugs Dermatol* 2004; 3:377.
24. Bonifaz A. *Micología Médica Básica.* Mexico, City, Mendez Editores, 2000.
25. Velasco O, González-Ochoa A. Tiña imbricata en la Sierra de Puebla, México. *Rev Inv Salud Pub* 1975;35:109.
26. Hay RJ. Tinea imbricata: The factors affecting persistence. *Int J Dermatol* 1985; 24:562.
27. Ravine D. Genetic inheritance of susceptibility to tinea imbricata. *J Med Genet* 1980;17:342.
28. Saúl A. Tiña imbricata: Recidiva después del tratamiento con griseofulvina. *Dermatol Rev Mex* 1962;5:2.
29. Bout G, Lavalle P, Mariat F, et al. Etude épidémiologique de Mycétome au Mexique: A propos de 502 cases. *Bull Soc Pathol Exp* 1987;80:329.
30. Lavalle P. Nuevos datos sobre la epidemiología del Micetoma en México. *Gac Med Mex* 1996;96:545.
31. Maghoub ES, Murra IG. *Mycetoma.* London, Heinemann Medical Books, 1973.
32. Novales J. Contribución de la dermatopatología al conocimiento de los micetomas. *Med Cu ILA* 1995;23:248.
33. Welsh O. Current concepts in treatment of mycetoma. *Int J Dermatol* 1991;30:387.
34. Gomez TA, Saul A, Bonifaz A. Amoxacilin and clavulanic acid in the treatment of actinomycetoma. *Int J Dermatol* 1993;32:218.
35. Gonzalez-Benavides J. La esporotricosis enfermedad ocupacional de los alfareros. *Rev Hosp Univ Monterrey Mexico* 1952; 2:215.
36. Jaramillo O. Esporotricosis: Aspectos clínicos y epidemiológicos en México y Costa Rica. Thesis, Universidad Nacional Autónoma de México, México City, 1964.
37. Lavalle P, Mariat F. Sporotrichosis. *Bull Inst Pasteur* 1983;81:295.
38. González-Ochoa A, Soto-Figueroa E. Polisacáridos de S. Schenkii. Intradermorreacción para el diagnóstico de esporotricosis. *Rev Inst Enf Tropicales Mex* 1947;8:143.
39. Saul A. Sporotrichosis, in Jacobs PH, Nail L (eds), *Antifungal Drug Therapy.* New York, Marcel Dekker, 1990.
40. Fair S. Tuberculosis in the world today. JAAPA, May 2003.
41. Garcia-Garcia L, Valdespino-Gomez J, García-Sancho C, et al. *Mycobacterium tuberculosis* infection in HIV-infected subjects using reactivity to tuberculin and anergy panel. *Int J Epidemol* 2000;29:369-375.
42. Saul A. La tuberculosis ayer y hoy. *Dermatol Rev Mex* 1996;40:249-250.
43. Arenas R. *Dermatología: Atlas, diagnóstico y tratamiento.* México City, McGraw Hill, 1987, pp 345-350.
44. Villa B, Estrella P, Franco A, et al. Tuberculosis verrugosa: Comunicación de tres casos. *Rev Cent Dermatol Pascua* 1998;7:143-147.
45. Rodríguez M, Aguilera V. Tuberculosis cutánea verrugosa: Presentación de un caso. *Rev Cent Dermatol Pascua* 2003;12: 71-74.
46. Nachbar F, Cassen V, Nachbar T, et al. Orificial tuberculosis: Detection by polimerase chain reaction. *Br J Dermatol* 1996;135:106-109.
47. Cabrera E, Cancela R. Tuberculosis nodular profunda: Reporte de un caso. *Rev Cent Dermatol Pascua* 1998;6:45-47.
48. Jurado F, Pérez J, Novales J, et al. Tuberculosis cutánea: Tb nodulo necrótica. *Rev Centro Dermatol Pascua* 1992;1:65-66.
49. Fuentes P, Hernández B, Jimenez H, et al. Tuberculide micronodular: Comentarios a propósitos de los casos. *Rev Cent Dermatol Pascua* 1998;7138-142.
50. Lopez-Cepeda D, Beirana A. Diagnóstico de tuberculosis: Revisión del tema. *Rev Cent Dermatol Pascua* 1999;8:130-132.
51. Chan Y, Yosipovitch G. Suggested guidelines for screening and management of tuberculosis in patients taking oral glucocorticoid: An important but often neglected issue. *J Am Acad Dermatol* 2003; 49:91-95.
52. Margall N, Basega E, Coll P. Detection of *Mycobacterium tuberculosis* complex DNA by the polymerase chain reaction for rapid diagnosis of cutaneous tuberculosis. *Br J Dermatol* 1996;135:231-236.
53. Senturk N, Sedef S, Kocagoz T. Polymerase chain reation in cutaneous tuberculosis: Is it a reliable diagnostic method in paraffin-embedded tissues? *Int J Dermatol* 2002;41:863-866.
54. Joplin WH. *Handbook of Leprosy.* London, Heinmann, 1978.
55. Languillon J. Précis de Leprologie. *Acta Leprologica,* 1999.
56. Terencio de las Aguas J. *Lecciones de Leprología.* Fontilles, 1999.
57. Kerdel Vega F. American leishmaniasis, in Cañizares O (ed), *Clinical Tropical Dermatology.* Oxford, England, Blackwell Scientific, 1975.
58. Canizares O. Epidemiology of dermatosis in Latin America, in Marshall J (ed), *Essays on Tropical Dermatology.* Amsterdam, Excerpta Medica, 1972.
59. Canizares O. *Clinical Tropical Dermatology.* Oxford, England, Blackwell Scientific, 1975.
60. Stone OJ, Mullins JF. Thiabendazol. *Arch Dermatol* 1965;95:427.
61. Peniche J. Tumores de la Piel, in Saul A (ed), *Lecciones de Dermatologia.* México City, Mendez Editores, 2001, p 650.
62. Registro Histopatológico de Neoplasias en México, DGE, Secretaria de Salud, 1998.
63. Miller S, Moresi JM. Actinic keratosis, basal cell carcinoma and squamous cell carcinoma, in Bologna J, Jorisso J, Rapini

R (eds), *Dermatology*, Vol 2. St Louis, MO, Mosby, 2003, p 1677.
64. Peniche J. *Carcinoma Basocelular in Oncología Cutánea: PAC-Dermatología.* Mexico City, Intersistemas, 2000, p 32.
65. Peniche A. *Carcinoma epidermoide in Oncología Cutánea: PAC-Dermatología.* Mexico City, Intersistemas, 2000, pp 40-47.
66. Boyd A. Tumors of the epidermis, in Barnhill R (ed), *Textbook of Dermatopathology.* New York, McGraw-Hill, 1998, p 522.
67. Peniche J, Arellano I. *Melanoma Maligno in Oncología Cutánea: PAC-Dermatología.* Mexico City, Intersistemas, 2000, pp 48-56.
68. Alfeiran A, Escobar G, De la Barreda F, et al. Epidemiología del melanoma de piel en México. *Rev Inst Nacional Cancerolog* 1998;44:168.
69. Arellano I, Peniche J. Melanoma maligno: Estudio epidemiológico de 214 casos observados en el Hospital General de México en los años 1975-1985. Postgraduate thesis, Hospital General de México, 1989.
70. De la Barreda F, Alfeiran A, Escobar G. Melanoma cutáneo. *Rev Inst Nacional Cancerolog* 1998;44:201.
71. Gonzalez J, Mora A, Beltrán A. 261 casos de melanoma cutáneo: Características generales y factores de valor pronóstico. *Rev Inst Nacional Cancerolog* 1990;36: 1103.
72. Pineda J, Peniche J, Leon G. Factores de riesgo en el melanoma acral lentiginoso: Estudio de casos y controles (1987-1996). Postgraduate thesis, Hospital General de México, 1997.
73. Balch CM, Buzaid, Soong SJ. Final version of the American Joint Committee on Cancer staging for cutaneous melanoma. *J Clin Oncol* 2001;19: 3635-3648.

CHAPTER 82

Common Skin Diseases and Treatments in Latin America: Brazil

Marcia Ramos-e-Silva
Gabriela Munhoz-da-Fontoura
Dóris Hexsel

Key Points

- Indigenous Indians, Portuguese, and Africans were the three primary groups that formed the Brazilian population.
- Currently, Brazil has an ethnically diverse population composed of Indians; blacks; descendants of Europeans from Portugal, France, Spain, Holland, Italy, and Germany; and descendants of Asians from Japan and Korea.
- Brazil is presently the country with the largest black population outside of Africa.
- The Brazilian black and Mestizo populations experience cutaneous disorders similar to those of individuals of African descent throughout the world.
- Typical skin disorders include dyschromias, tropical infectious diseases, hair disorders, scarring, and skin cancer.

Brazil is a country known for its natural beauty, as well as for its diversity of ethnicities. Black skin in Brazil has the same characteristics as in other parts of the world, and therefore, data found in the literature may be applied here. About 6% of the current population belongs to the black race, according to the Brazilian Institute of Geography and Statistics, with a very large percentage of Mestizos, whose skin behaves similar to black skin. Indians, Portuguese, and Africans were the three primary groups that formed the Brazilian population; however, it is difficult to identify an ethnicity whose genetic heritage is not represented in the DNA of Brazilians. Brazilian geneticists and pharmacologists anticipate high hopes using pharmacogenomics as an instrument for improving treatment of many diseases; in this case, focus should be on the individual and not on skin color.[1] In Brazil, miscegenation and cultural "transfusions" have shaped the population, as well as the virtually insurmountable social barriers imposed by slavery. "Brazil's body is in America, but its soul is in Africa" (Father Antonio Vieira, seventeenth century).[2]

Brazil, discovered officially in 1500 by the Portuguese, had a population made up of countless indigenous tribes. The native population was small and dispersed as compared with the "Spanish America," where Mayas, Incas, and Aztecs had well-organized socioeconomic societies. The first contact of Brazil's indigenous Indian population with whites was friendly, but this relationship deteriorated rapidly with the onset of the colonization process and ultimately resulted in slavery. Ethnic cleansing, whether by diseases introduced by the Europeans (e.g., smallpox, grippe, sexually transmitted diseases, etc.), hunger, or cultural marginalization, occurred. The Indian population was forced to abandon its culture and religion and to adopt Christianity. As a result of these factors, the native population, estimated at 10 million in 1500, was reduced to the current 200,000.[3]

After 1550, the Europeans transported blacks from Africa to Brazil as part of the slave trade. It is uncertain how many actually arrived at Brazilian ports, but estimates range from 3 to 18 million. Owing to the number of African slaves who arrived in Brazil, coupled with widespread miscegenation, Brazil is presently the country with the largest black population outside of Africa. The black slaves who arrived in Brazil had common characteristics: dark skin and eyes and very curled hair. The genetic blood diseases of some African populations resulted in a high incidence of hematologic disorders (e.g., falciform anemia), as well as other blood disorders possibly related to malaria resistance. Additionally, blacks were victims of unfavorable conditions in Brazil, including poor socioeconomic conditions, exposure to chronic and fatal disease, poor housing, lack of education, and malnutrition. Mortality rates were very high even during their transportation from Africa to Brazil, when only the fittest survived; fortunately, those conditions improved gradually with the end of slavery in 1888.

In the nineteenth and twentieth centuries, a great influx of immigrants from diverse regions of the world occurred. As a consequence, Brazil now is ethnically diverse, with a population composed of Indians, blacks, and descendants of Europeans, especially Portuguese but also French, Spanish, Dutch, Italian, Japanese, German, Arab, Slovak, Korean, among many other groups. Thus 500 years after the discovery of Brazil, immense ethnic and cultural variety prevails, which is reflected in the many skin hues and cultural identities of its people.

The Brazilian black and Mestizo populations experience cutaneous problems specific to the black race, and often diseases or skin lesions assume different characteristics from those found in the skin of white individuals. We will discuss some of the problems that commonly affect this important segment of the Brazilian population.[2,4]

HYPERTROPHIC SCARS AND KELOIDS

Keloids are a very frequent problem in Brazil owing to the large black and miscegenated population.[5,6,7] Both keloidal and hypertrophic scarring occur equally in men and women in Brazil as a result of trauma, burns, surgical excision, vaccination. and/or acne.[6] Young blacks and Mestizos are more prone to this type of scar development, often presenting with keloids in the presternal region.[8] These scars also can be observed among the Asian population, but they are uncommon in Brazilian whites. Patients seek treatment to relieve pain, itching, and restriction to movement, but the aesthetic aspect is invariably the most important factor.[9,7]

Keloids are firm, elevated lesions presenting shiny, often flat, uniform surfaces, sometimes with a hypochromic aspect. Lesions can be pedunculated or sessile depending on the location. In blacks, keloids may reach large dimensions. Some keloids present more clinical activity than others. Among the most resistant to treatment are those with a tendency to show prolongations with peripheral extensions in the form of a claw or a dumbbell.

Familial predisposition occurs, especially in cases of multiple lesions. They have been reported to be more common in individuals with blood type A, and the familial predisposition seems to be related to gene histocompatibility. Prevention is fundamentally important in patients with a history of keloid formation.

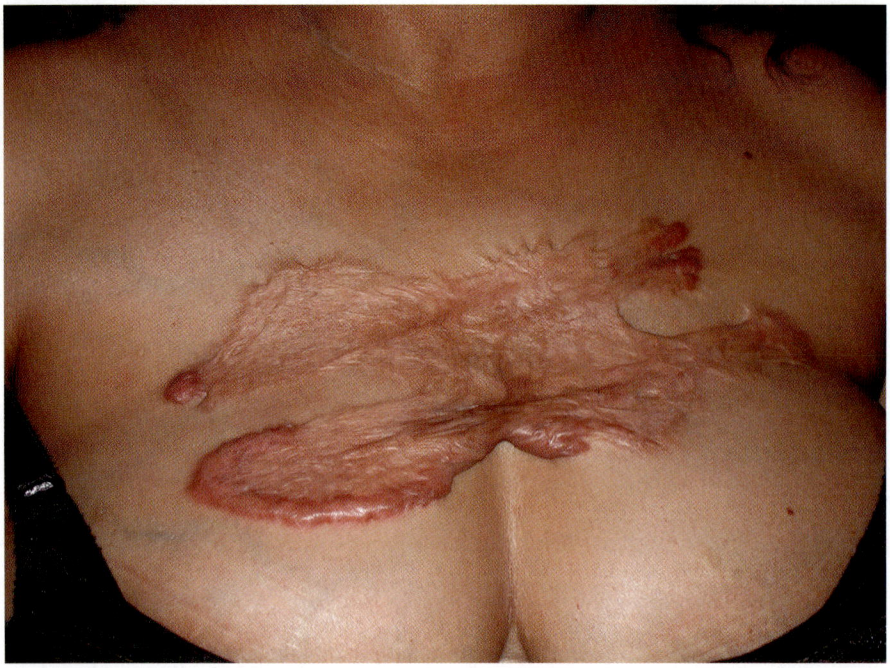

▲ **FIGURE 82-1** Keloids.

Keloids and hypertrophic scars represent abnormal scar formation with excessive production of extracellular matrix materials and high rates of division of dermal fibroblasts[5] (Figures 82-1 and 82-2). It is felt that tension plays an important role in scar formation owing to trauma. Keloids are the result of an imbalance between fibroblast proliferation and production and extracellular matrix degradation.

DRY SKIN

Dry skin, or xerosis, is a skin condition caused by a reduction of the lipid mantle that constitutes the barrier of the stratum corneum, which results in an increase in cutaneous water loss[10–12] (Figures 82-3 and 82-4). Dry skin presents with scaling and a loss of corneocyte flexibility and elasticity, with cracking, fissuring, itching, and formation of other lesions.[13] Dry, fragile skin is more common in the elderly, most likely owing to a reduction of sebum production and the diminished functioning of the cutaneous appendices.[14,15]

In Brazil, xerosis occurs in individuals of both sexes regardless of age and is a frequent complaint among blacks. In this population, especially when xerosis occurs on the lower limbs and face, the skin becomes grayish (ashy skin) owing to the dryness. Often the use of inappropriate emollients and moisturizers, oils, and comedogenic products, as well as inadequate bathing habits, worsens this skin condition and precipitates allergies and acneiform eruptions, among other disorders.

Dry skin may be constitutional or acquired. Constitutional, or intrinsic, dry skin is genetically determined or, alternatively, may be related to disorders such as atopic dermatitis,[16–18] hypothyroidism,[19,20] hypoparathyroidism,[21] uncontrolled diabetes, and renal disease,[12] among others. Acquired xerosis occurs as a result of external factors such as climate, pollution, exposure to chemical products that dissolve the lipidic mantle, and exposure to hot water or air conditioning, among others. In Brazil, complaints about dry skin among blacks are very frequent, and in most, the xerosis is either constitutional or related to systemic disorders. External factors worsen xerosis, and in Brazil, climatic factors are frequently involved.

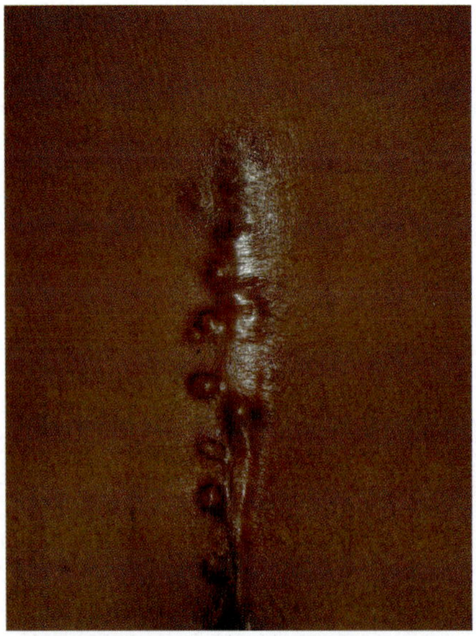

▲ **FIGURE 82-2** Hypertrophic scar.

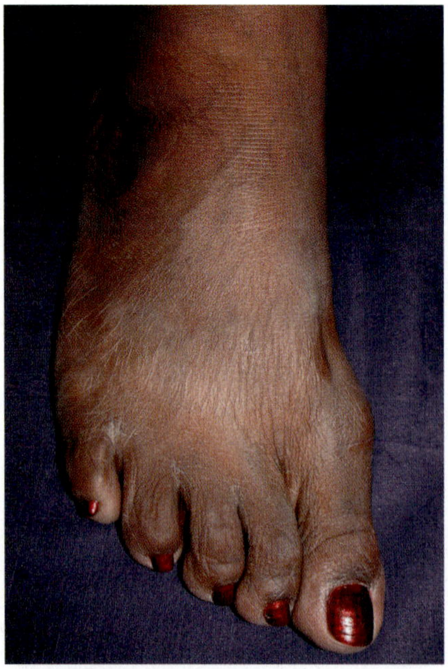

▲ **FIGURE 82-3** Xerosis.

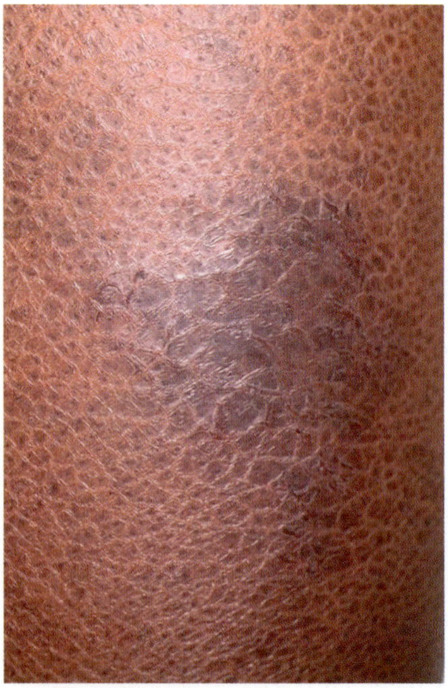

▲ **FIGURE 82-4** Xerosis.

DYSCHROMIA

Dyschromias in black skin may be classified as melanotic (with a melanocytic component) and nonmelanotic (of other origin). Melanotic dyschromia may be subdivided into hyperpigmentation and hypopigmentation. Hyperpigmentation may be caused by natural factors (linked to the race), primary factors (acquired hyperpigmentation, idiopathic, or familial), and secondary factors (a postinflammatory process).[22–25]

Examples of natural hyperpigmentation of black skin include hyperpigmentation of the oral mucosa (which often can be confused with diseases that cause areas of dark pigmentation),[26] palmoplantar hyperpigmentation, melanonychia striata, Mongolian spots (observed in 40–90% of newborns), and dermatosis papulosa nigra (extremely common in Brazil). The main type of primary hyperpigmenation is melasma, which is discussed below. Secondary hyperpigmentation may be caused by trauma, allergy, acne vulgaris, eczema, psoriasis, pytiriasis rosea, lichen planus, seborrheic dermatitis, atopic dermatitis, keratosis pilaris, intertiginous mycoses, and topical or systemic medications, among others, all of which may lead to postinflammatory hyper-pigmentation.

Black skin can be affected by natural hypopigmentation, such as the hypochromic mask in the middle of the face, the hypochromic triangle of the trapeze, and hypopigmentation of the median line. Primary hypopigmentation examples are vitiligo (very common in Brazil), albinism, hypopigmented sarcoidosis (almost exclusively in blacks), achromatic pityriasis versicolor, pityriasis alba, hypochromic fungal mycosis, and idiopathic guttate hypomelanosis (common in blacks living in tropical countries).

Examples of secondary hypochromia include iatrogenic hypochromia and hypochromia caused by face makeup (owing to the presence of depigmenting agents). Among the examples of nonmelanotic dischromias are angiomas, varicosities and telangiectasia, tattoos, and hemosiderotic deposits.[25]

Dyschromias occur quite frequently in the black population of Brazil, and most of the disorders of hyperpigmentation become even darker with the intense, year-round sun exposure, whereas the disorders characterized by hypochromia or achromia often result in serious sunburns.

Melasma

Melasma is a commonly occurring chronic, symmetric facial hyperpigmentation that manifests as irregularly shaped brownish patches on the skin[27,28] (Figure 82-5). It occurs on areas exposed to sunlight, particularly the face, with involvement of the upper lip, nose, cheeks, chin, and forehead being most common.[29–31] Extrafacial melasma is a little-described entity, typically affecting postmenopausal women, 40 years of age and older, using hormonal replacement.[32–35]

The factors responsible for melasma are not yet completely clarified, but they almost always appear as a result of and are aggravated by exposure to sun light.[36,37] In addition to ultraviolet (UV) light, genetic and hormonal factors also may be involved. Other causes of melasma are pregnancy[38,39] and use of oral contraceptives[40] and other medications.[29–31] Women with darker skin types (Fitzpatrick phototypes III–VI) are more often affected.

In Brazil and in other South American countries, there is racial miscegenation with a resulting high prevalence of darker phototypes. In most of the Latin American countries, exposure to sunlight occurs during the entire year owing either to employment (e.g., farming) or to leisure activities. Furthermore, culturally, a tan is considered to be healthy and beautiful by most of the population. These reasons explain the high incidence of melasma in tropical regions.[31]

Postinflammatory Hyperpigmentation

Postinflammatory hyperpigmentation (PIH) is the most frequent form of residual hyperpigmentation, being a consequence of increased melanin synthesis in response to an inflammatory processes[30] (Figure 82-6). In PIH, a localized increase of skin color occurs in areas affected by physiologic or pathologic processes. It occurs more frequently

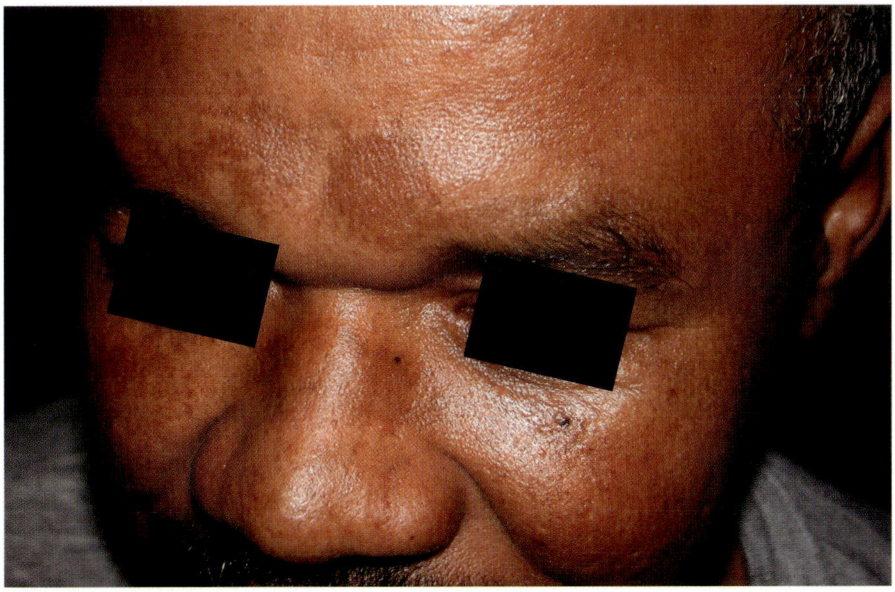

▲ **FIGURE 82-5** Melasma.

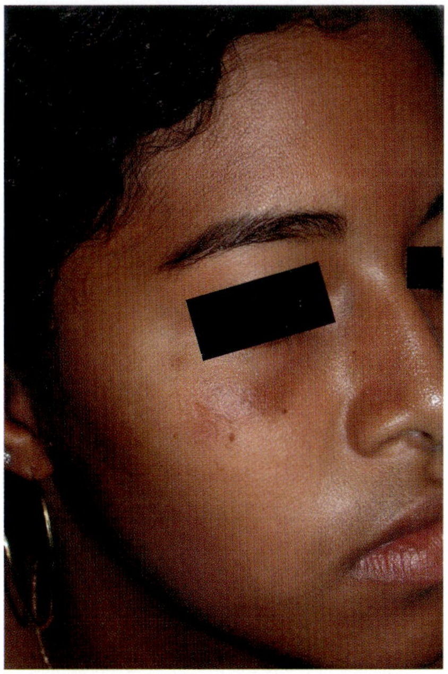

▲ **FIGURE 82-6** Postinflammatory hyperpigmentation.

in patients with Fitzpatrick skin phototypes III–VI.[41]

PIH may appear as a result of a myriad of disease, including but not limited to eczema, contact dermatitis, acne, pseudofolliculitis barbae, and insect bites.[42] It also occurs after allergic processes induced by chemicals or other external agents, as well as after surgical procedures such as chemical peels, cryotherapy, and laser therapy.

TRACTION ALOPECIA

Traction alopecia is very common in Brazilian black and Mestizo women who wear hairstyles that unduly pull the hairs, causing hair traction. Alopecia is more common in the temporal region or in scalp margins, called *marginal alopecia* (Figure 82-7).

Also recognized are the cosmetic-induced alopecias, which may be caused by vigorous brushing, straightening by application of heat, excessive massage, and processes that make the hair curly.[43] In addition, in Brazil it is very common to use chemical products such as phorbal, to straighten curly hair almost indiscriminately.

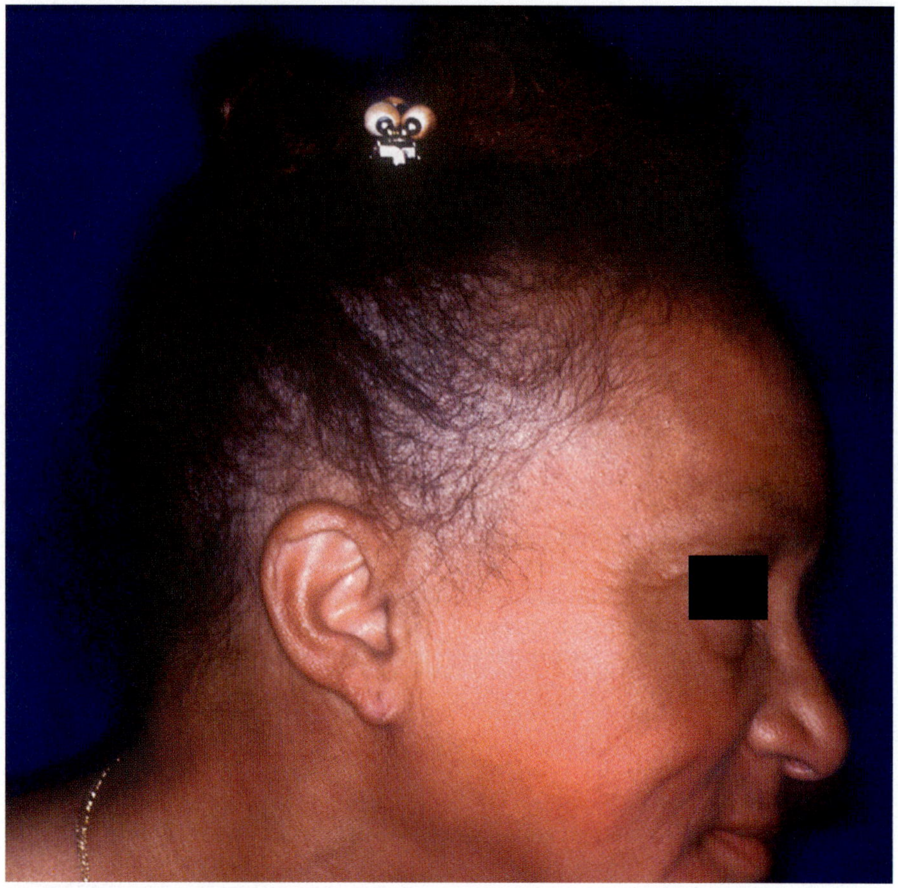

▲ **FIGURE 82-7** Traction alopecia.

PSEUDOFOLLICULITIS OF THE BEARD AND GROIN

Pseudofolliculitis of the beard occurs in blacks and Mestizos who shave frequently and who have curly hair (Figure 82-8). The hair penetrates the skin, leading to folliculitis. Since the hair in whites is not as curly, pseudofolliculitis is infrequent among them.

In recent years, pseudofolliculitis has been observed in the inguinal area of women and also occasionally on the thighs and legs. This is due to the use of ever-shorter bathing suits on Brazilian beaches, necessitating hair removal in these areas, a widespread practice among Brazilian women. To avoid this condition, more permanent methods of hair removal such as lasers are increasingly in demand.

TROPICAL DISEASES

Scabies

Scabies, a common disease in developing countries, mainly among the poorer populations, is caused by *Sarcoptes scabiei*. It is transmitted through personal contact without preference for age, sex, or race.[44,45] In blacks, it often becomes a diagnostic challenge because the classic erythematous papules are hardly visible, and the diagnosis then is based on intense itching. Itching occurs primarily at night and often involves other family members. In Brazil, scabies occurs commonly in the setting of shelters, day-care centers, prisons, and other environments with poor hygiene.

Syphilis

Syphilis is a contagious venereal treponemal disease that has systemic and cutaneous manifestations. Syphilis, caused by *Treponema pallidum,* occurs frequently in Brazil without preference

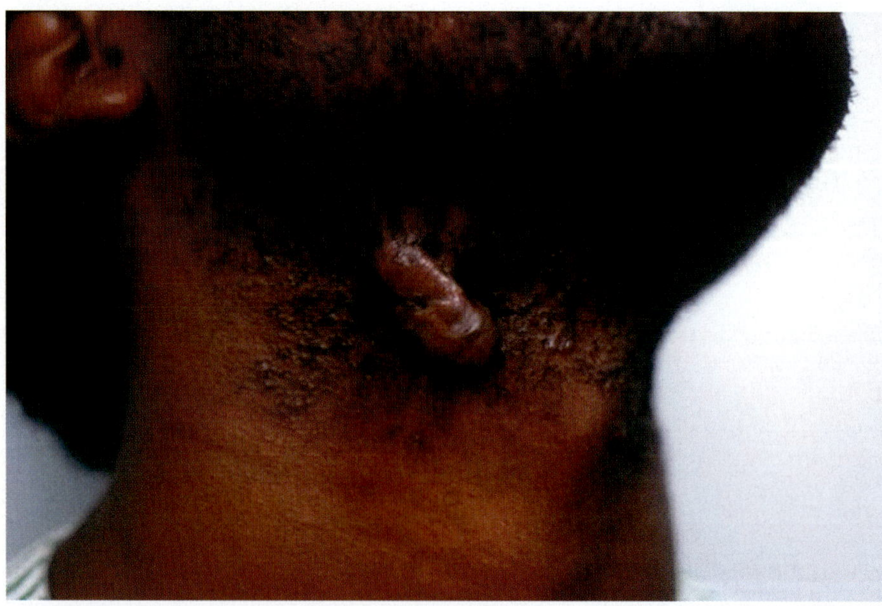

▲ **FIGURE 82-8** Pseudofolliculitis of the beard and keloid.

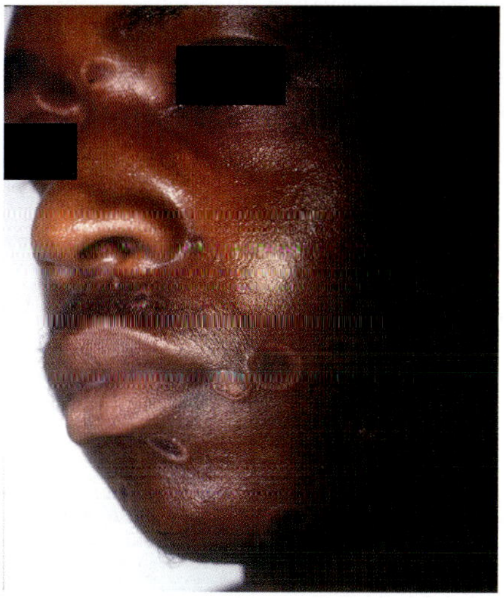

▲ **FIGURE 82-9** Elegant syphilides.

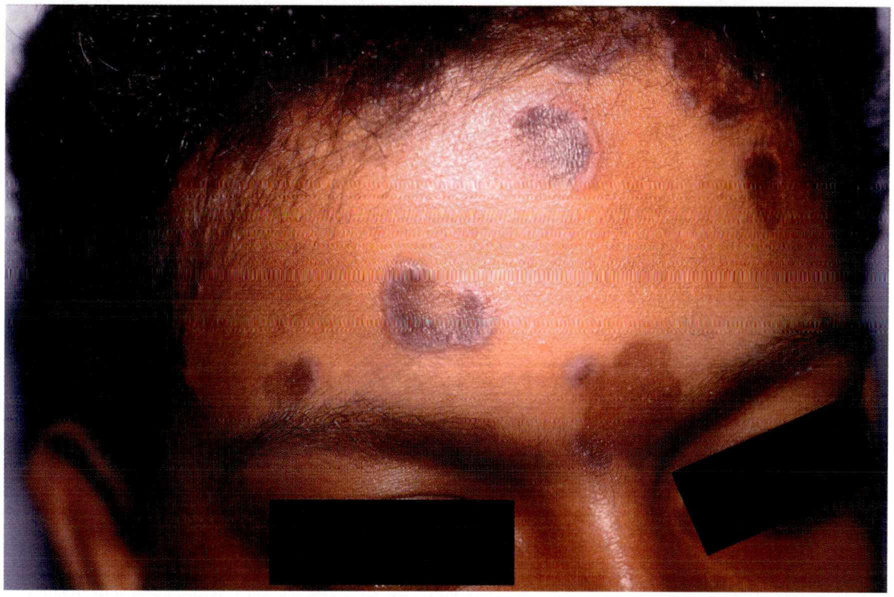

▲ **FIGURE 82-10** Elegant syphilides.

for race or sex. The disease can be congenital or acquired through sexual contact or transfusions and develops in phases (i.e., recent and late or primary, secondary, and tertiary). The secondary phase, with onset 2–3 months after infection, is characterized by a generalized monomorphous eruption of small lesions, called *syphilides*. In this asymptomatic phase, polyadenopathy, muscular pain, and fever may occur. Additionally, patients may present with migraine headaches, pharyngitis, palmarplantar lesions, and later, alopecia areata, madarosis, and paronychia. In black patients, cutaneous lesions may be circinate or have a ring configuration or even assume geometric forms called *elegant syphilides* (Figures 82-9 and 82-10).

Pityriasis Versicolor

Pityriasis versicolor is a superficial mycosis caused by *Malassezia furfur*. Asymptomatic, of universal distribution, and found more frequently in countries with hot and humid tropical climates, such as Brazil, it affects both genders from childhood to old age, with predominance in young adults. The disorder is evidenced, in general after solar exposure, and in Brazil, for this reason, it is known popularly as "beach mycosis." Pityriasis versicolor presents with various shades or hues from white to brown and is the reason the disorder is called *versicolor*. In individuals with white skin, brown, erythematous or hypochromic macules are frequently observed, whereas in dark or black skin, the lesions are, in general, hypochromic and often less visible. This makes the diagnosis more difficult in this population and often leads to involvement of the fungus over large areas of the skin.

Tinea

Dermatophytosis is caused by a group of keratinophylic fungi called *dermatophytes* that infects skin, hair, nails, and mucous membranes. In Brazil, the term *tinea* is used frequently. More common in summer and autumn, its distribution is influenced by geographic and population factors. The name varies according to the area of the body affected: Tinea capitis (scalp) *tinea cruris* (groin), *tinea corporis* (body), and *tinea pedis* (foot). Tinea corporis, very common in Brazil, can involve large areas if it is not diagnosed and treated (Figure 82-11).

MELANOMA AND OTHER SKIN CANCERS

In Brazil, melanoma incidence is estimated at approximately 4 cases per

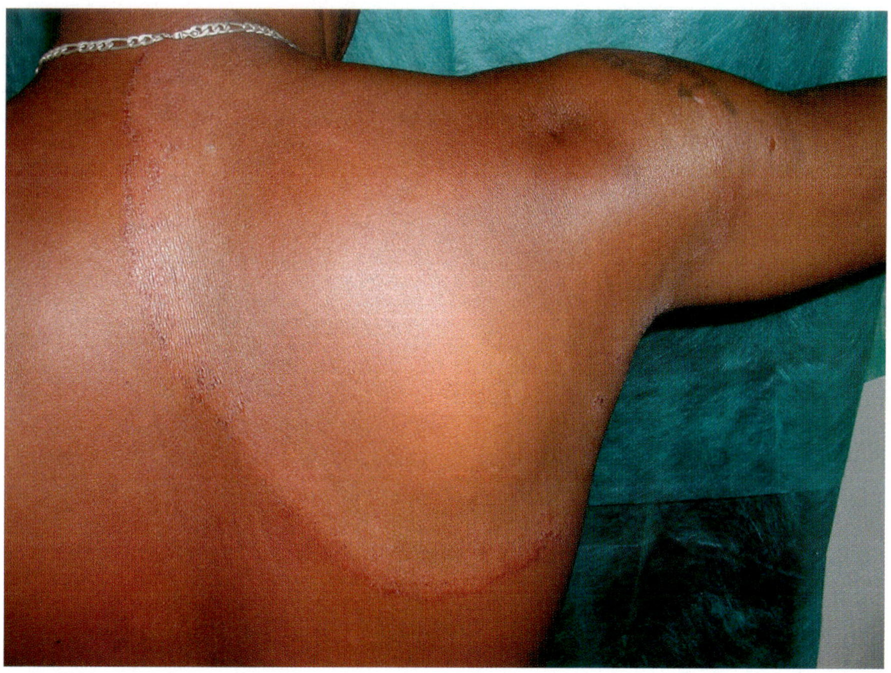

▲ **FIGURE 82-11** Tinea corporis.

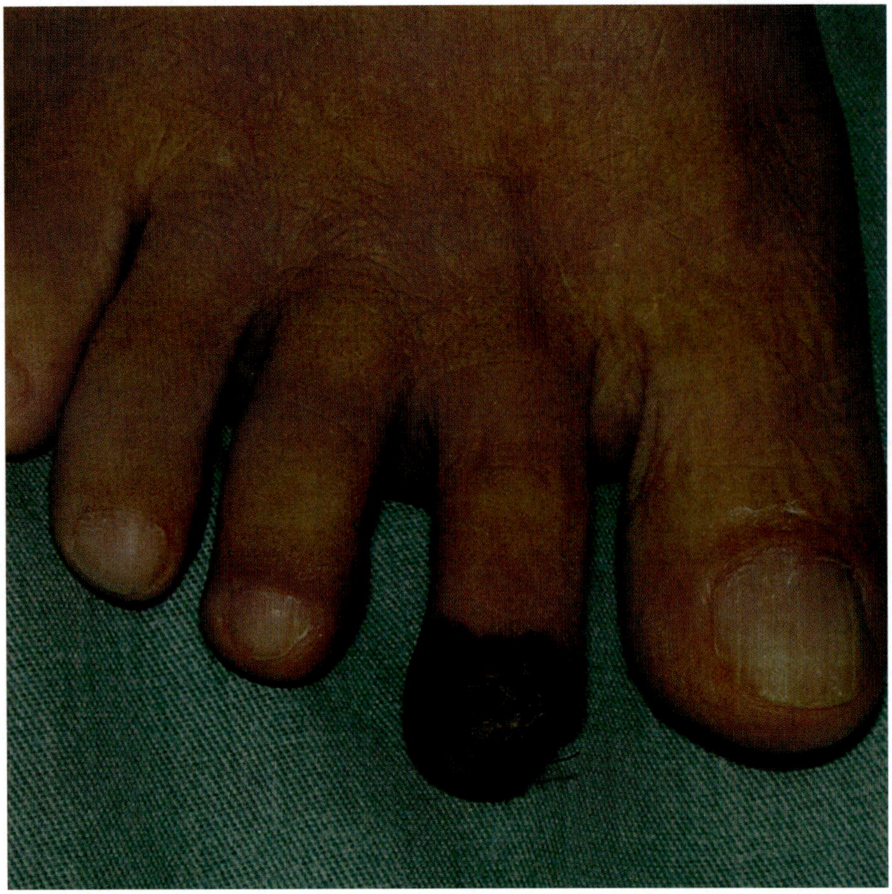

▲ **FIGURE 82-12** Melanoma.

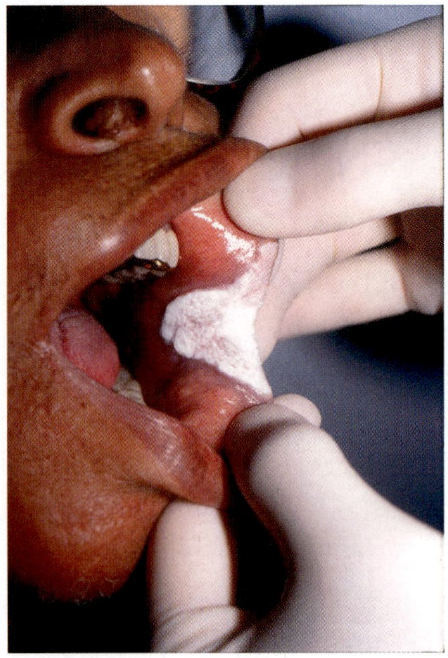

▲ **FIGURE 82-14** Squamous cell carcinoma.

100,000 inhabitants. It has increased 30% from 1978–1991. Brazilian patients who seek public health services for the treatment of melanoma often present with advanced disease (vertical growth phase) or metastases. A study of patient demographics performed in 2002 demonstrated that in public hospitals, significantly more patients were nonwhite, of older age, and had a high percentage of acrolentiginous melanoma, in contrast to those from private clinics, which had a predominance of white patients who were younger and who had a low percentage of acrolentiginous melanoma.

In November 2003, a national campaign for the prevention of skin cancer, sponsored by the Brazilian Dermatology Society, was completed[46] (Figures 82-12 through 82-14). The results are detailed in Table 82-1.

Furthermore, the survey revealed that the northern and northeastern regions of Brazil had the lowest rate of skin cancer, perhaps owing to the greater number of blacks in those regions.

The incidence of skin cancer in Brazil is relatively high, and it is therefore a significant public health problem. The campaign for skin cancer prevention needs to emphasize the importance of sun protection, particularly in blacks and Mestizos, as it had done for the white population.

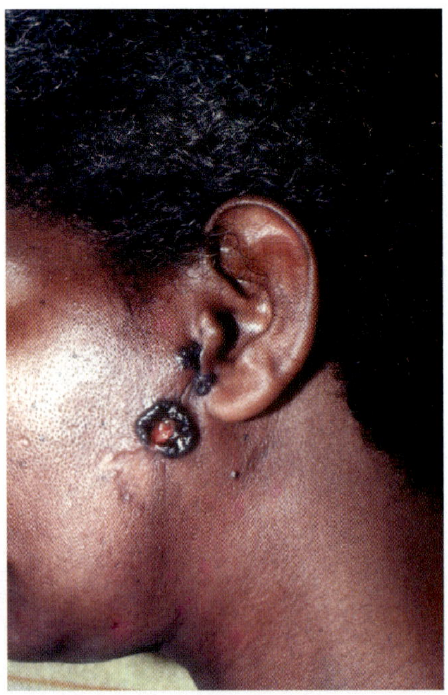

▲ **FIGURE 82-13** Basal cell carcinoma.

SPECIFIC COSMETIC PRODUCTS FOR BLACK SKIN AND HAIR IN BRAZIL

Brazil has a large population of individuals with darker skin tones, including Mestizos and blacks, who search the marketplace for cosmetics appropriate for their skin.[47] In countries with major black populations, such as Brazil and the United States, more studies on differences between the skin and hair of whites and blacks are needed. Furthermore, there is a need and a demand for the development of specific products for the skin and hair of blacks. The cosmetics industry today is beginning to invest in products for the skin of all races.[48]

TABLE 82-1
Brazilian Dermatology Society Skin Cancer Survey

37,853 total number subjects surveyed
69.9% reported sun exposure without protection
3108 (8.2%) new cases of skin cancer detected
209 (0.5%) cases of melanoma
2448 (6.4%) cases of basal cell carcinoma
446 (1.2%) cases of squamous cell carcinoma (1.2%)
2591 blacks surveyed
78.7% of blacks reported sun exposure without protection
1.7% of blacks presented skin cancer

In Brazil, medical and cosmetic products specifically for black skin are increasingly arriving in the marketplace and include those for keloids, xerosis, hair damage (caused by frequent hair straightening and relaxing), hypo- and hyperpigmentation, and conditions that require camouflage. Additionally, since the skin and hair characteristics of Brazilian black individuals are similar to those of blacks in other parts of the world, the products of other countries can be used, taking into account some differences, such as the climate of the country. The sun's intensity in Brazil needs adequate photoprotection of black skin to avoid photoaging and skin cancer, as well as melasma and other disorders of hyperpigmentation.[49] The use of broad-spectrum sunscreens containing both chemical and physical blockers (such as titanium dioxide[28,30,31]) is important in this population. Individuals with black skin also must be made aware of the need for daily, ongoing use of photoprotection to maintain clearance of their pigmentation disorders and for their prevention as well.[50]

REFERENCES

1. Azevedo AL. Todas as cores do mundo. *Revista O Globo* 2004 ;1:42-45.
2. Bueno E. *Brazil: uma história—a incrível saga de um país.* São Paulo, Atica, 2003, pp 112-123.
3. Caceres F. Os primeiros habitantes do Brazil, in Caceres F, *História do Brazil.* São Paulo, Editora Moderna, 1995, pp 21-24.
4. Caceres F. O mundo do açúcar, in Caceres F, *História do Brazil.* São Paulo, Editora Moderna, 1995, pp 42-49.
5. Carneiro SCS, Ramos-e-Silva M. Cicatrização, in Kede MP, Sabatovich O (eds), *Dermatologia Estética.* Rio de Janeiro, Atheneu, 2003, pp 11-20.
6. Sampaio S, Rivitti EA. Tumores mesenquimais e neurais, in Sampaio S, Rivitti EA (eds), *Dermatologia,* 2nd ed. São Paulo, Artes Médicas, 2001, pp 847-868.
7. Martins S. Manejo dos quelóides, in Gadelha AR, Costa IMC (eds), *Cirurgia Dermatológica em consultório.* São Paulo, Atheneu, 2003, pp 219-222.
8. Barr RJ, Stegman SJ. Delayed skin test reaction to injectable collagen implant (Zyderm): The histopathologic comparative study. *J Am Acad Dermatol* 1984; 10:652-658.
9. Fitzpatrick RE. Treatment of inflamed hypertrophic scars using intralesional 5-FU. *Dermatol Surg* 1999;25:224-232.
10. Mazereeuw J, Bonafe JL. Xerosis. *Ann Dermatol Venereol* 2002;129:137-142.
11. Baumann L. Dry skin, in Baumann L, *Cosmetic Dermatology: Principles and Pratice.* New York, McGraw-Hill, 2002, pp 29-32.
12. Magalhaes L, Hofmeister H. Avaliação e classificação da pele sã, in Kede MPV, Sabatovich O (eds), *Dermatologia Estética.* São Paulo, Atheneu, 2003, pp 23-42.
13. Norman RA. Xerosis and pruritus in the elderly recognition and management. *Dermatol Ther* 2003;16:254-259.
14. Cestari TF, Trope BM. The mature adult, in Parish LC, Brenner S, Ramos e Silva M (eds), *Women's Dermatology from Infancy to Maturity.* Lancaster, PA, Parthenon, 2001, pp 73-80.
15. Maibach HI. Pele seca e envelhecimento: o que é verdade e o que não é. *Cosmet Toiletries* 1991;3:15-16.
16. Uehara M, Miyauchi H. The morphologic characteristics of dry skin in atopic dermatitis. *Arch Dermatol* 1984;120:1186-1190.
17. Linde YW. Dry skin in atopic dermatitis: I. A clinical study. *Acta Dermatol Venereol* 1989;69:311-314.
18. Tagami H. Causas da pele seca. *Cosmet Toiletries* 1992;4:26-28.
19. Westphal SA. Unusual presentations of hypothyroidism. *Am J Med Sci* 1997;314:333-337.
20. Heymann WR, Gans EH, Manders SM, et al. Xerosis in hypothyroidism: A potencial role for the use of topical thyroid hormone in euthyroid patients. *Med Hypoth* 2001;57:736-739.
21. Jabbour AS. Cutaneous manifestations of endocrine disorders: A guide for dermatologists. *Am J Clin Dermatol* 2003;4: 315-331.
22. McDonald CJ. Structure and function of the skin: Are there differences between black and white skin? *Dermatol Clin* 1988;6:343-347.
23. Grimes PE, Davis LT. Cosmetics in blacks. *Dermatol Clin* 1991;9:53-68.
24. Westerhof W. A few more grains of melanin. *Int J Dermatol* 1997;36:573-574.
25. Kede MPV, Britz M. Discromias em pele negra, in Kede MPV, Sabatovich O (eds), *Dermatologia Estética.* São Paulo, Atheneu, 2003, pp 269-299.
26. Ramos-e-Silva M, Fernandes NC Afecções das mucosas e semimucosas. *J Bras Med* 2001;80:50-66.
27. Grimes PE. Melasma. *Arch Dermatol* 1995;131:1453-1457.
28. Pandya AG, Guevara IL. Disorders of hyperpigmentation. *Dermatol Clin* 2000;18:91-98.
29. Choi HJ, Hann SK. Diseases of pigment changes, in Parish LC, Brenner S, Ramos-e-Silva M (eds), *Women's Dermatology from Infancy to Maturity.* Lancaster, PA, Parthenon, 2001, pp 174-186.
30. Baumann L. Disorders of pigmentation, in Baumann L, *Cosmetic Dematology: Principles and Practice.* New York, McGraw-Hill, 2002, pp 63-71.
31. Sacre RC. Melasma, in Kede MPV, Sabatovich O (eds), *Dermatologia Estética.* São Paulo, Atheneu, 2003, pp 255-264.
32. O'Brien TJ, Dyall-Smith D, Hall AP. Melasma of the forearms. *Australas J Dermatol* 1997;38:35-37.
33. Johnston GA, Sviland L, McLelland J. Melasma of the arms associated with hormone replacement therapy. *Br J Dermatol* 1998;139:932.
34. Varma S, Roberts DL. Melasma of the arms associated with hormone replacement therapy. *Br J Dermatol* 1999; 141:592.
35. O'Brien TJ, Dyall-Smith D, Hall AP. Melasma of the arms associated with hormone replacement therapy. *Br J Dermatol* 1999;141:592-593.
36. Sanchez NP, Pathak MA, Sato S, et al. Melasma: A clinical, light microscopic, ultrastructural, and immunofluorescence study. *J Am Acad Dermatol* 1981; 4:698.
37. Mosher DB, Fitzpatrick TB, Ortonne JP, Hori Y. Hypomelanoses and hypermelanoses, in Freedberg IM, Eisen AZ, Wolff K, et al (eds), *Fitzpatrick's Dermatology in General Medicine,* 5th ed. New York, McGraw-Hill, 1999, pp 945-1017.
38. Martin AG, Leal-Khouri S. Physiologic skin changes associated with pregnancy. *Int J Dermatol* 1992;31:375-378.
39. Mazaffar F, Hussain I, Haroon TS. Physiologic skin changes during pregnancy: A study of 140 cases. *Int J Dermatol* 1998;37:429-431.
40. Deharo C, Berbis P, Privat Y. Dermatological complications caused by oral contraceptives. *Fertil Contracept Sex* 1988;16:299-304.
41. Lobão A. Hiper e hipopigmentação pós-inflamatória, in Kede MPV, Sabatovich O (eds), *Dermatologia Estética.* São Paulo, Atheneu, 2003, pp 265-268.
42. Halder RM, Richards GM. Management of dyscromias in ethnis skin. *Dermatol Ther* 2004;17:151-157.
43. Bakos L, Bakos RM, Dzulay DR. Afecipes dose pêlos, in Azulay R, Dzulay DR (eds) Dermatolgie. Rio de Janeiro, Gvansbara, Koogan, 2006, pp. 628-638.
44. Sampaio SAP, Rivitti EA. Piodermites e outras dermatoses por bactérias, in Sampaio SAP, Rivitti EA, *Dermatologia,* 2nd ed. São Paulo, Artes Medicas, 2001, pp 435-452.
45. Cardoso AC. Dermatoses zooparasitárias, in Talhari S, Neves RG (eds), *Dermatologia Tropical.* Rio de Janeiro, Medsi, 1995, pp 1-21.
46. Campanha Nacional de Pervenção ao Câncer de Pele, November 2003, www.sbd.org.br/medicos/atualidade/noticia.asp?cod_noticia=50 & Ano=2004 & Pg_Id=3, accessed on September 25, 2008.
47. Schlossman ML. Formulação de produtos étnicos para maquilagem. *Cosmet Toiletries* 1996;8:60.
48. Rocha Filho PA. Cosméticos étnicos: Aspectos fisiológicos. *Cosmet Toiletries* 1996:8:34-38
49. Verallo-Rowell VM. Protecting brown skin: Q&A, in Verallo-Rowell VM, *Skin in the Tropics: Sunscreens and Hyperpigmentation.* Pasig City, Philippines, Anvil Publishing, 2001, pp 35-46.
50. Verallo-Rowell VM. The tropics: Q&A, in Verallo-Rowell VM, *Skin in the Tropics: Sunscreens and Hyperpigmentation.* Pasig City, Philippines, Anvil Publishing, 2001, pp 1-14.

CHAPTER 83

Immunizations for International Travel

Jasmine H. Yun

Key Points

- In the last 30 years, international travel has become increasingly popular, posing a threat to the prevention of infectious diseases.
- As a medical practitioner, one will often be asked about travel immunizations and prevention of infectious diseases. Travel vaccines are classified into three categories: routine immunizations, required immunizations when traveling to specific countries, and recommended immunizations.
- Physicians should refer to the most recent recommendations on travel-related infections.

Spawned by Jenner's use of the smallpox vaccine in the 1700s, vaccination has been ranked as the greatest public health achievement, contributing the most to decreased global morbidity and mortality.[1] However, in the last 30 years, international travel has become increasingly popular, posing a threat to the prevention of infectious diseases. With the improvement of commercial airline operations, reduction of airfares, and expansion of flight schedules, travel to exotic locales has become less daunting. Also, first-generation immigrants to the United States have increasingly been able to visit their families in their countries of origin. With this rise in travel, the risk of travel-related infections and the introduction of new diseases from travelers returning from an endemic area have become prominent public health problems. However, since vaccinations for smallpox have been discontinued in the general population, the incidence of cutaneous reactions to vaccines is now low.[2]

As a medical practitioner, one will often be asked about travel immunizations and prevention of infectious diseases. Travel vaccines are classified into three categories: routine immunizations, required immunizations when traveling to specific countries, and recommended immunizations (Table 83-1).

Because vaccines are not available for all infectious diseases, physicians must stay abreast of the current recommendations on how to prevent travel-related diseases. Physicians must evaluate patients on a case-by-case basis, learn the current information on travel vaccines, the time before departure, medical conditions of patients, and possible contraindications and adverse effects of a vaccine. Travelers should consult a physician at least 4 weeks before departure because some vaccinations require a precise schedule of doses to obtain proper immunity. Patients at high risk for travel-related infections (patients who are above age 65, who are immunocompromised, who plan to stay abroad for over 30 days, or who plan to travel to rural areas or participate in outdoor activities) may need further consultation with a physician specializing in travel medicine (Table 83-2).

Physicians should refer to the most recent recommendations on travel-related infections given by the Centers for Disease Control and Prevention (CDC) at *www.cdc.gov/travel* and the World Health Organization at *www.who.int/ith*.[3] Other resources that may be helpful are MD Travel Health (*www.mdtravelhealth.org*) and American Society of Tropical Medicine and Hygiene (*www.astmh.org*) (Table 83-3).

Immunization can be either active or passive. Active immunization can be provided by attenuated live organisms, by killed organisms, or by modified toxin. Passive immunizations may be by relatively unpurified human immunoglobulin, by specific human immunoglobulins, or by antisera produced in animals.[4]

TABLE 83-1
Travel Vaccines

- Routine immunizations
- Required immunizations when travelling to specific counties
- Recommended immunizations

TABLE 83-2
Patients at High Risk

- Above age 65
- Immunocompromised
- Stay more than 30 days
- Travel to rural areas

TABLE 83-3
Information Regarding Vaccinations and Travel-Related Infection.

- CDC at *www.cdc.gov/travel*
- WHO at *www.who.int/ith*
- MD Travel Health at *www.mdtravelhealth.org*
- American Society of Tropical Medicine Hygiene at *www.astmh.org.*

ROUTINE IMMUNIZATIONS

When evaluating a patient for travel immunizations, the physician should update all routine immunizations. Measles, a highly virulent virus owing the low number of virions needed to produce infection, is still a large problem in underdeveloped countries. More than 1 million children die each year from measles.[5] A booster of measles-mumps-rubella (MMR) vaccine should be given to any patient born after 1956 who has not had two doses of the vaccine or cannot demonstrate immunity by serum antibody. Infants 6–11 months of age should receive one dose of MMR vaccine when traveling to high-risk areas; in addition, they must receive two doses after the age of 12 months to achieve full immunity (Table 83-4). Adverse effects from the MMR vaccine are mild, usually consisting of low fever, viral exanthem, and arthralgias.

Tetanus and diphtheria (Td) boosters should be given to patients who have not been vaccinated within the last 5 years who are traveling to areas where postexposure tetanus immunizations may not be available.

Poliomyelitis is endemic to seven countries: Afghanistan, Niger, Somalia,

TABLE 83-4
Measles-Mumps-Rubella (MMR) Vaccine

- Born after 1956 and not had two doses of vaccine
- Unable to demonstrate immunity
- Infants 6–11 months of age = 1 dose MMR
  - Before traveling to high-risk areas
- Two doses of MMR after 12 months
  - For full immunity

TABLE 83-5
Varicella Vaccine

- Immunity not proven by serum antibody titers
  - Children 12 years of age and younger = single dose of vaccine
  - Over age 13 = double dose of vaccine
    - 4–8 weeks apart
  - Avoid contact with immunosuppressed patients for 6 weeks
  - Avoid contact with high-risk patients for 6 weeks
  - Vaccine contraindicated for infants younger than 12 months of age
  - Vaccine contraindicated in pregnant women

Egypt, Pakistan, India, and Nigeria.[6] Those traveling to these countries should receive a single booster of inactivated polio vaccine (IPOL) if the primary doses have already been given.

If the patient cannot demonstrate immunity to varicella by serum antibody titers, children 12 years and younger should receive a single dose of vaccine, and patients over the age of 13 should receive two doses of the vaccine 4–8 weeks apart. The patient should avoid contact with immunosuppressed or high-risk patients for up to 6 weeks after vaccination. The vaccine is contraindicated in infants younger than 12 months of age and pregnant women (Table 83-5).

The influenza vaccine is recommended in all patients traveling during the influenza season. Influenza season occurs during November through March in the northern hemisphere and during April through September in the southern hemisphere. The pneumococcal vaccine is recommended for patients who are over age 65 and for all patients with cardiac or pulmonary disease, asplenia, diabetes mellitus, or liver cirrhosis.

REQUIRED IMMUNIZATIONS

Yellow fever is caused by a flavivirus transmitted by a mosquito vector via horizontal and vertical transmission. It is a potentially fatal illness that is endemic to equatorial Africa and South America. The symptoms range from mild fever to acute renal failure, hepatitis with jaundice, and death. Yellow fever vaccine must be given to patients over 9 months of age who are traveling to endemic areas or to rural areas of countries that do not officially report yellow fever but are within the endemic zone. Most endemic countries require documentation of immunization on entry. Also, many nonendemic countries require immunization on entry if one is traveling from an endemic country. The vaccine is a live-attenuated virus and must be repeated every 10 years. For proper documentation, the vaccine must be given at an approved yellow fever vaccination center. Most local health departments are approved centers. The vaccine is not recommended in pregnant women, and travel should be delayed if a patient is pregnant. If a pregnant woman must travel to a high-risk area, vaccination is recommended because the risk of infection with yellow fever outweighs the adverse effects of the vaccine to the mother and the fetus.[7]

RECOMMENDED VACCINATIONS

Hepatitis A

The hepatitis A vaccine is recommended for travelers to all international countries except the United States, Canada, Japan, Australia, New Zealand, and countries in western Europe. The inactivated vaccine is available in the United States. Immunization entails two doses given 6–12 months apart in patient 2 years of age and older. After the first dose, 97–99% of patients develop protective levels of antibodies 1 month, and 99–100% are fully protected 1 month after the second dose.[8] Travelers who need protection earlier than 2 weeks after the first dose of hepatitis A vaccine should receive immunoglobulin with the first dose at a different injection site.[9] If the patient is younger than 2 years of age, pregnant, or allergic to the vaccine, the patient may receive immunoglobulin (at a dose of 0.2–0.6 mL/kg) and achieve 80–90% protection for 3–5 months.[10] Hepatitis A vaccine may be given at the same time as other vaccines. The incidence of hepatitis A in Hispanics is twice that in non-Hispanics. Cutaneous reaction may include hives or paleness. These reactions may be present in any severe reaction secondary to vaccination.

Hepatitis B

Before the introduction of the hepatitis B vaccine, 200,000–300,000 new cases of hepatitis B infection were reported each year.[11] Plasma-derived hepatitis B vaccine was first introduced in 1982, vastly decreasing the rate of infection. Children are vaccinated routinely in the United States for hepatitis B, but many adults in the United States have never been immunized. Travelers to endemic areas (e.g., South America, Africa, Southeast Asia, and the South Pacific), those in close contact with high-risk populations, and those born overseas traveling to their country of origin should receive the vaccine. In adults 20 years of age or older, the hepatitis B vaccine should be given at 0, 3, and 6 months. It is not contraindicated in pregnancy. People should not be given hepatitis B vaccine if they have ever had a severe allergic reaction to baker's yeast.

Combined Hepatitis A and B

This combined vaccine can be used in patients 18 years of age and older. It is given at 0, 3, and 6 months and is as effective as the monovalent vaccines.

Typhoid Fever

Typhoid fever is endemic to Central and South America, India, and Africa. Vaccination against typhoid fever should be considered for persons planning short- or long-term travel to high-risk areas. The vaccine is also recommended for travelers who will be exposed to contaminated food and drink. Two vaccines are available (a live-attenuated oral Ty21a vaccine and Typhim VI), and they are both 50–80% effective.[12] Careful selection of food and drink and practicing good hygiene are essential to further preventing infection. Primary vaccination with the oral vaccine consists of taking one enteric-coated tablet every other day for four doses. Immunity is achieved 14 days after the last dose. A booster dose, consisting of the same regimen, is taken every 5 years as needed. The vaccine is contraindicated in pregnancy, in children under 6 years of age, and in immunocompromised patients. It should not be taken with antibiotics, which will decrease the efficacy of the vaccine.

Primary vaccination with Typhim VI is achieved with a 0.5-ml intramuscular dose, with immunity achieved 14 days after the dose. It may be given to patients above the age of 2 years, and no data have been shown of its effects in pregnant women and immunocompromised patients.

Meningococcus

Meningococcal disease owing to serogroup A or C is an epidemic disease in sub-Saharan Africa from December to June. The vaccine is recommended for those traveling to that area, as well as pilgrims traveling to Saudi Arabia during the religious holidays. The Menomune vaccine is effective only against serogroups A, C, Y, and W-135. Primary immunization consists of a 0.5-ml dose given subcutaneously to patients 2 years of age and older. Two meningococcal vaccines are available in the United States:

- Meningococcal polysaccharide vaccine 4 (MPSV4) has been available since the 1970s.
- Meningococcal conjugate vaccine was licensed in 2005.

Both vaccines work well and protect about 90% of those who get meningitis; however, MCV4 is expected to give better, longer-lasting protection and should be better at preventing the disease from spreading from person to person.[13]

Japanese Encephalitis

Japanese encephalitis is caused by a mosquito-borne arbovirus and is endemic to India, China, Korea, Japan, and Southeast Asia. The majority of infections are subclinical, but in rare instances, the virus can cause severe encephalitis. The vaccine is recommended for travelers to endemic areas who are staying longer than 30 days during the transmission season or if outdoor activities in rural areas are anticipated. The immunization schedule consists of a 1.0-ml subcutaneous dose at 0, 7, and 30 days. Immunity is conferred after the second dose with an efficacy of 91%.[14] A booster dose may be given 3 years after the primary vaccine schedule.

Adverse reactions to the vaccine manifesting as generalized urticaria and angioedema have occurred within minutes to as long as 2 weeks after vaccination. Epinephrine and other medications and equipment to treat anaphylaxis should be available in case this reaction occurs. The patient should be observed for at least 30 minutes after administration of the vaccine and should have medical care readily accessible for 10 days following vaccination. No specific information on the safety of the vaccine in pregnant women or in infants younger than 1 year of age is available. However, pregnant women staying in high-risk areas for long periods of time should receive the vaccine because the risk of the infection outweighs the theoretical risk of the vaccine.[15]

TABLE 83-6
Vaccines for Travel-Related Infections

Vaccine	Primary Vaccination	Booster
Hepatitis A	1.0 ml IM	1.0 ml IM 6–12 mos after first dose
Hepatitis B	1.0 ml IM at 0, 1, 6 mos	Not routine
Combined hepatitis A/B	1.0 ml IM at 0, 1, 6 mos	Not routine
Japanese encephalitis	1.0 ml SQ on days 0, 7, 30	1.0 ml SQ every 3 years
Meningococcus	0.5 ml SQ	0.5 ml SQ every 3–5 years
Rabies	1.0 ml IM on days 0, 7,21, 28	1.0 ml IM every 2–5 years
Typhoid fever PO	1 capsule PO qod × 4 capsules	Repeat regimen every 5 years
Typhoid fever IM	0.5 ml IM	0.5 ml IM every 2 years
Yellow fever	0.5 ml SQ	0.5 ml SQ every 10 years

IM = intramuscularly; SQ = subcutaneously; PO = per oral; QOD = every other day.

Rabies

Rabies virus causes acute encephalitis in all warm-blooded hosts, including humans; the outcome without treatment is almost always fatal. Rabies virus is transmitted through the bite and virus-containing saliva of an infected host. The first symptoms of rabies may be nonspecific flulike signs—malaise, fever, or headache—which may last for days. There may be paresthesias at the site of exposure, progressing within days to symptoms of ataxia, confusion, and agitation. Postexposure prophylaxis is effective but may not be available in underdeveloped countries.

Canine rabies is endemic to China, Southeast Asia, Indonesia, Latin America, Africa, India, and parts of the former Soviet Union. Patients who plan to stay in endemic areas for longer than 30 days and those who plan to participate in outdoor activities or activities that involve interactions with animals should receive the vaccine. The vaccine consists of three 1.0-mL doses given intramuscularly on days 0, 7, and 21 or 28. If the patient has received the vaccine and gets a high-risk bite, two additional doses of the vaccine should be given on the day of the bite and on postbite day 3. Immunoglobulin administration is not required if the patient has received preexposure prophylaxis[16] (Table 83-6).

REFERENCES

1. Centers for Disease Control and Prevention. Ten great public health achievements: United States, 1990-1999. *MMWR* 1999; 48:241-243.
2. McMahoon BJ, Helminiak C, Wainwright RB, et al. Frequency of adverse reactions to hepatitis B vaccine in 43,618 persons. *Am J Med* 1992; 92:254-256.
3. Lo V, Gluckman S. Travel immunizations. *Am Fam Physician* 2004;70:89-99.
4. Hay RJ, Champion RH, Greaves MW. Vaccinations and immunizations, in Champion RH, Burton JL, Ebling FJG (eds), *Rook/Wilkinson/Ebling Textbook of Dermatology*, 5th ed. London, Blackwell Scientific, 1992, Chap 73, pp 2959-2960.
5. Murray C, Lopez A. Mortality by cause for eight regions of the worlds: Global burden of disease study. *Lancet* 1997;349: 1269-1276.
6. Progress toward global eradication of poliomyelitis, 2002. *MMWR* 2003; 52: 366-369.
7. Yellow fever vaccine: Recommendations of the Immunization Practices Advisory Committee (ACIP). *MMWR* 1990;39:1-6.
8. Westblom TU, Gudipati S, DeRousse C, et al. Safety and immunogenicity of an inactivated hepatitis A vaccine: Effect of dose and vaccination schedule. *J Infect Dis* 1994;169:996-1001.
9. Wolfe MS. Protection of travelers. *Clin Infect Dis* 1997;25:177-186.
10. Prevention of hepatitis A through active or passive immunization: Recommendations of the Immunization Practices Advisory Committee (ACIP). *MMWR* 1999; 48:1-37.
11. Armstrong GL, Mast EE, Wojczynski M. et al. Childhood hepatitis B virus infections in the United States before hepatitis B immunizations. *Pediatrics* 2001;108:1123-1128.
12. Typhoid immunization: Recommendation of the Immunization Practices Advisory Committee (ACIP). *MMWR* 1994; 43:1-7.
13. Control and prevention of meningococcal disease: Recommendations of the Immunization Practices Advisory Committee (ACIP). *MMWR* 1997; 46:1-10.
14. Hoke CH, Nisalak A, Sangawhipa N, et al. Protection against Japanese encephalitis by inactivated vaccines. *N Engl J Med* 1988;319:608-614.
15. Inactivated Japanese encephalitis vaccine: Recommendations of the Immunization Practices Advisory Committee (ACIP). *MMWR* 1993; 42:1-15.
16. Wilde H, Briggs, Meslin FX, et al. Rabies update for travel medicine advisors. *Clin Infect Dis* 2003;37:96-100.

SECTION 15

Atlas for Skin of Color: Africa, Asia, and Latin America

CHAPTER 84

Atlas for Skin of Color: Africa, Asia, and Latin America

Special Atlas Editor: Allison Nicholas Metz

Barbara J. Leppard
Rashmi Sarkar
Marcia Ramos-e-Silva

ACNE

Definition

Acne vulgaris is a self-limiting disease of the sebaceous glands that occurs mainly during adolescence and presents with pleomorphic lesions such as comedones, papules, pustules, nodules, and cysts that can leave behind severe scarring (Figures 84-1 through 84-6).

Etiology

Acne vulgaris is multifactorial in origin. The factors involved in its pathogenesis are increased sebum production, hypercornification of the pilosebaceous duct, abnormality of the microbial flora (especially colonization of the duct with *P. acnes*), and the production of inflammation.

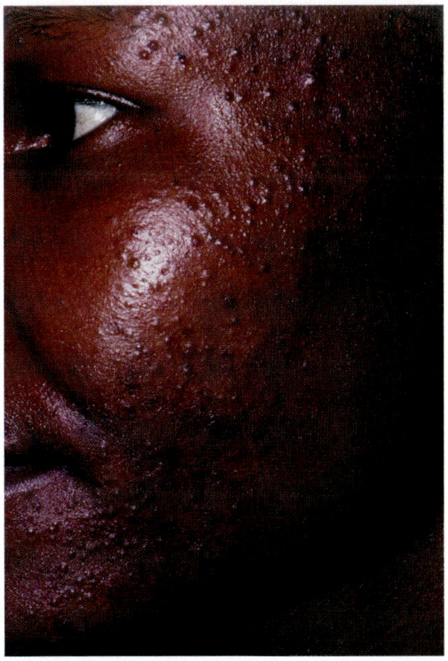

▲ **FIGURE 84-1** Africa. Greasy skin with open and closed comedones. Courtesy of Dr. Barbara J. Leppard.

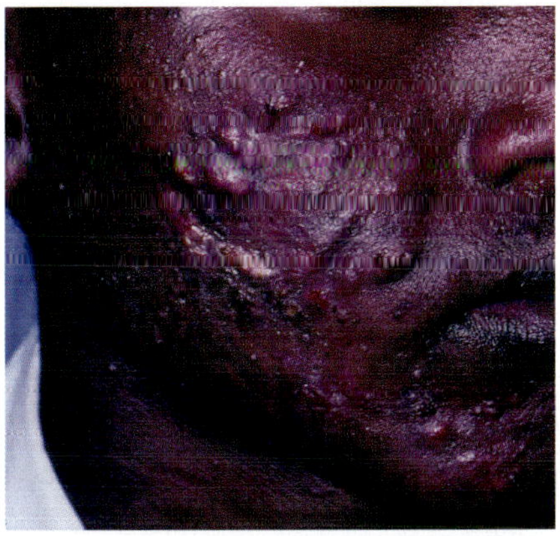

▲ **FIGURE 84-2** Africa. Comedones, papules, pustules, nodules, and cysts. Courtesy of Dr. Barbara J. Leppard.

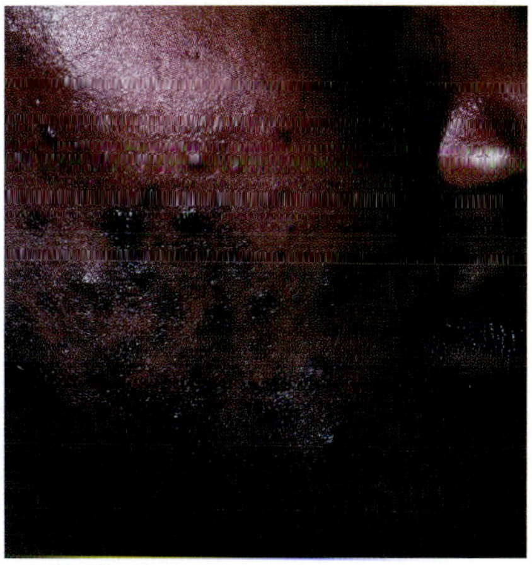

▲ **FIGURE 84-3** Africa. Papules and pustules with postinflammatory hyperpigmentation. Courtesy of Dr. Barbara J. Leppard.

Clinical Perspective

The lesions of acne vulgaris are seen on the sebaceous gland–rich body areas, mainly the face, midchest, back, shoulders, and upper arms. There are two types of lesions: inflammatory and noninflammatory lesions. Comedones are the pathognomic lesions and are conical raised lesions with a broad base and plugged apex and may be black or white. The inflammatory lesions are papules, pustules, nodules, and cysts. Pustular and nodular lesion are seen commonly in Asian patients. The sequelae of acne, which include hyperpigmentation and scarring, are more socially and psychologically distressing for the patient than the disease itself. The scars can be hypertrophic and keloidal scars owing to increased collagen or "ice pick," depressed fibrotic, macular atrophic, or follicular atrophic scars owing to loss of collagen.

Differential Diagnosis

Rosacea may be considered in the differential diagnosis (papules and erythema are prominent on the flush areas of the face and chin; comedones and scars are absent). Drug-induced acne has monomorphic lesions. Folliculitis presents with pustules as predominant lesions.

Treatment

Patient education is important. For mild cases, topical benzoyl peroxide or retinoic acid is used. For moderate cases, topical antibiotics can be given in addition. In severe cases, in addition to topical therapy, systemic antibiotics and isotretinoin may be used. For cystic acne, aspiration, intralesional steroids, and dapsone have to be given. Antiandrogens are given in selected patients. Scars may be treated surgically, and for postacne pigmentation, adapalene or azelaic acid cream can be used.

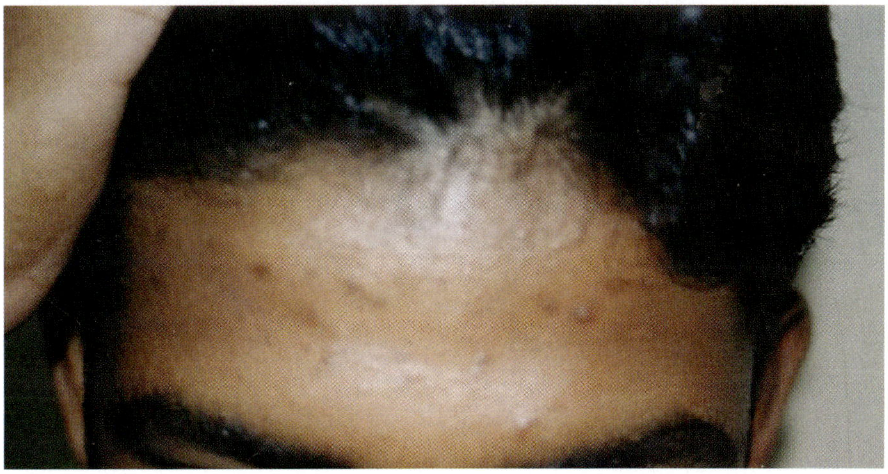

▲ **FIGURE 84-4** Asia. Mild acne with postacne hyperpigmentation. Courtesy of Dr. Rashmi Sarkar.

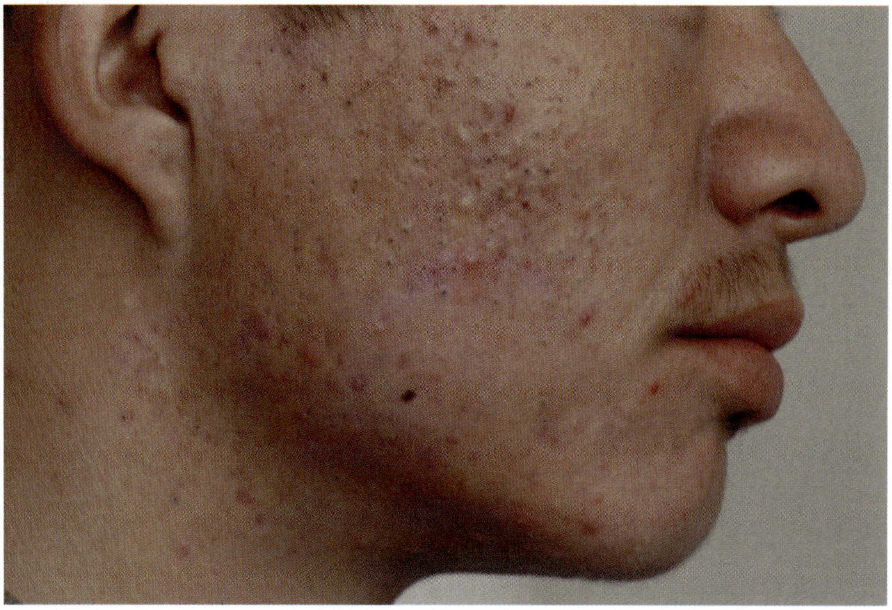

▲ **FIGURE 84-5** Asia. Acne with pustules and nodules in a Chinese man. Courtesy of Dr. Diqing Luo.

ATOPIC DERMATITIS

Definition

Atopic dermatitis (AD) is a common chronic or relapsing dermatitis characterized by severe pruritus occurring primarily in infants and children. A personal or family history of asthma, allergic rhinitis, or atopic dermatitis may be present.

Etiology

The disease arises as a result of a complex interplay between various genetic and immunologic factors. It is triggered or exacerbated by interactions between a genetic predisposition and environmental factors. The environmental factors include physical factors such as sweating, climate, warm surroundings, detergents and soap, synthetic or woolen fabrics, cigarette smoke; food items such as tomato, orange, and citrus fruits; and allergens such as house dust mite, animal hair, pollens, plants, and *Staphylococcus aureus*.

Clinical Perspective

The prevalence of AD varies from 10–15.6%. In India, it has been reported to comprise 28.46% of the total pediatric diseases. It is usually seen in the mild and moderate forms; severe forms are seen less commonly. Xerosis can be found shortly after birth. In dark-skinned individuals, the lesions may have a follicular distribution, or the seemingly unaffected skin may have a dry, lackluster appearance. In the infantile phase, face and scalp involvement is common (Figures 84-7, 84-9 and 84-11), as well as, the extensor surfaces and trunk. In the childhood phase, 18–24 months onward, eczema is observed on the flexural surfaces, including the neck, antecubital and popliteal fossae, wrists, and ankles (Figures 84-8, 84-10 and 84-12). In the adult phase, lichenification of the flexures and hands commonly occurs.

Differential Diagnosis

Contact dermatitis and scabies have to be considered. Contact dermatitis would have a typical history, and in scabies, there is predilection of the lesions for finger web spaces, axillae, and periumbilical area and a history of similar lesions in close contacts and exacerbations of itching at night. Infantile seborrhoic dermatitis may have to be considered in the infantile stage, which has more well-defined lesions and lesions in the diaper area.

Treatment Options

General measures such as avoidance of provoking factors, bathing and moisturizers, antibiotics for secondary infection, and antihistamines are important part of therapy. Topical corticosteroids and

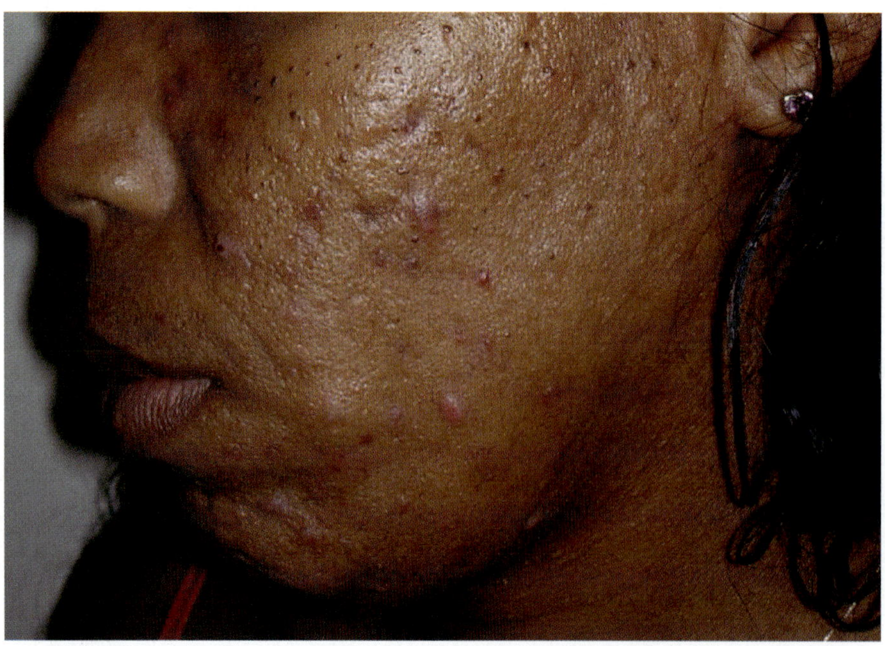

▲ **FIGURE 84-6** Latin America. Acne. Courtesy of Dr. Marcia Ramos-e-Silva.

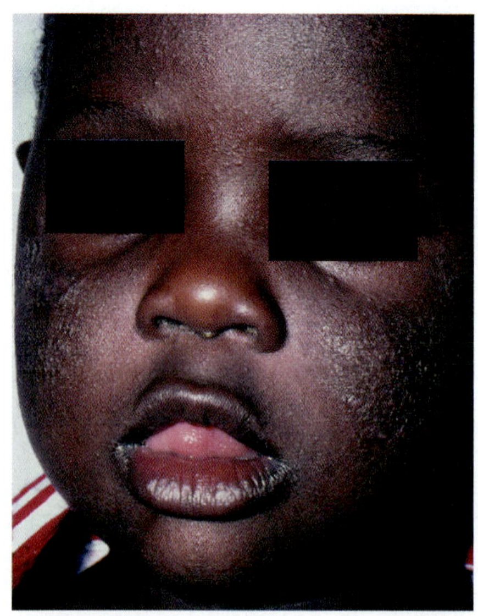

▲ **FIGURE 84-7** Africa. Atopic dermatitis on the cheeks of a 2-year-old. Courtesy of Dr. Barbara J. Leppard.

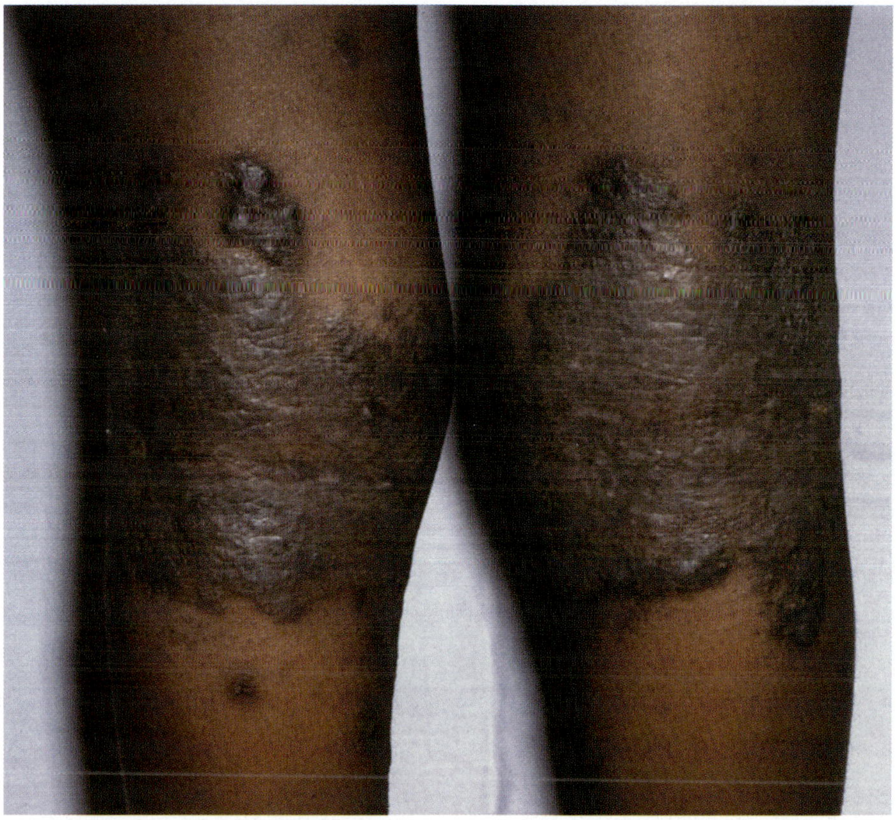

▲ **FIGURE 84-8** Africa. Lichenified eczema behind the knees in a 10-year-old girl. Courtesy of Dr. Barbara J. Leppard.

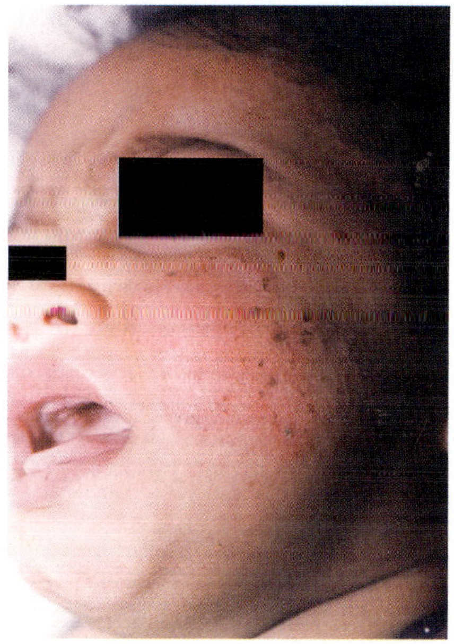

FIGURE 84-9 Asia. Atopic dermatitis on the cheeks. Courtesy of Dr. Rashmi Sarkar.

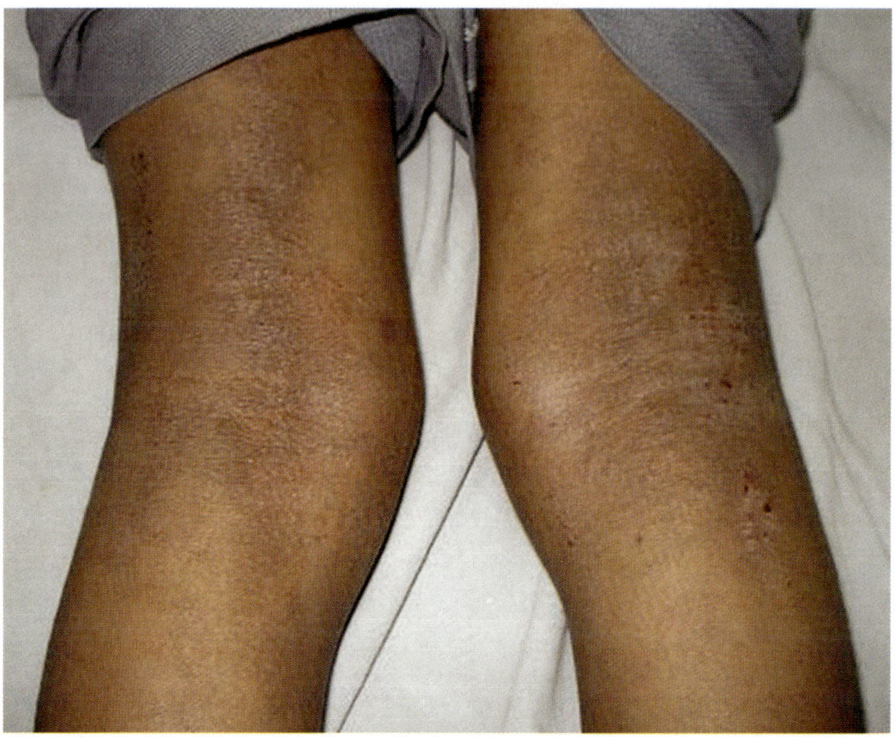

▲ **FIGURE 84-10** Asia. Atopic dermatitis. Flexural dermatitis with lichenification. Courtesy of Dr. Rashmi Sarkar.

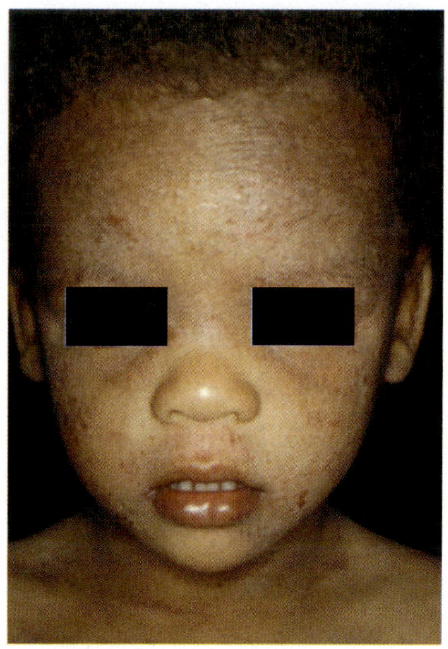

▲ **FIGURE 84-11** Latin America. Atopic dermatitis. Courtesy of Dr. Tania Cestari.

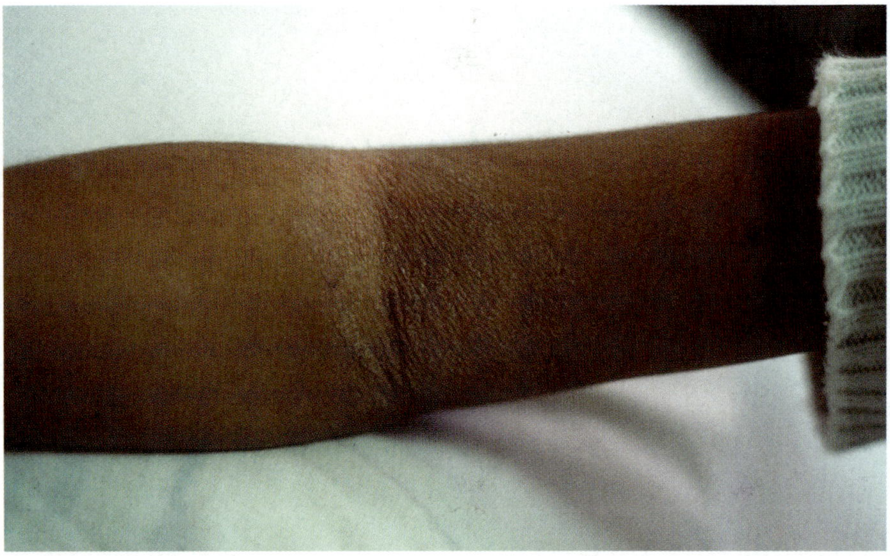

▲ **FIGURE 84-12** Latin America. Atopic eczema. Courtesy of Dr. Marcia Ramos-e-Silva.

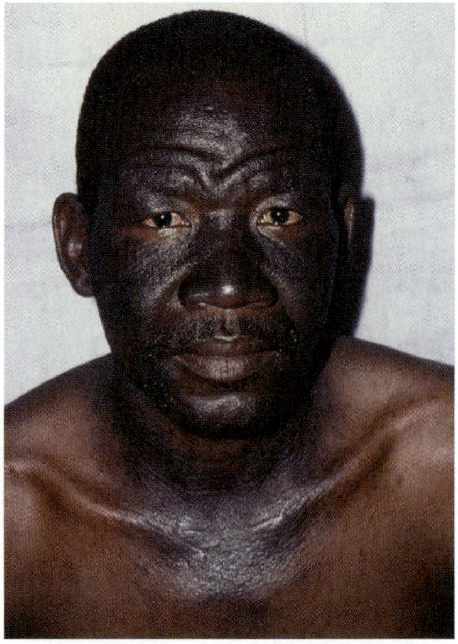

▲ **FIGURE 84-14** Africa. Photosensitivity reaction. Courtesy of Dr. Barbara J. Leppard.

topical calcineurin inhibitors such as tacrolimus and pimecrolimus are mainstays of therapy. Severe cases may require treatment with phototherapy, photochemotherapy, cyclosporine, azathioprine, or interferons.

DRUG-INDUCED PHOTOSENSITIVITY REACTION

Definition

Abnormal skin reactions to sunlight and artificial sources of ultraviolet (UV) and visible radiation induced by external or internally ingested photosensitizing drugs and other chemicals are known as *drug-induced photosensitivity reactions.*

Etiology

Most systemic photosensitizers are phototoxic in mechanism (exogeneous: antibiotics, antidepressants, diuretics, psoralens, dyes, coal tars, anthracene, and chemical sunscreens; endogeneous: porphyrins). Less common mechanisms include drug-induced lupus, pellagra, and photoallergy. Photoallergy occurs commonly owing to topical exposure to nonsteroidal anti-inflammatory drugs (NSAIDs), fragrances, and sunscreens. Photoallergic reactions are cell-mediated, whereas phototoxic reactions are nonimmunologic.

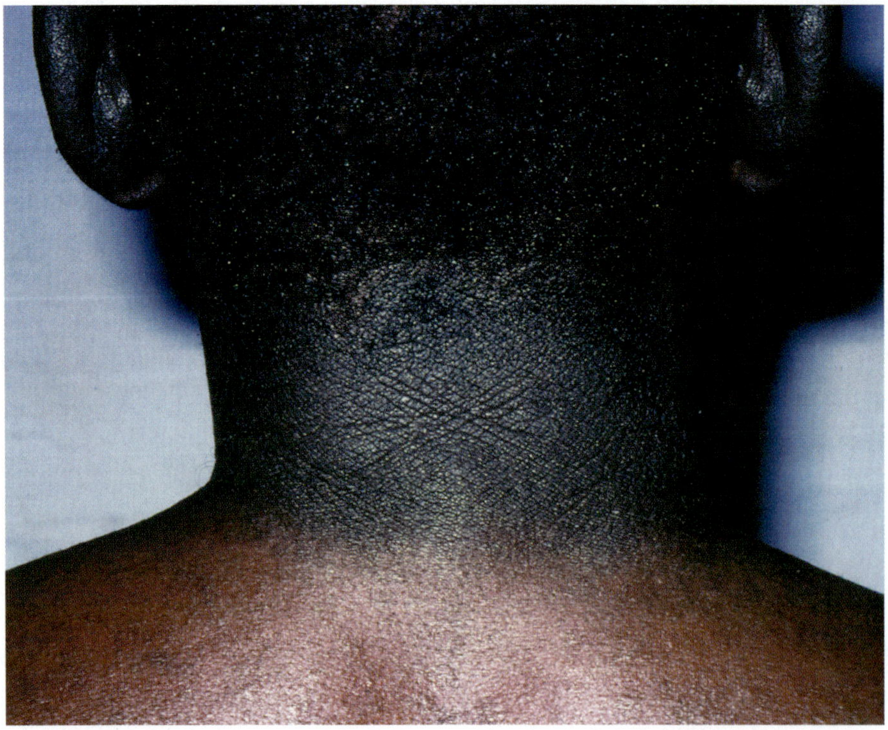

▲ **FIGURE 84-13** Africa. Photosensitivity reaction. Courtesy of Dr. Barbara J. Leppard.

Clinical Perspective

Acute phototoxic reactions to drugs and chemicals can produce an immediate erythema and burning sensation in light-exposed areas, followed sometimes by blistering. Common sites of involvement are the forehead, nose, malar region, neck, V of the chest, extensor forearms, and dorsal hands (Figures 84-13 through 84-15). The upper eyelids, nasolabial folds, upper lip, and submental regions are characteristically spared. Photoallergic eruptions are itchy, eczematous, or vesicular. In Asians, photoallergic reactions are more common than phototoxic reactions.

Differential Diagnosis

Photoallergic reactions may have to be differentiated from airbone contact dermatitis (involvement of the upper eyelid and submental region, typical history), atopic dermatitis (history of atopy), and polymorphous light reaction (absence of history of drug intake). Phototoxic reactions have to be differentiated from severe sunburn, which is common in Asians owing to their clothing.

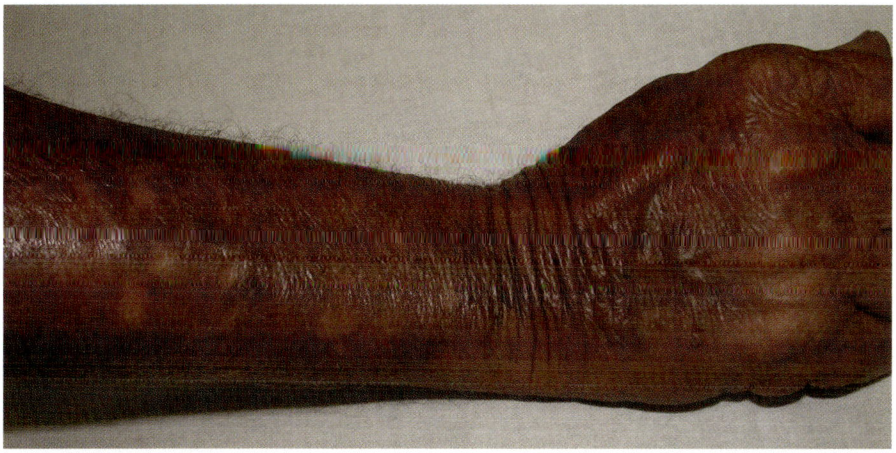

▲ **FIGURE 84-15** Latin America. Drug-induced photosensitivity. Courtesy of Dr. Marcia Ramos-e-Silva.

Treatment Options

The best option is to replace the offending drug with a nonphototoxic alternative. Sun avoidance and broad spectrum sunscreens are an important part of the treatment. Topical and oral corticosteroid, antihistamines, and UVB or psoralen with UVA (PUVA) desensitization may be required.

LEISHMANIASIS

Definition

Leishmaniasis is a protozoan disease whose diverse clinical manifestations dependent on both the infective species of *Leishmania* and the immune response of the host. The transmission of the disease occurs through the bite of a sandfly infected with *Leishmania* parasites.

Etiology

Post-kala-azar dermal leishmaniasis (PKDL) is a type of leishmaniasis that is endemic in East Africa and India and is caused primarily by *L.donovani.* It has been reported in 20% of Indian patients and 5% of East African patients. PKDL frequently follows an attack of kala-azar, or visceral leishmaniasis (VL), after 1–2 years and is considered to be a dermal extension of the disease after healing of VL either spontaneously or as a result of treatment.

Clinical Perspectives

In India, hypopigmented macules are usually the first manifestation. They begin as tiny macules that enlarge to form irregular patches, which are often bilateral and symmetric.

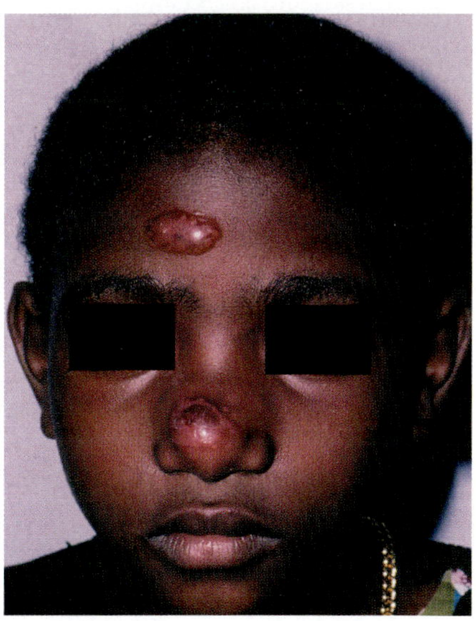

▲ **FIGURE 84-16** Africa. Cutaneous leishmaniasis. Two lesions on face of an 8-year-old boy. Courtesy of Dr. Barbara J. Leppard.

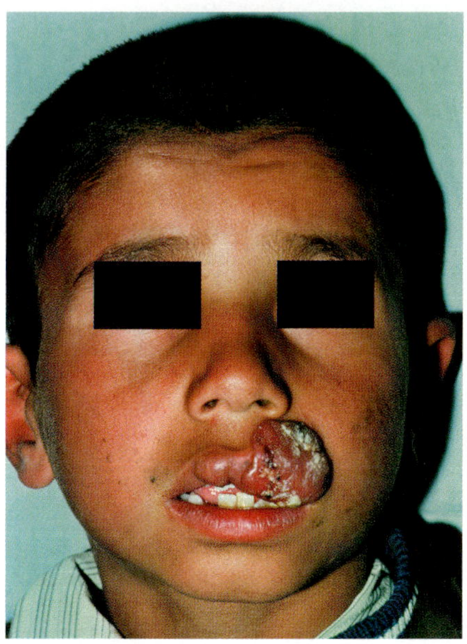

▲ **FIGURE 84-17** Africa. Cutaneous leishmaniasis on the lip of an 8-year-old boy. Courtesy of Dr. Barbara J. Leppard.

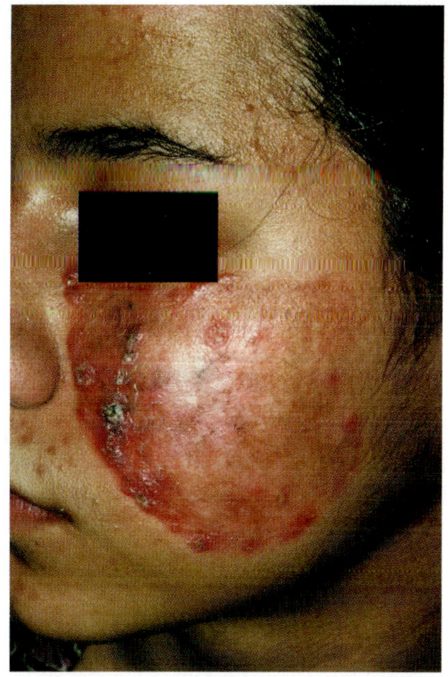

▲ **FIGURE 84-18** Africa. Cutaneous leishmaniasis on the cheek of a 12-year-old girl. Courtesy of Dr. Barbara J. Leppard.

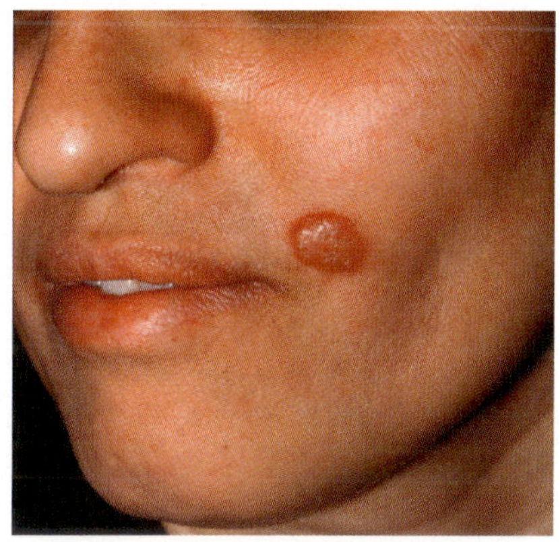

▲ **FIGURE 84-19** Africa. Cutaneous leishmaniasis. Early lesion—single red papule. Courtesy of Dr. Barbara J. Leppard.

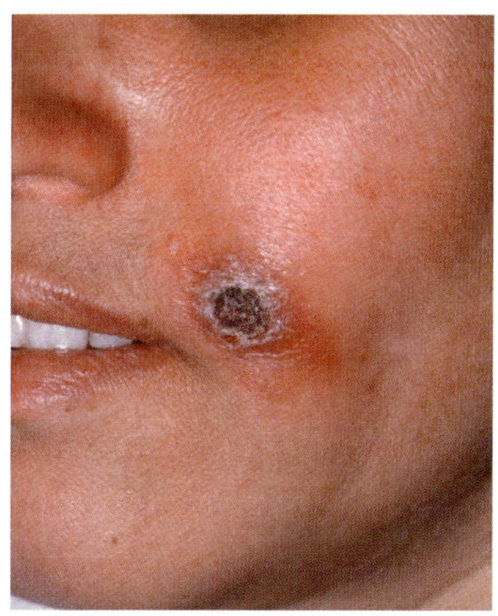

▲ **FIGURE 84-20** Africa. Cutaneous leishmaniasis. Same lesion 2 months later. Courtesy of Dr. Barbara J. Leppard.

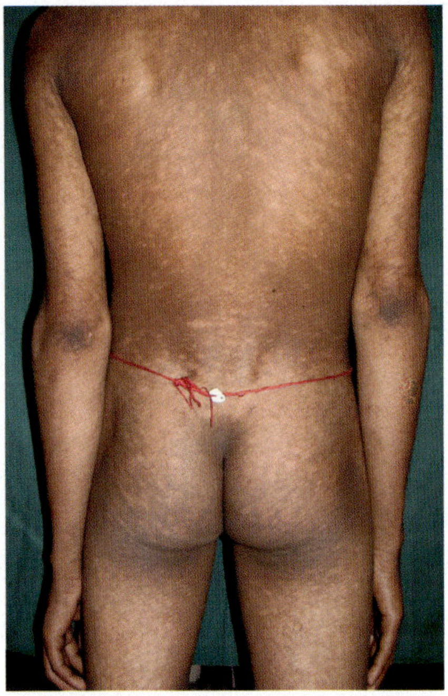

▲ **FIGURE 84-21** Asia. Post-kala-azar dermal leishmaniasis. Hypopigmented macules of PKDL. Courtesy of Dr. V. Ramesh.

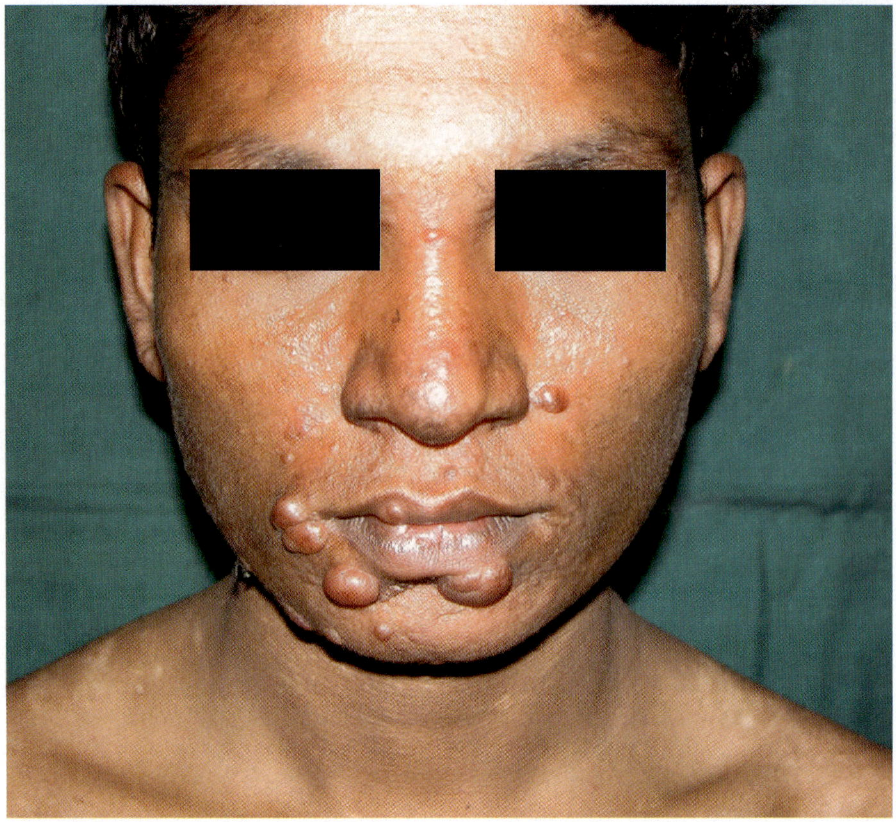

▲ **FIGURE 84-22** Asia. Post-kala-azar dermal leishmaniasis. Nodular lesions. Courtesy of Dr. V. Ramesh.

Widespread erythematous papules and nodular and noduloulcerative lesions involving skin, nasal, oral, oropharyngeal, and laryngeal mucosa are also seen. Unusual forms include annular, hypertrophic, and rarely, xanthomatous forms (Figures 84-16 through 84-24).

Differential Diagnosis

Leprosy, diffuse cutaneous leishmaniasis, secondary syphilis, and sarcoidosis can simulate PKDL. In those with macules, pityriasis (tinea) vesicolor and vitiligo should be ruled out. A history of kala-azar and clustering of lesions in the central part of the face will point to the diagnosis.

Treatment

PKDL is refractory to treatment. Sodium antimony gluconate, at a dosage of 20 mg/kg up to a maximum of 850 mg/day, is given intramuscularly for 4 months. Ketoconazole, allopurinol, and amphotericin B can be added to improve the response. The hypopigmented macules may persist for a long time and may require PUVASOL on psoralen plus ultraviolet A (PUVA) therapy to aid their resolution.

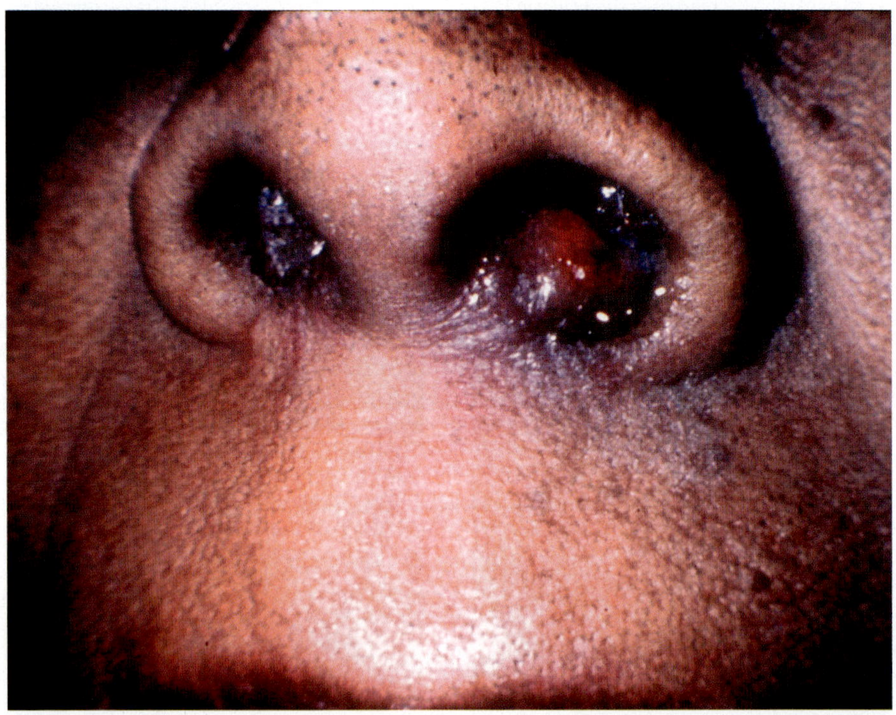

▲ **FIGURE 84-23** Latin America. Muco cutaneous leishmaniasis, early. Courtesy of Dr. Marcia Ramos-e-Silva.

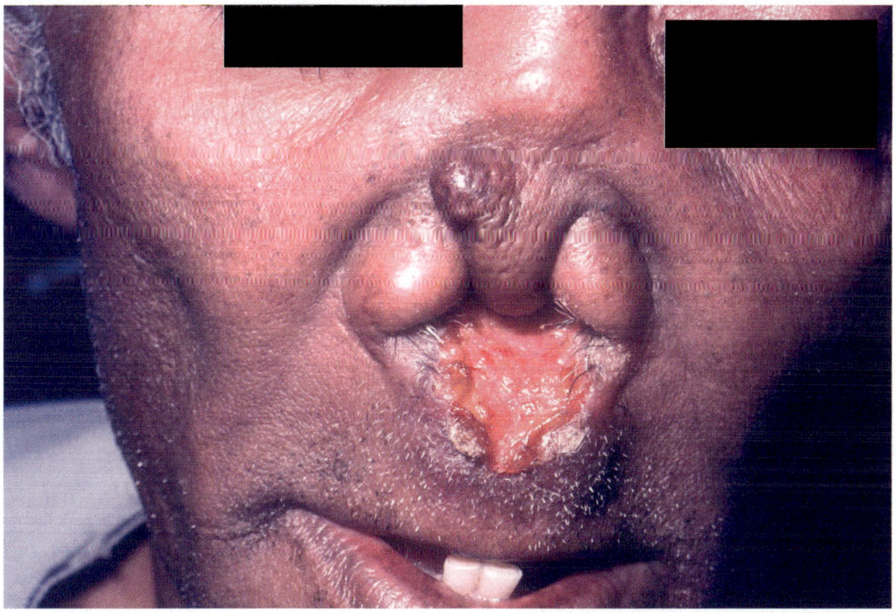

▲ **FIGURE 84-24** Latin America. Muco cutaneous Leishmaniasis, late. Courtesy of Dr. Marcia Ramos-e-Silva.

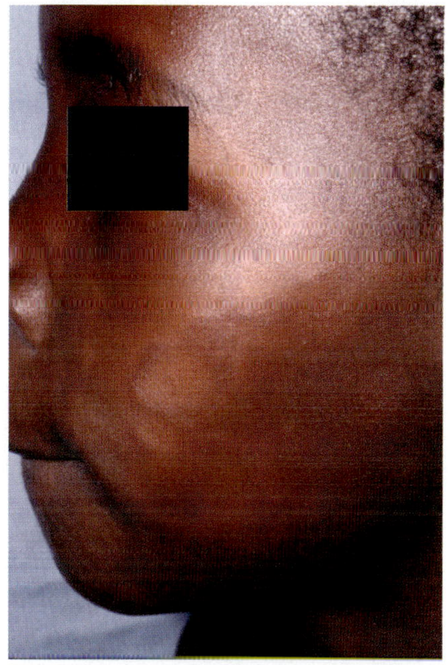

▲ **FIGURE 84-26** Africa. Mid-borderline leprosy. Multiple annular plaques. Courtesy of Dr. Barbara J. Leppard.

LEPROSY

Definition

Leprosy is a chronic granulomatous disease caused by *Mycobacterium leprae,* which affects primarily the peripheral nerves, skin, and other tissues such as the eye, the mucosa of the upper respiratory tract, the reticuloendothelial system, and the testes.

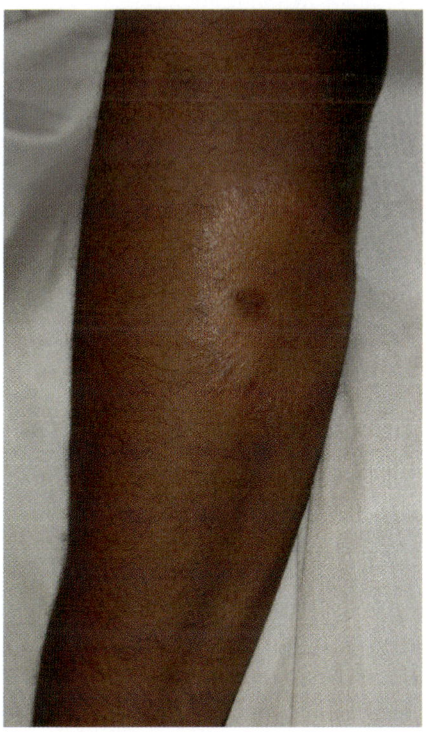

▲ **FIGURE 84-25** Africa. Tuberculoid leprosy. Single anesthetic plaque. Courtesy of Dr. Barbara J. Leppard.

Etiology

Leprosy is caused by *M. leprae,* and nasal discharges from untreated lepromatous leprosy patients who are often undiagnosed for several years are the main source of infection in the community. Leprosy has a long incubation period of up to 12 years. India dominates the global picture with one-third of the world's leprosy cases. Brazil, Myanmar, Indonesia, Madagascar, and Nepal are other countries where there are large numbers of leprosy cases.

Clinical Perspective

The characteristic clinical manifestations of leprosy are numb hypopigmented or

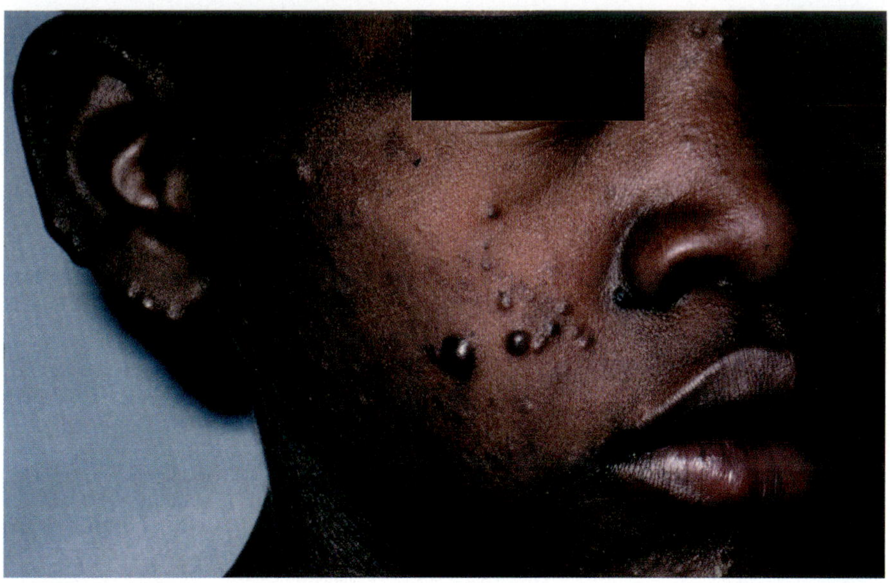

▲ **FIGURE 84-27** Africa. Lepromatous leprosy (LL). Multiple papules on the face and ears. Courtesy of Dr. Barbara J. Leppard.

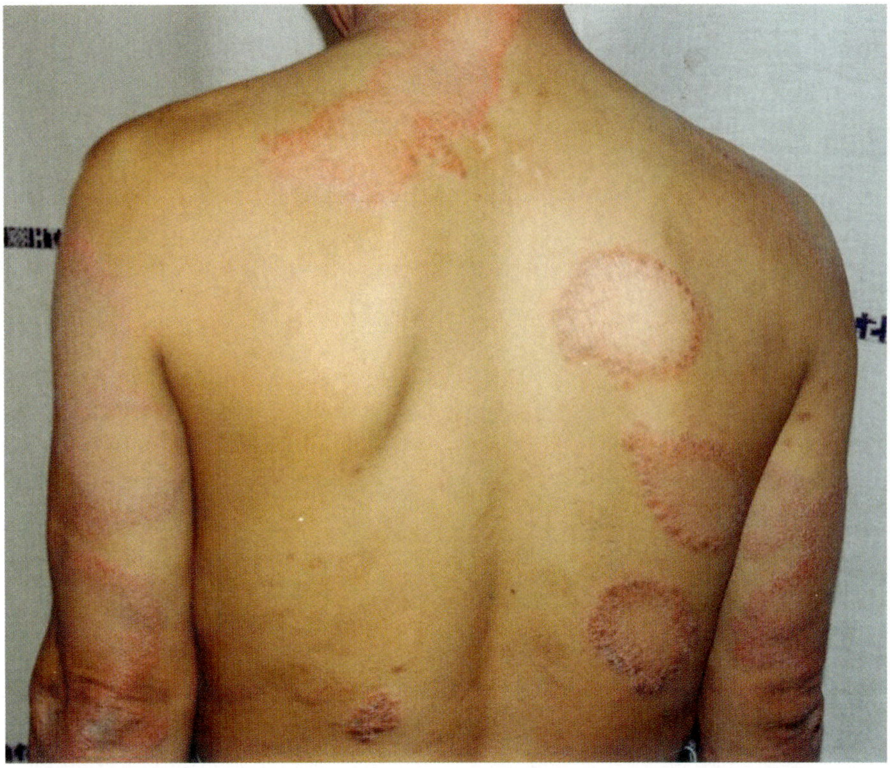

▲ **FIGURE 84-28** Asia. Borderline borderline leprosy. Courtesy of Dr. Rashmi Sarkar.

erythematous patches on the skin, thickened or enlarged peripheral nerves, and demonstration of acid-fast bacilli on slit-skin smear examination from skin lesions. It commonly presents as localized paresthesia in the hand or foot in the distribution of the nerve, shooting pains along the nerve, blisters on hands and feet, motor weakness or fatigue of grip of toes, nasal stuffiness, and epistaxis. According to the Ridley-Jopling classification of leprosy, tuberculoid and borderline tuberculoid lesions are hypopigmented or erythematous hypesthetic macules or plaques (Figures 84-25, 84-26, 84-29 and 84-32). Borderline borderline leprosy is unstable and has widespread bilateral but asymmetric erythematous infiltrated plaques with either a punched out appearance, geographic appearance, or irregular borders (Figure 84-28). Borderline lepromatous lesions are nodular, macular, or plaques. Lepromatous leprosy may have numerous uncountable, small, bilaterally symmetric, smooth, shiny, ill-defined macules that are hypopigmented, or there may be erythematous, progressive infiltration of the lesions, which may lead to formation of papules, nodules or plaques (Figures 84-27 and 84-33). If untreated, the skin becomes more infiltrated and shows a waxy appearance. Reactions in leprosy may present as type I, in which there is neuritis and sudden edema of existing lesions (Figure 84-30), or type II, erythema nodosum leprosum lesions, where there is sudden appearance of erythematous, evanescent lesions along with fever, arthritis, orchitis, and visual disturbances. In India, an Indian classification is followed because macular and maculoanesthetic lesions are seen throughout the spectrum; hence the subtypes are indeterminate, maculoanesthetic, tuberculoid, borderline, lepromatous and pure neuritic leprosy. Pure neuritic leprosy is a form of leprosy that has only nerve involvement and no skin lesions.

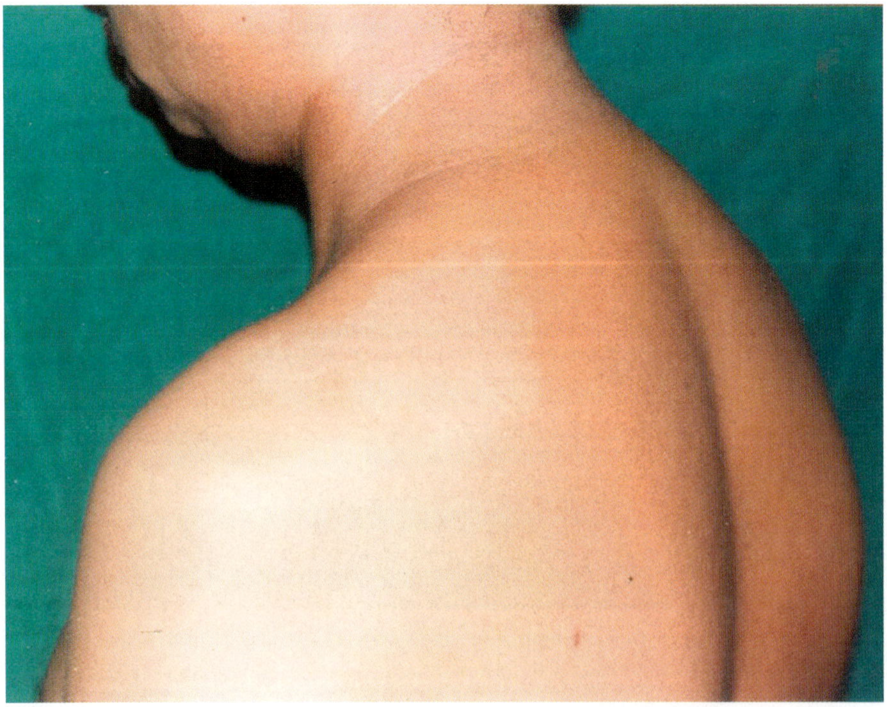

▲ **FIGURE 84-29** Asia. Borderline tuberculoid leprosy. Courtesy of Dr. Rashmi Sarkar.

Differential Diagnosis

Vitiligo can be differentiated by depigmented macules with normal sensation. Other granulomatous disorders, such as lupus vulgaris, sarcoidosis, syphilis, and leishmaniasis, have to be ruled out. Demonstration of acid-fast bacilli in slit-skin smear and skin biopsies, as well as loss of sensation or thickened nerves, points to the diagnosis.

Treatment Options

Multidrug therapy (MDT), introduced by World Health Organization (WHO) in 1982, is given for paucibacillary (PB) MDT as once-a-month rifampicin, 600 mg orally, and dapsone, 100 mg daily for 6 months, or as multibacillary (MB) MDT, in which clofazimine is given as 300 mg once monthly and 50 mg daily, in addition to the drugs of the PB MDT regime for 1 year. Reddish discoloration of skin owing to clofazimine is a condition that is difficult for dark-skinned patients to bear (Figure 84-31). Steroids, antimalarial agents, and thalidomide are given for reactions.

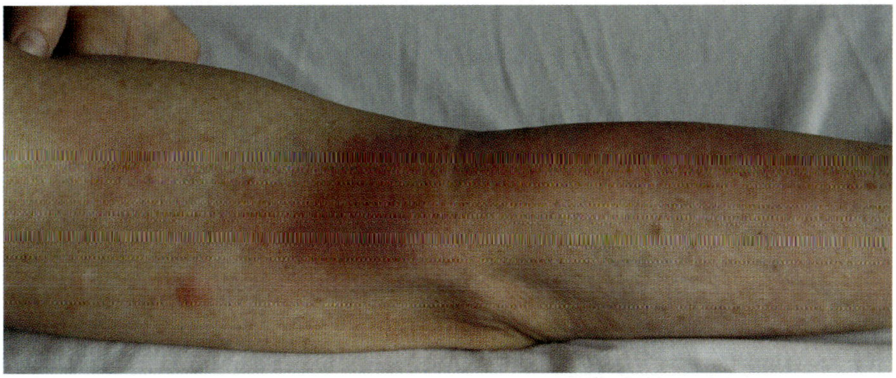

▲ **FIGURE 84-30** Asia. Borderline tuberculoid leprosy in reaction. Courtesy of Dr. Diqing Luo.

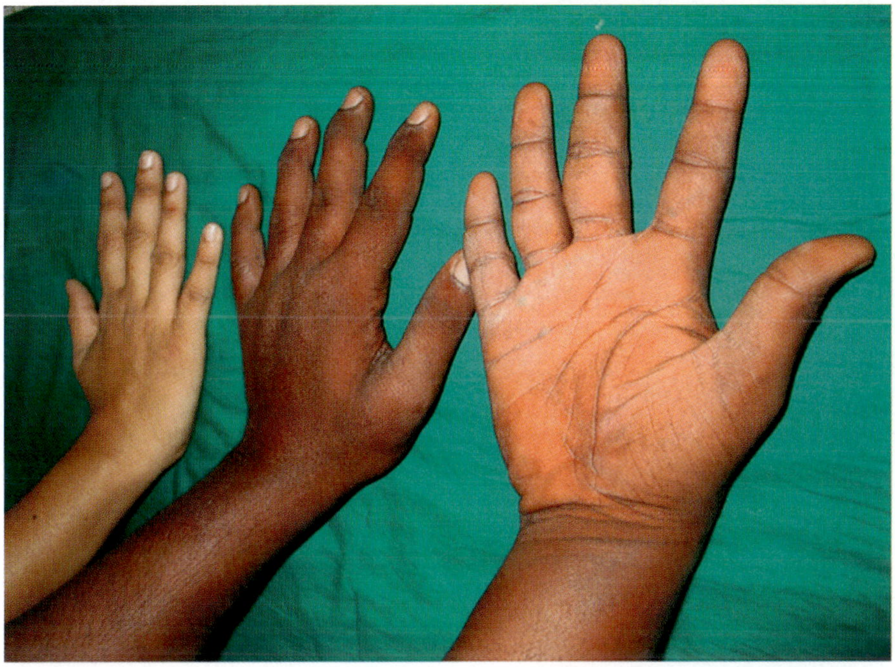

▲ **FIGURE 84-31** Asia. Sri Lankan patient on chofazimine. Courtesy of Dr. Prasad Kumarasinghe.

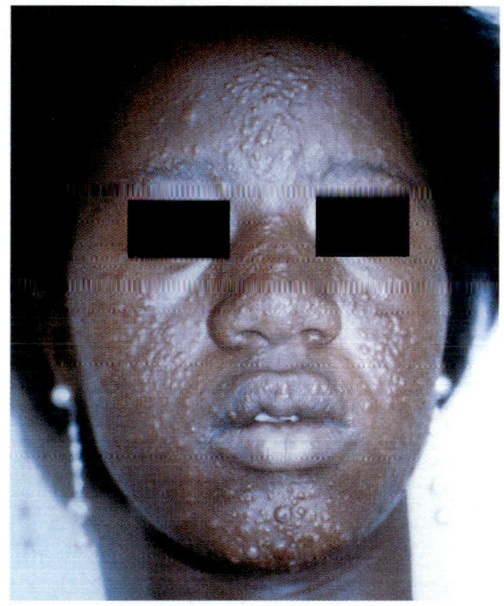

▲ **FIGURE 84-33** Latin America. Lepromatous leprosy. From Ramos-e-Silva M, Rebello P. Leprosy: Recognition and treatment. *Am J Clin Dermatol* 2001;2:203–211.

LEUKODERMA

Definition

Any condition characterized by hypomelanotic or amelanotic lesions is known as *leukoderma*. Vitiligo is a primary, usually progressive, symmetric disorder of depigmentation of unknown etiology.

Etiology

The highest incidence of vitiligo has been recorded in India and Mexico. The incidence is 3–4% in India. A genetic role is implicated in its pathogenesis. Familial incidence is from 20–30%. The mode of

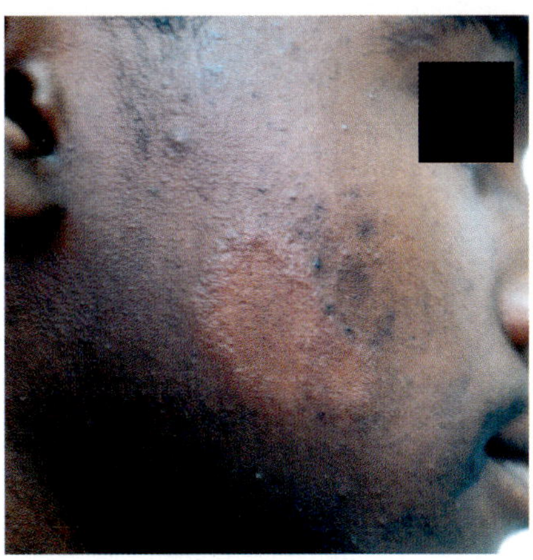

▲ **FIGURE 84-32** Latin America. Tuberculoid leprosy. From Ramos-e-Silva M, Rebello P. Leprosy: Recognition and treatment. *Am J Clin Dermatol* 2001;2:203–211.

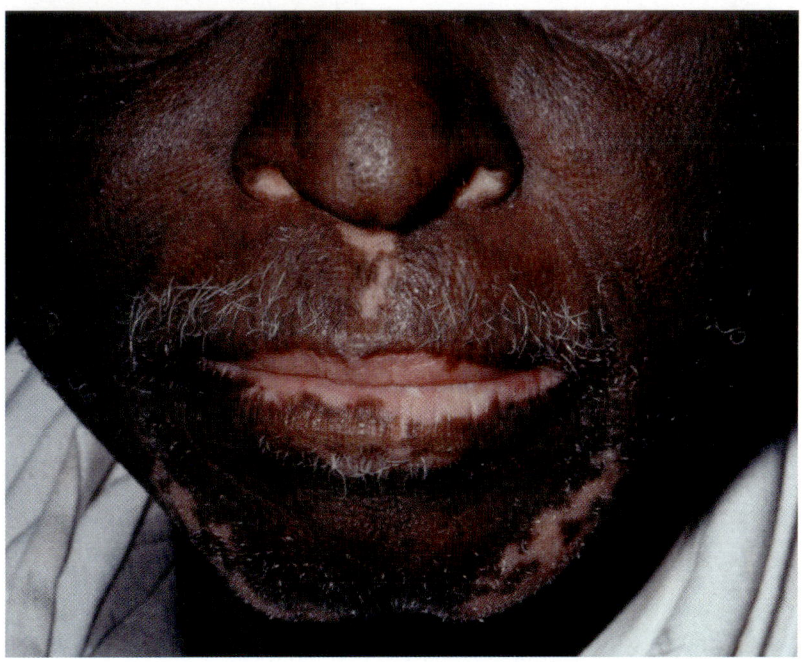

▲ **FIGURE 84-34** Africa. Vitiligo, face. This is a huge cosmetic problem. Courtesy of Dr. Barbara J. Leppard.

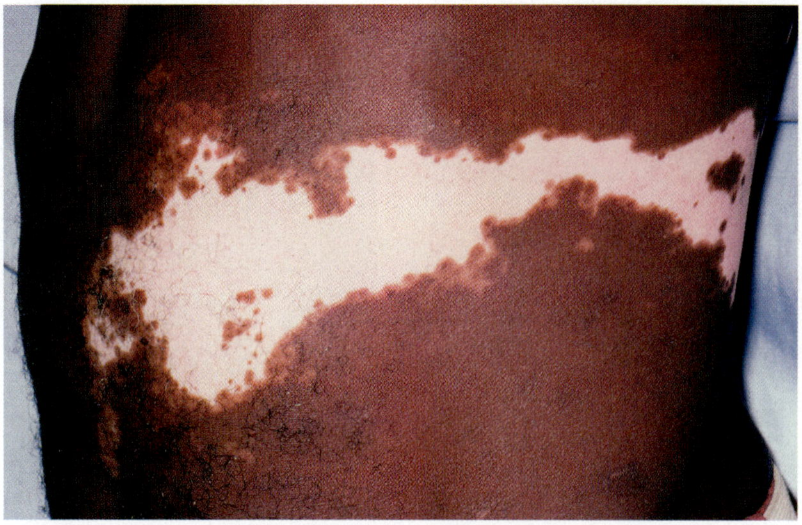

▲ **FIGURE 84-35** Africa. Segmented vitiligo. Courtesy of Dr. Barbara J. Leppard.

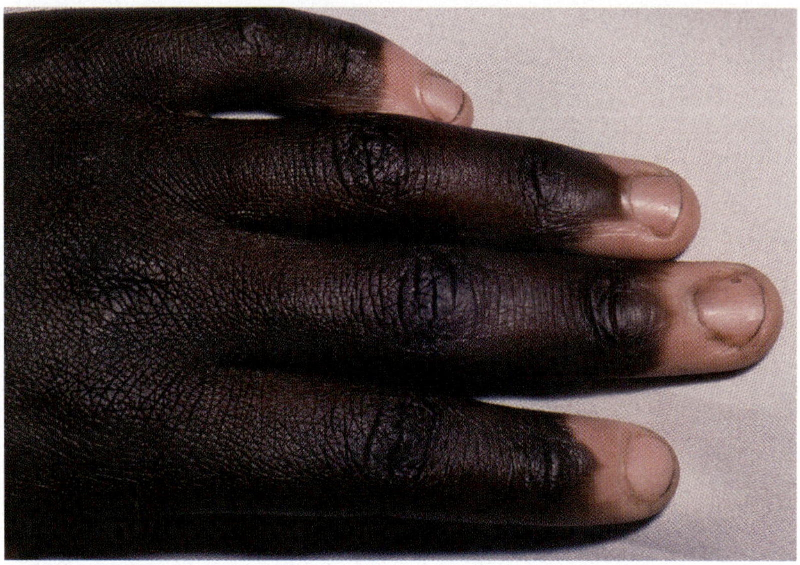

▲ **FIGURE 84-36** Africa. Vitiligo. Distal fingers will not repigment. Courtesy of Dr. Barbara J. Leppard.

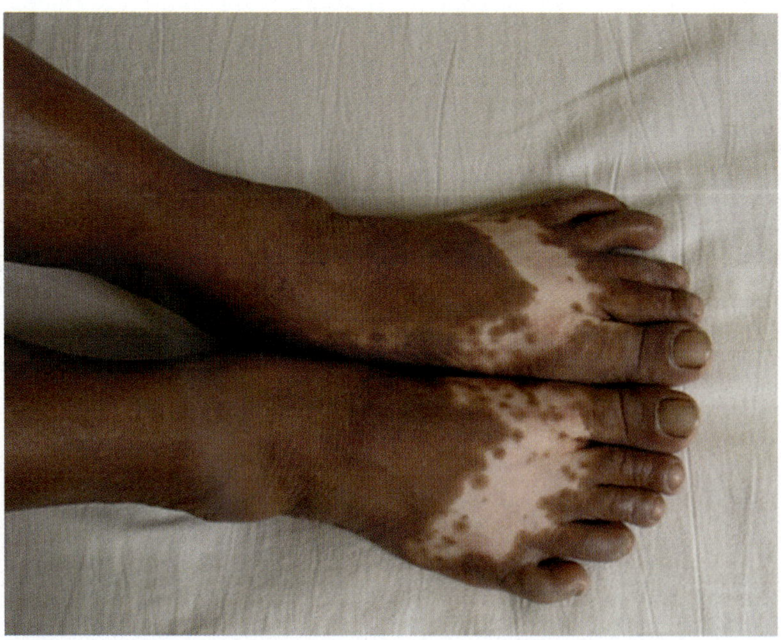

▲ **FIGURE 84-37** Asia. Chemical leukoderma. Courtesy of Dr. Prasad Kumarasinghe.

inheritance is autosomal dominant, although autosomal recessive or polygenic inheritance also has been suggested. An autoimmune etiology also has been suggested owing to associations with thyroid disease, diabetes mellitus, alopecia areata, and pernicious anemia. A neural autotoxic self-destructive hypothesis is also suggested. Onset of the unilateral dermatomal type is usually seen in childhood within the first 10 years, whereas the onset of vitiligo vulgaris is in the second to fourth decades of life.

Clinical Perspective

A typical lesion of vitiligo is a well-defined depigmented macule often associated with leukotrichia (Figures 84-34 through 84-36, Figures 84-39 and 84-40). Trichrome vitiligo discribes a depigmented area surrounded by a comparatively hypopig-mented zone that is separated from normal skin by a thin hyperpigmented rim. Vitiligo vulgaris is one of the common types of vitiligo seen in Asia. The disease is associated with a great deal of psychological and social stress in Asian patients.

Differential Diagnosis

Bilateral lesions of vitiligo have to be differentiated from piebaldism (white forelock present at birth). Chemical leukoderma can be differentiated because it will be confined to the area of contact with certain chemicals. Chemical leukoderma owing to bindi (a decorative mark worn on the forehead in Indian women) and footwear is common (Figures 84-37 and 84-38). Pityriasis alba affects primarily the face and is slightly scaly.

Treatment Options

The treatment of vitiligo will depend on the extent of clinical involvement. For localized vitiligo (<2% body surface area), topical corticosteroids and topical calcineurin inhibitors (e.g., tacrolimus or pimecrolimus) are usually given. For involvement of more than 2% body surface area or generalized vitiligo, oral pulse corticosteroids, narrow-band UVB, PUVA therapy, khellin therapy, phenylalanine, placental extract, cyclophosphamide, and levamisole can be used. In selected cases of stable vitiligo, surgery in the form of punch grafting, surgical excision, minigrafting, thin Thiersch grafting, and suction blister grafting may be attempted. Psychological counseling is an important part of therapy, along with cosmetic camouflage.

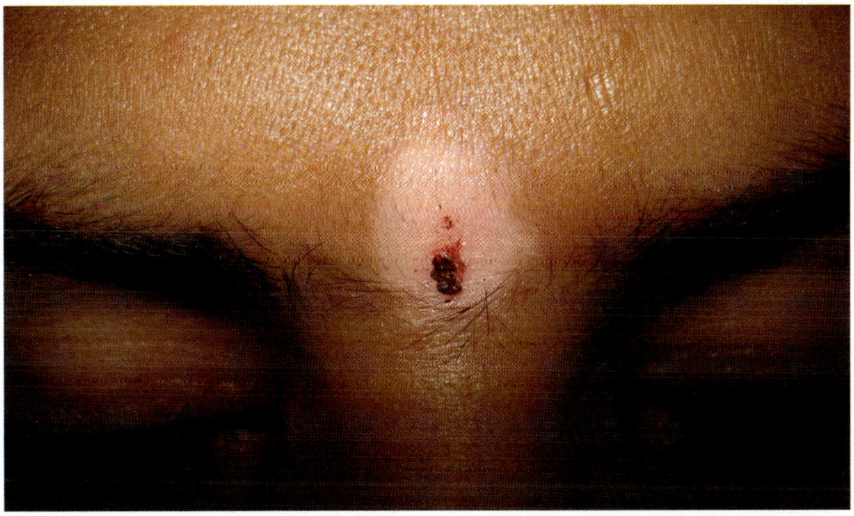

▲ **FIGURE 84-38** Asia. Chemical leucoderma owing Bindi application. Courtesy of Dr. Sudhanshu Sharma.

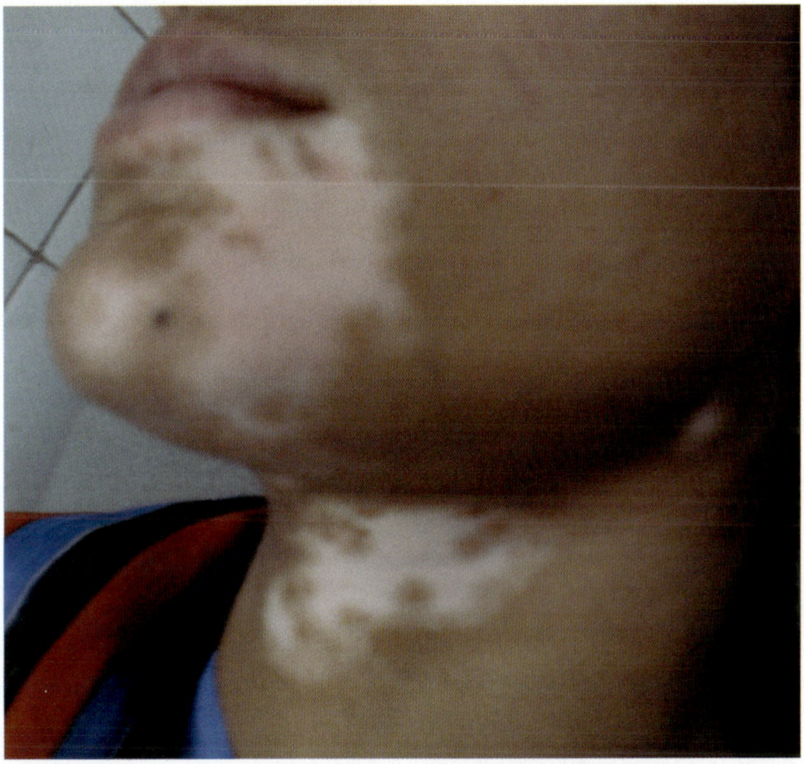

▲ **FIGURE 84-39** Asia. Segmental vitiligo. Courtesy of Dr. Sudhanshu Sharma.

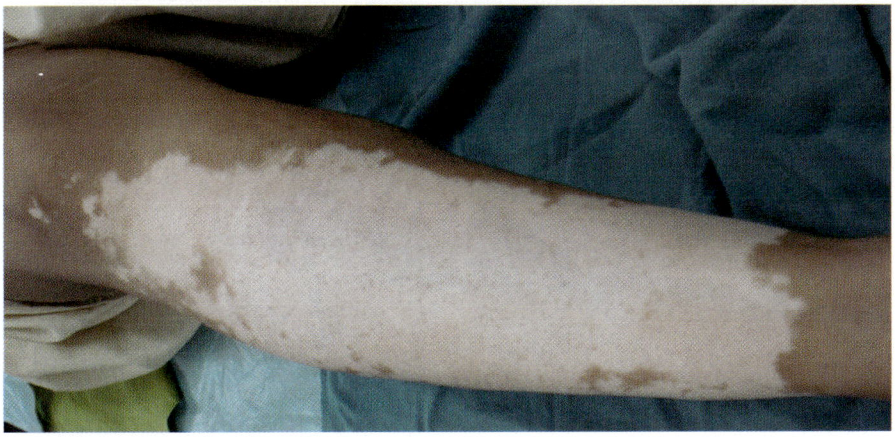

▲ **FIGURE 84-40** Asia. Vitiligo. Courtesy of Dr. Sudhanshu Sharma.

LICHEN NITIDUS

Definition

Lichen nitidus consists of tiny, nonpruritic, shiny flat-topped papules present on the arms, abdomen, and penis.

Etiology

Some believe lichen nitidus to be a variant of lichen planus, yet others believe it to be a distinct entity. Most cases occur in children and young adults. There are also reports of familial lichen planus. It seems to occur more frequently in dark-skinned patients. It also has been associated with Crohn disease and atopic dermatitis.

Clinical Perspective

Lichen nitidus consists of pinhead-sized, round or polygonal, skin-colored papules present on the shaft and glans of the penis, lower abdomen, groin, breasts, and flexor surfaces of the arms and wrists (Figures 84-41 through 84-43). Oral and nail lesions are rare.

Differential Diagnosis

Lichen planus can be differentiated by the presence of pruritic, violaceous papules. Keratosis pilaris has lesions on the extensor surfaces of the arms. Lichen scrofulosorum has both follicular and interfollicular lesions and a positive tuberculin test.

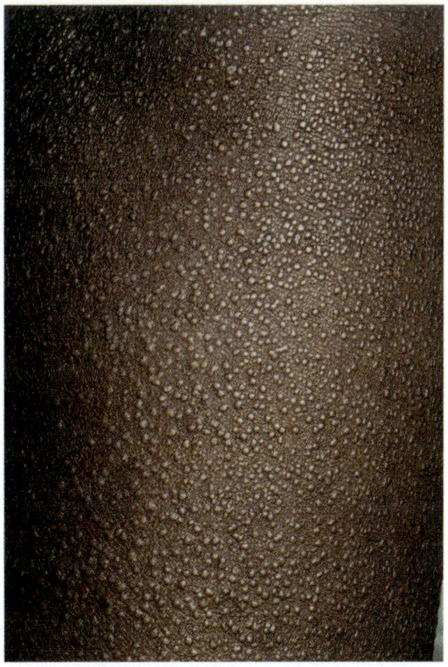

▲ **FIGURE 84-41** Africa. Tiny flat-topped papules of lichen nitidus. Courtesy of Dr. Barbara J. Leppard.

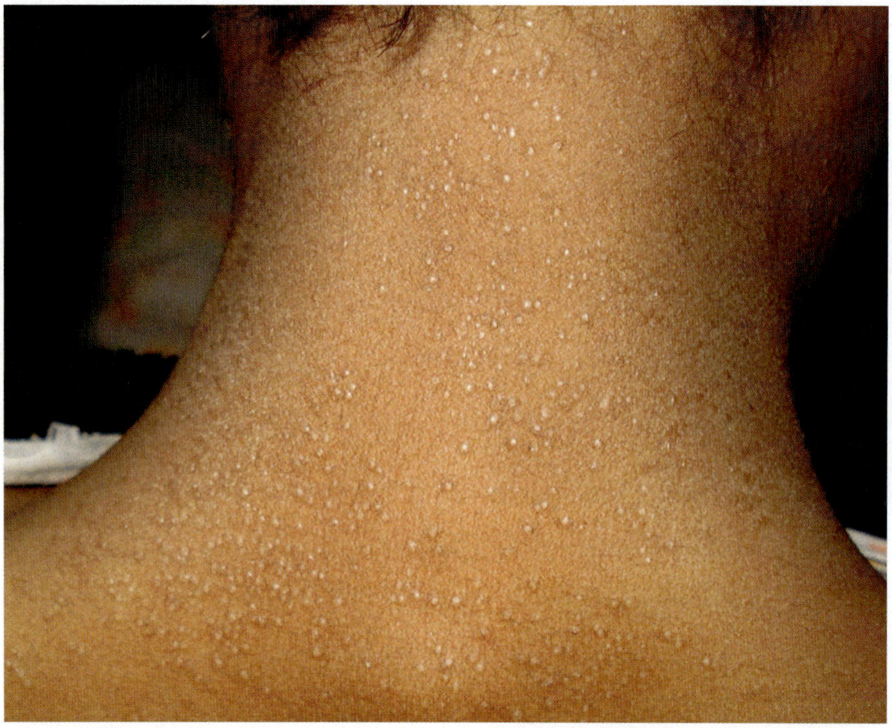

▲ **FIGURE 84-42** Asia. Lichen nitidus. Courtesy of Dr. Sudhanshu Sharma.

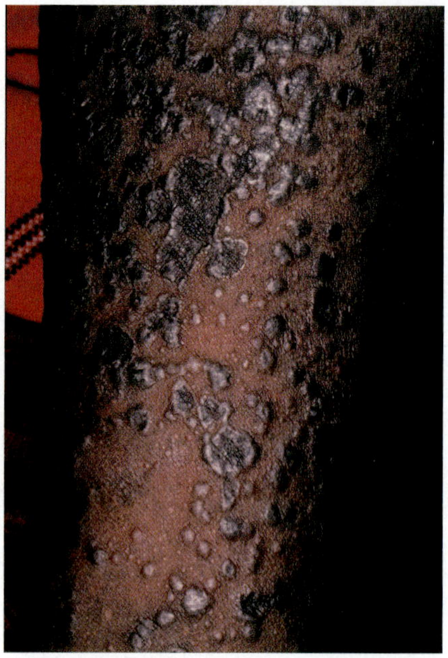

▲ **FIGURE 84-44** Africa. Lichen planus. Very distinctive navy blue hyperpigmentation. Courtesy of Dr. Barbara J. Leppard.

Treatment Options

Lichen nitidus can undergo spontaneous resolution after many years. No treatment is required in most cases. Topical steroids, photochemotherapy, astemizole, cetirizine, and levamisole are other treatment options.

LICHEN PLANUS

Definition

Lichen planus is a distinctive papulosquamous disorder characterized by pruritic, violaceous papular lesions involving the skin, mucous membranes, hair, and nails.

Etiology

The etiology of lichen planus is unknown. Viruses, drugs, and contact with certain chemicals such as color film developer may act as precipitating causes.

Clinical Perspective

The lesions are violaceous, polygonal, shining, flat-topped papules that are intensely pruritic (Figures 84-44 through 84-47 and Figure 84-50). They involve the flexural areas, the wrists, the lumbar region, and the ankles. The clinical variants are hypertrophic, actinic, linear, annular, atrophic, guttate, follicular, ulcerative, bullous, and Graham Little syndrome. Oral lichen planus is seen in 4–12% patients and nail lichen planus in 10% of patients. Two characteristic types seen in Asia are actinic lichen planus and lichen planus pigmentosus

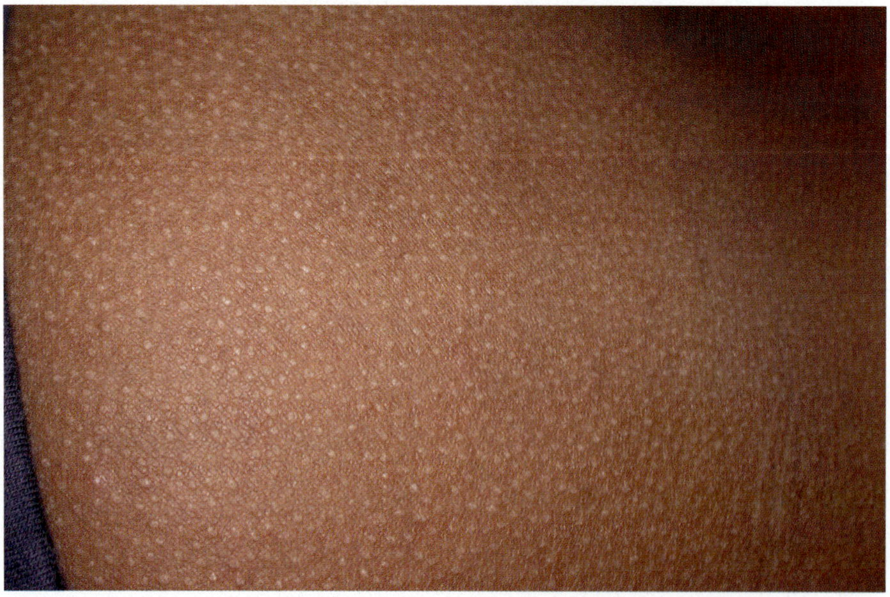

▲ **FIGURE 84-43** Latin America. Lichen nitidus. Courtesy of Dr. Marcia Ramos-e-Silva.

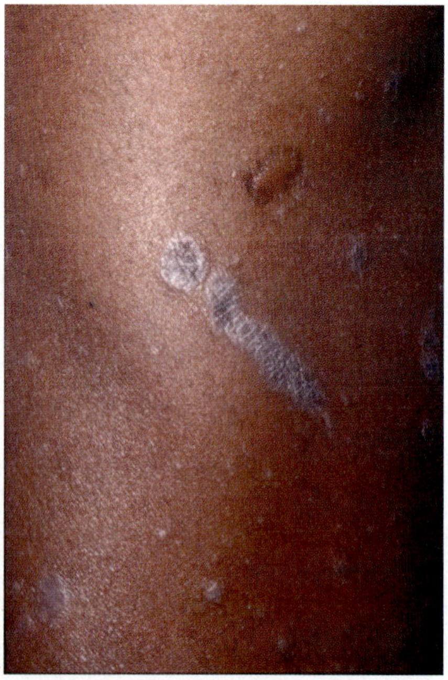

▲ **FIGURE 84-45** Africa. Koebner phenomenon. Courtesy of Dr. Barbara J. Leppard.

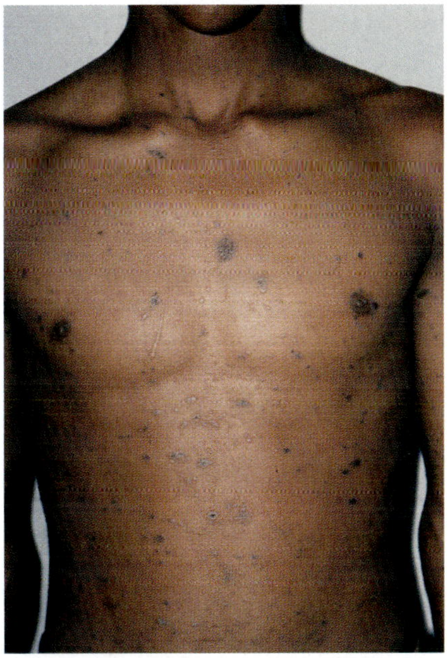

▲ **FIGURE 84-46** Africa. Lichen planus. Courtesy of Dr. Barbara J. Leppard.

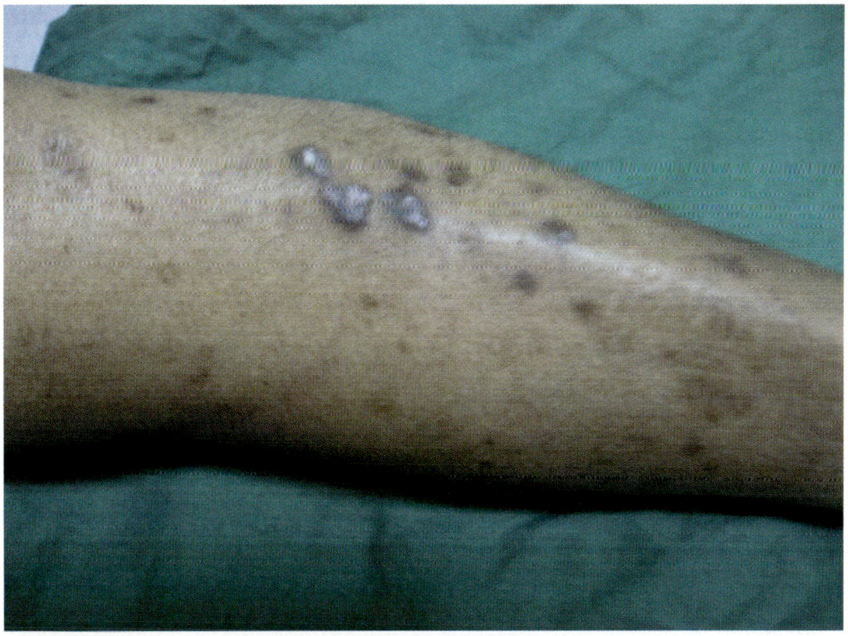

▲ **FIGURE 84-47** Asia. Classic lichen planus. Courtesy of Dr. Rashmi Sarkar.

(Figure 84-48). Actinic lichen planus has a predilection for the Middle East, India, and East Africa. Sunlight appears to be a precipitating factor. The lesions are well-defined, bluish brown, nummular patches with a fine, slightly raised, pale margin, giving them an annular appearance, and they are present on the lateral aspects of forehead, hands, forearm, lower lip, cheeks, and neck (Figure 84-49). Lichen planus pigmentosus, another variant, has been mainly reported from India. It presents as multiple, discrete, hyperpigmented macules on the trunk, upper limbs, and face (Figure 84-48).

Differential Diagnosis

Other papulosquamous disorders have to be ruled out. Psoriasis has a characteristic red color, has thick scales, and is seen more on extensors.

Treatment Options

Since the disease is benign and self-limited, treatment is symptomatic. Topical, intralesional, and systemic corticosteroids may be used. Retinoids, cyclosporine, PUVA, dapsone, and griseofulvin are other options.

LUPUS VULGARIS

Definition

Lupus vulgaris is the most common form of cutaneous tuberculosis caused by *Mycobacterium tuberculosis,* which is usually acquired by an exogenous source.

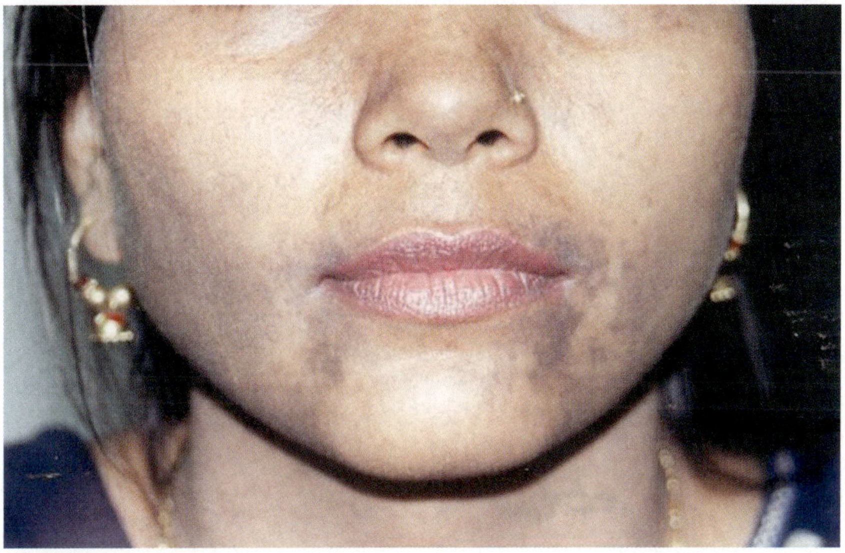

▲ **FIGURE 84-48** Asia. Lichen planus pigmentosus. Courtesy of Dr. Rashmi Sarkar.

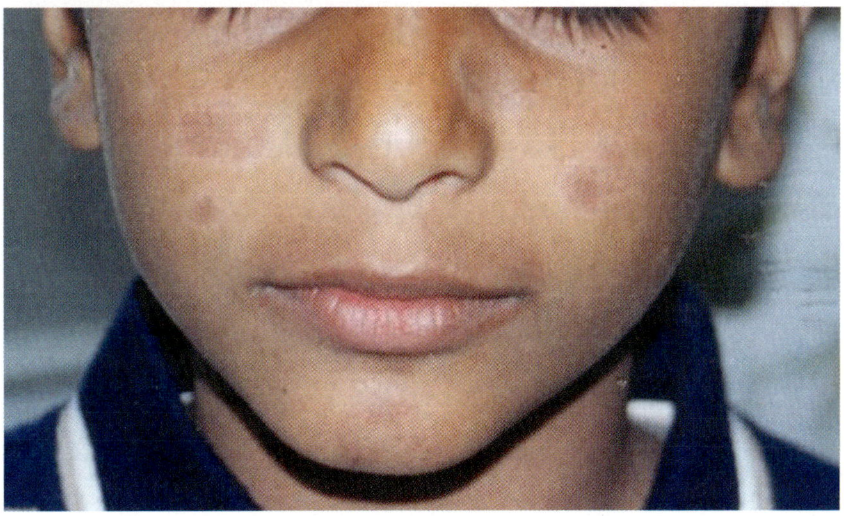

▲ **FIGURE 84-49** Asia. Lichen planus actinicus. Courtesy of Dr. Rashmi Sarkar.

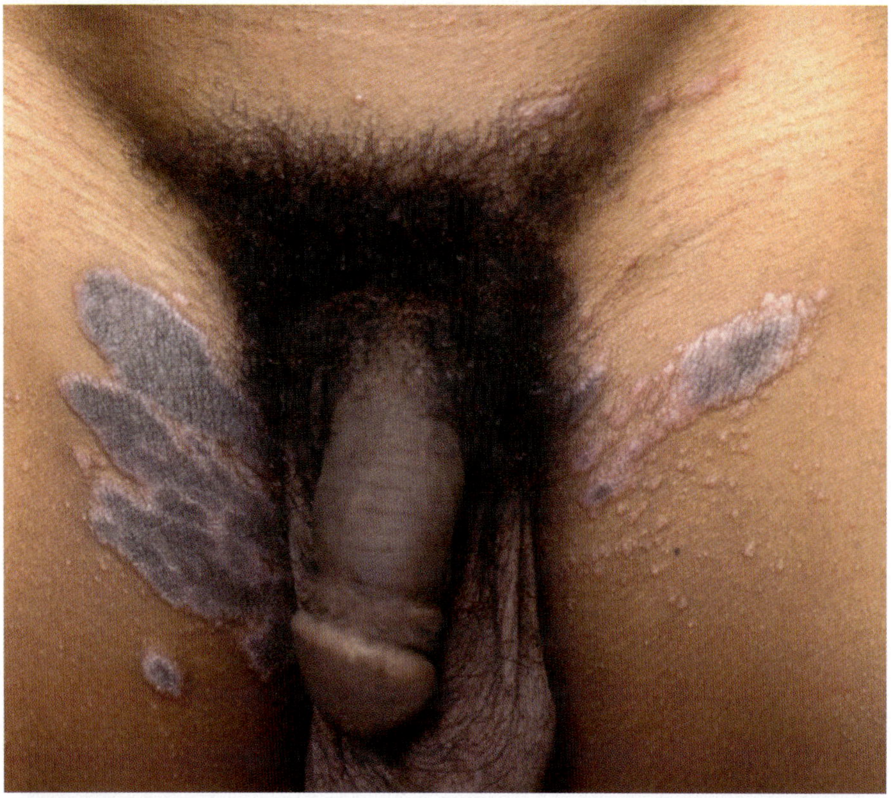

▲ **FIGURE 84-50** Latin America. Lichen planus. Courtesy of Dr. Marcia Ramos-e-Silva.

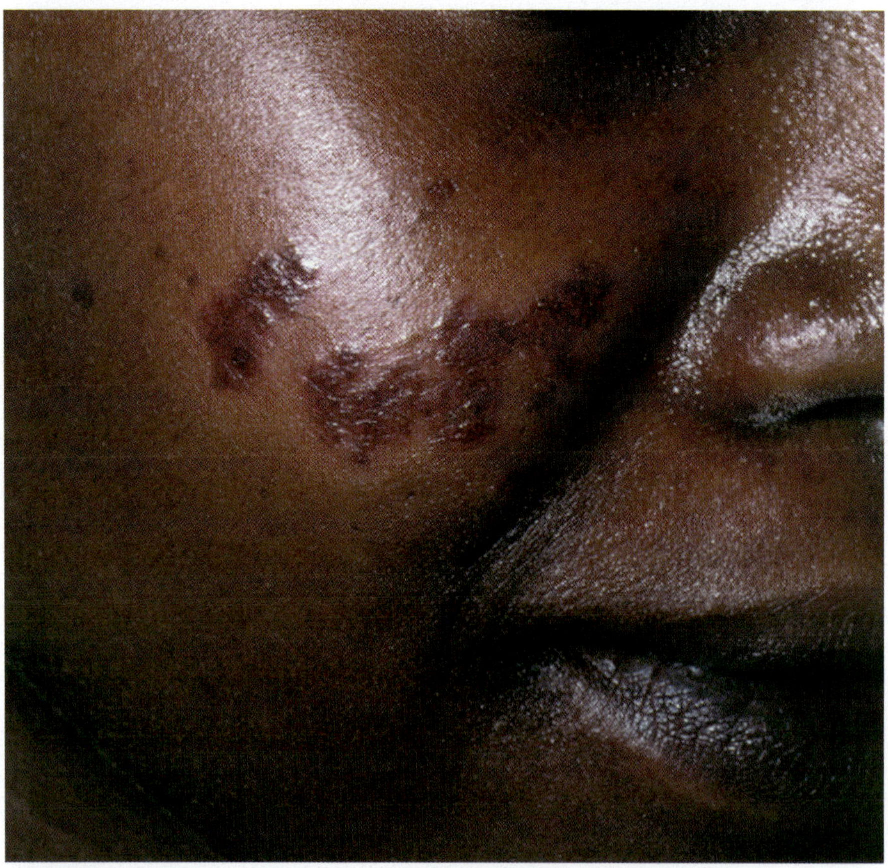

▲ **FIGURE 84-51** Africa. Lupus vulgaris. Courtesy of Dr. Barbara J. Leppard.

Etiology

This type of post–primary cutaneous tuberculosis is acquired from an exogenous source, although it also may arise from hematogenous dissemination of *M. tuberculosis* in the body. These patients have a moderate or high degree of immunity against tubercle bacilli. The disease also may be due to progress of tuberculosis, chance, or as a result of bacille Calmette-Guérin (BCG) vaccination, rarely.

Clinical Perspective

The face, buttocks, thighs, and legs are the most common sites of involvement (Figures 84-51 through 84-53). The lesion starts as a few soft nodules, which may coalesce to form a plaque. The typical "apple jelly" nodules cannot be appreciated in dark skin (Figure 84-51). The disease progresses with irregular extension of the plaque, which may heal with superficial scarring. Sometimes there can be ulceration, crusting, and scarring with destruction of underlying tissues and cartilage.

Differential Diagnosis

Lupus vulgaris has to be differentiated from other granulomatous conditions, for example, leprosy, leishmaniasis, sarcoidosis, and syphilitic gumma. The clinical features, tuberculin reaction, histology, and demonstration of acid-fast bacilli, as well as the presence of active tuberculosis elsewhere in the body, will lead to the suspicion of tuberculosis.

Treatment Options

Antitubercular therapy consisting of a 2-month initial phase of rifampicin, isonazid, pyrinamide, and ethambutol is given, followed by a 4-month continuation phase with isoniazed and rifampicin as a short-course regimen. The period of treatment also can be for 7–8 months.

MELASMA

Definition

This is a common, acquired, hyperpigmentation characterized by symmetrically distributed medium to dark patches on sun-exposed areas such as the forehead, cheeks, temples, and upper lip (Figures 84-54 through 84-56).

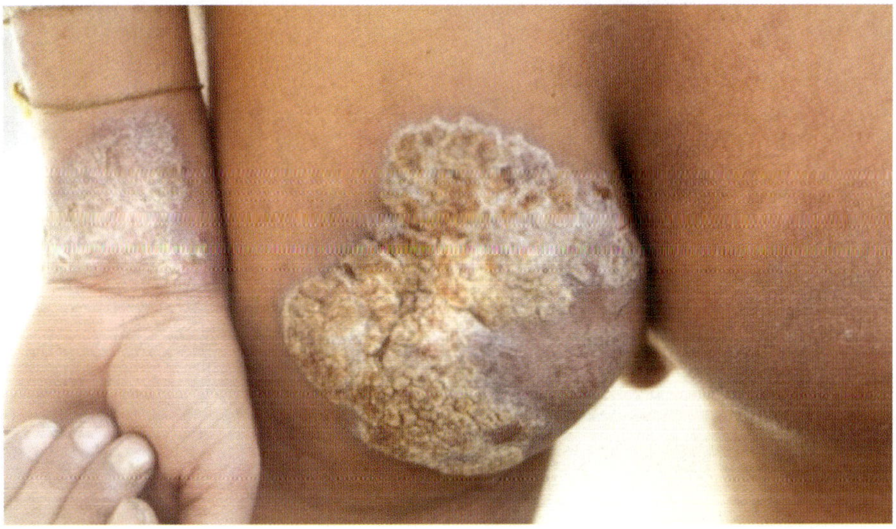

▲ **FIGURE 84-52** Asia. Lupus vulgaris. Courtesy of Dr. V. Ramesh.

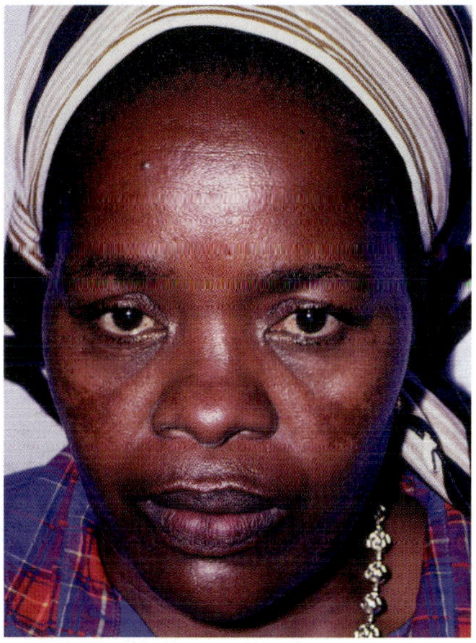

▲ **FIGURE 84-54** Africa. Melasma on the cheeks. Note the well-defined but irregular outline of the hyperpigmentation. Courtesy of Dr. Barbara J. Leppard.

Etiology

It is seen commonly in dark-skinned patients such as Asians, Hispanics, and blacks, though persons of any race may be affected. Women of childbearing age are affected predominantly (90%), but men also may be affected. Overall, in India, one in six patients may be affected with melasma. In Iraq, 33% patients are affected. Melasma occurs in genetically predisposed individuals. In addition, sunlight exposure, pregnancy, hormones, cosmetics, and drugs (e.g., phenytoin) are important factors in the development of melasma. Melasma is also seen frequently in persons residing in hilly regions of Nepal and Bhutan.

Clinical Perspective

The light to dark brown hyperpigmentation may be distributed in a centrofacial pattern (63%), with pigmentation confined to cheeks, forehead, upper lip, nose, and chin; a malar pattern (21%), affecting the cheeks and nose; and a mandibular pattern (16%), affecting the ramus of the mandible. Wood's lamp examination helps to identify the lesions as epidermal, dermal, mixed, or epidermal-dermal types. Histopathologically, the lesions are classified as epidermal, dermal, and mixed types.

Differential Diagnosis

This disease would have to be differentiated from other types of facial hyperpigmentation, such as lichen planus pigmentosus (violaceous or slate-gray color) and toxic melanosis (occurring in workers with tar, coal tar products, mineral oils, etc.), that occurs commonly in Asians.

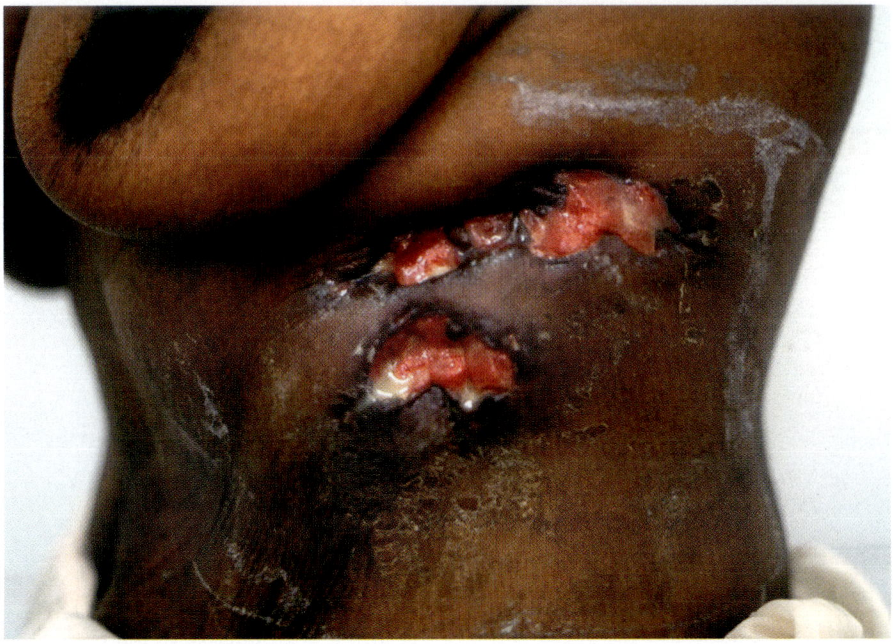

▲ **FIGURE 84-53** Latin America. Cutaneous tuberculosis. Courtesy of Dr. Marcia Ramos-e-Silva.

Treatment Options

The epidermal variety of melasma is readily responsive to treatment. Melasma of pregnancy (chloasma) also fades away within a few months of delivery. Discontinuation of provoking factors and the use of broad-spectrum sunscreens are cornerstones of treatment. Topical depigmenting agents such as hydroquinone, kojic aicd, azelaic acid, glycolic acid, tretinoin, arbutin, lactic acid, and fluorinated steroids have been used. Triple-combination therapy consisting of retinoic acid (0.025–0.05%), hydroquinone (2–4%), and hydrocortisone 1% or mometasone furoate is a popular form of treatment. Other modalities include chemical peels (e.g., glycolic acid and salicylic acid) either alone or in combination with topical therapy and fractional laser therapy.

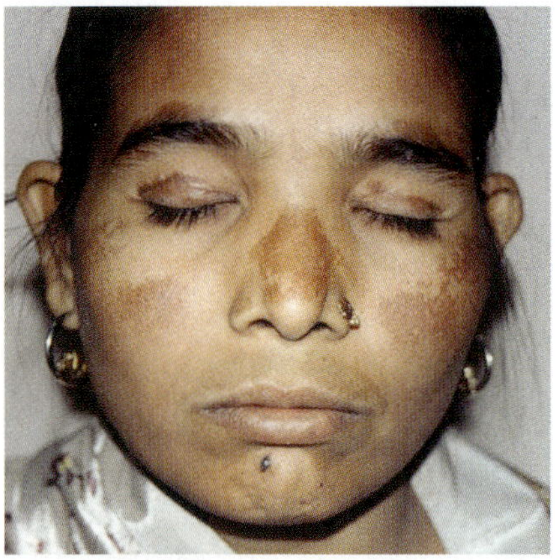

▲ **FIGURE 84-55** Asia. Melasma. Courtesy of Dr. Rashmi Sarkar.

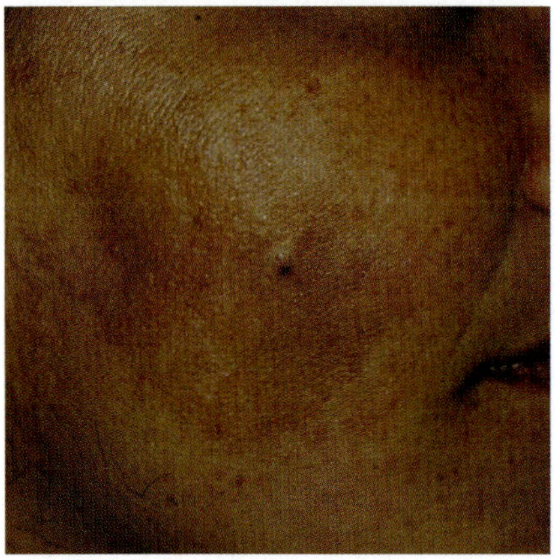

▲ **FIGURE 84-56** Latin America. Melasma. Courtesy of Dr. Marcia Ramos-e-Silva.

MONGOLIAN SPOT

Definition

The Mongolian spot is a congenital blue-gray patch usually located lumbosacrally (Figures 84-57 and 84-58).

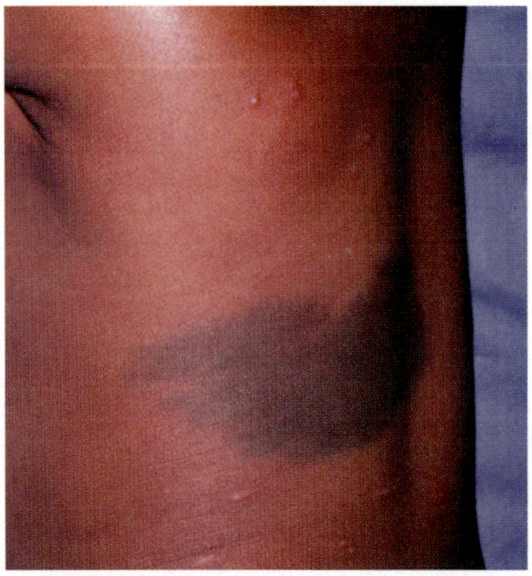

▲ **FIGURE 84-57** Africa. Mongolian spot. Courtesy of Dr. Barbara J. Leppard.

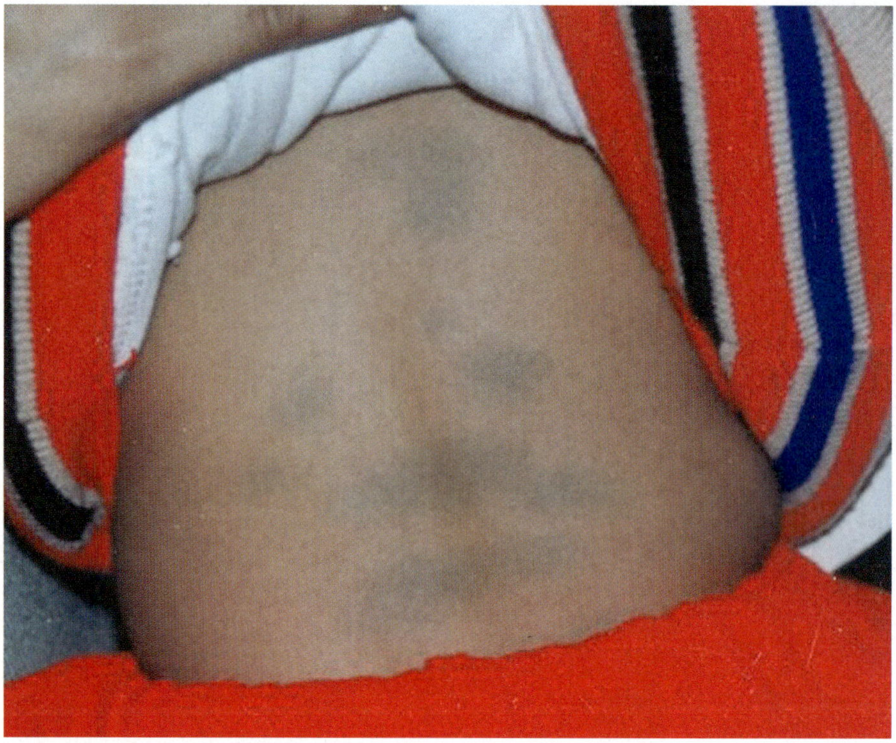

▲ **FIGURE 84-58** Asia. Mongolian spot. Courtesy of Dr. Rashmi Sarkar.

Etiology

The pigmentation is due to melanocytes in the dermis owing to failure of the melanocytes to complete their migration from the neural crest of the developing embryo to their proper location in the basal layer of the epidermis. The affected areas have a slate-brown or blue color (ceruloderma) owing to an optical effect from the pigment lying in the dermis. They are found in up to 90% of Asian babies.

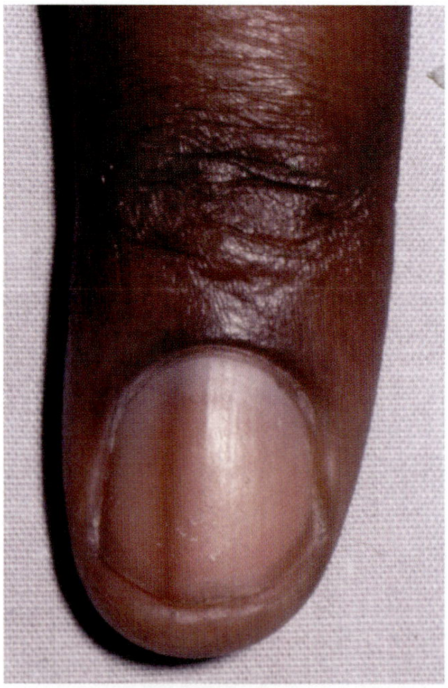

▲ **FIGURE 84-59** Africa. Junctional nevus of the nail matrix. Courtesy of Dr. Barbara J. Leppard.

Clinical Perspective

The lesions are poorly circumscribed areas of slate-brown or blue-black pigmentation that are sometimes extensive. Multiple lesions also may be located in sites other than the lumbosacral region. They may fade in early childhood, although aberrant extrasacral spots may persist.

Differential Diagnosis

Mongolian spot may have to be differentiated from a bruise.

Treatment Options

The parents have to be reassured that the lesions disappear with time.

NAIL PIGMENTATION

Definition

Modification of the color of the nail can be a normal variant in dark-skinned patients.

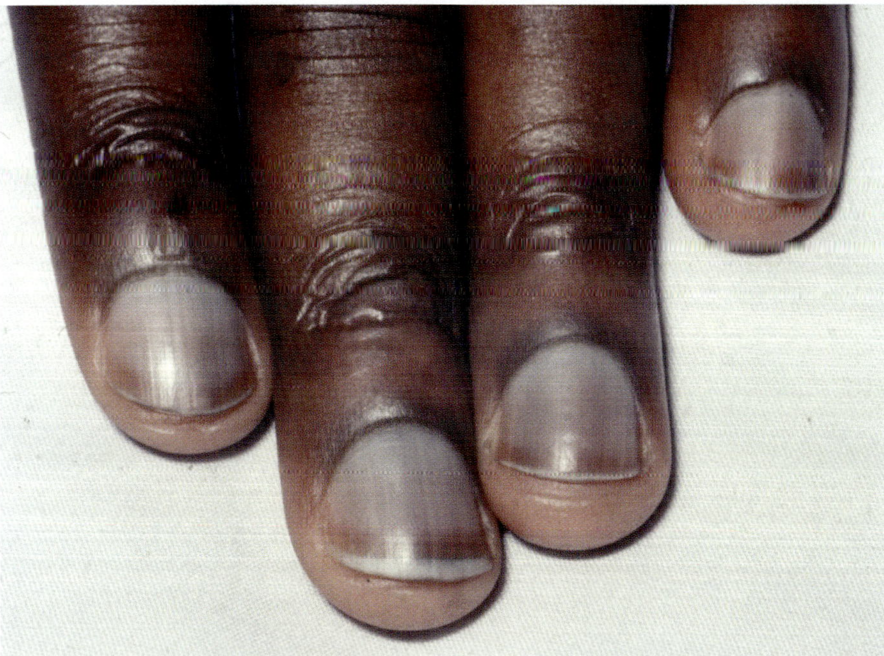

▲ **FIGURE 84-60** Africa. Diffuse blue discoloration of nails in this 32-year-old man was the first sign of human immunodeficiency virus (HIV) infection. He was on no drugs. Courtesy of Dr. Barbara J. Leppard.

Etiology

Nail pigmentation can be a normal pigment variation in Asians. It also can occur during pregnancy and menstruation.

Clinical Perspective

Nail pigmentation may be distributed as linear streaks of diffuse pigmentation of the nails, which may be bilaterally distributed. The nails on the thumb and index finger are mostly affected.

Differential Diagnosis

Nail pigmentation that occurs as a normal variant in dark-skinned patients must be differentiated from drug-induced nail pigmentation (e.g., zidovudine, antimalarials, and bleomycin), systemic diseases (Addison disease), and melanoma (single, unilateral lesion).

Treatment Options

The patient has to be reassured.

NEVUS OF OTA

Definition

Nevus of Ota is a benign hyperpigmentation that affects one side of the face in the region supplied by the ophthalmic and maxillary divisions of the trigeminal nerve (Figures 84-64 through 84-67).

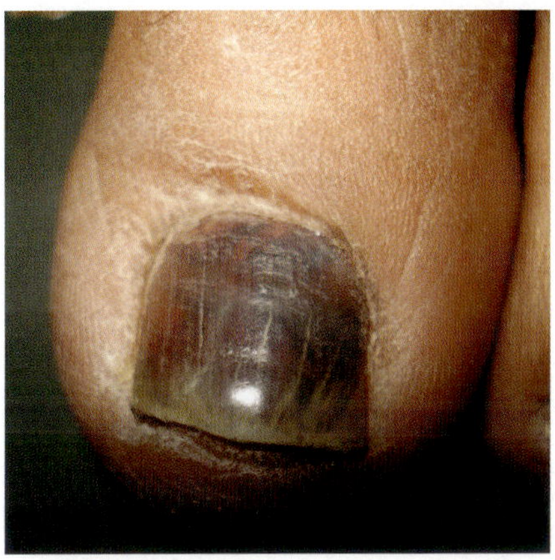

▲ **FIGURE 84-61** Asia. Nail pigmentation. Courtesy of Dr. Sudhanshu Sharma.

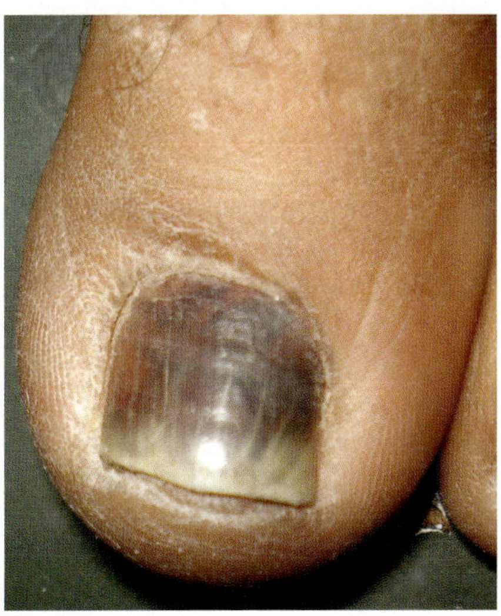

▲ **FIGURE 84-62** Asia. Nail pigmentation. Courtesy of Dr. Sudhanshu Sharma.

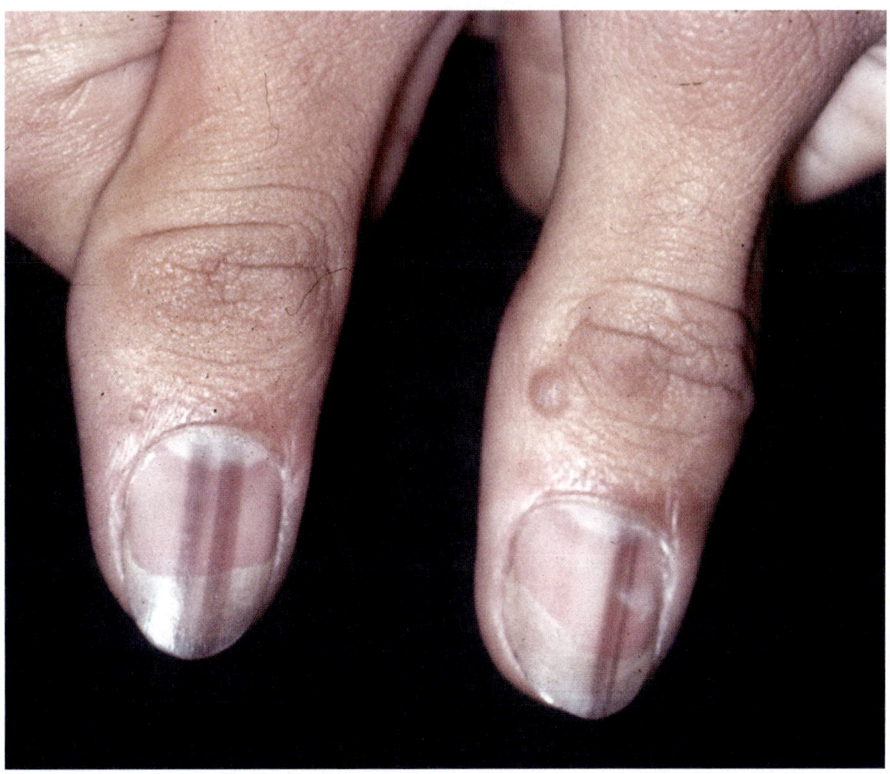

▲ **FIGURE 84-63** Latin America. Nail pigmentation. Courtesy of Dr. Marcia Ramos-e-Silva.

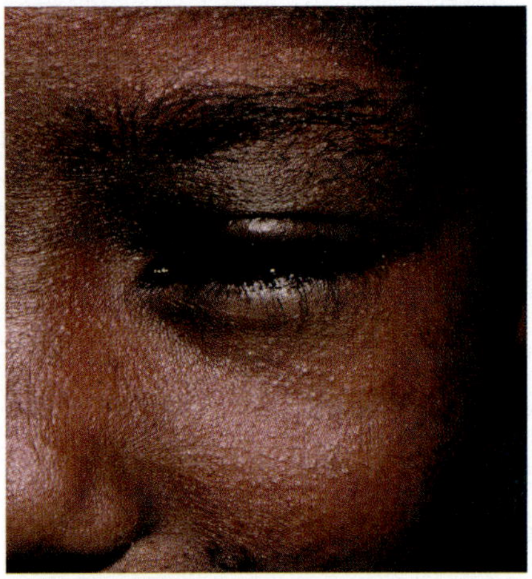

▲ **FIGURE 84-64** Africa. Nevus of Ota. Courtesy of Dr. Barbara J. Leppard.

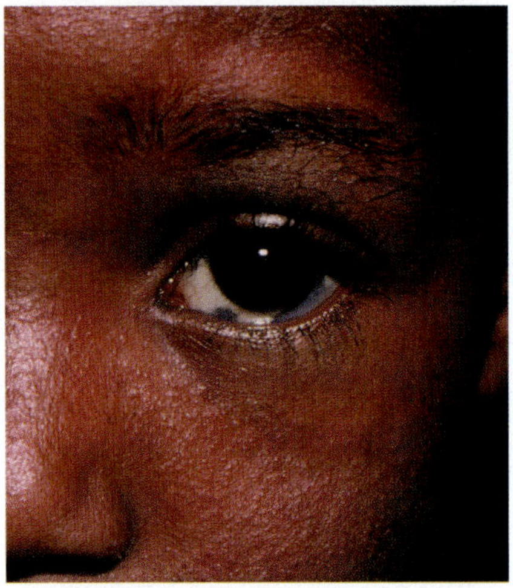

▲ **FIGURE 84-65** Africa. Nevus of Ota. Courtesy of Dr. Barbara J. Leppard.

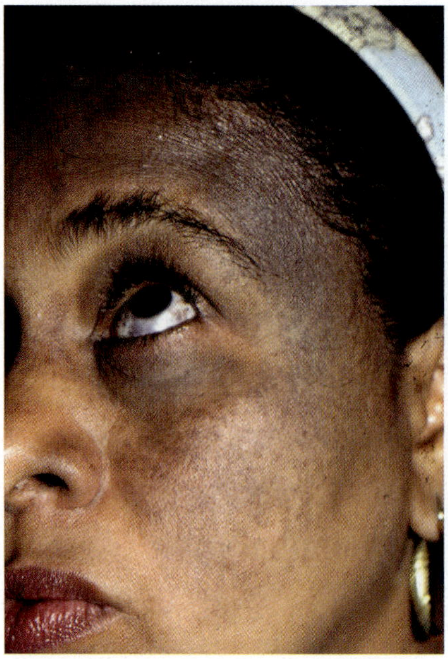

▲ **FIGURE 84-67** Latin America. Nevus of Ota. Courtesy of Dr. Marcia Ramos-e-Silva.

Etiology

The lesion occurs because of an arrest in migration of melanocytes from the neural crest to the epidermis. Most cases are congenital, although some may arise later on during life. It is more prevalent in the Japanese but can be observed in other races as well.

Clinical Perspective

The lesion is usually slate-brown or blue in color, although the color can be variable. It can be bilateral. Sclerae may be involved, and the cornea, iris, retina, ocular muscles, and orbit may be pigmented. It does not resolve with time. Although malignant change in the cutaneous lesion is rare, melanomas are common in the choroid, iris, orbit, and brain.

Differential Diagnosis

Bilateral acquired dermal melanosis of the face may have to be considered in the differential diagnosis.

Treatment Options

The Q-switched ruby laser shows good results in the treatment of this condition.

ORAL HYPERPIGMENTATION

Definition

Light brown to dark brown pigmentation of the gingiva, buccal mucosa, hard palate, and tongue in dark-skinned patients is known as *oral hyperpigmentation.*

Etiology

Oral hyperpigmentation represents a normal variant in dark-skinned patients, although it is seen less frequently in Asians than among blacks.

Clinical Perspective

Although the anterior gingiva may be predominantly involved, the buccal and

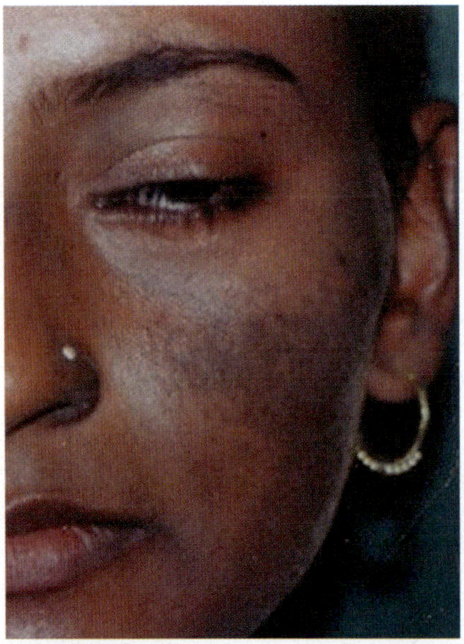

▲ **FIGURE 84-66** Asia. Nevus of Ota. Courtesy of Dr. Rashmi Sarkar.

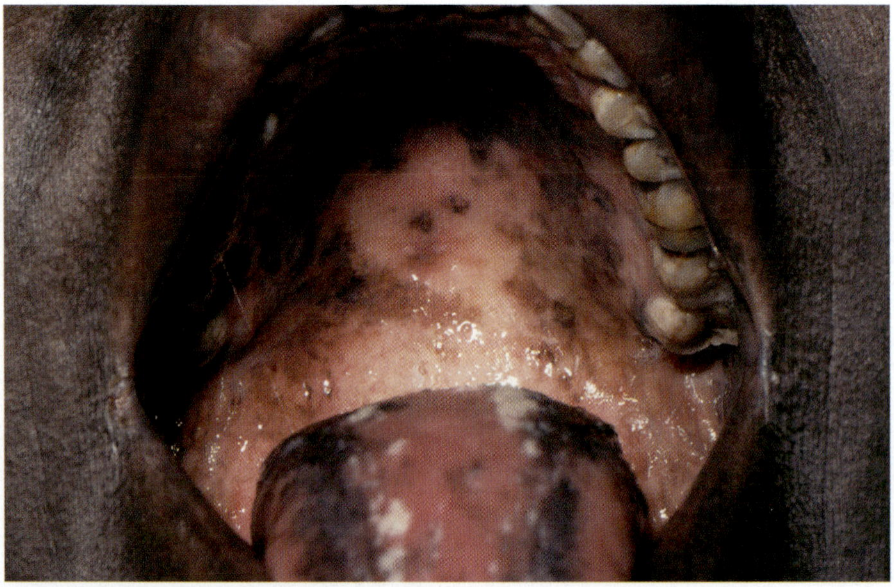

▲ **FIGURE 84-68** Africa. Normal racial hyperpigmentation on the palate. Courtesy of Dr. Barbara J. Leppard.

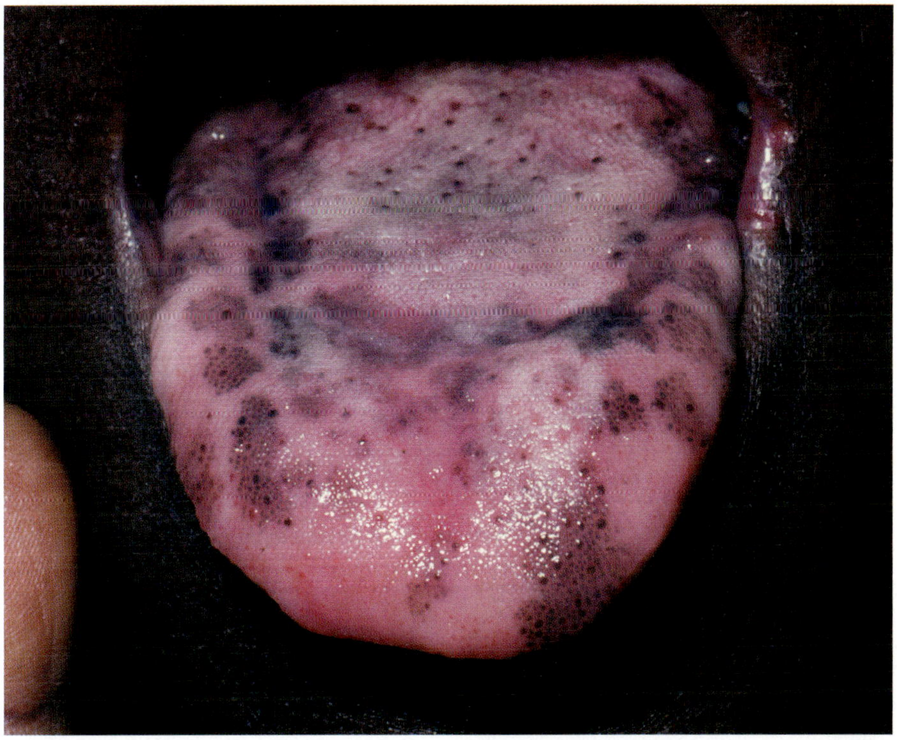

▲ **FIGURE 84-69** Africa. Normal racial hyperpigmentation on the palate. Courtesy of Dr. Barbara J. Leppard.

labial mucosae, hard palate, and tongue are also affected (Figures 84-68 through 84-70).

Differential Diagnosis

Endocrine disorders such as Addison disease, Peutz-Jegher syndrome, and hemochromatosis should be ruled out. Heavy metals that are components of indiginous drugs, antimalarials, and phenothiazines also may cause oral hyperpigmentation, which should be ruled out by a careful history. Oral lichen planus would have a violaceous color, and lesions would be present elsewhere on the body.

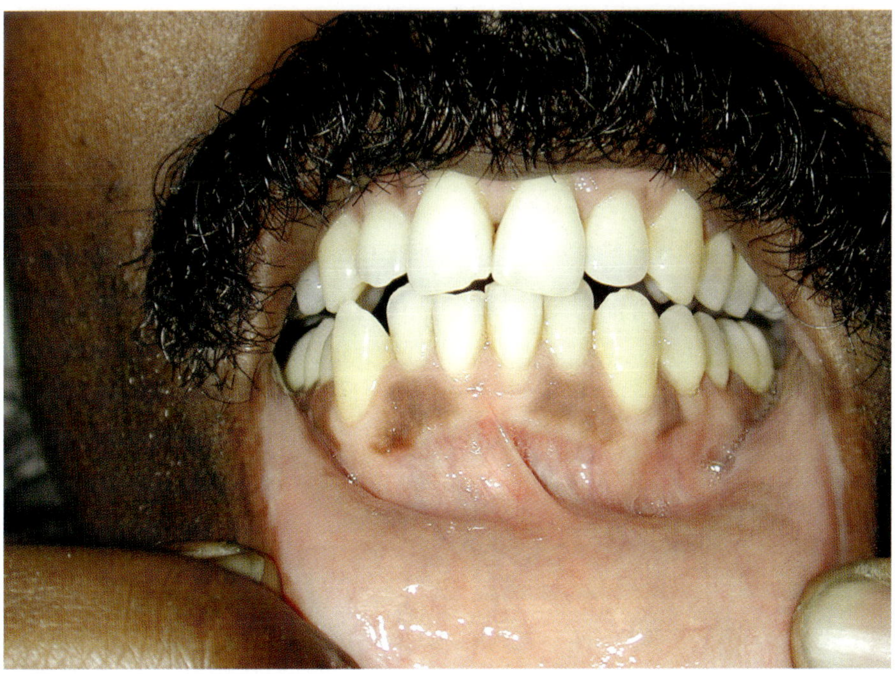

▲ **FIGURE 84-70** Latin America. Oral hyperpigmentation. Courtesy of Dr. Marcia Ramos-e-Silva.

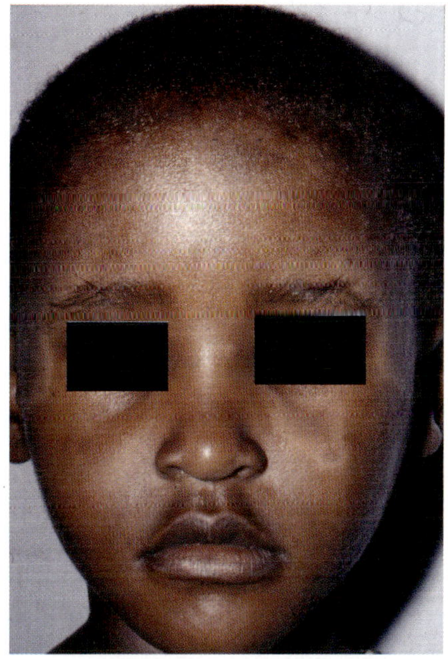

▲ **FIGURE 84-71** Africa. Pityriasis alba in an 8-year-old boy. Courtesy of Dr. Barbara J. Leppard.

Treatment Options

Reassurance is all that is needed owing to the benign nature of this condition.

PITYRIASIS ALBA

Definition

This is a pattern of dermatitis in which erythema and scaling usually precede the development of conspicuous hypopigmentation (Figures 84-71 through 84-73).

Etiology

Pityriasis alba is sometimes a manifestation of atopic dermatitis, but it may not be confined to only atopic individuals. It is believed to result either from a decrease in the number of active melanocytes or from reduced capacity of the epidermal cells to acquire melanin during inflammation. This condition is extremely common in Asian and black children.

Clinical Perspective

Pityriasis alba occurs commonly in children between 3 and 16 years of age. The lesion or lesions are round, oval, or irregular plaques that are red, pink, or skin-colored with fine, branny scaling. In dark-skinned patients, it presents mainly as persistent fine scaling and hypopigmentation (Figures 84-71 through 84-73). Lesions may be confined to face, but the neck, arms, and trunk also may be involved. Lesions may be

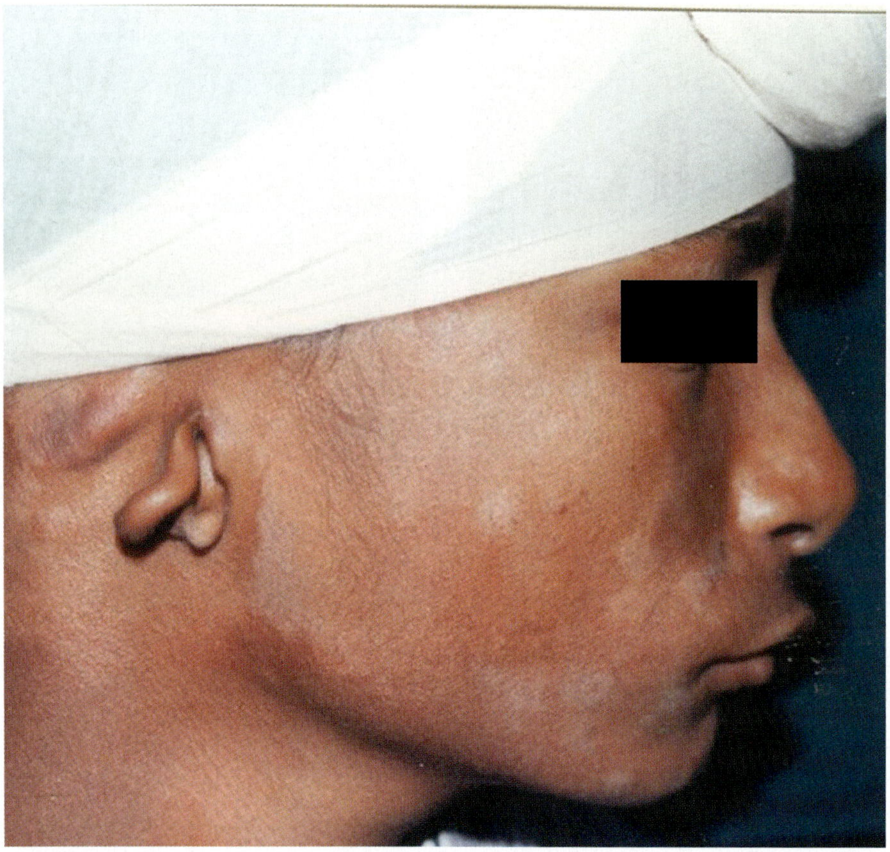

▲ **FIGURE 84-72** Asia. Pityriasis alba. Courtesy of Dr. Rashmi Sarkar.

persistent, and hypopigmentation may last for a year or more.

Differential Diagnosis

Conspicuous hypopigmentation may lead to the misdiagnosis of vitiligo, but the age at incidence, scaling, and distribution may point to the diagnosis.

Treatment Options

The scaling can be reduced by a bland emollient. Topical tar or topical corticosteroids are useful in the inflammatory phase. Topical tacrolimus and pimecrolimus are useful for facial lesions.

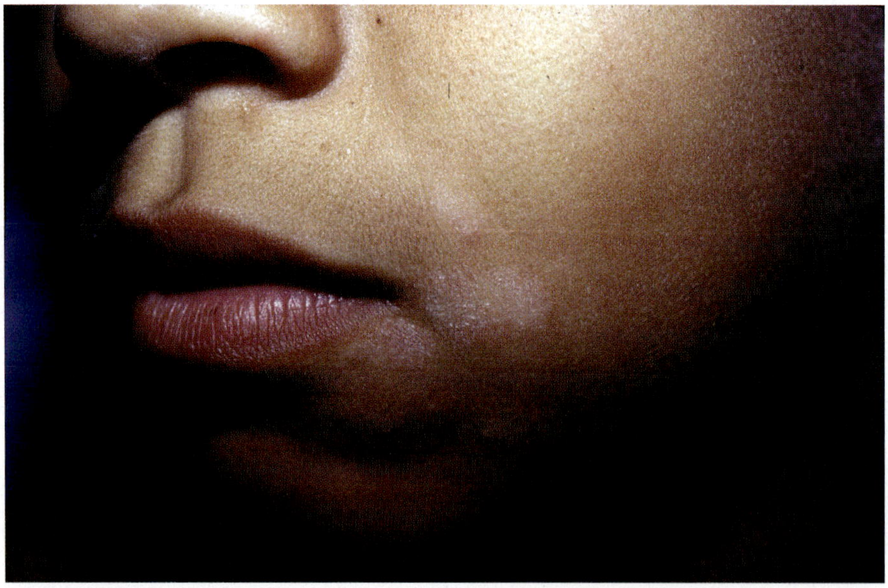

▲ **FIGURE 84-73** Latin America. Pityriasis alba. Courtesy of Dr. Marcia Ramos-e-Silva.

PITYRIASIS ROSEA

Definition

Pityriasis rosea is an acute self-limiting disease characterized by a distinctive eruption of oval scaly papules and plaques and minimal constitutional symptoms.

Etiology

Pityriasis rosea is common throughout the world, especially in tropical countries. Most cases occur between 10 and 35 years of age. An infective agent may be implicated in the pathogenesis, although the etiology is largely unknown. Occasional household outbreaks, seasonal and year-to-year fluctuations, statistical evidence for clustering in time and space, the natural history of the disease, and the infrequency of second attacks point to a viral etiology. Drugs (e.g., arsenic, bismuth, barbiturates, clonidine, and captopril) have been implicated in its pathogenesis.

Clinical Perspective

In Asians, pityriasis rosea presents as dull red or reddish brown scaly papular and oval-shaped medallions distributed on the trunk in a "Christmas tree" pattern (Figures 84-74 and 84-75). In black skin, it presents as a hyperpigmentated scaly eruption. Occasionally, slight fever, malaise, and lymphadenopathy may be present. Papulovesicular, vesicular, pustular, follicular, and erythema multiforme-like lesions may be seen commonly. The skin lesions fade in 3–6 weeks, leaving behind temporary hyperpigmentation or hypopigmentation.

Differential Diagnosis

Guttate psoriasis may have to be differentiated from pityriasis rosea by the presence of thick white scales, whereas the scales are peripherally attached and centrally free like a "collarette" in pityriasis rosea. Secondary syphilis may have to be excluded by a careful history and positive Venereal Disease Research Laboratory (VDRL) test.

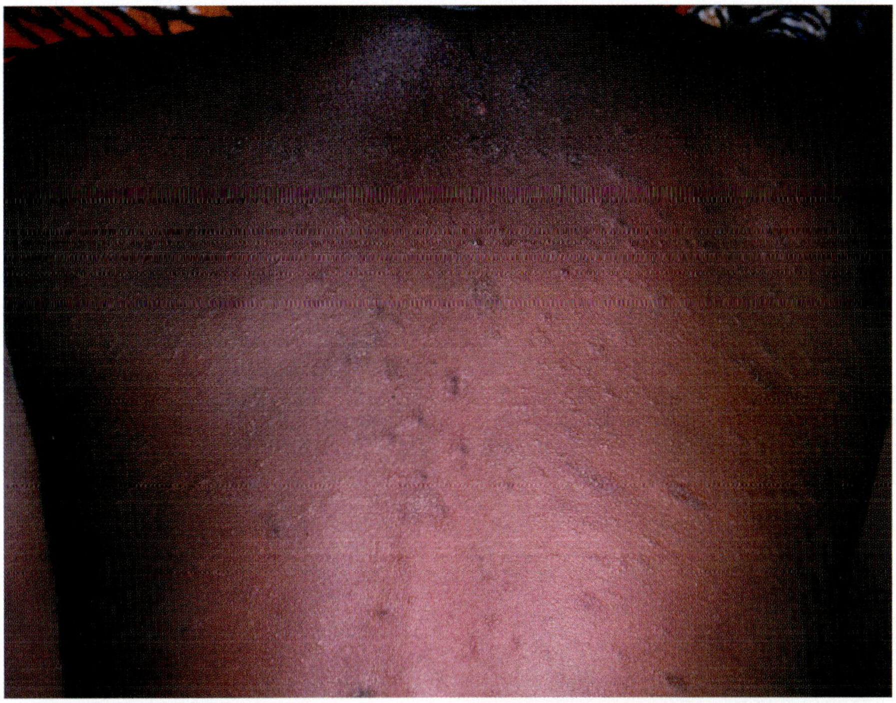

▲ **FIGURE 84-74** Africa. Pityriasis rosea. Courtesy of Dr. Barbara J. Leppard.

Treatment Options

Asymptomatic patients do not require treatment. A moderately potent topical steroid or UVB treatment may be useful. Oral erythromycin, given in a dose of 200 mg four times a day, may hasten clearance of the lesions.

POSTINFLAMMATORY HYPER-/HYPOPIGMENTATION

Definition

Postinflammatory hyperpigmentation/hypopigmentation is an acquired disorder of excess or decreased pigment deposition that follows resolution of various cutaneous disorders, as well as therapeutic interventions (e.g., laser therapy, chemical peels, and dermabrasion) (Figures 84-76 through 84-81).

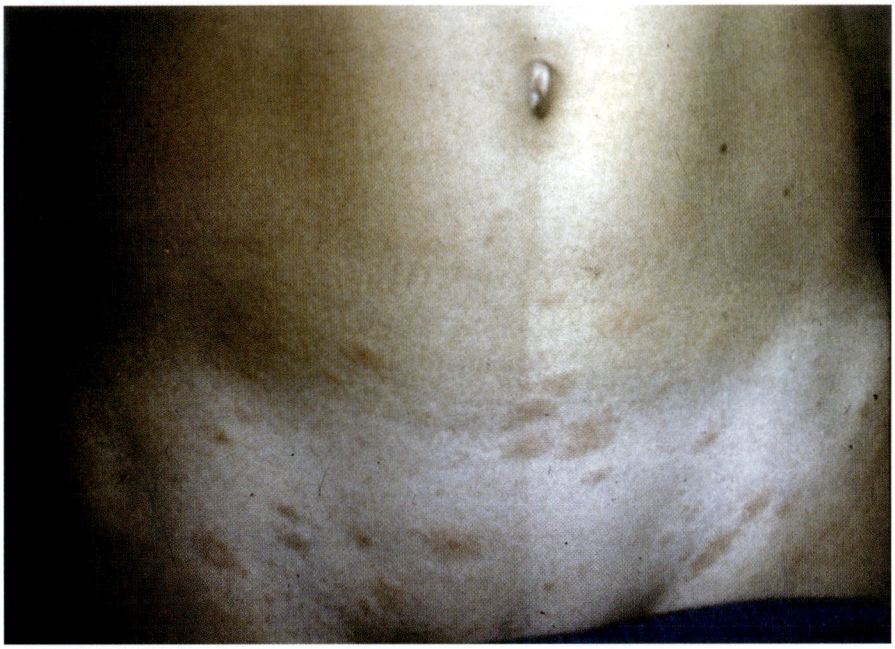

▲ **FIGURE 84-75** Latin America. Pityriasis rosea. Courtesy of Dr. Marcia Ramos-e-Silva.

Etiology

Postinflammatory hyperpigmentation/hypopigmentation is more severe in dark-skinned patients. Hyperpigmentation follows diseases such as contact dermatitis, lichen planus, phototoxic eruptions, acne vulgaris, atopic dermatitis, fixed drug eruption, pityriasis rosea, secondary syphilis, and sarcoidosis. In dark-skinned patients, the hyperpigmentation worsens with ultraviolet (UV) exposure. Hypopigmentation is caused by atopic dermatitis, contact dermatitis, seborrheic dermatitis, secondary syphilis, discoid lupus erythematous, pityriasis alba, scleroderma, and lichen striatus. Physical therapies such as chemical peeling, laser therapy, cryosurgery, and dermabrasion also may lead to hypopigmentation or hyperpigmentation. Hypopigmentation also may be a sequela of topical, intralesional, and intramuscular corticosteroid administration.

Clinical Perspective

Postinflammatory hyperpigmentation/hypopigmentation may be more noticeable and distressing to Asian patients than the actual disease itself. Many of these pigmentary disturbances normalize with time.

Differential Diagnosis

Postinflammatory hypopigmentation may need to be differentiated from vitiligo, but a history of the original skin lesions leading to pigmentary alterations may establish the diagnosis.

Treatment Options

Postinflammatory hypopigmentation may require treatment with topical steroids, topical calcineurin inhibitors, and topical PUVA therapy to cause repigmentation. Treatment of postinflammatory hyperpigmentation is often difficult and prolonged. A broad-spectrum sunscreen is an important part of the treatment. Epidermal postinflammatory hyperpigmentation may be treated with topical depigmenting agents such as hydroquinone,

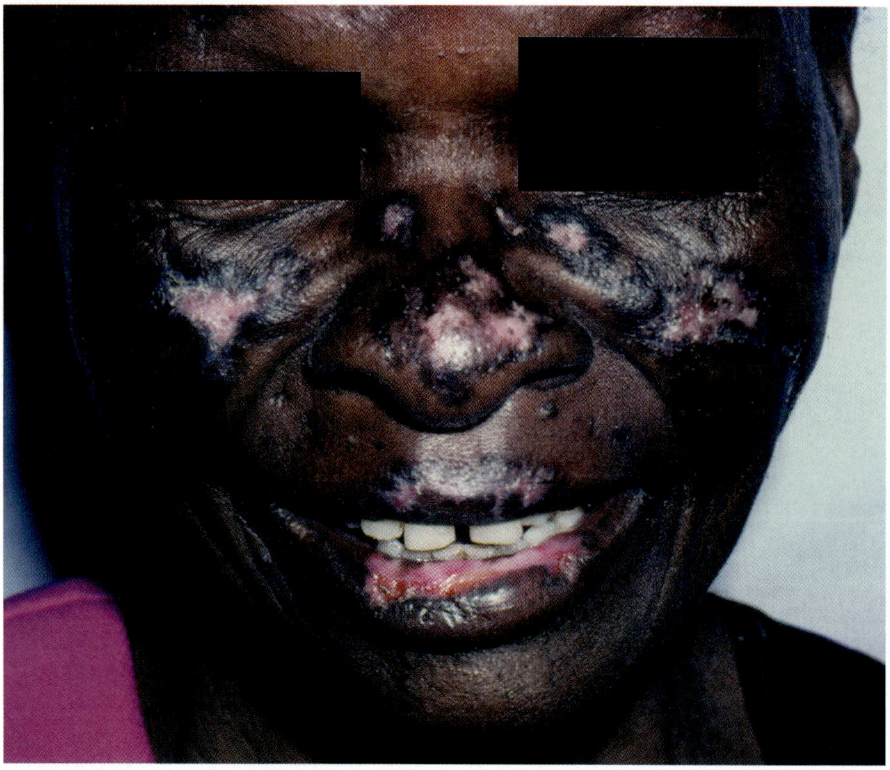

▲ **FIGURE 84-76** Africa. Postinflammatory hyper- and hypopigmentation of discoid lupus erythematosus. Courtesy of Dr. Barbara J. Leppard.

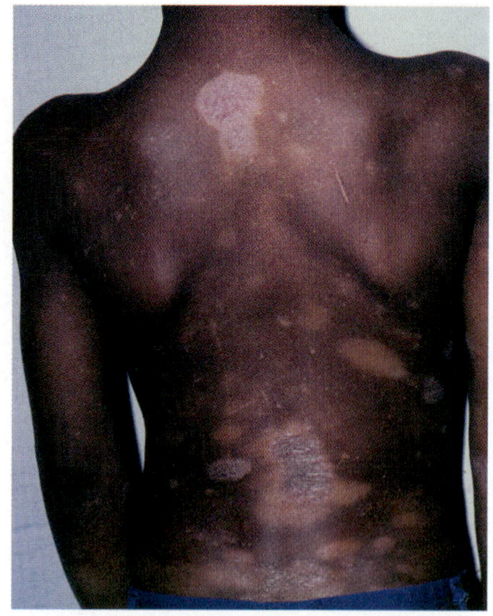

▲ **FIGURE 84-78** Africa. Postinflammatory hypopigmentation after resolution of eczema. Courtesy of Dr. Barbara J. Leppard.

corticosteroids, tretinoin cream, or combinations of these three agents, as well as azelaic acid and kojic acid. Dark-skinned patients also benefit from glycolic acid peels, especially when combined with topical tretinoin, hydroquinone, and topical steroids. However, laser treatment is not very effective in treating patients with postinflammatory hyperpigmentation.

PSORIASIS VULGARIS

Definition

Psoriasis is a common inflammatory disease of the skin, hair, and nails recognized by its characteristic red scaly plaques on the skin.

Etiology

It is probably genetically determined, but injury to the skin, streptococcal throat infection, certain drugs, and physical and emotional stress can trigger it.

Clinical Perspective

Well-defined red scaly plaques can appear anywhere on the body (Figures 84-82 through 84-88). If you scratch the surface of the plaques, the scale becomes more obvious. It is less likely to be located on the elbows and knees than in America. Thick scaly plaques occur in the scalp and may extend down onto the forehead (Figures 84-84 and 84-88). Nail changes such as

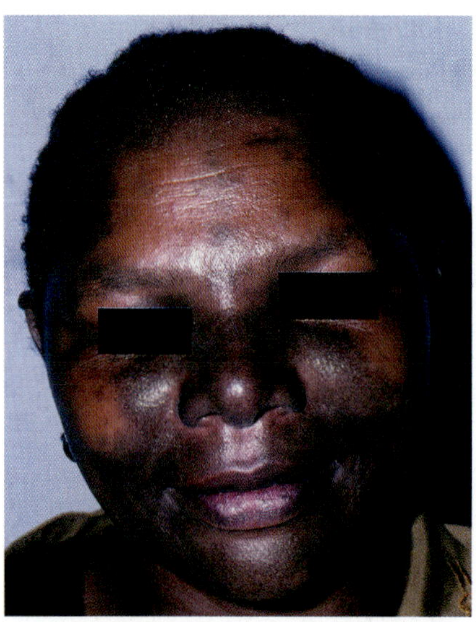

▲ **FIGURE 84-77** Africa. Postinflammatory hyperpigmentation on the face. Courtesy of Dr. Barbara J. Leppard.

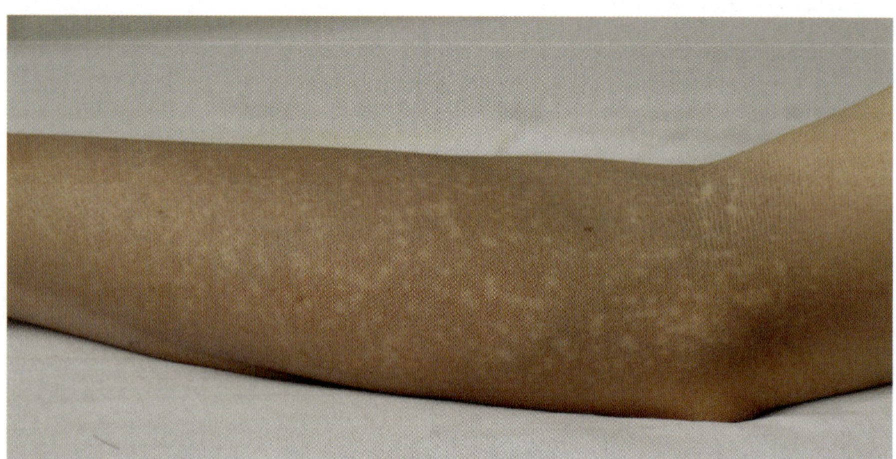

FIGURE 84-79 Asia. Postinflammatory hyperpigmentation in a Chinese man. Courtesy of Dr. Diqing Luo.

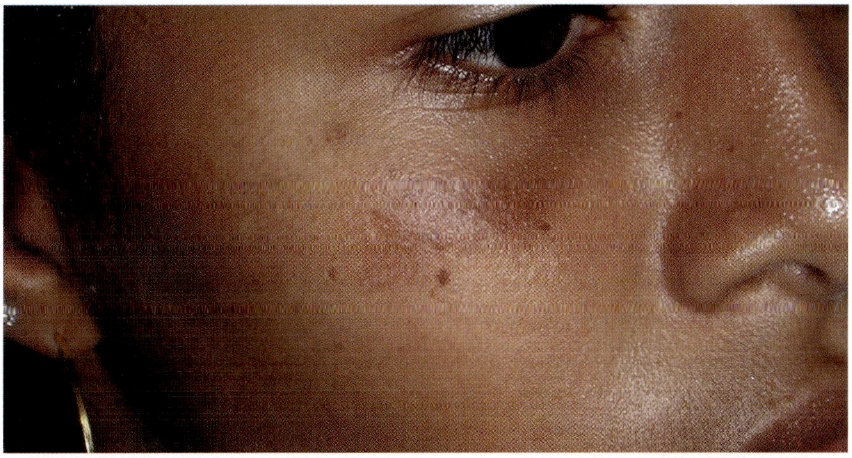

▲ **FIGURE 84-80** Latin America. Postinflammatory hyperpigmentation. Courtesy of Dr. Marcia Ramos-e-Silva.

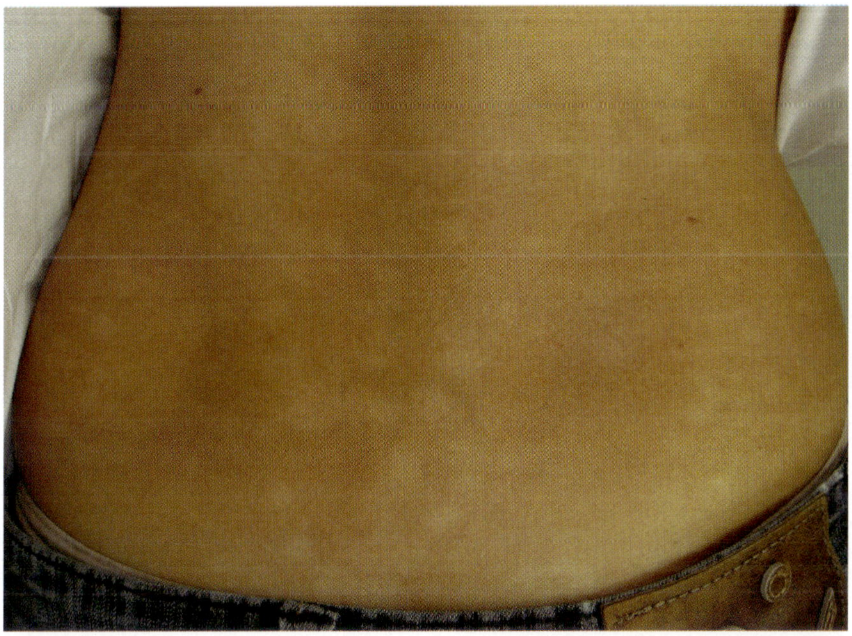

▲ **FIGURE 84-81** Latin America. Postinflammatory hypopigmentation. Courtesy of Dr. Marcia Ramos-e-Silva.

pitting (Figure 84-85), salmon patches, onycholysis, and subungual hyperkeratosis are identical to those seen in the West.

Differential Diagnosis

Include other scaly rashes such as eczema and tinea. The well-defined border, the erythema, and the prolific scale of psoriasis usually make the diagnosis easy.

Associations

Psoriatic arthritis, which is usually less severe than rheumatoid arthritis. It characteristically affects the distal interphalangeal joints. Rarely, it can cause a mutilating arthritis indistinguishable clinically from severe rheumatoid arthritis, but patients will not have a positive rheumatoid factor. In extensive or hyperkeratotic psoriasis, think of associated HIV/AIDS.

Treatment Options

Topical therapy such as emollients, coal tar, corticosteroids, dithranol, calcipotriol, PUVA therapy, and tazarotene can be used to treat psoriasis vulgaris. Phototherapy and photochemotherapy (e.g., UVB, PUVA, and PUVA sol), methotrexate, acitretin, and cyclosporine are required for extensive disease.

SARCOIDOSIS

Definition

Sarcoidosis is a disease characterized by the formation of epithelioid cell tuber-

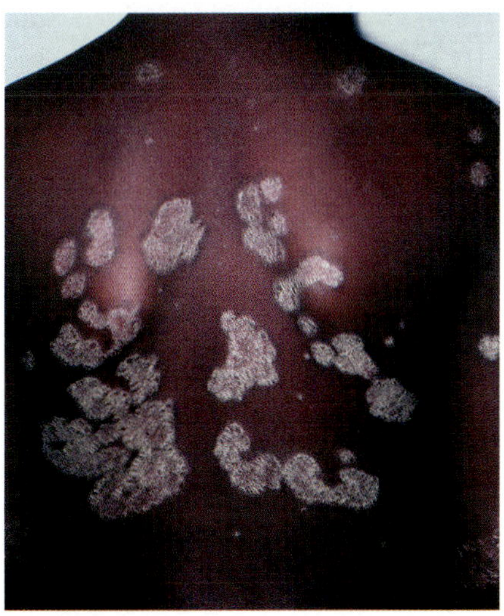

▲ **FIGURE 84-82** Africa. Psoriasis on the back of a 9-year-old girl. Courtesy of Dr. Barbara J. Leppard.

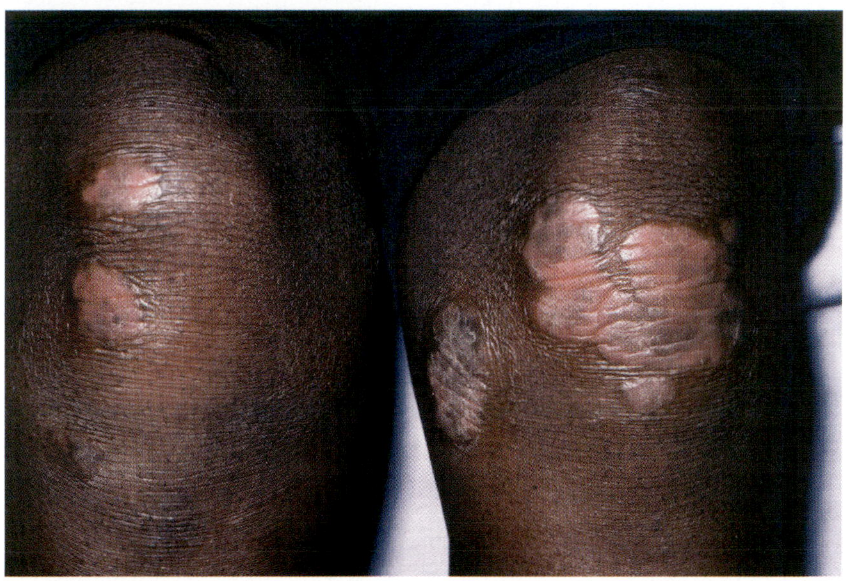

▲ **FIGURE 84-83** Africa. Psoriasis on the knees of a 13-year-old boy. Red color is obvious, even in African skin. Courtesy of Dr. Barbara J. Leppard.

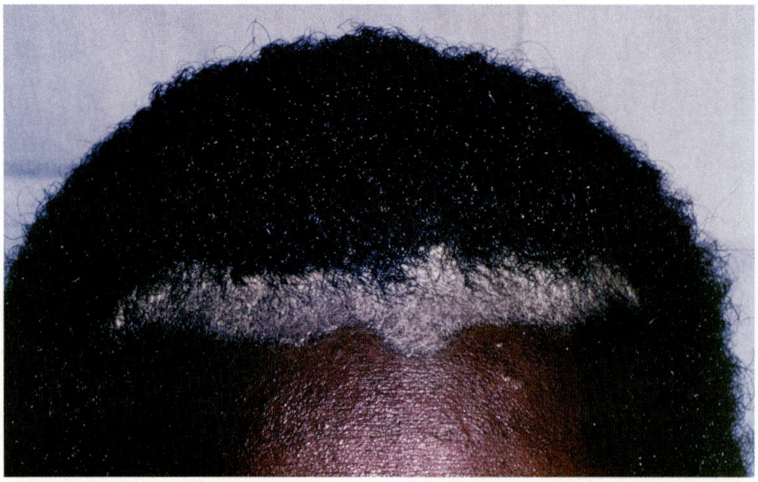

▲ **FIGURE 84-84** Africa. Corona psoriatica, psoriasis extending from the scalp onto the forehead. Courtesy of Dr. Barbara J. Leppard.

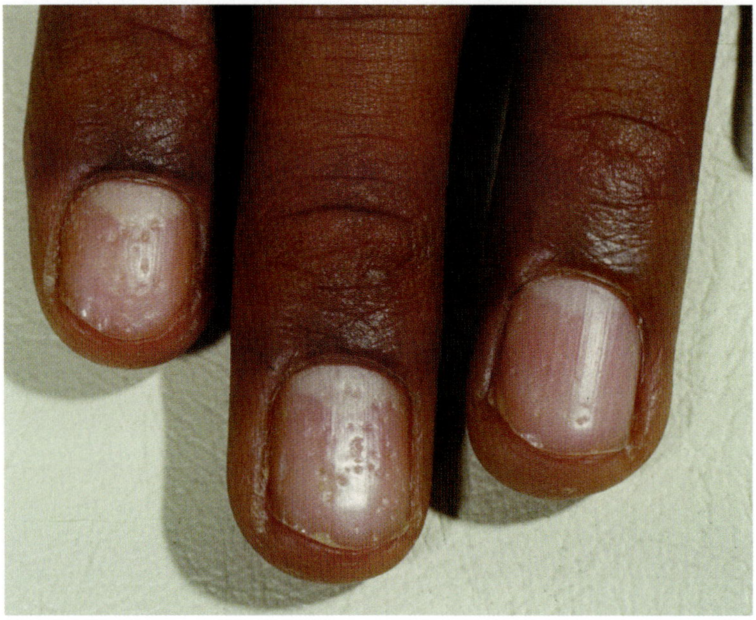

▲ **FIGURE 84-85** Africa. Pitting of the nails. Courtesy of Dr. Barbara J. Leppard.

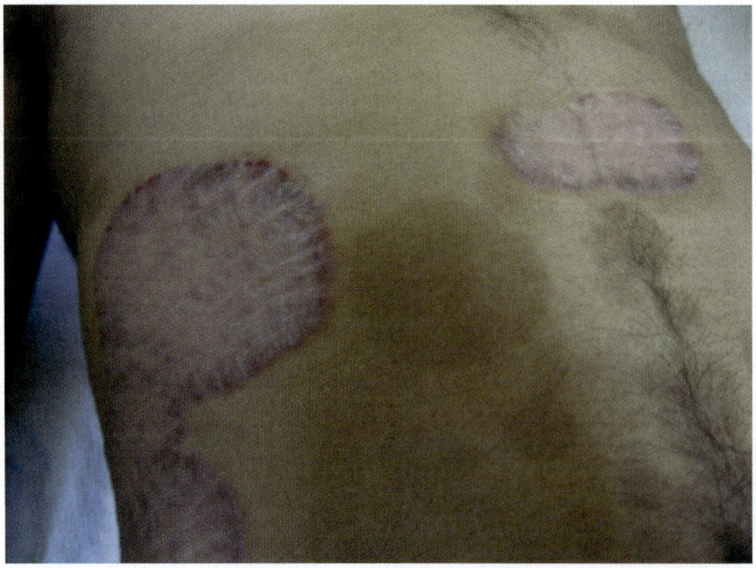

▲ **FIGURE 84-86** Asia. Psoriasis vulgaris. Courtesy of Dr. Rashmi Sarkar.

cles without caseation in all or several of affected organs, with cutaneous involvement in 10–30% patients. In Asia, sarcoidosis is less common than in African patients.

Etiology

The cause of sarcoidosis is unknown. It is believed that the disease possibly could represent an unusual host reaction to infectious agents. Genetic factors also appear to be linked with this condition. Depression of cell-mediated immunity is the hallmark of the disease.

Clinical Perspective

Two types of cutaneous lesions are recognized: specific cutaneous sarcoid lesions and nonspecific reactive lesions. Specific cutaneous lesions arise from a dense collection of epithelioid cell granulomas in the dermis. Papules, plaques, and nodules are the common specific lesions, where the color ranges from yellow ochre to a livid violaceous hue, and on diascopy, pale yellowish gray, dusky, violaceous, soft, doughy nodules and plaques are seen uncommonly (Figures 84-89 and 84-90). The plaques of sarcoidosis that are usually seen in Asian patients are irregular, infiltrated lesions that may be annular or serpiginous.

Differential Diagnosis

Lupus vulgaris, generalized granuloma annulare, secondary syphilis, and lymphoma all may mimic sarcoidosis. Histopathology would confirm the diagnosis.

Treatment Options

Treatment would depend on the extent of involvement. Corticosteroids are the mainstay of treatment. Topical and intralesional steroids are used for disfiguring cutaneous lesions. Cryotherapy also has been used occasionally. Cutaneous lesions in systemic sarcoidosis involving the eyes and lungs require oral steroids or cytotoxic drugs such as methotrexate, chlorambucil, and azathioprine. Allopurinol, antimalarials, and oxyphenbutazone have been used with limited success.

SCABIES

Definition

Scabies is a disease in humans characterized by intense itching and caused by the mite, *Sarcoptes scabiei* var. *hominis*.

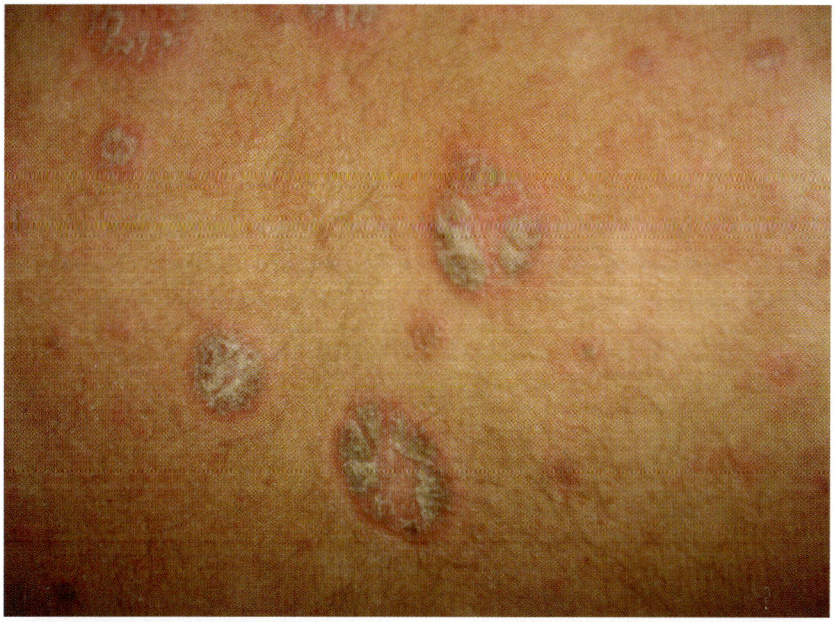

▲ **FIGURE 84-87** Asia. Psoriasis vulgaris. Courtesy of Dr. Rashmi Sarkar.

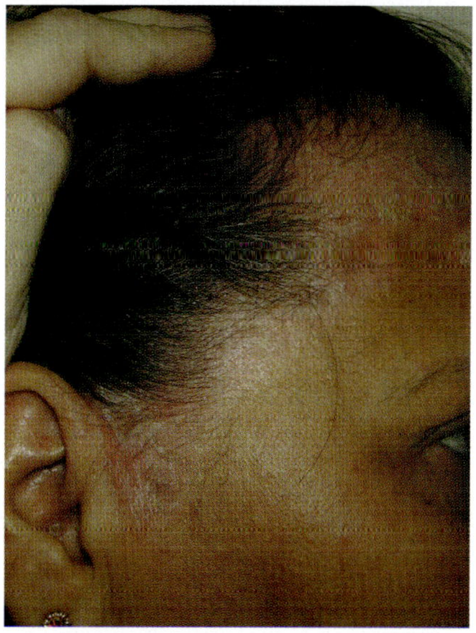

▲ **FIGURE 84-88** Latin America. Psoriasis vulgaris. Courtesy of Dr. Marcia Ramos-e-Silva.

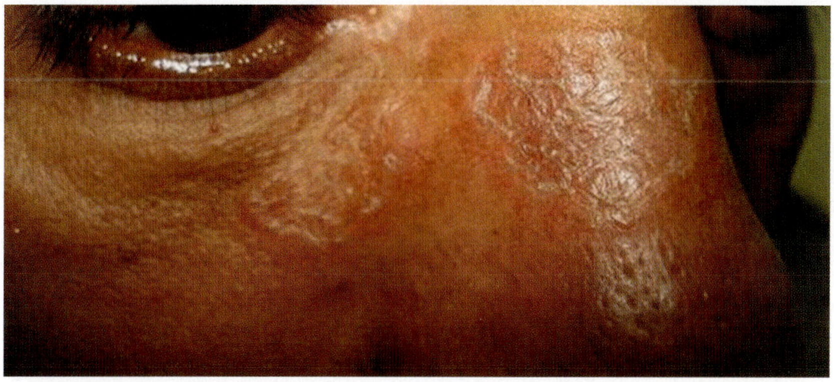

▲ **FIGURE 84-89** Asia. Sarcoidosis. Courtesy of Dr. Rashmi Sarkar.

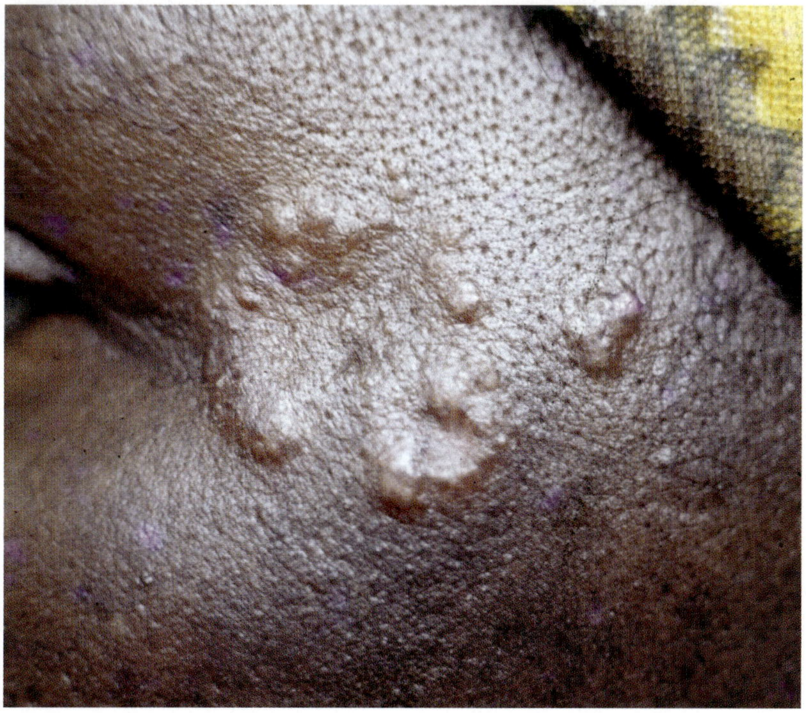

▲ **FIGURE 84-90** Latin America. Sarcoidosis. Courtesy of Dr. Marcia Ramos-e-Silva.

Etiology

Scabies affects all races and social classes worldwide. It is usually transmitted by close physical contact, such as prolonged bed sharing or hand holding. Indirect spread by clothing or bedding is unimportant. In Asia, in developing countries, overcrowding, poverty, and poor hygiene encourage the spread of scabies. Scabies epidemics occur in 30-year cycles and affect people commonly in India and other Asian countries.

Clinical Perspective

Intense itching is usually the main characteristic of scabies, and it is marked at night. The eruption consists of inflammatory papules, vesicles, excoriations, and crusting, and the onset occurs 3–4 weeks after the infection is acquired. The pathognomic lesion is the burrow, which appears as a slightly raised, brownish, tortuous lesion, with the point of entry of the mite being the most superficial part of the burrow. Burrows occur on the wrists, the finger web spaces, the sides of the fingers, the genitalia, and the feet (Figures 84-92, 84-93 and 84-95).

The pruritic papules occur predominantly around the axillae, the periareolar area, the periumbilical region, buttocks, and thighs. Postscabetic nodules may persist in the axillae, groin, scrotum, and penis (Figures 84-91 through 84-99). Eczematous changes and secondary infection are common. Vesiculopustular lesions on the hands and feet are common in India.

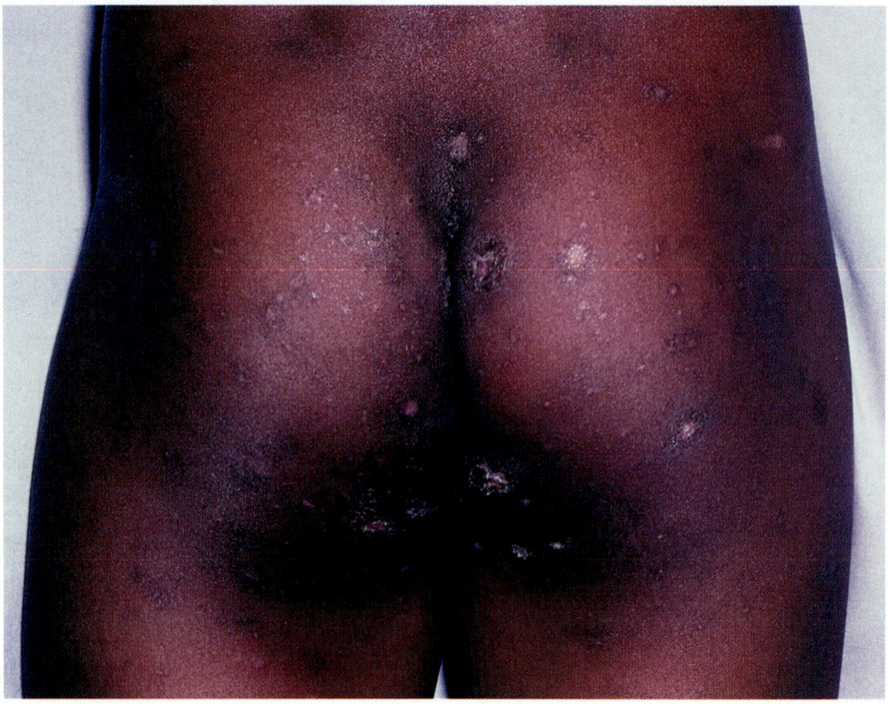

▲ **FIGURE 84-91** Africa. Scabies. Excoriated, crusted lesions on the buttocks. Courtesy of Dr. Barbara J. Leppard.

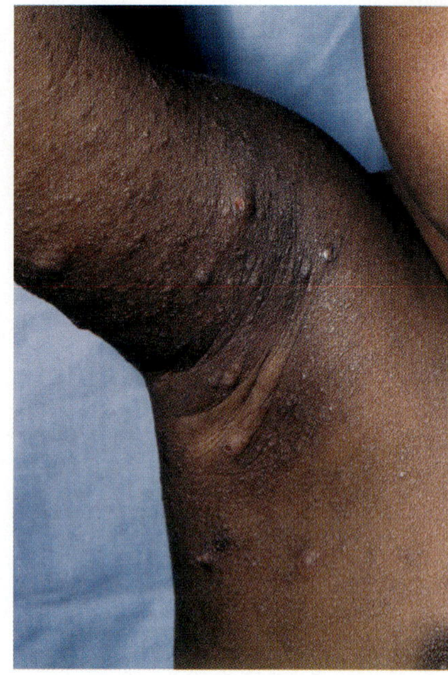

▲ **FIGURE 84-94** Africa. Scabies. Itchy papules with excoriations and erosions. Courtesy of Dr. Barbara J. Leppard.

Differential Diagnosis

In children, scabies with eczematization may be difficult to differentiate from atopic eczema. However, the presence of contact cases in the family, the lack of a history of atopy, and demonstration of a burrow may help in differentiating scabies from atopic dermatitis.

Treatment Options

Although there are several available scabicides, the choice of therapy will be determined by the efficacy, potential toxicity, cost, ease of application, secondary eczematization, and age of the patient. Permethrin 5% cream is an effective and safe scabicide and should be washed off after 8–12 hours, with a second application after an interval of 1 week. Other topical treatments

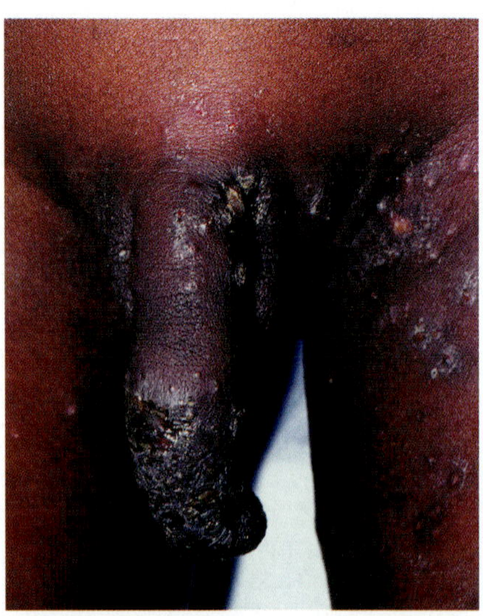

▲ **FIGURE 84-92** Africa. Scabies. In males, the genitalia are always involved. Courtesy of Dr. Barbara J. Leppard.

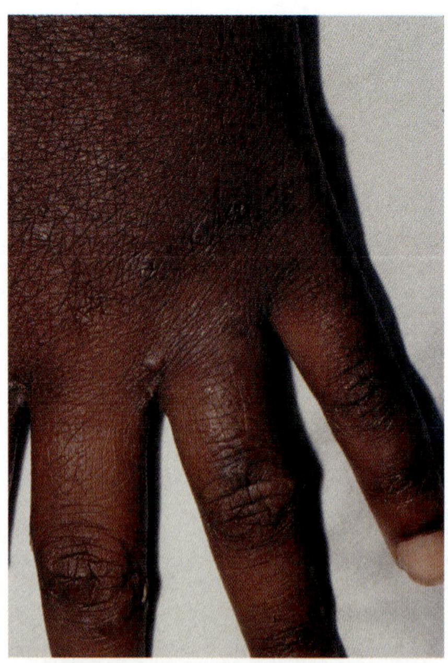

▲ **FIGURE 84-93** Africa. Scabies. Involvement of the hands and finger webs. Courtesy of Dr. Barbara J. Leppard.

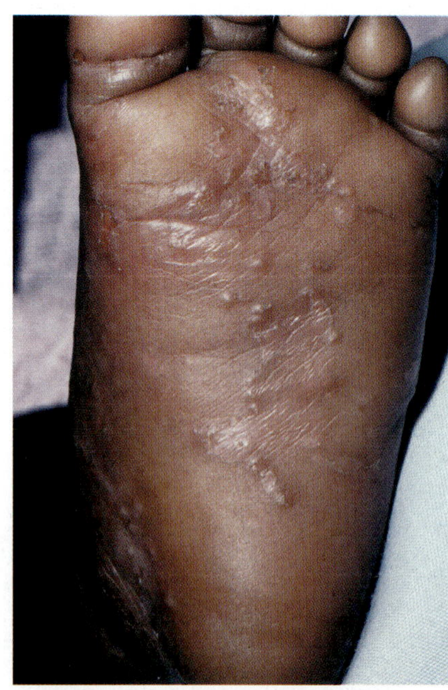

▲ **FIGURE 84-95** Africa. Scabies. Numerous borrows on the sole of a 3-month-old baby. Courtesy of Dr. Barbara J. Leppard.

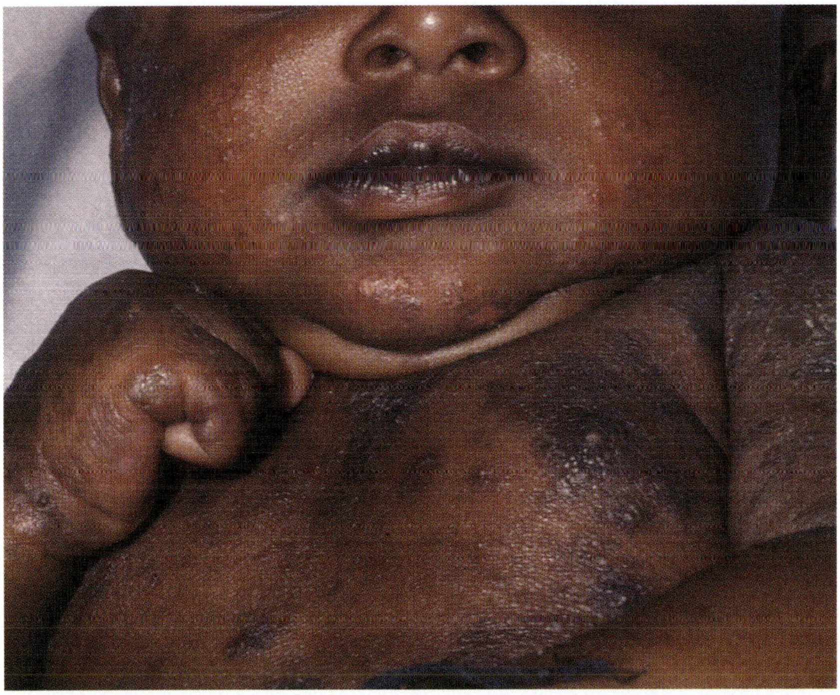

▲ **FIGURE 84-96** Africa. Scabies. Itchy rash in a 9-month-old boy. At this age, there can be involvement of the face. Courtesy of Dr. Barbara J. Leppard.

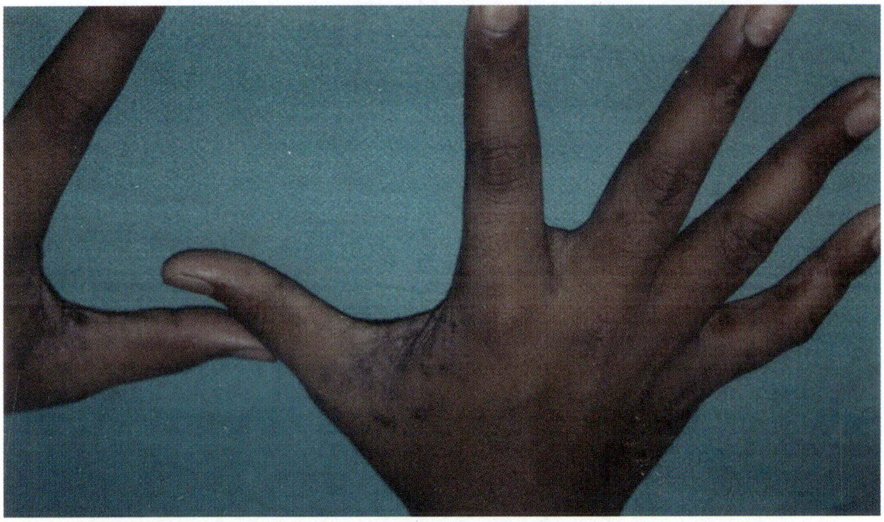

▲ **FIGURE 84-97** Asia. Scabies. Courtesy of Dr. Rashmi Sarkar.

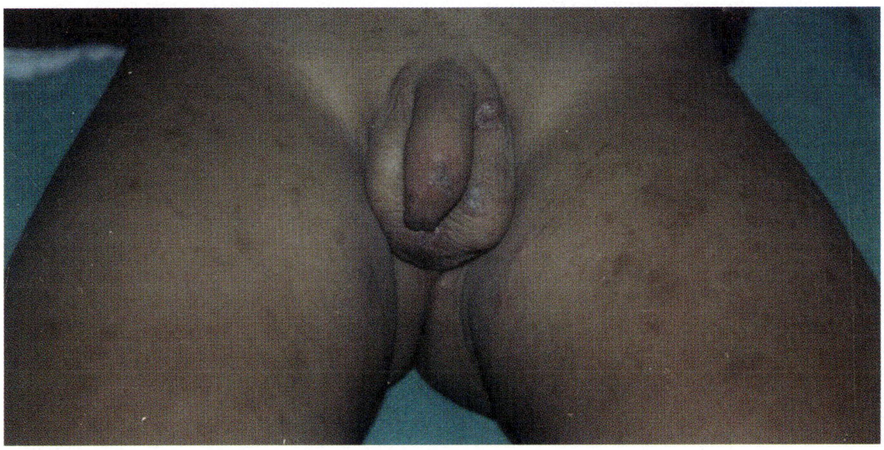

▲ **FIGURE 84-98** Asia. Scabies. Genital lesions. Courtesy of Dr. Rashmi Sarkar.

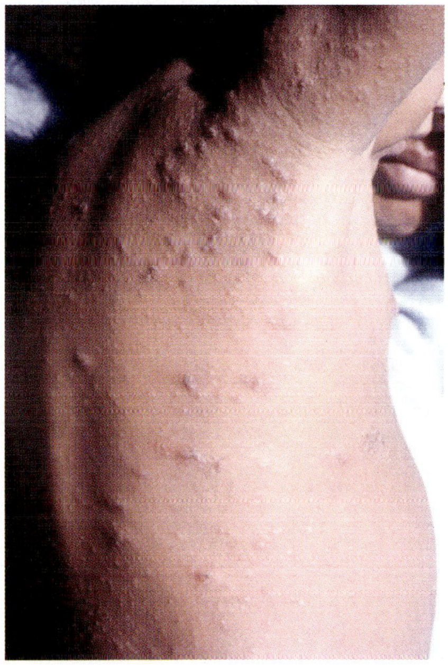

▲ **FIGURE 84-99** Latin America. Scabies in an 18-month-old child. Courtesy of Dr. Marcia Ramos-e-Silva.

include 1% gamma-benzene hexachloride lotion, 25% benzyl benzoate, monosulfiram, malathion, and crotamition. In infants, sulfur and crotamitan or permethrin cream is a safe choice. Systemic antihistamines should be given for the prolonged pruritus. Systemic antistaphylococcal antibiotics should be given for secondary infection. At present, oral ivermectin, in a dose of 200 μg/kg of body weight given 1 week apart, is useful for ordinary scabies and institutional outbreaks of scabies.

SYPHILIS

Definition

A sexually transmitted disease due to *Treponema pallidum*.

Etiology

Direct contact with an infected individual.

Clinical Perspective

PRIMARY SYPHILIS About 10–90 days after infection (usually 2–3 weeks), a firm, painless ulcer (primary chancre) occurs at the site of inoculation (Figure 84-100). At this stage, the diagnosis can be confirmed by finding the spirochetes on a smear taken from the ulcer and looked at under dark-field illumination (Figure 84-101). The ulcer heals spontaneously after 4–6 weeks if untreated.

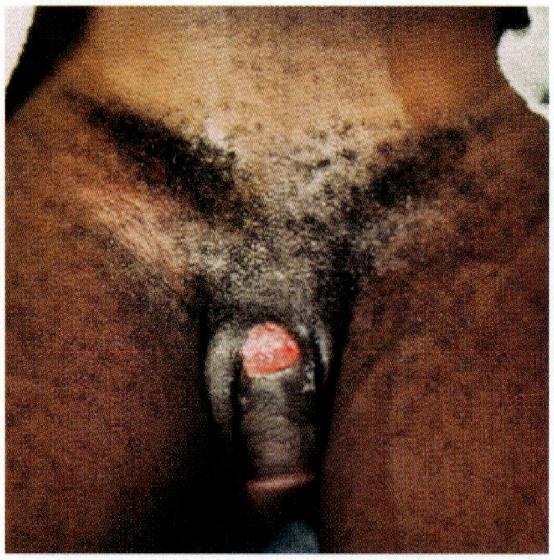

FIGURE 84-100 Africa. Primary chancre of syphilis. Courtesy of Dr. Barbara J. Leppard.

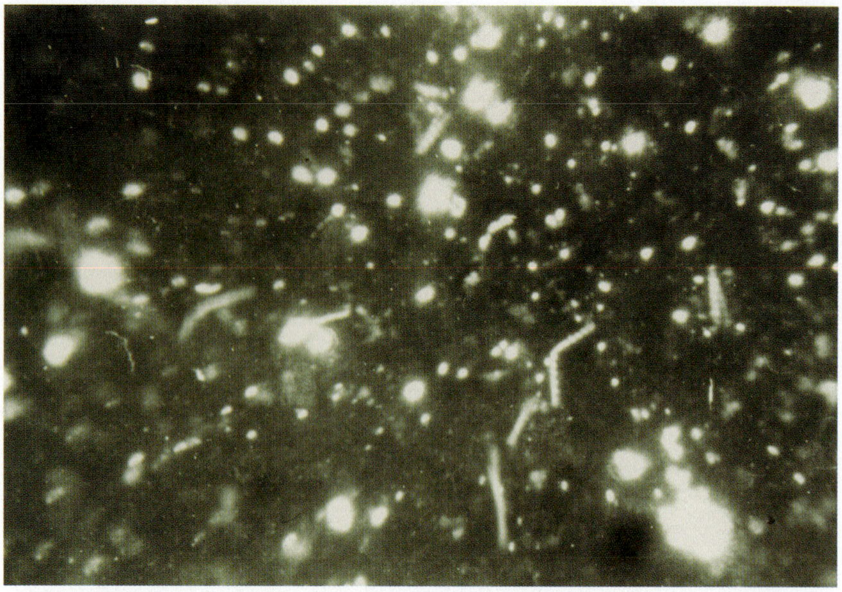

FIGURE 84-101 Africa. Dark-field examination of fluid taken from a primary chancre. Courtesy of Dr. Barbara J. Leppard.

SECONDARY SYPHILIS As the primary chancre (Figure 84-100) is healing or a few weeks later (can be up to 6 months later), the patient begins to feel unwell (e.g., general malaise, headache, sore throat, and widespread lymphadenopathy) and develops a rash. The nonitchy rash can be made up of macules, papules, or plaques (Figures 84-102 through 84-104 and Figure 84-109). Characteristically, the palms and soles are involved (Figure 84-105), and there also erosions in the mouth and on the genitalia. In addition, flat warty lesions (condylomata lata) are seen on the

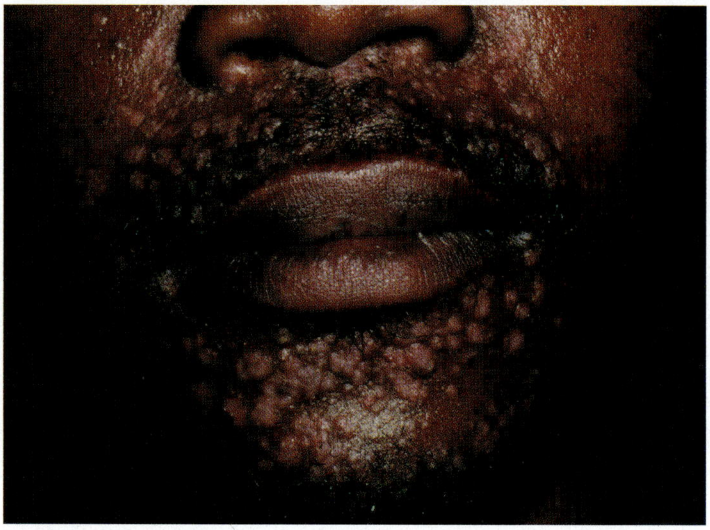

▲ **FIGURE 84-103** Africa. Secondary syphilis. Diffuse papular rash on face. Courtesy of Dr. Barbara J. Leppard.

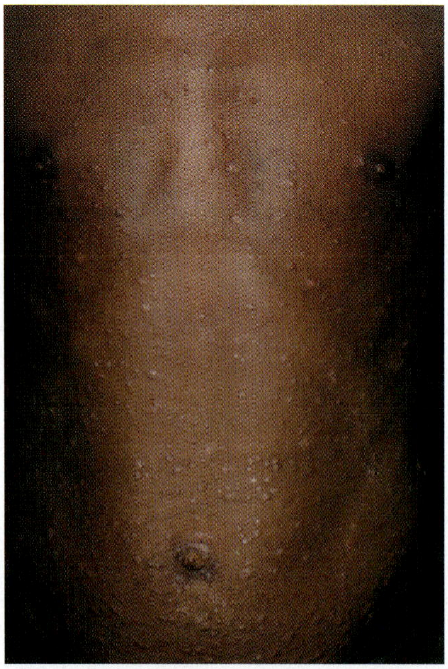

▲ **FIGURE 84-102** Africa. Secondary syphilis. Widespread nonitchy papular rash on trunk. Courtesy of Dr. Barbara J. Leppard.

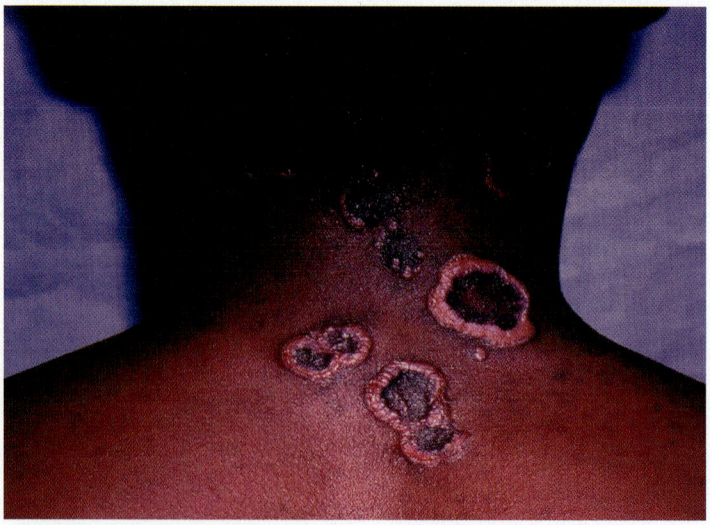

▲ **FIGURE 84-104** Africa. Secondary syphilis. Annular plaques on the back of the neck and upper back. Courtesy of Dr. Barbara J. Leppard.

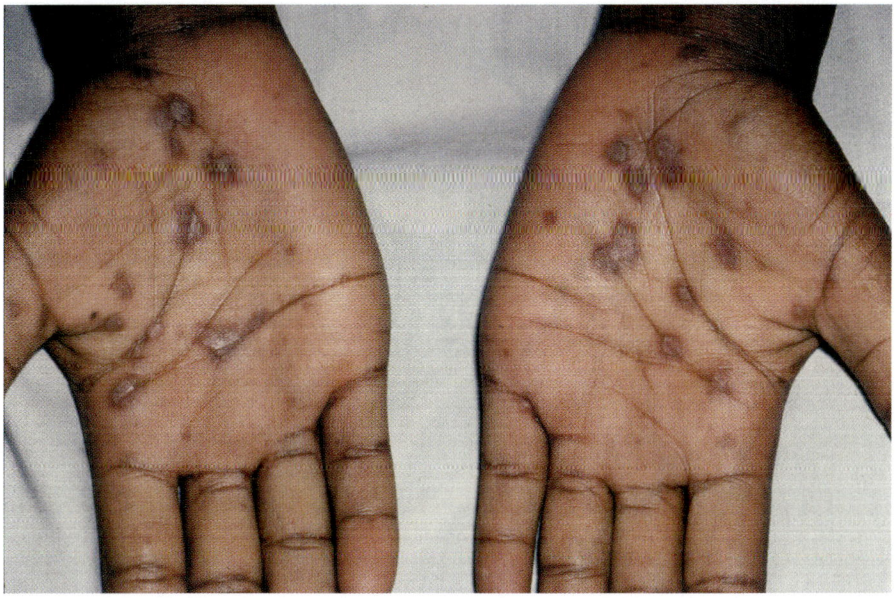

▲ **FIGURE 84-105** Africa. Secondary syphilis. Macules and papules on the palms. Courtesy of Dr. Barbara J. Leppard.

talia (Figures 84-106 and 84-108), and there is patchy hair loss (Figure 84-107).

The diagnosis can be confirmed by a positive serologic test, VDRL test, or the more specific TPHA or FTA-ABS. Without treatment, this stage also will pass after about 6 months.

Differential Diagnosis

PRIMARY SYPHILIS Other genital ulcers—herpes simplex and chancroid. Both of these have a short incubation period (<1 week) and cause painful ulcers. But remember that the patient may have more than one sexually transmitted disease at the same time.

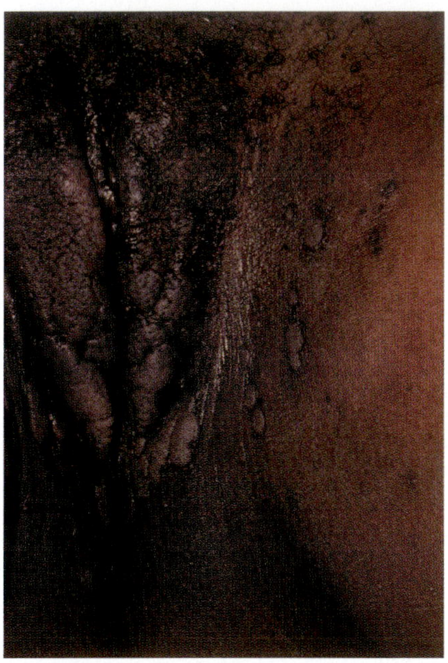

▲ **FIGURE 84-106** Africa. Secondary syphilis. Condyloma lata. Courtesy of Dr. Barbara J. Leppard.

SECONDARY SYPHILIS Other nonitchy rashes—guttate psoriasis (small red scaly papules, all the same size, following 2 weeks after a sore throat) and pityriasis rosea (the patient is not unwell). If in doubt, check the serology.

Associations

Any other sexually transmitted disease and HIV/AIDS.

Treatment Options

Single dose of benzathine penicillin 2.4 megaunits intramuscularly. If the patient is HIV-positive, give 3 weekly doses of benzathine penicillin 2.4 megaunits intramuscularly.

TINEA CAPITIS

Definition

Tinea capitis is a dermatophyte (fungal) infection of the hair and scalp. The infection is most commonly caused by *Trichophyton* and *Microsporum* species of dematophytes.

Etiology

In rural south India, tinea capitis has been found in up to 28.5% of children. Earlier, it was believed to occur more

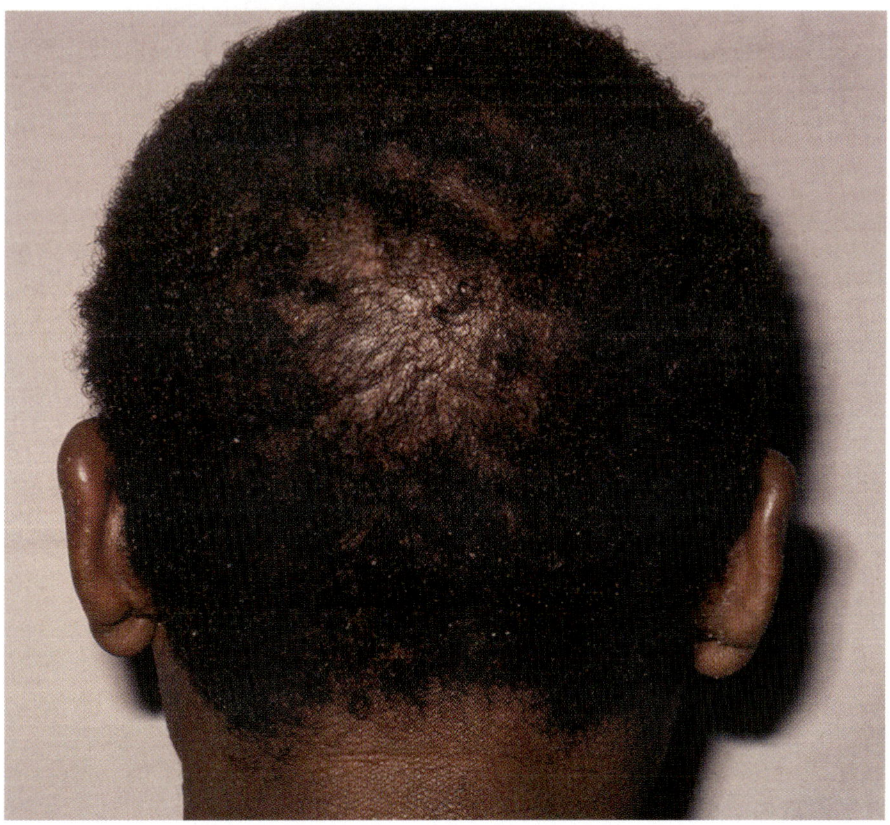

▲ **FIGURE 84-107** Africa. Secondary syphilis. Patchy alopecia, often described as "moth-eaten" in appearance. Courtesy of Dr. Barbara J. Leppard.

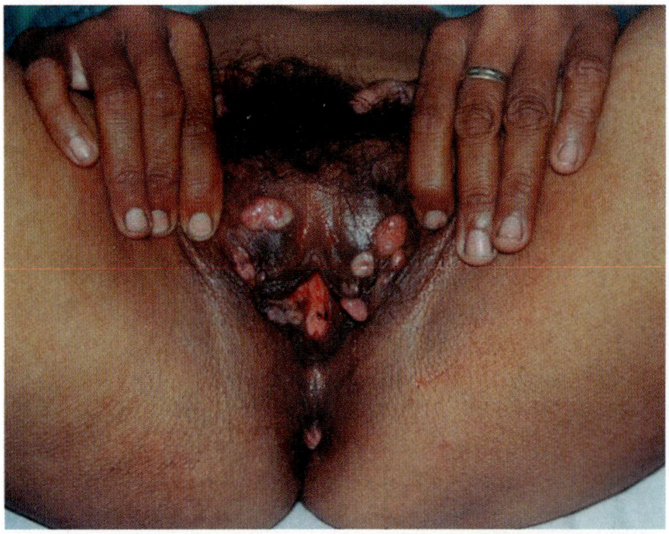

▲ **FIGURE 84-108** Asia. Syphilis. Condyloma lata of secondary syphilis. Courtesy of Dr. Rashmi Sarkar.

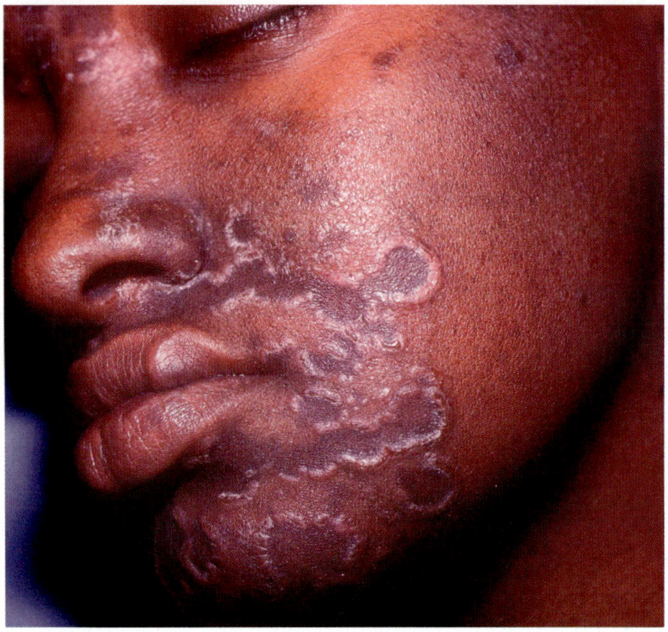

▲ **FIGURE 84-109** Latin America. Secondary syphilis. From Parish LC, Brenner S, Ramos-e-Silva M, Parish JL. *Atlas of Women's Dermatology.* London, Taylor & Francis, 2006.

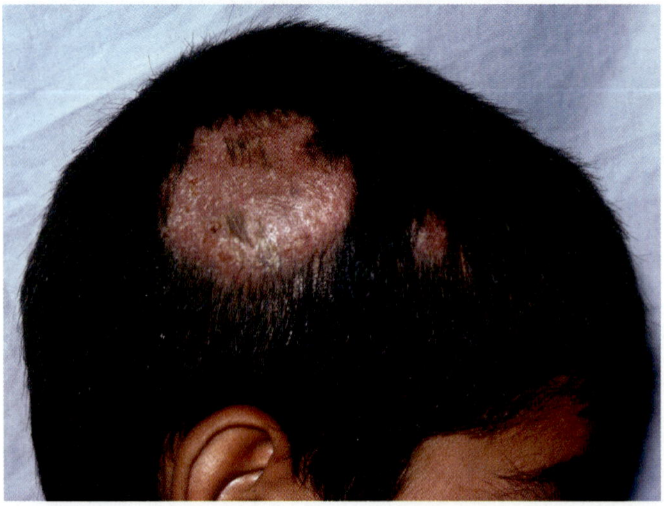

▲ **FIGURE 84-110** Africa. Kerion. Inflammatory tinea capitis due to *M. canis*. Courtesy of Dr. Barbara J. Leppard.

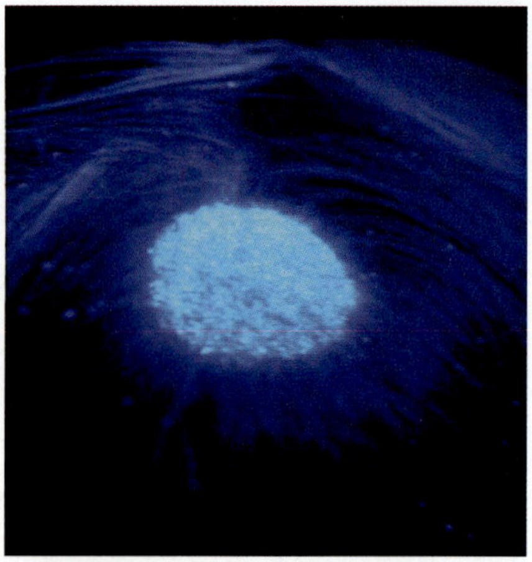

▲ **FIGURE 84-111** Africa. Wood's light examination of the scalp—green fluorescence if the tinea is due to *Microsporum* species. Courtesy of Dr. Barbara J. Leppard.

in India owing to the use of vegetable oils on the scalp for hair dressing, which is a traditional custom. *T. violaceum* has been found to be the main cause in Indian school children. Trauma to the scalp owing to shaving of the head for religious purposes seemed to be an important contributory factor. The disease mainly affects children from 4–14 years of age and can be transmitted from child to child as well as by infected combs, brushes, and caps.

Clinical Perspective

The clinical appearance of tinea capitis is extremely variable and determined by the species of dematophyte responsible for the infection, as well as by the immunity of the host. The appearance may vary from a few dull gray, broken-off hairs with little scaling known as

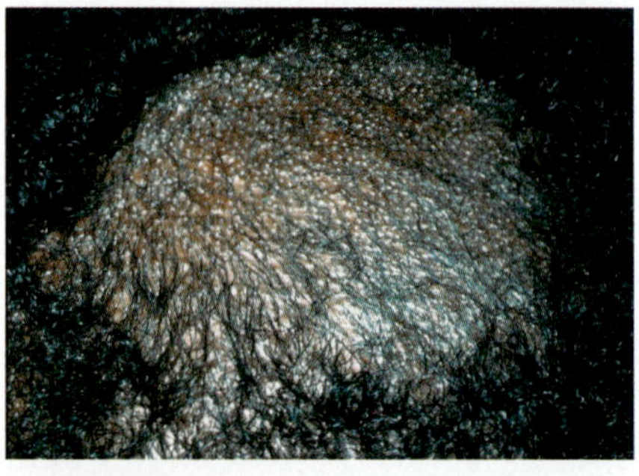

▲ **FIGURE 84-112** Africa. Tinea capitis. Short broken-off hairs rather than complete baldness in the affected patch. Courtesy of Dr. Barbara J. Leppard.

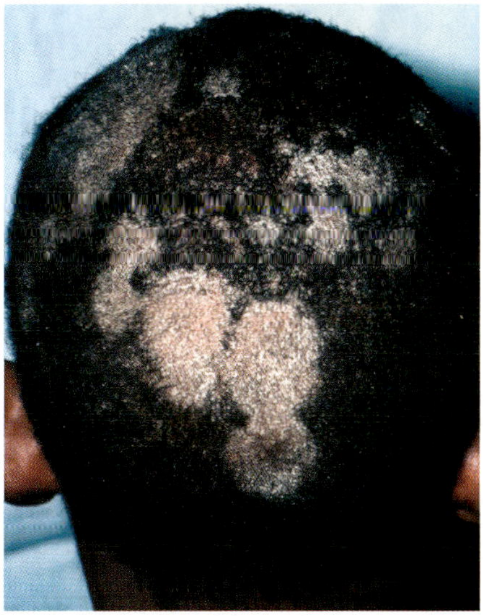

▲ **FIGURE 84-113** Africa. Tinea capitis. Multiple bald patches on a child's scalp. Courtesy of Dr. Barbara J. Leppard.

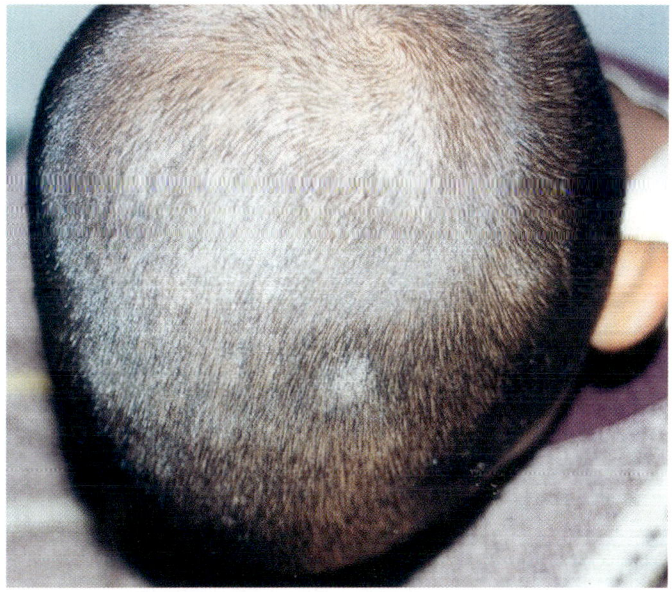

▲ **FIGURE 84-114** Asia. Gray patch of tinea capitis. Courtesy of Dr. Rashmi Sarkar.

gray patch (Figures 84-113 through 84-116), or an inflammatory type with a boggy, indurated swelling that is studded with broken or unbroken hairs, vesicles, and pustules known as *kerion* (Figure 84-110), or the *black dot* type consisting of broken hairs at the level of the scalp (Figure 84-112), or *favus*, which has yellow cup-shaped crusts pierced by hairs.

Differential Diagnosis

Alopecia areata, psoriasis, and seborrheiic dermatitis have to be differentiated. When in doubt, a potassium hydroxide (KOH) preparation and/or a fungal culture will aid in the diagnosis.

Treatment Options

Oral griseofulvin, ketoconazole, itraconazole, and terbinafine are the mainstays of treatment. Selenium sulfide and other topical antifungal shampoos are useful for getting rid of the carrier state.

TINEA VERSICOLOR

Definition

This is a superficial fungal infection of the skin characterized by discrete or confluent, scaly, discolored or hypopigmented areas on the upper trunk (Figures 84-117 through 84-120).

Etiology

The causative organism is a lipophilic yeast, *Malasezzia furfur.* It is seen commonly in tropical climates and in Asia.

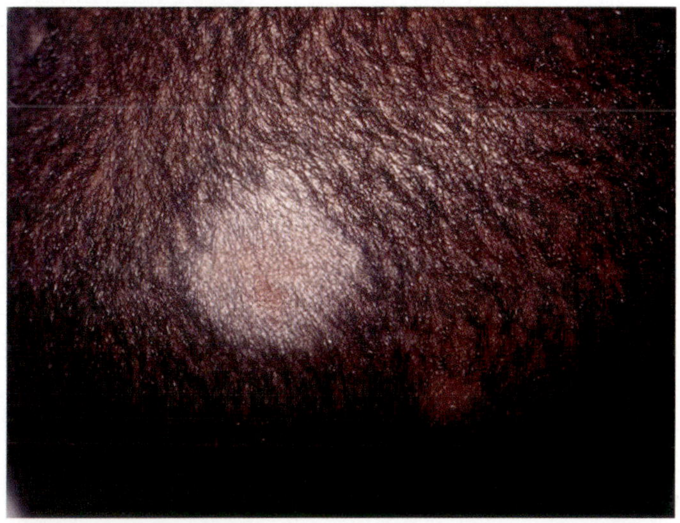

▲ **FIGURE 84-115** Latin America. Tinea capitis. Courtesy of Dr. Marcia Ramos-e-Silva.

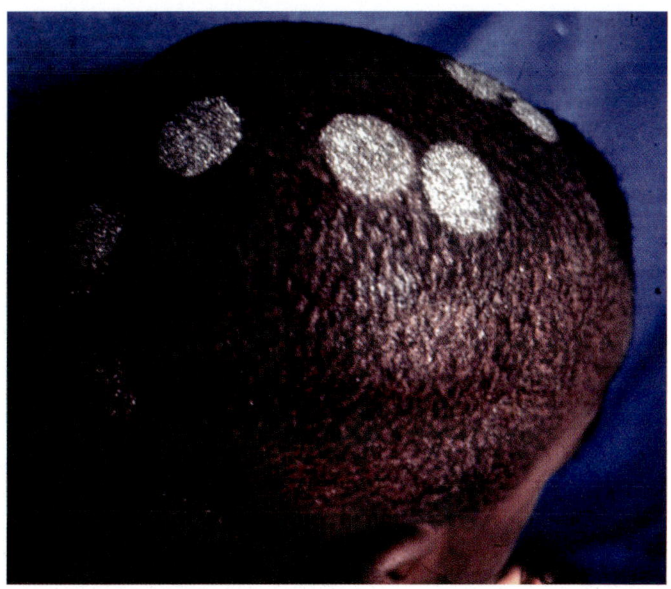

▲ **FIGURE 84-116** Latin America. Tinea capitis. Courtesy of Dr. Marcia Ramos-e-Silva.

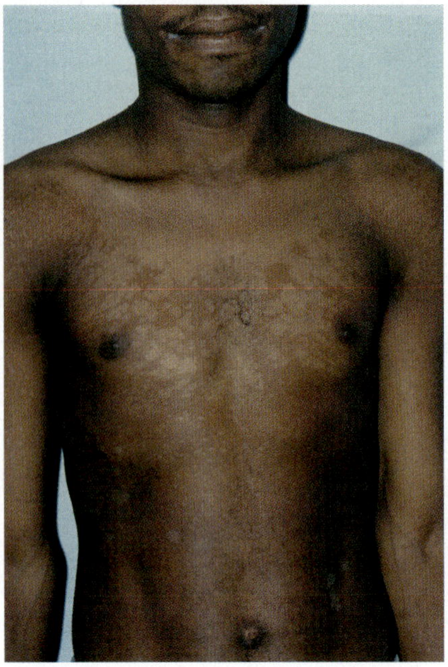

▲ **FIGURE 84-117** Africa. Tinea versicolor in a teenage boy. Courtesy of Dr. Barbara J. Leppard.

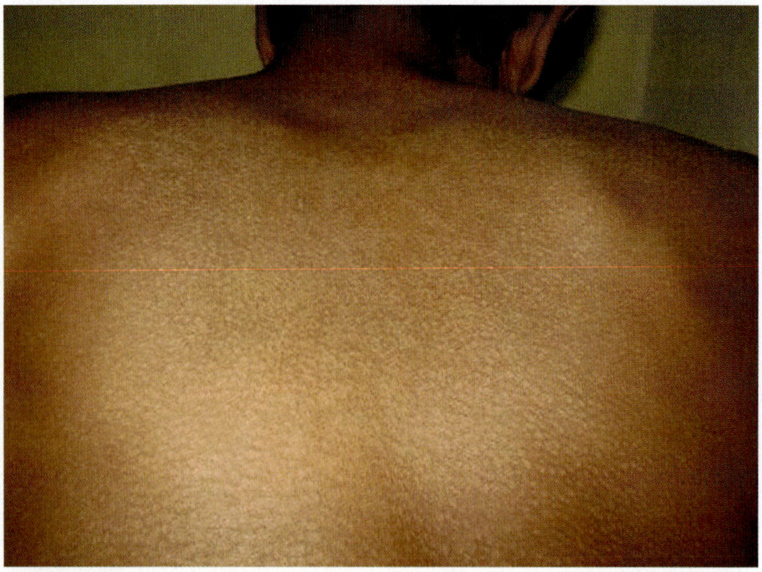

▲ **FIGURE 84-118** Asia. Pityriasis (tinea) versicolor. Courtesy of Dr. Sudhanshu Sharma.

Clinical Perspective

The primary lesions are sharply demarcated macules, which may be pink, tan, or white (versicolor) and covered by fine scaling. In dark-skinned patients, large confluent areas of gray-brown pigmentation with scaling may be seen on the upper trunk, upper arms, neck, and abdomen (Figure 84-117) or extending to the groin and thighs. Facial and scalp involvement is common in Indian patients. The residual hypopigmentation, without any scaling, may persist for months.

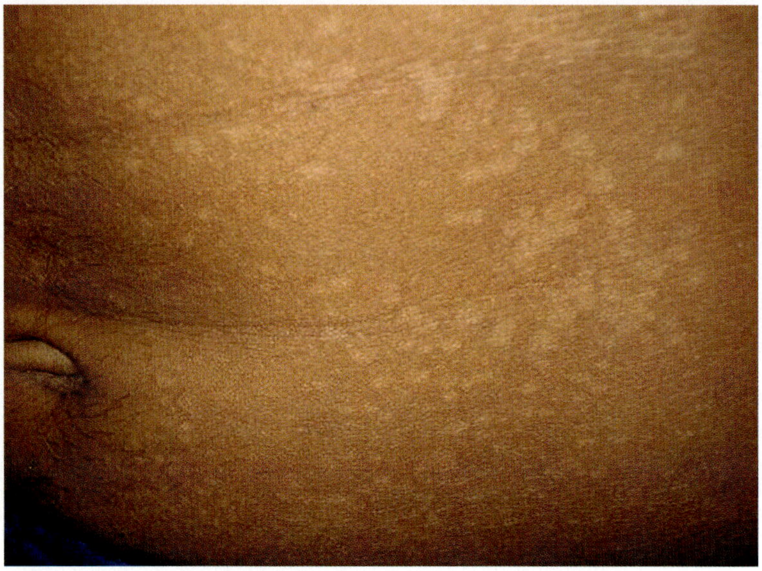

▲ **FIGURE 84-119** Asia. Tinea versicolor. Courtesy of Dr. Sudhanshu Sharma.

Differential Diagnosis

Vitiligo and melasma are differentiated owing to a lack of scaling. Seborrhoic dermatitis would have yellow greasy scales, and pityriasis rosea consists of papules with collarette of scales. Syphilis can be differentiated by frequent involvement of palms and soles and a positive VDRL test.

Treatment Options

The topical azole antifungals and 1% terbinafine cream work well in tinea versicolor, and recovery takes 2–3 weeks. Ketoconazole lotions and shampoos and 2.5% selenium sulfide are other alternatives. Oral ketaconazole and itraconazole are also effective in tinea vesicular. Itraconazole is given in a total dose of 800–1000 mg over 5 days.

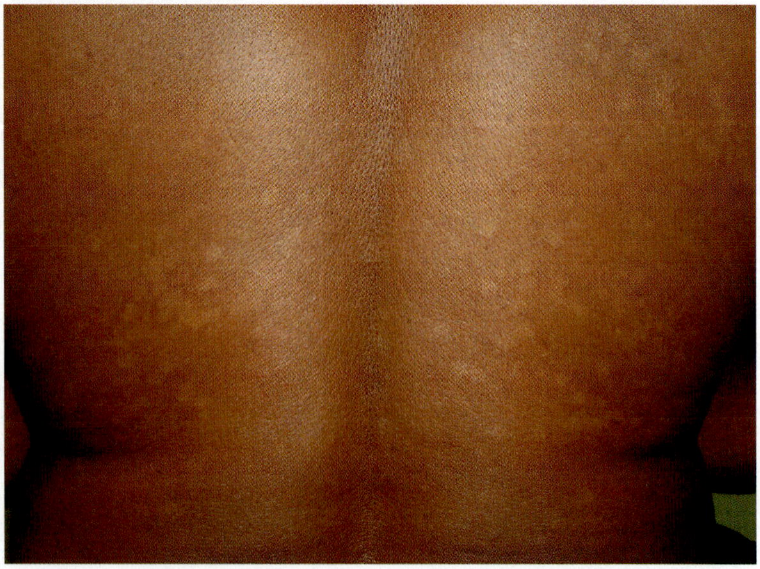

▲ **FIGURE 84-120** Latin America. Tinea versicolor. Courtesy of Dr. Marcia Ramos-e-Silva,

SECTION 16

A History of African-American Dermatologists: Nineteenth Century through the Present

CHAPTER 85

A History of African-American Dermatologists: Nineteenth Century through the Present

Angela D. Dillard
Frederick N. Quarles

In his 1963 "I Have a Dream" oration, the Reverend Dr. Martin Luther King, Jr., looked with longing and hope to the day when people would be judged according to the content of their character rather than the color of their skin. In attacking the causes and consequences of discrimination, inequality, and injustice, it was certainly not King's intent to play down the importance of the objective study of black skin itself. While many theorists locate the roots of racial prejudice in the color of skin, black skin also has generated a long and rich history of men and women who have dedicated their lives to the study, treatment, and care of dermatologic conditions and diseases. Race may only be skin deep—and not, that is to say, a matter of genetics and blood—but that skin holds many characteristics, oddities, benefits, and mysteries peculiar unto itself. What follows is a brief history of individuals—along with some of the institutions and organizations they have founded and influenced—dedicated to looking deeply and conscientiously into the layers of African-American skin, hair, and nails.

Today, African-American dermatologists practice across the country, hold positions in major research universities and corporate institutions, and serve as advocates in public health organizations. Institutionally, most belong to the American Academy of Dermatology, which has subsections for both skin of color dermatology and women's specialties, and many are also counted among the 25,000 members of the National Medical Association, the oldest and largest national organization of African-American physicians. The study and practice of skin of color dermatology and of ethnic skin in general is currently well established in a variety of medical schools and hospitals. But this was not always the case. Indeed, writing a history of African-American dermatology presents some interesting historical challenges, not the least of which is deciphering what "counts" as "dermatology" and who can be regarded as a "dermatologist." Doubtless "African-American dermatology" existed in various forms long before there were officially trained and board-certified practitioners.

The first phase of modern dermatology in the United States (as well as Continental Europe and Great Britain) dates from roughly 1850–1900, coinciding with periods of virulent racism and systemic racial exclusion in America. The first regional dermatologic associations began appearing in the United States at least as early as 1869, with the first national organization, the American Dermatology Association, holding its first annual meeting in 1877. Yet the specialty did not receive full official recognition until 1932 with the formation of the American Board of Dermatology as the first incorporated entity charged with setting and maintaining the standards for the practice of dermatology and syphilology. The American Academy of Dermatology made its appearance shortly after, in 1939, and is presently the largest member-based organization for dermatologists in America and worldwide. As was the case in other medical specialties and within the professions at large, African-Americans were pointedly excluded from these organizations and were forced to establish their own separate associations and networks.

The men who met during the Cotton States and International Exposition in 1895 to call the National Medical Association (NMA) into existence knew the power of racial prejudice even as they sternly rejected the badge of inferiority because of it. As was the case with other African-American professional and fraternal organizations founded during the "nadir" in African-American and American history, the NMA grew out of patterns of racism and segregation that made African-American professionals—indeed all African-Americans—marginal to the mainstream of American society. They were far from marginal inside their own communities, however. Dr. Charles V. Roman captured the spirit of this duality in a statement that has become the historical manifesto of the organization:

> Conceived in no spirit of racial exclusiveness, fostering no ethnic antagonism, but born of the exigencies of the American environment, the National Medical Association has for its object the banding together for mutual cooperation and helpfulness, the men and women of African descent who are legally and honorably engaged in the practice of the cognate professions of medicine, surgery, pharmacy and dentistry.[1]

They were collectively denied admission to the ranks of the American Medical Association, which maintained a strict policy of racial exclusivity, and in response, they turned inward to the mutual support and solidarity of their own association. Such professional, fraternal, and religious organizations founded on the broken shards of Reconstruction became the central components in the creation and maintenance of a vibrant African-American public sphere. Thus this era of gross discrimination also was the age of institution and community building that erected the infrastructure—the bones and muscle—of African-American communities.

And where there are bones and muscle, there is also skin—the human body's largest organ. A dermatologist was not among the charter members of the NMA, but the Dermatology Section (founded in 1940) has a distinctive history, and numerous dermatologists have served in various capacities within the NMA throughout the twentieth century. What follows is far from *the* definitive history of African-American dermatologists in America. Rather, it is a brief overview of some of the men and women who can be regarded—and celebrated—as pioneers in the field, as institution builders and educators, as trailblazers and mentors, and as those who are helping to shape the profession as we move into the twenty-first century.

THE PIONEERS

The first generation of African-American dermatologists included a handful of mavericks and pioneers. Among the earliest and most emblematic of this group was Dr. Theodore K. Lawless (1892–1971). Born in Thibodeaux, Louisiana, his parents were Alfred Lawless, Jr., and Harriet Dunn Lawless. Shortly after his birth, the family moved to New Orleans, at a time when members of the African-American community were struggling against the rising tide of racial segregation. Known by his friends as "T. K.," Lawless attended Straight College, a historically African-American college that operated between 1868 and 1934, when it merged with New Orleans University to form Dillard University. Years later, in 1955, he would remember these roots and honor his father by establishing the Lawless Chapel at Dillard with a $500,000 gift.[2]

After graduating from Straight, he received an A.B. degree at Talladega College in Alabama in 1914. Lawless attended the University of Kansas Medical School, earned an M.D. from Northwestern University in 1919 and an M.S. in 1920. After a 1-year fellowship in dermatology and syphilology at Massachusetts General Hospital, Lawless completed his postgraduate training at the University of Paris. Given the hostile racial climate within the United States, it was hardly unusual for aspiring African-American professionals to seek additional education in Europe.

By 1924, Dr. Lawless had returned to the United States and established a private practice in a predominantly African-American neighborhood on the southside of Chicago during the years of the "Great Migration" that drew thousands of African-American southern migrants to northern cities. In the same year, he began teaching dermatology at Northwestern's medical school, where he served until 1941. As an instructor and researcher, Lawless made a number of contributions to the field of dermatology. His research was published in such scholarly publications as the *American Journal of Dermatology,* the *Journal of Laboratory and Clinical Medicine,* and the *Journal of the American Medical Association.* He worked to find a cure for leprosy and made several strides in the treatment of both leprosy and syphilis. As a dermatologist, Lawless was often consulted by other doctors, and he was noted for his equal treatment of patients regardless of class or race. Dr. Lucius C. Earles, III, who trained with Lawless in the late 1960s after completing his residency at Howard, recalled that his patients included figures from "all walks of life, a heavy influx of folks from the lily white suburbs as well as African-Americans from Chicago."[3]

"Dr. Lawless was a doctor in the old sense of the word," recalled another associate. "He dealt in humanity." The more people he could see, the more he felt he accomplished, and at $3 a visit (a substantial discount at a time when others were charging between $10 and $15), he amassed a fortune owing to the sheer volume of patients he was able to accommodate.[4]

But Lawless was not alone, and Chicago emerges as one of the early hubs of the profession. Also in the city at this time was Paul Prince Boswell, M.D., a prominent southside dermatologist in private practice. A native of Pittsburgh and a graduate of Lincoln University in Pennsylvania, he received an M.D. at the University of Minnesota. While it is not clear where he did his residency in dermatology, he became a staff physician at Chicago's Provident Hospital and also was on the staffs of Michael Reese and Michigan Avenue hospitals. In 1947, he was elected as a member of the American Academy of Dermatology, becoming one of only three African-American members at the time. Dr. Boswell's first wife was a prominent figure in medical social work, and his second wife was a local activist and educator, Arnita Young Boswell, whose brother, Whitney Young, was head of the National Urban League. Dr. Boswell was for years a fixture in the black society pages of the *Chicago Defender* and was deeply engaged in civic work. In the mid-1960s, he even served a term in the Illinois legislature. He died, in Chicago, in 1982.[5]

Lawless and Boswell were joined by Harold Thatcher, M.D. A native of Kansas City, Kansas, and a1929 graduate of the University of Minnesota Medical School, Thatcher's dermatologic training included an internship at Provident Hospital in Chicago and 4 years of study at Billings Hospital with grants from both the Rockefeller and Rosenwald foundations, as well as a year at University and Bellevue hospitals in New York, where he worked in dermatology and syphilology.

In 1942, Dr. Thatcher volunteered for military service and entered the Army with the rank of major in the medical corps, serving his entire tenure as chief of medical services, regional and station hospitals, while based at Fort Huachuca in Arizona. In 1944, he was promoted to lieutenant colonel and in 1945 was awarded the Legion of Merit by the War Department. When he returned to civilian life, he returned to Chicago and entered private practice, with an affiliation with Provident Hospital's Department of Dermatology. He also was a member of the board of trustees of Cook County Hospital's nursing school and a member of numerous civic and civil rights organizations.

Thatcher and Lawless worked closely together in a variety of nonmedical ventures, most notably the Federal Savings and Loan, for which Lawless was founder and chairman and for which Thatcher served as vice chair, as well as the creation of the Theodore K. Lawless Gardens, a three-building, 24-story housing complex on Chicago's southside. After Lawless' death in 1971, Dr. Thatcher took over the chairmanship of the Federal Savings and Loan and served as the executor of Lawless' million-dollar estate. A tireless professional and a major philanthropist—his several donations included the establishment of a dermatology department at Belinson Hospital in Tel-Aviv, Israel—Lawless was also an educator, serving on the faculty of the University of Illinois.

One of his students, Homer E. Harris, Jr., M.D., was to become a pioneer in his own right. Born in 1916 in Seattle, Washington, Harris was the first African-American to venture into practice in the Pacific Northwest region. As a Garfield High School student, he excelled in athletics and graduated in 1933 as the captain of the school's football team. It was an accomplishment that aided his matriculation at the University of Iowa, where he was an All-Big Ten player. Had it not been for the racist policies of the National Football League (NFL), Harris would have been well placed to pursue a career as a professional athlete. Instead, he turned to medicine. Harris attended Meharry Medical College in Nashville, Tennessee, and interned in Kansas City, Missouri. He completed his dermatology residency at Illinois under Lawless' guidance.

Returning home to Seattle, he set up private practice in 1955 and remained there for over 40 years with a practice reputed to be the largest west of the Rockies. Dr. Harris became a fixture within Seattle's African-American community and found that the practice of dermatology "provides me a sense of independence in not having to rely on hospitals or physicians for referrals." He was well liked by his patients and highly regarded by the Seattle community, so much so that an anonymous donor contributed $1.3 million to be used for the creation of a half-acre park named in his honor.[6]

Within the category of pioneers and mavericks, one also could arguably include Madame C. J. Walker and the burgeoning hair and beauty industry. A self-made millionaire, Walker invented several hair care products, including Madame Walker's Wonderful Hair Grower and a hair softener that could be used with a hot comb. Bald patches and scalp diseases functioned as the scarlet letter of poverty for many women of this era, and the famous Walker System offered them relief. Not a trained professional in any conventional sense, she nonetheless revolutionized the ways African-American women styled and cared for their hair and went on to open a school—Lelia College, in Pittsburgh—where hundreds of "beauty culturists" were trained. This would have been one of the only major institutions where large numbers of women received any sort of training in the care of hair and skin. While Madame Walker eventually would relocate to New York, her empire was firmly rooted in African-American Chicago community, giving that city a fair bid to be called the "home of African-American dermatology."[7]

The challenges of training African-American professionals in a climate of racial hostility and segregation were substantial. Many of our pioneers looked to Europe or to the ranks of the military for training, and most spent some amount of time at a historically African-American institution, either for their undergraduate or medical school education. Some came from other countries across the African-American diaspora to attend these institutions. Thomas Obadiah Senior, M.D., for example, was born in Broughton, Jamaica, in 1883 and came to New York from Havana, Cuba, in 1919. Dr. Senior graduated from Meharry Medical College in 1923 and spent the bulk of his career there as first an instructor and later a professor in the fields of dermatology, genitourinary diseases, and syphilodermatology. He died in 1937.[8]

There is one institution itself that deserves special mention for its pioneering role. The history of the Department of Dermatology of the Howard University College of Medicine and Howard University Hospital (formerly Freedmen's Hospital) stretches back to 1906, when Henry H. Hazen, M.D., conducted weekly dermatology clinics at Freedmen's Hospital and gave a regular course in dermatology to medical students. Hazen continued these efforts almost single-handedly until 1927, when C. Wendell Freeman, M.D., graduated from the Howard College of Medicine and began work in the dermatology clinic.

Freeman, a native of Washington, DC, traveled to Europe for advanced training in the specialty. From 1934–1935, he studied dermatology in Germany, Vienna, and other European medical centers as a fellow of the Oberlander Trust of Philadelphia. In subsequent years, Dr. Hazen's visits became less frequent, and Freeman's duties at the hospital expanded. By the early 1940s, he had become a clinical assistant professor at Howard and in 1941 was made a diplomate of the American Board of Dermatology and Syphilology after passing the board's examination. He also was widely known for his efforts to educate the general populace and specialists about the perils of syphilis. In 1942, for example, he embarked on a four-state lecture tour designed to bring the latest advancements to the general practitioner.[9] At various times over the next two decades or so, the division of dermatology at Freedmen's Hospital would be augmented by Drs. John C. Payne, Peter D. Johnson, Jocelyn Mitchell, and eventually, Jesse A. Kenne and Joseph G. Gathings.

Gathings, who also was among the earliest African-American diplomates of the American Board of Dermatology and Syphilology, had 2 years of special training, from 1941–1943, as a Rosenwald Fellow at the New York Skin and Cancer Hospital. He would serve for some 15 years in the Division of Dermatology at Freedmen's Hospital and the Howard University College of Medicine, first as a clinical instructor and later advancing to a clinical assistant professor. He also had been a president of the NMA. At the time of his death in 1965, he was conducting a research project, supported by the Shriners, in the skin condition known as *vitiligo*. Dr. Freeman left the program at the hospital and the college well provided for. In 1961, he had been instrumental in obtaining the services of John A. Kenney, Jr. (Figure 85-1), who, in continuing the work of these pioneers, would go on to leave a distinctive mark on the study and African-American practices of dermatology as one of the field's most noted institution builders.

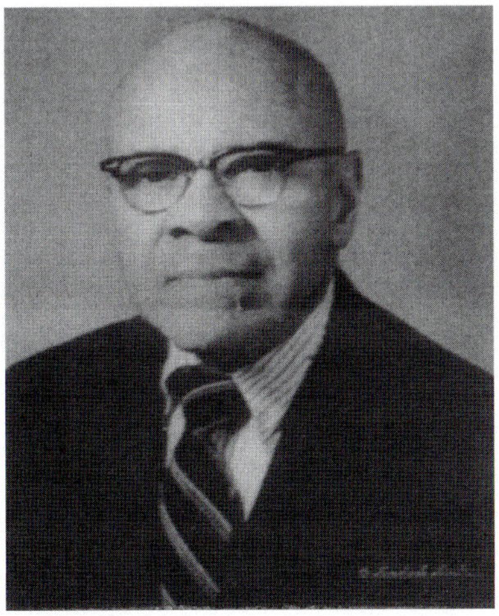

▲ **FIGURE 85-1** John A. Kenney, Jr., M.D. (deceased).

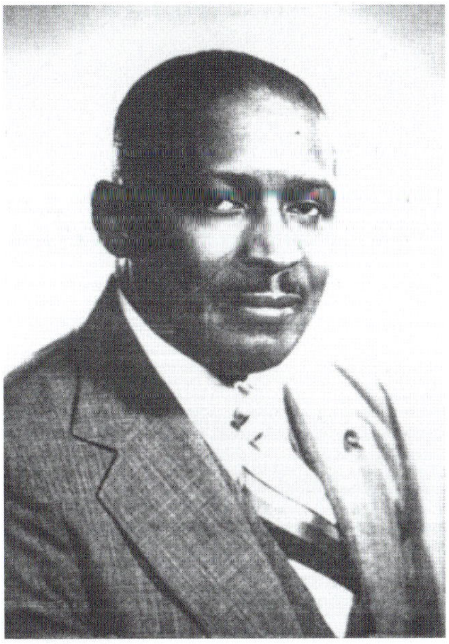

▲ **FIGURE 85-2** Vernal Cave, M.D. (deceased).

INSTITUTION BUILDING: AFRICAN-AMERICAN DERMATOLOGY COMES OF AGE

New fields of study, professional practice, and human endeavor need pioneers and trail blazers to search out new opportunities and to enlarge our sense of possibilities. As these avenues develop and grow and become more established, however, there must be a second generation willing to take on the vast responsibilities for building and sustaining institutions and networks. It is this generation, straddling the divide between pioneers and builders, that is awarded more official recognition than their predecessors and that contains members who were granted a wider arena in which to develop their talents and to practice their craft.

Vernal Gordon Cave, M.D. (Figure 85-2), was born in 1918 in Colon, Republic of Panama, and was raised primarily in Brooklyn, New York, reminding us that the "great migration" that brought thousands of African-Americans from the South to the North and dovetailed with the sizable wave of black immigration to urban centers such as New York. Cave earned a B.S. at City College (City University of New York) and an M.D. at Howard University College of Medicine in 1944. He served as a medical officer in the United States Army and Air Force for the renowned Tuskegee Airmen from 1947–1952 and was honorably discharged after obtaining the rank of captain. His postgraduate studies were pursued at a number of hospitals, including Harlem Hospital in New York City, Freedman's Hospital in Washington, DC, the North Carolina Sanatorium for the Treatment of Tuberculosis in Wilson, North Carolina, New York University Post-Graduate Medical School, and the New York Bellevue Medical Center. In 1956 he became a diplomate of the American Board of Dermatology and Syphilology, thus becoming the first board-certified African-American dermatologist in Brooklyn. The earliest black dermatologist across the river in New York City seems to have been Thomas L. Day, M.D., who had a practice in Harlem, followed by Gerald Spencer, M.D.

For 16 years ending in 1975, Dr. Cave served as deputy director, acting director, and director of the Bureau of Venereal Disease Control of the New York City Department of Health. During his tenure of leadership within the NYC Department of Health not only did the incidence of infectious syphilis in New York City decline,but he also implemented a policy of equal rights and opportunities for positions and promotion for women.

He has authored or coauthored some 35 scientific articles and chapters in scientific journals and medical textbooks. He was one of the original members of the board of directors at the inception of the New York City Health and Hospitals Corporation, exerting his efforts for improved health care for all Americans regardless of race or economic status. Dr. Cave was a career member of the National Medical Association, of which he was a past president, and was a member of the board of trustees of the Brooklyn Branch of the NAACP. He also was a member of the Ad Hoc Committee on the Tuskegee Syphilis Study appointed by the federal government and also was chairman of the National Medical Association Ad Hoc Tuskegee Syphilis Study Committee. It was through the investigative work of these committees that the atrocities of the Tuskegee Syphilis Study were exposed.

Born in Tuskegee, Alabama, in 1914, John A. Kenney, Jr., M.D., was a son of Dr. John A. Kenney, Sr., medical director and chief surgeon at the general hospital at the Tuskegee Institute and personal physician to the institute's founder, Booker T. Washington. Dr. Kenney, Sr., also was a cofounder of the National Medical Association. When his activities on behalf of African-American doctors and nurses led to a KKK-initiated cross burning on the Kenney family's lawn, Kenney, Sr., moved the family to Montclair, New Jersey, where Kenney, Jr., and his three siblings grew up and pursued their educations. He graduated from Bates College and was a member of the class of 1945 at the Howard University College of Medicine.

While interning at Cleveland City Hospital in Ohio (then one of the first white city hospitals to admit African-American residents), Kenney had a transformative experience. An influential white doctor at the hospital persuaded him to choose dermatology as his specialty. At the time, none of the other 80 African-American physicians in Cleveland were dermatologists, and many white dermatologists refused to treat African-American patients—a situation that was painfully ubiquitous in most regions of the country. Inspired by the older doctor, Kenney pursued dermatologic training at the University of Pennsylvania and the University of Michigan, returning in 1954 to Cleveland to join the staff at University Hospital and the faculty at Case Western Reserve. As the city's only African-American dermatologist, he also built a sizable practice, including many white patients as well. Despite this success, he felt the lure of academic medicine and the rigors of research and the training of new dermatologists. In accepting a teaching and administrative position at Howard, Kenney moved from the category of pioneer in the field to institution builder.

Kenney came to Freedmen's Hospital and the Howard College of Medicine in 1961 as associate professor of dermatology and was selected as chief of the division when Dr. C. Wendell Freeman retired from Howard in 1963. It was a position Kenney would hold until 1981. In these crucial decades in which the study and practice of African-American dermatology fully came of age, Dr. Kenney not only trained residents but also gave dermatology lectures to medical students. Indeed, many of the field's "next generation" would cite these lectures as one of the reasons they were attracted to the specialty. During his nearly four decades at Howard, he established a full dermatology department, a 3-year residency program, and a research laboratory in dermatology. Above all, he was instrumental in training numerous students pursuing careers in dermatology; by one reckoning, he trained and mentored one-third of all black dermatologists practicing at the time of his death in 2003.

But Dr. Kenney was not the only major figure at Howard during this period and not the only person responsible for the institutional growth and expansion of its dermatology program. There was also, among others, Dr. Harold E. Pierce, Jr. (1922–2006) (Figure 85-3), who served as an assistant professor of dermatologic surgery at Howard for 17 years. Pierce had been a graduate of Howard College of Medicine (in 1946) and had gone on to intern at Harlem Hospital in New York and to complete a residency in dermatology at the Philadelphia General Hospital. In 1951, he accepted a commission as a captain in what became the U.S. Air Force Medical Service and served with distinction until officially retiring from the Air Force National Guard in 1976. As a dermatologist, Dr. Pierce built his practice and reputation on his diagnoses and treatment of people of color with complex skin disorders that his fellow clinicians were unable to solve.

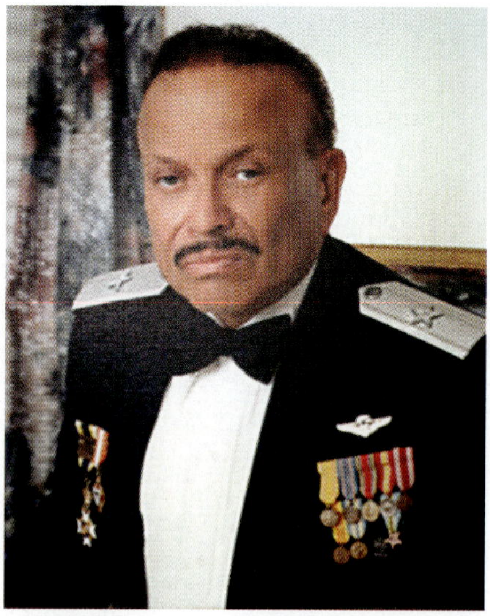

▲ **FIGURE 85-3** Harold Pierce, M.D. (deceased).

During his long and varied career, he preformed the first dermabrasion on an African-American patient, as well as hair transplants and scar revision surgery. Years later he participated in the first liposuction. He was among the first and most prominent African-American cosmetic surgeons in the country and is widely regarded as the "father of African-American cosmetic surgery." Author of more than 50 medical articles and editor of *Cosmetic Surgery in Nonwhite Patients* (New York, Grune & Stratton, 1982), Dr. Pierce trained numerous students, including Mershiler Allen, his medical-surgical assistant, at the Philadelphia College of Osteopathic Medicine and at Howard. His daughter, Sandra E. Vause, M.D., is a practicing dermatologist in New Jersey and has established the Harold E. Pierce, Jr., M.D. Scholarship Trust Fund to support

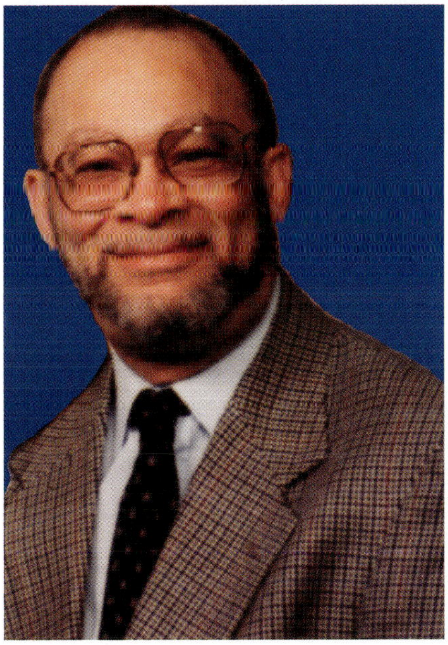

▲ **FIGURE 85-4** Harold Minus, M.D.

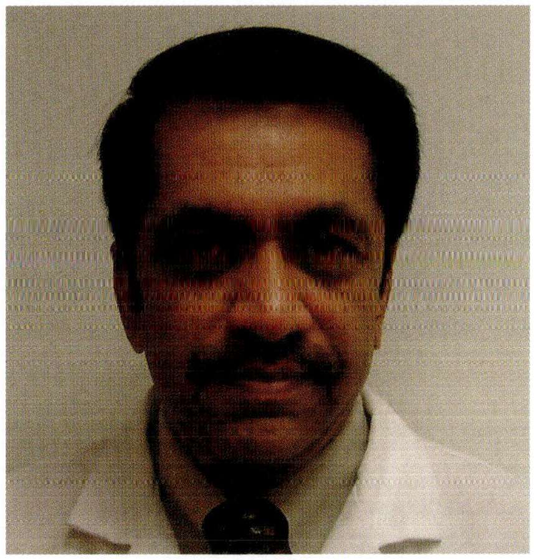

▲ **FIGURE 85-5** Rebat Halder, M.D.

resident doctors in the training and advancement of dermasurgery.[10] She is also the first African-American woman dermatologist with dual board certification in dermatology and cosmetic surgery. She completed the American Board of Dermatology certification in November 1989 and subsequently completed a 1-year fellowship in cosmetic surgery with Drs. Farber and Bridenstein and then sat for and successfully completed the written and oral boards in cosmetic surgery through the American Board of Cosmetic Surgery in November 1991.

Freedmen's Hospital, which changed its name to Howard University Hospital in 1975, and the College of Medicine also had the good fortune to secure the presence of Harold R. Minus, M.D. (Figure 85-4), who took over as chairman of the Department of Dermatology from Dr. Kenney in 1980. He served in this capacity until 1992, when the department's current chair, Rebat M. Halder, M.D. (Figure 85-5), succeeded him. While the next generation of dermatologists was trained at several different institutions, including predominantly white universities such as the University of Michigan and within the ranks of the U.S. armed forces, Howard nonetheless stands out as a virtual powerhouse in the field.

William Coffey, M.D., and Lucius C. Earles, M.D., were graduates of the Howard Medical School class of 1963, and both credit Dr. Kenney for influencing them in choosing careers in dermatology. Dr. William Coffey went on to help develop the dermatology program at King-Drew Medical Center in Los Angeles, which includes the Charles Drew University of Medicine and Science, incorporated in 1966 after decades of militant community-based advocacy for improved medical services. Dr. Earles has been in private practice in Chicago for over 40 years and is a past president of the National Medical Association.

Dr. Earles reflects on his residency training:

> When I began the program … the total number of those choosing dermatology in our class of about 88 at Howard University, 1963, was four. During that most interesting and informative two years, Charles Thurston, the second African-American at [the] University of Michigan, generally came to our Friday morning sessions. It was at that time that I discovered that Dr. Kenney was the first African-American dermatologist trained at the University of Michigan, and little did I have the slightest idea that I would in time be the third.… During my residency at HU, I had the pleasure also of first meeting Greta Clarke, then a student rotating through dermatology as one of her electives. It was during this time in the program at Howard, when we attended the American Academy of Dermatology convention, that I came to realize actually how miniscule the field of African-Americans was in dermatology. Present at the meeting were Dr. Kenney and his flock, John Carney from Los Angeles, John Butler of Detroit, Tommy Williams of DC, a dermatologist who worked at DC General Hospital, and of course our own Carnot Evans.… To sum things up, it was apparent that there was minimal representation at that meeting of those who look like us.

This situation, however, was dramatically altered by the increase in dermatology residents in the late 1960s and early 1970s. The field was forever changed.

THE NEXT GENERATION: AFRICAN-AMERICAN DERMATOLOGY IN THE 1960S AND 1970s

By 1965, the post–World War II Civil Rights Movement had accomplished at least two of its major legislative goals: the Civil Rights Act of 1964 and the Voting Rights Act of 1965. Secured at a painfully high price in terms of human life and nearly a decade of sustained organizing and activism, the social and political environment of the nation was forever changed. Legalized racial segregation was now a thing of the past, and despite the lingering effects of racism, African-Americans were granted an unprecedented level of access and opportunity in education and professional life. At this moment when change was in the air and a new militancy was gripping young African-Americans across the nation, Howard University College of Medicine enjoyed the "dermatology class" of 1965. Dr. Kenney was still relatively new to his post at Howard, and it was his first full year teaching. In 1966, dermatology became an elective, and during these years, the program was home to a group of students dubbed by Dr. A. Paul Kelly as the "Magnificent 7": Robert Heidelberg, Boyd Savoy, Ike Willis, O. G. Rodman, Fletcher Robinson, James Hobbs, and Dr. Kelly himself, who notes that when this group completed their residencies, they "almost doubled the number of practicing African-American dermatologists."[11]

Kelly, the son and grandson of physicians, was born in 1938 in Ashville, North Carolina, and arrived at Howard Medical School after earning an undergraduate degree at Brown. He was in his third-year clinical rotations when he heard a lecture on dermatology by Dr. Kenney and was inspired to choose dermatology as his area of specialization. "Close your eyes and stick a pin in a map of the USA," he recalls Dr. Kenney

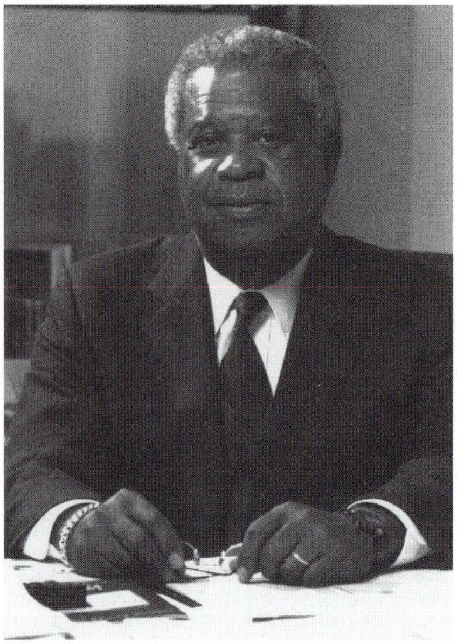

▲ **FIGURE 85-6** Charles McDonald, M.D.

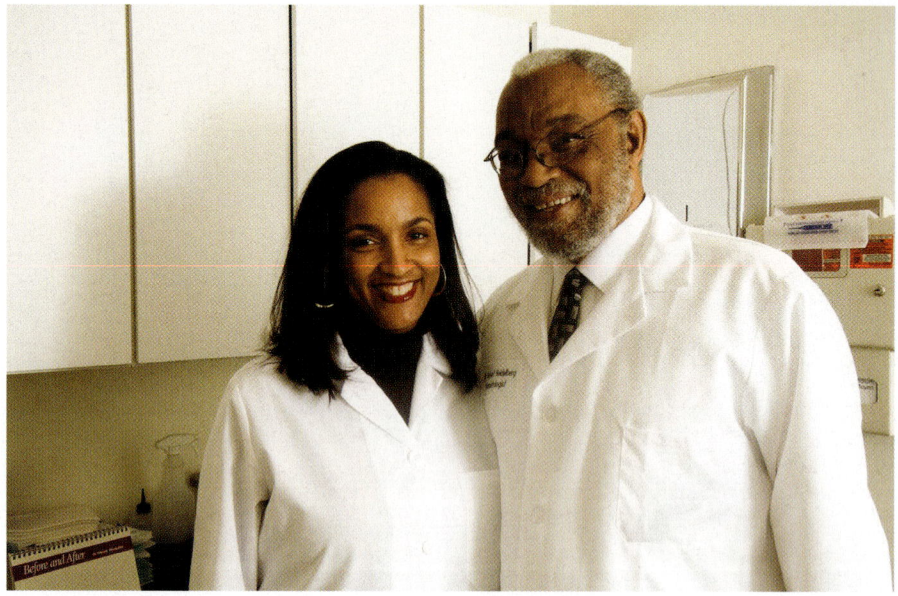

▲ **FIGURE 85-7** Robert P. Heidelberg, M.D., and Karen Heidelberg, M.D.

intoning. "Wherever the pin lands, you can go there and probably be the only African-American dermatologist." For Kelly and his classmates, the pins landed in several different locations, making them in many instances a "African-American first."

Dr. Kelly was the first African-American resident trained in dermatology at Henry Ford Hospital in Detroit, Michigan. His first faculty position was at Brown University Department of Dermatology from 1971–1973, chaired by Charles McDonald, M.D. (Figure 85-6), the first African-American chairman of a dermatology program at a majority white institution. Dr. McDonald remains the first and only chairman of dermatology at Brown University.

After leaving Brown University, Dr. Kelly went to Los Angeles and eventually became Chief of the Division of Dermatology at King-Drew Medical Center/Charles Drew University School of Medicine and Science from 1975– 2006. The dermatology program at King- Drew was the only program other than Howard's specifically developed for the training of minority dermatologists. Dr. Kelly is well known nationally and internationally for his keloid research and has enjoyed a career marked by several "African-American firsts." He was the first African-American president of the American Dermatological Association, the Pacific Dermatologic Association, and the Association of Professors of Dermatology. He is also active in the National Medical Association, having served as editor-in-chief of the *Journal of the National Medical Association* for 8 years (1997–2005).

Dr. Robert Heidelberg was not the first African-American dermatologist in Detroit—that distinction goes either to John Butler, M.D., or Edward W. Kelly, Jr., M.D.—but he has had one of the largest private practices in Detroit for over 40 years. His daughter, Karen Heidelberg, M.D. (Figure 85-7), is also a dermatologist and practices with her father and his classmate, L. Boyd Savoy, M.D. James Hobbs, M.D., has been in private practice in Los Angeles for over 40 years. He, too, has a daughter, Lori Hobbs, M.D., who is a dermatologist also practicing in Los Angeles (Figures 85-8). Orlando G. Rodman, M.D., was a member of Howard's "dermatology class" of 1965 but left school to join the Army in 1966, serving as a paratrooper until 1969. Following in the footsteps of Vernal Cave, Harold Pierce, Harold Thatcher, and others, he trained in dermatology

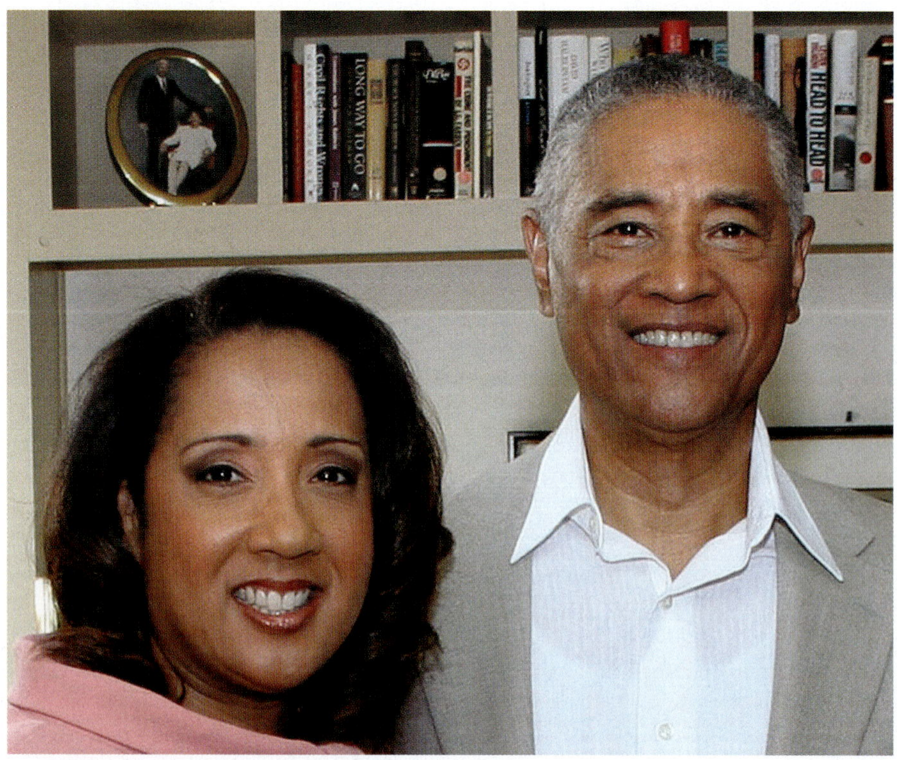

▲ **FIGURE 85-8** James Hobbs, M.D., and Lori Hobbs, M.D.

while in the armed services. Board-certified in dermatology and dermatopathology, in 1974 he was named chief of dermatology at Walter Reed Army Medical Center. After retiring from the Army as a colonel in 1987, he joined the American Academy of Dermatology's scientific program as director of its Gross and Microscopic Symposium and was vice chairman of the Department of Dermatology at Detroit's Henry Ford Hospital from 1987–1993. In 1993, he relocated to Macon, Georgia, where, until his retirement in 2005, he was part of the Georgia Dermatology Group in Macon.

Isaac (Ike) Willis, M.D., was trained in dermatology at the University of Pennsylvania, where he worked closely with Albert Kligman, M.D. Through their joint efforts, they developed the first combination fading cream that consisted of hydroquinone, retinoic acid, and corticosteroid. Today, this combination fade cream is patented as Triluma by Galderma Pharmaceutical Company. After completing his training at Penn, he relocated to his hometown of Atlanta, Georgia, joining the practice of Wesley Wilborn, M.D., who is credited as the first African-American dermatologist in the state of Georgia. Dr. Willis has written numerous scientific papers mainly pertaining to melanin metabolism and the treatment of dyschromia. He remained in private practice in Atlanta for over 30 years until his recent death in August 2007.

Leonard Boyd Savoy, M.D., is a faculty member within the Department of Dermatology at Wayne State University in Detroit and was chairman of the Dermatology Department at the VA Medical Center in Allen Park, Michigan, for several years. He has written numerous scientific papers mostly relating to the urticaria and the inflammatory and chemotactic response in atopic dermatitis. He practices part time with Drs. Robert and Karen Heidelberg. Fletcher Robinson, M.D., the last of the seven, is the first and only African-American dermatologist to have a dual private practice in both St. Thomas, U.S. Virgin Islands, and Washington, DC, for over 25 years.

Adding to the geographic diversity of the "magnificent seven" were a number of individuals who made their mark as the first to set up private practices in various locations, including Drs. Norman Walton (Alabama), Errol Quintal (Louisiana), Richard Gibbs (Tennessee), William Anderson (East Orange, New Jersey), and Raymond Blackburn (Texas), as well as Drs. Claude Vernon Caver (Hawaii) and, a little later, John H. Bocachica (Alaska).

As this generation came of age within the profession, they were both the cause and the beneficiaries of racial integration and the increased liberalization of American society in the late 1960s and 1970s. Educated and trained during the era of sit-ins, freedom rides, and civil rights marches, they entered the profession as calls for "Freedom Now" were replaced with the demands of "Black Power." Black was beautiful, and militant activists began to organize around community control and empowerment. By the late 1970s and early 1980s, the study and the practice of skin of color dermatology had truly come into its own. The program at Howard, which has been overseen by Rebat Halder since 1992, continued to turn out dozens of new dermatologists and was joined, in 1975, by the newly minted residency program at King-Drew in Los Angeles.

In many ways, and under very different circumstances, Dr. Kelly sought to do at Drew what Dr. Kenney and other pioneers had done at Howard. At the same time, black students were being increasingly admitted to programs at institutions such as Michigan, Pennsylvania, and Brown, where Charles McDonald, M.D., has been such an important presence since 1968. While Dr. McDonald and Dr. Algin Garrett (Figure 85-9), a specialist in Mohs' micrographic surgery and chair of the dermatology program at Virginia Commonwealth, are the rare African-American heads of programs at majority institutions, this generation has had the benefit of education and mentoring from across the lines of race and ethnicity. Many of those who went on to play leading roles in staking out new geographic territories, in engaging in new techniques, and in providing leadership for professional organizations such as the National Medical Association's Dermatology Section were educated during this expansive period.

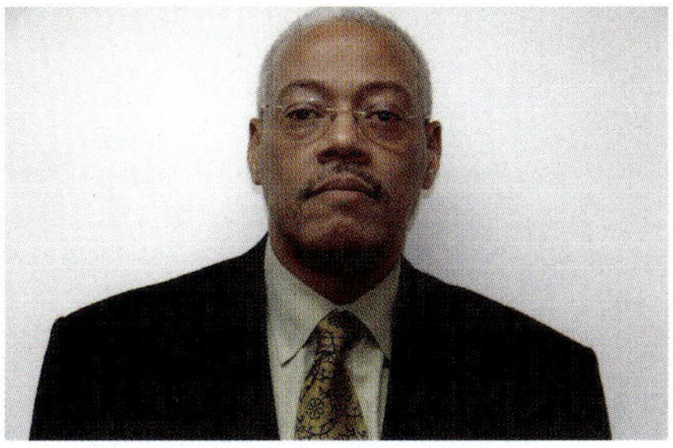

▲ **FIGURE 85-9** Algin Garrett, M.D.

The experiences of Dr. Frederick Quarles are to some extent emblematic of this expansive generation. Born in Detroit in 1955, he is old enough to have known pioneers and institution builders such as Vernal Cave, Harold Pierce, and John Kenney personally and young enough to have witnessed and helped to encourage the transformation of the field in terms of gender, setting up private practice in Norfolk, Virginia, with Dr. Katherine Treherne in 1985. Dr. Quarles received the M.D. degree from Howard in 1981 and completed the residency in dermatology at Howard under the guidance of Drs. Kenney, Minus, Pierce, Carnot Evans, and Halder, as well as Pearl Grimes and Cassandra McLaurin. His career has been shaped by both the liberalization of race relations in the United States since the mid-1960s and the continuing existence of our nation's racial polarization. His concern over the latter has propelled his involvement over the years with the Old Dominion Medical Society in Virginia (past president) and with the NMA, especially the Dermatology Section, of which he served as chairman in 2005–2207. Always a student of history and distressed by the lack of attention to African-American men and women in the histories of national organizations such as the American Dermatological Association, the American Academy of Dermatology, and the American Board of Dermatology, this present history project was initiated as part of his service to the NMA.

As the barriers of race became less daunting to black dermatologists and other professionals, so too did the traditional demarcations based on gender. With Harold Minus as chairman and Pearl Grimes and Cassandra McLaurin as assistant professors within the Dermatology Department at Howard, during the 1980s, the door for black women to enter into the field of dermatology was opened wide at old historic Howard and at a host of other institutions.

AFRICAN-AMERICA WOMEN IN DERMATOLOGY

Dr. Pearl Grimes (Figure 85-10) is fondly referred to by some as "Mother Pearl" for her leadership, mentoring, and encouragement for women in dermatology within the NMA and American Academy of Dermatology. Since 1990,

▲ **FIGURE 85-10** Pearl Grimes, M.D.

she has been the medical director of the Vitiligo and Pigmentation Institute of Southern California and maintains a full-time private practice in Los Angeles. Dr. Grimes is also a clinical professor of dermatology at the David Geffen School of Medicine, and she lectures extensively on issues pertaining to her research in the skin disease known as *vitiligo*—a topic she first developed an interest in from the direct mentoring received from Dr. Kenney while at Howard. Grimes completed her medical education at Washington University in St. Louis (1970–1974) and her residency training in dermatology at Howard University Hospital (1975–1978), where she was chief resident (1978–1979). Grimes credits much of her success to a number of pioneers and institution builders, including Dr. Kenney, "who recognized strengths that I did not recognize myself." Dr. Kenney, she continues, "built the walls for an academic foundation that was laid at Washington University," and her experiences with Dr. Harold Minus and Dr. A. Paul Kelly "were the mortar and wood that completed the process."[12]

Dr. Grimes has been an important mentor to men and especially women in dermatology in her own right. She was first an instructor and later an assistant professor at Howard's College of Medicine, as well as director of the Vitiligo Research Center. In 1984, she left Howard for a position at Charles R. Drew University of Medicine and Science, where she was an assistant professor until 1992 and an associate professor until 2005. As a teacher within and beyond the walls of academia, she also has played a leading role in broadly disseminating the histories of the profession, including such video productions as *The Women's Dermatologic Society: A Historical Perspective* (2005), *The Measure of a Great Man: The Life and Legacy of Dr. John A. Kenney, Jr.* (2004), and *History of the American Society of Dermatologic Surgery* (2006).

Greta Clark, M.D., was one of the first African-American women in private practice in Oakland, California, where she has been located for over 30 years and has served as a regional trustee for the NMA. Born in Detroit, Michigan, she received the M.D. degree in 1967 from Howard; she completed a residency in internal medicine at Harlem Hospital, followed by a residency in dermatology at New York University in 1972. She was greatly influenced by Dr. Kenney at Howard and by Dr. Thomas Day in New York, as well as by Hilda Germaine Straker, M.D., who maintained a private practice in Manhattan while heading the Division of Dermatology at Harlem Hospital.

Dr. Straker is more than likely the first African-American woman to be board-certified in dermatology. A native of New York and a 1940 graduate of Howard, she completed an internship at Harlem Hospital and further dermatologic training at NYU–Bellevue Medical Center. She was a member not only of the NMA but also of the American Medical Association, the American Academy of Dermatology, and the American Women's Medical Association. After she retired from private practice, she became a consultant to the Revlon Cosmetics Company.[13]

Cassandra McLaurin, M.D., has been at Howard for the past 30 years as an instructor (1978–1979), an assistant professor (1979–1984), and an associate professor (1984–present) in the Department of Dermatology. She chose an academic career initially because Dr. Kenney recruited her to Howard and has remained because of a dedication to the training and empowerment of the next generation of dermatologists. Specializing in pediatric dermatology, she has a long publications record on topics ranging from keloids to pediatric dermatoses. She claims Drs. Kenney and Minus as important mentors and has published studies with colleagues such as Dr. Grimes. As a student, she especially admired Burnett Johnson, M.D., "for his expertise in the arts and balanced approach to medicine and life"—a balance that she still seeks to help her own students and residents achieve.

Yvonne Knight, M.D. (Figure 85-11), heads the Aesthetic Clinique and the Medi Spa Clinic. She graduated from the University of Michigan in premedical studies and trained at Howard, is a board-certified dermatologist and is an assistant clinical professor in the Department of Dermatology of the VCU Medical Center. Margery Scott, M.D., completed the dermatology residency at Thomas Jefferson University Hospital and a dermatopathology fellowship at Temple University's Skin and Cancer Hospital in Philadelphia and then returned home to Norfolk, Virginia, becoming one of the first African-American female dermatologists to practice in Virginia—an honor she shares with Yvonne Knight, M.D. Dr. Scott was chief of the Division of Dermatology at the VA Medical Center in Hampton, Virginia, for over 30 years before retiring and accepting a full-time faculty position within the newly formed Department of Dermatology at Eastern Virginia Medical School (EVMS) in Norfolk, Virginia. Dr. Scott has a daughter, Dr. Kimberly Scott, who recently completed a dermatology residency at EVMS and is a faculty member within its department, making them the first mother-daughter dermatologists working in tandem.

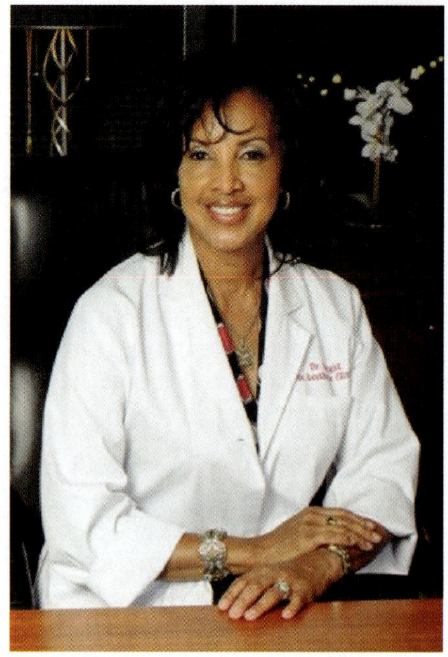

▲ **FIGURE 85-11** Yvonne Knight, M.D.

Outside strictly academic circles, Susan C. Taylor, M.D., has become a highly visible leader in the field. She serves on the board of directors for the American Academy of Dermatology, and she is also a founding board member for Skin of Color Society, established in 2004. Born in Philadelphia and educated at the University of Pennsylvania (B.A. 1979) and Harvard Medical School

(M.D. 1983), she completed an internship and residency at Pennsylvania Hospital and a residency in dermatology at Columbia Presbyterian Medical Center in New York. She holds certifications in both internal medicine and dermatology. In private practice in Philadelphia since 1989, in 1999 she was appointed as director of the Skin of Color Center at St. Luke's Roosevelt Hospital Center. The center, which is the first of its kind in the nation, is dedicated to the investigation, diagnosis, and treatment of diseases in individuals with skin of color, inclusive of those with African-American, Hispanic, and Asian ancestry.

Indeed, Dr. Taylor sits at the cusp of one of the major new trends in the field, one that involves the broadening of the category "black dermatology" in the direction of the science, study, and treatment of skin of color. Howard's medical school and hospital have a history of nonwhite and non-African-American students, particularly Indian students, and its present chair, Dr. Halder, is of Indian ancestry. A 1978 graduate of Howard University College of Medicine, he completed a residency at Howard University Hospital. He joined the faculty at Howard in 1982 and has been chairman of the Dermatology Department since 1992. Dr. Halder established and is the director of the Ethnic Skin Research Institute within the department and is an authority on pigmentary disorders of the skin and in ethnic dermatology. In 1999, he directed the first session in ethnic dermatology for an annual meeting of the American Academy of Dermatology and is the author of the first textbook on ethnic dermatology entitled, *Dermatology and Dermatological Therapy of Pigmented Skins* (2006). Dr. Kelly, moreover, has trained Hispanic, Asian, and Euro-American residents within the King-Drew program. Consciously working under the rubric "skin of color," promoting its study and care in societies, publications, Web sites and lecture tours, Dr. Taylor and her colleagues are helping to reconfigure the very idea of black skin. And Drs. Kelly and Taylor, editors of this textbook, *Dermatology for Skin of Color* (McGraw), seek to further develop awareness of cutaneous manifestations of skin diseases in people of color while giving young and more mature dermatologists a platform for writing about these subjects.

Black women have come to occupy the very center of black dermatology and are simply too numerous to mention and document in these pages. A representative sample drawn from academic and private practice, from national organizations such as the NMA and the Women's Dermatologic Society (WDS), and the continuing tradition of highlighting "African-American firsts" would include the following women: Lynn McKinley-Grant (Figure 85-12), a board-certified dermatologist, has 19 years' experience in private practice and academic medicine. McKinley-Grant is an associate clinical professor of dermatology and an attending physician at the Melanoma Center at the Washington Hospital Center. She attended Harvard Medical School, has a master's degree from Columbia University Teacher's College, and did her residency at New York University. She is a diplomate of both internal medicine and dermatology. Valerie Callender, M.D., who trained under Dr. Minus, lectures frequently nationally and internationally and has served as a past chairman of the Dermatology Section of the NMA. Positioning herself at the nexus of the NMA, the WDS, and the Skin of Color Society, of which she serves as treasurer and a member of the board, she also heads the Callender Skin and Laser Center in Mitchellville, Maryland. Cheryl Burgess, M.D., practices in the Washington, DC, area and also was trained at Howard under Dr. Minus. She received an M.D. degree from Howard in 1984 and completed her residency in 1988, during which time she was greatly influenced by Drs. Beverly Johnson, Katherine Treherne, and Frederick Quarles, all of whom allowed her to rotate with them and learn various aspects of running a dermatologic practice. Dr. Burgess is the founder, medical director, and president of the Center for Dermatology and Dermatologic Surgery, P.C., in Washington, DC, and an assistant clinical professor at Georgetown University Medical Center and George Washington Hospital. She is also the director of an Allegan-sponsored Botox Cosmetic Training Center, as well as author and senior editor of *Cosmetic Dermatology* (Springer-Verlag).

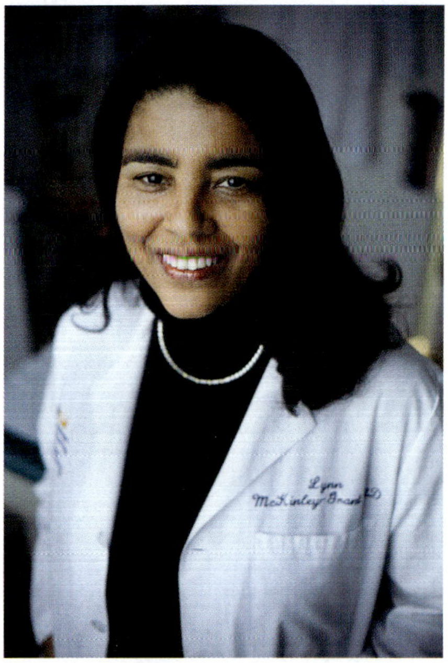

▲ **FIGURE 85-12** Lynn McKinley-Grant, M.D.

Wendy Roberts, M.D., who was trained at King-Drew by Dr. Kelly, is in private practice in Desert Palms, California, and serves as a regional trustee for the American Academy of Dermatology. Born in East Orange, New Jersey, she received an M.D. degree at Stanford in 1984 and completed her residency in 1991 and a dermatopathology fellowship at New York University Medical Center in 1993. She is the founding director of the Section of Dermatopathology, Loma Linda University Medical Center, Division of Dermatology, and is currently a clinical assistant professor of medicine at Loma Linda, the first African-American dermatologist on the faculty. In addition to her practice in cosmetic dermatology, geriatric dermatology, and dermatopathology, she is active in numerous regional associations and in the WDS. Presently the vice-president/president elect of the WDS, she is in line to be that organization's first African-American president in 2009.

Women who were the first to venture into private practice in various states include Denise Buntin, M.D. (Tennessee), who was also the first African-American resident in dermatology at the University of Tennessee, where she served as chief resident (1982–1983). Dr. Buntin was, in addition, one of the first women to chair the Dermatology Section of the NMA. Patricia Treadwell, M.D. (Figure 85-13), pediatric dermatologist (Indiana), became interested in dermatology during a residency in pediatrics at Riley Hospital. Spending time in the office of Dr. Arthur Sumrall solidified her devotion, and she completed her residency at Indiana School of Medicine in 1983. She continues to hold faculty positions at Indiana in the departments of pediatrics and dermatology. While attending a meeting of the American Academy of Dermatology as a resident, Dr. Treadwell met and befriended Gloria Campbell-D'Hue, M.D. (Georgia). A graduate of Emory University School of Medicine who did

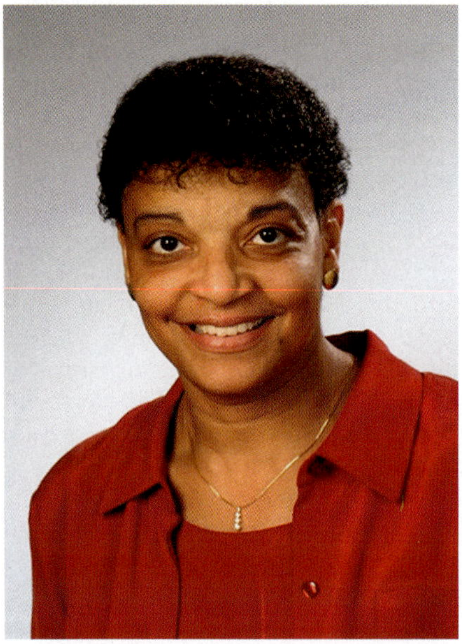

▲ **FIGURE 85-13** Patricia Treadwell, M.D.

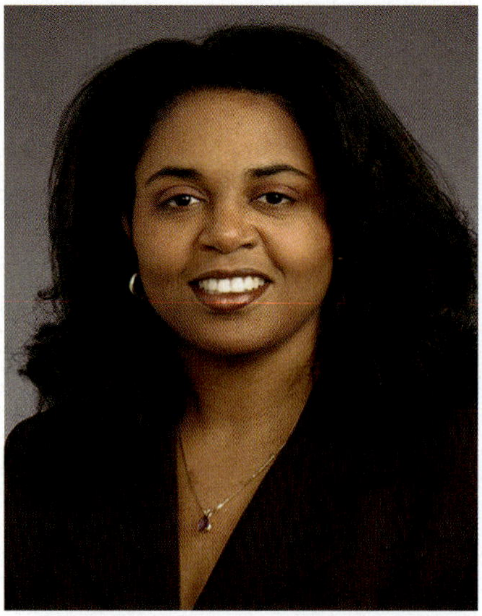

▲ **FIGURE 85-14** Amy McMichael, M.D.

her dermatology residency at Cincinnati Hospital, Dr. Campbell-D'Hue has been in private practice in Atlanta since 1983.

Lorna Lacen Thomas, M.D. (Michigan), received a medical degree from the University of Michigan and completed her internship and residency training at Detroit's Henry Ford Hospital. The first African-American president of the Michigan Dermatological Society and a member of numerous boards and associations, she maintains a thriving practice in Detroit. Katherine Treherne, M.D. (Virginia), is a graduate of Meharry Medical College (1980). She did dermatologic training at Howard University Hospital before moving to the Tidewater area in 1985, where she remains in private practice. Over the years, Dr. Treherne has served as president of the Tidewater Dermatological Society, which is just one of many regional associations, and as chairman of the Dermatology Section of the NMA (1993–1995). Jacquelyn B. Garrett, M.D. (Missouri), graduated at the top of her 1985 class at Howard. The first lecture in dermatology she attended was delivered by Dr. Grimes, and she benefited from the tutelage and support of Drs. Halder and Minus. She moved to St. Louis to intern at Barnes Hospital, where she also completed her residency in dermatology in 1989, serving as chief resident her last year. Dr. Garrett maintains a busy practice in the northern suburbs of St. Louis and has served as president of a regional medical society (Mound City Medical Forum) and as head of the Dermatology Section of the NMA (1999–2001).

To round out the field and this segment of our history, we have selected an additional academic, a leader in the arena of cosmetics and pharmaceuticals, and a woman committed to what might be called "dermatologic community service". Very few new-era women have chosen to pursue full-time careers in academic dermatology, unlike Amy McMichael, M.D. (Figure 85-14), who is assistant professor within the Department of Dermatology at Wake Forest University in Winston Salem, North Carolins. Born and raised in Philadelphia, she is a graduate of the University of Pennsylvania School of Medicine and did her residency training at the University of Michigan. Those professional experiences that she finds most memorable include becoming a faculty member, doing advanced training in epidemiology, and finishing her first book. She selected a university career over private practice in order to teach others and to encourage more people of color to enter into academia.

Victoria Holloway Barbosa, M.D. (Figure 85-15), is a graduate of the Yale University School of Medicine. She completed an internship in internal medicine at the Massachusetts General Hospital in Boston and her dermatology residency at Yale, serving as chief resident. While she has been an instructor at Johns Hopkins and a clinical assistant professor at Howard, Dr. Barbosa has spent the majority of her career as a vice president in research and development at L'Oreal USA, where she built and ran the L'Oreal Institute for Ethnic Hair and Skin Research in Chicago—the birthplace of the hair and beauty industry generated by Madam C. J. Walker in the early decades of the twentieth century. Board-certified since 1998, Dr. Barbosa specializes in general dermatologic conditions such as acne and eczema, as well as ethnic skin and hair disorders. In 2006, she decided to leave the industry and return to academia, accepting a

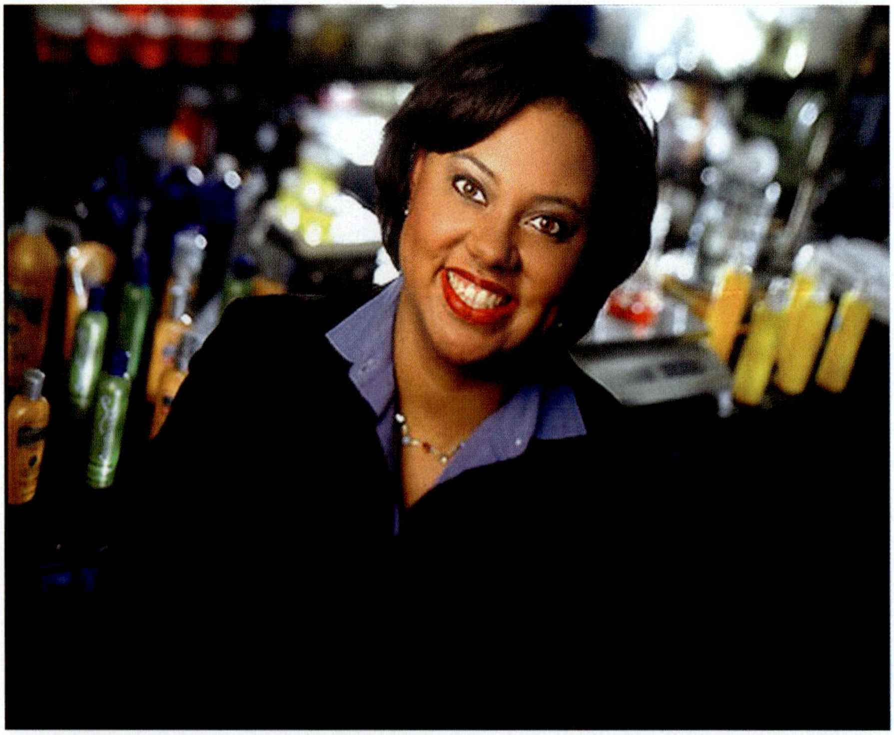

▲ **FIGURE 85-15** Victoria Holloway Barbosa, M.D.

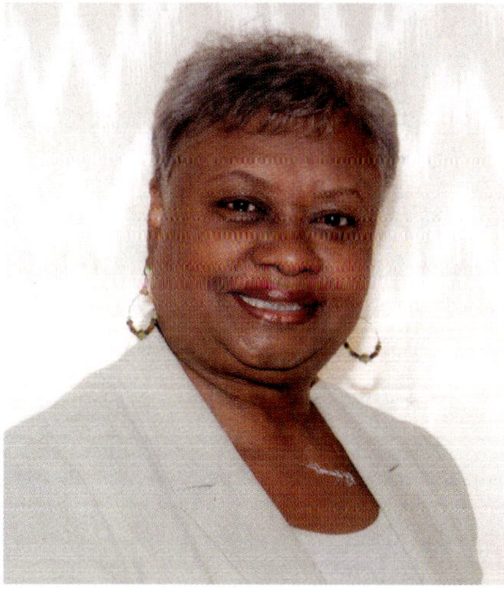

▲ **FIGURE 85-16** Allison Nicholas Metz, M.D.

position as an assistant professor and assistant attending for the Dermatology Department at Chicago's Rush University Medical Center.

Allison Nicholas Metz, M.D. (Figure 85-16), daughter the former dean of admissions at Meharry Medical College, was the first African-American female dermatologist in the Northern California Permanente Medical Group, where she practiced for over 30 years until her retirement in 2007. A native of Jamaica, West Indies, she moved to Nashville, Tennessee, and subsequently received an M.D. degree from Meharry Medical College in 1969. After an internship at Letterman Army Medical Center, Presidio, San Francisco, she completed a residency in dermatology at the University of California San Francisco Medical Center in 1976. Drs. Isaac Willis and Arthur Mayo certainly influenced her choice of dermatology as a specialty, but as a resident, she became greatly inspired by Drs. Kenny and A. Paul Kelly in training so many African-American dermatologists.

Stella Bulengo, M.D., received a B.A. and M.D. degrees and residency training from the University of Michigan, after finishing high school in Nairobi, Kenya. Board-certified in dermatopathology as well as dermatology, she has worked to educate others—both at home and abroad—about the prevention of skin diseases. Since 1996, she has worked with her father (who is also a physician) in Tanzania on HIV/AIDS prevention and has worked with that nation's Regional Dermatology Training Center, which trains doctors from Tanzania and other African countries. Over the years, she also has taught skin hygiene in Arusha and has participated in similar programs in the United States. Bridging cultures and continents, Dr. Bulengo's experiences and commitments are representative of the range of community and outreach efforts black dermatologists have been associated with for nearly a century.

FACING THE FUTURE: AFRICAN-AMERICAN DERMATOLOGY IN THE TWENTY-FIRST CENTURY

Many of the women and men—and the fathers and sons and mothers and daughters—highlighted in the preceding sections are helping to define the future of black dermatology at the close of the first decade of the twenty-first century. A quick survey of several practitioners identified a number of major trends. First and foremost is the shift from African-American dermatology to the study and care of skin of color discussed earlier. From Dr. Halder's Ethnic Skin Research Institute at Howard, to Rush University's Ethnic Skin and Hair Clinic under the direction of Drs. Ella Tooms and Victoria Holloway Barbosa, to the Skin of Color Society, whose executive officers include Drs. Taylor, Halder, Callender, Barbosa, Kelly, Grimes, and others, this shift is beginning to make itself felt in the training and practice of dermatologists across the nation and throughout the world.

Where black dermatologists train also has undergone a shift in more recent decades. The program at King-Drew trained roughly 60–64 residents of various ethnic backgrounds before recently closing, whereas Howard's program exists alongside programs at majority institutions with which it must compete. What the future holds for one of the other major sites for training black dermatologists—the U.S. armed services—remains an open question. As this history makes clear, many of the earliest black dermatologists, such as Drs. Harold Thatcher and Vernal Cave, served and practiced in the military, as did several second-generation specialists such as Dr. Orlando G. Rodman. So too did Charles S. Thurston, M.D., a 1958 graduate of Meharry Medical College, who did his internship at William Beaumont Army Hospital, a residency at the University of Michigan (1963–1966), and advanced training at the School of Aviation Medical School before going on to pursue an academic career in and out of the U.S Air Force. He is a retired colonel and remains a member of the Association of Military Dermatologists.

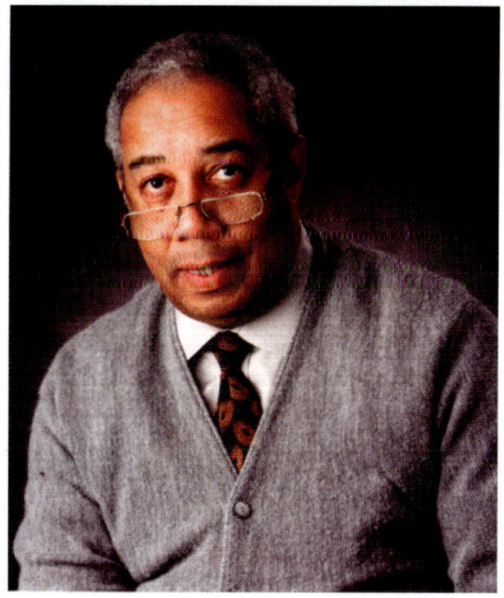

▲ **FIGURE 85-17** Bernett L. Johnson, Jr., M.D.

Bernett L. Johnson, Jr., M.D., (Figure 85-17), is also a graduate of Meharry. He did his dermatology residency at the University of Pennsylvania and the Naval Hospital in Philadelphia. He spent 23 years in the Navy's medical corps in a mixture of clinical, academic, and administrative positions before returning to civilian life. He is currently a professor of pathology and laboratory medicine at the University of Pennsylvania. Dr. Johnson's son, Brian Johnson, M.D., has followed in his father's footsteps, replicating something of a pattern of intergenerational pairings. Dr. Brian Johnson received his dermatological training in the Navy, and he is now in practice as a Mohs' surgeon in Norfolk, Virginia.

One also could point to the career of Norvell Vandervall Coots, M.D. Dr. (Colonel) Coots is the commander of the Keller Army Community Hospital at West Point, New York, and the fifty-second command surgeon for the United States Military Academy. He did part of his medical training at Howard but finished the M.D. degree at the Oklahoma College of Medicine. After performing a transitional internship at William Beaumont Army Medical Center in El Paso, Texas, and a 2-year tour as a general medical officer in Korea, he completed his dermatology residency at Brooke Army Medical Center in San Antonio. As mentors, he claims, among others, Drs. Rodman and Thurston, as well as Dr. Clarence Wiley, a civilian in private practice in Oklahoma. Dr. Coots' military assignments have included both clinical and operational positions and have taken him around the world in the service of the nation.

Dr. Coots is a highly decorated military man with numerous publications to his name. He is also the current chairman of the Dermatology Section of the NMA and is scheduled to become the assistant deputy for health policy for the Assistant Secretary of the Army for Manpower and Reserve Affairs in July 2008. Asked whether he had advice for persons considering a career in dermatology, he says

> It is the best career decision that one can make. It offers immense rewards in terms of scope of practice, personal time and family time management; in essence it is a lifestyle specialty, and it is financially rewarding as well. Being an Army dermatologist is an issue in-and-of itself, and it is particularly rewarding to be able to treat Service Members and their family members for both common dermatoses and the unusual diseases contracted from world-wide deployments and travel.[14]

As the United States continues to engage in battles on many fronts and in numerous, often exotic locations, the arena for dermatologists to serve the needs of men and women in the armed services seems destined to continue to attract new practitioners.

Another notable trend is the move from medical dermatology toward cosmetic dermatology. Facial contouring via the use of dermal fillers is being demonstrated and taught nationally and internationally by Pearl Grimes, M.D., and Cheryl Burgess, M.D. In terms of invasive procedures such as body contouring via liposuction, Ella Toombs, M.D., has been performing and lecturing on this procedure since first being introduced to liposuction by Dr. Harold Pierce in the mid-1980s. She is currently director of the Ethnic Skin and Hair Clinic at Rush University Medical Center in Chicago. Dr. Toombs also has been associated with an additional trend within the field: the development and testing of drug applications. Before joining the faculty at Rush, she followed in the footsteps of Carnot Evans, M.D., and served for years as a dermatology medical officer at the U.S. Food and Drug Administration (FDA), as had Dr. Evans. At the FDA, Dr. Toombs oversaw the approval of drug applications that have transformed the practice of dermatology, including Dovonex (for psoriasis), Ortho-tricyclen (the first birth control pill approved for acne), Doxepin (the first tricyclic antidepressent approved for pruritus), and Renova (the first and only FDA-approved "antiwrinkle" cream).

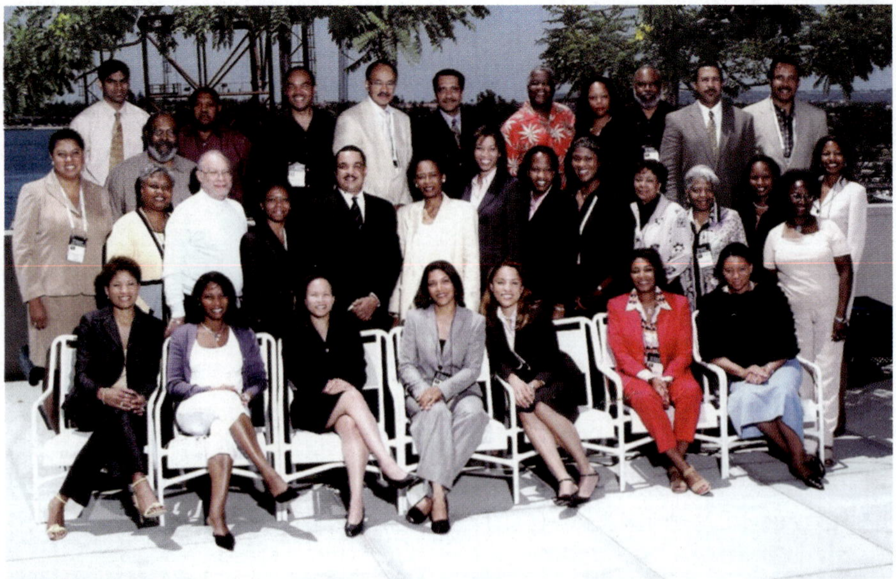

▲ **FIGURE 85-18** National Medical Association Section of Dermatology, San Diego, CA 2004. *First row seated from left to right:* Katherine Treherne, Cheryl Burgess, Dawna Shabazz, Shari Hicks-Graham, Kim Nichols, Tina Baisden-Pickett, Jacquelyn Garrett. *Second row from left to right:* Victoria Barbosa, Allison Nichols Metz, Harold Minus, Yolanda Holmes, Eliot Battle, Terry Dunn, Nicole DeYampert, Yolanda Lenzy, Denise Buntin, Brenda Vaughn, Cassandra McLaurin, Kimberly Scott, Denise Cook. *Third Row from left to right:* Pavan Nootheti, William Coffey, Roland Hart, Moses Elam, A. Paul Kelly, Rebat Halder, George Cohen, Valerie Callender, Sidey Thompson, Fred Quarles, A. Melvin Alexander.

In the growing field of laser surgery technology in skin of color, trendsetters include Arthur Sumrall, M.D. (Indiana), who was one of the first eight American physicians to travel to France to learn the liposuction process from a French creator; Clarence Wiley, M.D. (Oklahoma), who specializes in dermatologic, cosmetic and laser surgery, photomedicine, and cosmetic products research; Seymour Weaver, M.D. (Texas), who studied dermatologic surgery with Dr. Harold Pierce in Philadelphia during his residency at Martin Luther King, Jr., General Hospital in Los Angeles; and Eliot Battle, M.D. (Washington, DC). Dr. Battle did his dermatology fellowship at Howard and his pioneering laser research at Harvard's Wellman Laboratories of Photomedicine under the tutelage of Rox Anderson, M.D., who helped to invent the new generation of noninvasive cosmetic lasers that are safe and effective on skin of color. A past chairman of the Dermatology Section of the NMA, he is also cofounder and director of laser surgery for Washington, DC's Cultura Cosmetic Medical Spa, a medical practice that merges dermatology, laser surgery, plastic surgery, and spa therapy.

The rise of "medi-spas" such as Cultura and Odyssey Medispa in Marina del Rey, owned by Marcia Glenn, M.D., represents yet another important developing trend in the field—one that will no doubt continue to offer new challenges and opportunities, new advancements in patient care (and comfort), and new avenues of research and innovation.

CONCLUSION

Whether a pioneer, an institution builder, an academic, or a head of a department, center, institute, organization, board, or section, black dermatologists in all fields and subspecialties continue to contend with misconceptions about black skin and skin of color in terms of both diagnosis and treatment. While the dark days of exclusion and marginalization are happily over, the profession—and the nation—still struggle with the legacy of racial and gender discrimination. The men and women of the National Medical Association still have an important role to play in moving us toward a future in which all forms of discrimination and prejudice are consigned to the distant past.

Many of the women and men who have served as chairs of the NMA Dermatology Section have met this challenge head on. Some of their accomplishments have been noted in this historical overview, including those of Drs. McDonald, Willis, Grimes, Wilborn,

Wiley, Kelly, Treadwell, Buntin, Treherne, Garrett, Callender, Battle, Quarles, and Coots. To this list we also would like to add Thomas Johnson, former chief of dermatology at Meharry College of Medicine, and Lindley Mordicai of San Francisco, and we would like to thank Drs. Earl Walker and Oscar Saffold.

No history is ever completely written, and the process of "making history" (in the dual sense of the phrase) is an ongoing one. Above all, as Dr. Jacquelyn B. Garrett so nicely expressed the sentiment, "Given the increasing percentage of Americans with brown skin, there will be an increasing need for dermatologists who are sensitive and knowledgeable about the special needs of those patients" (Figure 85-18). We hope that the past and the future of those dedicated dermatologists will continue to be chronicled and shared.[15] The authors would like to thank the many members of the Dermatology Section of the National Medical Association for their assistance in the collection of materials needed to complete this phase of our historical project, and we welcome their continued participation as the project grows and develops.

REFERENCES

1. Roman, quoted in "Introduction," National Medical Association Web site, *www.nmanet.org*. Roman was a founding member and first editor of the *Journal of the National Medical Association*.
2. "Dillard Names Chapel for Lawless, Dad," *Chicago Defender*, October 1, 1955.
3. Lucius C. Earles, III, to Fredrick Quarles, November 20, 2005; in possession of the author.
4. Quoted in Jack Mabley's profile on Lawless, *Chicago Tribune*, October 10, 1957; see also Theodore K. Lawless, Black Biography, Answers.com.
5. On Boswell, see "Dr. Paul Boswell Honored," *Chicago Defender* (National Edition), December 27, 1947; and "GOP Picks Negro in W. Side Purge," *ibid*, June 3, 1964, which has a brief profile.
6. Christine Clarridge, "Donor Honors Seattle Legend with $1.3 Million Park," *Seattle Post-Intelligencer*, November 12, 2002; Craig Smith, "Homer Harris, 1916–2007: Dermatologist a Sports Pioneer," *Seattle Times*, March 27, 2007.
7. For a good overview of Walker's early career in Chicago and an excellent study of the city's post–World War I black community, see Davarian L. Baldwin, *Chicago's New Negroes: Modernity, The Great Migration, and Black Urban Life* (Chapel Hill, University of North Carolina Press, 2007).
8. The information on Thomas Senior, M.D., was provided by Dr. Fern Nelson and the public service librarian at Meharry Medical College, fax transmission, January 13, 2008; in possession of author.
9. "Howard Instructor Passes Skin Specialist Exams," *Chicago Defender* (National Edition), January 11, 1941, p. 3; "Dermatologist," *Pittsburgh Courier*, March 7, 1942, p. 14.
10. Obituary of Dr. Harold E. Pierce, Jr., MD, Brigadier General (USAF, PANG, ret.), October 2006; in possession of the author.
11. Quoted in Dr. George Dawson, "A Quiet Pioneer: An Interview with A. Paul Kelly, M.D." (2004). Noteworthy is that Dr. Kelly is the son and grandson of physicians and felt that his services to the academic dermatology community were a continuation of his father's and grandfather's services in their own communities as family practice physicians. E-mail correspondence with Dr. A. Paul Kelly, April 29, 2008; in possession of the author.
12. E-mail correspondence with Dr. Pearl Grimes, January 8, 2008; in possession of the author.
13. "Dr. Hilda Straker Fashions Enviable Career as New York Skin Specialist," *Chicago Defender* (National Edition), July 29, 1950, is a profile of Dr. Straker. See also Valerie D. Callender, "Dermatology Section of the National Medical Association," *Women's Dermatologic Association Newsletter* 2002;6:8, which has a brief mention of Straker. Information on Straker also was provided by Greta Clarke, e-mail correspondence, August 1, 2007; in possession of the author.
14. Norvell Vandervall Coots, correspondence, January 13, 2008; in possession of the author.
15. E-mail correspondence with Frederick Quarles with A. Paul Kelly, editor, April 28, 2008; in the possession of the author; he sent a partial list of noteworthy African-American Dermatologists: A. Melvin Alexander, M.D., William Anderson, M.D., Saundrette G. Arrindell, M.D., Tina Baisden-Pickett, M.D., Victoria Holloway Barbosa, M.D., Eliot Battle, M.D., Michael Bigby, M.D., Mavis V. Billups, M.D., Raymond Blackburn, M.D., John H. Bocachica, M.D., Paul Prince Boswell, M.D., Khari Bridges, M.D., Stella Bulengo, M.D., Cheryl Burgess, M.D., Denise Buntin, M.D., John Butler, M.D., Valerie Callender, M.D., Gloria Campbell-D'Hue, M.D., John Carney, M.D. (deceased), Claude Vernon Cave, M.D. (deceased), Greta Clark, M.D., Earl Claiborne, M.D. (deceased), William Coffey, M.D., Fran Cook-Bolden, M.D., Denise Cook, M.D., George Cohen, M.D., Norvell Vandervall Coots, M.D., Linda Davis, M.D., Thomas L. Day, Jr., M.D., Thomas L. Day, Sr., M.D., Kwame Deniake, M.D., Nicole DeYampert, Angela Dillard, Ph.D., Terri Dunn, M.D., Lucius C. Earles, III, M.D., Rene Earles, M.D., Moses Elam, M.D., Roselyn E. Epps, M.D., Carnot Evans, M.D., C. Wendell Freeman, M.D., Madeleine E. Gainers, M.D., Algin Garrett, M.D., Jacquelyn B. Garrett, M.D., Raechele Gathers, M.D., Joseph G. Gathings, M.D., Yvette George, M.D., Richard Gibbs, M.D., Marcia Glenn, M.D., William Grier, M.D., Pearl Grimes, M.D., Rebat M. Halder, M.D., Jennifer Haley, M.D., Roland Hart, M.D., Carla Herriford, M.D., Homer E. Harris, Jr., M.D., Candrice Heath, M.D., Karen Heidelberg, M.D., Robert P. Heidelberg, M.D., Shari Hicks-Graham, M.D., Stacey Hunt, M.D., James Hobbs, M.D., Lori Hobbs, M.D., Yolanda Holmes, M.D., Robert Jackson, M.D., Bernett L. Johnson, Jr., M.D., Beverly Johnson, M.D., Brian Johnson, M.D., Bernett Johnson, M.D., Peter D. Johnson, M.D., Thomas Johnson, M.D., William D. Keith, M.D., Jesse A. Kenne, M.D., A. Paul Kelly, M.D., Edward W. Kelly, Jr., M.D., John A. Kenney, Jr., M.D., Yvonne Knight, M.D., Theodore K. Lawless, M.D. (1892–1971) (deceased), Yolanda Lenzy, M.D., Charles McDonald, M.D., Lynn McKinley-Grant, M.D., Cassandra McLaurin, M.D., Amy McMichael, M.D., Arthur Mayo, M.D., Allison Nicholas Metz, M.D., Harold R. Minus, M.D., Jocelyn Mitchell, M.D., Lenley Mordecai, M.D., Fern Nelson, M.D., Lamar Nelson, M.D., Kim Nichols, M.D., Pavan Nootheti M.D., John C. Payne, M.D. , Sherri Peace, M.D., Harold E. Pierce, Jr., M.D. (deceased), Frederick N. Quarles, M.D., Chemene R. Quinn, M.D., Errol Quintal, M.D., Wendy Roberts, M.D., Fletcher Robinson, M.D., Orlando G. Rodman, M.D. (deceased), Charles V. Roman, M.D., Oscar Saffold, M.D., Darlene Sampson, M.D., Leonard Boyd Savoy, M.D., Kimberly Scott, M.D., Margery Scott, M.D., Thomas Obadiah Senior, M.D., Dwana Shabazz, M.D., Ralph Skull, M.D. (deceased), Silvan Soden, M.D., Gerald Spencer, M.D., Hilda Germaine Straker, M.D., Antoinette Stockton, M.D., Pamela Summers, M.D., Arthur Sumrall, M.D., Susan Taylor, M.D., Harold Thatcher, M.D., Lorna Thomas, M.D., Sidney Thompson, M.D., Charles S. Thurston, M.D., Ella Toombs, M.D., Patricia Treadwell, M.D., Katherine Treherne, M.D., Andrea Trowers, M.D., Phillip Valentine, M.D., Sandra E. Vause, M.D., Earl Walker, M.D., Norman Walton, M.D., Carl V. Washington, M.D., Seymour M. Weaver, III, M.D., Wesley Wilborn, M.D., Clarence Wiley, M.D., Isaac Willis, Sr., M.D., Vernon Wilson, M.D., Johnnie Woodson, Jr., M.D., Linda Woodson, M.D., Dakara Wright, M.D.

INDEX

C

D

M

Q

R

S

W

Y

Z